RE
65
.P75
1995

Primary eyecare in
systemic disease.

Do Not Special Loan

5/30/96 JP

$95.00   No Checkout

DATE			

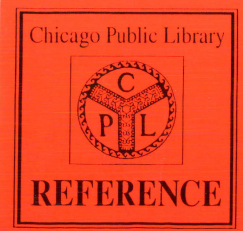

PRIMARY EYECARE IN SYSTEMIC DISEASE

PRIMARY EYECARE IN SYSTEMIC DISEASE

Edited by

Esther S. Marks, OD, FAAO
Director of Optometric Residency and
 Externship Program
Optometry Section
Department of Veterans Affairs Brooklyn Medical
 Center/St. Albans Extended Care Center
Brooklyn, New York
Assistant Clinical Professor
Department of Clinical Sciences
State College of Optometry
State University of New York
New York, New York

Diane T. Adamczyk, OD, FAAO
Assistant Professor
Chief, Primary Care Optometry Service
Department of Clinical Sciences
State College of Optometry
State University of New York
New York, New York

Kelly H. Thomann, OD, FAAO
Supervisor of Optometric Residency and
 Externship Program
Optometry Service
Franklin Delano Roosevelt Veterans Affairs Hospital
Montrose, New York
Adjunct Assistant Clinical Professor
State College of Optometry
State University of New York
New York, New York
Adjunct Assistant Professor
Indiana University College of Optometry
Bloomington, Indiana

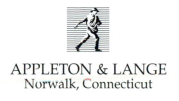

APPLETON & LANGE
Norwalk, Connecticut

Notice: The authors and the publisher of this volume have taken care to
make certain that the doses of drugs and schedules of treatment are correct
and compatible with the standards generally accepted at the time of
publication. Nevertheless, as new information becomes available, changes in
treatment and in the use of drugs become necessary. The reader is advised to
carefully consult the instruction and information material included in the
package insert of each drug or therapeutic agent before administration.
This advice is especially important when using new or infrequently used drugs.
The publisher disclaims any liability, loss, injury, or damage incurred as
a consequence, directly or indirectly, of the use and application of any of
the contents of this volume.

95 96 97 98 99 / 10 9 8 7 6 5 4 3 2 1

Prentice Hall International (UK) Limited, *London*
Prentice Hall of Australia Pty. Limited, *Sydney*
Prentice Hall Canada, Inc., *Toronto*
Prentice Hall Hispanoamericana, S.A., *Mexico*
Prentice Hall of India Private Limited, *New Delhi*
Prentice Hall of Japan, Inc., *Tokyo*
Simon & Schuster Asia Pte. Ltd., *Singapore*
Editora Prentice Hall do Brasil Ltda., *Rio de Janeiro*
Prentice Hall, *Englewood Cliffs, New Jersey*

Library of Congress Cataloging-in-Publication Data

Primary eyecare in systemic disease / edited by Esther S. Marks, Diane
    T. Adamczyk, Kelly H. Thomann.
        p.   cm.
    ISBN 0-8385-7997-3
    1. Ocular manifestations of general diseases. I. Marks, Esther
S. II. Adamczyk, Diane T. III. Thomann, Kelly H.
    [DNLM: 1. Eye Manifestations.   WW 475 P952 1994]
    RE65.P75 1994
    617.7—dc20
    DNLM/DLC
    for Library of Congress   94-10704
                                                CIP

Acquisitions Editor: Cheryl L. Mehalik
Production Editor: Jennifer Sinsavich
Designer: Elizabeth A. Schmitz

PRINTED IN THE UNITED STATES OF AMERICA

ISBN 0-8385-7997-3
90000
9 780838 579978

To the events and people,
who in the course of writing this book,
gave us perspective as to what is truly important in life.

To our families
Dean Novelli, Mom and Dad Adamczyk, Sean and Carly Thomann,
whose encouragement, patience, and constant support,
along with some gentle prodding, made it all possible.

Contributors

Diane T. Adamczyk, OD, FAAO
Assistant Professor
Chief, Primary Care Optometry Service
Department of Clinical Sciences
State College of Optometry
State University of New York
New York, New York

Elizabeth B. Aksionoff, OD, FAAO
Assistant Clinical Professor
Department of Clinical Sciences
State College of Optometry
State University of New York
New York, New York

Sherry J. Bass, OD
Professor
Ocular Disease and Special Testing Service
Department of Clinical Sciences
State College of Optometry
State University of New York
New York, New York

Debra Bezan, MEd, OD, FAAO
Professor
Director of Clinics
College of Optometry
Northeastern State University
Tahlequah, Oklahoma

Bernard H. Blaustein, OD
Associate Professor
The Eye Institute
Pennsylvania College of Optometry
Philadelphia, Pennsylvania

Tanya L. Carter, OD
Director of Optometry Services
Coler Memorial Hospital
Assistant Professor
Department of Clinical Science
State College of Optometry
State University of New York
New York, New York

Jerry D. Cavallerano, OD, PhD
Staff Optometrist
Beetham Eye Institute
Joslin Diabetes Center
Associate Professor
New England College of Optometry
Boston, Massachusetts

Michael A. Chaglasian, OD
Assistant Professor
Illinois Eye Institute
Illinois College of Optometry
Chicago, Illinois

Connie L. Chronister, OD, FAAO
Associate Professor
Department of Basic Sciences
Staff Optometrist
Department of Clinical Sciences
The Eye Institute
Pennsylvania College of Optometry
Philadelphia, Pennsylvania

John Elliott Conto, OD
Associate Professor
Attending Module Chief
Division of Primary Care
Illinois Eye Institute
Illinois College of Optometry
Chicago, Illinois

Bernard J. Dolan, OD, MS
Staff Optometrist
Department of Veterans Affairs Medical Center
San Francisco, California
Associate Clinical Professor
School of Optometry
University of California at Berkeley
Berkeley, California

Mitchell W. Dul, OD, MS, FAAO
Chief, Optometry Service
Franklin Delano Roosevelt Veterans Affairs Hospital
Montrose, New York
Adjunct Assistant Clinical Professor
Department of Clinical Sciences
State College of Optometry
State University of New York
New York, New York
Adjunct Assistant Professor
Indiana University College of Optometry
Bloomington, Indiana

Christine M. Dumestre, OD
Assistant Clinical Professor
Department of Clinical Sciences
State College of Optometry
State University of New York
New York, New York

Charles Haskes, OD, MS
Staff Optometrist
Eye Clinic
Department of Veterans Affairs Medical Center
West Haven, Connecticut

Lloyd P. Haskes, OD
Assistant Clinical Professor
Department of Clinical Sciences
State College of Optometry
State University of New York
New York, New York

Brian Patrick Mahoney, OD
Chief, Optometry Section
Department of Veterans Affairs Medical Center
Wilmington, Delaware
Adjunct Professor
The Eye Institute
Pennsylvania College of Optometry
Philadelphia, Pennsylvania
Adjunct Assistant Clinical Professor
Department of Clinical Sciences
State College of Optometry
State University of New York
New York, New York

Esther S. Marks, OD, FAAO
Director of Optometric Residency and Externship Program
Optometry Section
Department of Veterans Affairs Brooklyn Medical
   Center/St. Albans Extended Care Center
Brooklyn, New York
Assistant Clinical Professor
Department of Clinical Sciences
State College of Optometry
State University of New York
New York, New York

Taryn Mathews, OD
Attending Optometrist
Eye Clinic Gouverneur Hospital
New York, New York

Margaret McNelis, OD
Staff Optometrist
Eye Surgeons and Consultants Limited
Chicago, Illinois

Leonard V. Messner, OD
Associate Professor
Director, The Center for Advanced Ophthalmic Care
Illinois Eye Institute
Illinois College of Optometry
Chicago, Illinois

Holly Myers, OD
Assistant Professor
Department of Clinical Sciences
Chief, Primary Care Module
The Eye Institute
Pennsylvania College of Optometry
Philadelphia, Pennsylvania

Susan C. Oleszewski, OD, MA
Assistant Dean, Department of Clinical Sciences
The Eye Institute
Pennsylvania College of Optometry
Philadelphia, Pennsylvania

Leonard J. Oshinskie, OD, FAAO
Chief, Optometry Section
Department of Veterans Affairs Medical Center
Newington, Connecticut
Adjunct Clinical Professor
New England College of Optometry
Boston, Massachusetts
Adjunct Assistant Clinical Professor
Department of Clinical Sciences
State College of Optometry
State University of New York
New York, New York

Joan Katherine Portello, OD, FAAO
Assistant Clinical Professor
Department of Clinical Sciences
State College of Optometry
State University of New York
New York, New York

Susan P. Schuettenberg, OD, FAAO
Assistant Clinical Professor
Department of Clinical Sciences
State College of Optometry
State University of New York
New York, New York

Jerome Sherman, OD, FAAO
Distinguished Teaching Professor
Ocular Disease and Special Testing Service
Department of Clinical Sciences
State College of Optometry
State University of New York
New York, New York

Kelly H. Thomann, OD, FAAO
Supervisor of Optometric Residency and Externship
  Program
Optometry Service

Franklin Delano Roosevelt Veterans Affairs Hospital
Montrose, New York
Adjunct Assistant Clinical Professor
Department of Clinical Sciences
State College of Optometry
State University of New York
New York, New York
Adjunct Assistant Professor
Indiana University College of Optometry
Bloomington, Indiana

William J. Tullo, OD
Assistant Clinical Professor
Contact Lens Service
Department of Clinical Sciences
State College of Optometry
State University of New York
New York, New York

Roger Wilson, OD
Associate Professor
Chair, Department of External Clinical Programs
New England College of Optometry
Associate Director of Eye Care Services
Dorchester House Multi-Service Center
Boston, Massachusetts

Contents

Foreword

Optometry is a unique profession that is evolving before our very eyes. Changes that have taken place over the past two decades are extraordinary. Everything from the educational curriculum to the scope of practice is different. One clear sign that the profession has evolved is its library of publications. Optometry's catalog of textbooks has grown, reflecting changes that have occurred within the profession. Two decades ago, texts written by optometrists centered around topics pertaining to contact lenses, refraction, ophthalmic optics, and low vision. Ophthalmologic and medical texts were used in the areas that pertained to ocular or systemic disease. As the optometric profession has expanded into "primary eyecare," books written by optometrists have appeared that deal with the peripheral retina, the posterior segment, the anterior segment, glaucoma, and primary eyecare procedures. All these topics signify our profession's growth and expansion in its scope and breadth of practice and our emergence as members of the health care team. With the publication of *Primary Eyecare in Systemic Disease*, a further evolution and growth has occurred, and it is my honor to write the foreword introducing this textbook.

With the expansion in the scope of optometric practice, an awareness of the "total patient" has developed that has changed how we assess our patients. Simply put, we no longer focus specifically on the eye during the "ocular examination." A host of systemic conditions may involve the eye. Abnormal signs detected during an eye examination might be due to a systemic cause that can have diagnostic or therapeutic significance. Also, clinical signs found throughout the body might be associated with ocular involvement. Just as importantly, therapeutic treatment of ocular conditions with topical or systemic medications may have adverse sequelae on certain systemic conditions. *Primary Eyecare in Systemic Disease* is a text that reviews these areas of concern.

I have had the opportunity to work alongside Drs. Marks, Adamczyk, and Thomann in their roles as faculty members at the SUNY College of Optometry and at the VA hospitals where two of the authors are now located. Each of the authors is emblematic of the "new breed" of optometrist and exemplifies the changes that have occurred in optometry. All are residency-trained and decided to go into optometric education after finishing their training. Each has taken an interest in systemic disease and its ocular involvement, and has taught courses at the SUNY College of Optometry in this area. Most importantly, all practice in either a hospital or multidisciplinary setting where the principles of practice outlined in this text are performed on a daily basis. The authors have assembled a talented pool of optometrists from around the country to help in the creation of this book. With all their expertise, *Primary Eyecare in Systemic Disease* is a book that will aid us in our role as viable members of the health care team.

Murray Fingeret, OD
Chief, Optometry Section, St. Alban's Veteran's
Administration Extended Care Center
Brooklyn VA Medical Center
Brooklyn, New York

Preface

Primary Eyecare in Systemic Disease is a text which is meant to serve as a bridge between systemic diseases and their ocular manifestations. This bridge underscores the important role the eyecare practitioner plays in patient care. Our goal has been to produce a clinically oriented textbook providing a concise, user friendly guide for students, the emerging practitioner, and seasoned clinicians. This is not intended to be an all inclusive compendium of every systemic disease with ocular manifestations. Rather, we chose to focus on systemic diseases commonly encountered by the eyecare practitioner (eg, diabetes and hypertension), as well as less frequently encountered conditions with important ocular manifestations (eg, myasthenia gravis). Finally, we chose to include some rarely encountered disorders whose ocular manifestations are crucial for the systemic diagnosis (eg, Wilms tumor).

Section I provides the reader with an overview of patient assessment. This includes history taking, selected examination techniques (eg, cranial nerve evaluation), and diagnostic laboratory and imaging tests.

Sections II through XVI are the "heart" of the textbook. These organized sections cover 80 systemic diseases with ocular manifestations. To maintain continuity throughout this section, each chapter discusses systemic and ocular manifestations with a similar format by introducing the disorder, providing epidemiological data, explaining the natural history, equipping the clinician with keys to diagnosis, and finally discussing treatment and management. Consistent throughout each chapter are easy-to-use reference tables highlighting systemic manifestations, ocular manifestations, and treatment and management protocols. Many chapters have additional tables which include pertinent information regarding the disorder.

Finally there are 3 important appendices. Appendix I is a useful table cross referencing ocular manifestations to systemic diseases. Appendix II provides the normal reference ranges for common diagnostic laboratory tests. Appendix III is a guide to common medical abbreviations.

It is our hope that this textbook, through the integration of ocular and systemic disorders, will be a valuable resource for practitioners intent on providing their patients with the highest quality eyecare possible.

Esther S. Marks
Diane T. Adamczyk
Kelly H. Thomann

Acknowledgments

We would like to thank Murray Fingeret, whose support and faith in us made this book possible. Many others contributed to the completion of this book, especially Barry Barresi, Mitch Dul, Melissa Dempsey, and the Library and Media Department at the SUNY State College of Optometry.

PRIMARY EYECARE
IN SYSTEMIC DISEASE

SECTION I

INTRODUCTION

1
Chapter

Patient Assessment

Kelly H. Thomann ▪ Esther S. Marks ▪ Diane T. Adamczyk

Primary eyecare encompasses more than simply an ocular evaluation. Although addressing a patient's chief complaint is vital, as well as assessing refractive, binocular, and ocular health status, the examination becomes comprehensive only if the patient's systemic health is integrated into the eye evaluation. As primary healthcare providers, eyecare clinicians must understand how a patient's overall health can significantly affect and interact with visual functioning.

The ocular assessment often follows a problem-oriented medical approach. This approach was delineated in the 1960s by Lawrence Weed, a physician, to provide optimal, consistent care and record-keeping. This approach has subsequently become an underlying feature of the eyecare evaluation.

PATIENT HISTORY

The patient history is probably the most important part of the examination, because a thorough and correctly pursued history often provides the diagnosis, relying on the physical examination for confirmation of the clinician's initial impressions. During this initial interaction, various aspects of the patient's speech, demeanor, and overall presentation can be assessed, providing useful information for diagnosis and management.

The case history should begin with the patient's age, sex, and race. These immediately establish a basis for potential differential diagnoses throughout the examination, and allow the clinician to begin sorting the differential diagnoses into logical order. For example, sarcoidosis is more likely to be suspected in an African-American patient, Reiter syndrome more often in young men, or giant-cell arteritis in an older population.

The case history may be delineated into chief complaint, ocular history, and medical history. The chief complaint (CC) establishes the reason for the patient's visit, and is best recorded in the patient's own words. This helps to prevent the clinician from making an erroneous initial diagno-sis. For example, a complaint of a "burning" sensation should not be recorded as dry eye symptoms, or the clinician may fail to look beyond dry eyes. Once the chief complaint is established (eg, "red eyes"), the clinician must then become a fact finder, in order to gain more information regarding the problem. Clues or descriptive information should be elicited from the patient (how long have the eyes been red, what alleviates the redness, and so forth; see Table 1–1). This narrative paragraph is often referred to as the history of the present illness (HPI).

A complete ocular history should follow. This includes date of last eye examination, refractive history (spectacles and contact lenses), eye health, and family eye history (Table 1–2). Once again, symptom descriptors should be elicited with any positive aspect of the history.

The complete medical history includes last medical examination, medical history (Table 1–3), family medical history, current medications, and allergies. Personal and social history may also be useful. A comprehensive medical history includes a review of systems (Table 1–4). Such a detailed history is not always warranted; rather, it is dependent on the individual case.

Throughout the examination, additional information regarding the patient should be elicited when indicated. For

TABLE 1–1. SYMPTOM DESCRIPTORS

Location
Quality
Quantity or intensity
Chronology: onset, frequency, duration
Provocative factors
Palliative or alleviative factors
Associated factors and symptoms

example, a patient with evidence of uveitis may be further questioned regarding past or current medical history for rheumatologic disorders, infections, or inflammatory disorders not typically asked about during the initial history. The patient history is an ongoing process throughout the entire encounter.

OCULAR EXAMINATION

A comprehensive ocular examination evaluates the patient's refractive, binocular/ accommodative, and eye health status. A variety of tests may be done to reach this end, with a basic battery of testing procedures used to comprise the minimum database. The problem-oriented approach uses the minimum database as a foundation to be built upon, which may then require additional testing (Table 1–5).

TABLE 1–2. OCULAR HISTORY

Last Eye Examination

When
Where, by whom

Eye History

Trauma
Surgery
Disease
Strabismus or amblyopia or both
Flashes or floaters or both
Diplopia
Loss of vision (monocular or binocular)
Headaches, pain
Burning, itching, redness, tearing
Photophobia
Contact lens history, if applicable: type, age of lenses, wearing time, disinfection method, solutions, enzymes

Family Eye History

Disease (eg, glaucoma, macular degeneration)
Strabismus or amblyopia or both
Surgery
Blindness (from what)

PHYSICAL EXAMINATION

In order to completely assess the patient, systemic testing procedures are often required to provide important specific information regarding overall health and its interrelationship with the visual system.

Vascular Testing
Several tests may be done by the eyecare practitioner when the diagnosis of a vascular disease is suspected. These may

TABLE 1–3. MEDICAL HISTORY[a]

Last Medical Exam

When
Where, by whom

Medical History

Diabetes
    IDDM (type I)
    NIDDM (type II)
Hypertension
Heart disease
Chronic obstructive pulmonary disease (COPD)
    Asthma
    Emphysema
Pregnancy
Other:
    Sickle-cell disease
    Syphilis
    Cancer
    HIV/AIDS
    Thyroid
    Arthritis
Hospitalizations
Operations
Serious injuries

Family Medical History

Diabetes
    IDDM (type I)
    NIDDM (type II)
Hypertension
Heart disease
Chronic obstructive pulmonary disease (COPD)
    Asthma
    Emphysema
Cancer

Medications

Prescription
Over the counter (OTC)

Allergies

Medications
Other

[a]If any of the above are positive, follow up with duration, control, last examination, next appointment for follow-up.

TABLE 1–4. REVIEW OF SYSTEMS

General

Usual state of health
Fever
Chills
Usual weight
Change in weight
Weakness
Fatigue
Sweats
Hot or cold intolerance
History of anemia
Bleeding tendencies
Blood transfusions and
    possible reactions
Exposure to radiation

Skin

Rashes
Itching
Hives
Easy bruisability
History of eczema
Dryness
Changes in skin color
Changes in hair texture
Changes in nail texture
Changes in nail
    appearance
History of previous skin
    disorders
Lumps
Use of hair dyes

Head

"Dizziness"
Headaches
Pain
Fainting
History of head injury
Stroke

Eyes

Use of eyeglasses
Current vision
Change in vision
Double vision
Excessive tearing
Pain
Recent eye examinations
Pain when looking at light
Unusual sensations
Redness
Discharge
Infections
History of glaucoma
Cataracts
Injuries

Ears

Hearing impairment
Use of hearing aid
Discharge
"Dizziness"
Pain
Ringing in ears
Infections

Nose

Nosebleeds
Infections
Discharge
Frequency of colds
Nasal obstruction
History of injury
Sinus infections
Hay fever

Mouth and Throat

Condition of teeth
Last dental appointment
Condition of gums
Bleeding gums
Frequent sore throats
Burning of tongue
Hoarseness
Voice changes
Postnasal drip

Neck

Lumps
Goiter
Pain on movement
Tenderness
History of "swollen
    glands"
Throid trouble

Chest

Cough
Pain
Shortness of breath
Sputum production
    (quantity, appearance)
Tuberculosis
Asthma
Pleurisy
Bronchitis
Coughing up blood
Wheezing
Last x-ray
Last test for tuberculosis
History of BCG
    vaccination

Cardiac

Pain
High blood pressure
Palpitations
Shortness of breath with
    exertion
Shortness of breath when
    lying flat
Sudden shortness of breath
    while sleeping
History of heart attack
Rheumatic fever
Heart murmur
Last ECG
Other tests for heart
    function

Vascular

Pain in legs, calves, thighs,
    or hips while walking
Swelling of legs
Varicose veins
Thrombophlebitis
Coolness of extremity
Loss of hair on legs
Discoloration of extremity
Ulcers

Breasts

Lumps
Discharge
Pain
Tenderness
Self-examination

Gastrointestinal

Appetite
Excessive hunger
Excessive thirst
Nausea
Swallowing
Constipation
Diarrhea
Heartburn
Vomiting
Abdominal pain
Change in stool color
Change in stool caliber
Change in stool
    consistency
Frequency of bowel
    movements
Vomiting up blood
Rectal bleeding
Black, tarry stools
Laxative or antacid use
Excessive belching

Food intolerance
Change in abdominal size
Hemorrhoids
Infections
Jaundice
Rectal pain
Previous abdominal x-rays
Hepatitis
Liver disease
Gall bladder disease

Urinary

Frequency
Urgency
Difficulty in starting the
    stream
Incontinence
Excessive urination
Pain on urination
Burning
Blood in urine
Infections
Stones
Bed wetting
Flank pain
Awakening at night to
    urinate
History of retention
Urine color
Urine odor

Male Genitalia

Lesions on penis
Discharge
Impotence
Pain
Scrotal masses
Hernias
Frequency of intercourse
Ability to enjoy sexual
    relations
Fertility problems
Prostate problems
History of venereal disease
    and treatment

Female Genitalia

Lesions on external
    genitalia
Itching
Discharge
Last Pap smear and result
Pain on intercourse
Frequency of intercourse
Birth control methods
Ability to enjoy sexual
    relations

Fertility problems
Hernias
History of veneral disease
    and treatment
History of DES exposure
Age at menarche
Interval between periods
Duration of periods
Amount of flow
Date of last period
Bleeding between periods
Number of pregnancies
Abortions
Term deliveries
Complications of
    pregnancies
Description(s) of labor
Number of living children
Menstrual pain
Age at menopause
Menopausal symptoms
Postmenopausal bleeding

Musculoskeletal

Weakness
Paralysis
Muscle stiffness
Limitation of movement
Joint path
Joint stiffness
Arthritis
Gout
Back problems
Muscle cramps
Deformities

Neurologic

Fainting
"Dizziness"
"Blackouts"
Paralysis
Strokes
"Numbness"
Tingling
Burning
Tremors
Loss of memory
Psychiatric disorders
Mood changes
Nervousness
Speech disorders
Unsteadiness of gait
General behavioral
    change
Loss of consciousness
Hallucinations
Disorientation

Reprinted, with permission, from Swartz MH: *Textbook of Physical Diagnosis, History and Examination.* Philadelphia: Saunders, 1989.

TABLE 1–5. AUXILIARY OCULAR TESTING

Anterior Segment

Gonioscopy
Tear breakup time
Iris transillumination
Rose bengal testing
Jones dye testing
Schirmer testing
Lacrimal dilation and irrigation
Punctal implants
Corneal sensitivity
Cultures and smears
Exophthalmometry
Forced ductions
Orbital auscultation

Posterior Segment

Interferometry or potential acuity
Ultrasonography
Scleral indentation
Fluorescein angiography
Three mirror fundus evaluation
Amsler grid
Contrast sensitivity
Brightness comparison
Red desaturation

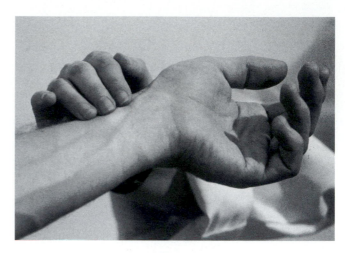

Figure 1–1. Radial pulse measurement.

include the assessment of arterial pulses, sphygmomanometry, auscultation, and ophthalmodynamometry.

There are various indications for evaluating pulses. They may be taken as part of blood pressure measurement, prior to and after initiating ophthalmic medications with systemic side effects (eg, β-blockers for glaucoma), and in patients suspected of having carotid artery or cerebrovascular disease. When evaluating the pulse, several factors are taken into account. These include rate (most accurately measured by counting the full 60 seconds), rhythm (regular versus irregular), volume/strength (normal/full versus weak/thready), and the condition of the vessel wall (palpable, tender, or rigid). The results are recorded; for example, "R carotid 55 thready." The average pulse rate for adults is between 60 and 100 beats/minute (although the elderly may have slower pulses), and for children between 90 and 140 beats/minute. If the pulse rate is high, the clinician should recheck it at the end of the examination. It may be temporarily elevated for reasons other than disease (eg, nervousness).

The radial pulse is located on the wrist (Figure 1–1) just below the ball of the thumb. It is tested with the second, third, and fourth fingers placed firmly on the radial artery. The thumb should not be used because the pulse in the thumb may be confused with the radial pulse due to their anatomic proximity. To evaluate the brachial pulse, the patient's arm should be resting palm up, with the elbow at the level of the heart. The examiner places his or her first two fingers over the brachial artery, located medially at the antecubital fossa just under the tendon of the biceps.

In order to evaluate the carotid pulse, the first two fingers are placed at the angle of the jaw and then slid down between the sternocleidomastoid muscle and the trachea. Each carotid is palpated gently to avoid stimulating the carotid sinus, which may cause a drop in blood pressure and heart rate. To prevent obstruction of blood flow to the brain, simultaneous palpation of both carotids should be avoided.

The carotid artery is often further evaluated because it is commonly affected by atherosclerosis. Palpation and auscultation of the carotid artery are indicated in patients with symptoms of amaurosis fugax, transient ischemic attacks, reversible ischemic neurologic deficits, or signs of emboli, retinal occlusive disease, asymmetric diabetic retinopathy, ocular ischemic syndrome, or previous history of carotid artery or vertebrobasilar disease.

Palpating the pulse initially can give an indication if there is any asymmetry, in addition to providing a gross assessment of the integrity of the carotid arteries. Auscultation is done to detect bruits, caused by turbulent blood flow due to blockage within the arteries. A bruit is usually audible with a stethoscope if the vessel is more than 50% occluded. This occlusion will cause a rushing or "whooshing" sound.

To auscultate the carotid arteries, the patient should elevate the chin slightly and turn away from the side to be auscultated first. The bell (or diaphragm) position of the stethoscope is placed just below the angle of the jaw where the common carotid bifurcates. The patient is told to take a breath and hold it, while the examiner listens for a bruit. The stethoscope can be moved up and down the artery. Care should be taken not to exert excess pressure on the artery while auscultating. The same procedure should be repeated over the other carotid. The absence of a bruit does not rule out carotid artery disease, because it will not be heard once the occlusion exceeds 90%. Any patient suspected of occlusive arterial disease, with or without a bruit, requires a vascular workup.

Blood pressure assessment has become routine for many eyecare practitioners. Sphygmomanometry may be performed to screen for hypertension and monitor known hypertensives, as well as to monitor the effects of some ophthalmic medications (eg, topical sympathomimetics, β-blockers) and diagnose certain ocular conditions (eg, hypertensive retinopathy). The technique for blood pressure measurement (Figure 1–2) is described in Table 1–6 and the expected values are listed in Table 1–7.

Ophthalmodynamometry (ODM) is another in-office technique that can aid in the detection of carotid artery disease. It measures the relative ophthalmic artery pressure between the two eyes. This procedure has the same indications as carotid artery auscultation. ODM is contraindicated in patients with a history of retinal detachment or tears, recent intraocular surgery, recent penetration or blunt injury to the globe, ectopia lentis, and neovascularization.

Compression ODM is the most commonly used technique. The ODM instrument has a scale (usually a dial) at one end and a footplate at the other. The ODM footplate is placed on the anesthetized sclera and gentle pressure is applied to the globe (Figure 1–3). The amount of pressure (read off the dial) required to pulsate and then collapse the central retinal artery corresponds to its systolic and diastolic pressures, respectively. Although the absolute numerical values provide useful information, the presence of asymmetry between the eyes is particularly important, indicating asymmetric carotid artery disease. A difference of 15 to 20% between the two eyes is considered clinically significant.

If an ophthalmodynamometer is unavailable, a modified ODM technique may be performed by gently pressing on the globe with a finger while visualizing the central retinal artery through a direct ophthalmoscope. As the intraocular pressure increases and becomes greater than the diastolic arterial pressure, the veins will collapse and the artery will begin to pulsate. The procedure is repeated on the other eye, noting any significant difference in the pressure required to cause the artery to pulsate.

Nervous System Testing

If a patient presents with signs or symptoms suggestive of neurological dysfunction, further evaluation may be necessary. Astute observation skills and in-office screening tests can provide valuable information regarding the nervous system, along with directing the examination. A cranial nerve evaluation (Table 1–8 and Figures 1–4 and 1–5) is a logical starting point, because four of the six cranial nerves are routinely assessed in a comprehensive eye examination. The complete neurological examination requires the evaluation of six more areas: mental status, motor function, sensory function, station and gait, cerebellar function, and reflexes.

TABLE 1–6. SPHYGMOMANOMETRY[a]

Choose appropriate cuff size (cuff bladder must be 20% wider than arm circumference)

Choose appropriate environment (relaxed atmosphere)

Patient should be seated erect or lying supine
The arm should be bare, extended, and well supported at the level of the heart

Check the pulse (radial or brachial)
Place the cuff over biceps (approximately 1 inch above the elbow crease) and turn the valve screw clockwise to close the valve
Pump air into the bladder while palpating the radial or brachial artery
When the pulse is no longer palpable, pump at least 20 mm Hg more
Center the diaphragm of the stethoscope over the brachial artery and hold in place with one hand

Slowly deflate the cuff (no faster than 5 mm Hg/sec)
Note the reading at the first audible beat (systolic pressure) and at the last audible beat (diastolic pressure)
Rapidly deflate the cuff

Wait at least 30 seconds and repeat
If there is a discrepency of greater than 5 mm Hg, recheck

False high readings may result from the following

Cuff too small
Cuff wrapped too loosely
Cuff deflation too slow (causing venous congestion)
Tilted mercury column
Anxious patient
Tobacco use or caffeinated beverage just prior to reading

False low readings may result from the following

Arm not level with the heart
Failure to hear beats
Cuff too large
Constrictive clothing
Auscultatory gap

[a]Be certain to periodically calibrate aneroid sphygmomanometers against a mercury manometer of known accuracy.

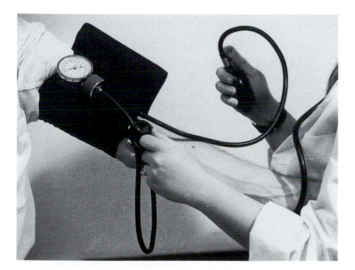

Figure 1–2. Blood pressure measurement.

TABLE 1–7. SPHYGMOMANOMETRY—EXPECTED VALUES

Blood Pressure Range (mm Hg)	Category	Management
Diastolic		
<85	Normal	Recheck within 2 years
85–89	High normal	Recheck within 1 year
90–104	Mild hypertension	Confirm within 2 months
105–114	Moderate hypertension	Confirm or refer within 2 weeks
>115	Severe hypertension	Immediate referral
Systolic, When Diastolic <90		
<140		Recheck within 2 years
140–199		Confirm within 2 months
>200		Confirm or refer within 2 weeks

Reprinted with permission from Good GW, Aughburger AR: Role of optometrists in combatting high blood pressure. JAOA 1989; 60:352–355.

Mental status can be screened for by using the mnemonic "FOGS." The patient's level of awareness (alert and attentive versus "foggy" or lethargic) is noted primarily. Other factors to evaluate include *F*amily history, *O*rientation, *G*eneral information and *S*pelling. The family history utilizes input from family members about changes in the patient's mental status, which include characteristics such as intellect, mood, affect, and attention. Orientation may be assessed by asking the patient to recall the day, date, time, and location of examination. Minor inaccuracies may occur with normal patients; however, grossly incorrect responses may indicate mental dysfunction. Lastly, to screen mental function, a simple spelling test can be done in which the patient is asked to spell the word WORLD forwards and backwards (a five-number sequence may be used with an illiterate patient). The inability to do either part of this test may indicate a decrease in mental ability.

Motor function is another aspect of the neurological evaluation. Muscle tone, strength, and bulk are assessed. Also any abnormal movements (tremor, tics, dyskinesia) are noted (Table 1–9). To screen, the patient can be asked to hold the arms straight out, directly in front of his or her body. The clinician looks for symmetry/asymmetry, the ability to maintain position, and any drifts or weakness. Resistance may be added, again noting symmetry/asymmetry.

Sensory testing in a complete neurological examination includes the assessment of light touch, pain, vibration, and position (primary sensory modalities) along with stereognosis, graphesthesia, and two-point discrimination (secondary sensory modalities). Primary sensory modalities are generally not tested in a screening of neurological function; however, if dysfunction is suspected, specific modalities (light touch, pain) may be individually assessed in the appropriate dermatome. Secondary sensory modalities offer more information in the screening of neurological function because they are integrative, providing information regarding primary sensory modalities and higher cortical (parietal lobe) function. The identification of common objects through touch (eg, by placing a paper clip in the patient's hand) will assess stereognosis. The inability to identify a number traced on the hand may indicate agraphesthesia (the inability to identify traced figures on the skin of a limb in the

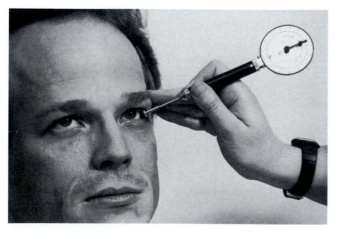

Figure 1–3. Ophthalmodynamometry.

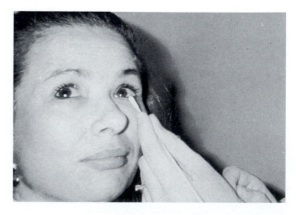

Figure 1–4. The blink reflex tests the fifth (corneal sensation) and seventh (lid closure) cranial nerves.

TABLE 1–8. CRANIAL NERVE EXAMINATION

Cranial nerve I—Olfactory nerve

Key test: Smell—Have the patient occlude one nare and close eyes. Present an aromatic substance (ie, coffee, vanilla, chocolate). Ask if they can smell or identify it. Repeat with the other nare.

Pearl: Do not use substances such as ammonia or alcohol. These stimulate a portion of the trigeminal nerve located in the nasal mucosa which responds to painful or noxious odors. This may give the false impression of smell if the olfactory nerve is not functional.

Cranial nerve II—Optic nerve

Key tests: Best corrected visual acuity; optic nerve assessment; visual field testing; pupil testing (afferent component).

Cranial nerves III, IV, and VI—Oculomotor, trochlear, and abducens nerve

Key tests: Eye movements in all positions of gaze; pupil testing (efferent component via cranial nerve III); note any symmetry or asymmetry of lid position—follow up with family album tomography (FAT) scan.

Pearl: Follow up with diplopia workup if eye movement dysfunction is found.

Cranial nerve V—Trigeminal nerve

Key tests: Corneal reflex—Use a cotton tip swab with a wisp of cotton pulled out. With the patient looking up and away (to avoid the lashes and reflex blink), touch the center of the cornea with the wisp. Look for prompt, complete lid closure of *both* eyes (afferent = cranial nerve V; efferent = cranial nerve VII). Compare with the other side.
   Pain and light touch in all three sensory divisions of cranial nerve V. Use the dull and sharp ends of a pin. Have the patient close eyes, and alternate each end in all three divisions on the left and right sides. Have the patient report if a sharp or dull sensation is felt.
   To test the motor division, have the patient open his or her jaw and note any deviation (it will deviate *toward* the weak side with dysfunction). Have the patient clench teeth and palpate the masseter muscle (located about 2 cm above the angle of the jaw). Check for symmetry. Have the patient push the jaw against your hand and compare strength on each side.

Cranial nerve VII—Facial nerve

Key tests: Instruct the patient to "look up with your eyes only" or "wrinkle up the skin of your forehead" (tests the frontalis muscle). Compare the symmetry of wrinkles on each side.
   Ask the patient to close eyes as tightly as possible and resist as you attempt to pry them open (tests the orbicularis oculi muscles). Compare strength on each side.
   Ask the patient to "smile and show all your teeth" (tests the buccinator and orbicularis oris muscles). Look for weakness or asymmetry.

Cranial nerve VIII—Acoustic nerve

Key tests: Begin at 40 cm and slowly move a ticking watch or vibrating tuning fork toward the patient's ear while his or her eyes are closed. Ask the patient to tell you when a sound is first heard and on which side.
   Use an otoscope to assess each auditory canal and ear drum.

Pearl: If there is decreased hearing on one side, follow up with the Rinne test. This takes advantage of the fact that air is a better conductor of sound than bone is. A faintly vibrating tuning fork is placed on the mastoid process behind the ear. Ask the patient to tell you when he or she stops hearing it. Next put it beside the ear. Under normal circumstances, the patient will still hear the fork. With blockage, (ie, cerumen of the lumen) it will *not* be heard when placed beside the ear.
   When decreased hearing is found also perform the Weber test. Place a faintly vibrating tuning fork in the center of the forehead. Ask the patient if it is heard more loudly on either side. If it is heard more loudly on the *same* side as the decreased hearing, this suggests a bone conduction deficit. If it is heard more loudly on the contralateral side, this suggests a neural deficit.

Cranial nerves IX and X—Glossopharyngeal and vagus nerves

Key tests: Gag reflex—Examine the palatial arches for symmetry. Touch one arch with a tongue depressor. The normal response is a brisk elevation of both arches and the sensation of gagging (afferent = cranial nerve IX; efferent = cranial nerve X).

Pearl: If dysfunction is suspected, ask if the patient has trouble swallowing or has noticed changes in his or her voice recently. Speech and swallowing dysfunction go together with cranial nerve IX and X lesions.

Cranial nerve XI—Accessory nerve

Key test: Have the patient elevate his or her shoulders against your resistance, and have the patient turn his or her head to each side against your resistance. Note strength and symmetry.

Cranial nerve XII—Hypoglossal nerve

Key test: Have the patient stick out his or her tongue. If there is weakness, it will protrude *toward* the weak side. Also note any wasting, atrophy, or fasciculation.

(Reprinted with permission from Thomann KH, Dul MW. The optometric assessment of neurologic function. J Am Optom Assoc *1993;64:421–431.)*

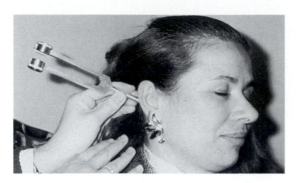

Figure 1–5. The Rinne test uses bone versus air conduction of sound, differentiating hearing loss secondary to a conduction as opposed to a neural etiology.

TABLE 1–9. SELECTED NEUROLOGICAL SCREENING TESTS

Abnormal Involuntary Movements: Important observations and inquiries during exam

1. History of abnormal movement: when it began, under what conditions does it manifest or disappear.
2. Extent of dyskinesia (abnormal movement): part of body involved, location and distribution of movement.
3. Pattern, rhythmicity, course, speed, and frequency of each particular movement.
4. Relationship to posture, rest, voluntary activity or exertion, involuntary movement and fatigue.
5. Response to heat, cold, emotional tension, and excitement.
6. Degree increased or controlled by attention; presence or absence during sleep.

Romberg Test

The patient stands with the feet together and eyes open. Any imbalance is noted. If there is imbalance *with* the eyes open, the test is stopped. This is *not* a positive test, but implies cerebellar dysfunction. If no sway is noted with eyes open, have the patient shut the eyes. Sway with eyes shut is a positive test and implies vestibular or proprioceptive dysfunction. Follow up a positive test with tests of vestibular and proprioceptive senses.

Tests of Cerebellar Function

1. *Nose to finger to nose test:* The patient touches the tip of his or her index finger alternately to his or her nose and to the tip of the examiner's finger, which is placed at approximately arm's length in the facial plane. The examiner moves his or her finger in eight cardinal positions during the test. Left and right sides are tested separately. Tremor or accuracy is noted.
2. *Finger to nose test:* The patient fully extends the arm at the elbow so the upper arm is at a horizontal plane with the eyes closed. The patient then touches his or her nose with the index finger, and returns to the starting position. This is repeated with the other arm. Tremor or dysmetria is noted.
3. *Knee pat test:* The patient is seated and pats his or her knees alternately with the palm and dorsum of one hand then the other, slowly and gradually increasing the rate to its maximum. Abnormalities in rate, rhythm, and position are noted.

Babinski Test

The bottom of the foot is stroked on the lateral aspect with a sharp object (eg, handle end of a reflex hammer). A normal response is plantar (downward) flexion of the toes. An abnormal or positive response is dorsiflexion (upgoing) of the great toe and a fanning or separation of the small toes.

(Reprinted with permission from Thomann KH, Dul MW. The optometric assessment of neurologic function. J Am Optom Assoc 1993;64:421–431.)

presence of normal primary sensory modalities). Simultaneous confrontation visual field will assess two-point discrimination.

Station (the position assumed in standing) and gait are easily assessed by scrutinizing the patient as he or she enters the examination room. Walking is a highly complex task, requiring the integration of a number of neural mechanisms involving different levels of the nervous system. The examiner should note any deficiencies of station (such as swaying to one side), balance (which can also be tested by the Romberg test; see Table 1–9), and gait (ataxic gait, Parkinsonian gait).

The function of the cerebellum is to integrate senses, primarily vision, vestibular sense, and proprioception. Cerebellar dysfunction is characterized by awkwardness of intentional movements. Cerebellar function can be assessed through specific tests (see Table 1–9) and the Romberg test.

The final portion of the neurological examination tests the patient's reflexes. The most commonly tested are the muscle-stretch reflexes (eg, patellar, biceps, Achilles, and triceps). Asymmetry is the most useful sign, indicating either hypo- or hyper-reflexia. The Babinski reflex (see Table 1–9) is probably the most useful sign in clinical neurology. This looks for a pathologic reflex (one that should not normally be present). A positive test indicates disease of the pyramidal system at any level from the motor cortex through the descending corticospinal pathways.

Lymph Node Evaluation

Patients presenting with anterior ocular segment inflammation or infection may have involvement of the lymphatic drainage system of the head and neck. It is a relatively straightforward examination procedure requiring simultaneous palpation of both sides of the head and neck. Starting over the occipital area, the examiner should feel for palpable occipital and postauricular lymph nodes (Figure 1–6). The clinician should then examine the posterior cervical chain located behind the sternocleidomastoid muscle, followed by the superficial and deep cervical chains over and under the sternocleidomastoid muscle, and then up to the

angle of the jaw for tonsillar nodes, running the fingers under the jaw for submaxillary nodes (Figure 1–7), to under the tip of the chin in search of submental nodes. The fingers should next palpate up in front of the ears for preauricular nodes (Figure 1–8). Finally, the examiner should stand behind the patient and palpate for supraclavicular nodes just behind the clavicles as the patient inhales deeply. Any palpable node should be noted for consistency, mobility, and tenderness. Inflammation or infection is usually indicated by tender, enlarged nodes. Fixed, hard nodes may indicate a malignancy.

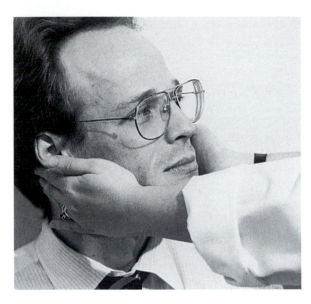

Figure 1–6. Occipital and postauricular lymph node evaluation.

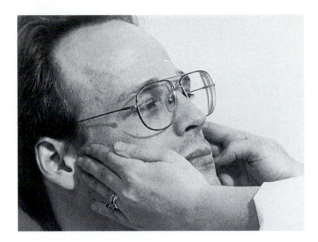

Figure 1–8. Preauricular lymph node evaluation.

Sinus Evaluation

The maxillary and frontal sinuses may be grossly evaluated in patients with suspected sinus infection, congestion, or mass. The examination room must be as dark as possible. A lighted transilluminator should be gently placed up under the superior nasal orbital rim of the right orbit. The light should be directed up into the frontal sinus, and may be moved around gently for full transillumination. A red glow may be observed on the forehead if the sinus is unobstructed. Repeat the procedure with the left orbit. The maxillary sinuses may be transilluminated by tilting the patient's head back, and asking the patient to open the mouth. The transilluminator should be placed inside the center of the infraorbital rim, and moved around gently for full sinus transillumination. The

clinican should observe the red glow in the roof of the patient's mouth. Repeat the procedure with the left orbit. Any asymmetry in transillumination should be noted. The involved sinus may be further evaluated by gently tapping over the sinus (forehead for frontal, cheekbone for maxillary). Tapping on an infected or congested sinus will cause discomfort or pain. Sinus transillumination and tapping are gross evaluations. Any suspected pathology warrants further evaluation (eg, x-rays of the paranasal sinuses).

Thyroid Palpation

Thyroid palpation should be performed on patients with suspected thyroid eye disease, or with notable thyroid gland enlargement. The thyroid is most easily palpated by standing behind the patient. The examiner should place the fingers of both hands just below the thyroid cartilage (cricoid) on the slightly extended neck of the patient (Figure 1–9). The patient should be asked to swallow in order to feel the thyroid isthmus as it rises and falls with the swallowing action. Next, the examiner's fingers should be rotated to either side (down and out) to palpate the lateral lobes as the patient swallows. The normal thyroid consistency is rubbery or muscle-like, without palpable nodules. A firm thyroid gland may indicate a neoplastic process or scarring.

LABORATORY DIAGNOSTIC TESTING

Laboratory tests are useful as a clinical tool in the diagnosis, management, and treatment of a variety of ocular diseases. Later chapters on specific diseases discuss the indications for certain tests; Table 1–10 lists laboratory tests to rule out diseases that may be causing selected ocular conditions. Appendix 2 contains an overall summary with

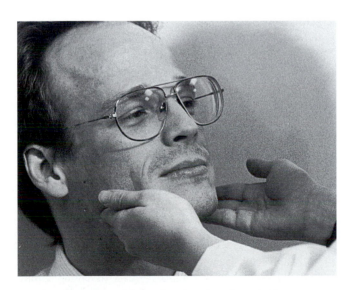

Figure 1–7. Submaxillary lymph node evaluation.

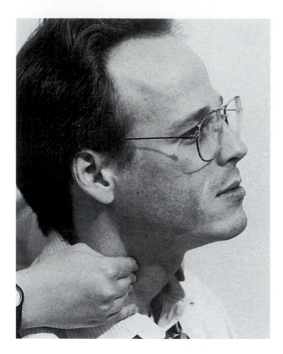

Figure 1–9. Thyroid palpation.

expected values for selected diagnostic tests. Normal values vary from laboratory to laboratory. The present discussion will be limited to the more commonly used diagnostic tests: hematologic testing, serum/blood chemistries, urinalysis, endocrine function tests, serologic tests, skin tests, microbiologic studies, and cerebrospinal fluid testing.

Hematologic Testing

Hematologic tests usually include a complete blood cell count with differential white cell count (CBC with diff). This provides a measure of bone marrow health or competency, with information on several categories of disease processes (eg, hematopoietic, infectious, and hemostatic problems). A CBC with diff includes a hematocrit (Hct; the percentage of total blood volume comprised of cells); hemoglobin (Hgb/Hb; the concentration of oxygen-carrying protein); red blood cell count (RBC); RBC morphologic indices (the average values for size and hemoglobin content); white blood cell count (WBC) and differential (percent of neutrophils, lymphocytes, monocytes, eosinophils, and basophils); and platelet count.

Other tests include clotting times (eg, prothrombin time, or PT, and partial thromboplastin time, or PTT). If a hemoglobin disorder is suspected, hemoglobin electrophoresis will determine the amount and types of hemoglobin present (eg, hemoglobin S in sickle-cell disease). The erythrocyte sedimentation rate (ESR or sed rate) is a nonspecific test that measures the settling of RBCs. The ESR becomes elevated in any inflammatory, infectious, or neoplastic disorder. In normals, the ESR is higher in females and increases

with age. On average, institutionalized and hospitalized patients have a higher sedimentation rate than that expected based on age. Several scales are available for the ESR, with elevated laboratory values not always coincident with clinical standards.

Serum/Blood Chemistries

Serum/blood chemistries provide information concerning numerous chemical constituents in the blood or serum. Usually, more than one parameter will be abnormal in a disease process. Therefore, several parameters must be measured in order to demonstrate the pattern of abnormalities characteristic for the disease. Standard batteries/profiles of selected tests are ordered, which are usually organized for interpretation into logical categories (eg, lipid disorders, electrolytes).

A lipid profile is used to diagnose, manage, and treat lipid disorders and their sequelae (eg, atherosclerosis). This profile usually includes total lipids, cholesterol, triglycerides, and lipoproteins (classified by density: HDL = high-density lipoprotein, LDL = low-density lipoprotein, and VLDL = very-low-density lipoprotein). The National Heart Blood and Lung Institute developed guidelines for determining the risk of developing coronary heart disease in adults over 20 years of age. It is based upon three categories: total cholesterol level, LDL cholesterol level, and the atherosclerosis risk ratios (LDL/HDL and total cholesterol/HDL).

Angiotensin-converting enzyme (ACE) catalyzes the reaction of angiotensin I to the vasoconstrictor, angiotensin II. ACE is produced by granulomas, and is therefore elevated in granulomatous disorders such as sarcoidosis, tuberculosis, leprosy, and histoplasmosis. Serum lysozyme levels also may be elevated in these disorders, as well as in chronic infections and leukemia.

Glucose Testing

Glucose testing is rapidly becoming a routine test ordered by the eyecare practitioner. Glucose levels are important not only in assessing the patient's overall physical status, but also because of their role in ocular manifestations. The most common test is the fasting blood sugar (FBS). The FBS reflects the blood glucose status of the patient that day, in contrast to the glycosylated hemoglobin test (HbA$_{1c}$), which reflects the level of blood glucose over approximately the past 1 to 3 months. Both tests are particularly important in the evaluation of diabetics. The oral glucose tolerance test is done in those with suspected diabetes who have normal FBS. The patient must fast 8 to 12 hours prior to the test. The test begins with a fasting blood sugar and urine glucose test. The patient then ingests an oral glucose load (75 mg, standard for nonpregnant adults) with the blood and urine glucose levels checked at 30 minutes, 1, 2, and 3 hours later (see Appendix 2 for normal

TABLE 1–10. SUGGESTED LABORATORY EXAMINATIONS FOR SELECTED OCULAR CONDITIONS

Ocular Findings	Laboratory Tests	Disease to Rule Out
Episcleritis or scleritis	RF	Rheumatoid arthritis
	ANA	Lupus
	ESR	Nonspecific
	FTA-ABS, RPR	Syphilis
	Serum uric acid	Gout
Anterior uveitis	CBC	Nonspecific
	ESR	Nonspecific
	ANA	Lupus
	FTA-ABS, RPR	Syphilis
	PPD/anergy panel	Tuberculosis
	Chest x-ray	Tuberculosis, sarcoidosis
	ACE, serum lysozyme	Sarcoidosis
	Lyme IFA, ELISA[a]	Lyme disease
Posterior uveitis	Toxoplasma titers	Toxoplasmosis
	ACE, serum lysozyme	Sarcoidosis
	FTA-ABS, RPR	Syphilis
Periphlebitis	FTA-ABS, RPR	Syphilis
	ACE, serum lysozyme	Sarcoidosis
	Hb electrophoresis	Sickle-cell disease
Cotton-wool spot	FBS	Diabetes
	Blood pressure	Hypertension
	ANA	Collagen vascular diseases
	CBC	Anemia, leukemia
	HIV ELISA	AIDS
Retinal neovascularization	Hb electrophoresis	Sickle-cell disease
	ACE, serum lysozyme	Sarcoidosis
	FBS	Diabetes
	CBC	Hematologic disorders
Low-tension glaucoma or optic atrophy	ESR	Giant-cell arteritis, nonspecific
	ANA	Lupus
	FTA-ABS, RPR	Syphilis
	ACE, serum lysozyme	Sarcoidosis
	FBS	Diabetes
	Blood pressure	Hypertension
	Skull films, CT, MRI	Compressive lesions

[a]Endemic areas only.

Reprinted, with permission, from Roberts SP: Optometric utilization of clinical laboratory tests. In Abplanalp PL, ed: Problems in Optometry: Modern Diagnostic Technology. Philadelphia: Lippincott, 1991.

values). The 2-hour postprandial glucose test is a useful screening test for diabetes. Unlike diabetics, nondiabetic patients do not have elevated blood glucose levels 2 hours after a meal.

Endocrine Testing

In suspected thyroid disease, a standard profile often includes thyroid-stimulating hormone (TSH), triiodothyronine radioimmunoassay (T_3RIA), triiodothyronine resin uptake (T_3RU), thyroxine (T_4), and a free thyroxine index (FTI). Hyperthyroidism is usually characterized by elevated T_3RIA, T_3RU, T_4, and FTI, and depressed TSH; whereas hypothyroidism usually results in depressed T_3RIA, T_3RU, T_4, and FTI, and elevated TSH. Disorders of the hypothalamic–pituitary axis may require further endocrine testing (eg, prolactin, growth hormone, follicle-stimulating hormone, luteinizing hormone).

Urinalysis

Urinalysis is a specific measure of kidney function, as well as an indicator of liver, cardiovascular, and/or metabolic disorders. Abnormal test results may occur with certain diseases, diets, and medications. The standard urinalysis measures several parameters. Specific gravity is a measure of the kidneys' ability to concentrate urine. The appearance of urine should be clear to slightly hazy. The normal color of urine (indicating the concentration) is yellow to pale amber, and varies with its specific gravity. Medications can alter the color of urine (eg, sodium fluorescein used in fluorescein angiography will discolor urine to orange-yellow). The pH of urine is between 4.6 and 8, with the average being about 6. The presence of protein or albumin is an indication of a kidney disorder because the kidney filter spaces are normally too small to allow the passage of protein. If glucose is present in urine, it indicates that the renal glucose threshold was exceeded. Ketones or acetone are not normally found in the urine. In uncontrolled diabetes (in particular, Type I), the body turns to stored fat to burn for fuel, and ketones (or acetone), formed as byproducts, are spilled into the urine. The presence of blood, leukocyte esterase, nitrite, and bacteria may indicate infection of the urinary tract. The presence of bilirubin and urobilinogen indicate liver dysfunction. Sediment analysis (looking for trace cells, casts, and crystals in the urine sediment) may be done if urinary tract infections or kidney disorders are suspected.

Serologic Testing
Serologic tests look for the presence of immunologically active proteins (antibodies, immunoglobulins, and antigens). Antinuclear antibodies (ANA) are a group of antibodies that the body produces against its own tissue. They are rarely found in normal patients. The ANA test is useful to screen for autoimmune disorders (eg, systemic lupus erythematosus, rheumatoid arthritis, Sjögren syndrome). Rheumatoid factor (RF) may be present in rheumatoid arthritis, systemic lupus erythematosus, and sarcoidosis. Serum acetylcholine receptor antibodies may be present in patients with myasthenia gravis. Serologic testing utilizing immunofluorescent assays (IFA) or enzyme-linked immunosorbant assays (ELISA) may determine the presence of various infectious diseases (eg, toxocariasis, toxoplasmosis, cytomegalovirus, HIV, syphilis, and Lyme disease; see Table 1–10).

Histocompatibility locus antigen (HLA) typing was originally developed for tissue typing for organ transplantation. However, it was discovered that different HLA antigens are associated with certain diseases (eg, HLA B27 has been associated with ankylosing spondylitis). HLA typing is not routinely indicated, as it is a costly procedure and not necessarily diagnostic of a specific disease.

Skin Testing
Skin testing is often used to determine if a patient has been exposed to an infectious disease. The tuberculin skin test looks for a hypersensitivity reaction (wheal) on the forearm skin to purified protein derivative (PPD) of the mycobacterium tuberculosis. An intradermal injection is given, and 48 hours later the site is inspected for induration (usually 10 mm or more is considered positive). A positive result indicates exposure only and must be followed by a chest x-ray to determine if active disease is present. Other diseases also may be diagnosed via skin testing (eg, sarcoidosis). The Kveim–Siltzbach skin test for sarcoidosis uses human sarcoidal tissue for intradermal injection. The injection site is examined 4 to 6 weeks later for induration.

Microbiological Studies
Microbiological studies include several classes of laboratory tests for the diagnosis of infectious diseases. These include smears and cultures of blood, sputum, cerebrospinal fluid (CSF), and other bodily fluids; tissue biopsy; and serologic and skin testing.

Cerebrospinal Fluid Testing
A lumbar puncture allows evaluation of the cerebrospinal fluid (CSF) (eg, color, protein, glucose, cells, immunoglobulins) as well as the measurement of intracranial pressure (ICP) in mm of H_2O.

IMAGING TECHNIQUES

Imaging studies may be necessary to aid in the diagnosis of certain ocular conditions. This discussion will be limited to the more frequently used diagnostic imaging tests. Common radiographic studies include plain films, computerized tomography, and radiography with contrast media (eg, angiogram, venogram, pyelogram, barium enema). Other imaging studies include ultrasonography (eg, duplex scan), magnetic resonance imaging, and nuclear medicine studies.

Radiography
Radiographs use electromagnetic waves of very short wavelength (x-rays). As the x-rays pass through the body, their intensity is reduced by absorption. Denser tissue, such as bone, absorbs more and therefore appears whiter on the film, whereas soft tissue, which is less dense, absorbs less and therefore appears darker on the film. Contrast media may be used to enhance or highlight detail not normally seen on plain film. These may be radiopaque (fully block x-ray transmission) or radiolucent (partially block x-ray transmission). Potential contraindications to contrast media include allergic reaction, which may be mild (hives) to severe (anaphylactic death).

Angiography and Venography
Angiography and venography involve a rapid series of x-ray films obtained after an injection of contrast dye in order to study major arteries, branches, tumors, and venous drainage. Angiography may be used to study the cardiac, cerebral, carotid, and pulmonary arterial systems. Digital subtraction angiography (DSA) enhances an angiogram by eliminating the surrounding anatomy from the view. Venography may be used to study peripheral venous and orbital drainage. Angiography and venography are associated with a certain amount of morbidity and mortality, due both to the contrast media employed and the injection procedure itself.

Computed Tomography
Computed tomography (CT) is an x-ray procedure that allows for the examination of a single layer or plane of

tissue. A computer performs rapid calculations to eliminate the multiple x-rays not absorbed by the plane of tissue in focus, thus providing better visualization of tissue not ordinarily viewed on routine x-rays. CT with contrast further highlights details not normally revealed. CT (with and without contrast) may be employed for viewing any part of the body, but it is especially useful for visualizing the brain, chest, and retroperitoneum.

■ Nuclear Medicine Studies

Nuclear medicine studies or scans are used to visualize organs and regions within organs that cannot be seen with regular x-ray. Various radiopharmaceuticals may be injected or ingested depending upon the tissue or structure being imaged (eg, thyroid, bone, brain). A scanning device is passed over the tissue or body part to be examined to pick up emitted radiation in order to determine the distribution of the substance. Abnormal tissues (necrosis, tumors, granulomas) readily take up excessive amounts of the radioisotope and show up as hot spots on the scan. Contraindications to nuclear scans include certain prosthetic devices in the body, which can absorb radioisotopes and distort the scanning process; and a history of allergies to radioisotopes.

■ Radiation Hazard

There is a radiation hazard with radiographic studies and, to a lesser degree, nuclear scans. Therefore, pregnant or nursing mothers should not undergo these procedures unless absolutely necessary. Genetic and somatic damage (tissue burn) may occur, depending on the type and length of exposure.

■ Magnetic Resonance Imaging (MRI)

Magnetic resonance imaging (MRI) scans have fast become one of the most useful imaging tests available. However, due to the cost and time factors, MRI scans are not routine. Images obtained by MRI scans are usually at least equal to CT scans. In brief, MRI is based upon the principle that atomic nuclei with an odd number of protons or neutrons will act like magnets when placed in a magnetic field. In the human body, hydrogen is the most abundant element satisfying this definition. When the body is placed in a strong magnetic field, the hydrogen nuclei align describing a net magnetic vector. A radiofrequency pulse is then introduced, which displaces the net magnetic vector. When the pulse is removed, the nuclei return to their original orientation while emitting the absorbed energy in the form of a radiofrequency signal. It is this signal that is used to generate the image. MRI is particularly useful for delineating soft tissue (eg, demyelinating plaques in the central nervous system, aneurysms, tumors). Contraindications include metallic foreign bodies (pacemakers, metallic

vascular clips, metallic plate) and claustrophobia. Unlike other imaging techniques, MRI requires up to an hour to complete and is particularly loud as it generates the magnetic field. Therefore, patients should be educated prior to this test about the length of time, as well as the intensity of noise the instrument produces during the test. It is unknown whether pregnancy is a contraindication for MRI; therefore, it should be done only when absolutely necessary. Contrast medium (gadolinium) may now be used to enhance the MR image.

■ Ultrasonography

Ultrasonography (echography) is a noninvasive procedure used to visualize soft tissue structures. An ultrasound beam is directed into the body part to be examined. Propagated by vibration, the sound waves are reflected differently depending upon tissue density. The reflected sound waves, or echoes, are electronically processed and imaged. The reflected ultrasound waves are interpreted by the instrument and displayed on a screen. Photography and videotaping are two common methods available to record the displayed image. There are several different procedure methods and display techniques depending on the structure to be imaged. A-mode ultrasonography (amplitude modulated) gives information regarding time and amplitude of the structure studied (eg, length of the eyeball for determination of the power of an intraocular lens). A-mode does not provide an image; however, it is from this which all other modes of ultrasound are derived. B-mode (brightness modulated) provides two-dimensional or cross-sectional information, thus forming an image of the structure studied as well as the movement of tissues. To study the movement of blood flow through vessels and cardiac valves, the Doppler principle is applied. This interprets the change in frequency in the movement of objects (red blood cells through the vessels or valves). Duplex scans are used to evaluate occlusive vessel disease (eg, carotid arteries). This method combines doppler ultrasound and B-mode sonography into one instrument. Echocardiograms utilize this method to assess the vessels and valves of the heart.

CONCLUSION

Primary eyecare in systemic disease mandates an overall evaluation of the patient. Incorporation of ocular and physical examinations, laboratory diagnostic tests, and imaging studies is vital for comprehensive evaluation of the patient. Referrals to or consultations from other specialties should be used in the management of a patient with ocular manifestations of a systemic disease.

REFERENCES

Barresi BJ, Nyman NN. Implementation of the problem-oriented system in an optometry teaching clinic. *Am J Optom Physiol Optics.* 1978;55:765–770.

Bates B. *A Guide to Physical Examination and History Taking.* 5th ed. Philadelphia: Lippincott; 1991.

Classe JG. Clinicolegal aspects of practice record keeping and documentation in clinical practice. *Southern J Optom.* 1987;5:11–25.

Fingeret M, Casser L, Woodcombe HT. *Atlas of Primary Eyecare Procedures.* Norwalk, CT: Appleton & Lange; 1990.

Fischbach F. *A Manual of Laboratory Diagnostic Tests.* 3rd ed. Philadelphia: Lippincott; 1988.

Gomella LG, ed. *Clinician's Pocket Reference.* 6th ed. Norwalk, CT: Appleton & Lange; 1989.

Ravel R. *Clinical Laboratory Medicine: Clinical Application of Laboratory Data.* 5th ed. Chicago: Yearbook; 1989.

Roberts SP. Optometric utilization of clinical laboratory tests. In: Abplanalp PL, ed. *Problems in Optometry: Modern Diagnostic Technology.* Philadelphia: Lippincott; March 1991.

Sloan PG. A "problem-oriented" optometric record? *Am J Optom Physiol Optics.* 1978;55:352–357.

Swartz MH. *Textbook of Physical Diagnosis: History and Examination.* Philadelphia: Saunders; 1989.

Thomann KH, Dul MW. The optometric assessment of neurologic function. *J Am Optom Assoc.* 1993;64:421–431.

Weed LL. Medical records that guide and teach. *N Engl J Med.* 1968;278:593–599, 652–657.

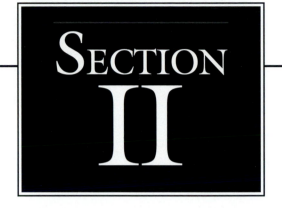

SECTION II

CARDIOVASCULAR DISORDERS

2

Chapter

Hypertension

Mitchell W. Dul

Hypertension accounts for the greatest number of office visits to healthcare providers in the United States. In a given individual, blood pressure can vary with the time of day, level of anxiety, and a host of other factors. It is therefore advisable to reserve the diagnosis of hypertension for those individuals who, in a relaxed atmosphere, demonstrate diastolic pressure exceeding 90 mm Hg or whose systolic pressure exceeds 140 mm Hg on two or three separate occasions. Hypertension can be divided into two general categories: primary (essential), accounting for approximately 95% of all cases; and secondary hypertension. Although a common ailment, the etiology of primary hypertension is not fully understood. Secondary hypertension is generally a sequela of kidney or endocrine disorders. Ocular complications may occur in the presence of long-standing systemic hypertension or may result from acute severe episodes. The vasculature of the retina, choroid, and optic nerve are affected differently by hypertension.

EPIDEMIOLOGY

■ Systemic

Hypertension is present in approximately 57 million Americans, roughly 30% of the adult population in the United States over the age of 40. The risk factor for stroke is four times greater in those persons having hypertension, and the risk of stroke increases with the elevation of the systolic pressure.

■ Ocular

It is difficult to calculate the actual incidence of hypertensive retinopathy, but it is second only to diabetic retinopathy as the most common retinal vascular disease seen in general practice. Its clinical presentation will vary with the severity, degree of control, and duration of the hypertension. Hypertension is the most commonly associated systemic disease in the presence of a branch retinal vein occlusion.

NATURAL HISTORY

■ Systemic

The etiology of essential hypertension is unknown and probably no singular mechanism accounts for its development. It is likely to result from a combination of causes whose cumulative effect results in poor blood pressure control. Risk factors include male sex, increased age, family history, the affects of the renin–angiotensin system, and sympathetic nervous system overactivity. Alcohol abuse, obesity, sedentary life style, and cigarette smoking also may contribute to hypertension. Salt intake, while commonly associated with an increased risk, applies primarily to patients with established hypertension or those with a family history of the disease.

The renin–angiotensin system and sympathetic nervous system overactivity, although not primarily implicated in the pathogenesis of essential hypertension, are noteworthy in order to better understand both treatment options and the etiology of the more common types of secondary hypertension.

The renin–angiotensin system serves to maintain normal regulation of blood pressure via its influence on peripheral resistance. The interaction between peripheral resistance to blood flow and cardiac output determines the arterial pressure (arterial pressure = cardiac output × total peripheral resistance). Therefore, any increase or decrease in either of these variables will produce a corresponding increase or decrease in arterial pressure.

Peripheral resistance is provided primarily by the arterioles. It varies as they dilate or constrict as a result of the effects of neural and hormonal influences. Peripheral resistance is also increased in the presence of arteriolosclerosis, which decreases the size of the lumen through which blood must flow.

The release of renin by the juxtaglomerular cells may be triggered by any number of conditions including decreased renal perfusion pressure, decreased intravascular volume, circulating catecholamines, and increased sympathetic nervous system activity. The release of renin precipitates a sequence of biochemical reactions that result in the formation of angiotensin II, a potent vasoconstrictor. Vasoconstriction increases peripheral resistance, which correspondingly increases arterial pressure. This effect is short lived. A prolonged effect results from the direct effect of angiotensin II on the kidneys and the adrenal glands. Its presence causes the kidneys to retain salt and water and causes the adrenal glands to release aldosterone, which also directly causes kidney salt and water retention. This increases extracellular fluid volume, which ultimately results in increased arterial pressure and causes an increase in blood flow from the heart to the tissues of the body, producing local vasoconstriction. Vasoconstriction in turn increases peripheral resistance, which further increases the arterial pressure. Translated to the kidneys, this increase in arterial pressure will increase the glomerular filtration rate, thus promoting the release and subsequent excretion of salt and water. This is called pressure diuresis or pressure natriuresis. This will decrease the extracellular fluid volume and, by means of the previously reported cascade of events, normalize the blood pressure.

Sympathetic nervous system overactivity increases the heart rate up to 250 beats per minute and causes up to a 100% increase in the strength of ventricular contractions. At the same time it decreases the duration of systolic contractions to allow for greater filling time during diastole. Direct stimulation of blood vessels under sympathetic control leads to vasoconstriction, which results in increased peripheral resistance, thereby increasing arterial pressure.

The systemic manifestations of hypertension vary with the severity of the condition and the affected organs. Although most patients are asymptomatic and are diagnosed as an incidental finding, acute hypertension is often associated with headaches, nausea, vomiting, and loss of consciousness. Prolonged, poorly controlled hypertension will compromise the ability of the cardiovascular system to transport oxygenated blood to vital organs (especially the heart, brain, and kidneys). The clinical picture will therefore be variable.

Heart

Left ventricular hypertrophy is a common sequela of prolonged hypertension and results in a significant increase in risk of mortality and morbidity at any level of blood pressure. The contraction of the ventricles must create enough force to move blood out of the ventricle and into the circulation. It is resisted by the pressure of the blood already in the arteries. The greater this peripheral resistance, the harder the ventricles must work. Like skeletal muscle, one way in which the myocardium responds to a prolonged increased workload is to increase in size (hypertrophy). Muscle hypertrophy causes an increase in oxygen demand and, particularly in the presence of concurrent atherosclerosis or previous myocardial infarct with subsequent tissue necrosis, this new demand may not be adequately met. This is clinically manifested as angina, myocardial infarct, or sudden death. In addition, there are other limitations to ventricular hypertrophy. If the arterial pressure is high enough, the ventricle, despite its increased mass, may be unable to pump out its full load of blood with each beat. This results in a given amount of blood remaining in the heart (referred to as forward failure) at the expense of both the oxygen demand of the body's tissues and the ventricular capacity (which cannot adequately hold all of the new blood arriving from the atria). The latter causes a hematologic log jam (backward failure), which backs up the pulmonary vein (on the left side) or the vena cava (on the right). Left ventricular failure is characterized by difficult or labored breathing (dyspnea) and low cardiac output. This may be exacerbated when the patient lies down, due to further increases in pulmonary blood volume. Some patients may have difficulty breathing, except in the upright position (orthopnea). Long- standing pulmonary venous hypertension, in a manner analogous to the development of collaterals between the central retinal vein and choroidal circulation in the presence of a central retinal vein occlusion, can promote anastomoses between the pulmonary and bronchial veins in the form of bronchial submucosal varices (enlarged and tortuous vessels), which often rupture, producing the expectoration of blood or blood-stained sputum (hemoptysis). In the presence of left ventricular hypertrophy, rales (any abnormal respiratory sound) and gallop rhythms (an accentuated extra cardiac sound) may be audible with the stethoscope. Right ventricular failure, which backs-up the vena cava, predictably results in peripheral edema, distended neck veins, abdominal distension, and hepatomegaly.

Brain

The effects of hypertension and associated atherosclerosis are responsible for the majority of cerebral vascular accidents (CVAs) by hemorrhagic, thrombotic, or embolic causes, and account for a significant amount of patient mortality and morbidity (see Chapter 5). Intracerebral hemorrhage almost always occurs secondary to sustained, elevated systolic blood pressure. In addition, approximately 40% of all CVAs, whether hemorrhagic or not, can be attributed to systolic blood pressure greater than 140 mm Hg.

Hypertensive encephalopathy is associated with a rapid rise in blood pressure and presents with symptoms of headache, nausea, vomiting, or loss of consciousness as well as severe hypertensive retinopathy and renal insufficiency. It probably results from acute capillary congestion and exudation, which causes cerebral edema. These changes are usually reversible as blood pressure is brought under control. In general, diastolic blood pressure exceeds 130 mm Hg, although there are often exceptions to this.

Kidneys
Prolonged hypertension is also commonly implicated in the pathogenesis of renal artery stenosis. It may also lead to renal insufficiency.

In general, when under stable control, the incidence of complications as a result of elevated blood pressure are minimized. Most treated patients will occasionally experience a mild to moderate increase in blood pressure that is either short lived or responsive to modifications in therapy. Complications do not typically occur without a prolonged period of increased pressure that directly impacts the heart (left ventricular hypertrophy), the vessels, and their respective end organs (formation of aneurysms or hemorrhage). Indirect complications may occur as a result of atherosclerosis, which is often accompanied and exacerbated by unchecked hypertension. The degree of pressure increase leading to end- organ damage varies from patient to patient.

A small percentage (5%) of patients with essential hypertension will develop malignant hypertension, which is defined as a systolic pressure greater than or equal to 200 mm Hg and a diastolic pressure greater than or equal to 120 mm Hg with concurrent evidence of end-organ damage (systemic: renal failure, left ventricular failure; ocular: disc edema, hemorrhage, exudate, hypertensive encephalopathy). These patients are typically males in their late 30s to early 40s with high levels of renin, angiotensin II, and aldosterone. An association may exist between this condition and human leukocyte antigen (HLA) B15. The etiology of malignant hypertension is unknown.

Secondary Hypertension
Hypertension may develop secondary to oral contraceptive use, renal disease, coarctation of the aorta, pregnancy, hyperparathyroidism, hypercalcemia, and diseases associated with increased intracerebral pressure (Table 2–1). The most common specific cause of secondary hypertension is the use of oral contraceptives (estrogen), which increases the activity of the renin–angiotensin system. Most women will experience some rise in blood pressure when taking these medications;

however, approximately 5% will have an increase above 140/90. This is more common in obese women and in those over the age of 35. This phenomena is not known to occur in postmenopausal women on estrogen therapy.

Another common cause of secondary hypertension is stenosis of the renal artery either from atherosclerosis (generally in patients over the age of 50) or fibromuscular hyperplasia (generally in women under the age of 50). Fibromuscular hyperplasia accounts for approximately 30% of renal disease. Stenosis of the renal artery causes decreased renal blood flow and perfusion pressure. This triggers the release of renin, which results in increased blood pressure. Less commonly, adrenal tumors may produce secondary hypertension. Primary hyperaldosteronism (usually a result of an adrenal adenoma with subsequent hypersecretion of aldosterone) is present in less than 0.5% of all cases of hypertension. Pheochromocytoma, a rare condition, is usually the result of an adrenal tumor with subsequent hypersecretion of catecholamine. The typical clinical picture includes fluctuating blood pressure with headache, palpitations, pallor, sweating, orthostatic hypotension, and hyperglycemia. Despite this, patients often present with relatively stable pressure and any one or a combination of these signs.

■ Ocular
The retina, optic nerve, and choroidal vasculature are differentially affected by hypertension (summarized in Table 2–2).

Retinal Vasculature
The retinal vasculature (the central retinal artery and its tributaries) provides blood to the inner portion of the retina. Zonular occludens between cells create a blood–tissue barrier similar to that of the circulatory system of the brain. Anterior to the lamina cribrosa, they are not under sympathetic nervous system control. These vessels respond to increases in blood pressure by autoregulation.

The initial response to increased pressure inside a retinal artery is vasoconstriction. This is accomplished by myogenic and metabolic autoregulation and is not under autonomic nervous system control. The myogenic autoregulatory system is regulated by pacemaker cells in the walls of the vessels that are stimulated by changes in perfusion pressure (a function of transmural pressure and the intraocular pressure). Vasodilation occurs, for instance, in the presence of increased intraocular pressure or low retinal arterial transmural pressure, and is a compensatory response intended to maintain a steady flow of uninterrupted blood under manageable pressure. Metabolic autoregulation is a function of the balanced concentration of metabolites and nutrients (excess O_2 produces vasoconstriction, whereas excess CO_2 produces vasodilation). Retinal vascular autoregulation is negatively impacted by age, hypertension, hyperglycemia, and other systemic conditions—so much so that a patient may have difficulty adapting to even normal changes in retinal perfusion pressure.

TABLE 2–1. CAUSES OF SECONDARY HYPERTENSION

Renal Disorders

Volume overload secondary to renal failure
Chronic renal failure (parenchymal disease)
    Polycystic kidneys
    Chronic glomerulonephritis
Obstructive uropathy
Primary abnormality in salt excretion
    Gordon syndrome
    Liddle syndrome
Renovascular disease
    Atherosclerosis
    Fibromuscular dysplasia
    Other (aortic arch syndrome, polyarteritis nodosa)
Tumors
    Renin-secreting (pericytoma)
    Wilms'
    Adenocarcinoma

Endocrine Disorders

Adrenal disease
    Mineralocorticoid excess
    Primary hyperaldosteronism
    11,17-hydroxylase deficiency
    Cushing syndrome
    Pheochromocytoma
Pituitary disease
    Acromegaly
    Cushing syndrome
Thyroid disease
    Hypothyroidism
    Hyperthyroidism

Hyperparathyroidism (hypercalcemia)

Drug Use

Hormonal
    Estrogen/progestogen contraceptive
    Exogenous ACTH
    Anabolic steroids
    Glucocorticoids
Nonhormonal
    Licorice
    Cocaine/crack
    Amphetamines

Other Causes

Excess ethanol intake
Ethanol or drug withdrawal
Pregnancy
Aortic coarctation
Neurologic disorders
    Increased intracranial pressure
    Familial dysautonomia
    Quadriplegia
    Guillain–Barré syndrome
Pain
Acute stress
Porphyria
Endothelin-producing tumor

Reprinted with permission from Nasir M, Eisner GM: Reversible hypertension in adults. Hospital Med 1992;28:23.

TABLE 2–2. OCULAR MANIFESTATIONS OF HYPERTENSION

■ **RETINAL VASCULATURE**
- Vasoconstriction
- Sclerosis
- Exudation
- Complications of sclerosis

■ **OPTIC NERVE VASCULATURE**
- Bilateral disc edema
- Variable concurrent retinal vascular changes
- Exudation

■ **CHOROIDAL VASCULATURE**
- Elschnig spots
- Siegrist spots
- Fluorescein leak in late phase
- Possible serous RD or macular star

Appreciation of constricted retinal arteries relies on accurate and dependable knowledge of the normal retinal arterial caliber. Using the caliber of the retinal veins and describing the two vessels as a ratio is a common practice that can be misleading, because the caliber of retinal veins are variable. Furthermore, this technique offers poor interobserver reliability. It is also not uncommon to see arterial attenuation and even arterial–venous crossing changes in elderly patients with no evidence of hypertension.

It would better serve the practitioner to develop an appreciation for normal retinal vascular caliber and use this as a reference when assessing vasoconstrictive changes in the retina. Retinal arterial vasoconstriction is best appreciated beyond the second branch of the central retinal artery. In fact, the primary site of vasoconstriction is the precapillary arterioles. The goal of retinal vasoconstriction is to stabilize the intraluminal pressure, thereby supplying the tissue that is fed by the retinal capillary beds with a constant source of oxygenated blood under pressure that will not damage the vessel walls. Prolonged elevated hypertension will result in retinal arterial damage—specifically, intimal hyalinization, medial hypertrophy, and endothelial hyperplasia. This translates to a thickening of the arterial wall and is clinically appreciated as attenuation of the arteries, widening of the arterial light reflex, and nicking/banking changes at arterial–venous crossings. This phase of hypertensive retinopathy is considered the sclerotic phase (Figure 2–1), and it is clinically and histopathologically indistinguishable from arteriolosclerotic retinal arterial changes described in chapter 3.

Over the years, several grading systems were established in an effort to judge the efficacy of treatment and the progression of hypertension. However, many of the clinical signs are found in a nonhypertensive population and may represent normal age-related changes. For instance, debris accumulating in the perivascular sheath, a normal age-related phenomena, may appear clinically as a widening of the arterial reflex. Most grading systems also do not consider the dynamics of the retinal arterial response to increased intraluminal pressure. For example, focusing upon the sclerotic component alone (as in previous classification systems) narrows the clinical utility of this examination. When the clinician is familiar with the dynamic response of the retinal vasculature to increased pressure, more useful information can be generated from a retinal examination. For instance, the presence of recurrent vasoconstriction in a patient with "stable" hypertension suggests that the condition is in fact not consistently controlled. This is useful information to a practitioner who is basing the success of treatment in large part on an in-office reading of blood pressure, which is often an inaccurate measure of long-term stability. Hypertensive retinopathy has also been classified by several clinical grading systems that, in many cases, supply the clinician with little if any useful information that might affect the treatment of the patient. It would be more useful to incorporate what is known about the physiologic response of the retinal vasculature to increased blood pressure into a classification system that would provide practitioners with some degree of evidence of improper control of hypertension. Such a classification system has been postulated by Tso and associates (1991) and is summarized in Table 2–3.

If the pressure of blood inside the retinal artery acutely rises or remains elevated over a prolonged period of time, it may exceed the limits to which vasoconstriction and sclerosis can compensate. This leads to a compromise in the integrity of the endothelial zonular occludens, which results in the vessel leaking blood products. The leaking of red blood cells is seen clinically as flame-shaped (on the precapillary side) or dot/blot hemorrhages (on the postcapillary side). Plasma lipoprotein, phospholipid, cholesterol, and triglycerides may leak, and are clinically seen as hard exudates. In the case of acute or severe hypertension, the change is so rapid that the response of the vessel progresses from the vasoconstrictive phase directly to this exudative phase (Figure 2–2). If the hypertension is not brought under control, the vessel wall becomes necrotic. This results in loss of autoregulation and a resultant dilation of the vessel. Without the benefit of the protection afforded by vasoconstriction, the capillary beds are subject to the high pressure. The result is capillary damage and leakage, which impairs the flow of blood to the retina. This is seen clinically as retinal nerve fiber layer ischemia (cotton-wool spots). If the

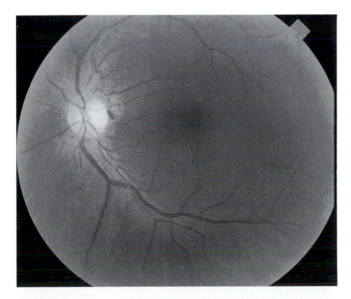

Figure 2–1. The sclerotic phase of hypertensive retinopathy, which is clinically and histopathologically indistinguishable from arteriolosclerotic retinal arterial changes (Chapter 3).

TABLE 2–3. STAGES OF RESPONSE OF RETINAL ARTERIAL SUPPLY TO INCREASES IN BLOOD PRESSURE

Vasconstriction

Initial response to HTN
Transient
Controlled by autoregulation
Beyond second branch of CRA

Sclerosis

Results from prolonged HTN
Irreversible
Damage and thickening of arterial wall
May mimic normal age-related changes

Exudation

Results from prolonged HTN or abrupt acute
Integrity of tight junctions compromised
Blood produces leak into retina

Complications of Sclerosis

Branch retinal vein occlusion, central retinal vein occlusion (ischemic and nonischemic)
Central retinal artery occlusion, branch retinal artery occlusion
Retinal macroaneurysm

underlying hypertension is brought under control during the "vasoconstrictive" or "exudative" phase, the arterial supply returns to its normal caliber and the retinal hemorrhages, exudates, and ischemia eventually resolve.

Retinal arterial sclerosing is not thought of as a reversible pathologic change. Sclerosing may be segmental, which is evident as retinal arteries of irregular caliber. This may be particularly apparent during subsequent vasoconstriction of the retinal arteries (in response to a rise in blood pressure). Complications of the sclerotic phase include central and branch artery occlusion (Figure 2–3), retinal

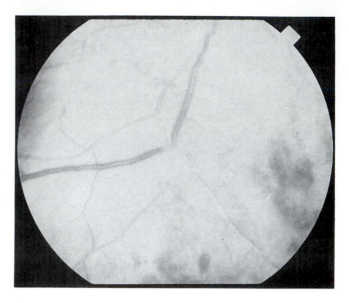

Figure 2–3. Branch artery occlusion (note the concurrent vasoconstriction of adjacent arteries).

macroaneurysm (outpouching of the compromised vessel wall in the presence of high intraluminal pressure; Figure 2–4), and central and branch retinal vein occlusion (Figure 2–5). The latter results from the compression of the venous branch at an arterial–venous crossing.

Retinal ischemia resulting from either central or branch vein and arterial occlusions may produce retinal, optic nerve, and/or anterior segment neovascularization as well as vitreal hemorrhage and rhegametogenous retinal detachment. The probability of neovascularization, and in particular of rubeosis irides secondary to central retinal artery occlusion, may be as high as 20% (approximating that of

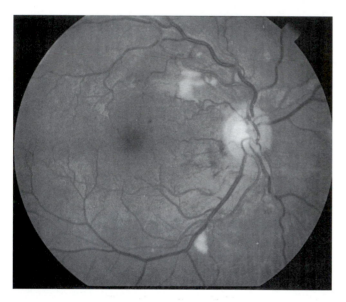

A

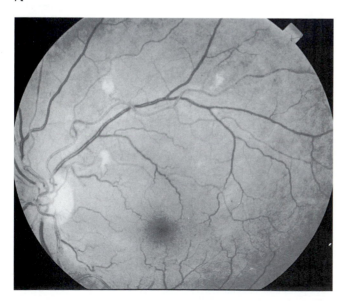

B

Figure 2–2. The vasoconstrictive and exudative phases concurrently present due to a prolonged episode of acute hypertension. **A.** Right eye. **B.** Left eye.

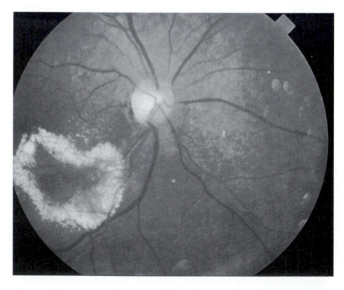

Figure 2–4. A complication of the sclerotic phase: retinal macroaneurysm.

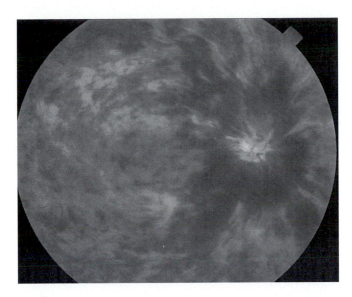

A

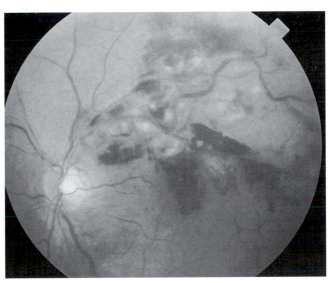

B

Figure 2–5. Complications of the sclerotic phase. **A.** Central retinal vein occlusion. **B.** Branch retinal vein occlusion.

central retinal vein occlusion). When it does occur, its peak incidence is approximately 4 weeks following the occlusion versus the average of 5 months following a central retinal vein occlusion. Panretinal photocoagulation has proven to be beneficial in some of these patients, although those who go on to develop neovascularization generally require additional treatment modalities such as cyclocryotherapy or YAG laser cyclophotocoagulation.

Optic Nerve Vasculature

The blood supply of the optic nerve head is composed of a complex network of vessels derived from the posterior ciliary, retinal, and pial circulations. The latter is primarily composed of branches of the ophthalmic artery or recurrent branches from the posterior ciliary arteries. These three sources, in addition to their individual contributions, anastomose, and in some individuals form an incomplete intrascleral circle that surrounds the optic nerve known as the circle of Zinn–Haller. Because the optic nerve receives a blood supply from sources regulated by sympathetic tone and autoregulation, it is subject to each of these forms of intraluminal pressure regulation. Like the blood–retinal barrier in the retinal vasculature, the blood supply to the optic nerve is characterized as having tight endothelial junctions, muscular walls, and thick basement membranes that provide an effective blood–nerve barrier. Although it is unlikely that direct anastomoses exist between the choriocapillaris and the capillaries of the optic nerve, the border tissue of Elschnig, which separates these two systems, does not offer an effective blood–nerve barrier. It is capable of leaking choroidal fluid, which may contribute to disc edema. In secondary hypertension, the release of renin leads to the production of angiotensin II. It is theorized that this potent vasoconstrictor is able to pass through the fenestrations of the choriocapillaris to produce vasoconstriction of the muscular arteriolar walls of the choroid. From the choriocapillaris, it may also be able to cross the border tissue of Elschnig to produce vasoconstriction in the vessels of the optic nerve.

The vasculature of the optic nerve head is most prominently affected in the presence of acute, severe hypertension. The ocular presentation of malignant hypertension is characterized by bilateral disc edema (Figure 2–6), with or without hypertensive retinal vascular changes, and venous engorgement. Visual acuities may be unaffected or dramatically reduced. Retinal exudation may appear in the macula in the form of a star pattern (consistent with the architecture of the Henle layer) and hypertensive encephalopathy may be present. In animal models, the order of appearance of fundus lesions is (1) focal intraretinal periarteriolar transudates; (2) acute focal retinal pigment epithelial lesions, macular edema, and disc edema; and (3) focal nerve fiber layer ischemia (cotton-wool spots).

Disc edema may be secondary to the ingress of choroidal fluid or angiotensin II through the border tissue of Elschnig, direct damage of the vascular supply of the optic nerve with secondary ischemia, or in the presence of hypertensive encephalopathy, the corresponding elevation of cerebral spinal fluid pressure. It is important to note that, contrary to previously held assertions, disc edema can be present in the absence of encephalopathy, and the extent of disc edema is not an indication of the patient's visual or general prognosis. Generally, these patients are concurrently treated for the underlying increase in blood pressure. However, if the blood pressure is brought down too abruptly, the perfusion pressure to the nerve may become so low as to cause further irreparable damage. The same is true regarding the perfusion pressure to the brain.

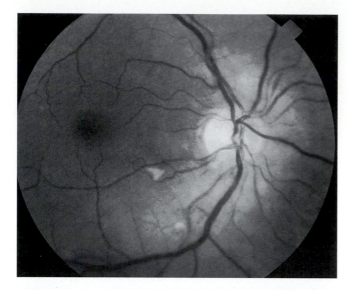

A

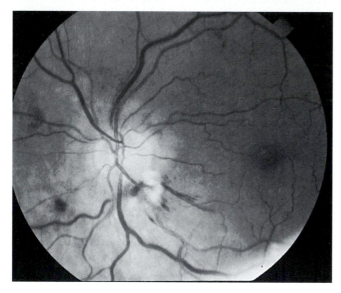

B

Figure 2–6. Bilateral disc edema secondary to malignant hypertension. **A.** Right eye. **B.** Left eye.

Choroidal Circulation

The choroidal circulation is a fenestrated system that lacks a tight blood–tissue barrier. It is derived primarily from the short posterior ciliary arteries. There is also some lesser contribution from the peripapillary blood vessels. Its response to changes in intraluminal pressure is regulated by the sympathetic nervous system.

Unlike the retinal vasculature, the choroid responds to sympathetic stimulation. In addition, the fenestrated choriocapillaris may allow angiotensin II and/or other substrates to pass into the choroidal stroma to stimulate choroidal arteriolar muscular walls. The choroidal circulation is also influenced by the intraocular pressure. Elevation of intraocular pressure increases choroidal vascular resistance possibly due to pressure translated to the vortex veins as they pass through the oblique scleral canal.

The majority of cases of hypertensive choroidopathy (HC) are found in young patients and result from acute hypertension (pregnancy induced, renal diseases, pheochromocytoma, malignant hypertension). Ocular signs include RPE disruption and retinal vascular changes.

The choriocapillaris is vulnerable to increased blood pressure due to the relatively short course and scant branching of the choroidal arteries. Vasoconstriction of these arteries protects the nearby choriocapillaris but may produce local ischemia to the RPE. The result is focal necrosis of the RPE in a pattern corresponding to the structural arrangement of the choriocapillaris. The ensuing window defect will typically leak fluorescein during the late phase. There may also be a corresponding serous retinal detachment and/or macular star formation.

The structural arrangement of the choriocapillaris varies with its location. In the posterior pole, an arteriole supplies oxygenated blood to the center of a lobular network of capillaries, which is drained circumferentially. The benefit of this lobular arrangement appears to be greater blood flow to this region. In the posterior pole, the RPE disruption is termed an Elschnig spot and the pattern is lobular in shape. This suggests that each lobule is an independent functioning vascular unit. In time, these areas will develop a pigmented center surrounded by a depigmented halo, and there will no longer be fluorescein leakage in the late phase.

In the equator, the medium-sized choroidal arteries travel anteriorly and join the choroidal veins, which are traveling in the same direction toward the vortex veins. This results in choriocapillaries that travel a relatively straight course in a spindle-shaped arrangement. Here, the lesion is termed a Siegrist spot (Figure 2–7). It is typically larger in area. Multiple spots may follow the course of a choroidal vessel.

In the periphery, the choroidal arteries and veins are relatively parallel and travel perpendicular to the ora serrata. They are connected by a network of capillaries that run between them at right angles. The result is a ladder-shaped configuration. These spots are generally triangular in shape with the base toward the ora serrata.

DIAGNOSIS

■ Systemic

An exhaustive workup is not required in the diagnosis of hypertension. Systolic pressure greater than 140 mm Hg or diastolic greater than 90 mm Hg on at least two (preferably three) occasions (taken in as stress-free an environment as possible) constitutes high blood pressure. Clinical findings

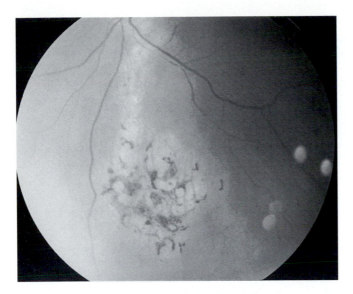

Figure 2–7. Siegrist spot.

suggestive of primary or secondary hypertension are summarized in Table 2–4. Tests for renal function (creatinine levels), complete blood count (to detect anemia or polycythemia), serum potassium (to assist in ruling out hyperaldosteronism), urinalysis (to rule out hematuria, proteinuria, and casts—signs of primary renal disease and/or renal artery sclerosis), fasting blood glucose (to assess for diabetes and evidence of pheochromocytoma), plasma lipids (to assess risk for atherosclerotic disease), and ECG (which is highly specific but not sensitive in ruling out left ventricular hypertrophy), assist in differentiating essential from secondary hypertension by focusing on various target end-organs. Unfortunately, most tests for renal vascular hypertension are not highly sensitive and lack specificity. Renal hypertension should be suspected if the age of onset is less than 20 years or greater than 50, in the presence of concurrent atherosclerotic disease elsewhere, or if renal function is dramatically compromised following angiotensin-converting enzyme inhibitor (ACE) therapy.

■ Ocular

The diagnosis of the ocular manifestations of hypertension are based on the funduscopic and fluorescein angiographic appearance previously described (see Table 2–2).

TREATMENT AND MANAGEMENT

■ Systemic

Until fairly recently, diuretics were used almost exclusively as the initial form of treatment of hypertension. Evidence now shows that four classifications of medications have approximately equal chance of controlling hypertension as a sole therapy. The selection of the initial drug of choice is

TABLE 2–4. CLINICAL FINDINGS SUGGESTIVE OF HYPERTENSION

Primary Hypertension

History
Age at onset 30–50 years
Presence of family history

Physical Examination
Diastolic pressure exceeding 90 mm Hg or systolic exceeding 140 mm Hg on two or three separate occasions

Secondary Hypertension

History
Age at onset <20 or > 50 years
Absence of family history
Poor BP control on 3-drug regimen
Uncontrolled BP after period of good control
Palpitations, tremors, excessive sweating, weight loss, glucose intolerance
Peripheral vascular disease, cerebrovascular disease, or myocardial infarction
Ethanol intake >3 drinks /day
Hormonal contraceptive use
Use of cocaine, amphetamines, or similar drugs
Genitourinary or renal disease
Possible malignancy
Deterioration in renal function induced by ACE inhibitors
Muscle pain or weakness, especially after diuretic use
Symptoms of Cushing syndrome

Physical Examination
Difference in BP in upper extremities
Difference in BP and pulse in upper and lower extremities
Abdominal bruit
Abdominal mass
Peripheral cyanosis or gangrene
Peripheral edema
Needle marks
Perforated nasal septum
Thyroid enlargement
Immature secondary sex characteristics

BP, Blood pressure.
Modified with permission from Nasir M, Eisner GM: Reversible hypertension in adults. Hospital Med 1992;28:26.

made based upon patient characteristics that make one classification preferable to another. The four classifications are diuretics, β-blockers, ACE inhibitors, and calcium channel blockers. The indications for use, side effects, and mechanism of pressure control are summarized in Table 2–5. Central sympatholytics (clonidine, methyldopa), peripheral sympatholytics (guanethidine, reserpine), and arteriolar dilators (hydralazine, minoxidil) are classifications of

TABLE 2–5. TREATMENT AND MANAGEMENT OF HYPERTENSION

	■ DIURETICS	■ β-BLOCKERS	■ ACE INHIBITORS	■ CA CHANNEL BLOCKERS
• Patient Type Best Suited for	• African-Americans • Elderly • Obesity	• Caucasians • Younger age	• Caucasians • Younger age • (Less effective in blacks and elderly)	• All demographic groups
• Effectivity	• 50-60% effective as a single drug	• Cardioprotective	• Combination with diuretic or Ca^{++} channel blocker is potent	• 50–60% effective as a single drug • Peripheral vasodilation with less reflex tachycardia (myocardial contractility increases; fluid retention)
• Pressure-lowering Effects	• Initially decreases plasma volume • Subsequent reduction of peripheral vascular resistance by unknown mechanism	• Decreases heart rate • Decreases cardiac output • Decreases renin release • Therefore, good for concurrent use to treat angina pectoris, previous MI, migraine, age-related tremor, somatic manifestations of anxiety	• Inhibition of renin angiotensin–aldosterone system • Inhibits bradycardia • Stimulates vasodilating prostaglandin synthesis • May decrease sympathetic nervous system	• Inhibits the influx of Ca^{++} during membrane depolarization
• Secondary or Side Effects	• Lowers K^+, Mg^{++} • Increases glucose • Increases CO^{++} • Increases LDL • Increases uric acid (may precipitate gout) • May aggravate diabetes but acceptable if monitored closely	• Bradycardia • Fatigue • Bronchospasm • Sleep disturbance • Impotence • Increased triglycerides • Decreased HDL	• Few side effects: Dry cough secondary to bronchial laryngeal irritation in 5–10% Skin rash (Captopril) Taste alterations (Captopril) Angioneurotic edema is an uncommon but potentially dangerous side effect of all ACE inhibitors	• Positive Antianginal (good if concomitant angina contraindicates β-blocker) Not contraindicated with peripheral vascular disease or bronchioconstriction (asthma) • Negative: Headache Peripheral edema Bradycardia Constipation (Verapamil)
• Contraindications	• Reasonably safe drug	• Congestive heart failure • Symptomatic bronchospasm • Peripheral vascular disease (PVD) • Relative contraindication: IDDM (inhibits gluconeogenesis and may increase hypoglycemic episodes)	• Reasonably safe drug	• BID, TID, QID dosages • Concomitant paroxysmal supraventricular tachycardia

TABLE 2–5. CONTINUED

	■ DIURETICS	■ β-BLOCKERS	■ ACE INHIBITORS	■ CA CHANNEL BLOCKERS
• Comments	• Major criticism is failure to reduce incidence of myocardial infarction in Medical Research Council trial; this showed no significant reduction in deaths or MI with β-blockers either (but no comparative study for ACE or Ca⁺⁺)	• May better prevent coronary artery disease in men		
• Combinations	• ACE and β-blockers good combination, but CAUTION with the combination of ACE and a potassium-sparing diuretic; it causes reduced aldosterone secretion (ACE inhibition), which can lead to hyperkalemia	• Ca⁺⁺ hannel blockers good combination with associated decrease in angina • α-blocker lowers peripheral resistance	• Ca⁺⁺ channel blocker good combination • Diuretics should be used with caution	• Can be used with ACE inhibitors, β-blockers • Less of an additive effect with diuretic • β-blocker

antihypertensive drugs that are less often used in the management of hypertension.

In general, patients with increased plasma volume and/or low plasma renin activity tend to respond more favorably to diuretics and calcium channel blockers. This group usually includes African-Americans, geriatric patients, and obese patients. These drugs adequately manage increased blood pressure as a single medication in 50 to 60% of patients. Diuretics and calcium channel blockers, taken in combination, are less additive than if either is combined with an ACE inhibitor or β-blocker. The common use of these medications for these populations should not preclude a practitioner from prescribing other classifications of medications for these patients. For example, β-blockers have additional benefits in the presence of concurrent disease. Because they lower both the cardiac output and heart rate, they are often used for patients with previous myocardial infarcts and angina, and they may better prevent coronary artery disease. They are also useful for patients with migraine headaches and the somatic manifestations of anxiety. Calcium channel blockers might also be beneficial for patients with concurrent angina and in those instances where the use of other classifications of drugs are contraindicated. For instance a hypertensive patient with angina and chronic obstructive pulmonary disease (COPD) would not be a candidate for a β-blocker. This would likely exacerbate the COPD due to its vasoconstrictive and bronchospasm effects. This patient could benefit from the antihypertensive and antianginal effects of a calcium channel blocker without adversely impacting the COPD.

Patients who generally have elevated plasma renin activity (young, Caucasian) tend to benefit more from the use of ACE inhibitors and β-blockers. As a single therapy, either is effective in controlling hypertension in 40 to 50% of cases. ACE inhibitors are generally preferred in this population due to their relative lack of adverse side effects.

There are generally two schools of thought regarding the approach to drug therapy for hypertension. One advocates the use of low doses of multiple drugs, while the other advocates the use of a single drug in increasing dosage until the pressure is stabilized. Although the side effects of these medications are generally dose related, multiple medications, despite a low dose, could produce multiple side effects, both individually and interactively. Compliance problems also increase with multiple medications.

Clearly, there is no one drug or cookbook approach to the treatment of hypertension. Each drug has its unique properties and each patient unique characteristics that require an individualized plan.

■ Ocular

The management of the ocular complications of hypertension is summarized in Table 2–6 and, in general, centers around the treatment of the underlying systemic hypertension. Treatment specific to the eye is generally limited to the complications of the sclerotic phase of the retinal vasculature.

TABLE 2–6. MANAGEMENT OF THE PATIENT WITH KNOWN OR SUSPECTED HYPERTENSION[a]

Retinal Finding	Clinical Suggestion	Management
Vasoconstriction	**_Known Hypertensive_**	
	Suggests noncompliance or failure of current treatment regimen	Take blood pressure Consult with internist
	Undiagnosed hypertensive	
	Suggests hypertension	Hypertension history: risk factors; family history; signs/symptoms (although generally none) Take blood pressure: if elevated, reschedule patient and repeat in a relaxed atmosphere or consult with internist; if "normal," schedule follow up in 3–6 months for repeat blood pressure, fundoscopy, and photos Photodocument
Exudative phase	Suggests rapid, prolonged, significant elevation of blood pressure (if concurrent vasoconstriction present, this suggests a relatively recent onset; if vasoconstriction absent, this suggests the onset was greater than 1–2 months)	Take blood pressure Hypertension history including recent headaches, vomiting, nauseousness Consult with internist Return in 3 months for follow-up
Sclerotic phase	Suggests prolonged, uncontrolled hypertension	Take blood pressure Consult with internist Photodocument
Complications of the sclerotic phase	Suggests prolonged, uncontrolled hypertension	Take blood pressure Consult with internist Photodocument Monitor as indicated for complications of ocular ischemia (eg, neovascularization)

[a] Based on fundus findings.

CONCLUSION

Undoubtedly, many patients live a long and "healthy" life with undiagnosed hypertension. It is clear however, that high blood pressure poses a significant risk factor for disease that is easily reduced with proper intervention. Hypertension is implicated in the pathogenesis of atherosclerotic disease, stroke, heart disease, and a host of other conditions, but despite its potentially deleterious effects, most patients with hypertension in the United States die as a result of complications of atherosclerosis.

While in the overwhelming majority of cases the cause of a patient's hypertension is unknown (primary hypertension), a small but significant percentage of patients will have a definable underlying cause (secondary hypertension). Patients with hypertension are generally asymptomatic, which complicates compliance with follow-up. Also, medications are costly, must be used chronically, have side effects, and are disruptive of a patient's daily routine. Much of the problem with hypertension is in identifying undiagnosed patients and maintaining them on proper treatment. The measurement of blood pressure should, therefore, be as publicly accessible as possible and should be incorporated into the routine assessment of all patients. The ocular effects of hypertension are a function of the amplitude and duration of the increased blood pressure, are easily assessed by a trained eyecare practitioner, and provide valuable clinical information regarding the status of these patients.

REFERENCES

Alexander L. *Primary Care of the Posterior Segment.* 2nd ed. Norwalk, CT: Appleton & Lange; 1994:171–276.

Casser-Locke L. Ocular manifestations of hypertension. *Optom Clin.* 1992;2:47–76.

Nasir M, Eisner GM. *Reversible hypertension in adults. Hospital Med.* 1992;28:22–44.

Robbins SL, Cotron RS, Kumar V. *Pathologic Basis of Disease.* 3rd ed. Philadelphia: Saunders; 1984:1041–1048.

Schroeder SA, Krupp MA, Tierney LM, McPhee SJ, eds. *Current Medical Diagnosis and Treatment.* Norwalk, CT: Appleton & Lange; 1991:244–256.

Schwartz GL. *Diagnosis, Pathogenesis and Management of Essential Hypertension. Optom Clin.* 1992;2:31–46.

Tso. In: Singerman LJ, Jampol LM, eds. *Retinal and Choroidal Manifestations of Systemic Disease.* Baltimore: Williams & Wilkins; 1991:79–127.

Williams HW. The eye in malignant hypertension. *Clin Eye Vision Care.* 1990;2:172–185.

Chapter

Arteriosclerosis

Mitchell W. Dul

Arteriosclerosis is a general term used to define the process of progressive narrowing of the arterial lumen. This may prevent an adequate blood supply from reaching various tissues and manifest clinically as ischemia or ischemic atrophy. In addition to a chronic progressive narrowing of the arterial lumen, there are other mechanisms through which this disease can cause damage to the human body. Arteriosclerosis also causes the loss of elasticity of arterial walls, which increases peripheral resistance and arterial pressure. It can also be responsible for the abrupt occlusion of a vessel lumen by thrombus formation or from hemorrhage internally into an atheromatous plaque. The fibrin–platelet covering of a plaque may be compromised, resulting in the exposure of its cholesterol-rich contents to the arterial circulation. These emboli are then free to travel downstream and potentially occlude the arterial supply of a tissue. Arteriosclerosis can also damage the vessel itself, with subsequent aneurysm formation or frank rupture. The clinical manifestations of arteriosclerosis will vary with the end organ affected. Evidence of this disease is common in the heart, brain, abdomen, and legs.

In general, there are two important variations of arteriosclerosis based upon differing pathophysiology. One variation, atherosclerosis, is an intimal disease characterized by, as the name implies, atherosis and sclerosis. The second general type of arteriosclerosis is arteriolosclerosis. This is characterized by hyalinization of the walls of small arteries and arterioles. Arteriolosclerosis is implicated in nephrosclerosis and the intraocular manifestations of arteriosclerotic disease. In the eye, arteriolosclerosis negatively affects retinal vessel autoregulation, exacerbates retinal ischemic disease, and contributes to occlusions of retinal veins.

EPIDEMIOLOGY

■ Systemic

Atherosclerosis is pervasive in the western world. By the fifth decade, the majority of the population has some form of this disease.

Atherosclerosis-related disease accounts for approximately 50% of all deaths in the United States. Myocardial infarction, a condition in which atherosclerosis is implicated in the majority of cases, accounts for 20 to 25% of deaths in the United States.

■ Ocular

The prevalence of arteriolosclerosis in the ocular vasculature is difficult to assess because the clinical signs of a widening of the arterial reflex also occur as normal age-related changes in the retinal vasculature. However, it does appear to be more prevalent and more severe in patients with long-standing hypertension and/or diabetes irrespective of age.

NATURAL HISTORY

The pathogenesis of atherosclerosis is not completely understood; however, specific risk factors associated with

31

this disease as well as its characteristic morphologic changes and predilection for certain locations in the cardiovascular system must be considered. No one theory accomplishes this. Probably the most sound explanation is that the lesions associated with arteriosclerosis are a response to injury to the vessel endothelium or the smooth muscle layer of the arterial media. This injury may result from prolonged exposure to subtle abuse such as turbulence of blood flow created at a bifurcation, or moderately elevated hypertension. In addition to arterial injury, risk factors such as hypertension, cigarette smoking, diabetes and most notably high serum lipid (cholesterol) levels play key roles in the pathogenesis of an atheroma. Other "soft" risk factors include lack of exercise, obesity, and stress.

Cholesterol is an integral component in the formation of nerve tissue, bile, and some hormones. The body receives cholesterol from two general sources: the ingestion of cholesterol-containing foods, and the cholesterol produced by the liver. If the dietary intake of cholesterol is too low, the liver manufactures an additional amount in order to fulfill the body's requirement. A diet high in cholesterol will suppress endogenous production and may create a surplus, which will circulate in the bloodstream bound to protein. Plasma lipoproteins are generally divided into four categories: chylomicrons (present only after a meal), very-low-density (VLDL) (used primarily to transport liver-synthesized triglycerides), low-density (LDL), and high-density lipoproteins (HDL). The latter two are used to transport endogenous cholesterol to the cells of the body. LDLs are the richest in cholesterol, and high serum levels of this lipoprotein have been associated with atherosclerosis. HDLs are believed to provide a vehicle by which cholesterol is removed from arterial walls and transported to the liver to be metabolized. Therefore, the ratio between the serum levels of these two lipoproteins is thought to be an indicator of risk for atherosclerotic-related disease (eg, ischemic heart disease).

The evidence for a link between serum lipid levels and atherosclerosis is compelling. Atherosclerosis can be induced in most normal species when fed diets rich in cholesterol. Symptomatic atherosclerosis rarely develops, even when other risk factors are present, unless plasma cholesterol levels are high. When these levels are high due to genetic disorders (eg, cholesteryl ester storage disease), atherosclerosis develops even in the absence of other risk factors. Furthermore, even in the presence of overt endothelial damage in animal models, atheroma formation will only occur if accompanied by elevated serum cholesterol levels. In these cases, lipids will then be deposited beneath the endothelial wall as the precursors to atheromatous plaques.

The endothelial cells of an artery normally provide a relatively smooth surface that hinders the adherence of blood cells (monocytes and platelets) to its surface. At the same time, the surface selectively allows for the passage of nutrients into the arterial wall. Low-density lipoproteins (LDLs) circulating in the blood modify the surface of both the endothelium (by making it more permeable) and the circulating monocytes and T lymphocytes (by making them more adhesive). While these cells are adhering to the endothelial surface, the lipid and lipoproteins are being actively transported through this layer and deposited between the endothelial cells and their basement membrane. From here, lipid particles are filtered through the basement membrane. During this process the lipoproteins are chemically altered and now assist in drawing the monocytes through the endothelial wall into the intima, where they are converted into macrophages. The macrophages then take up the lipids and lipoproteins. These ingested lipid-laden macrophages are converted to "foam cells," which accumulate in the intima. This accumulation creates a bumpy and irregular surface to the normally smooth endothelium. Macrophages are also capable of forming growth-regulatory molecules (platelet-derived growth factor) that chemotactically attract smooth muscle cells from the media into the intima, where they proliferate. The combination of exposed foam cells (as they pass through the endothelium) and the irregular surface created by their subendothelial accumulation sets the stage for thrombogenesis. As platelets aggregate, many will release growth factors that serve as powerful stimulators of connective tissue. The result is a dense covering of fibrous connective tissue over a bolus of ingested lipid-laden macrophages and smooth muscle cells. The contents of this bolus varies considerably from plaque to plaque as well as within an individual plaque. In general, however, it resembles a thin porridge or gruel. The term atheroma is derived from the Greek word for gruel, "athere."

Soft atheromas and hard collagenous plaques are generally present concurrently and probably represent different expressions of the same disease. This variability in plaque composition may be a result of the age of the plaque, although it is not clear whether plaques soften as they age (due to increased production of lipid laden gruel) or if they harden as a result of sclerosing. Sclerosing, which may represent episodic thrombosis and healing of a previously soft atheroma, results in a hard collagenous plaque that occupies a large percentage of the volume of a vessel lumen. These variations in plaque morphology play a significant role in the risk of developing acute clinical manifestations of atherosclerotic disease. In general, small- to medium-sized, soft atheromas with a high lipid content are more likely to rupture—particularly if the concentration of the lipid is eccentrically located in the intima, where hemodynamic forces may further contribute to plaque disruption (Figure 3–1).

■ Systemic

Atherosclerosis generally affects large and medium-sized muscular arteries (coronary artery, carotid artery, and arteries of the lower extremities) and the large elastic arteries

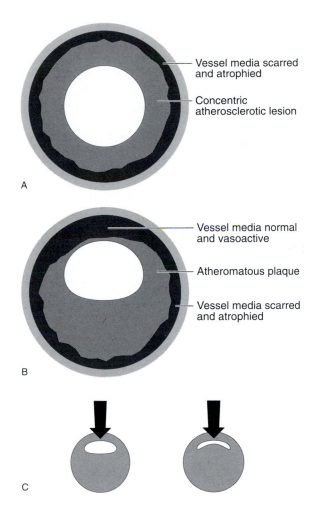

Figure 3–1. Concentric and eccentric atheroma. **A.** Concentric plaque. Concentric intimal disease; the adjacent media is thinned due to scarring and atrophy. **B.** Eccentric plaque. Eccentric intimal disease; the media adjacent to the plaque is similar to the media in concentric plaque. Media adjacent to normal intima is normal and vasoactive. **C.** Arterial spasm, particularly in the presence of eccentrically located plaques, is able to significantly reduce blood flow and may play a role in acute ischemic events. Vasoactive mediators are cold temperatures, emotional stress, cigarette smoking, and vasoconstrictive drugs.

aneurysm formation. Aneurysms are one type of complication associated with atherosclerosis. Other complications include calcification, thrombus formation, hemorrhage, and ulceration.

Atherosclerosis has many detrimental consequences. In general, progression is slow and chronic (Figure 3–2); therefore, patients may remain asymptomatic for prolonged periods of time. With continued progression, patients may only be symptomatic upon exertion, when the oxygen demands of the tissues surpass the available means to transport oxygenated blood. In some instances, the progression of the disease is accelerated. This is thought to be a result of fissures forming in existing plaques, which are quickly sealed by thrombosis. Plaques may undergo many of these episodes during the normal course of their natural history. This type of progression is known to be associated with unstable angina, acute myocardial infarction, and sudden ischemic death. This process provides a basis for the use of antiplatelet therapy in the treatment of atherosclerotic disease. Acute clinical symptoms are generally a consequence of a ruptured plaque with subsequent occlusive thrombus formation.

Arterial spasm may also play a role in acute ischemic events. Many vasoactive mediators from endogenous and exogenous sources (eg, cold exposure, emotional stress, cigarette smoking, vasoconstrictive drugs) are capable of producing vessel spasm sufficient to reduce blood flow. As the severity of the stenosis increases, the degree of vasomotor tone necessary to yield a clinically significant event decreases. This is even more problematic in cases of eccentrically located plaques. Concentric plaques represent concentric intimal disease in which the adjacent media is thinner than normal as a result of scarring and atrophy. Eccentrically located plaques also show a thinned media adjacent to the plaque but have relatively normal vasoconstrictive media where the intima is free of disease (see Figure 3–1). As a result, eccentrically located plaques pose a greater risk in the presence of vasospasm. Pathologic studies show that approximately 70% of coronary arteries of patients who die as a direct result of coronary artery disease have eccentrically oriented atheromata. This type of atheroma may cause underestimation of disease when viewed angiographically.

The clinical manifestations of atherosclerotic disease vary with the degree of compromise of blood flow and the oxygen demands of the target organ(s) as well as its location in the systemic circulation. Symptoms usually develop when the oxygen demands of a particular organ are unmet. Patients with atherosclerotic occlusive disease of the aorta, iliac, femoral, and popliteal arteries generally present with complaints of intermittent claudication in the buttocks, thighs, knees, calves, or feet, depending on which vessel is occluded. The effects of this disease on the cerebrovascular system are detailed in Chapter 5. Its effects on the arteries of the eye, heart, abdomen, and feet are summarized in Table 3–1.

(aorta and iliac artery). Early in the disease the atheromata are widely distributed in relatively predictable locations throughout the circulatory system. They are most likely to appear in the following arteries in descending order: the abdominal aorta (especially near the ostia of its major branches), the coronary arteries (especially within the first 6 cm), the popliteal arteries (supplying blood to the calf and foot), the descending thoracic aorta, the internal carotids and the vessels of the circle of Willis. The vessels of the upper extremities, mesenteric, and renal arteries (except at their ostia) are less often affected. As the disease progresses, the number and size of these plaques increases. This progressively encroaches upon the lumen of the vessel and also weakens it, which sets the stage for subsequent

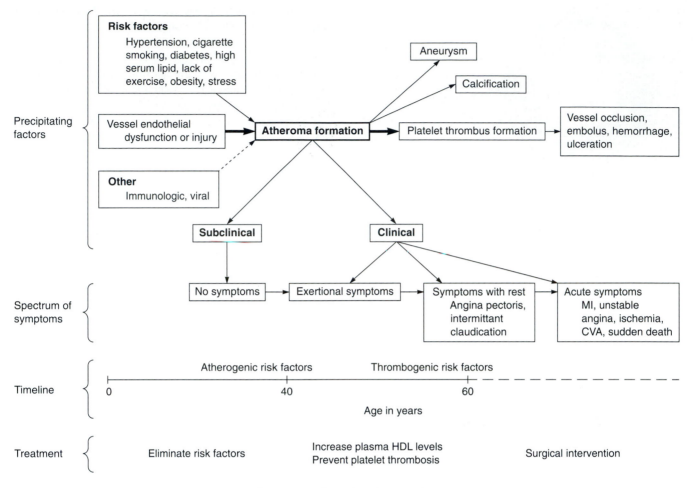

Figure 3–2. Atherosclerosis progression.

Atherosclerotic Heart Disease

Symptoms. In the heart, the most common clinical symptoms are angina pectoris (stable and unstable), acute myocardial infarct, or sudden death (which unfortunately is the first clinical manifestation of atherosclerotic coronary disease in approximately 25% of all cases). Angina pectoris is defined as chest discomfort associated with myocardial ischemia. Although other causes of arterial obstruction are capable of producing angina (vasospasm, arteritis, coronary dissection), in most cases it is secondary to atherosclerotic heart disease. Angina pectoris is generally precipitated by emotional stress or exertion (especially lifting or fast-paced walking). It is often described as a tightness or gripping sensation (as if someone were standing on the patient's chest). It has also been variably described as indigestion, burning, or vague discomfort. In the majority of cases (80 to 90%) the sensation can be localized to the midsternum or immediately to the left of the sternum. It will often radiate from this central location to the left shoulder and upper arm then down the arm to the fourth and fifth fingers. It may also radiate to the jaw and the back of the neck. The pain of angina is not sharp; if a patient points to the source of pain with a single finger, the odds are it is not angina.

Angina rarely lasts for more than 30 minutes. Angina lasting longer than 30 minutes is suggestive of unstable angina. This type is precipitated by less exertion or at rest, is less responsive to medication, and is of longer duration than previously stable angina. Most angina attacks dissipate within 3 minutes of rest unless precipitated by anger or following a large meal, in which case a 15- to 20-minute delay is more likely. The etiology of the sensation of pain that characterizes angina pectoris is unknown. It may be a sequelae of the buildup of lactic acid or other pain-producing substances (histamine, kinins, cellular proteolytic enzymes) in the presence of myocardial ischemia. In many instances, even in almost completely stenosed coronary arteries, patients remain asymptomatic. Therefore, clinical symptoms, although providing some indication of the presence of disease, are generally poor indicators of the degree of disease.

■ Ocular

The effects of arteriosclerosis on the eye are most significant when the disease affects the cerebral vascular system

TABLE 3–1. SYSTEMIC AND OCULAR MANIFESTATIONS OF ARTERIOSCLEROSIS

CORONARY ARTERY
- Location: Within first 6 cm
- Symptoms: Angina pectoris following stress or exertion, relieved by resting
- Signs: Significant elevation of both systolic and diastolic blood pressure; gallop rhythm; apical systolic murmur

AORTA/ILIAC ARTERY
- Location: Just distal to the bifurcation (aorta), just proximal to the bifurcation of the common iliac
- Symptoms: Intermittent claudication (especially calf muscle)
- Signs: Possible bruit over aorta, iliac, or femoral artery

FEMORAL/POPLITEAL ARTERY
- Location: Distal portion of superficial femoral (common and deep generally patent)
- Symptoms: Intermittent claudication limited to calf/foot
- Signs: Affected area: hair loss, thinning of skin, decreased muscle mass, coolness to touch; good to fair femoral pulses (possible bruit); no popliteal or pedal pulse

OCULAR
- Widening of the arterial reflex
- Copper-wire appearance of retinal arteries
- Silver-wire appearance of retinal arteries
- Loss of autoregulation of retinal arteries
- Contributing factor in ischemic retinal diseases
- Retinal vein or artery occlusion
- Atheromatous emboli (carotid) in retinal vasculature

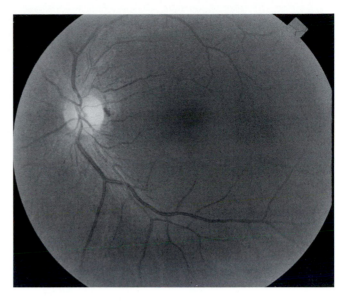

Figure 3–3. Hyalinization secondary to arteriolosclerosis.

(producing a myriad of signs and symptoms, such as amaurosis fugax, retinal artery occlusion, and visual field loss).

Arteriolosclerosis results from a leakage of plasma components through the vessel endothelium. This process is presumably augmented by the chronic hemodynamic stresses of hypertension or the metabolic stresses of diabetes. The result is an irregular thickening of basement membrane with deposition of amorphous extracellular substances and smooth muscle cells within the vessel wall with intimal and medial collagenization. In histologic section, the lesion appears homogenous and pink with thickening of the arteriolar walls, loss of structural detail, and a narrowing of the vessel lumen. The descriptive term for this histologic presentation is hyaline, and the process is called hyalinization (Figures 3–3 and 3–4).

The walls of normal retinal arteries are transparent, which allows the practitioner to view the column of blood within the vessel. The retinal arterial light reflex is produced by the reflection of light off of this blood column, which normally occupies the center one fifth of the width of the column. The progressive hyalinization of the vessel

walls (as well as the normal deposition of basement membrane materials and other debris in the perivascular sheath) serve to make the vessel less transparent and the arterial light reflex appear to broaden. Previous clinical assessments of the degree of hyalinization in the retinal vasculature relied upon estimations of the arterial reflex width. This approach offers poor interobserver reliability, lacks specificity (because it includes normal age-related arterial changes), and provides little or no prognostic value. The blood column, viewed through the hyalinized vessel deposits, may appear copper in color (hence the term "copper-wire" appearance). Further hyalinization of the wall will cause a loss of vessel transparency and a resultant appearance of a "silver wire." This is indicative of severe

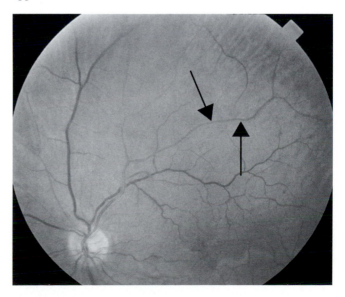

Figure 3–4. Hyalinization and sectorial sclerosis (arrows).

will cause a loss of vessel transparency and a resultant appearance of a "silver wire." This is indicative of severe hyalinization. Even so, fluorescein angiography may reveal that these vessels remain patent. Complications associated with intraocular arteriolosclerosis include compromise of vessel autoregulation and vein occlusion (at arterial–venous crossings when the vessels share a common adventitial sheath), particularly if accompanied by high intraocular pressure. The condition may also exacerbate retinal ischemic disease (hypoperfusion retinopathy).

In the eye, atheromas are rarely present in the intraocular retinal vessels. They may form at the entrance of the artery into the optic nerve or at the lamina cribrosa, but even this is relatively uncommon. Most of what could be confused for intraocular atheromas are actually emboli from either carotid or cardiac origins.

DIAGNOSIS

■ Systemic

The diagnosis of arteriosclerosis is based upon history, clinical presentation, and physical examination (Table 3–2). For example, patients may experience chest pain (angina) or leg cramps when walking (intermittant claudication). Bruits may be heard over the affected arteries and pulses may be weak or absent. Doppler ultrasound and angiograms assess the extent of the occlusion.

Electrocardiogram stress tests, thallium-201 perfusion testing, and echocardiography are noninvasive tests that provide beneficial diagnostic information, particularly in asymptomatic patients.

TABLE 3–2. DIAGNOSIS OF ARTERIOSCLEROSIS

Coronary

ECG
Exercising ECG
Thallium-201 scintigraphy
Radionuclide angiography
Echocardiography
Coronary angiography
Left ventricular angiography

Aorta/Iliac

Doppler ultrasound
Aortography

Femoral/Popliteal

Ultrasound
Arteriogram

Noninvasive Testing

Exercise Electrocardiogram (ECG) Stress Tests are beneficial in confirming the diagnosis of angina because the patient's symptoms and/or characteristic ECG patterns are elicited in a controlled environment. The test is less helpful in assessing asymptomatic patients because the rate of false positives are high (often exceeding true positives). It becomes much more reliable when conducted in tandem with thallium-201 scintigraphy, which through the process of uptake of this radionuclide is able to demonstrate and differentiate hypoperfused versus infarcted tissue. This test is generally able to identify 75 to 90% of patients with significant coronary artery disease. The exercise ECG and thallium-201 tests are also able to provide insight into the subclinical limits of physical activity as well as the patient's response to therapeutic interventions (both medical and surgical). Echocardiography is used primarily to assess left ventricular function, which is an important prognostic indicator and assists in the course of therapy.

Invasive Testing

Coronary angiography is generally reserved for presurgical cases and assists in determining the surgical procedure of choice (percutaneous transluminal coronary angioplasty, or PTCA, versus coronary bypass surgery). Coronary angiography has an overall mortality rate of 1 in 500 (Collaborative Study of Coronary Artery Surgery, 1979). In addition, it provides a two-dimensional representation of atheromatous disease, a three-dimensional process. The results of angiography rely upon the degree to which an atheroma encroaches upon the lumen of a vessel, irrespective of its depth, centricity, or composition. Therefore, angiography tends to underestimate the degree of atherosclerotic disease. In addition, angiography poorly assesses plaque fractures, arterial dissections, composition of the plaque, depth of the plaque, presence of intracoronary thrombi, and degree of residual stenosis following surgical intervention. The extent of atherosclerotic disease can only be inferred based upon the extent to which the atheroma encroaches upon the arterial lumen. Eccentrically located atheroma pose a particular problem when viewed angiographically, because this procedure is unable to localize the arterial lumen relative to the external arterial wall. Such a lumen may appear angiographically open (in two dimensions), but may in fact be a lesion of particular risk. These limitations decrease the sensitivity and specificity of this procedure in assessing intracoronary pathology. The clinical utility of angiography is augmented by the use of ultrasonography of the coronary arteries.

Ultrasound of the coronary arteries is accomplished using intravascular ultrasound devices in tandem with high- frequency transducers. Although an invasive procedure, it is capable of producing images of the various histologic layers of the artery. In general, there are two types of intracoronary ultrasound, Doppler and B-mode ultrasound. Doppler ultrasound, like angiography, provides an image of the lumen of the vessel. It provides useful information in addition to the findings of an angiogram because it does not use an injected contrast medium, which may itself be capable of dilating an artery. B-mode ultrasound, which relies upon differences in acoustic impedance of various tissues, is capable of imaging the walls of arteries as well as their lumen. The relatively high acoustic impedance of collagenous and calcified tissue provide for clear boundaries of the arterial collagenous tunica adventitia, of collagenous atherosclerotic lesions, and of the intima-lumen boundary. The use of this technology may provide a means to assess atheromas that, based upon the morphology, location, or composition, are more likely to carry a high risk of acute disease. The technique may also prove helpful in assessing the effects of treatment.

■ Ocular
The diagnosis of intraocular arteriolosclerosis is based upon ophthalmoscopic findings (see Table 3–1).

TREATMENT AND MANAGEMENT

■ Systemic
Treatment of atherosclerotic disease should address the control of risk factors associated with the condition (especially plasma lipid levels), the removal of lipids from arterial walls (eg, increase plasma HDL levels), and prevention of conversion of chronic events to acute events (antithrombotic therapy; Table 3–3).

Controlling Risk Factors
Epidemiologic evidence suggests that controlling risk factors such as smoking, elevated cholesterol levels, and elevated blood pressure may decrease the risk of mortality and morbidity from coronary artery disease. In addition, stress management (eg, through meditation, yoga), a purely vegetarian diet (with only 10% of calories from fat), moderate exercise, and support groups to assist in this change of life style, has recently been advocated by Dean Ornish, director of the Preventive Medicine Research Institute in Sausalito, California. This form of management was the first nonsurgical, nonpharmaceutical treatment for heart disease to qualify for insurance reimbursement. Evidence suggests that this approach can both retard and even reverse atherosclerotic heart disease. Reversal of the disease has been difficult to assess, due in part to the limits of diagnostic assessments, which are often poor indicators of the actual pathology. Coronary artery ultrasonography has demonstrated promising evidence of disease regression.

TABLE 3–3. TREATMENT AND MANAGEMENT OF ARTERIOSCLEROSIS

CORONARY
- Acute attack: Nitroglycerin (sublingual)
- Preventive maintenance:
  Eliminate exacerbating conditions
  Nitroglycerin
  Long-acting nitrates
  β-blockers
  Calcium channel blockers
  Platelet inhibitors
  Bypass grafting
  Percutaneous transluminal angioplasty

AORTA/ILIAC
- Endovascular:
  Balloon angioplasty
  Atherectomy
- Prosthetic graft

FEMORAL/POPLITEAL
- Walking (develop collateral circulation)
- Arterial graft
- Thromboendarterectomy
- Endovascular surgery

OCULAR
- Monitor for secondary complications
- Maintenance of normal intraocular pressure

Medical Management
Evidence from recent National Institutes of Health epidemiologic reports suggest that for every decrease of 1 mg/dL in HDL cholesterol, there appears to be an approximately 3% increase in the risk of coronary artery disease—independent of risk factors. Gemfibrozil (Lopid), a lipid-regulating agent, and niacin, are capable of producing a 10 to 15% increase in HDL level. Bile-acid-sequestrant resins (cholestyramine resin powder; Questran) and HMG-CoA reductase inhibitors (lovastatin; Mevacor) are also capable of increasing the HDL level, but to a lesser extent.

Even though agents to prevent platelet thrombosis probably do not reduce either total mortality or, specifically, total cardiovascular mortality, aspirin (acetylsalicylic acid) is the most frequently employed and generally least toxic antiplatelet medication. It is effective in unstable angina, acute myocardial infarct, and possibly secondary prevention of cardiovascular and cerebrovascular disease. Heparin and other anticoagulants partially interfere with the coagulation system and may be of some benefit. In addition, calcium channel blockers and ACE inhibitors may also be effective in the prevention of acute events.

In general, the indications for surgical intervention of the coronary artery, in an otherwise healthy individual, include

(1) the use of maximum medications failing to relieve patient symptoms, (2) greater than 50% stenosis of the left main coronary artery (even if the patient is asymptomatic), (3) the presence of three-vessel disease with moderate left ventricular dysfunction, (4) patients successfully treated for unstable angina who continue to show ischemia on exercise testing or monitoring, and (5) patients with previous heart attack and persistent symptoms or evidence of ischemia. The two most popular forms of coronary artery surgical intervention are percutaneous balloon angioplasty and coronary bypass surgery.

Percutaneous balloon angioplasty is a palliative procedure in which a balloon catheter is inserted via the femoral artery and used to mechanically enlarge the lumen of the narrowed vessel. It does not remove atheromatous plaques, but compresses them within the walls of the vessel. This residual compressed material remains and may contribute to subsequent restenosis. Angioplasty is best suited for patients with single-vessel disease with recent angina pectoris. Approximately 30 to 40% of all patients with coronary artery disease are appropriate candidates for this procedure. The procedure is less effective in completely occluded arteries (approximately 50% success rate), diffuse disease, and in cases of restenosis (which occurs in up to 40% of cases).

The success rate is influenced by many factors (including the extent of the patient's disease, the ability of the surgeon to obtain and accurately assess a presurgical image of the affected artery, and the experience of the surgeon). Angioplasty should be performed in a setting where open heart surgery is available should bypass surgery be immediately necessary. This occurs in approximately 5% of all cases.

The expansion of the balloon is also capable of fracturing a plaque at a weak point. If the fracture extends into the media of the artery, an arterial dissection may ensue, which is capable of occluding the vessel lumen. Catheters are also capable of stimulating the smooth muscles of the arterial media, causing vasospasm. This potentially deleterious effect may be minimized with the presurgical use of calcium channel blockers and intracoronary nitroglycerine. Vasovagal attacks (with bradycardia, hypotension, and possibly loss of consciousness) also occur with enough regularity that IV atropine is often used as a routine presurgical medication. Percutaneous balloon angioplasty is less invasive than coronary bypass surgery (and less expensive). Its application in the presence of coronary atherosclerosis has some clear benefits, although it is not without risk. The overall mortality rate secondary to coronary balloon angioplasty is approximately 1%. There are other, newer surgical catheter devices currently being used in the treatment of coronary atherosclerosis, but the success rates and long-term outcomes of these procedures have yet to be determined.

Coronary bypass surgery involves grafting up to five segments of a vein (usually the saphenous vein) or prefer-

ably an artery (especially the internal mammary arteries) from the aorta to a coronary artery past the locus of the obstruction. The internal mammary arteries are generally the vessels of choice due to the decreased long-term closure rate. Approximately 10 to 20% of grafts will close within the first 6 months, beyond which the annual failure rate is approximately 4%. If risk factors for atherosclerotic disease are not controlled following surgery, the risk of graft closure increases. Aspirin, used solely or in combination with dipyridamole, improves the overall failure rates of grafts.

Mortality rates are higher for patients with preexisting left ventricular dysfunction, those over 70 years of age, and patients with significant concurrent noncardiac disease. In general, for otherwise healthy patients, this procedure has traditionally had a relatively low mortality rate (1 to 3%). In recent years, this rate has increased to 5 to 10%, reflecting an increase in high-risk and older patients and a decrease in the number of younger patients with focal lesions who instead pursue percutaneous balloon angioplasty as the treatment of choice. If a repeat procedure is required, the rate of success is generally less favorable.

■ Ocular

Treatment of intraocular arteriolosclerosis is limited to regular observation for complications of the disease (eg, vein occlusion) and proper monitoring and maintenance of intraocular pressure. Concurrently, the patient should be treated systemically.

CONCLUSION

Arteriosclerosis, especially atherosclerosis accounts for a tremendous amount of morbidity and mortality throughout the world. In the United States, approximately $18 billion was spent on coronary bypass surgery in 1992. This figure makes it the most expensive item on the nation's healthcare expenditure list. The American Heart Association estimates that if work loss is added to the cost of hospitalization, pharmaceutical and surgical intervention, the figure approximates $117.4 billion per year.

Patients with atheroclerosis may remain asymptomatic for decades or experience sudden death as the presenting sign. The goal of the practitioner is to identify patients at risk for atherosclerosis and to eliminate the risk factors before the onset of adverse effects of the disease. Ideally, this should occur prior to the onset of symptoms. Atherosclerosis is a disease that is influenced, to a great extent, by the life style of the patient. Poor dietary habits, poor control of blood pressure, and cigarette smoking all contribute to this disease, and unless they are corrected, will continue to contribute even after surgical intervention. Unfortunately, many patients do not seek the care of practitioners until such symptoms occur. No amount of healthcare reform will be of benefit if patients do not contribute to their own health and well-being.

REFERENCES

Atherosclerosis: Quantitative imaging, risk factors, prevalence and change. *Circulation.* 1993;87(suppl):1–81.

Davis K, Kennedy JW, Kemp HG, et al. Complications of coronary arteriography from the Collaborative Study of Coronary Artery Surgery (CASS). *Circulation.* 1979;59:1105–1112.

Gomez CR. Carotid plaque morphology and risk for stroke. *Stroke.* 1990;21:148–151.

Progression–regression of atherogenesis: Molecular, cellular, and clinical bases. *Circulation.* 1992;86(suppl):1–123.

Robbins SL, Cotran RS, Kumar V. *Pathologic Basis of Disease.* 3rd ed. Philadelphia: Saunders; 1984:506–518.

Schroeder SA, Krupp MA, Tierney LM, McPhee SJ. *Current Medical Diagnosis and Treatment.* 30th ed. Norwalk, CT: Appleton & Lange; 1991:256–266, 316–320.

Sokolow M, McIlroy MB, Cheitlin MD. *Clinical Cardiology*, 5th ed. Norwalk, CT: Appleton and Lange; 1990:87–224, 333–436.

Tobis JM, Yock PG. *Intravascular Ultrasound Imaging.* New York: Churchill Livingstone; 1992.

4

Chapter

Cardiogenic Emboli and Valvular Heart Disease

Mitchell W. Dul ■ Charles Haskes

Cardiogenic emboli have been increasingly recognized as a significant etiology of ischemic stroke and are clearly implicated in the genesis of retinal ocular disease. The mitral and aortic valves are the most common sources of cardiac emboli. Valvular emboli, due to their relatively small size, are responsible for many cases of amaurosis fugax (transient monocular blindness) and highly focal transient ischemic attacks.

In the retinal vasculature, cardiogenic emboli can be symptomatic or asymptomatic, and may be clinically differentiated from emboli of carotid origin. Clinical evidence suggesting their presence should prompt the eyecare practitioner to pursue a comprehensive cardiovascular workup, because prophylactic treatment with antithrombotic agents make this one of the most preventable forms of ischemic cerebrovascular accidents.

EPIDEMIOLOGY

■ Systemic

Valve disease may remain hemodynamically insignificant or well tolerated for decades; therefore, it is difficult to meaningfully assess its incidence and prevalence in the general population. More than two thirds of the patients are female, and a family incidence may be striking in some individuals. Mitral valve prolapse occurs in up to 5% of the adult population. Congenital malformation of the aortic valve occurs in approximately 2% of the general population. Mitral and aortic valve disease most often occurs as a sequela of acute rheumatic fever, although only 50% of patients with recognized mitral stenosis recall a history of the disease. When secondary to rheumatic fever, or its postinfectious sequelae, the mitral valve is involved exclusively in 40 to 50% of cases, the aortic in 34 to 40%, and a three-valve combination of mitral, aortic, and tricuspid valves in 2 to 3%. Approximately 9 to 28% of patients with mitral valve stenosis produce emboli from calcific or thrombotic material. Approximately 30% of all cases of valvular infection result in embolization. More than half are cerebrovascular accidents involving the middle cerebral artery.

■ Ocular

Ocular emboli of cardiac origin account for approximately 5 to 10% of all embolic retinal disease.

NATURAL HISTORY

■ Systemic

Valve Dysfunction
The heart valves function to prevent backflow of blood into the chambers or vessels of the heart. The tricuspid valve separates the right atrium and ventricle, the mitral valve separates the left atrium and ventricle, and the aortic valve separates the left ventricle from the ascending aorta. Valve dysfunction may either be the result of failure of the valve to completely close, which results in the backflow of blood (regurgitation, insufficiency, or incompetence); or to completely open, which results in the impedance of blood flow (stenosis). These two disorders frequently occur concurrently in varying degrees in the same valve and differentially affect the heart chambers.

Valvular disease generally occurs as a sequela of congenital anomalies (eg, Marfan syndrome), infection or resultant postinflammatory scarring (eg, acute rheumatic fever), autoimmune disease (eg, systemic lupus erythematosus), or cardiac tumors (eg, myxomas; Table 4–1). It is manifested clinically as stenosis or regurgitation and may be complicated by degenerative changes associated with aging (calcification) or infection (infectious endocarditis). Valvular disease is a source of emboli (eg, calcific, infectious, tumor) that may travel to the cerebrovascular or retinal vascular systems, with potentially vision-threatening and even life-threatening complications.

The clinical manifestations of valvular dysfunction vary in degree from barely perceptible signs or symptoms to severe disease and potentially sudden death. Approximately 50% of patients diagnosed as having severe stenosis with or without symptoms die within 5 years.

Rheumatic Fever

The effects of rheumatic fever on the heart valves account for a large percentage of all cases of valvular disease (especially involving the aortic and mitral valves). Rheumatic fever is an acute, recurrent inflammatory disease, generally found in children, although adults comprise approximately 20% of new cases. Approximately 3% of patients having a pharyngeal infection with group A beta-hemolytic streptococci will develop rheumatic fever (a result of a cross-reaction between streptococci antigens and tissue antigens, especially in the heart). Cardiac symptoms generally develop in the fourth and fifth decades.

Target tissues and cells of rheumatic fever include cardiac myofiber–smooth muscle, heart valves, connective tissue, and neurons in the subthalamic and caudate nucleus. The mitral valve is involved exclusively in almost half of the cases, and a combination of both mitral and aortic valves in about one third of cases, with the aortic valve only or aortic and tricuspid valves comprising the remainder. Postinflammatory scarring of valves generally occurs several decades after the resolution of the acute disease. Many patients, therefore, have no recollection of prior streptococcal infection. Following active inflammation, the valvular leaflets become thickened, fibrotic, shortened, and blunted, and the commissure between them is bridged by connective tissue. The result is valve stenosis, regurgitation, or some combination of the two.

Cardiac Tumors

Cardiac tumors can be a source of emboli to any part of the body. The most common benign primary tumor of the heart is a myxoma, which is usually found in the left atrium. Atrial myxomas account for approximately 1% of strokes in young adults. Myxomas are generally slow growing, mobile, and surgically treatable. Symptoms of cardiac myxoma correspond to their impact on normal heart and valve function. Right-sided myxomas cause right-sided heart signs and symptoms (eg, increased pulmonary or venous congestion, pulmonary hypertension or right heart failure). Left-sided myxoma may cause right-sided heart signs and symptoms due to its effect on the pulmonary circulation (impeding the flow of blood from the lungs into the left atrium) or left-sided heart signs and symptoms (left ventricular hypertrophy, left atrial hypertrophy). The severity of symptoms associated with cardiac myxoma varies as the tumor moves and grows in size. Myxomas can result in sudden death from total obstruction of the mitral valve.

Mitral Stenosis

Mitral stenosis is the resistance to flow through the mitral valve during diastolic filling of the left ventricle. Echocardiographic studies demonstrate thickened cusps and a narrowed opening into the left ventricle. The thickened valves produce an audible snap as they open in early diastole. This is followed by a low-pitched murmur during mid-diastole. If the opening of the valve is less than normal, the left atrial pressure must increase in order to maintain normal flow across the valve and normal cardiac output. This creates a pressure differential between the left atrium and ventricle during diastole. In cases of severe stenosis, the left atrial pressure may be high enough to back up the pulmonary system, which is reflected to the pulmonary veins, capillaries, and eventually to the pulmonary arteries and right

TABLE 4–1. MAJOR RISK SOURCES FOR CARDIOGENIC EMBOLI

Valves

Mitral
   Rheumatic mitral stenosis
   Infectious endocarditis
   Prosthetic valve
Aortic
   Infectious endocarditis
   Calcific stenosis
   Prosthetic valve

Left Atrium

Atrial fibrillation
Myxoma

Iatrogenic Emboli

Postcardiac catherterization
Prosthetic valves

Other Sources

Nonischemic dilating cardiomyopathy (eg, rheumatic myocarditis, contusion, crack cocaine use, sarcoid, alcohol)
Paradoxical emboli (eg, atrial septal defects, patent foramen ovale, ventricular septal defects)
Left ventricle (acute myocardial infarction)

heart, causing pulmonary venous congestion at rest, reduced cardiac output, and, potentially, right heart failure. Many of these patients will also develop paroxysmal or chronic atrial fibrillation (clinically manifested as palpitations; Table 4–2).

Pulmonary venous congestion causes difficult and labored breathing (dyspnea). This is common as the presenting complaint in the symptomatic patient. It may only manifest when the patient lies down, due to the secondary increase in pulmonary blood volume in this position (orthopnea). In the presence of long-standing pulmonary edema, anastomoses may develop between bronchial veins and pulmonary veins in the form of bronchial submucosal varices, which often rupture. Rupture of these varices can cause the patient to cough up blood from the lungs (hemoptysis).

Secondary changes associated with mitral stenosis include calcification of leaflet tissue and thrombosis due to adherence of blood and blood products to the roughened valve surfaces. Fragmentation of calcific or thrombotic material introduces this material to the systemic circulation. This should always be considered as a possible mechanism of systemic embolization especially in young females.

Neurologic symptoms from a cerebral embolus can sometimes be the presenting manifestation of mitral stenosis.

Mitral valve stenosis can result from rheumatic valvulitis, congenital stenosis, thrombus formation, atrial myxoma, bacterial vegetations, and calcification in the valve. The most common cause of mitral stenosis remains rheumatic fever, in which the leaflets and chordae tendineae are scarred and contracted.

Mitral Regurgitation

Mitral regurgitation occurs when contraction of the left ventricle ejects blood into the left atrium as a result of abnormalities in the mitral valve apparatus. For many years rheumatic fever was considered the most common etiology for mitral regurgitation, but in recent years mitral valve prolapse and coronary artery disease have become the predominant mechanisms and are probably the most common cause of mitral regurgitation in the adult population today. Less common etiologies of chronic mitral regurgitation include calcification of the annulus and connective tissue disorders such as Marfan syndrome, Ehlers–Danlos syndrome, and pseudoxanthoma elasticum. Papillary muscle

TABLE 4–2. SYSTEMIC MANIFESTATIONS OF VALVE DISEASE

MITRAL STENOSIS
- Thickened, less mobile valves
- Increased atrial pressure
- Atrial fibrillation
- Hyperplasia and hypertrophy of the pulmonary vessels
- Pulmonary venous congestion
- Right heart failure

- **Signs and Symptoms**
- Dyspnea (most common)
- Fatigue
- Palpitation
- Hemoptysis
- Cerebrovascular accident secondary to embolus

EMBOLI
- Amaurosis fugax
- Transient ischemic attacks
- Cerebrovascular accident
- Peripheral vascular disease

AORTIC STENOSIS
- Left ventricular hypertrophy
- Increased left ventricular end-diastolic pressure
- Decreased cardiac output
- Pulmonary hypertension

- **Signs and Symptoms**
- Chest pain
- Syncope
- Palpitations
- Fatigue
- Left ventriculur heart failure

MITRAL REGURGITATION
- Left ventricular hyperplasia (chronic)
- Pulmonary edema (acute)

- **Signs and Symptoms**
- Palpitations
- Chest pain
- Fatigue
- Anxiety
- Orthostatic hypotension
- Asymptomatic

AORTIC REGURGITATION
- Left ventricular volume overload

- **Signs and Symptoms**
- Left ventricular failure
- Fatigue
- Dyspnea
- Edema

INFECTIOUS ENDOCARDITIS
- Infectious vegetations on the surface of damaged valves and local infection
- Embolization of infected vegetation to peripheral locations
- Mitral valve stenosis
- Aortic regurgitation
- Embolization

- **Signs and Symptoms**
- Fever of 1–2 week duration
- Heart murmur
- Nonspecific complaints of coughing, diarrhea, and malaise

dysfunction and congenital heart disease have also been associated with mitral regurgitation. Acute mitral regurgitation can be created from mechanical disturbances such as disruption of the chordae, rupture of the papillary muscle, or perforation of the mitral valve leaflet (as in bacterial endocarditis). Calcification of the mitral ring is commonly found in the elderly, particularly in the elderly female, and regurgitation occurs when the posterior mitral leaflet adheres to the calcific mass.

The compensatory mechanism of the left ventricle in chronic mitral regurgitation is dilatation to accommodate the increased left ventricular stroke volume necessary to maintain the forward systemic stroke volume. This is accompanied by an increase in wall thickness and hypertrophy to maintain mechanical function. Compliance of the left ventricle and left atrium increases and thereby minimizes the extent of pulmonary venous hypertension. Because of increased left ventricular compliance, systolic regurgitation into the left atrium and pulmonary venous bed can be tolerated without severe elevation of the pulmonary capillary arterial pressure in chronic mitral regurgitation. This ventricular compensatory mechanism is compromised in the presence of coronary artery disease (especially following myocardial infarction), which results in impaired muscle function and loss of ventricular wall motion.

In acute mitral regurgitation (see Table 4–2), sudden regurgitation of blood into the left atrium and pulmonary veins is not accompanied by immediate dilatation of the left atrium or ventricle. These abrupt hemodynamic alterations produce marked elevation of the left ventricular end-diastolic pressure, left atrial pressure, and pulmonary capillary pressure. This creates a pressure overload on the pulmonary vascular tree and produces acute pulmonary edema.

In the mitral leaflet prolapse syndrome, the abnormalities consist of thinning of the leaflet, elongation of the chordae, and dilatation of the mitral annulus. Abrupt deceleration of blood beneath the prolapsed mitral leaflet and the increased tension on the chordae produce a systolic click.

Although many patients with mitral valve prolapse are asymptomatic, symptoms can develop, including palpitations, chest discomfort, fatigue, and anxiety. There are suggestions of abnormal changes in heart rate and blood pressure from the lying to sitting position (orthostatic hypotension). A small percentage of patients will develop endocarditis, rupture of the chordae, progressive mitral regurgitation, or sudden death.

Aortic Stenosis

Aortic stenosis is the obstruction of flow across the aortic valve during left ventricular systolic ejection. It can be caused by a congenital malformation (eg, the normally tricuspid valve develops as a unicuspid or bicuspid valve), postinflammatory (eg, following rheumatic fever), or degenerative calcification of the valve in the elderly. In general,

aortic stenosis is either fibrous or calcific. The fibrous type is usually of rheumatic origin. Recurrent rheumatic carditis causes fibrous contracture with shortening of the cusps and a tendency for fusion of adjacent cusps. If the adhesion occurs between two of the three cusps, the valve becomes bicuspid (one normal valve and one valve produced by the fusion of the remaining two valves). Such valves create, as do congenital bicuspid valves, a tendency for acquired calcification of the cusp. However, the primary basis for the stenosis resides in adhesions of one cusp to another.

Aortic valve stenosis (the valve between the left ventricle and the aortic arch) increases the pressure inside the left ventricle because, although the volume of blood in the ventricle is essentially normal, it must pass through an impeded opening on the way to the aortic arch. This resistance increases the workload of the ventricle, which, like its response to increased peripheral resistance in atherosclerosis and hypertension, stimulates ventricular hypertrophy to meet the new demands. This is accompanied by an elevation of the left ventricular end-diastolic pressure. A sustained pressure overload on the ventricle could eventually depress its contractile properties. As a result, forward cardiac output is compromised, which could advance to left-sided heart failure. Unfortunately, most symptoms associated with aortic stenosis tend to occur late in the course of the disease, when critical reduction of valve size has already developed. Angina pectoris is the most common clinical manifestation of aortic stenosis. It occurs in 50 to 70% of affected individuals. Additional symptoms attributed to severe aortic stenosis include palpitations and general fatigue (see Table 4–2).

Life expectancy averages 5 years after the development of exertional chest discomfort. Exertional syncope is also a frequent symptom that probably results from cerebral ischemia. Survival after syncope due to aortic stenosis has been estimated at 3 to 4 years.

Although patients examined at autopsy usually have had a history of symptoms, approximately 15% of patients with aortic stenosis at autopsy died suddenly without previous symptoms.

Aortic Regurgitation

Aortic regurgitation is due to incompetence of the aortic valve, allowing the flow of blood from the systemic circulation into the left ventricle. Aortic incompetence (regurgitation) increases the workload of the left ventricle by increasing the volume of blood in the chamber (its normal volume plus the backflow of the incompetent valve during diastole). In general, the left ventricle can better compensate for increases in volume by increasing its stroke volume. Therefore, stenosis of the aortic valve is generally more clinically significant than regurgitation.

Incompetent closure of the aortic valve can result from intrinsic disease of the cusp or from diseases affecting the aorta. In the past, rheumatic fever and syphilis were major causes. But these diseases have diminished in frequency in recent years due to effective antimicrobials. As these two infectious conditions have diminished, diseases of the connective tissue and anatomic abnormalities of the valve have become more frequent causes. Marfan syndrome includes aortic dilatation often accompanying incompetence of the valve, and myxomatous changes in the leaflets may further exaggerate the condition. Changes are also seen with rheumatoid arthritis, systemic lupus erythematosis, ankylosing spondylitis, Reiter syndrome, osteogenesis imperfecta, and trauma.

Long-standing vascular disorders such as hypertension and atherosclerosis can also produce mild incompetence of the aortic valve. Finally, any primary cause of aortic stenosis frequently results in regurgitation across the fixed stenotic leaflets. Acute disturbances such as aortic dissection, bacterial endocarditis, and acute rheumatic fever can create sudden regurgitation across the valve.

The two principal congenital causes of aortic regurgitation are a bicuspid aortic valve and a ventricular septal defect. Myxomatous change within the valve can also be a cause of aortic incompetence in the absence of other Marfan syndrome features. Aortic regurgitation from a congenital bicuspid valve is often not detected until early adult life. Infectious endocarditis may involve a normal tricuspid aortic valve, but frequently the valve is bicuspid from congenital or acquired mechanisms.

Regurgitation of diastolic flow across the incompetent aortic valve increases filling of the left ventricle and imposes a volume overload on the myocardium. Chronic aortic regurgitation gradually increases left ventricular end-diastolic volume, because the chamber receives blood from the left atrium and the systemic circulation. This causes compensatory left ventricular wall hypertrophy. As the compliant properties or elasticity of the ventricle decline, the left ventricular end-diastolic pressure will increase. The increased end-systolic volume and decrease in diastolic compliance elevate left atrial pressure and eventually produce pulmonary venous hypertension (see Table 4–2).

Compensatory mechanisms of the volume-overloaded left ventricle enable the patient to remain asymptomatic for many years with aortic regurgitation.

Infectious Endocarditis

Infectious endocarditis may be divided into two classifications: (1) subacute, which generally occurs in patients with preexisting cardiac anomalies (eg, postrheumatic scarring in 70%, congenital anomaly in 10%); and (2) acute, which occurs primarily as a result of intravenous drug use or cardiovascular surgery (a preexisting cardiac anomaly need not be present).

This potentially devastating infection is often associated with cardiac valvular disease. Incompetent valves cause blood regurgitation and stenotic valves cause jet streams of rapidly flowing blood. Hemodynamically, the blood surrounding the opening to these defective valves is relatively idle. This pooled blood provides an excellent medium for deposition of fibrin and aggregation of agglutinated organisms. This promotes the development of infected vegetations on the surface of the damaged valve. Damage from this infection may be confined locally to the valves, or embolization of the infected vegetation may introduce the infectious bolus to peripheral locations. Virtually every form of microbiological agent has been implicated in the development of these infections, although *Streptococcus viridans* (50%) and *Staphylococcus aureus* (20%) are most common.

In the face of advances in antibiotic therapies, surgical correction of cardiac valve lesions, and the declining incidence of rheumatic fever and rheumatic heart disease, it would be expected that the incidence of infectious endocarditis would be declining. In fact, this is not the case. Advances in treatment appear to be offset by the increase in the prevalence of foreign substances introduced to the systemic circulation. This can be self-inflicted (intravenous drug use represents 5 to 15% of all cases), or iatrogenically induced during surgical or exploratory procedures. Replacement heart valves, catheters, pacemakers, and other devices all provide a potential port of entry for infectious agents. Although this has had little impact on the number of new cases of infectious endocarditis, the average age at onset has changed significantly.

Although previously occurring more frequently in young adults, currently the vast majority of cases (90%) occur over the age of 20, with a peak incidence in the fourth to fifth decades. Nearly one quarter of new cases have had previous cardiovascular surgery. In particular, if a valve was replaced, the infection occurred shortly after surgery in approximately one third of patients. Infection in the remainder occurred more than 5 years later. In approximately 25 to 50% of all cases of infectious endocarditis, no apparent cardiac disease or evidence of predisposing cardiovascular anomaly could be found.

■ Ocular

Valve disease is a source of emboli that may dislodge from the heart and travel anywhere in the body, including the eye. Ocular emboli of valvular origin are potentially sight threatening, because they can cause branch or central retinal artery occlusions. The differential diagnosis of these emboli provides useful clinical information that assists in directing the clinician's attention to alternative origins (carotid, lungs). In general, emboli originating from the cardiac valves are small in size. When introduced to the systemic circulation, these patients often present with episodes of transient monocular blindness (amaurosis fugax) or with a highly focal transient ischemic attack. The

TABLE 4–3. OCULAR MANIFESTATIONS OF CARDIOGENIC EMBOLI AND VALVE DISEASE

EMBOLI TRAVERSING THROUGH THE RETINAL ARTERIES
- **Signs**
  May be visualized in retinal arterioles
- **Symptoms**
  Amaurosis fugax or asymptomatic

EMBOLI LODGED IN RETINAL ARTERIES
- **Signs**
  Visualized in branch or central retinal artery
  Central or branch retinal artery occlusion
- **Symptoms**
  Asymptomatic or loss of vision/blurred vision

INFECTIOUS RETINAL EMBOLI
- **Signs**
  Central retinal artery occlusion
  Branch retinal artery occlusion
  Roth spot
  Optic neuritis
- **Symptoms**
  Loss of vision, blurred vision, metamorphopsia

OTHER OCULAR MANIFESTATIONS OF INFECTIOUS ENDOCARDITIS
- **Signs**
  Conjunctival petecchiae
  Cranial nerve III, IV, or VI dysfunction
- **Symptoms**
  Diplopia

left atrium and ventricle are sources for larger emboli (dislodged tumor, thrombus) that often produce cortical branch artery syndromes (especially homonomous hemianopsia and Wernicke aphasia).

Along with ocular retinal emboli and their manifestations, infectious endocarditis can also cause conjunctival petechiae, superficial retinal hemorrhages surrounding focal accumulations of white blood cells (Roth spots), and single or multiple cranial nerve dysfunction (including nerves II, III, IV, and VI; Table 4–3).

Diagnosis

■ Systemic

Patient History and Physical Examination
Patient history along with physical examination may reveal signs and symptoms characteristic of valve disease. The patient should be questioned regarding past history of rheumatic fever, congenital disorders, infectious diseases, and past drug use. The most common symptoms of mitral

valve stenosis (in approximately 80% of all patients) is shortness of breath on exertion. Many patients with mitral regurgitation are asymptomatic; however, history may elicit signs and symptoms such as chest pain, syncope, palpitations, and fatigue.

Detection of aortic stenosis in a patient under the age of 30 suggests a congenitally stenotic aortic valve as the etiology. Between the ages of 30 and 70 years, rheumatic disease may still play a role, but beyond 70 years degenerative calcification of the cusps of the aortic valve is the most common cause. Symptoms of angina pectoris, palpitations, fatigue, and visual disturbances may be present. Patients with aortic regurgitation may experience similar symptoms.

The variety of symptoms associated with cardiac tumors creates an often-complicated clinical picture, which poses diagnostic challenges. Patients may present with dyspnea, chest pain, pulmonary edema, fever, and other symptoms that may be confused with other clinical entities (eg, infectious endocarditis).

The diagnosis of infectious endocarditis can be clinically challenging. The most common presenting sign is fever of 1- to 2-week duration and heart murmur (present in 90 to 95% of patients). There may be concurrent, nonspecific complaints of coughing, diarrhea, and malaise. In the elderly, fever may not be present, and because heart murmurs in this population are common, the diagnosis may be overlooked. Unfortunately, the longer the disease is left untreated, the greater the potential damage to the heart (especially the valves) and the greater the risk of embolization. In addition, the disease often accompanies other chronic or acute diseases (such as heart failure), and as such it is often undetected until postmortem studies are conducted. The signs and symptoms associated with embolization may be the presenting sign of infectious endocarditis.

The physical examination in mitral stenosis may show distended neck veins, and auscultation may reveal an accentuated first heart sound, opening snap, or diastolic rumble. Chronic mitral regurgitation can be tolerated for many years without clinical evidence of a reduction in cardiac reserve. Fatigue and dyspnea are initial symptoms that can gradually progress to orthopnea, paroxysmal nocturnal dyspnea, and peripheral edema. Other symptoms include palpitations, chest discomfort, fatigue, and anxiety. In acute mitral regurgitation, physical findings are often those of acute pulmonary edema and left ventricular failure. In mitral valve prolapse, the majority of patients are female and orthostatic hypotension is present. Characteristic auscultatory finding is an early-, mid-, or late-systolic click and late apical murmur. In acute mitral regurgitation, sudden disruption of the mitral valve apparatus results in symptoms of congestive heart failure or acute pulmonary edema.

In aortic stenosis, the physical examination may show delayed upstroke of the peripheral pulse, systolic murmur, or hypertrophy of the left ventricle. Auscultation may reveal delayed closure of the aortic valve or ejection click after the first sound. Common clinical manifestations of aortic incompetence include symptoms of left ventricular failure, fatigue, dyspnea, and edema.

A diagnostic clue suggestive of myxomas, which are typically mobile, is change in the sound of an associated murmur as the patient changes posture from one position to another (eg, standing versus supine). The tumor may also produce an audible sound during early diastole if it contacts the mitral valve.

Diagnostic Imaging

Echocardiography is a noninvasive method of cardiac examination that provides direct information about cardiac anatomy and physiology. As such, this procedure provides useful diagnostic and functional information. Its main use is as a preliminary screening test. Indications for echocardiography are ocular and/or cerebral ischemic events (eg, transient weakness in arms or legs), chest pain, palpitations, dyspnea, and syncope. In addition, amaurosis fugax in a patient under age 45 is also an indication for echocardiography (due to the increased probability of cardiac origins).

The mitral valve is one of the structures that registers most clearly and consistently on echocardiography. In mitral stenosis, the valve is thickened and less mobile. The thickened adherent mitral valve leaflets move together. Although anterior valve motion may be less than normal, the posterior leaflet may in some cases move more than normal. Thickened chordae tendineae are also diagnostic of mitral stenosis. The orifice size in a patient with a stenosed mitral valve can be determined. Echocardiography will show a narrowed orifice at the tip of the valve leaflets.

A definitive diagnosis of mitral valve insufficiency cannot be made using echocardiography. Abnormalities in other structures of the heart secondary to mitral insufficiency can aid in diagnosis. For example, an enlarged left atrium and excessive left atrial and ventricular wall motion due to volume overload are seen in this condition. Echocardiography is useful in determining the etiologic basis of mitral insufficiency. Mitral prolapse, papillary muscle dysfunction, vegetative endocarditis, and calcified annulus are all associated with echocardiographic abnormalities.

The clinical significance of mitral valve prolapse demonstrated on the echocardiogram is unclear and the criteria for making the diagnosis are controversial. Echocardiography has been primarily responsible for the great increase in the frequency of the diagnosis. Normally, the mitral valve echoes gradually move anteriorly without interruption during systole. In mitral prolapse, there is a sudden posterior motion in mid-systole as the leaflets prolapse toward the left atrial wall. The sudden change in direction of motion is often associated with a sudden simultaneous auscultatory click, and a murmur may accompany the period of prolapse. The prolapse begins immediately after mitral valve closure and has the appearance of a "hammock." The clinical significance of an echocardiographic diagnosis of mitral valve prolapse must await further clinical research. Very few of the thousands of persons with this diagnosis die suddenly or suffer other serious consequences. The diagnosis is clinically useful in explaining systolic clicks and murmurs. It may also provide an explanation for atypical chest pain or cardiac arrhythmias.

Most adults with aortic stenosis, regardless of its cause, have thickened aortic valve leaflets with calcification detected on the echocardiogram as multiple dense echoes in the valve area. The leaflet separation is less than normal. Additional echocardiographic evidence for significant aortic stenosis includes left ventricular hypertrophy and an abnormal mitral valve pattern suggestive of a compliant left ventricle.

Echoes from the aortic valve leaflets are not useful in the diagnosis of aortic insufficiency. Leaflet separation is usually normal and the valve leaflets may appear either normal or thickened. The mitral valve echocardiogram is useful in detecting aortic insufficiency because the regurgitating blood produces a characteristic fluttering of the mitral valve leaflets. Mitral valve closure in aortic insufficiency may be prolonged owing to an elevated left ventricular end-diastolic pressure; or in patients with severe acute aortic insufficiency, the mitral valve may close prematurely because of the rapid increase in left ventricular pressure during diastole. The left ventricular volume overload in aortic insufficiency causes an increase in the echocardiographic left ventricular internal dimension at end-diastole.

Echocardiogram with myxoma may reveal multiple, dense echoes adjacent to the mitral valve leaflet in diastole; however, two-dimensional echocardiogram (with Doppler) is more sensitive. Angiography may be the most useful diagnostic test in cardiac tumors. In these studies, the tumor, particularly myxoma, will be generally visible.

Despite the diagnostic value of echocardiography in the assessment of valve disease, diagnoses generally should not be made based on abnormalities uncovered in a single test, especially if the patient is asymptomatic and otherwise normal. The electrocardiogram and chest x-ray are two important procedures to consider in addition to echocardiography. Electrocardiographic and x-ray findings consistent with various forms of valve disease are summarized in Table 4–4.

Cardiac catheterization is generally reserved as a preoperative study, but provides useful information regarding the differential diagnosis of valve disease, including the extent to which the valves are damaged and the likelihood of a favorable surgical outcome.

Blood culture and sensitivity studies provide the backbone for diagnosis and subsequent treatment with infectious endocarditis.

TABLE 4–4. ELECTROCARDIOGRAM AND CHEST X- RAY IN VALVE DISEASE

	ECG	X-ray
Mitral valve stenosis	Decreased diagnostic assistance if low pulmonary resistance If right ventricular hypertrophy is found, pulmonary resistance is probably elevated May reveal left atrial abnormalities	If normal pulmonary resistance, heart size will be normal Useful for assessing the degree of pulmonary congestion Left atrium enlarged, pulmonary artery enlarged if pulmonary pressure >45 mm Hg
Mitral incompetence (regurgitation)	Evidence of left ventricular hypertrophy (acute) If untreated, right ventricular hypertrophy (secondary to pulmonary vascular resistance) Atrial arrhythmias (especially atrial fibrillation) develop over time	Normal heart size, if hemodynamically insignificant Acute incompetence: Initially normal heart but marked pulmonary congestion and edema Within about 2 weeks, enlarged left atrium/ventricle hemodynamically significant; left atrium/ventricle enlarged proportionate to severity of lesion
Aortic stenosis	Moderately severe: gross evidence of left ventricular hypertrophy (75%); left/right or complete bundle branch block (10%) Some cases where little or no evidence of abnormality	Left ventricular hypertrophy (rounded shadow on left border of heart), but may not be present early on
Aortic incompetence (regurgitation)	Chronic hemodynamically significant incompetence: Left ventricular hypertrophy (unless masked by left bundle block) 10% with bundle blocks (left and right complete)	Cardiac silhouette shows: Both left ventricular dilatation and hypertrophy (in severe disease) Aortic dilatation Linear calcification of ascending aorta suggests aortitis, strongly suggests syphilitic origin Acute episodes: Ventricle may be initially normal Evidence of pulmonary edema

■ Ocular

In the eye, cardiogenic emboli may be difficult to differentiate from those of other origins (eg, carotid). In general however, carotid emboli are typically yellow-golden in color, refractile, small, and multiple, and are typically located at branch retinal artery bifurcations. Cardiac emboli of valvular origin tend to be whiter and larger, and are therefore more likely to be located in the central retinal artery prior to its branching. As such, these emboli are also more likely to cause a secondary retinal artery occlusion (Figures 4–1, 4–2, and 4–3).

TREATMENT AND MANAGEMENT

■ Systemic

Mitral Stenosis

Because medical management of mitral stenosis cannot reduce obstruction through the valve, efforts are directed at prevention of recurrent rheumatic fever and bacterial endocarditis. Rheumatic fever prophylaxis should continue until 35 years of age (Table 4–5). Systemic embolization requires anticoagulation for an indefinite period. If the embolus is to an extremity or in the mesenteric system, surgery should be considered. However, a systemic embolus is not an absolute indication for mitral valve surgery, because the embolic phenomena can occur in milder forms of mitral stenosis. Symptoms of dyspnea and fatigue due to pulmonary venous congestion require evaluation for surgical intervention in mitral stenosis.

Atrial fibrillation in mitral stenosis should be treated concurrently with antiarrhthymic medications (eg, digoxin) and anticoagulation therapy (eg, warfarin) to prevent coagulation and thrombus formation (potentiated by the pooling of blood in the atrium, which during fibrillation is no longer an effective pump).

Valve replacement is associated more with late complications than are reconstructive procedures. Presently, mitral valve surgery is offered to patients with symptoms that interfere with their daily activities, such as dyspnea and

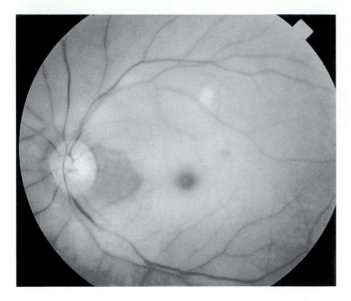

Figure 4–1. Central retinal artery occlusion, commonly secondary to cardiogenic emboli.

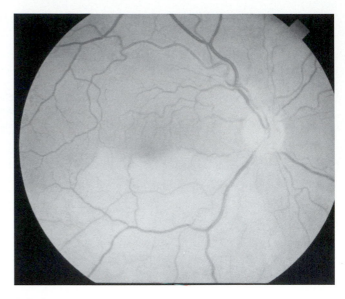

Figure 4–3. Branch retinal artery occlusion with retinal ischemia visible.

effort intolerance, and later, fluid retention, paroxysmal dyspnea, and finally, weight loss.

A mitral reconstructive procedure in mitral stenosis is based on preoperative assessment indicating a pliable mitral valve (the presence of an opening snap, little or no calcification noted on the echocardiography, absence of mitral insufficiency). These patients are less than 50 years old and most often have slight to moderate functional restrictions. Patients with unpliable mitral valve leaflets and patients who have had previous valve surgery will require mitral valve replacement. Most patients will qualify for a

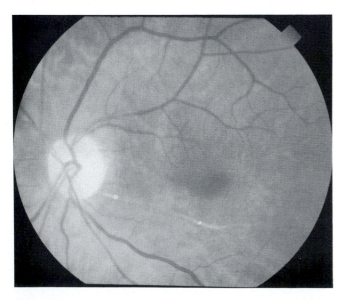

Figure 4–2. Branch retinal artery occlusion with evidence of emboli visualized.

porcine valve but younger patients should have a mechanical valve.

Patients will require digitalis or propranolol after mitral valve surgery to prevent rapid ventricular response if atrial fibrillation persists. If a prosthetic valve has been inserted, long-term anticoagulation will be required, unless a porcine valve has been inserted.

Mitral Regurgitation

As is the case in mitral valve stenosis, when rheumatic fever is the basis for the mitral regurgitation, prophylaxis is recommended until 35 years of age (see Table 4–5). Atrial fibrillation will require digitalis to slow the ventricular response. The incidence of embolism varies from 10 to 20% in chronic atrial fibrillation. Thus, anticoagulation should be considered. Dyspnea, fatigue, and orthopnea indicate impaired left ventricular function and require digitalis as well as diuretics.

Surgical replacement of the valve should be performed before clinical evidence of impaired contractility of the ventricle becomes manifest. An echocardiographic left ventricular end-diastolic dimension greater than 60 mm has been suggested by some studies as an indicator for surgery whether symptoms have developed or not.

Most patients with mitral leaflet prolapse syndrome are asymptomatic and merely require assurance. Beta-blocking agents and calcium channel blocking drugs may be required in patients with chest pain even though coronary anatomy is normal. These patients should be advised of the need to prevent infectious Endocarditis with antibiotics prior to dental work.

A reparative surgical procedure is done whenever the pathological condition of the valve permits (eg, in

TABLE 4–5. TREATMENT AND MANAGEMENT OF VALVULAR DISEASE

MITRAL STENOSIS
- Prophylactic antibiotics
- Anticoagulant medication
- Surgery: valve replacement or reconstruction
- Antiarrhythmics if atrial fibrillation exists

MITRAL REGURGITATION
- Prophylactic antibiotics
- Digitalis if atrial fibrillation exists
- Anticoagulants
- Surgery: valve replacement
- Mitral valve prolapse:
  Patient reassurance
  May require ß-blockers or calcium channel blockers

AORTIC STENOSIS
- Asymptomatic: prophylactic antibiotics
- Symptomatic/severe: valve replacement

AORTIC REGURGITATION
- Prophylactic antibiotics
- Heart failure: digitalis, diuretics, vasodilators
- Surgery

PROPHYLAXIS FOR INFECTIOUS ENDOCARDITIS FOR ADULTS AND CHILDREN OVER 60 LBS[a]
- Penicillin V:
  Adults: 2 g 1 hour prior to surgery and then 1 g 6 hours later
  Children < 60 lbs: 1 g 1 hour prior and 500 mg 6 hours later
- Patients with prosthetic valves (or others with a high risk of endocarditis):
  Adults: Ampicillin 1–2 g, either IM or IV, 1/2 hour prior and 1 g oral penicillin V 6 hours later (or the injected regimen once, 8 hours later)
  Children: Ampicillin, 50 mg/kg either IM or IV 1/2 hour prior and 1 g oral penicillin V 6 hours later (or the injected regimen once, 8 hours later)
- Allergy to penicillin:
  Adults: Erythromycin, 1 g orally 1 hour prior then 500 mg 6 hours later
  Children: Erythromycin 20 mg/kg 1 hour prior then 10 mg/kg 6 hours later

[a]From A Statement for Health Professionals by the Committee on Rheumatic Fever and Bacterial Endocarditis of the Council on Cardiovascular Diseases in the Young of the American Heart Association, 1985.

involvement, mitral stenosis with loss of pliability of the leaflets, and infectious Endocarditis.

If the patient remains in atrial fibrillation after hospital discharge, chronic digitalis administration will be required to control the ventricular response. Antibiotic coverage for dental work and elective surgical procedures remains important for prevention of infectious endocarditis. Depending on the type of prosthetic valve inserted, long-term anticoagulation therapy may be necessary. Echocardiographic studies can be obtained every 6 to 12 months.

Aortic Stenosis
In the asymptomatic state, aortic stenosis requires prophylactic antibiotics to prevent bacterial endocarditis (see Table 4–5). In patients with a suspected rheumatic basis for the aortic stenosis, prophylaxis should be continued until 35 years of age. Orifice size less than 0.8 cm² warrants serious consideration for valve replacement.

The natural history of the disease must be weighed against the results achieved by surgical intervention. With respect to valve disease, those with aortic stenosis have the poorest prognosis. Approximately 50% of patients diagnosed with severe stenosis (with or without symptoms) die within 5 years of the time of diagnosis. Aortic stenosis usually results in well-maintained ventricular function except in far-advanced situations. Patients with congestive heart failure, angina, or exertional syncope should undergo aortic valve replacement promptly. Asymptomatic patients with significant aortic valvular stenosis should be advised to have surgery.

The current operative mortality for primary isolated aortic valve replacement is less than 3 to 4% in most cases and is most closely related to the degree of left ventricular failure, with most deaths occurring in patients with end-stage disease. Actuarial survival at 5 years with various types of valve prosthesis is approximately 80%.

Aortic Regurgitation
A primary responsibility in the care of the asymptomatic patient with aortic regurgitation is prophylaxis against bacterial endocarditis (see Table 4–5). Heart failure can be treated with digitalis, diuretics, and vasodilating agents. However, the primary defect is mechanical, and medical therapy alone cannot modify the impaired or defective valve. Ideally, valve replacement should be proposed before clinical symptoms of heart failure develop or before dilatation of the ventricle has developed. Echocardiograms should be taken every 3 to 6 months when end-systolic chamber dimensions are 50 to 54 mm. Surgery should be considered when the dimension exceeds 55 mm even when symptoms are absent. Controversies persist regarding indications for surgery prior to symptoms.

Chronic aortic regurgitation may be well tolerated for several years before causing evidence of left ventricular dysfunction and symptoms. Acute aortic regurgitation resulting

myxomatous degeneration, in cases secondary to ischemic heart disease). These procedures have the advantage of avoiding the long-term risk of devices used to replace the mitral valve and the need for long-term anticoagulant therapy that accompanies many of them.

Calcification and immobility of the leaflets are indications for valve replacement. Such cases include rheumatic from bacterial endocarditis, acute dissection of the ascending aorta, and tearing of the aortic cusp is poorly tolerated and usually requires urgent or emergency surgical intervention.

Patients with chronic aortic regurgitation who are symptomatic are advised to have surgery, as are asymptomatic patients who show evidence of left ventricular dysfunction at rest as measured by echocardiography, and those patients who show ventricular dysfunction only with exercise. Patients with an end-systolic dimension greater than 55 mm have a poorer result in terms of longevity than those operated before this degree of left ventricular enlargement occurs.

In general, due to the increased likelihood of thrombogenesis, most mechanical prostheses require long-term anticoagulation; tissue prostheses do not, but these prostheses will probably prove less durable than most mechanical prostheses. The early mortality for aortic valve replacement for patients with aortic regurgitation is generally about the same as those having the operation for aortic stenosis, and is approximately 2 to 3%. Mechanical prostheses are associated with a 2 to 3% per year incidence of thrombotic complications and an equal incidence of bleeding complications. Tissue valves have a failure rate of 15 to 20% in 10 years.

Postoperative management is similar to aortic stenosis. Anticoagulation is determined by the valve type used. Prophylactic antibiotics are indicated during periods of increased susceptibility to bacteremia (see Table 4–5).

Infectious Endocarditis

Prophylaxis. The American Heart Association recommends pharmacologic prophylaxis for patients at risk for infectious endocarditis. Dental surgery (eg, tooth extraction), genitourinary surgery, gastrointestinal tract surgery, and other similar procedures are strong indications for prophylaxis. Table 4–5 contains the standard regimen (as per "A Statement for Health Professionals by the Committee on Rheumatic Fever and Bacterial Endocarditis of the Council on Cardiovascular Disease in the Young").

Treatment of Active Infection. Treatment of active infectious Endocarditis should begin once two positive culture and sensitivity studies have been conducted. The medication of choice is based upon the sensitivity studies and should be bactericidal. Treatment should continue until the infection is completely eliminated.

Surgery may be required especially in the case of fungal infections or when valvular function has been dramatically compromised. The benefits of anticoagulant therapy concurrent with treating the infection is not clear.

■ Ocular

When faced with retinal emboli of either cardiac or carotid origin, particularly in the presence of neurologic signs or symptoms (amaurosis fugax, hemianopsia, tingling or numbness of the extremities) or signs or symptoms suggestive of cardiac origins (angina, pulmonary edema), the most appropriate treatment is referral to an internist, cardiologist, or neurologist for a comprehensive cardiovascular workup.

The management of the ocular manifestations of cardiogenic emboli and valve disease centers around treatment of the underlying systemic disease. Acute arterial occlusion secondary to emboli can be managed aggressively in an effort to dislodge the emboli (eg, digital massage of the globe, paracentesis); however, this is rarely successful.

CONCLUSION

When faced with retinal emboli, it is important to remember that a significant percentage are of cardiac origin. This is particularly true in younger patients. Timely referral is indicated because cerebrovascular accidents secondary to cardiogenic emboli are one of the most preventable forms of stroke. As such, this information is potentially life-saving. The patient may appear otherwise healthy. This should not deter from an appropriate referral. Retinal emboli should be differentiated by their source (eg, carotid versus cardiac) in order to appropriately manage the patient. Emboli of carotid origin warrant a carotid workup (see Chapter 5) in tandem with a comprehensive cardiovascular workup (recall that the leading cause of mortality in patients with significant carotid stenosis is myocardial infarction). Care should also be taken, particularly in patients with known valve replacement or other invasive cardiac procedures, to rule out ocular signs of infectious endocarditis.

REFERENCES

Abernathy WS, Willis PW. Thromboembolic complications of rheumatic heart disease. *Cardiovasc Clin.* 1973;5:131.

Bonow RO. Left ventricular structure and function in aortic valve disease. *Circulation.* 1989;79:966.

Braunwald E. Valvular heart disease. In: Braunwald E, ed. *Heart Disease.* Philadelphia: Saunders; 1992:1007.

Braunwald E. Mitral regurgitation: Physiologic, clinical, and surgical consideration. *N Engl J Med.* 1969;281:425.

Chun PK, Gertz E, Davia JE, et al. Coronary atherosclerosis in mitral stenosis. *Chest.* 1982;81:36.

Cogan DG, Wray SH. Vascular occlusions in the eye from cardiac myxomas. *Am J Ophthalmol.* 1975;80:396–403.

Davison ET, Friedman SA. Significance of systolic murmurs in the aged. *N Engl J Med.* 1968;279:225.

Eiden SB, Olivares G. Transient vision loss associated with Barlow's syndrome. *J Am Optom Assoc.* 1986;57:446–447.

Gallo I, Ruiz B, Duran CMG. Five to eight year follow-up of patients with the Hancock cardiac prosthesis. *J Thorac Cardiovasc Surg.* 1983;86:897.

Grayburn PA, Smith MD, Handshow R, et al. Detection of aortic insufficiency by standard echocardiography, pulsed Doppler echocardiography and auscultation. *Ann Intern Med.* 1986;104:599.

Hart RG. Cardiogenic embolism to the brain. *Lancet.* 1992;339:589–594.

Jampol EM, Wong AS, Alber DM. Atrial myxoma and central retinal artery occlusion. *Am J Opthalmol.* 1973;75:242–249.

Marcus RH, Sareli P, Pocock WA, et al. Functional anatomy of severe mitral regurgitation in active rheumatic carditis. *Am J Cardiol.* 1989;63:577.

Nutter DO, Wickliffe C, Gilbert CA, et al. The pathophysiology of idiopathic mitral valve prolapse. *Circulation.* 1975;52:297.

Oh WMC, Taylor TR, Olsen EGJ. Aortic regurgitation in systemic lupus erythematosus requiring aortic valve replacement. *Br Heart J.* 1974;36:413.

Perloff JK, Roberts WC. The mitral apparatus: functional anatomy of mitral regurgitation. *Circulation.* 1972;46:227.

Pomerance A. Pathogenesis of aortic stenosis and its relation to age. *Br Heart J.* 1972;34:569.

Rackley CE, Karp RB, Edwards JE. Mitral valve disease. In: Hurst JW, Schlant RC, eds. *The Heart.* 7th ed. New York: McGraw-Hill; 1990:820.

Rackley CE, Wallace RB, Edwards JE, et al. Aortic valve disease. In: Hurst JW, Schlant RC, eds. *The Heart.* 7th ed. New York: McGraw-Hill; 1990:795.

Selzer A. Changing aspects of the natural history of valvular aortic stenosis. *N Engl J Med.* 1987;317:91.

Skulman ST, Amren DP, Bisno AL, et al. Prevention of bacterial endocarditis: A statement for health professionals by the Committee on Rheumatic Fever and Bacterial Endocarditis of the Council on Cardiovascular Diseases in the Young of the American Heart Association. *Am J Dis Child.* 1985;139:232–235.

Sokolow M, McIlroy MB, Cheitlin MD. *Clinical Cardiology.* 5th ed. Norwalk, CT: Appleton & Lange; 1990:377–435.

Wrobleroski E, James F, Spann JF, et al. Right ventricular performance in mitral stenosis. *Am J Cardiol.* 1981;47:51.

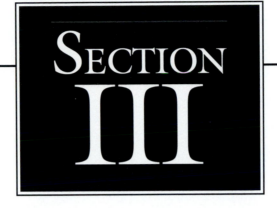

SECTION III

NEUROLOGICAL DISORDERS

5
Chapter

Cerebrovascular Disease

Bernard H. Blaustein

Cerebrovascular disease defines any pathologic process affecting the blood vessels that supply blood to the brain. The underlying pathologic process may be an occlusive lesion of the vessel, such as a thrombus or embolus, or rupture of a vessel wall leading to hemorrhage. Of singular importance in cerebrovascular disease is the potential for cerebral ischemia.

The threat of stroke is the major concern regarding cerebrovascular disease. Stroke is frequently a devastating event. There is an initial mortality of 20 to 30%. Moreover, for survivors, the residual disability is often considerable. Results of the Framingham study (Greshan et al, 1975) indicate that 16% of the survivors remain institutionalized, 31% need long-term assistance in self-care, and 71% have a reduced capacity to earn a living.

Eyecare practitioners may play a vital role in the reduction of stroke, because many cases of cerebrovascular disease present with characteristic eye signs and symptoms. By identifying these patients and referring them to the appropriate healthcare practitioner, interventional therapy may be instituted, and stroke may be averted.

EPIDEMIOLOGY

■ Systemic

The incidence of cerebrovascular disease has declined significantly during the past 30 years. The public has acquired an increasing awareness of stroke risk factors: hypertension, smoking, elevated serum lipids, diabetes mellitus, and cardiac disease (Table 5–1). However, cerebrovascular disease is still the third leading cause of death in the United States after heart disease and cancer. About 70 to 80% of all strokes are due to thromboembolism, 10% to subarachnoid hemorrhage, and 4% to intracerebral hemorrhage. The American Heart Association estimates that there will be in excess of 500,000 new cases of stroke each year in the United States, with most cases occurring in persons over age 55.

The incidence of stroke is rare before the age of 55. However, it tends to double with each successive decade. Males are slightly more prone to stroke than females, with the male preponderance being greater in the younger age groups. In the United States, rates of cerebrovascular disease in African-Americans are higher than in Caucasians in all ages and in both sexes. However, worldwide, stroke is less common in African-Americans than Caucasians. Asians have higher rates of cerebral hemorrhage.

■ Ocular

Transient visual loss (TVL) or amaurosis fugax, is a sudden, transient, monocular alteration of vision. TVL is the most common symptom of transient ischemia within the carotid vascular system, occurring in about 40% of cases. The incidence of transient ischemia that results in TVLs has been reported at 31 in 100,000 among the residents of Rochester, Minnesota, and 110 in 100,000 for the retirement community of Seal Beach, California. The incidence of TVLs increases with each decade between 45 and 75 years, with the mean age of onset in the seventh decade. Between 40 and 80 years of age men experience more episodes of TVL than women by a 2.3 to 1.0 margin.

TABLE 5–1. INCREASED RISK FACTORS FOR CEREBROVASCULAR DISEASE

Hypertension
Increased serum lipids
Diabetes mellitus
Cardiovascular disease
Atherosclerosis
Smoking
Oral contraceptives (?)
Increased age, male

Thromboembolic phenomena account for approximately 70 to 80% of all strokes. Most of the remainder are caused by intracerebral or subarachnoid hemorrhage.

The majority of this chapter will be devoted to thromboembolic vascular disease. This entity may lead to ischemic stroke and is apt to present with ocular manifestations that herald its onset.

NATURAL HISTORY

■ Systemic

Stroke is defined as a sudden, nonconvulsive, neurologic deficit caused by a reduction in blood flow below that which is necessary for the viability of brain cells. The term "cerebrovascular accident" (CVA) often is used interchangeably with the term "stroke." In its most severe form, the patient may become hemiplegic or comatose. In its mildest form, the stroke may cause a trivial neurological disorder. All gradations exist between these two extremes. However, it is the abruptness with which the neurological deficit develops—seconds, minutes, hours, or at most a few days—that marks the disorder as vascular. Embolic strokes characteristically begin suddenly, and the deficit reaches its peak almost at once. Thrombotic strokes also usually have an abrupt onset. However, in many the onset is somewhat slower, occurring over a period of several minutes, hours, or days in a steplike fashion.

In cerebral hemorrhage, the deficit may be sudden or may occur as a gradual, steadily progressive deterioration. Hemorrhagic strokes are almost always caused by severe, uncontrolled hypertension. Blood leaks from the vessel directly into the brain, one of the ventricles, or the subarachnoid space. The subsequent compression and displacement of brain tissue within the narrow confines of the closed cranial vault almost always results in significant neurological damage. Hemorrhagic strokes do not usually present with any warnings or prodromal symptoms.

Cerebral ischemia is a regional reduction in blood flow below that which is required for the normal function of brain tissue. It is usually caused by either a thrombus or an embolus. A thrombus may lead to cerebral ischemia by the obstruction of a larger vessel with an aggregation of platelets, fibrin, calcium, and other cellular elements. An embolus, a small portion of the clot, may break off from the parent thrombus and travel downstream to occlude a smaller vessel. If the reduction in blood flow is transitory or is not intense enough to result in cell death, neuronal function may return to normal.

Cerebral infarct is a histological term denoting the end result of sustained local ischemia to a particular part of the brain. The affected brain tissue undergoes irreversible ischemic necrosis and death. Lacunar infarctions are very small necrotic cavities and are caused by occlusions of small penetrating arterioles in the deeper, noncortical portions of the brain. In many instances the lacunae are so small that no clinically recognizable neurological deficit manifests. Indeed, lacunar infarcts are often discovered incidentally on CT or MRI scans.

Atherosclerosis is the major pathologic process underlying ischemic cerebrovascular disease. It is characterized by the deposition of lipids in the innermost layer of medium and large arteries in areas of bifurcations and curves. Atherosclerotic lesions are found most frequently at the origin of the internal carotid artery (ICA). The next most common site is the proximal portion of the vertebral arteries just after they branch off the subclavian arteries.

The pathophysiology of atherosclerosis has been under intense study for many years. It is felt that elevated levels of cholesterol, particularly with a concomitant elevation of low-density lipoproteins (LDL), encourage the deposition of lipids in the intima of medium and large arteries. Smooth muscle cells ultimately proliferate into the intimal layer, causing the formation of a plaque. These plaques contain a central core of extracellular LDL, necrotic cell debris, and calcium salts. Subsequently, a narrowing of the arterial lumen occurs resulting in a relative stasis and turbulence of blood flow in that area.

The continual deposition of lipids onto the intimal surface encourages the breakdown of the endothelial cells that make up the intima and leads to ulcer formation. The injured endothelium and turbulent blood flow encourage platelets to agglutinate and stick to the altered site.

The roughened ulcerative surface, presence of agglutinated platelets, and relative stasis of blood flow encourages the development of a thrombus. Subsequent bleeding into the thrombus from the vasovasorum greatly enlarges the thrombus and can lead to occlusion of the parent vessel. In addition, small particles may break off and embolize to smaller vessels distally.

Hypertension, increased serum lipids, diabetes mellitus, and cardiac disease are risk factors known to increase the patient's liability for cerebrovascular disease. Some of these factors contribute to the development of atherosclerosis.

Hypertension is present in up to 30% of the American adult population over the age of 40 and is the major risk factor for stroke. It is stongly related to atherothrombotic brain infarction as well as intracerebral and subarachnoid hemorrhage.

It has been estimated that hypertensives have a stroke risk four times that of normotensives. The risk of stroke increases in direct relationship to elevation of both diastole and systole, but the strongest association is with systolic pressure. Furthermore, several studies have shown that effective treatment of hypertension will reduce stroke incidence and mortality.

The major plasma lipids, including cholesterol and triglycerides, are transported in the form of lipoprotein complexes. The most important lipoproteins with regard to atherogenesis are the low-density (LDL) and high-density (HDL) lipoproteins. LDL is thought to transport cholesterol to the tissues, and in particular to the intimas of medium and large-sized arteries. HDL is thought to transfer cholesterol to the liver for degradation.

Tell and colleagues (1988) reviewed the literature and concluded that there was a positive relationship between cerebral atherosclerosis and elevated LDL and triglyceride levels. However, it is not presently known whether the reduction of serum lipids will reduce the risk of cerebral infarction.

Several epidemiological studies have implicated cigarette smoking as a significant risk factor for stroke. Data from the Framingham study (Sacco et al, 1984) indicate that the relative risk for stroke in those who smoke more than 40 cigarettes per day is twice that of those who smoke less than 10 per day.

Diabetes is a specific risk factor for thromboembolic brain infarction. It is felt that diabetes increases the LDL level within the serum and thus accelerates the production of atherosclerosis. When associated with hypertension, the risk is even stronger.

Impaired cardiac function, including coronary artery disease, congestive heart failure, left ventricular hypertrophy, valvular disease, and atrial fibrillation, is a major risk factor for stroke. At any level of blood pressure, persons with cardiac disease have more than twice the risk of stroke than those with normal cardiac function.

The role of oral contraceptives in stroke remains unclear. Some studies have suggested that oral contraceptives are associated with an increased risk of ischemic stroke. Others reveal a significant risk for subarachnoid hemorrhage. Nevertheless, it seems that the risk of stroke is increased if users of oral contraceptives are older than 35 years, are smokers, are migraineurs, or are diabetics.

Anatomic Correlates

A review of the cerebral vascular supply explains the sequelae of compromised blood flow. The major blood supply to the brain arises from the aortic arch and involves two vascular systems: the anterior circulatory system, fed by the carotid artery system; and the posterior circulatory system, fed by the vertebrobasilar artery system. Except for the origins and proximal portions of these systems, the blood supply is identical on each side (Figures 5–1 and 5–2).

The major derivative of the common carotid artery is the internal carotid artery (ICA). As it emerges from the cavernous sinus, the ICA gives off its first large branch, the ophthalmic artery, which supplies the ipsilateral globe and orbit. The ICA ends by dividing into the anterior and middle cerebral arteries. Most of the ipsilateral frontal, temporal, and parietal lobes are supplied by these arteries.

Carotid artery disease or a decreased perfusion within the ICA may result in decreased ophthalmic artery pressure with a concomitant ipsilateral decrease in vision. When the middle cerebral artery or its branches are specifically involved, a contralateral hemiplegia results, with the motor deficit being more pronounced in the upper extremities. The hemiplegia is frequently associated with a hemisensory deficit and a homonymous hemianopsia. When the anterior cerebral artery is involved, a contralateral hemiplegia and an occasional hemisensory deficit result. The defect is greater in the lower extremity.

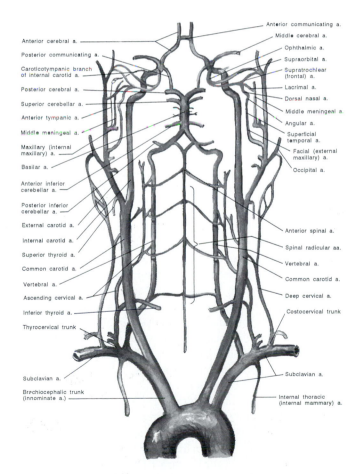

Figure 5–1. Cerebrovascular circulation.

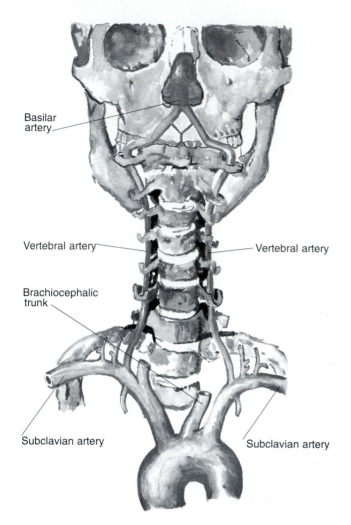

Figure 5–2. Course of the vertebral arteries.

most often caused by an atherosclerotic stenosis of the subclavian artery just proximal to the origin of the vertebral artery. As a pressure gradient develops between the exercised arm and the stenosed vessel, blood is diverted from the vertebrobasilar circulation to supply the arm.

Not all of the above signs and symptoms need occur with vertebrobasilar insufficiency. Moreover, vertigo and/or dizziness alone, without other symptoms, are often observed in older patients and do not necessarily indicate posterior circulatory ischemia.

Transient ischemic attacks (TIAs) refer to temporary episodes of cerebral dysfunction of vascular origin. They are rapid in onset, variable in duration, and commonly last from 2 to 15 minutes but occasionally last for as long as a day. Signs and symptoms that last for 24 hours are called reversible ischemic neurologic deficits (RIND). After the attack the patient returns to preattack status with no apparent clinical evidence of an infarct or permanent damage. Neuroimaging, however, may reveal evidence of minor cerebral infarct. The transient nature of the attack is explained by a temporary blockage of a vessel by a small embolus of fibrin–platelet material from a distant atherosclerotic site. The rapid fragmentation and dissolution of these microemboli preclude permanent neurologic dysfunction.

Carotid territory TIAs can be broadly divided into two categories: TVL and transient hemispheric attacks. TVL is the only feature distinguishing the extracranial carotid syndrome from that of an intracranial obstruction of the middle cerebral artery.

TVL is a brief alteration of vision in one eye ipsilateral to the carotid disease. Patients will occasionally describe the phenomenon as a temporary mist or cloud before the eye. More frequently, the patient will describe the vision loss as altitudinal, as though a curtain had been pulled over one eye.

The clinical manifestations of transient hemispheric attacks vary depending upon the location and severity of the cerebral ischemia. However, most symptoms are referable to the territory supplied by the middle cerebral artery. The most common symptoms include short-lived motor and sensory disturbances of the contralateral limbs. Depending on which hemisphere is involved, dysphasia and confusion due to spatial disorientation may occur. A less frequent occurrence is episodic limb shaking, a manifestation that may be mistaken for a focal seizure.

With vertebrobasilar TIAs, short-lived episodes of vertigo, unsteadiness, tunnel vision (bilateral hemianopsia), diplopia, dysarthria, nausea, headache, and vomiting are common.

The natural history of patients who experience TIAs is not precisely known. The general consensus is that persons who experience TIAs have a stroke risk of about 5 to 6% per year. The risk of subsequent infarction is greatest within the first month following a TIA; 36% of infarcts occur within this period. As a general rule, following a TIA about one third of patients will have no further symptoms,

Because the basilar artery is a single midline vessel with branches to both sides, the signs and symptoms that result from ischemia to the vertebrobasilar system may show considerable variation (Table 5–2). Unilateral, bilateral, or alternating involvement of cranial nerves III to VII may result in abnormal ocular motility, diplopia, or motor or sensory deficits in the face. Bilateral involvement of the medulla may impact on descending and ascending nerve tracts resulting in motor and sensory deficits in the limbs. If the descending sympathetic fibers that run along the lateral medulla are compromised, Horner syndrome may result.

Cranial nerves housed in the medulla may be involved resulting in dysphagia and dysphonia. Cerebellar defects may result in vertigo or ataxia. Ischemia to the occipital cortex may result in bilateral hemianopsia, which the patient often will interpret as a bilateral dimming of vision. Finally, headache, vomiting, and syncope may occur.

Symptoms of vertebrobasilar insufficiency in conjunction with claudication of the exercised arm constitutes the subclavian steal syndrome. This syndrome is

TABLE 5–2. SYSTEMIC AND OCULAR MANIFESTATIONS OF CEREBROVASCULAR DISEASE

■ **VERTEBROBASILAR DISEASE**

SYSTEMIC
- Transient ischemic attacks
- Reversible ischemic neurological deficits
- Unilateral, bilateral, alternate cranial nerve deficits III to VII
- Motor sensory deficits in limbs
- Dysphagia/dysphonia
- Vertigo/ataxia
- Headache /vomiting/syncope
- Claudication of exercised arm (subclavian steal syndrome)
- Dizziness
- Unsteadiness
- Dysarthria

OCULAR
- Ocular motility abnormalities
- Diplopia
- Horner syndrome
- Bilateral hemianopsia (bilateral dimming of vision/tunnel vision)

■ **CAROTID ARTERY DISEASE**

SYSTEMIC
- Transient ischemic attacks/transient hemispheric attacks (short-lived motor/sensory disturbances of the contralateral limbs)
- Dysphagia
- Spatial disorientation
- Episodic limb shaking

OCULAR
- Transient visual loss (ipsilateral/one eye/temporary mist or cloud/altitudinal vision loss or curtain)
- Ocular ischemic syndrome
     Engorged episcleral vessels
     Corneal edema
     Striate keratopathy
     Mild anterior uveitis

Carotid artery disease—ocular (cont'd)
     Irregular pupil
     Iris neovascularization
     Hypotony (initial)
     Orbital pain
     Cataracts
     Iris atrophy
- Retina
     Plaques (Hollenhorst/calcific)
     Infarcts
     Cotton-wool spots
     Asymmetric retinopathy
     Hypoperfusion retinopathy (venous stasis retinopathy)

■ **INTRACRANIAL HEMORRHAGE**

SYSTEMIC
- Severe headache
- Coma
- Death

■ **RUPTURED SACCULAR ANEURYSM**

SYSTEMIC
- Severe headache
- Transitory unilateral weakness, numbness, and tingling
- Speech disturbance
- Unconsciousness

■ **AV MALFORMATION**

SYSTEMIC
- Nondescript headache (may mimic migraine with visual aura)
- Audible cranial bruit
- Progressive neurological impairment
- Hemiparesis
- Hemiplegia
- Mental decline
- Death

one third will have recurrent TIAs, and one third will go on to have a stroke. It is significant to note that about 50% of patients suffering a cerebral infarction from occlusive carotid disease will have experienced a carotid TIA sometime beforehand.

Intracranial Hemorrhage
Spontaneous intracranial hemorrhage may involve bleeding into the parenchyma of the brain, the pituitary gland, the ventricular system, the subarachnoid space, or the epidural or subdural spaces. In many instances the hemorrhage involves several of these compartments. A discussion of

pituitary hemorrhage and isolated subdural or epidural hematomas is not included in this chapter.

Intracerebral hemorrhage (ICH), also known as primary hypertensive hemorrhage, almost always occurs as a result of sustained, elevated systolic blood pressure. The patient presents with an abrupt onset and rapid evolution of symptoms usually occurring over minutes or hours. Usually, there are no warnings or prodromal signs, although approximately 50% of patients report a severe headache as the stroke is evolving.

The hemorrhage occurs within brain tissue, forming an oval mass that disrupts the tissue and grows in volume as the bleeding continues. Adjacent brain tissue may be displaced and compressed. If the hemorrhage is very large, midline structures may be displaced to the opposite side and vital centers may be compromised. Coma and death will usually result. The vessel involved is usually a small penetrating artery. The hemorrhage is thought to arise from an arterial wall that has become weakened from being impregnated with a hyaline-lipid material as a result of the sustained hypertension. In order of frequency, the most common sites of hypertensive hemorrhage are (1) the putamen and adjacent internal capsule; (2) various parts of the central white matter of the temporal, parietal, or frontal lobes; (3) the thalamus; (4) the cerebellar hemisphere; and (5) the pons.

Ruptured Saccular Aneurysm

Saccular aneurysms (berry aneurysms) take the form of small, thin-walled blisters protruding from the arteries of the circle of Willis or its major branches. As a rule, the aneurysms are located at bifurcations and branchings, and are presumed to result from developmental defects in the tunica media or internal elastic membrane. The resultant weakness in the arterial walls causes the intima to bulge outward, covered only by adventitia. The sac gradually enlarges and finally ruptures.

Prior to rupture, the saccular aneurysms are usually asymptomatic. However, some patients will have had an episode of severe headache or transitory unilateral weakness, numbness and tingling, or speech disturbance in the days or weeks preceding the major event. These prodromal symptoms are generally attributed to minor leakage from the aneurysm. Rupture of the aneurysm usually occurs while the patient is active, and in many cases sexual intercourse or other exertion is the precipitant.

When the rupture occurs, blood under high pressure is forced into the subarachnoid space since the circle of Willis lies within this space. The resulting clinical events assume one of three patterns: (1) the patient may experience an excruciating headache and fall unconscious; (2) the patient may be stricken with a severe headache but remain relatively lucid; or (3) the patient may lose consciousness quickly without any preceding complaint.

Arteriovenous Malformation

An arteriovenous malformation (AVM) consists of a tangle of dilated vessels that form an abnormal communication between the arterial and venous systems. AVMs may occur in all parts of the brain, brainstem, and spinal cord, but the larger ones are more frequently found in the posterior half of the cerebral hemispheres. AVMs are about one tenth as common as saccular aneurysms and somewhat more common in males than in females.

The tangled blood vessels that are interposed between the arteries and veins are abnormally thin, and their walls do not possess the structural integrity of normal arteries or veins. Although most AVMs are clinically silent for a long time, most will eventually bleed. When hemorrhage occurs, blood may enter the subarachnoid space but is more likely to be partly intracerebral, causing a hemiparesis, hemiplegia, or even death.

Before rupture, a chronic nondescript headache is a frequent complaint. Occasionally, these headaches mimic migraines, and if the AVM is located in the occipital cortex, visual auras may accompany the headache. Typically, the visual auras do not flicker as do the auras of classic migraine. Other symptoms of AVMs include audible cranial bruit, convulsions, progressive neurological impairment, or mental decline.

■ Ocular

The nature of the ocular signs and symptoms that occur in cerebrovascular disease depends on whether the ischemia occurs in the carotid territory or the vertebrobasilar territory (see Table 5–2). It is important to ascertain the etiology of the ischemia, because the associated ocular findings and the subsequent treatment are different.

Ischemia of the anterior segment and the retina define the carotid territory syndrome. If the patient experiences TVL, he or she often feels as though a shade has been pulled over one eye.

Prolonged generalized ischemia to the anterior portion of the eye presents a constellation of signs and symptoms known as the ocular ischemic syndrome. The anterior manifestations of this syndrome are characterized by engorged episcleral vessels, corneal edema and striate keratopathy secondary to poor oxygen perfusion, mild anterior uveitis with flare and cells, irregular pupil, and iris neovascularization around the pupil and in the anterior chamber angle. Initially, hypotony occurs because of impaired ciliary body function. Ultimately, neovascular glaucoma may occur secondary to the iris neovascularization. In addition, the patient reports deep orbital pain and photophobia. In time the iris atrophies and diffuse cataracts develop.

The presence of plaques, infarcts, cotton-wool spots, or evidence of venous stasis imply retinal ischemia. Retinal arteriolar plaques may appear as bright and glistening. These crystalline particles, known as Hollenhorst plaques, tend to lodge at arteriolar bifurcations (Figure 5–3). They are thought to originate from the inner layers of carotid atheromas and represent cholesterol deposits. They may rarely cause transient visual loss but more often will fragment and pass through the retinal circulation without incident. Solid, white, nonrefractile plaques that lodge in the larger vessels around the optic nervehead originate from calcification of cardiac valves. These calcific emboli are often occlusive and may cause retinal infarcts.

Long dull-white plugs represent platelet emboli from the surface of atheromas. They are mobile and will undergo

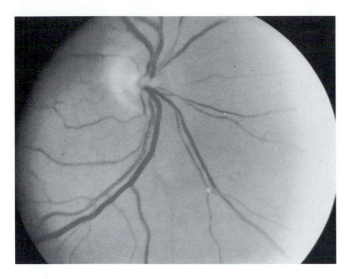

Figure 5–3. Hollenhorst plaque in an arteriolar bifurcation.

fragmentation and dissolution but can cause transient obstruction to retinal blood flow. TVL may occur. Linear white deposits within arterioles probably represent fibrin or thromboembolic material from the walls of the heart. They are less friable than platelets and may result in retinal artery occlusions and subsequent infarcts.

Asymmetric retinopathy may occur with carotid insufficiency to the eye. On the ipsilateral side there may be cotton-wool spots, indicating generalized retinal hypoxia, or frank retinal neovascularization. In addition, midperipheral blot and dot hemorrhages, microaneurysms, and dilated tortuous veins may be noted. This entity represents hypoperfusion retinopathy (venous stasis retinopathy, or nonischemic central retinal vein occlusion), and is an important hallmark of carotid insufficiency. Gay and Rosenbaum (1966) implied that unilateral carotid artery disease with a resultant decrease in ocular perfusion led to less diabetic retinal neovascularization. However, studies by Browning (1988), Ducker (1990), and their associates were unable to confirm Gay and Rosenbaum's findings.

The characteristic ocular symptomatology of vertebrobasilar insufficiency is associated with ischemia to the posterior portions of the brain: the occipital lobes, cerebellum, and brainstem. Bilateral disturbance of vision results from insufficiency of the posterior cerebral arteries that supply the visual cortex. Visual symptoms are described as being a bilateral dimming, graying, or blurring of vision. Total blindness may occur transiently. Attacks of vertigo and diplopia may also occur.

Diagnosis

The diagnosis of cerebrovascular disease is often made by integrating ocular clinical data with systemic clinical data.

■ Systemic

After the appropriate workup by the ocular clinician, the patient may be referred to the vascular specialist for further evaluation and management. The physician will attempt to reduce the risk factors associated with cerebrovascular disease, particularly hypertension, hypercholesterolemia, and impaired cardiac function. In addition, noninvasive and/or invasive tests will be performed to more completely evaluate the status of cerebral blood flow.

Noninvasive Tests

Noninvasive diagnostic techniques for the evaluation of carotid occlusive disease may be divided into those that indirectly assess the hemodynamics of the ICA distal to the bifurcation and those that directly assess the carotid bifurcation (Table 5–3).

Oculoplethysmography (OPG) combines some of the principles of ODM and the old techniques of ocular plethysmography. The procedure is performed by applying small vacuum cups to both anesthetized sclerae. Intraocular pressure is increased in each eye simultaneously by the application of a vacuum. Subsequently, the ocular pulse disappears. The vacuum pressure is then reduced simultaneously until the pulsations just return. A delay in the pulse in one eye indicates decreased flow to that eye and implies obstruction in the ICA ipsilaterally. Gee and co-workers (1974) developed a conversion table relating the intracranial ICA pressure to the level of vacuum at which the first ocular pulse appears.

Periorbital directional Doppler ultrasonography uses high-frequency sound waves to ascertain the direction of blood flow in the periorbital arteries. The transducer is placed just below the supraorbital notch, and high-

TABLE 5–3. TESTS FOR CAROTID ARTERY DISEASE

Systemic

Noninvasive assessment distal to the bifurcation
    Oculoplethysmography
    Periorbital directional Doppler
Noninvasive assessment at the bifurcation
    B-scan ultrasonography
    Doppler ultrasonography
    Duplex scanning
    Phonoangiography
Invasive
    Arteriography
    Digital venous subtraction angiography

Ocular

Auscultate extracranial arteries
Palpate pulses (superficial temporal artery)
Ophthalmodynamometry
Blood pressure (difference in systolic right arm/left arm >20 mm Hg)

frequency sound waves are transmitted to the area. The frequency of the reflected sound waves is a function of the direction of blood flow relative to the source. If red blood cells are moving toward the transducer, the frequency is increased. A hemodynamically significant stenosis at any point along the ICA will cause a reversal of blood flow in the supraorbital and supratrochlear arteries (Figure 5–4).

High-resolution B-scan ultrasonography provides a cross-sectional image of the carotid bifurcation by means of sound wave reflection from the interfaces of tissues of different acoustic impedances. Each point in the field being studied corresponds to a dot on the oscilloscope screen. The brightness of the dot is proportional to the amplitude of the reflected sound wave. This technique is capable of identifying subtle plaques and small ulcers as well as delineating the residual lumen diameter. Real-time ultrasonography has an accuracy approaching 90% when compared to carotid angiography. It is better than angiography for detecting small lesions, that is, with 1 to 25% luminal stenosis. However, with stenosis greater than 75%, B-mode images begin to suffer and become less reliable than angiograms. In addition, the presence of calcium within atheromatous plaques may degrade the image.

Doppler ultrasonography assesses carotid function by projecting high-frequency sound waves into the ICA at the bifurcation. The frequency of the reflected sound waves from the moving red blood cells is dependent upon the velocity of blood flow. When a stenosis is present, blood flow velocity increases in the stenotic portion of the vessel. The increased flow velocity results in an increase in the frequency of the reflected sound waves. The examiner may use an amplifier to audibly analyze the reflected signals as the probe is advanced along the carotid vessel. Additionally, the reflected waves may be displayed on an oscilloscope screen and plotted against time. This technique has an accuracy of 90% when compared to carotid angiography.

Duplex ultrasonography is a combination of B-scan ultrasonography with Doppler flow studies. In this technique there is a rapid alternation of B-scan and Doppler signals. The result is an image of the bifurcation and a quantitative estimate of the blood flow. Studies using the Duplex system followed by arteriography indicate a 95% agreement between the two methods in identifying carotid stenosis of greater than 50%.

Quantitative spectral phonoangiography analyzes the audible frequency–intensity components of a bruit via computer analysis. This technique provides an automatic auscultation of the bifurcation, and the sound is recorded and displayed on an oscilloscope. The residual lumen diameter is estimated from the intensity and frequency of the displayed bruit.

A number of newer methods have recently become available for the noninvasive determination of cerebral blood flow. These include xenon clearance techniques,

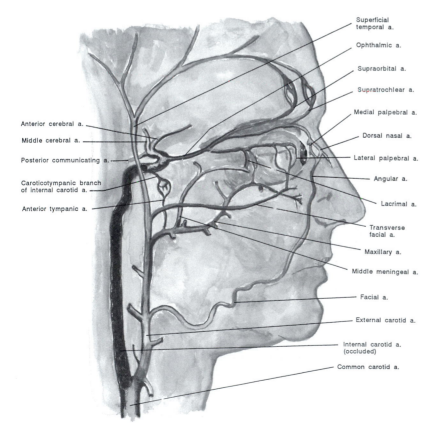

Superficial temporal a.
Ophthalmic a.
Supraorbital a.
Supratrochlear a.
Medial palpebral a.
Dorsal nasal a.
Lateral palpebral a.
Angular a.
Lacrimal a.
Transverse facial a.
Maxillary a.
Middle meningeal a.
Facial a.
External carotid a.
Internal carotid a. (occluded)
Common carotid a.

Anterior cerebral a.
Middle cerebral a.
Posterior communicating a.
Caroticotympanic branch of internal carotid a.
Anterior tympanic a.

Figure 5–4. Retrograde blood flow from the superficial temporal artery to the ophthalmic artery.

single photon emission computed tomography (SPECT), positron emission tomography (PET), and magnetic resonance imaging (MRI).

Radioactive xenon may be administered into the general circulation by either intravenous injection or by inhalation of xenon gas. By an indicator dilution technique, regional cerebral blood flow can be determined. SPECT requires the use of iodine, thallium, or technetium-labeled tracers whose distribution is proportional to cerebral blood flow. PET has enabled study of both hemodynamic and metabolic changes in the brain by providing accurate quantitative measurements of regional blood flow for both deep and superficial structures. MRI has an advantage over ultrasound studies in that it is capable of imaging deeper vessels, such as the basilar artery, and origins of both the common carotids and the vertebral arteries. Angiographic-type images can also be generated, because MRI can differentiate between a moving blood column, which has high signal strength, and stationary tissue in the blood vessel, which has a low signal strength.

Invasive Tests
Arteriography is the most definitive test for both the extracranial and the intracranial vasculature, and has traditionally been considered the "gold standard" for evaluation of patients with cerebrovascular disease. The technique is performed by inserting a catheter trans-femorally and advancing it into the aortic arch. From there, selective cannulization of the extracranial cerebral vessels can be achieved. An iodinated contrast agent is injected, and a fluoroscopic picture is taken.

Arteriography, like many other invasive procedures, is associated with certain risks. In several large series, neurologic complications developed in 2.4 to 4.2% of patients with cerebrovascular disease. Most of the neurological complications were transitory, but permanent neurological deficits occurred in 0.15 to 0.6% of the patients, and from 0.15 to 0.5% died. The neurological complications may develop from the embolization of fragile atheromatous material that becomes dislodged by the catheter. Because of the potential for neurological complications, clinicians must be concerned about performing unnecessary angiographies.

Digital venous subtraction angiography (DVSA) is a safer means of examining the extracranial and intracranial vasculature. Radiopaque contrast agent is injected into the brachial vein or superior vena cava. Before the arrival of contrast material at the region of interest, a fluoroscopic picture is taken, digitalized, and stored. The subsequent images with the dye are digitalized, and the original image is subtracted from them. The resultant images are viewed in real time.

DVSA is safer than conventional angiography because there is no catheter manipulation within the arterial system.

Thus the risk of embolism is decreased. The major limitations of DVSA are related to spatial resolution and motion artifacts. The spatial resolution is inferior to that of conventional angiography, and the images are degraded if the patient moves or swallows during the extracranial studies.

■ Ocular

In addition to a careful history, biomicroscopy, ophthalmoscopy, and visual fields, the clinician can perform several clinical procedures in the office to further aid in the diagnosis of cerebrovascular disease.

Auscultating the extracranial arteries in the neck may reveal an abnormal sound associated with turbulent blood flow through narrowed vessels. The abnormal sound, known as a bruit, commonly is located over the carotid bifurcation, but may be heard in the supraclavicular fossa in vertebral insufficiency (Figure 5–5). These bruits suggest a hemodynamically significant arterial stenosis, that is, a narrowing of the lumen in excess of 50% of the original diameter. Placing the bell of the stethoscope over the closed lids may reveal an orbital bruit, indicating a carotid–cavernous fistula. Finally, auscultating over the occipital cortex may reveal a bruit suggestive of an occipital cortical AVM.

Palpating the pulses through the superficial temporal arteries on each side and comparing their intensities may reveal reduced flow through one of the ICAs. Under normal circumstances, blood flows up the ICA into the ophthalmic artery. Flow then continues, via anastomatic channels, into the supraorbital and supratrochlear arteries and into the superficial temporal artery. If one of the ICAs is compromised, blood flow may be reversed. Blood may then flow retrograde from the superficial temporal artery to the ophthalmic artery (see Figure 5–4). The pulse in the superficial temporal artery ipsilateral to the blocked ICA will be stronger than its fellow.

Ophthalmodynamometry (ODM) is performed by increasing the intraocular pressure through an external force on the sclera. The force is applied via a calibrated instrument known as an ophthalmodynamometer. The clinician notes the amount of pressure needed to induce arterial pulsations at the nervehead in one eye, and compares this finding with that in the other eye. A reduced ODM reading in one eye implies reduced perfusion through the central retinal artery. Because the central retinal artery is derived from the ophthalmic artery, which is the first branch of the ICA, a lower ODM implies occlusive disease in the ipsilateral ICA. A 20% difference in ODM between the two eyes is considered significant.

A difference in systolic blood pressure of greater than 20 mm Hg between the arms suggests reduced flow in the subclavian artery to the arm with lower blood pressure. Symptoms of claudication of the exercised arm accompanied by symptoms of vertebrobasilar insufficiency

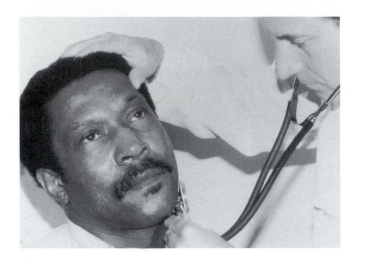

A

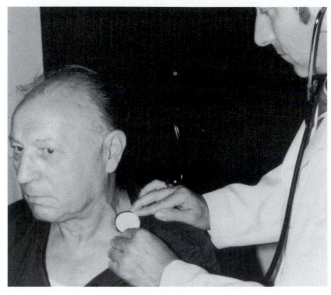

B

Figure 5–5. A. Auscultation of the carotid bifurcation. **B.** Auscultation of the vertebral artery in the supraclavicular fossa. (*Reprinted with permission from Blaustein BH. The subclavian steal syndrome. Clin Eye Vision Care. 1991;3:25–28.*)

constitute the subclavian steal syndrome. Other significant findings in this syndrome include a diminished radial pulse and a supraclavicular bruit on the affected side.

TREATMENT AND MANAGEMENT

Table 5–4 gives an overview of treatment and management, which is discussed in the following sections.

■ Systemic

The medical approach to cerebrovascular disease concentrates on reducing the risk factors for stroke and administering specific prophylactic medications. If possible, all risk factors should be reduced or eliminated, but as the predominate precurser of stroke, hypertension control is particularly important. Indeed, prevention of atherosclerosis and its complications is the best management for ischemic brain disease. In addition, treating cardiac dysfunction is of major importance.

Aspirin, a platelet aggregation inhibitor, results in a 25 to 30% reduction in the incidence of stroke after TIAs. The optimal dose of aspirin is debated, but one study indicated that low doses, such as 40 mg, may be as effective as larger doses. The addition of sulfinpyrazone (Anturane) or dipyridamole (Persantine) does not offer any advantage over aspirin alone for the prevention of stroke. Ticlopidine, a new antiplatelet aggregant, is currently undergoing clinical trials.

The most common surgical procedure for the remediation of reduced perfusion through the carotid

vasculature is carotid endarterectomy. Since 1971 there has been an increase of more than 500% in the use of this procedure in the United States.

In this procedure a longitudinal incision is made in the carotid artery and extended to the bifurcation to include the ICA. The atheromatous plaque is dissected and removed. The arterial incision is then closed with suture material. Often a patch graft can be made from either a leg vein or a polymer patch. Ott and co-workers (1990) have described a promising new procedure using the argon laser to cleave the atheroma from the vessel wall.

In the past, carotid endarterectomy was fraught with considerable risk. Fields and associates (1970) reported on a large controlled prospective study between 1962 and 1968. The combined perioperative stroke and death rate varied from 2.5 to 24.4%. Brott and Thalinger (1984) indicated that the risks of carotid endarterectomy were a function of the surgeon's skill.

The North American Symptomatic Carotid Endarterectomy Trial (NASCET) and the European Carotid Surgery Trial (ECST) were conducted to evaluate the efficacy of carotid endarterectomy as compared to medical therapy in the prevention of stroke. The data indicated that carotid endarterectomy was highly beneficial in preventing stroke in patients who had had recent cerebrovascular symptoms in the carotid territory and who had had severe carotid stenosis (70 to 99%). The risk of ischemic stroke over 2 or 3 years after surgery was reduced by 75%. On the basis of the results of NASCET and ECST, the following recommendations can now be made: Patients who have had recent symptoms within the carotid artery territory, have

TABLE 5–4. TREATMENT AND MANAGEMENT OF CEREBROVASCULAR DISEASE

- ■ **SYSTEMIC**
  - ● Prophylactic medications:
    Aspirin, 40 mg QD
    Sulfinpyrazone (Anturane)
    Dipyridamole (Persantine)
    Pentoxifylline (Trental)
  - ● Decrease the risk factors
  - ● Carotid endarterectomy

- ■ **OCULAR**
  - ● Treatment of systemic condition
  - ● Iris and/or retinal neovascularization
    panretinal photocoagulation

severe carotid stenosis, do not have cardiac disease or refractory hypertension, and who are otherwise fit for surgery should undergo carotid endarterectomy. Patients with mild stenosis, that is, less than 30%, should be treated medically. Patients with moderate stenosis (30 to 69%) should be randomized within ongoing carotid surgery trials.

■ Ocular

The treatment of the ocular manifestations of cerebrovascular disease depends on the specific ocular stigmata that are present. Generalized ischemia to the anterior portion of the eye as well as emboli in the retinal artioles may be ameliorated by the successful recanalization of the carotid artery via endarterectomy.

If iris neovascularization and/or retinal neovascularization is present, panretinal photocoagulation is the treatment of choice. It consists of the application of several hundred burns 500 μm in diameter to each quadrant of the fundus. The treatment extends posteriorly to two disc diameters from the center of the macula in the temporal quadrants and one-half disc diameter from the border of the optic nerve nasally. The total number of burns may vary between 1200 and 1600. Additionally, focal treatment using moderate-intensity confluent burns may be applied directly to the new vessels on the retina.

Panretinal photocoagulation is often followed by regression of the retinal neovascularization and the rubeosis iridis in several days. The beneficial effects of scatter photocoagulation stem from the ablation of retinal tissue sufficient to decrease retinal metabolic demands. It is believed that it is the decreased perfusion to the retina as a result of carotid artery disease that stimulates the formation of new vessels on the retina and on the iris.

Antiplatelet drugs or anticoagulants are the treatment of choice for vertebrobasilar insufficiency to the occipital cortex or brainstem. Treatment of the subclavian steal

syndrome is aimed at restoring normal blood flow by balloon angioplasty or by various surgical anastomoses.

CONCLUSION

The very nature of cerebrovascular disease is apt to result in ocular manifestations. An understanding of the applied vascular anatomy and sequelae of impaired cerebrovascular blood flow will enable the eyecare practitioner to diagnose cerebrovascular disease and participate in its management.

REFERENCES

Abernathy M, Brandt NM, Robinson C. Noninvasive testing of the carotid system. *Am Fam Physician.* 1984;29:157–168.

Adams HP Jr, Kassell NF, Wisoff HS, Drake CG. Intracranial saccular aneurysm and moyamoya disease. *Stroke.* 1979;10:174–179.

American–Canadian Cooperative Study Group. Persantine aspirin trial in cerebral ischemia. 2. Endpoint results. *Stroke.* 1985;16:406–415.

Blackwood W, Hallpike JF, Kocen RS. Atheromatous disease of the carotid arterial system and embolism from the heart in cerebral infarction: A morbid anatomical study. *Brain.* 1969;92:897–908.

Blaustein BH. The subclavian steal syndrome. *Clin Eye Vision Care.* 1991;3:25–28.

Brott T, Thalinger K. The practice of carotid endarterectomy in a large metropolitan area. *Stroke.* 1984;15:950–955.

Brott T, Thalinger K, Hertzberg V. Hypertension as a risk factor for spontaneous intracerebral hemorrhage. *Stroke.* 1986;17:1078–1083.

Brown MM, Humphrey PR. Carotid Endarterectomy: Recommendations for management of transient ischaemic attack and ischaemic stroke. *Br Med J.* 1992;305:1071–1074.

Brown GC, Magargal LE. The ocular ischemic syndrome: Clinical, fluorescein angiographic, and carotid angiographic features. *Int Ophthalmol.* 1988;11:239–251.

Browning DJ, Flynn HW, Blankenship GW. Asymmetric retinopathy in patients with diabetes mellitus. *Am J Ophthalmol.* 1988;105:584–589.

Cromwell RM, Ojemann R. Surgical management of extracranial occlusive disease. In: Barnett HJ, Stein B, Mohr JP, Yatsu F, eds. *Stroke: Pathophysiology, Diagnosis and Management.* New York: Churchill Livingstone; 1986;1014–1024.

Dorsch N. Cerebral aneurysms and subarachnoid hemorrhage. *Med J Aust.* 1966;1:651–657.

Duker JS, Brown GC, Bosley TM, et al. Asymmetric proliferative diabetic retinopathy and carotid artery disease. *Ophthalmology.* 1990;97:869–874.

Dyken ML, Wolf PA, Barnett HJM, et al. Risk factors in stroke. A statement for physicians by the Subcommittee on Risk Factors and Stroke of the Stroke Council. *Stroke.* 1984;15:1105.

Earnest F, Forbes G, Sandok BA, et al. Complications of cerebral angiography: Prospective assessment of risk. *AJNR.* 1983;4:141–159.

Faught E, Trader SD, Hannah GR. Cerebral complications of angiography for transient ischemia and stroke: Prediction of risk. *Neurology.* 1979;29:4.

Feussner JR, Matchar DB. When and how to study the carotid arteries. *Ann Intern Med.* 1988;109:805.

Fields WJ, Maslenikov V, Meyer JS. Joint study of extracranial arterial occlusion, 5. Progress report of prognosis following surgery or nonsurgical treatment of transient ischemic cerebral attacks and cervical carotid artery lesions. *JAMA.* 1970; 211:1993–2003.

Fisher CM. Clinical syndrome in cerebral thrombosis, hypertensive hemorrhage and ruptured saccular aneurysm. *Clin Neurosurg.* 1975;22:117–147.

Fisher CM, Roberson GH, Ojemann RG. Cerebral vasospasm with ruptured saccular aneurysm. The clinical manifestation. *Neurosurgery.* 1977;1:245–248.

Gautier JC. Clinical presentation and differential diagnosis of amaurosis fugax. In: Bernstein EF, ed. *Amaurosis Fugax.* New York: Springer-Verlag; 1988;24–42.

Gay AJ, Rosenbaum AL. Retinal artery pressure in asymmetric diabetic retinopathy. *Arch Ophthalmol.* 1966;75:758–762.

Gee W, Smith CA, Hinson CE, et al. Ocular pneumoplethysmography in carotid artery disease. *Med Instrument.* 1974; 8:244–248.

Gresham GE, Fitzpatrick TE, Wolf PA, et al. Residual disability in survivors of stroke: The Framingham study. *N Engl J Med.* 1975;293:954.

Hijdra A, van Gijn J. Early death from rupture of an intracranial aneurysm. *J Neurosurg.* 1982;57:765–768.

Johnston ME, Gonder JR, Canny CLB. Successful treatment of the ocular ischemic syndrome with panretinal photocoagulation and cerebrovasular surgery. *Can J Ophthalmol.* 1988;23: 114–121.

Kartchner MM, McRae LP, Morrison FD. Noninvasive detection and evaluation of carotid occlusive disease. *Arch Surg.* 1973;106:528.

Kearns TP, Hollenhorst RW. Venous stasis retinopathy of occlusive disease of the carotid artery. *Mayo Clin Proc.* 1963;38:304–312.

Kistler JP, Buonanno FS, De Witt LD, et al. Vertebral–basilar posterior cerebral territory stroke—delineation by proton nuclear magnetic resonance imaging. *Stroke.* 1984;15:417.

Kurtzke JF. Epidemiology and risk factors in thrombotic brain infarction. In: Harrison MJG, ed. *Cerebral Vascular Disease.* London: Butterworths; 1983:27–45.

Ljunggren B, Saveland H, Brandt L, Uski T. Aneurysmal subarachnoid hemorrhage. Total annual outcome in a 1.46 million population. *Surg Neurol.* 1984;22:435–438.

Moosey J. Cerebral atherosclerosis: Morphology and some relationships with coronary atherosclerosis. In: Zulch KJ, Kaufman W, Hossman KA, Hossman V, eds. *Brain and Heart Infarction.* New York: Springer-Verlag; 1977:253–260.

North American Symptomatic Carotid Endarterectomy Trial Collaborators. Beneficial effect of carotid endarterectomy in symptomatic patients with high-grade carotid stenosis. *N Engl J Med.* 1991;325:445–453.

O'Donnell TF, Erdoesl, Mackey WC, et al. Correlation of B-mode ultrasound imaging and arteriograph with pathologic findings at carotid endarterectomy. *Arch Surg.* 1985;120:443.

Ojemann RG, Heros RC. Spontaneous brain hemorrhage. *Stroke.* 1983;14:468–475.

Ott RA, Nudelman KL, Eugene J, et al. Initial clinical evaluation of carotid artery laser endarterectomy. *J Vasc Surg.* 1990;12:499–503.

Riles TS, Lieberman A, Kopelman I, et al. Systems, stenosis, and bruit. Interrelationships in carotid artery disease. *Arch Surg.* 1981;116:218.

Ross R, Glomset JA. The pathogenesis of atherosclerosis. *N Engl J Med.* 1976;295:369–377.

Sacco RL, Wolf PA, Bharucha NE, et al. Subarachnoid and intracerebral hemorrhage. Natural history, prognosis, and cursive factors in the Framingham study. *Neurology* (Cleveland). 1984;34:847–854.

Schroeder T. Hemodynamic significance of internal carotid artery disease. *Acta Neurol Scand.* 1988;77:353.

Sekhar LN, Heros RC. Origin, growth and rupture of saccular aneurysms. A review. *Neurosurgery.* 1981; 8:248–260.

Stroke statistics from the American Heart Association. *Stroke.* 1988;19:547.

Tell GS, Crouse JR, Furberg D. Relation between blood lipids, lipoproteins and cerebrovascular atherosclerosis. *Stroke.* 1988;19:423.

6

Chapter

Primary Intracranial Tumors

Leonard V. Messner

Intracranial tumors include primary neoplasms, which arise from either the brain or meninges, and metastatic tumors to the brain from distant body sites. Tumors of the central nervous system (CNS) typically exhibit slow, insidious growth with a progression of clinically related signs and symptoms. Although 40% of all CNS tumors are benign, their growth and spread to adjacent structures may render them inoperable, and death may result from damage to vital brain centers. Ocular manifestations of intracranial tumors may result from increased intracranial pressure or damage to adjacent structures.

EPIDEMIOLOGY

■ Systemic

Tumors of the central nervous system constitute 1.6% of all cancers reported in the United States, with an annual incidence of 14,000 new cases. Of these, 10,000 are tumors of the brain. CNS tumors are responsible for 1.7% of all cancer related deaths. There is a bimodal distribution of intracranial tumors, with one peak associated with children (3 to 12 years) and the other among older individuals (50 to 70 years). Regarding pediatric neoplasms, brain tumors are second only to leukemia among children younger than 10 years, and are approximately equal to leukemia between the ages of 10 and 14 years. Nearly two thirds of all pediatric central nervous system tumors are infratentorial in presentation, preferentially affecting the cerebellum, brainstem, midbrain, and thalamus.

Approximately 80% of all brain tumors are primary, while the remaining 20% develop elsewhere with intracranial metastases. Among primary tumors, gliomas are the most common accounting for 50% of all intracranial tumors followed by meningiomas (15%), schwannomas (10%), and pituitary tumors (10%). The incidence of metastatic tumors increases proportionately according to patient age.

Intracranial tumors may present at any time. Embryonic tumors, such as medulloblastomas, typically develop early in life. Gliomas can occur at any age, with an increasing frequency of presentation up to age 65. Gender specificity reveals a slightly higher incidence of central nervous system tumors among males (6.3 per 100,000 population) versus that seen in females (4.4 per 100,000). Astrocytomas are more common among men whereas meningiomas occur more frequently in women.

■ Ocular

Approximately 60% of patients with early developing brain tumors will manifest ocular signs or symptoms as the initial finding. Approximately 75% of all cases of papilledema are due to intracranial tumors. The prevalence of papilledema among individuals with brain tumors ranges from 59.5 to 80%.

NATURAL HISTORY

Although a precise mechanism cannot be defined for most individuals, several etiologic factors have been reported within the literature regarding brain tumors. These include heredity, environmental factors, and viral causes.

There is no direct correlation between primary brain tumors and environmental factors. Nevertheless, chemical and radiation factors have been implicated in the development of both astrocytomas and meningiomas. Transplant recipients show a profound increase in the risk for the development of primary lymphoma of the brain.

A familial history of cancer may predispose some individuals toward the development of some primary brain tumors. Included among specific genetic disorders with intracranial complications are neurofibromatosis, von Hippel–Lindau disease, Turcot syndrome, and Li–Fraumeni syndrome.

The expression of certain chromosomal elements known as oncogenes has been shown to result in neoplastic cell proliferation with some primary tumors. Additionally, the loss of specific tumor suppressor genes has been implicated in the pathogenesis of retinoblastoma, osteosarcoma, meningiomas, acoustic neuromas, von Hippel–Lindau disease, and astrocytomas.

Angiogenic factors may also play a role in tumor development and progression. Many malignant tumors are capable of producing chemical mediators (eg, acidic fibroblastic growth factor) that allow for new vessel growth with subsequent tumor-cell proliferation and invasion.

Although no conclusive evidence exists linking brain tumors with a viral etiology, tumors have been produced in animals by viral inoculation. Hochberg and Miller (1988) have shown that patients with primary CNS lymphomas exhibit a high incidence of seropositivity to Epstein–Barr virus.

■ Systemic

Intracranial tumors may present with a variety of signs and symptoms (Table 6–1). The clinical presentation is dependent on tumor size, location, effect on intracranial pressure, compression of cranial nerves, and invasion of adjacent structures. Patient signs and symptoms may be general or focal depending on the time course and position of the lesion. General signs and symptoms include headache, nausea and vomiting, vertigo, mental changes, circulatory and respiratory disturbances, papilledema, double vision, and seizures.

The clinical presentation of an intracranial tumor is determined by the following tumor induced factors: increased intracranial pressure, irritation of electrically sensitive neural tissue, functional impairment or destruction of brain tissue, and endocrine effects.

Increased intracranial pressure is most commonly induced by tumor impaired cerebrospinal fluid (CSF) flow. Other causes of increased intracranial pressure are venous compression with reduced CSF absorption and increased CSF production.

The evolution of increased intracranial pressure is multifactorial. Tumors within the cranial vault act as space-occupying lesions leading to increased intracranial volume. This

TABLE 6–1. SYSTEMIC MANIFESTATIONS OF PRIMARY INTRACRANIAL TUMORS

- Increased intracranial pressure
- Irritation of electrically sensitive neural tissue
- Functional impairment or destruction of brain tissue
- Endocrine changes
- Headache
- Nausea/vomitting
- Vertigo
- Mental changes
- Circulatory disturbances (tachycardia, arrhythmia)
- Respiratory disturbances (Cheyne–Stokes breathing)
- Seizures

may be augmented by cerebral edema caused by the mass lesion. Brain tumors can block or impede the flow of CSF as well as stimulate production of CSF.

Headache
The most common symptom of increased intracranial pressure is headache. The pain is of notable intensity and may awaken the patient from sleep. It is continuous and typically diffuse in nature although some patients report a localized quality to the headache. The latter may be of some localizing value regarding tumor position, especially with dural tumors affecting the bone. The headache is often paroxysmal with the pain being most intense upon awakening with some remission as the patient assumes an upright position. Coughing, vomiting, defecation, and other valsalva-like maneuvers also exacerbate the headache.

Nausea and Vomiting
Although both nausea and vomiting are associated with increased intracranial pressure, the presentation of vomiting alone is highly suggestive of acute pressure rise. Vomiting in conjunction with elevated intracranial pressure is due to compression of area postrema situated in the floor of the fourth ventricle.

Mental Changes
Changes in personality and mental ability may result from increased intracranial pressure. Patient symptomatology includes depression, irritability, indifference, loss of attention, and a dulling of intellectual function.

Circulatory and Respiratory Disturbances
Circulatory disturbances caused by increased intracranial pressure are tachycardia and arrhythmia with progression toward bradycardia. Increased respiration rate with altered respiration depth (Cheyne–Stokes breathing) may be coupled with circulatory defects among individuals who exhibit a prolonged course of acute pressure rise and is indicative of a poor prognosis.

Neuronal Irritation

Tumor invasion of cerebral cortex may irritate neurons evoking seizure and related cortical disturbances. Seizures in an apparently healthy individual over the age of 20 years should alert the clinician to the possibility of brain tumor. Seizures and convulsions are frequently associated with rapidly evolving tumors. The seizure pattern can be generalized or focal. Focal seizures that become generalized have a higher predictive value for an intracranial mass lesion.

Endocrine Effects

Endocrine disturbance is commonly associated with tumors affecting the pituitary gland and is discussed in Chapter 20.

■ Ocular

Careful ocular examination of a patient harboring an intracranial tumor is of paramount importance regarding the diagnosis and localization of the lesion. Given the extensive list of ocular manifestations (Table 6–2) associated with space-occupying lesions, this chapter will limit discussion to those conditions most commonly encountered in clinical practice.

Papilledema

The term papilledema should be reserved for those cases of optic disc edema secondary to increased intracranial pressure. It is generally accepted that papilledema presents as a bilateral clinical entity, although some degree of asymmetry is common. Truly unilateral papilledema is exceedingly rare and may be caused by an ocular or orbital mass lesion. The presence of optic atrophy prohibits subsequent disc swelling from increased intracranial pressure. The presentation of papilledema in one eye with optic atrophy in the fellow eye is termed Foster–Kennedy syndrome and is typically associated with tumors of the frontal lobe. True Foster–Kennedy syndrome is quite rare and may be mimicked by anterior ischemic optic neuropathy in one eye and optic atrophy in the other.

Although the pathogenesis of papilledema remains a topic of debate, it appears likely that as intracranial pressure rises, this pressure elevation is transmitted throughout the subarachnoid space of the brain and optic nerve. The increased pressure within the vaginal sheaths of the optic nerve leads to axoplasmic stasis at the level of the lamina

TABLE 6–2. OCULAR MANIFESTATIONS OF INTRACRANIAL TUMORS

- Papilledema (increased blind spot)
- Ocular motility dysfunction (3rd, 4th, 6th cranial nerves; diplopia)
- Pupil abnormality (Horner, dilated pupil)
- Color vision defects
- Visual field defects

cribrosa. This produces leakage of water, protein, and other axoplasmic contents into the extracellular spaces of the prelaminar portion of the optic nerve. In addition to the mechanical disruption of axoplasmic flow, there is compression of the central retinal vein within the intraorbital portion of the optic nerve, further compounding the exudative response (Figure 6–1).

Many patients remain asymptomatic in the early stages of papilledema. Exceptions to this include individuals with profound disc leakage into the macula, resulting in macular edema. Chronic macular edema can progress toward further retinal disintegration with subsequent macular hole formation. Visual field defects are variable and many patients demonstrate normal field studies. Enlargement of the blind spot, contraction of the peripheral field, and arcuate bundle defects are possible. However, none of these field defects are diagnostically specific for papilledema.

Individuals with well-developed papilledema may report "gray-outs" or "black-outs" that are often precipitated by postural changes. These visual disruptions may be unilateral or bilateral, or may alternate between eyes. The episodes typically last for several minutes with complete visual recovery.

With prolonged axoplasmic stasis, the neurons of the optic nerve become atrophic resulting in permanent vision loss. The presence of an afferent pupillary defect is to be expected with asymmetric optic atrophy.

Dysfunction of Ocular Motility

In addition to papilledema, elevated intracranial pressure often leads to compression of the cranial nerves and nuclei that govern ocular movement. The possibility of an intracranial tumor must be considered in patients who present with acquired diplopia that is progressive in nature along with other neurologic symptoms.

Of the cranial nerves that control ocular motility, the abducens nerve is most susceptible to increased intracranial pressure. Sixth-nerve palsies associated with brain tumors are commonly unilateral and offer little localizing information regarding tumor position. Bilateral abducens palsies, less frequent than unilateral palsies, are nevertheless highly indicative of a neoplastic etiology and have been reported by Keane (1976) to have an associated tumor incidence of 25%. In children, tumors account for 33% of all cases of sixth-nerve palsies, with the majority of cases related to primary brainstem gliomas.

From the point where the sixth nerve leaves the brainstem to its insertion within the lateral rectus, it is most vulnerable to insult from increased intracranial pressure where it crosses the petrous apex of the temporal bone. Downward displacement of the brainstem compresses the nerve between the brain and bone, resulting in a sixth-nerve paresis with an abduction deficit of the ipsilateral eye. Although unilateral defects are most common, both abducens nerves can be affected, producing a bilateral abduction deficit.

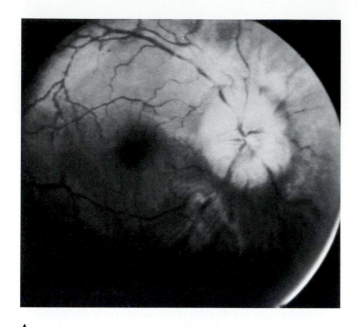

A

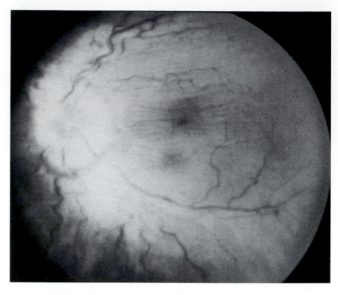

B

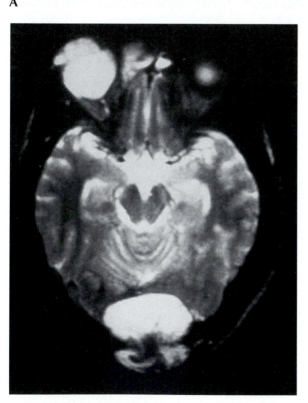

C

Figure 6–1. Funduscopic presentation of the right (**A**) and left (**B**) eyes of a patient with papilledema secondary to an intracranial soft tissue sarcoma. T_2-weighted MRI (**C**) demonstrates hyperdense signals, corresponding to sarcomatous lesions of the occipital lobe with extradural extension and of the left orbit. *(Reprinted with permission from: Conto JE. Soft tissue sarcoma metastatic to the orbit. Clin Eye Vision Care 1991;3:126–34.).*

In addition to the petrous ridge, the sixth-nerve can also be compressed between the branches of the basilar artery as it emerges from the brainstem.

Elevated intracranial pressure frequently causes intermittent episodes of abducens impairment related to variances in intracranial pressure. Patients may or may not complain of diplopia depending on the magnitude and duration of sixth-nerve insult. It must be remembered that an abduction deficit due to sixth-nerve paresis is suggestive only of increased intracranial pressure and has no localizing value with regard to tumor position.

Tumor compression of the third nerve along its course produces a progressive third-nerve palsy evidenced as a ptosis with a fixed dilated pupil associated with ipsilateral deficits of adduction, elevation, and depression. Tumors of the cavernous sinus are particularly unique in that combinations of third-, fourth-, and sixth-nerve palsies are common along with an ipsilateral Horner syndrome (Figure 6–2).

■ Primary Intracranial Tumors

Table 6–3 lists the primary intracranial tumors, which are described below.

Meningiomas

The most common form of benign intracranial tumor, meningiomas account for 10 to 15% of all primary brain tumors. Meningiomas arise from mesodermal tissue and develop from the arachnoid layer of cells of the meninges. Intracranial meningiomas most commonly arise in the parasagittal areas, sphenoid ridges, and falx cerebri (Figure 6–3). Middle-aged women are most commonly affected by these tumors.

Ocular meningiomas typically develop within the intraorbital portion of the optic nerve sheath. At this location, they can remain confined to the orbit or spread intracranially to occupy the middle cranial fossa. Patient signs and symptoms consistent with optic nerve sheath meningiomas include visual field cuts, reduced vision, disc edema, optocilliary shunt vessels, proptosis, optic atrophy, afferent pupillary defects, and color desaturation. Disc edema may

result from either direct compression of the optic nerve by the tumor or from increased intracranial pressure (papilledema). Intrapapillary refractile bodies may be observed in some cases of chronic disc congestion, although their precise composition remains speculative. Optocilliary shunt vessels of the optic nervehead frequently evolve from meningiomas due to the compression of the central retinal vein and often mimic those collaterals associated with central retinal vein occlusion. These vessels are known to regress after surgical excision of the tumor. Ipsilateral proptosis may develop with some optic nerve sheath meningiomas and often precedes profound vision loss.

The presentation of optic atrophy with ipsilateral anosmia and contralateral papilledema has been termed the Foster–Kennedy syndrome. Although exceedingly rare, this constellation of findings is pathognomonic for a tumor growing at the base of the frontal lobes. Meningiomas occupying the olfactory grooves are the most common cause of the Foster–Kennedy syndrome. Although many maladies have been reported as "masquerades" of the true syndrome, it is most important to note that ischemic optic neuropathy is capable of producing similar ocular findings and must be considered in the differential diagnosis.

Treatment of meningiomas remains controversial. Tumors of the optic nerve sheath with good vision and no evidence of intracranial extension are frequently followed.

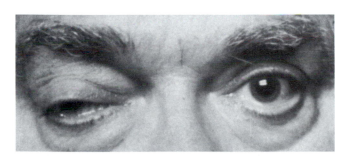

A

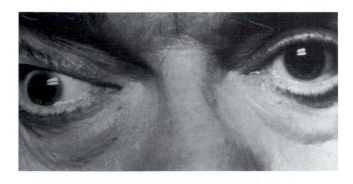

B

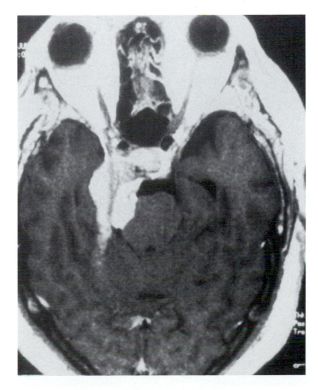

C

Figure 6–2. An incomplete right third nerve palsy **(A, B)** caused by a meningioma of the cavernous sinus. MRI with enhancement **(C)** reveals a hyperintense lesion involving the right cavernous sinus *(courtesy of Dr. Jeffrey M. Augustine).*

TABLE 6–3. PRIMARY INTRACRANIAL TUMORS

Meningiomas
Gliomas
    Astroglial tumors: astrocytomas, anaplastic astrocytoma,
      glioblastoma
    Oligodendroglioma
    Ependymoma
    Medulloblastoma
    Ganglioglioma
Craniopharyngiomas
Pineal-area tumors
Primary CNS lymphomas
Hemangioblastomas
Schwannomas
Colloid cysts
Choristomas

If vision is lost or if there is invasion of the middle cranial fossa, surgical excision is the treatment of choice. Tumor resection is more difficult if the meningioma involves the cavernous sinus, orbital apex, or superior orbital fissure. Radiotherapy holds promise as a lone therapeutic modality as well as an adjunct to surgery. Recent studies have documented the presence of estrogen and progesterone receptors on meningioma cells. It has also been established that pregnancy can exacerbate tumor growth. Therefore, it is reasonable to assume that hormonal therapy may play a role in the future management of meningiomas.

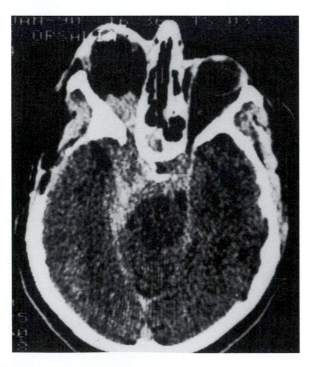

Figure 6–3. Axial CT scan of a sphenoid ridge meningioma that has spread to involve the left orbit and optic nerve. The left globe appears proptotic due to intraorbital tumor extension.

Gliomas

Glial cells provide the supportive matrix for the central and peripheral nervous systems. Tumors of neuroglial origin are collectively termed "gliomas." Gliomas are of neuroectodermal origin and constitute the most common primary CNS tumors, accounting for 40 to 60% of these neoplasia. Gliomas display significant genetic tendencies and represent 60 to 90% of all childhood primary intracranial tumors. Adult-presenting gliomas generally involve the cerebral hemispheres, while the brainstem and cerebellum are most commonly affected in children. The classification of gliomas includes those tumors of astroglial origin (astrocytomas), tumors arising from oligodendrocytes (oligodendroglia), tumors derived from ependymal cells (ependyomas), tumors of cerebellar origin (medulloblastomas), and those tumors with glial and neuronal precursors (gangliogliomas).

Astroglial Tumors. The subclassification of astroglial tumors according to histologic composition and location has proven to be somewhat difficult with regard to ultimate prognosis. Consequently, a "three-tiered" system has been devised to classify these neoplasms.

1. *Astrocytomas* are relatively benign, slow-growing tumors that demonstrate mild hypercellularity and pleomorphism with no evidence of vascular proliferation or tissue necrosis. The term "low-grade astrocytomas" is commonly used to describe these tumors.
2. *Anaplastic astrocytomas* exhibit moderate hypercellularity and pleomorphism with vascular proliferation.
3. *Glioblastomas* demonstrate all of the characteristic features of anaplastic astrocytomas along with tissue necrosis and hemorrhage. Additionally, glioblastomas differ from other astroglial tumors in that they usually occur later in life, with a peak incidence in the fifth and sixth decades. The multidimensional cellular organization of these tumors has lead to the descriptive term "glioblastoma multiforme" in reference to these neoplasms.

Astrocytomas are considered to be fairly nonaggressive, while anaplastic astrocytomas and glioblastomas demonstrate increasing malignant tendencies.

The term "optic glioma" is used to describe astroglial tumors of the anterior visual pathways. Involved structures include the optic nerves, chiasm, and optic tracts. Optic gliomas are found almost exclusively among younger individuals, with 80% occurring before age 10 and over 90% occurring before age 20. They present as low-grade astrocytomas with malignant transformation occurring in only about 1% of affected children. Rare cases of malignant optic nerve glioma in adults have been reported. These patients often exhibit early visually evoked potential (VEP) abnormalities that are followed by rapid visual deterioration. Optic nerve gliomas may be unilateral or bilateral with the latter often being associated with neurofibromatosis. The clinical presentation includes reduced vision, proptosis, and optic atrophy.

Magnetic resonance imaging (MRI) has proven to be superior to computed tomography (CT) in the evaluation of optic gliomas, because of its high-resolution characteristics that are relatively unaffected by surrounding bone.

Pontine gliomas can produce ocular motility abnormalities that mimic spasmus nutans (see Chapter 13). The triad of head tilt, head nod, and low-amplitude, high-frequency horizontal nystagmus is pathognomonic of spasmus nutans, and presents as a benign, self-limiting disorder of young children. Deviations from this constellation of signs should alert the clinician to the possibility of a brainstem tumor, necessitating neuroradiologic evaluation. It is generally recommended that acquired nystagmus in childhood be investigated by neuroimaging techniques, especially if the criterion for spasmus nutans are not met with precision.

The management of optic glioma remains a topic of debate. Many optic nerve gliomas remain relatively stable and do not merit treatment. In the event of progressive vision loss or intracranial tumor extension, surgical resection or radiation treatment may be warranted. If the tumor is confined to one optic nerve and vision is severely reduced, total resection of the tumor and nerve is recommended. The preservation of a nerve stump connected to the eye will also preserve the globe due to collateral anastomoses between the short posterior ciliary arteries and the central retinal artery. Radiation for optic nerve and chiasmal gliomas has proven effective with regard to the stabilization or improvement of vision in many cases.

Anaplastic astrocytomas and glioblastomas by definition represent malignant astroglial tumors and afford an extremely poor prognosis.

Newer surgical resection techniques, radiation, chemotherapy, and brachytherapy (the stereotactic implantation of radioactive seeds or plaques with subsequent removal) have improved the survival rate somewhat, although not overwhelmingly. Younger patients tend to fare better after surgery and radiation treatment. The Brain Tumor Cooperative Group (Shapiro, 1989) report that individuals under the age of 40 had a 64% survival rate after 18 months compared to only 8% over age 60, after surgery and radiation/chemotherapy.

Interferon and other methods of immunotherapy have not proven successful in the management of malignant astrocytomas. There is optimism that monoclonal antibodies directed against tumor-specific antigens may hold promise in the treatment of some patients with these tumors.

Oligodendrogliomas. Oligodendrocytes are the myelin-producing cells of the central nervous system. Histologically, the cells have a "halo" or "fried-egg" appearance. Oligodendrogliomas are typically slow-growing tumors with varying degrees of calcification that appear as hypodense lesions with CT and MRI. The frontal and parietal lobes represent the most common tumor locations with the presenting signs and symptoms consistent with lesions of these areas.

Although usually benign, oligodendrogliomas may be malignant and can present in conjunction with astrocytomas. Surgical resection is the most common form of treatment; however, radiation and chemotherapy are also useful in the management of malignant oligodendrogliomas.

Ependymomas. Ependymal cells line the ventricular cavities and canals of the central nervous system. Ependymomas arise from these cells, and are deeply situated within the spinal cord and brain. Children are most frequently affected, with the spinal cord being the most common site of tumor growth. The cerebral hemispheres are rarely affected by ependymomas. Ependymomas bear a strong resemblance to medulloblastomas with neuroimaging, but a circular growth pattern may be of some diagnostic value.

The treatment of choice for ependymomas is surgical resection followed by radiation unless tumor location obviates a surgical approach.

Medulloblastomas. Medulloblastomas are rare tumors arising from primitive neuroepithelial cells of the roof of the fourth ventricle that grow to involve the cerebellum. The exact cellular origin of these tumors remains unknown. These are malignant tumors of childhood with very aggressive growth patterns. The tumor is appreciated as a hyperdense lesion with MRI that is enhanced with gadolinium.

Although invasive in nature, medulloblastomas are amenable to surgical resection followed by radiation.

Gangliogliomas. Gangliogliomas are unique tumors of both astrocytic and neuronal origin (ganglion cells). These are tumors that afflict children and young adults, usually involving the temporal and frontal lobes. The most common clinical presentation is seizure. Rarely, gangliogliomas can manifest as intrinsic tumors of the optic nerve or chiasm, and as such can mimic optic gliomas. CT and MRI demonstrate low-density lesions that enhance with contrast; however, histologic examination is required for absolute diagnosis. Surgery remains the most acceptable mode of treatment.

Craniopharyngiomas
Craniopharyngiomas are tumors derived from the colloid–cystic remnants of the Rathke pouch, and constitute 3% of all intracranial tumors and up to 13.5% of all CNS tumors found in children. Younger individuals are most commonly affected by these neoplasms, which typically develop in the suprasellar region. Craniopharyngiomas liberate a viscous fluid of cholesterol composition that is highly irritating to the CNS. Although craniopharyngiomas are represented histologically as benign lesions, they nevertheless can exhibit malignant tendencies. Because of their location, progressive vision loss is the most frequent presenting symptom of these tumors. Unless treated, continued compression of the anterior visual pathway

structures leads to permanent vision loss. In addition to visual symptomatology, individuals can present with growth failure and sexual dysfunction.

CT of craniopharyngiomas depicts a hyperintense lesion with the triad of contrast enhancement, calcification, and cyst formation. Although CT is acceptable for the diagnosis of many of these tumors, there are reports of craniopharyngiomas that were not observed by CT but were ultimately discovered through MRI (Figure 6–4).

If vision is affected, surgical resection followed by radiation therapy appears to be the treatment of choice for most tumors. Postoperative visual prognosis is not as good for craniopharyngiomas as for pituitary adenomas or suprasellar meningiomas. This is probably because craniopharyngiomas are more tightly adherent to visual structures and are located more posteriorly, making removal more difficult. Complete tumor resection is imperative for optimal postoperative success. Concomitant radiation therapy has proven to be effective for increased patient survival as opposed to surgery alone. If treated effectively, vision loss can often be stabilized and in some cases improved. Progressive vision loss after treatment frequently denotes tumor exacerbation.

Pineal-area Tumors

Tumors of the pineal region include neoplasms of germ-cell origin (germinoma, teratoma, embryonal carcinoma, choriocarcinoma, and endodermal–sinus tumor) as well as pinealomas, astrocytomas, cysts, and vascular lesions.

Pinealomas can be subdivided into the poorly differentiated pinealoblastomas and pineocytomas, which are composed of mature pineal gland cells. There is a strong incidence of retinoblastoma among patients with pinealomas.

Although rare, pineal-area tumors often present with ocular consequences. In addition to the general pressure affects due to obstructive hydrocephalus, these tumors compress the dorsal midbrain structures, producing the constellation of pupillary and ocular motility abnormalities referred to as Parinaud syndrome.

Parinaud syndrome (dorsal midbrain syndrome, sylvian aqueduct syndrome) is characterized by a vertical-gaze palsy that is evident on attempted upgaze due to compression of the rostral interstitial nucleus of the medial longitudinal fasciculus (riMLF) fibers in the vicinity of the posterior commissure. Associated with the gaze palsy is convergence and (rarely) divergence retraction movements of the eyes into the orbits due to co-firing of muscle fibers. These unusual eye movements are most evident when upward saccadic movements are attempted. Additionally, lid retraction (Collier sign) is produced with attempted supraduction. Pupillary manifestations of mesencephalic compression include bilateral middilated pupils that do not react to light but become miotic when presented with a near target (light-near dissociation). With progressive compression of the Edinger–Westphal subnucleus, the pupils become fixed to both light and near stimuli. Also, convergence and downgaze pareses can develop. Along with oculomotor dysfunction, tumors of

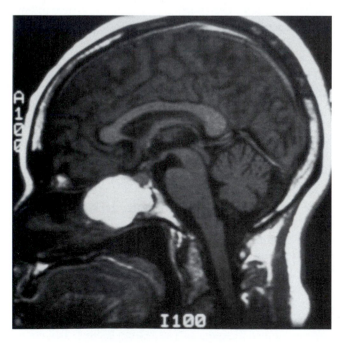 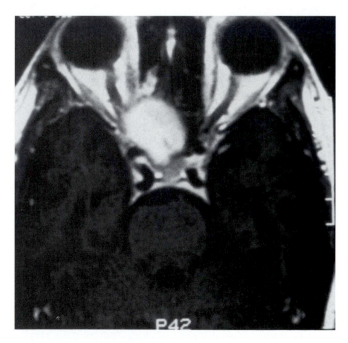

A   B

Figure 6–4. T$_1$-weighted coronal (**A**) and axial (**B**) MRI sections with gadolinium enhancement showing a hyperintense right-sided sphenoid mass with compression of the right optic nerve. Histologic examination of the lesion revealed cholesterol clefts and giant cells with fibrous tissue consistent with a craniopharyngioma *(courtesy of Dr. Ruth Trachimowicz).*

the pineal region may compress the trochlear nerve as it decussates within the superior medullary velum, resulting in a contralateral superior oblique palsy.

The presentation of a dorsal midbrain syndrome is often accompanied by headache and papilledema, and warrants immediate investigation by CT or MRI. Germ-cell tumors respond nicely to radiation, while resection along with radiation is the treatment of choice for most other pineal-area tumors.

Primary CNS Lymphomas

Lymphoma is a malignant, nonencapsulated neoplasm that originates from the precursor cells of B and T lymphocytes. There are two categorical divisions of lymphoma: (1) Hodgkin disease and (2) the non-Hodgkin lymphomas. Non-Hodgkin lymphoma is also referred to as reticulum cell sarcoma, diffuse histiocytic lymphoma, microgliomatosis, and diffuse large-cell lymphoma. It is the non-Hodgkin variant that is responsible for primary brain and eye involvement. See Chapter 72, Non-Hodgkin Lymphoma and Intraocular Lymphoma.

Hemangioblastomas

Vascular tumors of the brain include hemangiomas, hemangioblastomas, and arteriovenous malformations. Of particular interest to the eyecare practitioner are hemangioblastomas, which present along with retinal angiomatosis as the syndrome of von Hippel–Lindau (see Chapter 47).

Schwannomas (Neuromas, Neurinomas, Neurilemomas)

Along with oligodendrocytes, Schwann cells are responsible for the production of myelin. Schwann cells cover cranial nerves III through XII, the spinal roots, and most peripheral nerves.

As the name implies, schwannomas arise directly from Schwann cells and represent 8 to 10% of all intracranial tumors. They are almost always benign, but can coexist along with neurofibromatosis, often in association with meningiomas and gliomas. The vast majority of these tumors involve the eighth cranial nerve and are known as acoustic schwannomas. The peak incidence for acoustic schwannomas is the fourth to fifth decade of life. There is a slight female predilection.

Acoustic schwannomas typically arise within the internal auditory canal and spread to occupy the cerebellopontine angle. The initial presentation is progressive or sudden hearing loss, along with vestibular dysfunction and vertigo. Concomitant compression of cranial nerve VII (facial) results in a progressive facial paralysis that includes difficulty of attempted lid closure and loss of taste sensation to the anterior two thirds of the tongue. Involvement of the trigeminal nerve is common with these tumors, and results in the loss of corneal and facial sensation and weakening to the muscles of mastication. It is important to note that the triad of (1) unilateral deafness, (2) corneal hypoesthesia, and (3) incomplete facial palsy is highly indicative of a cerebellopontine angle mass lesion that is usually an acoustic schwannoma. As neoplasia of this region enlarge, there is further compression of brainstem structures and cerebellum, with associated neurologic dysfunction. Neuro-ophthalmic manifestations include skew deviations and nystagmus.

Abduction deficits from acoustic schwannomas may be due to either direct tumor compression of the abducens nerve or from elevated intracranial pressure. Exceptionally large acoustic schwannomas can compress the trochlear nerve producing a superior oblique palsy with vertical diplopia. Oculomotor involvement by these tumors is exceedingly rare.

Progressive unilateral deafness should be considered to be highly suggestive of acoustic schwannoma, necessitating appropriate auditory and vestibular investigation. CT and MRI with contrast enhancement are both useful in the identification of cerebellopontine angle mass lesions. MRI is relatively unaffected by surrounding bone, and is particularly useful for the visualization of small tumors that are located in the internal auditory canal.

Surgical resection is extremely effective in the management of these tumors. Early tumor detection and removal is essential for postoperative preservation of hearing and facial nerve function. Care must be taken to ensure removal of the entire tumor to minimize the chance of recurrence.

Colloid Cysts

Colloid cysts are rare (representing less than 1% of all intracranial tumors) neoplasms of neuroepithelial origin that invariably arise within the third ventricle. These circular tumors are attached to the ventricular wall by a fibrous stalk. Most cysts exhibit some degree of motility that is affected by body position and movement. This allows the tumor to function in a "valve-like" fashion, producing intermittent occlusion of the foramen of Monro, resulting in the obstruction of cerebrospinal fluid flow between the third and fourth ventricles. The ultimate consequence of this action is a paroxysmal rise in intracranial pressure with subsequent headache, hydrocephalus, and (rarely) sudden death.

Neuro-ophthalmic manifestations of colloid cysts are compatible with pressure-related signs and symptoms, and may include papilledema, optic atrophy, abduction deficits, and variants of the dorsal midbrain syndrome.

The diagnosis of these tumors is easily obtained with the use of neuroimaging studies. CT scanning and MR imaging reveal a well-delineated, circular mass lesion within the midline of the third ventricle.

The treatment of choice is surgical resection. Because of the risk of sudden death, these tumors always require immediate removal even in the absence of profound symptomatology or hydrocephalus. Recently, the use of CT-guided stereotactic cyst aspiration has gained favor among neurosurgeons due to the relatively low risk associated with the procedure. Shunting procedures are reserved only for those cases where hydrocephalus persists following surgery.

Choristomas

Choristomas are congenital, usually benign tumors that are composed of normal tissues that develop in abnormal locations. These tumors can develop in many anatomical regions including the brain, eye, and orbit. The most common types of intracranial choristomas are epidermoids and dermoids. Both are cystlike tumors of ectodermal origin.

Epidermoids usually develop within the cisterns at the base of the brain as well as on the tela choroidae of the ventricles. As opposed to colloid cysts, epidermoids tend to exhibit a more lateral position away from the midline. The most common anatomic substrate for these tumors is the cerebellopontine angle. Histologically, they are encapsulated, cystic tumors that contain an amorphous, granular material that is laden with cholesterol crystal. The latter has lead to the rubric "cholesteatomas" to describe these types of tumors.

Although congenital, epidermoids are extremely slow growing and may remain asymptomatic for many years. Seizure is the most commonly reported presenting symptom. Other nonspecific neurologic signs include dementia, cranial nerve abnormalities, and hydrocephalus. The neuro-ophthalmic signs and symptoms of epidermoids are dependent on tumor location. Suprasellar epidermoids can produce visual field defects often associated with hypothalamic dysfunction. Parasellar tumors can invade the cavernous sinus producing a painful ophthalmoplegia along with other aspects of cavernous sinus syndromes. Tumors of the cerebellopontine angle can produce ipsilateral deafness, facial paralysis, and trigeminal dysfunction, and mimic acoustic schwannoma.

Intracranial dermoids demonstrate a gross and histologic composition similar to epidermoids, with the inclusion of hair follicles and secretory glands within the capsular wall. As with epidermoids, the clinical signs and symptoms are slow to evolve, and depend on tumor location and involvement of associated structures.

The diagnosis of intracranial choristomas is best achieved by CT or MRI. Both epidermoids and dermoids exhibit a hypodense internal core surrounded by an enhanced capsular rim. Treatment is surgical removal of the entire tumor, with care taken not to rupture the tumor wall, as spillage of the internal contents can result in aseptic meningitis.

■ Metastatic Tumors

Approximately 20 to 30% of all systemic cancers result in intracranial metastases. Primary systemic cancers with reported brain metastases include melanoma, breast carcinoma, lung carcinoma, pelvic–abdominal tumors, renal-cell carcinoma, and non-Hodgkin lymphoma. These extracranial tumors metastasize to the brain usually as arterial emboli that most commonly lodge within the cerebral cortex of the frontal and parietal lobes. Among individuals with cerebral metastases, one half exhibit CNS involvement as the only metastatic site. Chapter 71 discusses metastasis of systemic malignancies to the eye and orbit.

DIAGNOSIS

There is no substitute for a careful case history and physical examination of the patient who is suspected of harboring an intracranial tumor. The ocular examination of these patients is particularly critical given the plethora of ophthalmic signs and symptomatology associated with brain tumors. Once a tumor is suspected, it is imperative to order the correct test to ensure proper diagnosis and management.

■ Systemic

Neuroimaging

The advent of CT and MRI has virtually eliminated the need for conventional brain scanning and pneumoencephalography in the investigation of suspected intracranial mass lesions. It is important to be aware of the salient attributes and drawbacks of specific neuroimaging techniques so as to maximize the diagnostic potential for the case at hand while at the same time minimizing the expense and trouble incurred by the patient for unnecessary studies.

CT employs an x-ray technique to image the cranial vault and its contents. The intensity and resolution of the scan is dependent upon the relative tissue densities being studied, with high-density structures displaying a high degree of appreciation. This feature makes CT particularly effective for visualization of the skull and bony defects (Figure 6–5). Because of the low tissue density of cortex and other brain structures, an intravenous contrast agent is required to elicit anatomic detail, tumor structure, hemorrhage, infarction, and abscess.

MRI uses a high-intensity magnetic field to align the free protons of hydrogen atoms throughout the body. A pulsed electromagnetic field is then applied to disrupt this alignment, and the resultant energy changes are detected as the protons are permitted to reassume their alignment. The relaxation times incurred during realignment are termed T_1- and T_2-weighted images. Because most hydrogen atoms are confined to water molecules, MRI, simply put, images the water content of a particular structure. This property makes MRI the method of choice for soft tissue investigation, and results in greater sensitivity and accuracy in the detection of many tumors when compared to CT. Bone, because of its low water content, appears dark with MRI, thus affording greater resolution of tumors in close proximity to bone as well as lesions of the posterior fossa. Small tumors that are difficult to image with standard MRI techniques may be readily visualized by employing the contrast agent gadolinium-DTPA, because of the breakdown of the blood–brain barrier associated with these lesions (Figure 6–6).

Angiography

Vascularized intracranial tumors can be appreciated with angiographic techniques. Although digital subtraction

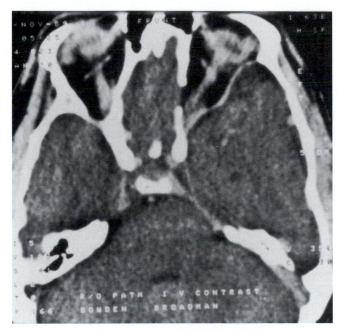

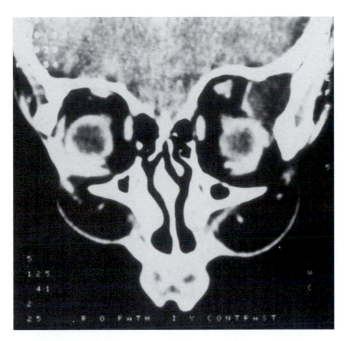

A

B

Figure 6–5. Axial **(A)** and coronal **(B)** sections of a meningoencephalocele produced by sphenoid wing defects. Note the total absence of the greater wing of the left sphenoid allowing for herniation of the frontal lobe into the orbit resulting in direct apposition with the globe. Such bony defects are commonly associated with neurofibromatosis.

intravenous angiography has shown much value for visualization of the major extracranial vessels of the neck, intracranial vascular resolution is markedly affected and degraded by the skull. Consequently, direct arteriography is the procedure of choice for intracranial angiography. Due to the inherent risks associated with arteriography, magnetic resonance angiography (MRA) holds great promise as a safe and effective alternative.

Metabolic Studies

Many tumors display an increased rate of protein synthesis and uptake of glucose and amino acids, making them amenable to identification by positron emission tomography (PET). Particularly effective in the imaging of astroglial tumors, PET can be used preoperatively to determine the degree of malignancy associated with these neoplasms. The implementation of radiotracer elements like *L*-3-iodo-alpha-methyl tyrosine (IMT) and thallium-201 (T_l) coupled with single photon emission computed tomography (SPECT) is extremely useful for the identification of high-grade malignant gliomas, due to the increased metabolic activity and growth rate associated with these tumors. Black and associates (1989) reported an 89% accuracy in the prediction of low-grade versus high-grade malignant gliomas using T_l-SPECT.

■ Ocular

Ocular testing includes evaluation of motilities, pupils, color vision, and visual fields. When papilledema is present, it should be considered as a sign of increased intracranial pressure secondary to a mass lesion until proven otherwise. Neuroradiologic evaluation should be ordered immediately to rule out a space-occupying intracranial process. If there is no evidence of a mass lesion, further investigation is in order to exclude pseudotumor cerebri and meningitis as the cause of papilledema. Lumbar puncture is mandatory for these cases where the diagnosis is inconclusive and serves as a measure of intracranial pressure as well as analysis of CSF. Ultrasonic examination of the optic nerve is useful both to measure nerve diameter and to detect the presence of hyaline bodies (buried drusen) that can mimic true papilledema. The 30-degree test, as described by Galetta and associates (1989), is a reliable procedure used to detect the presence of fluid engorgement of the intervaginal space of the optic nerve. The 30-degree test relies on the premise that the intraorbital portion of the optic nerve is somewhat sinusoidal in primary position and tends to straighten when the eye is abducted 30-degrees. Therefore conditions that result in the accumulation of fluid within the subarachnoid space (papilledema, optic neuritis, ischemic optic neuropathy) will produce maximal distention to the optic nerve in primary position, as measured through A-scan echography with abation as the eye is abducted, allowing for a more even distribution of subarachnoid fluid, with reduction of the optic nerve diameter. The "compression" of the optic nerve is termed a positive 30-degree test, and is pathognomonic for fluid engorgement for the nerve itself.

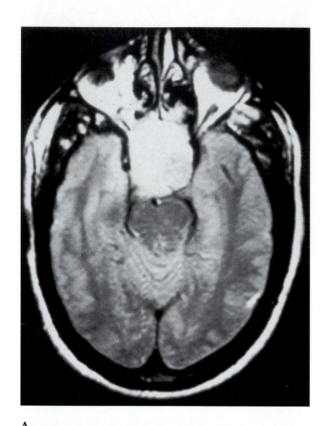

A

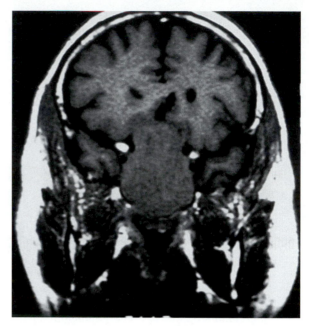

B

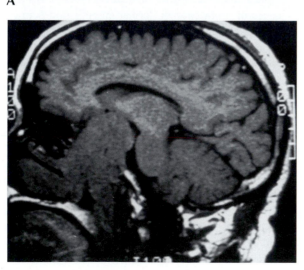

C

Figure 6–6. T$_1$-weighted axial **(A)**, coronal **(B)**, and sagittal **(C)** sections of a large pituitary adenoma taken before infusion with gadolinium. (continued)

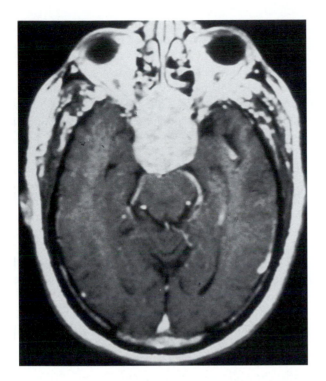

D

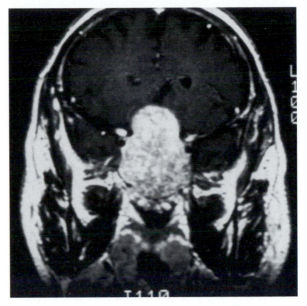

E

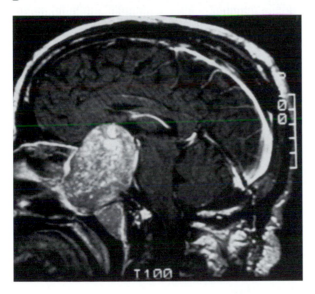

F

Figure 6–6 (continued). T₁-weighted axial (D), coronal (E), and sagittal (F) sections after infusion with gadolinium. Note the increased tumor blush and definition after contrast enhancement *(Courtesy of Dr. Dennis Cosgrove).*

TREATMENT AND MANAGEMENT

■ Systemic

Surgery

Surgery is the primary method of treatment for most benign, as well as malignant, brain tumors. Advances in surgical techniques, equipment, and imaging systems have led to the successful resection of tumors that were previously considered to be inoperable. The rate of success is determined largely by the location of the tumor and invasion of adjacent structures.

The evolution of microneurosurgery has greatly contributed to the effectiveness of tumor removal. The use of stereoscopic magnification allows for precise tumor dissection, with relative sparing of associated neuroanatomical structures. Microneurosurgery is particularly effective for tumors of the sellar and parasellar regions, cerebellopontine angle, ventricles, cavernous sinus, brainstem, odontoid process of the vertebral column, clivus, foramen magnum, and pineal region.

The use of CT- or MRI-guided surgery coupled with three-dimensional coordinates (stereotactic surgery) permits for the precise localization of intracranial lesions. In addition to a more controlled surgery, stereotaxis allows for the relatively safe biopsy of tumorous lesions. Approximately 10 to 12% of previously undiagnosed lesions have been accurately identified by this technique.

Intraoperative monitoring of evoked potentials (brainstem auditory, visual, and somatosensory) has enhanced the precision and safety involved with tumor resection and has resulted in improved postoperative neurologic function.

Laser

Laser therapy is beneficial for some brain neoplasms. The photocoagulation, vaporization, and tissue ablation features of various laser wavelengths can be coupled with stereotaxis for the treatment of certain tumors. The use of photosensitizing agents combined with laser therapy appears promising, in that this method allows for greater accuracy in the treatment of neoplastic tissue while preserving normal structures.

Radiation

Radiation therapy is useful both as a primary form of treatment as well as combined with surgical removal. Many malignant neoplasms are particularly sensitive to radiotherapy. Focal and limited-field radiation techniques allow for a more directed approach to tumor treatment and reduce the amount of radiation exposure to uninvolved brain areas. Brachytherapy is another method of precision-directed radiotherapy. Brachytherapy appears to hold promise in the treatment of highly malignant gliomas.

As has been described with laser treatment, the use of tissue-sensitizing agents (metronidazole, misonidazole, and etanidazole) can be used with stereotactic radiotherapy in the treatment of hypoxic tumor cells. The use of these agents is somewhat limited due to their neurotoxic side effects.

Due to the reported complications of developmental delays, pituitary dysfunction, and secondary tumor growth associated with radiation, this form of treatment is generally not recommended for children under the age of 2 years.

Chemotherapy

Chemotherapeutic (antineoplastic) agents are widely used in the treatment of many cancers. Categorically, these drugs work by suppression of tumor cell growth or through the inhibition of cellular reproduction. The mode of action is dependent on the mechanism by which these agents affect cell growth, and they are most effective in the treatment of actively mitotic tumors.

The alkylating agents carnustine (BCNU), lomustine (CCNU), and cisplantin (CDDP) replace hydrogen atoms with an alkyl group, resulting in abnormal DNA synthesis. The abnormal DNA molecules are unable to perform their normal function related to cellular reproduction. Alkylating agents are somewhat effective in the treatment of adult malignant gliomas.

Procarbazine is a chemotherapeutic agent whose exact mechanism remains speculative. It is thought that procarbazine inhibits both RNA and DNA synthesis, with positive results reported in the treatment of Hodgkin disease and gliomas.

Methotrexate (MTX) is an antimetabolite that competitively inhibits the enzyme dihydrofolic acid reductase required for DNA synthesis and cellular reproduction. MTX is particularly useful in the treatment of rapidly dividing tumors such as lymphomas and medulloblastomas.

Vincristine (VCR) is a mitotic inhibitor that is derived from the periwinkle plant. Its mode of action is related to the interference with intracellular tubulin (protein) function. Non-Hodgkin lymphomas are among the tumors most sensitive to vincristine.

A major complication of all antineoplastic agents is cytotoxicity. Normal tissues that are most adversely affected include bone marrow, hair follicles, and mucous membranes of the GI tract. Conservatively, 30% of all individuals committed to chemotherapy experience some degree of GI distress.

Due to the associated complications of radiation, chemotherapy is generally recommended as an alternative to radiotherapy for children under the age of 2 years.

Other Treatment Regimens

The role of immunologic therapy holds great promise for the treatment of many brain tumors. The development of monoclonal antibodies directed against specific tumor cells has already proven beneficial in the management of meningeal carcinomatosis. Corticosteroids have been shown to suppress lymphocyte production and have been used in the treatment of some lymphomas.

Hyperthermia has the effect of "sterilizing" tumor cells and has been used as an adjunct to enucleation for the treatment of malignant uveal melanomas. Microwave-induced hyperthermia has been employed coupled with surgical debulking in the management of certain brain tumors.

■ Ocular

Management of the ocular manifestations of intracranial tumors is primarily directed toward the treatment of the tumor itself, as delineated above. As needed, residual ocular motility dysfunctions may be managed with prismatic correction.

CONCLUSION

The ocular practitioner is frequently the first clinician consulted by a patient with an intracranial tumor. The recognition of associated ophthalmic signs and symptoms is paramount for early diagnosis and successful treatment. The evolution of neuroimaging technology along with other diagnostic studies permits earlier and more accurate diagnoses of intracranial lesions.

Advances in microneurosurgery have lead to more favorable postoperative outcomes with fewer associated complications among many individuals with tumors that were once considered to be inoperable. Radiation and chemotherapy used alone or in combination with surgery have resulted in higher treatment success rates, often with improved patient quality of life. Immunotherapy holds great promise as a future method of tumor management. As the understanding of the pathogenesis of tumor growth is expanded, the role of genetic, microbial, and environmental triggering mechanisms may significantly identify those individuals who are at risk for developing certain neoplasms, and allow for prophylaxis or early treatment.

REFERENCES

Ainbinder DJ, Faulkner AR, Haik BG. Review of orbital tumors. *Curr Opin Ophthalmol.* 1991;2:281–287.

Ammirati M, Vick N, Liao YL, et al. Effect of the extent of surgical resection on survival and quality of life in patients with supratentorial glioblastomas and anaplastic astrocytomas. *Neurosurgery.* 1987;21:201–206.

Anderson DR, Trobe JD, Taren JA, Gebarski SS. Visual outcome in cystic craniopharyngiomas treated with intracavitary phosphorus-32 . *Ophthalmology.* 1989;96:1786–1792.

Apuzzo ML, Chandrasoma PT, Cohen D, et al. Computed imaging stereotaxy: Experience and perspective related to 500 procedures applied to brain masses. *Neurosurgery.* 1987;20:930–937.

Atta HR. Imaging of the optic nerve with standardized echography. *Eye.* 1988;2:358–366.

Bailey P, Cushing H. *A Classification of the Tumors of the Glioma Group on Histogenetic Basis With a Correlated Study of Prognosis.* Philadelphia: Lippincott;1926.

Benedict WF, Murphree AL, Banerjee A, et al. Patient with 13 chromosome deletion: Evidence that the retinoblastoma gene is a recessive cancer gene. *Science.* 1983;219:973–975.

Biersack HJ, Coenen HH, Stocklin G, et al. Imaging of brain tumors with L-3-[123I]iodo-alpha-methyl tyrosine and SPECT. *J Nucl Med.* 1989;30:110–112.

Bigner SH, Mark J, Burger PC, et al. Specific chromosomal abnormalities in malignant human gliomas. *Cancer Res.* 1988;48:405–411.

Black KL, Hawkins RA, Kim KT, et al. Use of thallium-201 SPECT to quantitate malignancy grade of gliomas. *J Neurosurg.* 1989;71:342–346.

Black PMcL. Medical progress: brain tumors. N Engl J Med. 1991;324:1471–1476, 1555–1564.

Bowman CB, Farris BK. Primary chiasmal germinoma. *J Clin Neuro-ophthalmol.* 1990;10:9–17.

Brant-Zawadzki M, Norman D. *Magnetic Resonance Imaging of the Central Nervous System.* New York: Raven; 1987.

Brem S. The role of vascular proliferation in the growth of brain tumors. *Clin Neurosurg.* 1976;23:440–453.

Bullard DE, Rawlings CE III, Philips B, et al. Oligodendroglioma: An analysis of the value of radiation therapy. *Cancer.* 1987; 60:2179–2188.

Burde RM, Savino PJ, Trobe JD. *Clinical Decisions in Neuro-ophthalmology.* St. Louis: Mosby; 1985.

Burger PC, Vogel FS, Green SB, Strike TA. Glioblastoma multiforme and anaplastic astrocytoma: Pathologic criteria and prognostic implications. *Cancer.* 1985;56:1106–1111.

Cairncross JG, MacDonald DR. Successful chemotherapy for recurrent malignant oligodendroglioma. *Ann Neurol.* 1988;23:360–364.

Camel PW. Tumors of the third ventricle. *Acta Neurochir* (Wien). 1985;75:136–146.

Carr WA, Baumann RJ, Baker RS. Nuclear magnetic resonance imaging in neuro-ophthalmology. Demonstration of a pontine glioma. *Surv Ophthalmol.* 1984;29:79–83.

Castillo M, Davis PC, Takei Y, Hoffman JC Jr. Intracranial ganglioglioma: MR, CT, and clinical findings in 18 patients. *AJR.* 1990;154:607–612.

Chang CH, Horton J, Schoenfeld D, et al. Comparison of postoperative radiotherapy and combined postoperative radiotherapy and chemotherapy in the multidisciplinary management of malignant gliomas. *Cancer.* 1983;52:997–1007.

Cherninkova S, Tzekov H, Karakostov V. Comparative ophthalmologic studies on children and adults with craniopharyngioma. *Ophthalmologica.* 1990;201:201–205.

Chowdury CR, Wood CM, Samuel PR, Richardson J. Frontal bone epidermoid—A rare cause of proptosis. *Br J Ophthalmol.* 1990;74:445–446.

Chutorian AM. Optic gliomas in children. *Int Pediatr.* 1988;3:115–119.

Coleman DJ, Silverman RH, Iwamoto T, et al. Histopathologic effects of ultrasonically induced hyperthermia in intraocular malignant melanoma. *Ophthalmology.* 1988;95:970–981.

Coppeto JR, Monteiro MLR, Uphoff DF. Exophytic suprasellar glioma: A rare cause of chiasmal compression. *Arch Ophthalmol.* 1987;105:28.

DeAngelis LM, Yahalom J, Heinemann MH, et al. Primary CNS lymphoma: Combined treatment with chemotherapy and radiotherapy. *Neurology.* 1990;40:80–86.

Delattre JY, Krol G, Thaler HT, Posner JB. Distribution of brain metastases. *Arch Neurol.* 1988;45:741–744.

Del Regato JA, Harlan JS, Cox JD, eds. *Ackerman and del Regato's Cancer: Tumors of the Central Nervous System.* 6th ed. St. Louis: Mosby; 1985:119–154.

Doyle WK, Budinger TF, Valk PE, et al. Differentiation of cerebral radiation necrosis from tumor recurrence by [18F]FDG and 82Rb positron emission tomography. *J Comput Assist Tomogr.* 1987;11:563–570.

Dumanski JP, Carlbom E, Collins VP, Nordenskjold M. Deletion mapping of a locus on human chromosome 22 involved in the oncogenesis of meningioma. *Proc Natl Acad Sci USA.* 1987;84:9275–9279.

Eijpe AA, Koornneef L, Verbeeten B Jr, et al. Intradiploic epidermoid cysts of the bony orbit. *Ophthalmology.* 1991;98: 1737–1743.

Fine HA, Dear KBG, Loeffler JS, et al. Meta-analysis of radiotherapy with and without adjuvant chemotherapy for malignant gliomas in adults. *Proc Am Soc Clin Oncol.* 1991;10:125.

Folkman J, Klagsbrun M. Angiogenic factors. *Science.* 1987;235:442–447.

Frenkel REP, Spoor TC. Visual loss and intoxication. *Surv Ophthalmol.* 1986;30:391–396.

Friedman WA, Sceats JR, Nestok BR, Ballinger WE Jr. The incidence of unexpected pathological findings in an image-guided biopsy series: A review of 100 consecutive cases. *Neurosurgery.* 1989;25:180–184.

Fukuyama J, Hayasaka S, Setogawa T, et al. Foster Kennedy syndrome and optociliary shunt vessels in a patient with an olfactory groove meningioma. *Ophthalmologica.* 1991;202: 125–131.

Galetta S, Byrne SF, Smith JL. Echographic correlation of optic nerve sheath size and cerebrospinal fluid pressure. *J Clin Neuro-ophthalmol.* 1989;9:79–82.

Gans MS, Byrne SF, Glaser JS. Standardized A-scan echography in optic nerve disease. *Arch Ophthalmol.* 1987;105:1232–1236.

Garner A. Orbital lymphoproliferative disorders. *Br J Ophthalmol.* 1992;76:47–48.

Gelwan MJ, Seidman M, Kupersmith MJ. Pseudo-pseudo-Foster Kennedy syndrome. *J Clin Neuro-ophthalmol.* 1988;8:49–52.

Gilroy J. *Basic Neurology.* 2nd ed. New York: Pergamon; 1990:223–250.

Gittinger JW. To image or not to image. *Surv Ophthalmol.* 1988;32:350–356.

Glaser JS. Topical diagnosis: prechiasmal visual pathways. In: Glaser JS, ed. *Neuro-ophthalmology.* 2nd ed. Philadelphia: Lippincott; 1990:83–170.

Gonzalez CF, Becker MH, Flanagan JC, eds. *Diagnostic Imaging in Ophthalmology.* New York: Springer-Verlag; 1986.

Greig NH, Ries LG, Yancik R, Rapoport SI. Increasing annual incidence of primary malignant brain tumors in the elderly. *JNCI.* 1990;82:1621–1624.

Guidetti B, Gagliardi FM. Epidermoid and dermoid cysts: Clinical evaluation and late surgical results. *J Neurosurg.* 1977;47: 12–18.

Gum KB, Frueh BR. Transantral orbital decompression for compressive optic neuropathy due to sphenoid ridge meningioma. *Ophthalmic Plast Reconstr Surg.* 1989;5:196–198.

Haik BG, Saint Louis L, Bierly J, et al. Magnetic resonance imaging in the evaluation of optic nerve gliomas. *Ophthalmology.* 1987;94:709–717.

Hall WA, Lunsford LD. Changing concepts in the treatment of colloid cysts: An 11-year experience in the CT era. *J Neurosurg.* 1987;66:186–191.

Hardwig P, Robertson DM. Von Hippel–Lindau disease: A familial, often lethal, multi-system phakomatosis. *Ophthalmology.* 1984;91:263–270.

Hochberg FH, Miller DC. Primary central nervous system lymphoma. *J Neurosurg.* 1988;68:835–853.

Holman RE, Grimson BS, Drayer BP, et al. Magnetic resonance imaging of optic gliomas. *Am J Ophthalmol.* 1985;100:596–601.

Hoyt WF, Beeston D. *The Ocular Fundus in Neurologic Disease.* St. Louis: Mosby; 1966.

Huber A; Blodi FC, trans. *Eye Signs and Symptoms in Brain Tumors.* 3rd ed. St. Louis: Mosby; 1976.

Imes RK, Hoyt WF. Magnetic resonance imaging signs of optic nerve gliomas in neurofibromatosis, 1. *Am J Ophthalmol.* 1991;111:729–734.

Imes RK, Schatz H, Hoyt WF, et al. Evolution of optociliary veins in optic nerve sheath meningioma. *Arch Ophthalmol.* 1985;103:59–60.

Jakobiec FA, Depot MJ, Kennerdell JS, et al. Combined clinical and computed tomographic diagnosis of orbital glioma and meningioma. *Ophthalmology.* 1984;91:137–155.

Johnson LN, Hepler RS, Yee RD, et al. Magnetic resonance imaging of craniopharyngioma. *Am J Ophthalmol.* 1986;102:242–244.

Kalofonos HP, Pawlikowska TR, Hemingway A, et al. Antibody guided diagnosis and therapy of brain gliomas using radiolabeled monoclonal antibodies against epidermal growth factor receptor and placental alkaline phosphatase. *J Nucl Med.* 1989;30:1636–1645.

Kalyan-Raman UP, Olivero WC. Ganglioglioma: A correlative clinicopathological and radiological study of ten surgically treated cases with follow-up. *Neurosurgery.* 1987;20:428–433.

Keane JR. Bilateral 6th-nerve palsy. Analysis of 125 cases. *Arch Neurol.* 1976;33:681–683.

Kennerdell JS, Maroon JC, Malton M, Warren FA. The management of optic nerve sheath meningiomas. *Am J Ophthalmol.* 1988;106:450–457.

Kepes JJ. *Meningiomas: Biology, Pathology, and Differential Diagnosis.* New York: Masson; 1982.

Kernohan JW, Mabon RF, Svien HJ, Adson AW. A simplified classification of gliomas. *Proc Staff Meet Mayo Clin.* 1949;24:71–75.

King RA, Nelson LB, Wagner RS. Spasmus nutans: A benign clinical entity? *Arch Ophthalmol.* 1986;104:1501–1504.

Klein G. The approaching era of tumor suppressor genes. *Science.* 1987;238:1539–1545.

Kornblith PL, Walker MD, Cassady JR. Neoplasms of the central nervous system, In: DeVita VT Jr, Hellman S, Rosenberg SA, eds. *Cancer: Principles and Practice of Oncology.* 2nd ed. Philadelphia: Lippincott; 1985;2:1437–1510.

Kupersmith MJ, Warren FA, Newall J, Ransohoff J. Irradiation of meningiomas of the intracranial anterior visual pathway. *Ann Neurol.* 1987;21:131–137.

Larson DA, Gutin PH, Leibel SA, et al. Stereotaxic irradiation of brain tumors. *Cancer.* 1990;65:792–799.

Lashford LS, Davies AG, Richardson RB, et al. A pilot study of ^{131}I monoclonal antibodies in the therapy of lepto meningeal tumors. *Cancer.* 1988;61:857–868.

Lavery MA, O'Neill JF, Chu FC, Martyn LJ. Acquired nystagmus in early childhood: A presenting sign of intracranial tumor. *Ophthalmology.* 1984;91:425–435.

Leibel SA, Sheline GE. Radiation therapy for neoplasms of the brain. *J Neurosurg.* 1987;66:1–22.

Lesch KP, Schott W, Engl HG, et al. Gonadal steroid receptors in meningiomas. *J Neurol.* 1987;234:328–333.

Linden RD, Tator CH, Benedict C, et al. Electrophysiological monitoring during acoustic neuroma and other posterior fossa surgery. *Can J Neurol Sci.* 1988;15:73–81.

Lueder GT, Judisch GF, Wen BC. Heritable retinoblastoma and pinealoma. *Arch Ophthalmol.* 1991;109:1707–1709.

MacCarty CS, Leavens ME, Love JG, Kernohan JW. Dermoid and epidermoid tumors in the central nervous system of adults. *Surg Gynecol Obstet.* 1959;108:191–198.

Mahaley MS Jr, Mettlin C, Natarajan N, et al. National survey of patterns of care for brain-tumor patients. *J Neurosurg.* 1989;71:826–836.

Mahaley MS Jr, Urso MB, Whaley RA, et al. Immunobiology of primary intracranial tumors, 10. Therapeutic efficacy of interferon in the treatment of recurrent gliomas. *J Neurosurg.* 1985;63:719–725.

Mansour AM, Barber JC, Reinecke RD, Wang FM. Ocular choristomas. *Surv Ophthalmol.* 1989;33:339–358.

Masuyama Y, Kodama Y, Matsuura Y, et al. Clinical studies on the occurrence and the pathogenesis of optociliary veins. *J Clin Neuro-ophthalmol.* 1990;10:1–8.

Maxwell M, Black PMcL. Oncogenes, growth factors and brain tumors. In: Kornblith PL, Walker MD, eds. *Advances in Neuro-oncology.* Mount Kisco, NY: Futura; 1988:159–176.

McFadzean RM, McIlwaine GG, McLellan D. Hodgkin's disease at the optic chiasm. *J Clin Neuro-ophthalmol.* 1990;10:248–254.

McFadzean RM. Visual prognosis in craniopharyngioma. *Neuro-ophthalmology.* 1989;9:337–341.

McNab AA, Wright JE. Cysts of the optic nerve: Three cases associated with meningioma. *Eye.* 1989;3:355–359.

Mindel JS, Fetell MR. A pituitary adenoma with dilated ventricles. *Surv Ophthalmol.* 1985;30:59–61.

Mulvihill J, Parry DM, Sherman Jl, et al. Neurofibromatosis 1 (Recklinghausen disease) and neurofibromatosis 2 (bilateral acoustic neurofibromatosis): An update. *Ann Intern Med.* 1990;113:39–52.

Munden PM, Sobol WM, Weingeist TA. Ocular findings in Turcot syndrome (glioma-polyposis). *Ophthalmology.* 1991;98:111–114.

Nerad JA, Kersten RC, Anderson RL. Hemangioblastoma of the optic nerve: Report of a case and review of the literature. *Ophthalmology.* 1988;95:398–402.

Neumann HP, Eggert HR, Weigel K, et al. Hemangioblastomas of the central nervous system: A 10-year study with special reference to von Hippel–Lindau syndrome. *J Neurosurg.* 1989;70:24–30.

Neville RG, Greenblatt SH, Kollarits CR. Foster Kennedy syndrome and an optociliary vein in a patient with a falx meningioma. *J Clin Neuro-ophthalmol.* 1984;4:97–101.

O'Neill BP, Illig JJ. Primary central nervous system lymphoma. *Mayo Clin Proc.* 1989;64:1005–1020.

Patchell RA, Tibbs PA, Walsh JW, et al. A randomized trial of surgery in the treatment of single metastases to the brain. *N Engl J Med.* 1990;322:494–500.

Patronas NJ, Di Chiro G, Kufta C, et al. Prediction of survival in glioma patients by means of positron emission tomography. *J Neurosurg.* 1985;62:816–822.

Probst C, Gessaga E, Leuenberger AE. Primary meningioma of the optic nerve sheaths: Case report. *Ophthalmologica.* 1985;190:83–90.

Reifler DM, Holtzman JN, Ringel DM. Sphenoid ridge meningioma masquerading as Grave's orbitopathy. *Arch Ophthalmol.* 1986;104:1591.

Repka MX, Miller NR. Optic atrophy in children. *Am J Ophthalmol.* 1988;106:191–193.

Repka MX, Miller NR. Papilledema and dural sinus obstruction. *J Clin Neuro-ophthalmol.* 1984;4:247–250.

Repka MX, Miller NR, Miller M. Visual outcome after surgical removal of craniopharyngiomas. *Ophthalmology.* 1989;96:195–199.

Ridley M, Green J, Johnson G. Retinal angiomatosis: The ocular manifestations of von Hippel–Lindau disease. *Can J Ophthalmol.* 1986;21:276–283.

Rudd A, Rees JE, Kennedy P, et al. Malignant optic nerve gliomas in adults. *J Clin Neuro-ophthalmol.* 1985;5:238–243.

Russell DC, Rubinstein LJ. *Pathology of Tumors of the Nervous System.* 4th ed. Baltimore: Williams & Wilkins; 1977.

Ryder JW, Kleinschmidt-DeMasters BK, Keller TS. Sudden deterioration and death in patients with benign tumors of the third ventricle area. *J Neurosurg.* 1986;64:216–223.

Salcman M, Samaras GM. Interstitial microwave hyperthermia for brain tumors: Results of a phase-1 clinical trial. *J Neurooncol.* 1983;1:225–236.

Schanzer MC, Font RL, O'Malley RE. Primary ocular malignant lymphoma associated with the acquired immune deficiency syndrome. *Ophthalmology.* 1991;98:88–91.

Schatz H, Green WR, Talamo JH, et al. Clinicopathologic correlation of retinal to choroidal venous collaterals of the optic nerve head. *Ophthalmology.* 1991;98:1287–1293.

Schoenberg BS. Epidemiology of primary intracranial neoplasms: Disease distribution and risk factors. In: Salcman M, ed. *Neurobiology of Brain Tumors.* Vol 4 of *Concepts in Neurosurgery.* Baltimore: Williams & Wilkins; 1991:3–18.

Schrell UMH, Fahlbusch R. Hormonal manipulation of cerebral meningiomas. In: Al-Mefty O, ed. *Meningiomas.* New York: Raven; 1991:273–283.

Schwartz RB, Carvalho PA, Alexander E III, et al. Radiation necrosis vs high-grade recurrent glioma: Differentiation by using dual-isotope SPECT with ^{201}TI and ^{99}mTc-HMPAO. *AJNR.* 1991;12:1187–1192.

Seiff SR, Brodsky MC, MacDonald G, et al. Orbital optic glioma in neurofibromatosis: Magnetic resonance diagnosis of perineural arachnoidal gliomatosis. *Arch Ophthalmol.* 1987;105:1689–1692.

Seizinger BR, Rouleau GA, Ozelius LJ, et al. Common pathogenetic mechanism for three tumor types in bilateral acoustic neurofibromatosis. *Science.* 1987;236:317–319.

Shapiro WR, Green SB, Burger PC, et al. Randomized trial of three chemotherapy regimens and two radiotherapy regimens in postoperative treatment of malignant glioma. Brain Tumor Cooperative Group trial 8001. *J Neurosurg.* 1989;71:1–9.

Sibony PA, Kennerdell JS, Slamovits TL, et al. Intrapapillary refractile bodies in optic nerve sheath meningioma. *Arch Ophthalmol.* 1985;103:383–385.

Sibony PA, Krauss HR, Kennerdell JS, et la. Optic nerve sheath meningiomas: Clinical manifestations. *Ophthalmology.* 1984;91:1313–1326.

Slavin ML. Isolated trochlear nerve palsy secondary to cavernous sinus meningioma. *Am J Ophthalmol.* 1987;104:433–434.

Smith RW. Tumors. In: Wiederholt WC, ed. *Neurology for the Non-neurologist.* Philadelphia: Grune & Stratton; 1988:320–327.

Tan TJ. Epidermoids and dermoids of the central nervous system. *Acta Neurochir.* 1972;26:13–24.

Tator CH, Nedzelski JM. Preservation of hearing in patients undergoing excision of acoustic neuromas and other cerebellopontine angle tumors. *J Neurosurg.* 1985;63:168–174.

Tomita T, McLone DG. Medulloblastoma in childhood: Results of radical resection and low-dose neuraxis radiation therapy. *J Neurosurg.* 1986;64:238–242.

Vander JF, Kincaid MC, Hegarty TJ, et al. The ocular effects of intracarotid bromodeoxyuridine and radiation therapy in the treatment of malignant glioma. *Ophthalmology.* 1990;97:352–357.

Walker AE, Robins M, Weinfeld FD. Epidemiology of brain tumors: The national survey of intracranial neoplasms. *Neurology.* 1985;35:219–226.

Walker MD, Green SB, Byar DP, et al. Randomized comparisons of radiotherapy and nitrosoureas for the treatment of malignant glioma after surgery. *N Engl J Med.* 1980;303:1323–1329.

Wallner KE, Wara WM, Sheline GE, Davis RL. Intracranial ependyomas: Results of treatment with partial or whole brain irradiation without spinal irradiation. *Int J Radiat Oncol Biol Phys.* 1986;12:1937–1941.

Walsh FB, Hoyt WF: In: Miller NR, ed. *Clinical Neuro-ophthalmology.* 4th ed. Baltimore: Williams & Wilkins, 1988:3.

Walsh TJ, Garden J, Gallagher B. Obliteration of retinal venous pulsations. *Am J Ophthalmol.* 1969;67:954.

Wan WL, Geller JL, Feldon SE, Sadun AA. Visual loss caused by rapidly progressive intracranial meningiomas during pregnancy. *Ophthalmology.* 1990;97:18–21.

Wara WM. Radiation therapy for brain tumors. *Cancer.* 1985;55:2291–2295.

Weir B. The relative significance of factors affecting postoperative survival in astrocytomas, grades 3 and 4. *J Neurosurg.* 1973;38:448–452.

Weir B, Grace M. The relative significance of factors affecting postoperative survival in astrocytomas, grades one and two. *Can J Neurol Sci.* 1976;3:47–50.

Wilson WB, Lloyd LA, Buncic JR. Tumor spread in unilateral optic glioma. *Neuro-ophthalmology.* 1987;7:179–184.

Wright JE, McNab AA, McDonald WI. Primary optic nerve sheath meningioma. *Br J Ophthalmol.* 1989;73:960–966.

Young JL, Percy CL, Asire AJ, eds. *Surveillance, Epidemiology and End Results: Incidence and Mortality Data, 1973–77.* National Cancer Institute. Monograph. 57. Washington, DC: U.S. Government Printing Office; 1981.

Zhou XP, Zhao MY, Ma YJ. Blindness from intracranial tumors: A clinical analysis of 60 cases. *Am J Optom Physiol Optics.* 1987;64:329–332.

Zimmerman CF, Schatz NJ, Glaser JS. Magnetic resonance imaging of optic nerve meningiomas: Enhancement with gadolinium-DTPA. *Ophthalmology.* 1990;97:585–591.

7
Chapter

Pseudotumor Cerebri

Kelly H. Thomann

Pseudotumor cerebri (PTC), also known as idiopathic intracranial hypertension, is a disease most commonly found in young, obese females. It is characterized by increased intracranial pressure in the absence of a mass lesion or infection. Imaging studies and lumbar puncture, necessary to make the diagnosis, will reveal no abnormalities except increased intracranial pressure. Ocular involvement is a prominent component of PTC. Permanent visual loss is the most serious sequela of this disease, which is sometimes erroneously called benign intracranial hypertension.

EPIDEMIOLOGY

■ Systemic

Durcan and co-workers (1988) reported the annual incidence of PTC to be 0.9 per 100,000 in the general population. The incidence rises to 14 in 100,000 in women between the ages of 20 and 44 who are 10% over ideal weight, and almost 15 per 100,000 in those females who are 20% over ideal weight. Obesity is the most commonly associated condition, found in 50% of PTC patients.

Female-to-male ratio in PTC is eight to one, and men who are affected fall into the same age group as women. Digre and Corbett (1988) reported that men may be at a greater risk for visual loss, especially African-American males. Male and female children are affected equally, and also may be especially vulnerable to vision loss.

Among the initial symptoms of PTC, headache is the most common, found in 75 to 80% of patients. Nausea and vomiting are initially present in 21% of patients with PTC. Five percent of patients have no symptoms when the disease is diagnosed.

■ Ocular

Disturbances of visual acuity occur as initial symptoms in 68%, transient visual obscurations in up to 72%, diplopia is reported in 35%, and 22% have other visual complaints.

Papilledema is the most prominent sign in PTC and is found in almost every case. Visual loss is the major morbidity associated with this disorder as a sequela to papilledema. Visual acuity better than 20/25 was found initially in 89% of patients by Rush (1980) and abnormal visual fields in 93%. Final visual acuity worse than 20/30 was found in 11% of Rush's patients, and 46% of the patients had permanent visual field defects after resolution of the disease. According to Corbett and associates (1982), an enlarged blind spot is the most common type of visual field loss, followed by inferior nasal field loss. It was previously believed that duration of symptoms, degree of papilledema, and transient visual obscurations were indicative of a more severe visual outcome. However, many recent studies have found no relationship of these findings to the final visual outcome.

NATURAL HISTORY

■ Systemic

Intracranial pressure (ICP) is created by the cerebrospinal fluid (CSF), blood, and brain tissue, which are housed within the skull. The normal range of intracranial pressure is between 50 and 200 mm H_2O. The volume of each component can vary slightly without causing increased ICP, due to an internal mechanism that compensates for any changes. However, in PTC the ICP is above that which can be compensated for by this mechanism. The cause of the raised ICP in PTC remains unknown in about 90% of the cases.

Various mechanisms have been proposed to explain the etiology of the increased ICP. Dandy (1937) originally discussed 22 cases of PTC and thought it was due to increased cerebral blood volume. Diffuse cerebral edema (Sahs & Joynt, 1956) and abnormal CSF circulation (Symonds, 1931; Bercaw & Greer, 1970) have also been proposed. More recently, Johnston and Paterson (1974), and others have postulated an obstruction to the outflow of CSF within the venous sinus due to increased resistance of the arachnoid villi. Most speculate this to be the primary cause or it may be a mixed mechanism. Researchers felt current imaging techniques would prove the etiology, but to date they have not.

Many associated conditions have been proposed and studied as causes of PTC. Although a definite correlation has been found with some, the majority have not been proven with scientific documentation (Table 7–1). Endocrine abnormalities, menstrual irregularities, pregnancy, and the use of oral contraceptives have all been linked with PTC, although studies consistently have found no causal relationship. It is true that obesity is a common factor; however, endocrine and menstrual abnormalities are frequently found in obese women. Also, a relationship to hypertension and diabetes mellitus has been discussed, but these too are more common in obese persons.

Intracranial hypertension may be caused by any factor that causes a decrease in flow through the arachnoid villi or obstructs the venous pathway to the heart. Examples of conditions that can cause a state that resembles PTC are dural sinus thrombosis, which may occur following head trauma or secondary to radical neck dissection; or venous sinus thrombosis due to middle ear infection. Whether these are true cases of PTC or conditions resembling the idiopathic type is a semantic issue. However, PTC due to venous sinus thrombosis can only be diagnosed by visualization of venous sinus drainage. In cases where it is suspected, angiography is necessary.

Exogenous agents such as excessive doses of vitamin A, tetracyclines, lithium, and nalidixic acid all have a longstanding association with PTC in the literature. Although the causal relationship is not clear, a careful drug history may be important in those patients suspected of having PTC. It is unclear if steroids play a role in the pathogenesis of PTC, although there are reports of this disorder following steroid use and its resolution after discontinuation.

The most frequent presenting symptom in PTC is headache. The headache is described as severe, throbbing, nonlocalizable, episodic pain that occurs daily, usually lasting hours. It may be worse in the morning, exacerbated with head movement and the Valsalva maneuver. Patients may also complain of changes in vision, diplopia, neck stiffness, or pulsatile intracranial noises (Table 7–2).

Cerebral function remains normal in PTC. There is no change in consciousness or mentation. If focal neurologic deficits are found, the diagnosis of PTC may be incorrect.

TABLE 7–1. PSEUDOTUMOR CEREBRI AND POSSIBLE ASSOCIATED CAUSES

Highly Likely

Decreased flow through arachnoid granulations
    Scarring from previous inflammation (eg, meningitis, sequel to subarachnoid hemorrhage)
Obstruction to venous drainage
    Venous sinus thromboses, (hypercoaguable states, or contiguous infection such as middle ear or mastoid–otitic hydrocephalus)
    Bilateral radical neck dissection
    Superior vena cava syndrome
    Increased right heart pressure
Endocrine disorders
    Addison disease
    Hypoparathyroidism
    Obesity
    Steroid withdrawal
Nutritional disorders
    Hypervitaminosis A (vitamin, liver, or isotretinoin intake)
    Hyperalimentation in deprivation dwarfism
Arteriovenous malformations

Probable Causes

Anabolic steroids (may cause venous sinus thrombosis)
Chlordecone (Kepone)
Ketoprofen or indomethacin in Bartter syndrome
Systemic lupus erythematosus
Thyroid replacement therapy in hypothyroid children
Uremia

Possible Causes

Amiodarone
Diphenylhydantoin
Iron deficiency anemia
Lithium carbonate
Nalidixic acid
Sarcoidosis
Sulfa antibiotics

Causes Frequently Cited That Are Unproven

Corticosteroid intake
Hyperthyroidism
Hypovitaminosis A
Menarche
Menstrual irregularities
Multivitamin intake
Oral contraceptive use
Pregnancy
Tetracycline use

Reprinted with permission from Wall, M: Differential diagnosis of idiopathic intracranial hypertension. Neurol Clin 1988;9:76.

TABLE 7–2. SYSTEMIC MANIFESTATIONS OF PSEUDOTUMOR CEREBRI

- Headache[a]
- Nauseousness and vomiting[b]
- Vertigo[b]
- Pulsatile intracranial noises[c]
- Shoulder, arm or neck pain[c]
- Tinnitus[c]
- Paresthesias[c]

[a] Very common.
[b] Common.
[c] Rare, but reported in the literature.

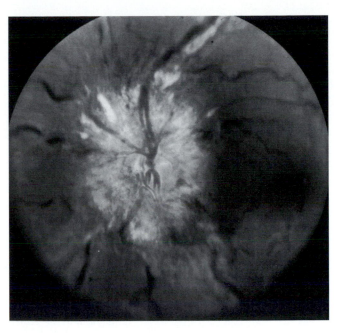

Figure 7–1. Papilledema in a 30-year-old female with intracranial pressure of 280 with normal imaging and laboratory studies. *(Courtesy of Dr. Scott Richter.)*

The increased intracranial pressure found in PTC causes papilledema, and occasionally sixth (abducens) cranial nerve palsies. These are the only clinical signs found with this disease (see the "Ocular" section below for discussion).

The course of PTC varies considerably from patient to patient. It is never fatal, and in many cases it will resolve on its own without treatment and leave no permanent damage. Most cases resolve in 3 to 9 months; however, in some cases, even with the most aggressive surgical treatment, vision loss may still ensue. Up to 37% of patients have recurrence of the disease, with the interval from onset to recurrence about 4 years.

■ Ocular

Papilledema (Figure 7–1) is the most prominent finding in PTC, although it may occasionally be absent. Visual symptoms secondary to papilledema vary considerably. They include transient visual obscurations (monocular or binocular) and blurred vision. Papilledema initially does not cause any visual symptoms or noticeable field defects unless it causes macula edema or hemorrhage. It is difficult to judge by the appearance of the papilledema the duration of the disease. The discs may remain elevated and unchanged for a number of years even after resolution of the disease. Signs that may be helpful in a gross estimate of duration include the presence of resolving hemorrhages, cotton-wool spots, vascular tortuosity, presence of optociliary shunt vessels, nerve fiber layer defects, horizontal choroidal folds, or gliosis of the discs. Prolonged or severe papilledema may cause optic atrophy and circumpapillary rings (which indicate the amount the disc had previously been elevated). It may also cause the disc margins to become more indistinct with time, creating a circumpapillary haze. Differential diagnosis includes other causes of papilledema, disc edema, or pseudopapilledema (such as disc drusen or oblique optic nerve insertion).

Visual loss may seem to occur quickly; however, the disease may go undiagnosed for some time without any sub-jective visual disturbance. Some patients experience gradual visual loss months to years after diagnosis; the rate and symptoms vary greatly in each case. Factors that appear to be related to a greater risk of visual loss are systemic hypertension, anemia, peripapillary subretinal neovascularization, older age, and high myopia. Patients with any of these factors should be watched more carefully and treated more aggressively to avoid visual loss.

Papilledema causes characteristic visual field defects, which are disc related (Table 7–3). An enlarged blind spot, seldom noticed by the patient, is almost always found. This defect may remain following resolution of the disease, and therefore is not used to evaluate the success of therapy. The enlarged blind spot is due to the displacement of the peripapillary nerve fibers as they exit the optic disc. Inferior nasal visual field deficits are second most commonly found, and are due to destruction of peripheral nerve fibers by progressive gliosis. The fibers subserving the inferior nasal visual field seem to be most at risk to mechanical compression and ischemic damage at the disc as in other causes of ischemia to the optic nerve (eg, anterior ischemic optic neuropathy). Glaucoma-like nerve fiber bundle defects and arcuate scotomas may also occur suggesting a similar mechanism at the level of the lamina cribrosa.

Patients may complain of diplopia, and motility disturbances in the form of sixth cranial nerve palsies may be found. The long intracranial course of the abducens nerve makes it vulnerable to any shifts in the brain, and one or both

TABLE 7–3. OCULAR MANIFESTATIONS OF PSEUDOTUMOR CEREBRI

PAPILLEDEMA
- Vision disturbances
    Decreased vision
    Transient visual obscurations
    Alterations of vision
- Visual field defects
    Enlarged blind spot
    Inferior nasal loss
    Nerve fiber layer defects
- Retro-ocular pain

SIXTH (ABDUCENS) CRANIAL NERVE PALSY
- Diplopia

nerves are especially susceptible as they course over the clivus (the bone that forms the foramen magnum in the skull). Paralysis of the other ocular motor nerves is not likely, and if found, a cause other than PTC should be suspected.

DIAGNOSIS

■ Systemic

PTC may be diagnosed by a practitioner during routine examination on an asymptomatic individual or on a patient who complains of headaches or visual symptoms. There are no systemic findings used to corroborate the diagnosis of PTC other than imaging studies and lumbar puncture. PTC is purely a diagnosis of exclusion made following ocular and neurologic examination, and rarely after the complaint of headaches alone. It should be emphasized that cerebral function remains intact in PTC. If neurological findings other than papilledema and sixth-nerve palsy are found, another diagnosis should be considered.

Indicated tests include lumbar puncture and brain scan by CT or MRI. Imaging studies must be performed before lumbar puncture. The CT or MRI will be normal in PTC, although small ventricles and an empty sella turcica are sometimes found. Lumbar puncture will reveal an opening pressure greater than 200 mm H_2O in PTC. The cerebral spinal fluid must show normal cell count, glucose, and protein, and negative VDRL for the diagnosis. The CSF protein concentration will typically be low in PTC.

Differential diagnosis of PTC includes brain lesions such as primary or secondary tumors that may cause increased ICP with or without other neurological localizing signs, hydrocephalus, and encephalopathies. Enlargement of the ventricles will be found in hydrocephalus, usually along with other neurological signs. Infections, toxins, and malig-

nant hypertension all may cause encephalopathy, and should be ruled out during the examination and by lumbar puncture. Blood tests to rule out systemic etiologies of swollen discs should include CBC, ESR, ANA, FTA-ABS, T_4, TSH, and Lyme titer.

■ Ocular

The ocular findings of papilledema and, less frequently, sixth-nerve palsy are the hallmarks in the diagnosis of PTC. Visual acuity will be reduced or normal. Automated perimetry is the preferred type of visual field test because of the ability to quantify defects for future follow-up of the patient. Defects range from mild loss to severe constriction of the visual field. Enlargement of the blind spot is almost always found, and will also vary with the patient's refractive error. Other visual field losses are similar to those found in any case of papilledema, and include decreased inferior nasal field, peripheral constriction, scotomas, and nerve fiber bundle defects.

Contrast sensitivity testing will show defects over all spatial frequencies. Color vision testing and pupil evaluation will not generally add helpful information unless the disc swelling is asymmetric. Visual evoked responses have limited use in the diagnosis and management of PTC.

TREATMENT AND MANAGEMENT

■ Systemic

Management of PTC ranges from monitoring the patient carefully to surgery (Table 7–4). A patient who has no vision loss and is not bothered by headaches or other symptoms is monitored monthly for any worsening of vision or new visual field loss and every 3 months if no change is found after the first 3 months. Many cases will resolve with no treatment, and patient follow-up is then tapered accordingly. Weight loss should be encouraged in all nonpregnant patients with PTC, although this alone is usually not sufficient to cure the disease. Standard analgesics, migraine medication, or β-blockers are used initially to control headaches.

Severe headaches and progression of visual loss are the primary reasons to initiate medical and surgical treatment. Options include dehydrating agents, corticosteroids, serial lumbar puncture, and surgery.

Carbonic anhydrase inhibitors (CAIs) have been shown to play a large role in the management of this disorder and are recommended as the initial means to control PTC. These medications cause a decrease in CSF production by inhibiting carbonic anhydrase. Acetazolamide (Diamox) has been suggested (Tomsak, 1985) as the initial drug of choice in the treatment of PTC. However, maximum doses of CAIs are often necessary to decrease CSF effectively,

TABLE 7–4. TREATMENT AND MANAGEMENT OF PSEUDOTUMOR CEREBRI

MANIFESTATION(S)	TREATMENT/MANAGEMENT
• No decrease in visual acuity • No visual field loss (except enlarged blind spot)	• Follow monthly for at least 6 months (must measure VA, VF, binocular optic nerve assessment with stereo photos, IOP) and if improvement, or no new symptoms, taper to every 3 months • Manage headaches with analgesics, β-blockers, migraine medications • Weight-reduction program
• Early (minimal) decrease in visual acuity or loss of visual field • Headaches not managed or relieved by above medications	• Oral acetazolamide (Diamox) 500 mg BID • If Diamox contraindicated or not tolerated, consider furosemide (Lasix) 40–160 mg BID • Manage as above
• Medical treatment not effective • Recent loss of acuity not secondary to macular edema • Progression of a pre-existing visual field defect • Persistent, intractible headache not relieved by oral medications • Anticipation of oral therapy likely to cause hypotension	• Lumbar peritoneal shunt • Optic nerve sheath fenestration (primarily used to treat vision loss, may be done if lumbar peritoneal shunt not efficaceous)

and this frequently leads to adverse side effects and poor patient compliance. Side effects include nauseousness, gastrointestinal upset, perioral and digital tingling, loss of appetite, tinlike taste in the mouth, electrolyte imbalance, renal stones, fatigue, and depression. Diamox Sequel (the long-acting form) may cause fewer side effects and be more efficacious.

Corticosteroids are used frequently in the management of the patient with PTC. However, today most advocate only a short dose in cases of progressive vision loss or debilitating symptoms. Long-term steroid use can increase IOP and aggravate vision loss. When steroids are discontinued, patients may also experience recurrence of PTC.

Repeated lumbar punctures were once used to treat PTC but they are no longer advocated, because lumbar punctures are difficult to perform on obese individuals and become more painful each time one is done. Also, their effect is short lived, as the CSF pressure can return to its previous level within 2 hours of the procedure.

Indications for surgery include recent or progressive visual loss not responding to medical treatment and not secondary to macula edema, debilitating headaches not responding to medications, and the anticipation of medical treatment that may lead to a hypotensive event and cause further damage to the disc (eg, the initiation of systemic antihypertensive medications).

Subtemporal decompression was the first form of surgery used in the treatment of PTC. However, it is rarely done today because it has a high incidence of complications such as strokes or seizures. It has been replaced by lumbar peritoneal shunt and optic nerve sheath decompression.

Lumbar peritoneal shunt remains the most common surgical technique used in the management of PTC. In this procedure, a catheter is placed in the subarachnoid space of the lumbar vertebrae and the tubing is passed to the abdominal region, where it empties into the abdominal cavity. It acts like a constant lumbar puncture. Problems include infection, blockage, or movement of the tube. Signs and symptoms of PTC can improve within 1 month of this procedure; however, over 50% of cases require shunt revision. There appear to be two types of lumbar peritoneal shunt patients—one group in which the initial shunt works very well, and another group where reshunting is required, often more than once.

■ Ocular

Ocular management (see Table 7–4) includes visual acuity measurement, quantitative perimetry, stereo optic nerve photographs, and intraocular pressure measurement. Contrast sensitivity and color vision offer some assistance in following these patients, and VEPs are generally not useful. Follow-up is monthly for at least 6 months, and if no changes are noted, every 3 months thereafter as long as the edema persists.

Optic nerve sheath decompression is the second form of surgery used in the management of patients with severe vision loss from the papilledema. It was first performed by DeWecker in 1872, but did not gain widespread acceptance until 1964 when Hayreh revived the procedure. There are two approaches used to fenestrate the optic nerve and each has its proponents. One involves a medial approach to the optic nerve and the other a lateral approach. If medially done, the medial rectus is disinserted and the globe is retracted. The exposed optic nerve sheath is incised. Some remove a single square-shaped portion (like a window) while others make multiple incisions to fenestrate the meninges. The lateral approach entails an incision from the lateral canthus toward the ear. The temporalis muscle is retracted, the orbital rim cut and removed, and the lateral rectus muscle retracted. The nerve is then exposed and fenestrated.

Proposed theories regarding the mechanism of optic nerve sheath decompression include local decompression of the optic nerve by filtration from the creation of a permanent fistula to drain CSF. Another theory proposes that scarring in the subarachnoid space around the optic nerve causes a shift of the pressure gradient from the back of the lamina cribrosa to the myelinated portion of the optic nerve, thus relieving the pressure on the anterior portion of the optic nerve.

Optic nerve sheath decompression is done unilaterally. The second eye may be operated on if worsening occurs in that eye. Most studies show improvement of papilledema in half of cases in the eye not operated on. Headaches are usually relieved, but should not be an indication for this type of surgery. Most advocate standard medical treatment of headache with analgesics and migraine medications and then lumbar peritoneal shunt for treatment of headache.

Several studies have shown improvement of visual acuity and visual field after surgery despite optic nerve pallor preoperatively. Therefore optic nerve pallor is not a contraindication to surgery, but vision may not return to 20/20. Pallor may indicate the need for more prompt, aggressive treatment to preserve the remaining visual fibers.

Results from optic nerve sheath fenestration surgery have shown sustained improvement of visual acuity and visual field along with frequent improvement of the opposite eye and headaches. There is less need for repeat surgery, and less intraoperative and postoperative complications when compared to lumbar peritoneal shunt. Some patients who have undergone optic nerve sheath decompression have shown vision improvement following unsuccessful lumbar peritoneal shunt. Postoperative complications include disturbances of ocular motility and irregular pupils.

CONCLUSION

The eyecare practitioner plays a major role in the diagnosis and management of the patient with PTC. Headaches, blurred vision, and loss of vision are frequent causes for patients to seek eyecare, and these are the most common symptoms of PTC. The eyecare practitioner must understand this disorder and be able to recognize it in the patient who may or may not fit the typical clinical picture (a young, obese female). Thus, when a patient presents with headaches or visual symptoms, and papilledema is found on examination, timely referral must be made to a neurologist, and lumbar puncture and brain imaging should be ordered. Careful monitoring of ocular health, visual acuity, and visual fields by an eyecare practitioner is the mainstay for long-term follow-up in patients with PTC.

REFERENCES

Ahlskog JE, O'Neill BP. Pseudotumor cerebri. *Ann Inter Med.* 1982;97:249–256.

Baker RS, Carter D, Hendrick EB, Buncic JR. Visual loss in pseudotumor cerebri of childhood: A follow-up study. *Arch Ophthalmol.* 1985;103:1681–1686.

Bercaw BL, Greer M. Transport of intrathecal 13 I RISA in benign intracranial hypertension. *Neurology.* 1970;20:787–790.

Brourman ND, Spoor TC, Ramocki JM. Optic nerve sheath decompression for pseudotumor cerebri. *Arch Ophthalmol.* 1988;106:1378–1383.

Bulens C, DeVries WA, Van Crevel H. Benign intracranial hypertension: A retrospective and follow-up study. *J Neuro Sci.* 1979;40:147–157.

Cody CM. Benign intracranial hypertension. *Am Fam Physician.* 1992;45:1671–1678.

Corbett JJ, Nerard JA, Tse DT, Anderson RL. Results of optic nerve sheath fenestration for pseudotumor cerebri. *Arch Ophthalmol.* 1988;106:1391–1397.

Corbett JJ, Savino PJ, Thompson HS, et al. Visual loss in pseudotumor cerebri: Follow-up of 57 patients from 5 to 41 years and a profile of 14 patients with permanent severe visual loss. *Arch Neurol.* 1982;39:461–474.

Corbett JJ, Thompson S. The rational management of idiopathic intracranial hypertension. *Arch Neurol.* 1989;46:1049–1051.

Dandy WE. Intracranial pressure without brain tumor. *Ann Surg.* 1937;106:492–513.

Digre KB, Corbett JJ. Pseudotumor cerebri in men. *Arch Neurol.* 1988;45:866–872.

Durcan FJ, Corbett JJ, Wall M. The incidence of pseudotumor cerebri—Population studies in Iowa and Louisiana. *Arch Neurol.* 1988;45:875–877.

Hupp SL, Glaser JS, Frazier-Byrne S. Optic nerve sheath decompression: Review of 17 cases. *Arch Ophthalmol.* 1987;105:386–389.

Ireland B, Corbett JJ, Wallace RB. The search for causes of idiopathic intracranial hypertension—a preliminary case-control study. *Arch Neurol.* 1990;47:315–320.

Johnston I, Paterson A. Benign intracranial hypertension—cerebral spinal fluid pressure and circulation. *Brain.* 1974;97:308–312.

Kelman SE, Sergott RC, Cioffi GA, et al. Modified optic nerve decompression in patients with functioning lumboperitoneal shunts and progressive visual loss. *Ophthalmology.* 1991;98:1449–1453.

Keltner JL. Optic nerve sheath decompression—How does it work? Has its time come? *Arch Ophthalmol.* 1988;106:1365–1369. Editorial.

Orcutt JC, Page NGR, Sanders MD. Factors affecting visual loss in benign intracranial hypertension. *Ophthalmology.* 1984;91:1303–1312.

Park S, Primo SA. Pseudotumor cerebri: Diagnosis and treatment. *Clin Eye Vision Care.* 1992;4:70–79.

Rush JA. Pseudotumor cerebri—clinical profile and visual outcome in 63 patients. *Mayo Clinic Proc.* 1980;55:541–546.

Sahs AL, Joynt RJ. Brain swelling of unknown cause. *Neurology.* 1956;6:791–803.

Sergott RC. Modified optic nerve sheath decompression provides long-term visual improvement for pseudotumor cerebri. *Arch Ophthalmol.* 1988;106:1391–1397.

Smith CH, Orcutt JC. Surgical treatment of pseudotumor cerebri. *Int Ophthalmol Clin.* 1986;26:265–275.

Sullivan JC. Diagnosis and management of pseudotumor cerebri. *J Nat Med Assoc.* 1991;83:916–918.

Susman JL. Benign intracranial hypertension. *J Fam Practice.* 1990;30:290–292.

Symonds CP. Otitic hydrocephalus. *Brain.* 1931;54:55–71.

Tomsak R. Treatment of pseudotumor cerebri with Diamox (acetazolamide). *J Clin Neuro-ophthalmol.* 1988;8:93–98.

Wall M. Idiopathic intracranial hypertension. *Neuro Clin.* 1991;9:73–95.

Wall M, George D. Visual loss in pseudotumor cerebri—incidence and defects related to visual field strategy. *Arch Neurol.* 1987;44:170–175.

Wall M, Hart WM, Burde RM. Visual field defects in idiopathic intracranial hypertension (pseudotumor cerebri). *Am J Ophthalmol.* 1983;92:654–669.

8

Chapter

Multiple Sclerosis

Susan C. Oleszewski

Multiple sclerosis (MS) is one of the most common acquired neurological diseases of young adults in the temperate zones. The disease probably accounts for more disability, more cost in care, and more lost income than any other neurological disease in this age group in Western Europe and in North America. Despite extensive research, the etiology remains unknown, treatment remains unsatisfactory, and the pathogenesis of the lesions is poorly understood. Neuro-ophthalmic signs and symptoms occur in virtually all patients some time during the course of the disease and are often critical in establishing a diagnosis.

EPIDEMIOLOGY

■ Systemic

Many aspects of the epidemiology of MS are controversial. However, a number of features, such as the overall geographic pattern, are clear and unequivocal. It is rare in the tropics and increases in frequency at higher latitudes north and probably also south of the equator. The prevalence in the United States is reported at 57.8 per 100,000, but increases in a somewhat continuous fashion with increasing latitude. Below the 37th parallel, the prevalence is reported at 35.5 per 100,000; above it, 68.8 per 100,000 (thus forming what is known as an "MS belt").

The risk of acquiring MS appears to be established around the time of puberty. Migration studies have found that persons less than 15 years of age migrating from high- to low-risk areas had a decrease in their risk of developing MS. Conversely, migration from low- to high-risk areas before age 15 resulted in an increased risk of acquiring MS. Presenting symptoms in MS vary according to what part of the brain or spinal cord is involved (Table 8–1).

■ Ocular

Neuro-ophthalmic signs and symptoms occur in virtually all MS patients some time during the course of the disease.

Poser and co-workers (1979) reported that 60% of the 1271 cases retrospectively studied during an 11-year period had an episode of optic neuritis, and 34% experienced diplopia. Poser also reported that optic neuritis was the initial symptom in 35% of the 1271 cases and diplopia the initial symptom in 13% of cases.

NATURAL HISTORY

The pathogenesis of MS is complex and at present poorly understood. Association between susceptibility and specific major histocompatibility complex (MHC) genes suggests a genetic predisposition. A widely considered hypothesis is that MS is the result of an immune reaction directed against self-myelin antigens. Another important hypothesis under consideration is that in MS the myelin is an "innocent bystander" that is destroyed as a consequence of an immune response triggered by a viral infection. To date, attempts to identify a single infectious agent as the cause of MS have been unsuccessful.

MS affects scattered areas of the central nervous system in the form of plaques, with a predilection for periventricular white matter, brainstem, spinal cord, and optic nerves. The plaques are characterized by primary demyelination

92

TABLE 8–1. INITIAL SYMPTOMS IN MS PATIENTS

Symptom	Percent[a]
Sensory disturbance in one or more limbs	33
Disturbance of balance and gait	18
Visual loss in one eye	17
Diplopia	13
Progressive weakness	10
Acute myelitis	6
Lhermitte symptom	3
Sensory disturbance in face	3
Pain	2

[a]Total is more than 100% because some patients presented with more than one major symptom.
Reprinted with permission from Poser S, The Diagnosis of Multiple Sclerosis. New York: Thieme; 1984:30.

(destruction of myelin sheaths with preservation of axons) and death of oligodendrocytes (myelin-producing cells) within the center of the lesion. During the early evolution of the plaque, perivascular inflammatory cells (lymphocytes, plasma cells, macrophages) invade the substance of the white matter and are thought to play a critical role in myelin destruction. This process is followed by extensive gliosis by astrocytes and aberrant attempts at remyelination, with oligodendrocytes proliferating at the edges of the plaque. In addition, immunoglobulins are deposited within each plaque.

The clinical course of MS can be classified as exacerbating–remitting, acute progressive, or chronic progressive. Exacerbating–remitting MS is the most common form in persons under age 40. It usually begins with the acute or subacute onset of focal neurologic signs and symptoms. The symptoms vary from mild to severe, and can result from involvement of any part of the brain or spinal cord.

Common presentations include blurred vision, diplopia, vertigo, weakness, and sensory symptoms. The focal symptoms and accompanying signs may come on rapidly over a few minutes, but more commonly progress gradually over several days. Symptoms typically evolve over 24 to 72 hours, stabilize for a few days, and then improve spontaneously. They may be followed months or years later by

new focal symptoms or signs, which again may remit either partially or completely. Patients commonly experience a recurrence of old symptoms with or without new ones.

Acute progressive MS, a rarer form of MS, has a relatively acute onset with a rapidly downhill course. This type involves multiple areas of the nervous system simultaneously and leads to severe impairment and death within a few weeks or months.

Chronic progressive MS advances in most patients with disease onset after age 35. The disease most often begins insidiously with slowly or intermittently progressive monoparesis, paraparesis, hemiparesis, or axial instability. A slowly progressive pattern is rare in patients below age 35 and usually indicates another etiology.

The long-term outcome of patients with MS is variable; some patients apparently remain asymptomatic throughout the course, and others (a minority) have a fulminant, rapid progression to death. Most patients have a course somewhere between these two extremes. At least 20% of the patients have a benign course for 15 years or more.

Several studies have attempted to determine the factors that have predictive value for the long-term outcome. Not all studies have reached the same conclusions, but there seems to be a consensus about certain factors (Table 8–2). The relapse rate does not seem to be a predictive value. The search for markers that have predictive value for the future course in MS patients continues.

■ Systemic

Multiple sclerosis is characterized by a myriad of neurological symptoms and signs (Table 8–3). The disease usually presents in patients under age 35 with the subacute onset of focal neurologic symptoms and signs indicative of disease in the optic nerve, pyramidal tract, posterior column, cerebellum, central vestibular system, or medial longitudinal fasciculus. Patients in the older age group more commonly present with an insidiously progressive myelopathy, manifesting as some combination of progressive spastic paraparesis, axial instability, and bladder impairment.

One of the most common clinical features in MS is the upper motor neuron syndrome. This consists of loss of motor control, spastic weakness, exaggerated tendon stretch reflexes, and extensor plantar responses (positive Babinski

TABLE 8–2. FACTORS WITH PREDICTIVE VALUE IN MS PATIENTS

Feature	Relatively Favorable	Relatively Unfavorable
Sex	Female	Male
Age at onset (yr)	< 40	> 40
Initial signs or symptoms	Optic nerve and sensory dysfunction	Motor dysfunction (cerebellar, corticospinal)
Disability	None after 5 yr	Rapidly progressive disease

Reprinted with permission from Swanson J, M.S.: Update in diagnosis and review of prognostic factors. Mayo Clinic Proc. 1989;64:578.

sign). Early in the course of the disease the patient complains of heaviness, stiffness, or clumsiness in one or both legs and a tendency to stumble. These symptoms are more prominent late in the day.

Fatigue, depression, and emotional lability are common symptoms of MS. Fatigue may be the most common single complaint of MS patients, and is often disabling. It usually comes on late in the afternoon, with strenuous activity, or in the heat. The etiology and mechanisms of depression in MS are unknown, but it appears to be more common in those with cerebral involvement than in those with predominantly spinal cord disease. Emotional lability may also be found in MS patients, ranging from a barely noticeable tendency to giggle or tear readily, to a very distressing and less common syndrome of powerful paroxysmal emotional outbursts.

Sensory symptoms in one or more extremities are common as initial symptoms and nearly universal in advanced stages of MS. These are most often described as "pins and needles" and less commonly as sensory loss. The paresthesias may be described as burning or hot. Defective postural, vibratory, and cutaneous sensations are common sensory signs in MS.

TABLE 8–3. PRESENTING SYMPTOMS IN MS BASED ON A STUDY OF 144 PATIENTS

Symptom	Patients	
	No.	%[a]
Paresthesia	53	37
Gait difficulty	50	35
Weakness or incoordination of one or both lower extremities	25	17
Visual loss (retrobulbar neuritis)	22	15
Weakness or incoordination of one or both upper extremities	15	10
Diplopia	14	10
Urinary difficulty	9	6
Dysarthria	8	6
Hemiparesis	7	5
Severe fatigue	5	3
Vertigo	4	3
Impotence	4	3
Convulsion	3	2
Severe emotionality	3	2
Lhermitte sign	2	1
Muscle cramps (legs)	2	1
Fecal incontinence	2	1
Dysphagia	1	<1
Severe movement tremor	1	<1
Hearing loss	1	<1

[a]Total is more than 100% because some patients presented with more than one major symptom.
Reprinted with permission from Swanson J, M.S.: Update in diagnosis and review of prognostic factors. Mayo Clinic Proc. *1989;64:585.*

Cerebellar involvement may occur concurrently, resulting in severe gait disturbance, a decreased facility of fine finger movements, and intention tremor.

Lower back, hip, and leg pain are common, are usually associated with significant gait disturbance or weakness, and may be caused in part by spasticity. Compensation for this weakness can further exacerbate the pain. Typical tic douloureux (usually bilateral) and atypical facial pain may be caused by disease in the pontine tegmentum.

On occasion, with plaque involvement of the cervical cord, flexing the neck gives rise to a sensation resembling an electric shock, which radiates through the neck and may extend to the trunk (Lhermitte sign). This is not specific for MS; other types of cervical cord lesions can also be associated with this sign.

Elevation in ambient temperature or endogenous temperature (eg, fever or exercise) can be associated with marked increases in symptoms and signs. These may include ataxia and weakness.

Bladder dysfunction, an autonomic nervous system disorder, is extremely common, occurring in two thirds of MS patients as a later manifestation. Patients may fail to empty urine adequately, leading to high urinary residual volumes and at times to frank urinary retention. MS may also be accompanied by severe constipation. Vascular congestion in the feet, or alternating pallor and congestion, are other autonomic nervous system dysfunctions, which occur most commonly in patients with moderate to severe paraparesis. Patients report a "hot and cold foot syndrome" in which their feet are either pale and cold or hot and flushed, but rarely comfortable.

Memory and learning impairment may occur frequently and early in MS. On rare occasions, MS appears to cause a progressive dementing illness, while at the other extreme it may have little if any cognitive or memory impairment, even in late stages of the disease.

Dysarthria, imperfect articulation, is a late occurrence in MS. This may present as a scanning speech pattern in which the words are measured or scanned with a pause after every slowly pronounced syllable. Dysarthria is reported to be present in approximately 6% of MS patients.

Sexual dysfunction was reported in 56% of women and 75% of men with MS in a population survey. This included fatigue, decreased sensation, decreased libido, erectile dysfunction, and a myriad of other symptoms. The sexual problems do not appear to be closely associated with motor system impairment.

■ Ocular

Neuro-ophthalmic signs and symptoms occur in virtually all patients some time during the course of the disease and are often critical in establishing a diagnosis (Table 8–4). The occurrence of acute optic neuritis in a previously healthy person immediately establishes a relatively high

TABLE 8–4. OCULAR MANIFESTATIONS OF MS

- Optic Neuritis
    - Visual loss
    - Visual field defect (central scotoma)
    - Afferent pupillary defect
    - Color desaturation
    - Nerve fiber layer defects
- Ocular Motility Dysfunction
    - INO/BINO (diplopia)
    - Impaired smooth pursuit
    - Impaired saccades
    - Ocular dysmetria
    - Conjugate gaze palsy
    - Nystagmus
- Other
    - Granulomatous uveitis
    - Uhtoff sign

BINO, bilateral internuclear ophthalmoplegia; INO, internuclear ophthalmoplegia.

risk of future demyelinating involvement of the central nervous system. Internuclear ophthalmoplegia (INO) in younger persons is almost pathognomonic of brainstem demyelination. Subtle disturbances of function of the visual or ocular motor systems may await the clinician searching for a diagnostic second lesion.

There is a well-established association of retrobulbar optic neuritis with demyelinating disease. Acute optic neuritis usually presents with the patient experiencing monocular loss of central vision, commonly associated with pain in, around, or behind the eye. Anterior lesions will cause optic disc swelling. In contrast, demyelination posterior to the optic nervehead (retrobulbar) will not cause a change in the appearance of the optic disc, but will cause the typical visual signs and symptoms (eg, impaired vision, visual field deficit, and color desaturation). The central scotoma is the hallmark of optic neuritis, although altitudinal defects in recent studies were the most commonly found. The onset of visual loss typically varies from a few hours to 7 days, with some cases progressing for weeks or months. The severity may range from mild impairment to complete blindness, more typically with peripheral vision preserved. The visual loss stabilizes, and then usually improves slowly over a period of weeks. The scotoma resolves more or less completely in 70% of patients. Less commonly, visual loss occurs abruptly or the patient may awaken with a maximal deficit. The extent of visual loss is highly variable, ranging from a small central scotoma to total loss of vision. Both extremes are less common than an intermediate syndrome.

Uhtoff sign is defined by a reduction or diminution of vision following exercise or any other cause of increased body temperature. This symptom is usually found in patients with chronic, rather than acute, optic nerve disease.

It has been reported that patients with a preexisting scotoma can get an enlargement of that scotoma following exercise. The pathophysiologic basis for Uhtoff sign is poorly understood. Other ocular manifestations of MS, such as diplopia, can also be exacerbated by heat.

MS is probably the most frequent cause of INO, resulting from lesions of the medial longitudinal fasciculus. It consists of a dysjunction of horizontal eye movements with a restriction of adduction on the side of the lesion, and a dissociated nystagmus, more marked in the abducting eye. Convergence is usually preserved. When bilateral (BINO), it is strong support for a diagnosis of MS.

Other abnormalities of eye movements include impaired smooth pursuit, acquired pendular nystagmus, ocular dysmetria, and less commonly, conjugate gaze palsy. Saccadic reaction times, velocities, and accuracies have been found to be reduced in MS patients.

There also seems to be an association between granulomatous uveitis and multiple sclerosis. Cases have also been reported in which MS patients have had pars planitis, foci of choroiditis, and sheathing of retinal veins with and without pars planitis.

DIAGNOSIS

■ Systemic

The diagnosis of MS is based primarily on the neurological history, findings on neurological examination, and to a lesser extent, results of special testing. The diagnosis is based on symptoms and objective evidence of white matter lesions of the central nervous system disseminated both temporally and spatially. Disturbances of sensation and gait and monocular loss of vision are the most common symptoms at the time of initial examination.

Although the diagnosis of MS is ultimately a clinical one, advances in laboratory, neurophysiologic, and neuroimaging techniques have aided in the diagnosis of this disorder. The emergence of these techniques led to the development of a new set of diagnostic criteria. These criteria (Table 8–5) were developed primarily to aid in the appropriate diagnosis of patients who are included in research protocols, but they can be helpful to the clinician.

Clinicians have long used spinal fluid changes to support the diagnosis of MS. However, it should be recognized that CSF abnormalities are not diagnostic, as they are also present in other neurological and inflammatory diseases. The cardinal features of the MS CSF profile include increased IgG levels, qualitative abnormalities in CSF IgG (IgG oligoclonal bands), mild pleocytosis, and occasionally an elevation of myelin breakdown products such as myelin basic protein (MBP).

Although computed tomography (CT) is not as sensitive as magnetic resonance imaging (MRI) in the detection of

TABLE 8–5. DIAGNOSTIC CRITERIA FOR MS[a]

CLASSIFICATION	NUMBER OF ATTACKS	CLINICAL EVIDENCE (OBJECTIVE SIGNS)	PARACLINICAL EVIDENCE (CNS LESION)	CSF OB/IGG
Laboratory-supported probable MS	2			+
Laboratory-supported definite MS	2	1 area involved	or 1 area involved	+
	1	2 areas involved		+
	1	1 area involved	and 1 area involved	+
Clinically probable MS	2	1 area involved		
	1	2 areas involved		
	1	1 area involved	and 1 area involved	
Clinically definite MS	2	2 areas involved		
	2	1 area involved	and 1 area involved	

[a]An attack is the occurrence of a neurological symptom, with or without objective confirmation, lasting for 24 hours.
Two attacks are said to have occurred when different parts of the CNS have been affected and the attacks were separated by at least 1 month.
In this classification, "clinical evidence" means objective neurologic signs demonstrated by neurological examination; "paraclinical evidence" refers to the demonstration of a CNS lesion in the central nervous system by means of special testing such as neuroimaging procedures (MRI and CT) along with evoked potentials. The lesion may have produced symptoms but not signs.
Reprinted with permission, Poser CM, et al, New diagnositic criteria for MS: Guidelines for research protocols. Ann Neur. 1983;13:227.

abnormalities in MS, it nevertheless may demonstrate a wide variety of findings. Cerebral atrophy is the most common and least specific abnormality. It usually is seen in patients with long-standing MS, although sometimes it is observed early and probably is related to widespread cerebral lesions. Increased size of ventricles, cisterns, and sulci are seen commonly in MS, particularly in later stages of the disease, and suggest loss of brain tissue.

MRI is currently the preferred imaging technique for obtaining diagnostic support of MS. The typical abnormalities on MRI are most commonly located in the supratentorial white matter, especially in the periventricular region. They may appear as multiple discrete lesions, or they may coalesce to form more homogeneous borders surrounding the ventricles. Less commonly, lesions can be detected in the cerebellum and brainstem (Figure 8–1).

MRI is positive in 70 to 95% of patients with clinically definite MS. Of more importance, MRI has been found to support a diagnosis of MS in a high percentage of patients in whom the diagnosis was suspected. With isolated optic neuritis at initial examination, MRI detects disseminated lesions in 61% of the patients. The lesions were primarily found in the periventricular white matter of the cerebral hemispheres, brainstem, and cerebellum.

■ Ocular

Ophthalmic testing that will delineate ocular involvement (optic neuritis) in MS includes visual acuity testing, visual field testing, pupillary reflex testing, color vision assessment, contrast sensitivity testing, and VEP (visual evoked potential) assessment. Common eye movement abnormalities (INO, BINO, nystagmus) will be evident on external evaluation.

The pattern shift VEP is currently the most useful evoked potential test in diagnosing optic nerve involvement of MS. VEPs can provide objective evidence of an optic nerve lesion, with or without associated visual symptoma-

tology. However, VEP testing is not specific for MS; therefore the data from VEP testing should be placed in the context of the overall clinical picture.

Slit-like defects (Figure 8–2) in the peripapillary nerve fiber layer and corollary defects in the field of vision occur frequently in MS, often before there is a change in the patient's visual acuity, color perception, or optic disc. Nerve fiber defects have been observed in two thirds of MS patients. These defects indicate retrograde degeneration of

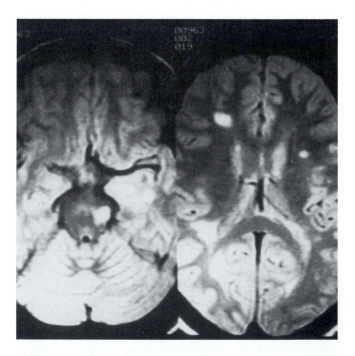

Figure 8–1. Plaque formation in MS. Left view shows plaque formation at the junction between the pons and midbrain; the right view shows a larger plaque in the white matter of the frontal lobe and a smaller plaque at the junction of the frontal and temporal lobes. (Courtesy of Dr. Lawrence Gray.)

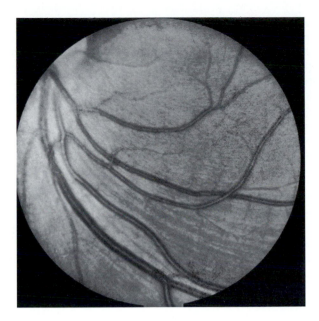

Figure 8–2. Slit-like defects in the peripapillary nerve fiber layer (NFL dropout).

scattered axon bundles from disease somewhere in the pregeniculate pathways.

TREATMENT AND MANAGEMENT

Because MS is thought by many to be an immunologically-mediated illness, immunosuppressive therapy may play a role in its management. The goals of immunosuppressive therapy in MS vary in accordance with the clinical stage of disease. The goals of therapy include (1) improving recovery from each exacerbation, (2) decreasing the number of future exacerbations, (3) decreasing the accumulation of additional disability, and (4) preventing the development of chronic progressive disease.

■ Systemic

The main therapy (Table 8–6) for acute exacerbations of MS has been adrenocorticotropic hormone (ACTH) or corticosteroids. Superior results have recently been found with high-dose intravenously administered methylprednisolone therapy. Both corticosteroid or ACTH therapy and IV administration of methylprednisolone produce a substantial decrease in the CSF IgG synthesis rate.

Beck and associates (1993) reported the results of a two-year study examining the risks of developing new demyelinating events following the treatment of acute optic neuritis with IV methylprednisolone followed by oral prednisone, or oral prednisone alone, or placebo. The results of this study have shown that those treated with IV methylprednisolone followed by oral prednisone had a reduction in

new clinical manifestations of MS over the next two years compared to the other two groups. This treatment strategy was most beneficial to those patients with multiple signal abnormalities on MRI at the time of diagnosis of optic neuritis. The value of treatment in those with normal MRI scans could not be adequately assessed.

Azathioprine and cyclophosphamide, agents with immunosupressive properties, also appear to play a role in the management of MS patients. The efficacy of cyclophosphamide and azathioprine in MS, however, is not universally accepted.

Other drug therapies in MS include anticholinergic drugs such as propantheline bromide for bladder function. Treatment for spasticity includes dantrolene, which acts at the level of the muscle, and diazepam and baclofen, which act centrally. Of all these therapies, baclofen, is the drug of choice for symptomatic spasticity in MS.

Patients with mild or transient depression may be managed with supportive measures. However, more severe depression is best managed with the addition of a tricyclic antidepressant such as amitriptyline.

A multidisciplinary approach to the care in MS is most effective because of the many systemic and neurological problems present. Physical and occupational therapy are often part of the comprehensive care required for the MS patient. A clinical psychologist also can play an important role in helping the patient deal with the depression that often accompanies this disease.

The use of recombinant interferon beta in patients with exacerbating–remitting MS has shown promising results, and in clinical trials it has been shown to decrease the frequency of flare-ups. Plasmapheresis, lymphoid irradiation, and cyclosporine A are other treatment modalities presently under investigation.

■ Ocular

The efficacy of corticosteroids and corticotropin as treatments for optic neuritis has been debated for many years.

TABLE 8–6. TREATMENT AND MANAGEMENT OF MS

■ **SYSTEMIC**
- ACTH
- Corticosteroids
- Anticholinergic drugs (bladder dysfunction)
- Muscle relaxants (spasticity)
- Tricyclic antidepressants (depression)
- Physical and occupational therapy
- Psychotherapeutic support

■ **OCULAR**
- Optic neuritis: no treatment or IV methylprednisolone followed by oral prednisone

The results of a multicenter, randomized clinical trial were reported in 1992 by Beck and associates. The results of this trial indicated that patients who received IV methylprednisolone followed by oral prednisone recovered vision faster than patients given placebo, but their visual outcome at the end of a 6-month follow-up period was only slightly better than that in the placebo group. Oral prednisone alone provided no benefit in terms of either the rate of recovery or the outcome at 6 months. However, Beck and associates (1993) reported the results of a study that found IV methylprednisone followed by oral prednisone as treatment for acute optic neuritis resulted in the reduction of subsequent new manifestations of MS. The authors report that these results justify the consideration of treatment of acute optic neuritis with IV methylprednisone followed by oral prednisone, even though the Optic Neuritis Treatment Trials results showed that this had only a marginal effect on visual recovery.

Counseling a patient who develops an acute unilateral idiopathic optic neuritis can be a complicated clinical dilemma. There may be a relatively long symptom-free interval between optic neuritis and the possible development of clinical MS. Therefore, some believe that it is not appropriate to inform the patient of this association. Speculating on the likelihood of developing MS is of no apparent benefit to the patient; however, the patient's right to know is a compelling argument in favor of disclosure. A varying spectrum of disclosure should be individually determined.

CONCLUSION

MS is a common neurological disorder whose ocular complications may be frequently encountered by the eyecare practitioner. With technological advances, the diagnosis of MS has become more definitive. However, this has done little to simplify management, patient apprehension, and prognosis. Rehabilitative and counseling services can provide improvement in quality of life for the MS patient. Ocular manifestations are common in MS; therefore, the eyecare practitioner is an integral part of the care and management of these patients.

REFERENCES

Archambean PL, Hollenhorst RW, Rucler CW. Posterior uveitis a manifestation of multiple sclerosis. *Mayo Clin Proc.* 1965;40:544.

Bachman DM, Rosenthal AR, Beckingsale AF. Granulomatous uveitis in neurological disease. *Br J Ophthalmol.* 1985;69:192.

Bamford CR, Ganley JP, Sibley WA, Laguna JF. Uveitis, perivenous sheathing and multiple sclerosis. *Neurology.* 1978;28:119.

Baum HM, Rothschild BB. The incidence and prevalence of reported multiple sclerosis in the United States. *Ann Neurol.* 1981;10:42.

Beck RW, Cleary PA, Anderson MM, et al. A Randomized, controlled trial of corticosteroids in the treatment of acute optic neuritis. *N Engl J Med.* 1992;326:581–588.

Beck RW, Cleary PA, Trobe JD, et al. The effect of corticosteroids for acute optic neuritis on the subsequent development of multiple sclerosis. *New Engl J Med.* 1993;329:1764–1769.

Bornstein MB, Miller A, Slagle S, Weitzman M. A pilot trial of Cop 1 in exacerbating–remitting multiple sclerosis. *N Engl J Med.* 1987;317:408.

Caroscio JT, Kochwa S, Sacks H, et al. Quantitative CSF IgG measurements in multiple sclerosis and other neurologic diseases. *Arch Neurol.* 1983;40:409.

Chiappa KG. Pattern-shift visual, brainstem auditory and short-latency somatosensory evoked potential in multiple sclerosis. *Ann NY Acad Sci.* 1984;436:315.

Chiappa KH. Evoked potentials in clinical medicine. In: Joynt RJ, ed. *Clinical Neurology.* Philadelphia: Lippincott; 1988;2:1–55.

Clifford DB, Trotter JL. Pain in multiple sclerosis. *Arch Neurol.* 1984;41:1270.

Cohen SR, Herndon RM, McKhann GM. Radioimmunoassay of myelin basic protein in spinal fluid: An index of active demyelination. *N Engl J Med.* 1976;295:1455.

Cox TA, Thompson HS, Clorbett JJ. Relative afferent pupillary defects in optic neuritis. *Am J Ophthalmol.* 1981;92:685.

Dailey FL, Brown JR, Goldstein F. Dysarthria in multiple sclerosis. *J Speech Hear Res.* 1972;15:229–245.

Durelli L, Cocito D, Riccio A, et al. High-dose intravenous methylpredisolone in the treatment of multiple sclerosis: Clinical–immunologic correlations. *Neurology.* 1986;36:238.

Farlow MR, Markand ON, Edwards MK, et al. Multiple sclerosis: Magnetic resonance imaging, evoked responses, and spinal fluid electrophoresis. *Neurology.* 1986;36:828.

Feinsod M, Hoyt WF. Subclinical optic neuropathy in multiple sclerosis. *J Neurol Neurosurg Psychiatr.* 1975;38:1190.

Frisen L, Hoyt WF. Insidious atrophy of retinal nerve fibers in multiple sclerosis. *Arch Ophthalmol.* 1974;92:91.

Gebarski SS, Gabrielson TO, Gilman S, Knake JE. The initial diagnosis of multiple sclerosis: Clinical impact of magnetic resonance imaging. *Ann Neurol.* 1985;17:469.

Grant I, McDonald WI, Trimble MR, et al. Deficient learning and memory in early and middle phases of multiple sclerosis. *J Neurol Neurosurg Psychiatr.* 1984;47:250.

Griffin JF, Wray SH. Acquired color vision defects in retrobulbar neuritis. *Am J Ophthalmol.* 1978;86:193.

Gyldensted C. Computer tomography of the cerebrum in multiple sclerosis. *Neuroradiology.* 1976;12:33.

Hauser SL, Bhan AK, Gilles F, et al. Immunohistochemical analysis of the cellular infiltrate in multiple sclerosis lesions. *Ann Neurol.* 1986;19:578.

Jensen TS, Rasmussen P, Reske-Nelsen E. Association of trigeminal neuralgia with multiple sclerosis: Clinical and pathological features. *Acta Neurol Scand.* 1982;65:182.

Kurtze JF, Beebe GW, Norman JE. Epidemiology of multiple sclerosis in U.S. veterans, 3. Migration and the risk of MS. *Neurology.* 1985;35:672.

Link H, Laurenze MA. Immunoglobulin class and light chain type of oligoclonal bands in CSF in multiple sclerosis determined by agarose gel electrophoresis and immunofixation. *Ann Neurol*. 1979;6:107.

Lukes SA, Crooks LE, Aminoff MJ, et al. Nuclear magnetic resonance imaging in multiple sclerosis. *Ann Neurol*. 1983;13:592.

Mastaglia FL, Black JL, Collins DWK. Quantitative studies of saccadic and pursuit eye movements in multiple sclerosis. *Brain*. 1979;102:817.

Mastaglia FL, Black JL, Thickbroom G, Collins DWK. Saccadic eye movements in multiple sclerosis. *Neuro-ophthalmol*. 1982;4:225.

Miller AE. Cessation of stuttering with progressive multiple sclerosis. *Neurology*. 1985;35:1341–1343.

Muri RM, Meienberg O. The clinical spectrum of internuclear ophthalmoplegia in multiple sclerosis. *Arch Neurol*. 1885;42:851.

Ormerod IEC, McDonald WI, duBoulay GH, et al. Disseminated lesions at presentation in patients with optic neuritis. *J Neurol Neurosurg Psychiatr*. 1986;49:124–127.

Paty DW, Oger JJF, Kastrukoff LF, et al. MRI in the diagnosis of MS: A prospective study with comparison of clinical evaluation, evoked potentials, oligoclonal banding, and CT. *Neurology*. 1988;38:180.

Paty DW, Poser CM. Clinical symptoms and signs of multiple sclerosis. In: Poser CM, ed. *The Diagnosis of Multiple Sclerosis*. New York: Thieme & Stratton; 1984:37.

Poser S, Wikstrom J, Bauer HJ. Clinical data and the identification of special forms of multiple sclerosis in 1271 cases studied with a standardized documentation system. *J Neurolog Sci*. 1979;40:159–168.

Poser S. *The Diagnosis of Multiple Sclerosis*. New York: Thieme; 1984.

Prineas JW. The neuropathology of multiple sclerosis. In: Vinken PG, Bruyn GW, Klawans HL, eds. *Handbook of Clinical Neurology*. Vol 47: *Demyelinating Diseases*. New York: Elsevier; 1985:213–257.

Rose AS, Kuzma JW, Kurtzke JF, et al. Cooperative study in the evaluation of therapy in multiple sclerosis: ACTH vs placebo; final report. *Neurology*. 1970;29:1–59.

Schiffer RB, Babigian HM. Behavior disorders in multiple sclerosis, temporal lobe epilepsy, and amyotropiclateral sclerosis. An epidemiologic study. *Arch Neurol*. 1984;41:1067.

Schiffer RB, Herndon RM, Rudick RA. Treatment of pathologic laughing and weeping with amitriptyline. *N Engl J Med*. 1985;312:1480.

Swanson J. M.S.: Update in diagnosis and review of prognostic factors. *Mayo Clinic Proc*. 1989;64:578–585.

Szasz G, Paty D, Maurice WL. Sexual dysfunctions in multiple sclerosis. *Ann NY Acad Sci*. 1984;436:443.

Thompson HS, Corbett JJ, Cox TA. How to measure the afferent pupillary defect. *Surg Ophthalmol*. 1981;26:39.

Tourtellotte WW, Baumhefner RW, Rotvin AR, et al. Multiple sclerosis de novo CNS IgG synthesis: Effect of ACTH and corticosteroids. *Neurology*. 1980;30:1155.

Troiano R, Hafstein M, Ruderman M, et al. Effect of high-dose intravenous steroid administration on contrast-enhancing computed tomographic scan lesions in multiple sclerosis. *Ann Neurol*. 1984;15:257.

Valleroy ML, Kraft GH. Sexual dysfunction in multiple sclerosis. *Arch Phys Med Rehabil*. 1984;65:125.

Weinshenker BG, Ebers GC. The natural history of multiple sclerosis. *Can J Neurol Sci*. 1987;14:255.

Whitaker JN, Gupta M, Smith OF. Epitopes of immunoreactive myelin basic protein in human cerebrospinal fluid. *Ann Neurol*. 1986;20:329.

9
Chapter

Alzheimer Disease

Susan C. Oleszewski

Alzheimer disease (AD), which becomes more prevalent with age, is a major cause of dementia in the older population. It is characterized by a progressive loss of memory, orientation, and other cognitive functions. As the population continues to become older, its incidence will increase further. Ocular manifestations of AD are not prominent and are usually the result of degeneration of the visual association areas of the cortex.

EPIDEMIOLOGY

■ Systemic

Alzheimer disease is a major cause of dementia; however, exact data on the prevalence of dementia or AD is not available. It is estimated that 4 to 5% of the U. S. population over age 65 has severe dementia, and that an additional 10% has mild to moderate impairment. In the 65- to 70-year age group, the prevalence of severe dementia is only 1% or less, but in those over 85, the fastest-growing segment of the population, the prevalence rises to over 15%. At this rate of increase, and as life expectancy extends into the late 90s (as anticipated by about the year 2040), an astonishing 45% of the population is likely to develop dementia.

Few studies exist on the incidence of AD in the general population. The most reliable data suggest an incidence rate of 0.7 and 0.5% for men and women, respectively, aged 70 to 79; and 1.9 and 2.5% for men and women aged 80 years and older.

■ Ocular

Although there is a broad range of visual system disorders in AD, data are not available on the percentages of patients who suffer from these disorders. At present it is known that AD patients vary considerably in extent of their visual system pathology. Most of the abnormalities are associated with the visual association cortex, rather than the retina and visual pathway.

NATURAL HISTORY

■ Systemic

Consistent changes are found in the brains of the AD patients. These include atrophy, especially a loss of synapses in the cortex; the presence of abnormally stained neurons, called neurofibrillary tangles; and the presence of numerous neuritic plaques (focal collections of degenerating nerve terminals that surround a core of an abnormal fibrillar protein, B-amyloid). Additionally, the cholinergic projection system to the neocortex is altered in AD, as indicated by decreased levels of choline acetyltransferase, a marker of cholinergic neurons. The decreased cholinergic function in the neocortex has been found to correlate well with the degree of dementia associated with AD. Many of the changes in the neocortex are part of the normal aging process; however, they seem to be markedly exaggerated in Alzheimer patients.

The course of AD is characterized by progressive cognitive and functional decline. It is important to stress that the course of the disease is quite variable. This may range from an individual with mild forgetfulness for a number of years, to a rapid decline.

The onset and details of the early course of the disease are often difficult to establish. The demented patient may be an unreliable witness, and the early symptoms are often so subtle as to escape the notice of even the most attentive family member or associate. Most often the initial symptoms are impaired memory, difficulty with problem solving, failure to respond to the environment with customary speed and accuracy, and easy distractibility. As the patient becomes more aware of the loss of mental efficiency, depression frequently occurs, taking a toll on mental function (Table 9–1).

Inability to recall acquired material of an impersonal nature is the most apparent memory defect in AD. Environmental disorientation is also common in AD. Patients are unable to find their way around familiar surroundings, including their own homes. They may have a tendency to wander and may become agitated, especially at night ("sundowning").

Language dysfunction is evident in AD patients, with dysnomia (incorrect naming of objects) usually the initial manifestation. This may lead to some form of dysphasia, which is encountered in almost every AD patient. This speech disorder usually progresses to a fluent aphasia, where there may be remarkable preservation of grammar and prose but the conversation is often devoid of ideas and can be called "empty speech." Alexia (inability to read), as well as agraphia (inability to write), are also common in AD patients.

Extrapyramidal signs, particularly rigidity and hypokinesia (decreased movements), frequently occur in patients with AD, especially those with severe dementia. Tremor is less prominent than in other degenerative disorders, as are other dyskinesias. Disorders of gait, limb paralysis, seizures, and urinary incontinence are less prominent and appear later than the dementia.

AD has three phases. In the initial phase, the patient becomes aware of intellectual or memory impairment, but the mild symptoms are not noticed by family and friends. As the disease progresses into the second phase, close family and friends begin to notice the patient's difficulties with memory, intellect, and judgment. Finally, in the third stage the patient loses awareness of the illness, but the symptoms are so advanced as not to be missed by those around the patient. The clinical and behavioral observations of patients in these three stages are further delineated in Table 9–2.

TABLE 9–1. COMMON SYSTEMIC MANIFESTATIONS OF AD

- Aphasia
- Impaired memory
- Difficulty with problem solving
- Dysphagia
- Alexia
- Agraphia
- Extrapyramidal signs (rigidity and hypokinesia)
- Prosopagnosia
- Environmental disorientation

TABLE 9–2. STAGES OF AD

Stage 1

Memory loss
Lack of spontaneity
Subtle personality changes
Disorientation to time and date

Stage 2

Impaired cognition and abstract thinking
Restlessness and agitation
Wandering, "sundowning"
Inability to carry out activities of daily living
Impaired judgment
Inappropriate social behavior
Lack of insight, abstract thinking
Repetitive behavior
Voracious appetite

Stage 3

Emaciation, indifference to food
Inability to communicate
Urinary and fecal incontinence
Seizures

Reprinted with permission from Matteson MA, McConnell ES, Gerontological Nursing: Concepts and Practice. *Philadelphia: Saunders; 1988:251.*

The progression of AD is a relentless process that occurs over 2 to 10 years or longer. The expected survival, following a diagnosis of AD, is between 5 and 15 years.

AD alone does not cause death. Rather, death usually results from a concurrent infection that is exacerbated by extreme weight loss, weakness, decreased metabolism, and dehydration. Bronchopneumonia is one of the major infections responsible for the death of AD patients. Stroke and myocardial infarction have also been identified as complications that may be associated with morbidity.

■ Ocular

Ocular manifestations of AD are not prominent. Findings consist of subtle disturbances of function that may or may not be noticed by the patient or family members. A broad range of visual disorders in AD may result from the involvement of the visual association cortex and optic nerves (Table 9–3).

Visuospatial difficulties are common. Agnosia, the inability to recognize familiar objects, is common, and is present in almost half of AD patients, resulting in a major source of disability. It may manifest as visuospatial agnosia (loss of visuospatial orientation), prosopagnosia (difficulty in facial recognition), simultanagnosia (inability to attend to more than one visual object at the same time), and topographagnosia (inability to follow a route).

TABLE 9–3. OCULAR MANIFESTATIONS OF AD

- Optic nerve degeneration
- Dyschromatopsia
- Depressed contrast sensitivity
- Impaired ocular motility/reading difficulty
- Visuospatial disorientation
- Agnosia
    Visual: visuospatial, prosopagnosia, simultanagnosia
    Spatial: Balint syndrome (simultanagnosia, oculomotor apraxia, optic ataxia)
- Apraxia, constructional
    Oculomotor
- Hallucinations
- Impaired saccades, pursuits, tracking, and scanning

Difficulties locating objects in space occur frequently, along with loss of the sense of "whereness" and clumsiness in attempts to reach for objects or avoiding bumping into them. This "spatial agnosia" is responsible for visual localization difficulties, a common complaint in AD. Spatial agnosia may also cause abnormalities in scanning, searching, and hand–eye coordination severe enough to constitute Balint syndrome in up to 20% of AD patients. Balint syndrome consists of simultanagnosia, oculomotor apraxia (inaccurate eye movements), and optic ataxia (inability to direct hand or other movements by visuospatial guidance). Constructional apraxia (inability to draw a design such as a circle, triangle, or clock face) may also occur in AD patients.

An early symptom of AD is the complaint of reading difficulty; specifically, losing one's place on the line or page, dancing of print, and blurred vision. Hallucinations may occur in up to 20% of patients with AD, and 80 to 90% of these are visual hallucinations.

Acuity is often difficult to confidently assess in Alzheimer patients because of their underlying dementia. Nonetheless, acuity of patients with AD appears to be normal, at least in the earlier stages of the disease.

There is both histological and clinical evidence that AD damages the retina and optic nerve. Degeneration has been noted in both the optic nerves and the retinas of mild and severe AD patients. Specific histological findings include widespread axonal degeneration, preferential loss of large-diameter axons, loss of retinal ganglion cells, and thinning of the nerve fiber layer. Optic nerve head pallor has been observed in AD patients.

Abnormal color vision has been reported and a significant percentage of errors fall in the tritan (blue) category. Dyschromatopsia may be one manifestation of the optic neuropathy of AD. Examination of the visual system in AD may reveal visual field defects, prolonged visual evoked potentials, abnormal eye movement recordings, and decreased contrast sensitivity. Contrast sensitivity studies

have yielded contradictory results that may reflect differences in patient selection.

Saccadic velocity, latency, and accuracy have been found to be abnormal with a higher frequency of ocular velocity arrests during smooth pursuits. Additionally, a significant correlation between the severity of the dementia and the frequency of velocity arrests during smooth pursuit has been found. Eye tracking (slow eye movements) and visual scanning have also been found to be abnormal in AD patients.

DIAGNOSIS

■ Systemic

Alzheimer disease is a clinical diagnosis of exclusion. The physical exam, including the detailed neurological examination, is usually normal. The definitive diagnosis is histopathologic. Nonetheless, there are several diagnostic tests that are helpful. The clinician must rule out other systemic diseases, organic or psychogenic brain disorders that might account for the impairment in memory and cognitive function. Clinical analysis must also include a detailed inventory of all medications that the patient may be taking, along with a study of their interactions and side effects. Any medications suspected of affecting memory and cognitive function should be discontinued if possible, and the patient observed without medication before the final diagnosis.

The following criteria support a clinical diagnosis of *probable AD*. The onset of cognitive and memory disturbances must occur between ages 40 and 90. There must be no systemic disorders or other neurologic disease that could account for the cognitive and memory deficits. Dementia must be established and documented through neuropsychologic testing. There must be deficits in two or more areas of cognition, and no disturbances of consciousness.

The diagnosis of *probable AD* is supported if there is progressive deterioration of specific cognitive functions such as language (aphasia), motor skills (apraxia), and perception (agnosia). Family history of similar disorders further assists an AD diagnosis. A diagnosis of AD will be further supported by impaired activities of daily living, as well as altered patterns of behavior.

Standard laboratory testing is often used to rule out other disorders, rather than to definitively diagnose AD. Electroencephalography (EEG) will either show normal patterns or nonspecific changes. Computerized tomography (CT) studies are essential to exclude intracranial structural disorders. CT also provides evidence of cerebral atrophy with progression documented by serial observation. Magnetic resonance imaging (MRI) has not been applied in a systematic way to aid in the diagnosis of AD. More recently, positron emission tomography (PET) has found

TABLE 9–4. COMPARISON OF DIAGNOSTIC CRITERIA FOR AD

Criteria	Possible	Probable	Definite
Dementia present			
Clinical evaluation	R	R	R
Mental status tests	R	R	
Cognitive deficit in two or more areas	+	R	
Impairment of function	+	+	
Onset age 40–90	+	R	
Insidious onset	+	+	
Progressive course	R	R	
Exclusive of systemic or brain disorders that may produce dementia	+	R	
Tests:			
Normal lumbar puncture	+	+	
EEG normal or slowing	+	+	
CT atrophy	+	+	
Absence of focal motor or sensory changes	+	+	
Histologic changes characteristic of AD			R

R, required; +, desirable/not required.
(Reprinted from Katzman R, Lasker B, Bernstein N. Advances in the diagnosis of dementia: Accuracy of diagnosis and consequences of misdiagnosis of disorders causing dementia. In: Terry RD, ed. New York; Raven: 1988, p 48.)

significant reductions in glucose metabolism in both cerebral hemispheres of Alzheimer patients.

After excluding other causes of dementia, clinical features consistent with the diagnosis of *probable AD* include associated symptoms of depression; insomnia; incontinence; delusions; hallucinations; verbal, emotional, or physical outbursts; sexual disorders; and weight loss. Other neurological abnormalities that occur in advanced disease include motor signs such as increased muscle tone, myoclonus, or gait disorder. Seizures are rare, but may be present in advanced disease.

A Work Group on the Diagnosis of Alzheimer's Disease was established by the National Institute of Neurological and Communicative Disorders and Stroke (NINCDS) and the Alzheimer's Disease and Related Disorders Association (ADRDA). Diagnostic criteria from the NINCDS–ADRDA Work Group are summarized in Table 9–4.

Advancing age and family history of AD are significant risk factors. There is some clinical evidence that prior head trauma may be a potential risk factor for AD. Identifying aluminum compounds in association with the neurofibrillary tangles and the core plaques that occur in the brains of AD patients has caused speculation that exposure to high levels of aluminum may be an additional risk in developing AD. Down syndrome or a family history of Down syndrome, and thyroid disease, are considered additional risk factors.

■ Ocular

Of special interest to eyecare practitioners is the prominence of visual symptoms at a time when the diagnosis is still uncertain. While there is nothing pathognomonic about visual symptoms of patients with AD, clinicians ought to be aware that early symptoms of patients with AD may be visual in nature.

TREATMENT AND MANAGEMENT

Drug treatment and other intervention strategies (Table 9–5) to prevent or delay progression of the disease have been limited, primarily because so little is known about the cause or risk factors for the disease. Ideally, treatment would either involve replacement therapy or drugs, which prevent or delay the pathologic changes that occur in AD.

Nerve growth factor (NGF) in rats is known to protect the cortical cholinergic system following experimental injury. Additionally, NGF improves the maze learning performance of impaired elderly rats. NGF is viewed by some as a potential experimental treatment that may play some role in future management modalities for AD patients.

Therapy with tetrahydroaminoacridine (tacrine), a cholinesterase inhibitor, may result in significant symptomatic

TABLE 9–5. TREATMENT AND MANAGEMENT OF AD

- Cholinesterase inhibitors
- Antipsychotics (haloperidol)
- Sedatives (chloral hydrate)
- Counseling:
  - Family counseling
  - Genetic counseling
  - Support groups
- Day care

improvement in mild to moderate AD. Presently there is no evidence that tacrine, or any other treatment, modifies the course of AD.

Drugs are useful primarily for symptomatic treatment of the depression, agitation, or sleep disorders associated with AD. In some cases, agitated or aggressive behavior may require administration of a neuroleptic agent (haloperidol) to allow the patient to remain within his or her family or social situation.

The most meaningful aspect of the care and management of AD should involve the maintenance of the patient's socialization and support for the family. Self-help groups that provide both educational and psychological support have proliferated during recent years. Daycare and respite centers can provide needed relief for the caregivers.

It appears that the earlier the onset and the more severe the disease, the higher the risk to the relatives. Geneticists differ in their interpretation of the data; some have suggested a predisposing autosomal dominant gene with age-related penetrance, reaching 40% at the age of 90 years. Heyman and associates (1984) postulated that the familial pattern is best explained by a single gene with typical autosomal dominant inheritance.

CONCLUSION

Alzheimer disease is the major cause of admission to nursing homes, and it is an important cause of chronic disability in the elderly. The emotional and socioeconomic price that society must pay for longevity is the tragic reality of caring for the AD patient. The visual system abnormalities contribute to the disability caused by AD, and may magnify the effects of other cognitive deficits.

The future challenges for those committed to research in AD are to understand its cause and to intervene to prevent the disease or halt its progression. Better diagnostic capabilities must be developed, along with improved treatment modalities.

REFERENCES

Barclay LL, Zemov A, Blass JP, Sansome J. Survival in Alzheimer's disease and vascular dementias. *Neurology.* 1985;35:834–840.

Cogan DG. Visual disturbances with focal progressive dementing disease. *Am J Ophthalmol.* 1985;100:68.

Corkin SH, Growdon JH, Nissen MJ, et al. Recent advances in the neuropsychological study of Alzheimer's disease. In: Wurtman J, Corkin SH, Growdon JH, eds. *Alzheimer Disease: Advances in Basic Research and Therapies.* Proceedings of the third meeting of the International Study Group on the Treatment of Memory Disorders Associated with Aging. Zurich: Center for Brain Sciences and Metabolism Charitable Trust; 1984:75.

Cronin-Golomb A, Corkin S, Rizzo JF, et al. Visual dysfunction in Alzheimer's disease: Relation to normal aging. *Ann Neurol.* 1991;29:41.

Eagger SA, Levy R, Sahakian BJ. Tacrine in Alzheimer disease. *Lancet.* 1991;337:989–992.

Evans DA, Scherr PA, Cook NR, et al. Impact of Alzheimer's disease in the United States population. In: Suzman R, Willis DP, eds. *The Oldest Old.* London: Oxford; 1992.

Fletcher WA, Sharpe JA. Saccadic eye movements dysfunction in Alzheimer disease. *Ann Neurol.* 1986;20:464.

Foster NL, Chase TN, Mansi L, et al: Cortical abnormalities in AD. *Ann Neurol.* 1984;16:649.

Henderson AS. The epidemiology of Alzheimer's disease. *Br Med Bull.* 1986;42:3.

Heyman A, Wilkinson WE, Hurwitz BJ, et al. Alzheimer's disease: A study of epidemiology aspects. *Ann Neurol.* 1984;15:335.

Hershey LA, Whicker L, Abel LA, et al. Saccadic latency measurements in dementia. *Arch Neurol.* 1983;40:592.

Hinton, DR, Sadun AA, Blanks JC, Miller CA. Optic nerve degeneration in Alzheimer's disease. *N Engl J Med.* 1986;315:485.

Hutton JT. Eye movements and Alzheimer disease: Significance and relationship to visuospatial confusion. In: Hutton JT, Kennedy AD, eds. *Senile Dementia of the Alzheimer Type.* New York: Liss; 1985:3–33.

Hutton JT, Nagel JA, Loewenson RB. Eye tracking dysfunction in Alzheimer-type dementia. *Neurology.* 1984;34:99.

Katz B, Rimmer S, Iragui V, Katzman R. Abnormal pattern ERG in AD: Evidence for retinal ganglion cell degeneration. *Ann Neurol.* 1989;26:221.

Katzman R. Alzheimer disease. *N Engl J Med.* 1986;314:964.

Larson EB, Kukull WA, Katzman RL. Cognitive impairment: dementia and Alzheimer's disease. *Ann Rev Pub Health.* 1992;13:431–449.

Lewis DA, Campbell MJ, Terry RD, Morrison JH. Laminar and regional distributions of neurofibrillary tangles and neuritic plaques in Alzheimer's disease: A quantitative study of visual and auditory cortices. *J Neurosci.* 1987;7:1799.

Matteson MA, McConnell ES. *Gerontological Nursing: Concepts and Practice.* Philadelphia: Saunders; 1988.

McKhann G, Drachman D, Folstein M, et al. Clinical diagnosis of the NINCDS-ADRDA Work Group under the auspices of Department of Health and Human Services Task Force on Alzheimer's Disease. *Neurology.* 1984;34:939.

Mendes MD, Mendez MA, Martin R, et al. Complex visual disturbances in Alzheimer's disease. *Neurology.* 1990;40:439.

Pearson RCA, Esiri MM, Hiorn RW, et al. Anatomical correlates of the distribution of the pathological changes in the neocortex in Alzheimer's disease. *Proc Natl Acad Sci USA.* 1985; 82:4531.

Sadun AA. The optic neuropathy of Alzheimer's disease. *Metab Pediatr Syst Opthalmol.* 1989;12:64.

Sadun AA, et al. Assessment of visual impairment in patients in AD. *Am J Ophthalmol.* 1987;104:113.

Sadun AA, Miao M, Johnson BM. Morphometric analysis of optic nerve axons in patients with Alzheimer's disease. *Invest Opthamol Vis Sci.* 1986;27(suppl):198. Abstract.

Terry RD, Katzman R. Senile dementia of the Alzheimer type. *Ann Neurol.* 1983;14:497.

Terry RD, Peck A, DeTeresa R, et al. Some morphometric aspects of the brain in senile dementia of Alzheimer type. *Ann Neurol.* 1981;10:184.

Trick GL, Barris ML, Bickler-Bluth M. Abnormal-pattern ERG in patients with senile dementia of ADT. *Ann Neurol.* 1989;26:226.

Wright CE, Drasdo N, Harding GF. Pathology of the optic nerve and visual association areas. Information given by the flash and pattern visual evoked potential and the temporal and spatial contrast sensitivity function. *Brain.* 1987;110:107.

10
Chapter

Parkinson Disease

Susan C. Oleszewski

Parkinson disease (PD), also known as parkinsonism or Parkinson syndrome, is a disorder consisting of tremor, rigidity, postural changes, and a decrease in spontaneous movement. This disorder is associated with several pathologic processes that damage the extrapyramidal system. It is considered Parkinson syndrome when etiologic causes such as infection, intoxication, vascular disease, and degenerative disease can be identified. However, this disorder is most commonly the degenerative or idiopathic type, in which case it is called Parkinson disease.

Although visual disturbances are not a major component of PD, a number of ocular motor abnormalities may be present, as well as loss in contrast sensitivity.

EPIDEMIOLOGY

■ Systemic

The worldwide prevalence of PD is between 90 and 100 per 100,000 population. There are approximately 200,000 patients with PD in this country, and approximately 40,000 new cases in the United States each year. The prevalence is similar in other countries. PD affects all ethnic groups and socioeconomic classes, with no sex predilection. Familial cases of PD are rare. It is estimated that PD makes up 1 to 2% of all neurological disorders.

PD usually begins in persons between 40 and 70 years of age, with the peak age of onset in the sixth decade. In the United States, about 1% of the population over 50 years of age is affected. It is infrequent before 30 years of age.

■ Ocular

Although ocular and visual disturbances associated with PD are commonly seen, prevalence and incidence data are not available.

NATURAL HISTORY

Most patients with PD have the degenerative or idiopathic type, and no clear cause can be demonstrated through diagnos-

tic testing. However, PD can be secondarily caused by infections (eg, encephalitis), intoxication (eg, carbon monoxide poisoning), vascular or arteriosclerotic disease, and brain tumors.

There is a loss of pigmented neurons in the substantia nigra of the midbrain in PD. Nigral neurons are a specialized population of nerve cells that contain neuromelanin and manufacture the neurotransmitter dopamine. Loss of neurons in the substantia nigra is a lifelong process that occurs in normal brains; however, when the number of dopaminergic neurons is reduced by 75 to 80%, PD occurs. Reduced levels of norepinephrine, serotonin, gamma-aminobutyric acid (GABA), and a number of neuropeptides and enzymes necessary for dopamine metabolism, have been reported as well.

Diffuse cortical atrophy may also be found in patients with idiopathic PD. These patients have more cortical degeneration and more dementia than other patients of similar age without PD, suggesting a diffuse degenerative brain disease. When dementia is marked, the changes in the brain outside the substantia nigra are similar to those found in Alzheimer disease, suggesting that some cases of PD may be variants of senile dementia.

■ Systemic

Parkinson disease is characterized by tremor, rigidity, and dyskinesia or difficulty with voluntary movement (Table

10–1). Any one of these signs may predominate. In the majority of patients, PD develops insidiously and progresses slowly. Initial symptoms may consist of aching pains in the neck, back, or limbs. Such pain may precede the appearance of motility disturbances by months or years. Although absent in about 30% of patients, tremor is usually the first feature that makes the patient aware of the disorder. This begins most commonly in one of the upper extremities. As the disorder progresses, the tremor worsens and spreads to other limbs.

The tremor of PD is characteristically regular and rhythmic. It is made noticeably worse with attention or in stressful situations. It may become so marked that patients are nearly disabled by it. The tremor is less severe or absent when relaxed. As rigidity increases, it may be dampened or even abolished. "Pill rolling" is a characteristic PD hand tremor that many patients with the disease manifest. In general, tremor is not as disabling as the rigidity and bradykinesia (sluggishness of movement).

When bradykinesia and rigidity are the initial manifestations, patients report difficulty in walking, attempting to stand, getting in and out of bed, and turning in bed. Patients feel as if they are walking or moving against great resistance. As rigidity becomes more prominent, postural changes become apparent. Patients develop a simian-like posture, with slight flexion of all joints, such as ankles, hips, back, and neck.

These patients often feel insecure walking in crowds, because they may lose their balance easily and fall forward. In an effort to restore balance, they may break into a small-stepped run or propulsive gait. Lack of postural reflexes thus leads to frequent falls due to the inability to correct the imbalance by appropriate arm or leg movements. Ambulatory patterns therefore may include difficulty starting to walk (start hesitation), shuffling, or taking many tiny steps and then walking faster and faster (festination). Decreased arm swing excursion typically accompanies the stride.

TABLE 10–1. SYSTEMIC MANIFESTATIONS OF PD

- Tremor
- Rigidity
- Bradykinesia
- Gait disturbances
- Postural changes
- Loss of facial expression (mask-like face)
- Infrequent blinking (reptilian stare)
- Micrographia
- Sialorrhea
- Dementia
- Sleep disturbances
- Depression

An early manifestation of hypokinesia is the loss of facial expression, which results in a mask-like face. Infrequent eye blinking also contributes to the staring look of PD (reptilian stare).

Changes in handwriting may be an early manifestation of PD. Writing is agonizingly slow and the script is often small (micrographia), letters are tightly bunched together, and the ends of lines tend to veer downward or upward.

Sialorrhea, or drooling, may be found in patients with PD. This is a loss of the autonomic process of clearing the throat and swallowing, rather than an excess production of saliva.

The speech patterns of PD patients are distinctive. Their voices lack volume and force. Their speech is monotonous and has a rapid, staccato quality. Enunciation is often impaired.

Dementia has been recognized as part of PD, with a prevalence of about 30 to 50%. The etiology of the dementia has yet to be determined. Sleep disturbances and depression may also be found in PD.

Characteristically, a gradual increase in all of the manifestations of PD occurs. Before L-dopa treatment was available, 25% of patients with symptoms of less than 5 years duration were severely disabled, while 75% of the patients with symptoms of 10 to 15 years duration who survived, were completely disabled. Patients with bradykinesia and rigidity have a poorer prognosis than those with tremor as their main manifestation. PD in itself does not lead to death, but increased mortality occurs because of debility, aspiration pneumonia, urinary tract infections, and decubitus ulcers.

■ Ocular

Ocular motor and visual abnormalities can occur at any stage of the disease process (Table 10–2). Blepharospasm occurs without apparent cause and it may be the earliest evidence of PD. It may be severe enough to impair vision. Blepharoplegia, real or apparent weakness of eyelid closure, may also be observed, and many patients show infrequency of blinking. Paradoxically, it has been observed that frequent blinking movements occur when quick thrusts are made toward the eyes with a finger. A more useful test is to tap on the glabella. This glabellar tap results in a blink that cannot be suppressed in a PD patient (Myerson sign) as it can in normals.

Patients with PD may manifest abnormalities in saccadic and pursuit movements. Saccades are characteristically hypometric, particularly in the vertical plane. Some patients cannot move their eyes laterally unless there is a preceding eyelid blink (Wilson sign).

Ocular motor abnormalities result in defective eye–head coordination. Patients may tend to move their head much later than normal individuals, in response to visual targets. Also, full lateral movements of the eyes may be obtained

TABLE 10–2. OCULAR MANIFESTATIONS OF PD

- Blepharospasm
- Blepharoplegia
- Myerson sign
- Wilson sign
- Abnormal saccades and pursuits
- Convergence insufficiency
- Decreased contrast sensitivity
- Abnormal VEPs

VEPs, visually evoked potentials.

only in association with parallel movement of the head (doll's-head phenomenon).

Convergence insufficiency is another physical finding in PD. Defective convergence or accommodation in PD patients can result in part from medication.

Although motor manifestations are the main PD sequelae, the generalized dopaminergic deficiency is also responsible for visual dysfunction. These include loss of contrast sensitivity and abnormal visually evoked potentials (VEPs). The site of the altered visual function in PD is still unknown.

DIAGNOSIS

■ Systemic
Diagnosis of PD is generally made on the basis of findings in the physical and neurological examinations, as well as general observation of the patient. The major motor signs such as tremor, rigidity, hypokinesia, bradykinesia, and abnormalities in gait are usually quite evident on neurologic examination.

Electroencephalography (EEG), computed tomography (CT), and magnetic resonant imaging (MRI) do not provide diagnostic information specific to PD, other than to rule out diseases that may mimic it, such as tumors affecting basal ganglia function.

■ Ocular
There are several ocular motor signs that present in PD. Although these signs are supportive of a diagnosis of PD, they are not generally diagnostic.

TREATMENT AND MANAGEMENT

■ Systemic
There is no known cure for PD. Treatment has been directed toward relieving symptoms and signs rather than altering the course of the disease (Table 10–3).

The earliest effective treatment for PD was with belladonna derivatives. These anticholinergic agents appear to relieve tremor and lessen rigidity. They provide only a modest improvement in symptoms, which progress despite medical therapy. The most commonly used anticholinergic drugs are trihexyphenidyl hydrochloride (Artane), procyclidine (Kemadrin), benztropine mesylate (Cogentin), and ethopropazone (Parsidol).

Since the introduction of L-dopa (levo-dopa) treatment, the course of PD has changed dramatically. L-Dopa is clearly the most effective medication available. L-Dopa greatly decreases hypokinesia, bradykinesia, rigidity, and tremor, even though postural instability may persist. In addition, some patients become more alert and have improved mental function. Administration of anticholinergic drugs may provide an additive effect when taken with L-dopa.

The side-effects of L-dopa are common and may be quite distressing. Nausea is the most common adverse effect encountered soon after initiating L-dopa therapy. Nausea tends to decrease during long-term therapy and is seldom a problem when L-dopa is given in conjunction with a decarboxylase inhibitor. Abnormal involuntary movements (dyskinesia) are the most striking side-effect of L-dopa. At least 80% of patients develop these movements at some time during treatment. The dyskinetic movements include lip smacking, tongue movements, grimacing, dystonic twisting of the trunk and the extremities, and motor restlessness. These abnormal movements are dose-related side effects, and can be relieved by reducing the dose; but they may reappear.

The mortality rate has been reduced by half since the introduction of L-dopa. Despite the potential for troublesome adverse effects with chronic L-dopa therapy, many patients continue to have a substantial response to the drug for a decade or more.

The use of dopa-decarboxylase inhibitors (eg, carbidopa) in conjunction with L-dopa has become the preferred therapy for PD patients. This combination (L-dopa/carbidopa) lowers the required total daily dose of L-dopa, which in turn markedly reduces or eliminates its side effects.

Amantadine hydrochloride (Symmetrel), an antiviral agent, also relieves symptoms. Amantadine is effective in approximately 60% of patients and partially relieves

TABLE 10–3. TREATMENT AND MANAGEMENT OF PD

- L-Dopa in conjunction with dopa-decarboxylase inhibitors (eg, carbidopa)
- Anticholinergic agents (eg, Cogentin)
- Amantadine hydrochloride (Symmetrel)
- Surgical implantation of fetal adrenal tissue (experimental)

rigidity, akinesia, and to a lesser extent, tremor. In patients who are responding to L-dopa, amantadine may potentiate the effect of L-dopa, prolonging the period of therapeutic benefit. Although levodopa and other drugs do not alter the progression of the disease, they do increase survival time because of improved functional capacity.

Surgical destruction of areas of the ventral thalamus has had some success in alleviating tremor in young patients with unilateral PD. Surgery is contraindicated for the elderly patient with advanced bilateral PD with predominant bradykinesia and rigidity. Surgical implantation of adrenal tissue into basal ganglia may benefit some patients. Implantation of human fetal dopaminergic cells, though controversial, has shown promising results. Tissue implantation techniques, however, are still being evaluated for efficacy.

■ Ocular

The eyelid and ocular motility deficits of PD patients are challenging problems that are rarely successfully addressed in isolation. In general, the nonocular problems in PD are considered much more serious, with management directed at alleviating them. Some of the ocular manifestations may be decreased with the use of systemic therapy.

CONCLUSION

The diagnosis of PD is usually based on the cardinal manifestations of bradykinesia, rigidity, tremor, and the characteristic disorder of posture and gait. Ocular motor disturbances are also frequent manifestations that reflect the affected extrapyramidal system in PD. Recognition of these signs, understanding the course of the disease, and medical co-management challenges the primary eyecare practitioner.

REFERENCES

Adams RD, Victor M. *Principles of Neurology.* 2nd ed. New York: McGraw-Hill; 1981;807–813.

Agid Y, Jovoy-Agid F. Peptides and Parkinson's disease. *Trends Neurol Sci.* 1985;8:30–35.

Bodis-Wollner I, Marx MS, Mitra S, et al. Visual dysfunction in Parkinson's disease. *Brain.* 1987;110:1675–1698.

Bodis-Wollner I, Yahr MD. Measurements of visual evoked potentials in Parkinson's disease. *Brain.* 1978;101:661–671.

Bulens C, Meerwaldt JD, van der Wildt GJ, Keemink CJ. Contrast sensitivity in Parkinson's disease. *Neurology.* 1986;36:1121–1125.

Corin MS, Elizan TS, Bender MB. Oculomotor function in patients with Parkinson's disease. *J Neurol Sci.* 1972;15:251–265.

Corin MS, Mones RJ, Elizan TS, Bender MB. Paresis of vertical gaze in basal ganglia disease. *Mt Sinai J Med.* 1972;39:330–342.

Hoehn MM, Yahr MD. Parkinsonism: Onset, progression, and mortality. *Neurology.* 1967;17:427–442.

Langston JW. Aging, neurotoxins, and neurodegenerative disease. In: Terry RD ed. *Aging and the Brain.* New York: Raven; 1988:149–164.

Lees AJ, Smith E. Cognitive deficits in the early stages of Parkinson's disease. *Brain.* 1983;106:257–270.

Lieberman A, Dziatolowski M, Kupersmith M, et al. Dementia in Parkinson's disease. *Ann Neurol.* 1979;6:355–359.

Lloyd K, Hornykiewicz O. Parkinson's disease: Activity of L-dopa decarboxylase in discrete brain regions. *Science.* 1970;170:1212–1213.

Lukes SA, Aminoff MJ, Crooks L, et al. Nuclear magnetic resonance imaging in movement disorders. *Ann Neurol.* 1983;13:690-691.

Mars H. Modification of levodopa effect by systemic decarboxylase inhibition. *Arch Neurol.* 1973;28:91–95.

Marsden CD, Parkes JD. Success and problems of long-term levodopa therapy in Parkinson's disease. *Lancet.* 1977;1:345–349.

Martin WR, Beckman JH, Calne DB, et al. Cerebral glucose metabolism in Parkinson's disease. *Can J Neurol Sci.* 1984;11:169–173.

McDowell FH, Cedarbaum JM. The extrapyramidal system and disorders of movement. In: Joynt RJ ed. *Clinical Neurology.* Philadelphia: Lippincott; 1988;3.

Pleet AB. Newly diagnosed Parkinson's disease: A therapeutic update. *Geriatrics.* 1992;417:24–29.

Rajput AH, Offord KP, Beard CM, Kurl LT. Epidemiology of parkinsonism: Incidence, classification and mortality. *Ann Neurol.* 1984;16:278–282.

Slatt B, Loeffler JD, Hoyt WF. Ocular motor disturbances in Parkinson's disease: Electromyographic observation. *Can J Ophthalmol.* 1966;1:267–273.

Villardita C, Smirni P, Zappala G. Visual neglect in Parkinson's disease. *Arch Neurol.* 1983;40:737–739.

White OB, Saint-Cyr JA, Sharpe JA. Ocular motor deficits in Parkinson's disease, 1. The horizontal vertibulo-ocular reflex and its regulation. *Brain.* 1983;106:555–570.

White OB, Saint-Cyr JA, Tomlinson RD, Sharpe JA. Ocular motor deficits in Parkinson's disease, 2. Control of the saccadic and smooth pursuit systems. *Brain.* 1983;106:571–587.

11
Chapter

Guillain–Barré Syndrome

John Elliott Conto

Guillain–Barré syndrome (GBS) is an acute, relatively symmetrical and progressive inflammatory polyneuropathy characterized by the loss of motor function of the limbs and areflexia. It has a transient course with spontaneous recovery in the majority of patients. Although the etiology and pathogenesis of GBS remain in debate, the disease is currently thought to be an autoimmunopathy that initiates a demyelination of the peripheral nerves. Both humoral and cellular mechanisms presumably contribute to the immune response. GBS often follows a preceding event, such as a viral or a bacterial infection, a surgical procedure, trauma, or exhaustion. The most common variant, Miller–Fisher syndrome (MFS), presents with acute ophthalmoplegia, ataxia, and areflexia.

The ocular findings in GBS are secondary to cranial nerve dysfunction. Paresis of the oculomotor, trochlear, or abducens nerve causes extraocular motility disturbances. Involvement of the trigeminal and facial nerves can lead to ocular surface abnormalities such as keratoconjunctivitis sicca or exposure keratitis.

EPIDEMIOLOGY

■ Systemic

The reported incidence of GBS is estimated to be 1.7 cases per 100,000 (Alter, 1990). It is the most common cause of acute generalized paralysis. In the United States, GBS seems to have increased in frequency since 1970. This may reflect an improved ability to recognize the disease. The incidence is higher in males (2.3 per 100,000) than females (1.2 per 100,000). GBS occurs in any age group, but the incidence increases with age, with 0.8 cases per 100,000 in individuals under age 18, as compared to 2.2 cases per 100,000 in individuals over age 60. There is a higher occurrence in Caucasians than other racial groups. There is no apparent seasonal fluctuation in incidence. An illness, usually viral, precedes the onset of GBS in one half to two thirds of cases.

The Miller–Fisher variant comprises about 5% of the cases of GBS. Males are affected twice as frequently as females, and the mean age at onset is about 44 years. Children represent about 14% of cases. Like GBS, the majority of MFS patients develop the acute neuropathy after a preceding event, most often a viral infection of the respiratory system.

■ Ocular

One or both facial nerves are involved in about 40% of GBS patients. The third, fourth, and sixth cranial nerves are affected, either as a solitary paresis or in combination, in about 10% of cases. Paralysis of accommodation is rarely reported. Papilledema is uncommon in adults, but occurs in 4 to 6% of cases in children (Farrell et al, 1981).

Complete ophthalmoplegia is the most common ocular finding in MFS, occuring in 49% of cases. Isolated external ophthalmoplegia has been reported in 32% of patients. Ptosis, either unilateral or bilateral, is present in 47% of the cases.

NATURAL HISTORY

■ Systemic

A history of a preceding event 5 days to 4 weeks before the onset of symptoms is common, but is not necessary for the

110

diagnosis of GBS. The most commonly associated disorder is a viral upper respiratory infection, followed by viral infection of the gastrointestinal tract. The herpes viruses, cytomegalovirus (CMV), Epstein–Barr virus (EBV), or varicella zoster, are commonly reported infectious agents. Other infectious agents include *Mycoplasma pneumoniae* and *Campylobacter jejuni/coli.* Five to ten percent of cases occur following a surgical procedure, trauma, or a period of exhaustion. GBS is not generally associated with vaccination, but there was an increased incidence in 1976 to 1977 after a mass immunization with the A/New Jersey swine influenza virus. It also presents more frequently in patients that have Hodgkin disease, lymphoma, lupus erythematosus, sarcoidosis, and HIV infection. It may also occur during pregnancy, usually in the third trimester or postpartum.

The disease course can be separated into three phases: progressive, plateau, and recovery. The progression of the illness from the onset of symptoms to plateau, or unchanging clinical signs, is typically 8 to 12 days, but may be as short as 2 to 3 days. About 90% of the cases will reach maximum disability within 3 to 4 weeks. Gradual improvement and recovery usually begin 2 to 4 weeks after the disease reaches a plateau. The duration of GBS is usually less than 12 weeks.

Typically, the disease onset is acute, with the presenting sensory symptoms of paresthesia and pain in the back or extremities in about 50% of the cases (Table 11–1). Fever is usually absent. These complaints are soon followed by dysesthesia of the hand and feet, with rapidly ascending weakness in the legs and in the arms. Rarely, the weakness may be confined to the arms. The peripheral neuropathy is usually symmetrical. Haymaker and Kernohan (1949) were the first to describe the perivascular infiltration of lymphocytes and macrophages that cause the demyelination of the peripheral nerve. The paresis may be mild or progress to total quadriparesis or respiratory paralysis. About 60% of patients are unable to independently walk. Respiratory

function is decreased in 50% of cases, and 15 to 20% require assisted ventilation. The facial nerve is involved in 40 to 50% of cases. Other cranial nerves affected include those that control the tongue, swallowing, and extraocular muscles. Sphincter muscles are usually intact.

About 10% of patients have a variable onset. In one group of patients, the onset is marked by a period of progression, followed by a plateau, and then another progressive phase before recovery. The recovery phase also shows periods of remission and relapse. Another distinct group demonstrates a slowly progressive onset that occurs over a period of several weeks.

Recovery begins in one third of patients within 2 weeks of onset, in one third of patients between 2 and 4 weeks of onset, and in one third of patients between 4 weeks to 3 months. Microscopically, abnormal Schwann cells are replaced by normal Schwann cells, with subsequent remyelination of the peripheral nerve. The majority of patients without assisted ventilation are able to recover to independent walking within 85 days. Those patients receiving assisted ventilation are able to independently walk on an average of 169 days. Relapses are seen in 2 to 3% of cases.

About 15% of patients have no residual deficits, while 65% have minor disabilities that do not interfere with daily activities. These mild deficits include digit numbness and foot drop. Permanent deficits, such as facial weakness, weakness of lower extremities, weakness and atrophy of hands, urinary retention, and impotence, occur in 5 to 10% of cases, and are usually seen in patients that suffer severe axonal damage and paresis during the acute phase of the disease. Other prognostic factors indicating a poor outcome include age over 50 years, long-term assisted ventilation, and a rapid progressive phase.

Pulmonary infection, urinary tract infection, and decubitus ulceration are common complications that usually respond to prompt treatment. Autonomic disturbances are also seen, such as cardiac arrhythmias, postural hypotension and impaired sweating. Decreased sodium levels (hyponatremia) may result from impaired antidiuretic hormone (ADH) secretion. The mortality rate has dropped from 33 to 5% with the development of modern artificial ventilation. Pneumonia, respiratory failure, cardiac arrest, or pulmonary emboli are common causes of death in GBS.

The onset of MFS occurs 10 days to 5 weeks after the preceding event. The two most frequent initial symptoms are diplopia and ataxia. Five to ten days after onset the disease usually peaks, with the triad of ataxia, areflexia, and ophthalmoplegia. Due to the finding of ataxia, and the symmetry of the ophthalmoplegia, there may be central nervous system involvement in the form of an encephalomyeloneuritis. Sensory symptoms are found in 44% of cases, and are described as paresthesia and dysesthesia of the extremities. Facial weakness is seen in the majority of cases. Paresis of the extremities occurs in 28% of patients, and is rarely

TABLE 11–1. SYSTEMIC MANIFESTATIONS OF GBS

SYMPTOMS
- Pain and burning of back and extremities
- Loss of touch sensation
- Weakness of the limbs
- Difficulty swallowing
- Diplopia
- Difficulty breathing

SIGNS
- Impaired vital capacity
- Areflexia
- Reduced motor amplitude
- Ataxia (in MFS)
- Mild pleocytosis
- Elevated CSF protein

CSF, cerebrospinal fluid.

quadriplegic in nature. Diminished sensation to vibrations (pallhypesthesia) was present in 18% of patients. Other less common findings include headache, incontinence, and psychological disturbances. Less than 5% of patients have respiratory insufficiency.

Recovery from MFS usually takes an average of 10 weeks, and over 50% of patients show no residual deficits. Persistent hyporeflexia and areflexia remain in 16% of cases. Residual diplopia and ataxia may be seen in 5% of patients, but are usually mild with minimal effect on daily activities. Relapse is rare. Mortality is about 5% and is due to secondary infections or pulmonary embolism.

■ Ocular

A painless rapidly progressive ophthalmoplegia, often mimicking a supranuclear or internuclear disorder of ocular motility, appears after the development of the peripheral neuropathy in only about 10% of cases. Rarely, the ophthalmoplegia precedes extremity involvement, and can cause delay in the diagnosis of GBS. It is usually bilateral. The third and sixth cranial nerves are most often involved, and the fourth cranial nerve less frequently.

Weakness of the orbicularis oculi muscle and the levator results in lagophthalmos, ectropion, or ptosis, with subsequent exposure of the globe. Paralysis of the seventh nerve can affect the secretion of tears from the lacrimal gland. These conditions may cause the drying of the ocular surfaces, and in severe cases, keratoconjunctivitis sicca or exposure keratitis may develop. An increased risk of infection is possible. Loss of corneal sensation from trigeminal nerve involvement is less common, but may lead to neurotrophic ulceration.

Pupils do not often become involved. However, pupil responses may show anisocoria or a sluggish response to light and near targets. Optic nerve involvement is limited to papilledema, which is thought to be the result of decreased cerebrospinal fluid (CSF) absorption due to elevated protein.

Most patients with GBS do not have residual ocular deficits, and recovery from ocular involvement is usually complete. Patients with severe disease may demonstrate persistent eyelid weakness or diplopia (Table 11–2).

Ophthalmoplegia is one of the hallmarks of MFS, and diplopia is a common presenting complaint. It is usually bilateral, but asymmetrical. Lid involvement is common, and the previously mentioned problem of ocular drying may occur. Like GBS, residual deficits are rare, and only occur in the most severe of cases.

DIAGNOSIS

■ Systemic

Asbury and Cornblath (1990) presented criteria for the diagnosis of GBS, which included clinical, laboratory, and elec-

TABLE 11–2. OCULAR MANIFESTATIONS OF GBS

SYMPTOMS
- Diplopia
- Increased tearing
- Irritation and foreign body sensation
- Burning
- Intermittent blurred vision

SIGNS
- Keratoconjunctivitis sicca
- Exposure keratitis
- Neurotrophic corneal ulceration
- Ectropion
- Ptosis
- Lagophthalmos
- External ophthalmoplegia
- Papilledema

trodiagnostic parameters. Variant features are occasionally seen with GBS. However, if the presence of two or more variant findings are found, the diagnosis of GBS is questionable.

Progressive motor weakness in more than one limb and areflexia is essential for the diagnosis of GBS. Other features that strongly support the diagnosis are rapid progression to plateau within 4 weeks, relative symmetry, mild sensory signs, involvement of cranial nerves, and recovery that begins 2 to 4 weeks after progression ceases. The presence of autonomic disturbances and the absence of fever at onset is also highly suggestive. Variant clinical features include fever at onset, painful severe sensory loss, progression exceeding 4 weeks, and central nervous system involvement.

Examination of the CSF will often demonstrate a protein level that is elevated after the first week of symptoms, but may be normal in about 20% of cases. CSF pressure is usually normal. There are usually less than 10 mononuclear leukocytes/mm^3. An elevated CSF cell count greater than 50 cells lends suspicion to the diagnosis, and suggests infection or neoplasm. CSF findings do not correlate with severity or prognosis of outcome.

Slowing or blockage of nerve conduction is seen in 80% of patients. Serial electromyography demonstrates segmental demyelination, with secondary axonal degeneration in most patients during the course of the disease. Electrophysiological studies can be useful in predicting the prognosis.

Boucquey and associates (1991) studied the serological findings in GBS. ELISA testing can demonstrate IgG and IgM antibodies to CMV, or herpes simplex virus (HSV). Testing for HIV should be considered when pleocytosis is present. Respiratory syncytial virus (RSV) and *Mycoplasma* can be discovered by complement fixation tests. IgG and IgM antibodies to EBV can be detected by indirect immunofluorescence techniques. Bacterial cultures may be useful in culturing strains of *Campylobacter jejuni/coli*.

TABLE 11–3. COMPARISON OF GUILLAIN–BARRÉ AND MILLER–FISHER SYNDROMES

Manifestations	GBS	MFS
Extremity weakness	Always	Occasionally
Respiratory insufficiency	Frequently	Rare
Areflexia	Always	Always
Ophthalmoplegia	Seldom	Always
Ataxia	Rare	Always

TABLE 11–4. TREATMENT AND MANAGEMENT OF GBS

- **SYSTEMIC**
  - Assisted ventilation
  - Plasmapheresis
  - IV gammaglobulin
  - Physical therapy and exercise

- **OCULAR**
  - Artificial tear supplements
  - Temporary lid patching
  - Diplopia occlusion
  - Levator resection for residual ptosis

Inquiries should be made regarding the previous abuse of hexacarbons or a history of recent diphtheritic infection. Other conditions that resemble GBS include lead neuropathy, poliomyelitis, botulism, and myasthenia gravis.

The diagnosis of MFS is dependent on the findings of ophthalmoplegia, areflexia, and ataxia. No other severe neurological signs should be present (Table 11–3). Laboratory findings include mildly elevated CSF protein level and occasional mild pleocytosis. Electroencephalography (EEG) may demonstrate generalized slowing, and electromyography findings show demyelination.

Radiological testing with computed tomography (CT) or magnetic resonance imaging (MRI) should be performed to rule out intracranial disease. Brainstem and pontine abnormalities have been reported in MFS (Giroud et al, 1990).

■ Ocular

Many patients with GBS are incapacitated, and are often not able to respond to subjective questioning. Objective ocular assessment will therefore be relied upon more heavily. Evaluation may include, if possible, visual acuities, externals, anterior and posterior segment evaluation, and ultrasonography.

TREATMENT AND MANAGEMENT

■ Systemic

Respiratory failure should be treated promptly by intratracheal tube or tracheostomy. Since paralysis may be prolonged, careful attention to pressure areas is important, especially the eyes, mouth, bowel, and bladder. Frequent repositioning to prevent ulceration is also indicated. Lung and urinary tract infections should be aggressively treated. Heparin may be given prophylactically to prevent deep venous thromboses and pulmonary emboli. Electrocardiogram (ECG) monitoring for cardiac arrhythmias, especially sinus bradycardia, is recommended. In severe cases with residual deficits, physical and occupational therapy may be helpful in restoring strength. Counseling may be indicated if the patient shows depression.

Corticosteroids are no longer considered to be an appropriate medical therapy for GBS. McKhann (1988) reported that plasmapheresis reduces the severity and shortens the duration of the disease, and is now the primary therapeutic measure in the management of GBS. Intravenous gammaglobulin may also be beneficial when administered in the early course of the disease, and does not carry the risks or limitations associated with plasma exchange (Table 11–4).

■ Ocular

When the facial or trigeminal nerve is involved, exposure to the cornea can occur, along with neurotrophic ulceration. The use of artificial tear supplements and ointments, as needed, along with temporary patching is advised in severe cases. Paresis or paralysis of the extraocular muscles may necessitate occlusion to relieve diplopic complaints. Surgery is not recommended until the deviation appears to be stable and irreversible. Residual ptosis may be corrected by levator resection techniques. Papilledema will spontaneously resolve, but should be monitored frequently (Table 11–4).

CONCLUSION

Guillain–Barré syndrome is thought to be an autoimmune disease that is characterized by paralysis of the extremities, impaired respiratory function, and cranial nerve dysfunction. Recovery of function is usually complete, although in severe cases residual deficits may persist. Diplopia and ocular surface drying are the most common ocular complications. The Miller–Fisher syndrome, the most common variant, is typified by ophthalmoplegia, loss of reflexes, and muscle coordination.

REFERENCES

Alter M. The epidemiology of Guillain–Barré syndrome. *Ann Neurol.* 1990;27:S7–S12.

Asbury AK, Cornblath DR. Assessment of current diagnostic criteria for Guillain–Barré syndrome. *Ann Neurol.* 1990;27:S21–S24.

Berlit P, Rakicky J. The Miller–Fisher syndrome: A review of the literature. *J Clin Neuro Ophthalmol.* 1992;12:57–63.

Boucquey D, Sindic CJM, Lamy M, et al. Clinical and serological studies in a series of 45 patients with Guillain–Barré syndrome. *J Neurol Sci.* 1991;104:56–63.

De Jager AEJ, Minderhoud JM. Residual signs in severe Guillain–Barré syndrome: Analysis of 57 patients. *J Neurol Sci.* 1991;104:151–156.

De Jager AEJ, Sluiter HJ. Clinical signs in severe Guillain–Barré syndrome: Analysis of 63 patients. *J Neurol Sci.* 1991;104:143–150.

Farrell K, Hill A, Chuang S. Papilledema in Guillain–Barré syndrome. *Arch Neurol.* 1981;38:55–57.

Giroud M, Mousson C, Chalopin JM, et al. Miller–Fisher syndrome and pontine abnormalities on MRI. *J Neurol.* 1990;237:489–490.

Haymaker W, Kernohan JW. The Landry–Guillain–Barré syndrome: A clinical pathological report of 50 fatal cases and a review of the literature. *Medicine.* 1949;28:59–141.

McFarlin DE. Immunological Parameters in Guillain–Barré syndrome. *Ann Neurol.* 1990:27:S25–S29.

McKhann GM, Griffen JW, Cornblath DR, et al. Plasmapheresis and Guillain–Barré Syndrome: Analysis of prognostic factors and the effect of plasmapheresis. *Ann Neurol.* 1988;23:347–353.

McLeod JG, Pollard JD: Inflammatory neuropathies In: Swash M, Oxbury J, eds. *Clinical Neurology*, Edinburgh: Churchill Livingstone; 1991:1189–1201.

Ropper AH. The Guillain–Barré syndrome. *N Engl J Med.* 1992;326:1130–1135.

12
Chapter

Chiari Malformations

John Elliott Conto

Chiari (1891, 1896) was the first to describe a group of disorders involving the hindbrain, skull base, and cervical spinal cord, which are also classified as Arnold–Chiari malformations in the literature. These anomalies varied from mild cerebellar displacement to hypoplasia of the cerebellar tissue. Currently, Chiari malformations (CM) consist of cerebellomedullary malformations without and with a meningomyelocele, known as CM Types I and II, respectively. Chiari malformations are usually congenital, but may not become apparent until later in life. Clinical presentations include various neurological features, such as head pain, extremity weakness, vertigo, and imbalance, which are similar to the symptoms seen in other cerebellopontine lesions. Although the specific etiology of these malformations remains unclear, it is thought to be either the result of trauma induced during birth, or a failure of development. Disturbances of ocular motility, such as nystagmus or internuclear ophthalmoplegia, are common, and are secondary to brainstem and cranial nerve dysfunction. Obstructive hydrocephalus may cause papilledema.

EPIDEMIOLOGY

■ Systemic

The actual incidence rate is unknown because the CM clinical presentation is so variable, and the symptoms and signs are often subtle. CM do not appear to occur more frequently in any specific racial group or in either gender. CM Type II appears to be more common than CM Type I.

One third of patients with Type I will have unilateral upper extremity pain (Eisenstadt et al, 1986; Paul et al, 1983). Trigeminal neuralgia will occur in about 10% of the cases. Weakness of the extremities occurs in 50% of patients, with the arms affected in 35 to 40% of cases and the legs in 20 to 50% of cases. Severe headaches are seen in 35% of patients.

■ Ocular

The oculomotor findings of CM have not been separately quantified, but a common presenting feature of CM Type I is oscillopsia, with nystagmus occurring in about 50% of cases.

NATURAL HISTORY

■ Systemic

The clinical presentation of CM is quite variable, and is dependent on the degree of cerebellum and lower brainstem displacement through the foramen magnum (Tables 12–1 and 12–2). A small posterior fossa with cerebellum tonsillar herniation is characteristic of patients with CM.

The signs and symptoms associated with CM result from the herniation and compression of the hindbrain at the foramen magnum. These include increased intracranial pressure, progressive cerebellar ataxia, and syringomyelia (fluid-filled cavities in the spinal cord). Symptoms may first appear during childhood, but are often delayed until adolescence or adulthood. Untreated cases of CM tend to slowly progress, and become more pronounced following exertion or Valsalva maneuvers. However, many patients have extended periods of relative stability.

CM Type I may be related to birth trauma that causes deformation or bony softening of the foramen magnum.

TABLE 12–1. SYSTEMIC MANIFESTATIONS OF CM

SYMPTOMS
- Headache and head pain
- Extremity pain or weakness
- Temperature sensation loss
- Pain sensation loss
- Tinnitus
- Vertigo
- Syncope
- Imbalance
- Deafness

SIGNS
- Hydrocephalus
- Lower cranial nerve palsies
- Syncope
- Central apnea
- Syringomyelia
- Meningomyelocele

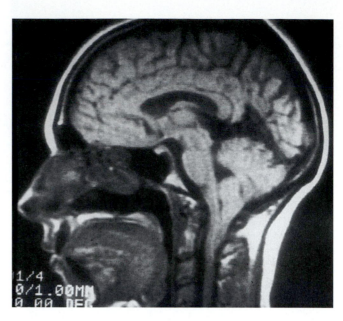

Figure 12–1. Sagittal MRI view of a CM Type I. Herniation of the cerebellar tonsils through the foramen magnum to the C-2 vertebra is evident. *(Reprinted with permission from Gilroy J.* Basic Neurology *2nd ed. New York: McGraw-Hill, 1990.)*

Findings suggestive of compressive birth injury include direct deformity of the occiput bones, caudal shifting of the brain from skull compression, local bleeding and edema, and transient hydrocephalus. The abnormal foramen magnum allows the cerebellar tonsils to bulge into the cervical spinal canal (Figure 12–1). However, the brainstem is usually not displaced, and the central cerebellar tissues are not elongated. Syringomyelia, present in about 40% of patients, often indicates a poor prognosis (Levy et al, 1983). About 25% of patients will have a "bull" neck appearance from arrested hydrocephalus (Figure 12–2). Meningomyelocele or myeloschisis (a cleft spinal cord) are usually not found in CM Type I. Patients with Type I are typically asymptomatic until late childhood or adult age, when mild brainstem or cerebellar symptoms become manifest. The onset of symptoms occurs between the third and fifth decades in the majority of cases, and about 50% of patients will report that the symptoms were present for 1 to 5 years (Mohr et al, 1977).

The most common presenting symptoms in patients with CM Type I are pain, weakness, and headache. The majority of patients complain of diffuse or burning pain of the head, particularly in the cervical and occipital regions. Upper extremity pain that is usually unilateral is common. Trigeminal neuralgia may also occur. Weakness of the extremities occurs, often accompanied by a loss in balance. Severe headaches are common, and are related to an increase in cerebrospinal pressure. They have a throbbing quality, and are typically located in the occipital area, often extending to the crown or temple region. The headaches may be precipitated by coughing, neck manip-

TABLE 12–2. COMPARISON OF CM TYPE I AND II CHARACTERISTICS

Characteristic	CM Type I	CM Type II
Age of onset	Late childhood to adult	Congenital
Meningomyelocele	Rarely	Always
Hydrocephalus	Arrested	Progressive
Nystagmus	Typically downbeat	Variable downbeat or upbeat

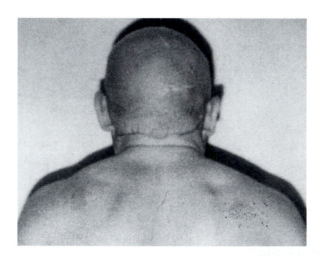

Figure 12–2. Short or "bull" neck appearance in a patient with CM Type I. *(Reprinted with permission from Pryse-Phillips W, Murray TJ.* Essential Neurology *4th ed. Norwalk, CT: Appleton & Lange, 1991.)*

ulation, exercise, or other Valsalva maneuvers. The onset is acute, and they usually resolve within an hour. Vomiting or disequilibrium may also accompany the headaches.

Patients with CM Type I often have dissociated sensory loss, which is characterized by the loss of pain and temperature sensation, with preservation of vibration and proprioception sense. The sensory loss is due to disruption of the crossed nerve fibers of the anterior and lateral spinothalamic tracts, with sparing of the uncrossed nerve fibers of the dorsal columns (Sclafani et al, 1990). Direct compression of the fibers at the base of the fourth ventricle, or at the central spinal cord, is usually the cause. Patients with dissociated sensory loss often suffer painless burns, distention and contraction of the fingers, and neuropathic (Charcot) osteoarthritis of the shoulder or elbow joints.

Neurotologic findings of hearing loss, tinnitus, disequilibrium, vertigo, and nystagmus also occur frequently, often developing prior to other neurological signs. These signs are believed to be caused by the compression of the vestibulocochlear nerve against the petrous portion of the temporal bone, or of the vestibular and cochlear nuclei by herniated cerebellar tissue. Ischemia from the distortion of the posterior inferior cerebellar artery or its tributaries may also play a role in the development of neurotologic symptoms (Bertrand et al, 1973; Rydell & Pulec, 1971).

Although not as common as other findings, palsies of cranial nerves V and VII through XII may cause difficulty with mastication, facial hypesthesia and hyperesthesia, dysphagia, and lateral vocal cord paralysis. Severe compression of the hindbrain and brainstem against the foramen magnum may result in syncope, central apnea, or sudden death.

CM Type II, which is usually obvious at birth, is generally considered to be a failure of development. However, it may become apparent later in infancy or childhood. Unlike Type I, spinal deformities such as meningomyelocele or spina bifida are almost always present. These deformities cause an abnormal pressure difference between the brain and the spinal cord in the embryo. The resultant higher pressure of the cranium produces hindbrain herniation through the foramen magnum, and distortion and inferior displacement of the medulla onto the cervical spinal cord (Figure 12–3). The fourth ventricle also becomes narrowed and shifted inferiorly into the cervical spinal column. The outlets of the fourth ventricle become obstructed, and hydrocephalus develops from the entrapped cerebrospinal fluid in the lateral ventricles. Although the reason is unclear, the hydrocephalus is compensated for prior to birth, but then progresses after delivery.

Many of the presenting findings of CM Type II are related to the progressive hydrocephalus. Sternomastoid paralysis, bilateral abducens palsies, facial weakness, deafness, laryngeal stridor, and tongue tremors are early signs of lower cranial nerve involvement. Cerebellar signs are generally not observed until after the first several months, and usually indicate a poor prognosis.

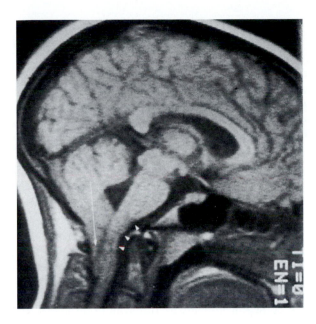

Figure 12–3. Sagittal MRI view of a CM Type II. Herniation of the cerebellar tonsils through the foramen magnum is visible (*single arrow*). Distortion of the brainstem is also characteristic (*small arrows*). (*Reprinted with permission from Bixenman WW, Laguna JF. Acquired esotropia as initial manifestation of Arnold Chiari malformation.* J Pediatr Ophthalmol Strabismus *1987;24:83–86.*)

■ Ocular

Patients with CM may commonly complain of diplopia, vision loss, or oscillopsia, which may become pronounced with head or neck movement (Table 12–3). The symptoms may be stable or become progressive over time. Oscillopsia is a common presenting complaint, especially in patients with CM Type I, and about 50% of cases will demonstrate nystagmus upon physical examination. Cogan (1968) reported that the nystagmus in CM Type II is typically downbeat on lateral gaze, but can be upbeat or rotary. The nystagmus associated with CM Type I is usually vertical, but may be variable in direction, frequency, and amplitude (Bertrand et al, 1973; Chait & Barber, 1979; Rydell & Pulec, 1971). It may be

TABLE 12–3. OCULAR MANIFESTATIONS OF CM

SYMPTOMS
- Oscillopsia
- Diplopia
- Loss of vision
- Foreign body sensation

SIGNS
- Nystagmus
- Papilledema
- Internuclear ophthalmoplegia
- Sixth-nerve palsy
- Exposure keratitis

constant or intermittent. Internuclear ophthalmoplegia may be seen in CM Type II if the medial longitudinal fasciculus is structurally malformed, or becomes damaged by the effects of hydrocephalus. Pursuits, saccades, and the optokinetic nystagmus response may also be impaired in either form. Involvement of the abducens nerve may result in an abduction deficit. Horner syndrome may develop when severe autonomic dysfunction occurs. Visual pathway involvement may result in vision loss due to decompensated papilledema or optic atrophy secondary to obstructive hydrocephalus. Exposure keratitis may result if the orbicularis muscle is weakened from facial nerve involvement.

DIAGNOSIS

■ Systemic

The presence of a meningomyelocele in an infant, along with characteristic signs and symptoms, often implies a diagnosis of a CM Type II. However, the diagnosis is more difficult in Type I malformations, particularly since the findings may mimic demyelinating disease or intracranial mass lesions. In these cases, magnetic resonance imaging (MRI) has become quite valuable in confirming the diagnosis of cerebellar tonsil herniation or hindbrain deformity.

■ Ocular

Most of the ocular manifestations of CM can be diagnosed through external examination and ocular motility testing. Nystagmus, usually vertical, will be evident with gross inspection, or on biomicroscopy. Internuclear ophthalmoplegia, as well as abnormal pursuits, saccades, or optokinetic nystagmus, will be revealed with motility testing. Although visual pathway involvement is rare, it may be diagnosed through optic nerve evaluation and visual field examination.

TREATMENT AND MANAGEMENT

■ Systemic

The management of CM depends on the severity of symptoms and the progression of clinical signs (Table 12–4). Stable or asymptomatic patients are usually monitored, while decompressive surgery is indicated when brainstem or cranial nerve dysfunction is present. The treatment of CM Type II in infants also includes surgical excision of the meningomyelocele, and placement of a shunt to relieve the hydrocephalus.

A surgical review by Levy and associates (1983) showed that symptoms improved in about 50% of adult patients after surgery, worsened in 20%, and remained unchanged in 30%. Eighty-five percent of patients with only cerebellar dysfunction or hydrocephalus improved, while only 33% of

TABLE 12–4. TREATMENT AND MANAGEMENT OF CM

- ■ SYSTEMIC
  - Surgical decompression
  - Meningomyelocele excision
  - Surgical shunt

- ■ OCULAR
  - Spectacle prism
  - Ocular lubricants
  - Eyelid taping or tarsorrhaphy

those with central cord involvement showed a reduction in symptoms. Operative mortality is about 3%.

■ Ocular

Treatment of the various oculomotility disorders with prism may be attempted, but is less than satisfactory. The visual fields should be monitored for involvement of the visual pathway, especially optic neuropathy. If lagophthalmos secondary to orbicularis oculi weakness is present, then protection against exposure is necessary. Artificial tears during the day and ointment at night are usually sufficient in mild cases. In severe cases, taping of the eyelid or tarsorrhaphy may be necessary (see Table 12–4).

CONCLUSION

Chiari malformations are uncommon cerebellomedullary malformations, which may present with or without a meningomyelocele. The most common ocular finding is nystagmus. Since the presenting signs and symptoms may imitate cerebellopontine lesions, radiological testing is necessary to confirm the diagnosis. Surgical intervention is reserved for symptomatic cases.

REFERENCES

Arnold AC, Baloh RW, Yee RD, Hepler RS. Internuclear ophthalmoplegia in the Chiari type II malformation *Neurology.* 1990;40:1850–1854.

Bertrand RA, Martinez SN, Robert F. Vestibular manifestations of cerebellar ectopia. *Adv Otorhinolaryngol.* 1973;19:355–366.

Chait GE, Barber HO. Arnold–Chiari malformation-some otoneurological features. *J Otol.* 1979;8:65–70.

Chiari H. Ueber Veranderungen des Kleinhirns infolge von Hydrocephalie des Grosshirns. *Deutsch Med Wschr.* 1891;17:1172–1175. English translation: Concerning alterations in the cerebellum resulting from cerebral hydrocephalus. *Pediatr Neurosci.* 1987;13:3–8.

Chiari H. Ueber Veranderungen des Kleinhirns, des Pons und der Medulla oblongata in Folge von congenitaler Hydrocephalous des Grosshirns. *Denschr Akad Wiss Wien.* 1896;63:71–116.

Cogan DG. Down-beat nystagmus. *Arch Ophthalmol.* 1968;80: 757–768.

Eisenstat DDR, Bernstein M, Fleming JFR, et al. Chiari malformations in adults: A review of 40 cases. *Can J Neurol Sci.* 1986;13:221–228.

Gardner WJ. Hydrodynamic mechanism of syringomyelia: Its relation to myelocele. *J Neurol Neurosurg Psychiatr.* 1965;28:247–256.

Haines SJ, Berger M. Current treatment of Chiari malformations types I and II: A survey of the Pediatric Section of the American Association of Neurological Surgeons. *Neurosurgery* 1991;28:353–357.

Harcourt RB. Ophthalmic complications of meningomyelocele and hydrocephalous in children. *Br J Ophthalmol.* 1968;52:670–676.

Levy WJ, Mason L, Hahn JF. Chiari malformation presenting in adults: A surgical experience in 127 cases. *Neurosurgery.* 1983;12:377–390.

MacManus D, Barlett P. The role of nuclear magnetic resonance imaging in the diagnosis of Arnold–Chiari malformation. *Radiography.* 1986;52:275–280.

Mohr PD, Strang FA, Sambrook MA, Boddie HG. The clinical and surgical features in 40 patients with primary cerebellar ectopia (adult Chiari malformation). *Q J Med.* 1977;46: 85–96.

Paul KS, Lye RH, Strang FA, et al. Arnold–Chiari malformation. Review of 71 cases. *J Neurosurg.* 1983;58:183–187.

Pillay PK, Awad IA, Little JR, Hahn JF. Symptomatic Chiari malformation in adults: A new classification based on magnetic resonance imaging with clinical and prognostic significance. *Neurosurgery.* 1991;28:639–645.

Rydell RE, Pulec JL. Arnold–Chiari malformation. Neuro-otologic symptoms. *Arch Otol.* 1971;94:8–12.

Sclafani AP, DeDio RM, Hendrix RA. The Chiari-I malformation. *Ear, Nose Throat J.* 1990;70:208–212.

Yee RD, Baloh RW, Honrubia V. Episodic oscillopsia and down-beat nystagmus in a Chiari malformation. *Arch Neurol.* 1984;102:723–725.

13
Chapter
Spasmus Nutans

John Elliott Conto

Spasmus nutans is an infantile syndrome characterized by the triad of nystagmus, head nodding, and abnormal head position. The etiology remains unknown, but is thought to be due to either an anatomic or developmental lesion of the ocular motor system. It is generally considered to be a benign and self-limiting condition, but can be difficult to distinguish from more serious disorders such as optic nerve and chiasmal gliomas or infantile nystagmus. Spasmus nutans usually presents before the age of 1 year and resolves by the age of 2.

EPIDEMIOLOGY

Hoyt and Aicardi (1979) reported that spasmus nutans has an incidence of 2 to 3 cases per 1000 infants. It affects males and females equally, and does not occur with increased frequency in any racial group. Familial cases are occasionally seen.

NATURAL HISTORY

Spasmus nutans was once thought to be caused by a variety of conditions, including epilepsy, malnutrition, and light deprivation. However, the etiology of spasmus nutans is still unclear. Gresty and associates (1982) suggested that a yoking abnormality of the ocular motor system, caused either by a distinct anatomic lesion of the oculomotor nuclei, or a delayed development of the conduction relays to the system, causes pendular nystagmus. Other studies have demonstrated that the nystagmus is not the result of an aberrant vergence or pursuit system (Weissman et al, 1987).

Spasmus nutans usually presents between 3 and 10 months of age. Although the majority of cases arise within the first year of life, onset may occur as late as 3 years of age. Recovery is typically spontaneous over a period of several months to 1 or 2 years. Exceptional cases can last as long as 8 years.

The classic features of spasmus nutans are nystagmus, head nodding, and abnormal head posture. When all three signs are present, the diagnosis is straightforward, but more difficult if only one or two components exist. Nystagmus appears to be the most frequent finding, and is usually the last to resolve. Head nodding also occurs in most cases, while abnormal head position, such as head turns and tilts, is the least seen of the three.

Although head nodding may be the most apparent sign, nystagmus is the first to develop and the most consistent feature of the syndrome. The oscillations are pendular and typically horizontal, although a vertical or rotary component may also be present. The nystagmus can be constant or intermittent. It tends to be bilateral, but asymmetric. Gresty and associates (1976) found that the nystagmus had a frequency between 6 and 11 cycles/second, and an amplitude of 2 degrees. Because the amplitude is small and the frequency is high, the eye appears to flutter.

Head nodding is usually the sign that alerts the parents or the pediatrician that a problem may exist. Like the nystagmus, it is variable in appearance and presentation. The direction of the head movement may be horizontal, vertical, or a combination of both. It has a frequency of 2 to 4

TABLE 13–1. SYSTEMIC AND OCULAR MANIFESTATIONS OF SPASMUS NUTANS

- ■ **SYSTEMIC MANIFESTATIONS**
  - Head nodding
  - Head turn or tilt

- ■ **OCULAR MANIFESTATIONS**
  - Pendular nystagmus
  - Strabismus
  - Amblyopia

cycles/second, and an amplitude of 3 degrees. Head nodding is believed to be a compensatory response to the nystagmus, because the eye movements decrease or disappear when the head motion occurs. Head nodding increases with visually related tasks, and ceases with eyelid closure or sleep.

Abnormal head position, or torticollis, is never seen in isolation with spasmus nutans, and is the most variable of the signs. About 50 to 60% of patients with spasmus nutans have a head tilt or turn. The head position is thought to stimulate the vestibular otoliths in an effort to lessen the nystagmus. The head turn or tilt is absent during periods of sleep.

Another frequent finding in spasmus nutans is strabismus, which tends to appear following the onset of the other signs, and often persists beyond recovery. Amblyopia may develop as a result (Table 13–1).

DIAGNOSIS

Although the triad of nystagmus, head nodding, and torticollis is distinctive for spasmus nutans, the diagnosis of spasmus nutans only requires that nystagmus and head nodding be present. If other neurological signs are evident—such as lethargy, see-saw nystagmus, headache, or visual field defects—the diagnosis becomes less certain, and other intracranial disorders must be considered, especially gliomas. When the diagnosis of spasmus nutans is suspected, further radiological assessment, with either computed tomography or magnetic resonance imaging, is indicated. Other conditions that have a similar clinical appearance include acquired pendular nystagmus and infantile nystagmus.

Spasmus nutans may be distinguished from acquired pendular nystagmus by the presence of oscillopsia. Unlike patients with acquired pendular nystagmus, children with spasmus nutans do not appear to suffer from oscillopsia.

Infantile nystagmus can be difficult to differentiate from spasmus nutans, but Gottlob and colleagues (1990) provided diagnostic criteria that assist in discriminating between the two conditions (Table 13–2). Infantile nystagmus is present at birth, whereas in spasmus nutans the nystagmus appears later, when the child is at least several months of age. Strabismus is more frequently found in spasmus nutans than infantile nystagmus. In spasmus nutans, the head nodding occurs more commonly, and is larger in amplitude. However, the nystagmus is smaller in amplitude and higher in frequency in spasmus nutans than in infantile nystagmus. The nystagmus can be intermittent in spasmus nutans, but is constant in infantile nystagmus. If bilateral, the nystagmus is often asymmetric in spasmus nutans, and symmetrical in infantile nystagmus. The nystagmus is characteristically pendular in spasmus nutans, but in infantile nystagmus it is a mixture of jerk and pendular waveforms.

Intracranial gliomas of the optic nerve and chiasm often present with clinical signs similar to those seen with spasmus nutans. Fifty percent of optic nerve and chiasmal gliomas are initially diagnosed as spasmus nutans, causing a mean delay of 15 months in the diagnosis of glioma. Because gliomas are life-threatening, any child presenting with nystagmus without head nodding must be further evaluated.

The presenting sign of optic nerve and chiasmal gliomas is often pendular nystagmus, which is bilateral in 50% of the cases. Like spasmus nutans, the nystagmus usually develops before 10 months of age. Head nodding and torticollis arise in 60% of patients. Features that are not found in spasmus nutans but are seen in intracranial gliomas include optic atrophy, increased intracranial pressure, and diencephalic syndrome.

Optic atrophy results from the direct compression of the optic nerve and chiasm from the glioma, or from chronic increased intracranial pressure. This may cause decreased visual acuities, afferent pupillary defects, and visual field deficits. Obstruction of the ventricles by the tumor may cause an increase in intracranial pressure, which produces papilledema, headaches, and hydrocephalus. The presence of diencephalic syndrome, failure to thrive, hyperactivity, and hyperhydrosis, is highly characteristic of optic nerve and chiasmal gliomas, and occurs in 50% of cases.

TABLE 13–2. COMPARISON OF SPASMUS NUTANS AND INFANTILE NYSTAGMUS

Clinical Features	Spasmus Nutans	Infantile Nystagmus
Age of onset	3–10 months	Congenital
Strabismus	Common	Less common
Head nodding	Common, larger amplitude	Less common, smaller amplitude
Nystagmus	Smaller amplitude, intermittent	Larger amplitude, constant
Waveform	Pendular	Pendular and jerky

TREATMENT AND MANAGEMENT

Because spasmus nutans is self-limiting, there is no direct treatment for the condition. Concurrent strabismus and amblyopia can be managed with visual therapy or surgery, when appropriate (Table 13–3).

CONCLUSION

Nystagmus, head nodding, and abnormal head position are the characteristic findings of spasmus nutans. Because it is self-limiting, there is no specific treatment for this condition. Because the presenting signs of optic nerve and chiasmal gliomas are similar to those in spasmus nutans, radiological assessment should be performed if the diagnosis of spasmus nutans is questionable.

TABLE 13–3. TREATMENT AND MANAGEMENT OF SPASMUS NUTANS

- Monitor
- Rule out other etiologies
- Vision training and/or strabismus surgery as needed

REFERENCES

Antony JH, Ouvrier RA, Wise G. Spasmus nutans, a mistaken identity. *Arch Neurol.* 1980;37:373–375.

Chrousos GA, Reingold DR, Chu FC, Cogan DG. Habitual head turning in spasmus nutans: an oculographic study. *J Pediatr Ophthalmol Strabismus.* 1985;22:113–116.

Farmer J, Hoyt CS. Monocular nystagmus in infancy and early childhood. *Am J Ophthalmol.* 1984;98:504–509.

Gottlob I, Zubcov A, Catalano RA, et al. Signs distinguishing spasmus nutans (with and without central nervous system lesions) from infantile nystagmus. *Ophthalmology.* 1990;97:1166–1175.

Gresty M, Leech J, Sanders M, Eggars H. A study of head and eye movements in spasmus nutans. *Br J Ophthalmol.* 1976;60:652–654.

Gresty MA, Ell JJ, Findley LJ. Acquired pendular nystagmus: Characteristics, localizing value and pathophysiology. *J Neurol Neurosurg Psychiatr.* 1982;45:431–439.

Hoyt CS, Aicardi E. Acquired monocular nystagmus in monozygous twins. *J Pediatr Ophthalmol Strabismus.* 1979;16:15–118.

King RA, Nelson LB, Wagner RS. Spasmus nutans: A benign clinical entity? *Arch Ophthalmol.* 1986;104:1501–1504.

Lavery MA, O'Niell JF, Chu FC, Martyn LJ. Acquired nystagmus in early childhood. *Ophthalmology* 1984;91:425–435.

Newman SA. Spasmus nutans—or is it? *Surv Ophthalmol.* 1990;34:453–456.

Norton EWD, Cogan DG. Spasmus nutans. *Arch Ophthalmol.* 1954;52:442–446.

Weissman BM, Dell'Osso LF, Abel LA, Leigh RJ. Spasmus nutans: A qualitative study. *Arch Ophthalmol.* 1987;105:525–528.

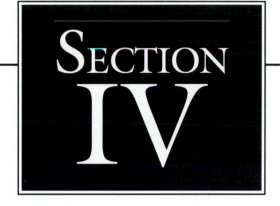

SECTION IV

MUSCULAR DISORDERS

14
Chapter

Myasthenia Gravis

Diane T. Adamczyk

Myasthenia gravis (MG) is an immunologic disorder that affects the neuromuscular junction. Myasthenia (Mys, Greek for "muscle," plus "asthenia," Greek for "weakness," and gravis, Latin for "heavy") manifests in the voluntary muscles, with the clinical characteristics of weakness and fatigability brought on by sustained or repeated muscle activity. Ocular involvement may occur in isolation or in association with generalized disease. It frequently occurs at some time during the course of the disease, often as the presenting sign.

Understanding of the pathophysiology of MG has grown over the past few decades. This, along with advances in treatment and management, have greatly improved both prognosis and quality of life.

EPIDEMIOLOGY

■ Systemic

MG occurs with an incidence between 1 in 20,000 and 1 in 40,000. The actual number of cases may be higher, because many go undiagnosed. These include mild cases, severe cases that result in sudden death, and paradoxical cases.

MG shows no racial preference and may be found at any age and in either sex. However, it occurs more commonly in females between the ages of 20 and 40 years, at a ratio of approximately 2 to 3 females to every male. It occurs equally in both sexes between 40 and 50 years and more commonly in males older than 50 years. The median age of onset is 20 years, with an overall mean age of 33 years. Onset in females is earlier, at the age of 28, versus the male onset of 42 years.

The mortality rate of MG is approximately 1 per million. This increases with age, reaching a peak of 6.4 per million in those between 75 and 84 years (Cohen, 1987).

■ Ocular

Ocular involvement occurs at some time during the course of the disease in up to 90% (Osserman, 1967). It is the initial presentation, along with other symptoms, in up to 84%, and is the sole presentation in approximately 50% of cases (Bever et al, 1983). Of those patients presenting with ocular involvement, 86% go on to develop generalized disease (Grob et al, 1987).

Ocular MG, which is limited to the ocular muscles, occurs in up to 14% of all MG patients, affecting older males more frequently. The mean age of onset is 38 years.

NATURAL HISTORY

In looking at the natural history of MG, the advancements in diagnosis and treatment must be considered, because both are now integral to the course of the disease. Prior to the use of anticholinesterase drugs for diagnosis, only severe cases of MG, which had a high mortality, were recognized. With the advent of anticholinesterase drugs in 1934, less severe forms have been recognized and subsequently treated, altering the course of the disease.

MG is divided into ocular and generalized disease. It may be further categorized according to sex; age of onset (neonatal, congenital, adolescent, or acquired); or according to the presence or absence of a thymoma (a tumor of the thymus, particularly the thymic epithelial cells). Osserman, in 1967, described a clinical classification of MG. Although this was prior to the increased understanding of the pathophysiology of the disease, it still provides a frequently used delineation of the natural history of the disease (Table 14–1). Compston and associates, in 1980, examined the relationship of various clinical, pathological, and immunologic characteristics found in MG. This subsequently led to a different categorization of patients, along with providing support for a multi-etiologic mechanism in MG (Table 14–2).

Neonatal, congenital, Lambert–Eaton myasthenic syndrome, and drug-induced MG all have a different pathophysiological basis than acquired MG. These will be briefly described, with the remainder of the chapter devoted to the more classic autoimmune-based MG.

Neonatal MG results from a transfer of maternal acetylcholine receptor antibodies through the placenta to the fetus. This occurs in 20% of infants born to MG mothers. Difficulty in sucking, ptosis, and extraocular muscle (EOM) involvement may occur. These transient symptoms, lasting 1 to 6 weeks, appear to coincide with decreasing antibody titers.

Congenital MG may be a genetically transmitted disease, characterized by weakness and abnormal fatigability. These rare congenital myasthenic syndromes may be the result of a defect in neuromuscular transmission, which differs from that found in acquired MG (Engel, 1984).

Lambert–Eaton myasthenic syndrome is characterized by weakness and fatigability of the proximal limb muscles,

TABLE 14–1. CLINICAL CLASSIFICATION OF MG

I. Pediatric Group

A. Neonatal: infants of mothers with MG
   Self-limited, lasting no more than 6 weeks
B. Juvenile: develops birth to puberty
   Siblings, close relatives (not mother) may have MG

II. Adult Group

Group I: Ocular myasthenia
   Excellent prognosis
Group IIA: Mild generalized MG
   Ocular involvement gradually generalizes
   Good prognosis
Group IIB: Moderate generalized MG
   Ocular involvement progresses to more severe generalized
      involvement, with dysarthria, dysphagia
Group III: Acute fulminating MG
   Rapid onset with severe ocular and skeletal weakness
   Progression of disease is complete within 6 months
   Involvement of respiratory muscles, thymomas
Group IV: Late severe MG
   Severe, with progression gradual or sudden
   Thymomas
   Poor prognosis

Adapted from Osserman KE, Ocular myasthenia gravis. Invest Ophthalmol. 1967;6:277–287.

TABLE 14–2. CATEGORIZATION OF MG BASED ON ASSOCIATED FINDINGS

Group 1
   No HLA antigen association
   High antibody titers
   Thymoma
   Males=females
Group 2
   HLA association (A1, B8, and/or DRw3)
   Intermediate antibody titers
   No thymoma
   Female patients younger than 40
Group 3
   HLA association (A3, B7, and/or DRw2)
   Low levels of antibodies
   No thymoma
   Males older than 40

Adapted from Compston DAS, et al, Clinical, pathological, HLA antigen and immunological evidence for disease heterogeneity in myasthenia gravis. Brain. 1980;103:579–601.

particularly the lower limbs, usually without ocular involvement. It affects males more frequently, and is often associated with carcinomas, particularly oat cell carcinoma of the lung. Other clinical features include a brief initial increase in strength after voluntary muscle contraction, followed by fatiguing, hyporeflexia, dry mouth, and impotence. Lambert–Eaton syndrome is believed to result from a defect in neuromuscular transmission, probably secondary to decreased acetylcholine release, at the presynaptic terminal (as opposed to true MG, in which the defect is postsynaptic). The pre- and postsynaptic mechanism appears to be normal. As compared to those with adult MG, these patients respond poorly to tensilon testing. Lambert–Eaton syndrome is suggestive of an autoimmune disorder. Therapies include tumor removal if present, steroids, other immunosuppressants, and plasmapheresis.

Drug-induced MG can result from a wide variety of medications. Some examples include D-penicillamine, β-blockers, antibiotics, lithium, steroids, and a few isolated cases of ophthalmic medications (eg, timolol, tropicamide, proparacaine) (Coppeto, 1984; Meyer et al, 1992). D-Penicillamine, used to treat rheumatoid arthritis and Wilson disease, may produce a presentation similar to acquired MG. This includes comparable antibody titers, electromyography results, and symptoms of muscle fatigue, which are usually mild and localized to the ocular muscles. These present after months of D-penicillamine treatment. Remission usually occurs within 1 year of discontinuing the drug. However, there are some cases that will continue on with the clinical presentation of acquired MG.

■ Systemic

MG is an autoimmune disease that affects the postsynaptic neuromuscular junction. Specifically, there is a decrease in acetylcholine receptors that alters neuromuscular transmission. Normally, acetylcholine is released from the presynaptic nerve terminal. It binds to the acetylcholine receptor (AChR) at the postsynaptic muscle fiber. This initiates a series of events that result in an action potential, with subsequent muscle fiber contraction. The acetylcholine then dissociates from the receptor and is degraded by acetylcholine esterase. The receptors degrade and rebuild in a normal cycle of 7 days.

In up to 90% of MG patients, antibodies to AChR, mostly IgG, are present. These appear to cause a decrease in the number of AChR. This decrease may result from decreased receptor cycle time, AChR being blocked from acetylcholine, and/or a damaged postsynaptic membrane. A defect in neuromuscular transmission then results.

Although the AChR antibody level does not always coincide with clinical severity or improvement, it may be higher in generalized MG and patients with thymomas, while being lower in ocular MG or in cases showing remission. In addition, 10 to 15% of MG patients are antibody negative. This inconsistency in antibody level may result from limitations in testing, such as the inability to test for bound antibodies or the presence of antibody variation.

A genetic predisposition for MG has been suggested, although it has not been substantiated. Support for a genetic factor includes the rare familial instances of MG, occasional EMG, and AChR antibody results suggestive of MG in asymptomatic relatives, and a possible HLA association.

The exact role of the thymus (an organ actively involved in immunologic functions, particularly in producing T cells) in MG has not been established, but its influence cannot be denied. This is substantiated by the clinical improvement and remission found after its removal. Thymic abnormalities may be present clinically in 70% of MG patients, and possibly all patients subclinically. Thymomas may occur in 10 to 15% of patients with MG and one third of the patients with a thymoma have MG. Thymomas are present more commonly in 40- to 60-year-olds, and are associated with a more severe clinical presentation and higher mortality rate.

In addition to thymomas, MG may be associated with other autoimmune diseases. These most commonly include Grave disease, rheumatoid arthritis, systemic lupus erythematosus, and sarcoidosis. Based on a number of associated findings, including the absence or presence of HLA, MG may be categorized into three groups (see Table 14–2).

A variety of triggering factors may precede the initial onset of MG. These may include childbirth, use of certain muscle relaxants with general anaesthesia, or an infection that results in respiratory failure.

The clinical presentation of MG (Table 14–3) includes muscle fatigue after repeated use of the muscle, with improvement seen after a period of rest. Signs and symptoms include muscle weakness (particularly limb, facial, and neck regions), slurred or nasal speech, and pharyngeal

TABLE 14–3. SYSTEMIC MANIFESTATIONS OF MG

- Difficulty swallowing or chewing
- Weakness of limb, neck, or facial muscles (myasthenic facies or "snarl")
- General fatigue
- Dysphagia
- Tingling and numbness (paresthesias)
- Slurred or nasal speech (dysarthria)
- Weight loss
- Pharyngeal weakness
- Nasal regurgitation
- Respiratory distress or failure
- Myasthenic tongue (longitudinal furrowing)
- Muscle atrophy
- Myasthenic crisis (loss of strength; difficulty talking, breathing, swallowing)

weakness. The severity usually peaks between 1 and 3 years after the onset of symptoms. This may be followed by a chronic form of the disease that has episodes of milder exacerbations and remissions. Usually clinical improvement occurs with spontaneous remission taking place in approximately 10%. Spontaneous remission is more likely to occur in patients with mild or localized muscle weakness.

Patients older than 50 years, with generalized MG, and with a greater risk for respiratory failure, have a poorer prognosis. Respiratory failure may develop after surgery, an upper respiratory tract infection, emotional stress, pregnancy, or certain drug use. The myasthenic crisis may occur, and is characterized by loss of strength and difficulty talking, breathing, and swallowing that may be severe. Myasthenic crisis and respiratory failure have a good prognosis if appropriate medical intervention is available.

Prior to the advancements in diagnosis and treatment, mortality was as high as 70%, with death resulting from respiratory failure or dysphagia. Medical therapy and intervention has decreased mortality for generalized disease to 7% (Grob et al, 1987). Today, morbidity and mortality usually result from an infection, a complicating illness, or therapy.

■ Ocular

Ocular involvement in MG (Table 14–4) may present as a clinically distinct entity, associated with generalized disease, or as a precursor to generalized disease. The majority of patients with initial ocular manifestations go on to develop generalized disease. Within the first year 87% will do so, and 94% within the third year of onset (Grob et al, 1987). Electromyography and drug testing may show the same changes seen in generalized disease in patients with only clinical ocular involvement.

The levator palpebrae is the most commonly involved ocular structure, with either a monocular or asymmetric

TABLE 14–4. OCULAR MANIFESTATIONS OF MG

- Ptosis
- Ophthalmoplegia
- Diplopia
- Blurred vision
- Lid twitch
- Orbicularis weakness
- Incomplete lid closure
- Nystagmus
- Pseudo-internuclear ophthalmoplegia (internuclear-ophthalmoplegia-like ocular motility disturbances secondary to MG)
- Convergence difficulties
- Saccadic quiver
- Anisocoria; sluggish and fatigueable pupillary responses
- Decreased corneal sensitivity
- Decreased accommodation

bilateral ptosis. It characteristically worsens with fatigue, sustained action, or in bright lights.

Extraocular muscle involvement is also common, with a variety of presentations. Diplopia, sometimes described as blurred vision, results from ophthalmoplegia secondary to MG. Often more than one muscle is involved. However, if only one muscle is involved, it is most commonly the medial rectus. Convergence difficulties resulting from EOM involvement have also been noted. Additionally, a quiver movement of the eye may occur during a rapid saccade of small excursion. The orbicularis oculi may also show signs of fatiguing, with a resultant incomplete lid closure. The EOMs may be more commonly affected in MG than other muscles because of fewer AChRs and lower acetylcholine concentrations, as well as a higher operating frequency of the motor unit (Kaminski et al, 1990).

Pupillary involvement in MG has not been firmly established. It is probably rare, but may include anisocoria, along with sluggish and fatiguable pupil responses. It has been speculated that pupillary involvement in MG is related to cholinergic innervation. Other clinical findings that may relate to cholinergic innervation include accommodative dysfunction and an increased corneal sensitivity threshold.

Ocular MG reaches peak severity in 70% of patients within the first year, and 85% within the first 3 years. Severity may vary over time. The majority of patients remain stable, with 14% going into remission (Grob et al, 1987). There may be a poorer prognosis in those with an older age of onset.

Diagnosis

■ Systemic
The diagnosis of MG may be made based on its clinical presentation, specific test results, and differentiation from

Lambert–Eaton syndrome, chronic progressive external ophthalmoplegia, and other neurologic disorders. A pattern suggestive of MG can be established through the history. This includes muscle weakness that varies with physical activity, rest, or time of day, and precipitating factors such as emotional stress, medications, or infection. A cranial nerve workup should be done to differentiate MG from other neurologic diseases. Specific testing includes the Tensilon test, determining the presence and level of acetylcholine receptor antibody, and electromyography. Other testing procedures previously utilized include curare and quinine. Both of these drugs increased myasthenic manifestations and the potential for respiratory or myasthenic crisis. Although quinine is no longer used in testing, precautions must be given to patients who drink tonic water, which contains quinine, or who use quinine to treat leg cramps.

The Tensilon (edrophonium) test is often the first diagnostic test used in MG. Tensilon acts by inhibiting acetylcholine esterase. This results in an increase of acetylcholine available to stimulate the receptors at the neuromuscular junction. The patient is observed in a quantitative and qualitative way before and after intravenous injection of Tensilon. Improvement in ptosis, diplopia, or ease of arm use is noted following injection of 2 mg of Tensilon. If there is no effect after 45 seconds, an additional 8 mg is injected. When a positive response occurs, it usually lasts a few minutes, but may last as long as 30 minutes. Adverse reactions to Tensilon include a cholinergic crisis, consisting of bradycardia, tearing, salivation, flushing, sweating, abdominal cramps, nausea, hypotension, and cardiopulmonary arrest. Atropine sulfate (5 mg or more) should be available for intravenous injection, to counteract an adverse reaction. The test should be performed in a clinical setting in which appropriate emergency care can be provided.

The Tensilon test has a sensitivity and specificity of 95% for generalized MG (Phillips & Melnick, 1990). False-positive results are possible. Although false negatives do occur, which on retesting may be positive, a negative result usually strongly indicates another diagnosis.

Various immunologic tests are used in the diagnosis of MG. These include AChR antibody titers, serum IgG concentrations, ELISA for AChR antibody detection, and measurement of the degradation rate of acetylcholine receptors. The most widely used test, AChR antibody testing, has a sensitivity of 89% and a specificity of 99% in generalized MG (Phillips & Melnick, 1990).

Electromyography (EMG) is used in questionable cases of MG. EMG measures the action potential generated by a muscle. In MG, the amplitude of the response declines over time. The sensitivity of the test is 76% , with a specificity of 90% (Phillips & Melnick, 1990). Single-fiber EMG is slightly more sensitive than regular EMG testing; however, it is more time consuming and often reserved for specific study purposes.

■ Ocular

When a patient presents with ocular signs and symptoms of MG, the eyecare practitioner can perform a number of in-office tests to assist in the diagnosis. These include the lid twitch sign, the sustained upgaze test, repeated lid opening and closure, the ice pack test, the peek sign, and the sleep test. A cranial nerve workup to assist in ruling out other etiologies should be performed.

The lid twitch sign, sustained upgaze test, and repeated lid opening and closure specifically evaluate the function of the levator palpebrae muscle. It is the most commonly affected muscle, and these tests will show the characteristic sequelae of fatigue.

The lid twitch sign or irritable lid phenomenon was first described by Cogan in 1965. It may be observed in the ptotic lid when the patient is instructed to look from the down position to primary gaze, or to blink. The lid shows an overshoot or upward twitch movement. This results as the levator, relaxing or recovering in the down position (or with the blink), elevates to the primary position, and then rapidly fatigues or falls, giving a flutter or twitch-like appearance.

In the sustained upgaze test, the lid position in primary gaze is observed before and after the test. The patient is instructed to look up, without blinking (which simulates a rest period), for approximately 1 minute, or until a normal fatigue onset is expected, and then back to primary gaze. If the lid position is lower than initially observed, a positive test is present. When the patient is instructed to repeatedly open and close their eyes, a fatiguing of the levator occurs. A positive result shows increased ptosis.

Other EOMs, like the levator, may show signs of fatigue. EOM fatigue may be seen when the position of the globe is observed as the patient looks in a sustained extreme lateral gaze. As the medial rectus fatigues, the eye slowly drifts toward primary position (Osher & Glaser, 1980).

In addition to the levator and EOMs, the orbicularis oculi may also be affected in MG. The resulting "peek" sign occurs when the patient's eyes are gently closed. Initially there will be no visible sclera because the lids are in apposition. However, after a couple of seconds, the orbicularis begins to weaken, with a separation of the lids, allowing the white sclera to "peek" through (Osher & Griggs, 1979).

Muscle function in MG can be improved by both rest and cold. Two tests that utilize rest and cold respectively are the sleep test and the ice pack test. The sleep test (Figure 14–1) may be used in cases of ptosis or ophthalmoplegia. The patient's palpebral apertures and EOMs are initially evaluated. The patient is then instructed to close the eyes in a dark, quiet room for 30 minutes and rest with an attempt to sleep. The palpebral apertures and EOMs are again evaluated for improvement. Improvement usually lasts for 2 to 5 minutes. The results of the sleep test are comparable to the Tensilon test in both time and magnitude. It therefore provides a safe, noninvasive alternative to the Tensilon test (Odel et al, 1991).

The ice pack test uses the improvement MG patients experience after muscle cooling. The initial lid position is evaluated. An ice pack, wrapped in either a towel or a surgical glove, is applied to the lightly closed, more ptotic lid for a period of 2 minutes, with the other eye serving as a control. The patient is then reevaluated for any improvement in lid position. Improvement in ptosis is usually greater with the cooling from ice than rest alone. The ice pack test is a good indicator of MG, with a positive response the result of decreased acetylcholinesterase activity and increased transmitter release (Sethi et al, 1987).

In addition to the tests an eyecare practitioner can perform in the office, confirmation of ocular MG can be made utilizing the same tests used for generalized disease. These include the Tensilon test, antibody titer determination, and

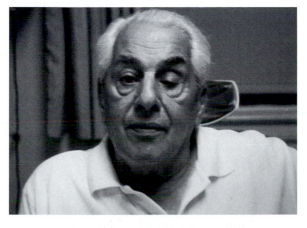

A

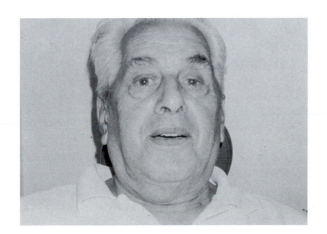

B

Figure 14–1. A. 70-year-old patient with ocular MG. **B.** The sleep test shows improvement in left ptosis following 30 minutes of sleep. *(Courtesy of Optometry Service, FDR VA Hospital, Montrose, NY.)*

EMG. However, in ocular MG, the sensitivity and specificity of these tests are often less than that found in generalized disease.

When using the Tensilon test to determine improvement of EOM function and diplopia, it is important to evaluate both subjective responses and objective findings (eg, use of prisms or Hess Lancaster screen). A patient may still report diplopia after the test, even if the EOMs show a measured improvement. The sensitivity of the Tensilon test in ocular MG is 86% and the specificity is 80% (Phillips & Melnick, 1990). A negative Tensilon test in ocular MG usually indicates another etiology, with further testing only indicated if there is a high suspicion of MG.

Many patients with ocular MG have a lower level or lack of AChR antibodies as compared to generalized MG. This may be the result of different antibodies present in ocular MG compared to generalized MG, which may not be detectable by present testing methods. AChR antibody testing has been found to have a sensitivity of 64%, but a specificity of 99% (Phillips & Melnick, 1990). Because antibody testing has a relatively low cost and a high specificity, it is a good choice of testing methods.

Treatment and Management

With the advancements in treatment and management, the morbidity and mortality rates of patients with MG have tremendously improved, particularly in the last 25 years (Table 14–5). Neurological consultation and co-management with the eyecare practitioner will provide optimal care. The goal of treatment in MG is to improve neuromuscular transmission and/or control the autoimmune involvement in MG with minimal side effects. Presently, however, the treatments are nonspecific and have side effects. Treatment may result in improvement in over 95% of patients (Drachman et al, 1988).

■ Systemic

Once the diagnosis of MG is made, management should include chest x-rays or computed tomography (CT) scan to rule out a thymoma, respiratory function tests, and appropriate testing to rule out associated diseases such as thyroid and collagen vascular disease (eg, rheumatoid arthritis and systemic lupus erythematosa).

Treatment in MG does not follow a specific protocol. In generalized disease it may include thymectomy, anticholinesterase drugs, immunosuppressive drugs, and plasmapheresis. Thymectomy may be done alone or in conjunction with other treatment modalities. Removal of the thymus is most often recommended to patients with generalized disease who have moderate to severe symptomatology or have a thymoma. It is not the preferred treatment in the older or younger population.

TABLE 14–5. TREATMENT AND MANAGEMENT OF MG

■ **SYSTEMIC**
- Co-management with neurologist
- Chest x-ray or CT scan (rule out thymoma)
- Respiratory function tests (lung volume and capacity)
- Testing to rule out associated diseases (eg, thyroid, collagen vascular—rheumatoid arthritis, systemic lupus)
- Thymectomy
- Cholinesterase Inhibitors
  Neostigmine 15 mg Q4H, increased to 30 mg Q3H if needed
  Pyridostigmine 60 mg Q6H, increased to 120 mg Q4H if needed
- Immunosuppressive Drugs (steroids, aziathoprine):
  Steroid: Prednisone 60–80 mg initial, 30–40 mg daily (taper, may have to continue on alternate-day schedule for several years)
  Azathioprine: 2–3.5 mg/kg per day (slow taper, continue 1–2 years)
- Plasmapheresis (4–8 exchanges, over 1–2 weeks)

■ **OCULAR**
- Steroids
- Possibly cholinesterase inhibitors or thymectomy
- Ptosis tape/crutch
- Dark tinted glasses
- Fresnel prism
- Patching
- Monitor decreased corneal sensitivity
- Lubricants for exposure keratitis
- Vision training for convergence problems

Clinical improvement may be found up to 96% of those treated by thymectomy (Younger et al, 1987). Although the reason for improvement is not completely understood, removal of the thymus may result in the elimination of the source of antibodies and antigens. The removal of the thymus may also decrease the occurrence of or improve the course of any associated autoimmune diseases. Evidence of improvement may not be seen for months or possibly years after treatment, but when it does occur, it may last for years. It is difficult to determine if the improvement is a result of the thymectomy or the normal course of the disease.

Cholinesterase inhibitor (CHEI) improves transmission at the neuromuscular junction by increasing acetylcholine. Dosage must be controlled because once patients reach a peak improvement, increased dosage may lead to muscle weakness and cholinergic crisis. Cholinergic crisis is similar to the manifestations of myasthenic crisis, and may include diarrhea, nausea, salivation, and lacrimation. Oral neostigmine and pyrodostigmine (Mestinon) are the CHEI drugs of choice, with pyrodostigmine preferred. Tensilon is used diagnostically, but is not used in treatment because of its potency and short half-life. CHEIs were formerly a major treatment modality for generalized disease. They have been used less because they provide only symptomatic relief, usually in mild cases, with some residual disability remaining.

Immunosuppressant therapy includes steroids, aziathoprine, plasmapheresis, and cyclosporin A (which has limited use in MG). Immunosuppressant therapy is nonspecific, consequently it can affect the entire immune system.

Steroids may be used alone or in conjunction with other therapies for MG. The action of steroids is to lower acetylcholine receptor antibodies. Steroids are often the first choice of therapy, causing a rapid improvement. However, side effects may occur in up to 67% of treated patients (Johns, 1987). These may include, but are not limited to, weight gain, cataracts, diabetes mellitus, gastric ulcer, and hypertension. Steroid therapy may be administered by oral or intravenous routes. Treatment schedules may vary, utilizing incremental dosage or alternate day administration. When improvement is noted, the dosage is slowly decreased; however, the patient may need to be on a maintenance dose. Once the patient begins treatment, it should continue for a minimum of 2 years. Improvement or remission may be seen in up to 80% of treated patients (Johns, 1987). It usually occurs within a few weeks to 6 months.

Azathioprine, another immunosuppressant drug, may be used alone or with other treatment modalities. Azathioprine is best used in difficult to treat, severe, late-onset MG patients, who have high AChR antibody titers. It is usually not the first drug of choice. Although the exact mechanism is not known, azathioprine decreases the level of acetylcholine receptor antibodies. Improvement or remission often occurs, between 3 and 12 months. Treatment should be continued for 1 to 2 years and slowly reduced.

Side effects of azathioprine may be seen in up to 33% of the patients (Genkins et al, 1987), thus precluding its use as a drug of first choice. These include but are not limited to bone marrow dysfunction, hepatic dysfunction, and gastrointestinal disturbances. The patient must be followed with complete blood counts and liver function/enzyme tests.

Plasmapheresis or plasma exchange may be used in severe cases of MG, along with other treatment modalities. Plasmapheresis removes toxins, metabolic substances, and plasma constituents (antibodies) from the blood. The blood is removed, with plasma separated from the formed elements. The formed elements and replaced plasma are then reinfused. It is not used as an initial treatment in MG because it is a complicated procedure with risks and high costs. Its mode of action in MG is thought to be related to the removal of acetylcholine receptor antibodies (Consensus Conference, 1986).

Improvement from plasmapheresis is usually rapid, transient, reaching a temporary peak, and then declining. It may occur after one exchange, but usually requires a few exchanges. Improvement may be seen in approximately 75% of treated patients, lasting days to months. Complications may include hypotension, hypocalcemia, sepsis, embolism, chest pain, and death (Seybold, 1987).

■ Ocular

Treatment and management of ocular MG may take a variety of forms. Dependent on the severity of the ocular disease, systemic treatment may be warranted, along with specific ocular management. Management may also include observation alone.

Treatment of ocular myasthenia may include those techniques mentioned for systemic disease; however, the responses may differ greatly from those found in generalized disease. Ocular MG appears to have the best response to steroids. It has a less favorable response to anticholinesterases and thymectomy. Thymectomy is usually not recommended for ocular MG alone, with the rare exceptions of disabling, nonresponsive cases.

Patients who suffer from ptosis may benefit from lid supports such as lid tape and ptosis crutches, along with darkly tinted glasses. Ptosis surgery should be considered only after a stable lid position is present for 3 to 4 years.

In cases of diplopia, occlusion of one eye (eg, via a patch or opaque lenses) or Fresnel prisms may used. Since the symptoms of diplopia may fluctuate, ground in prism should not be used. Vision therapy has been found to improve convergence dysfunction (Vogel & Soden, 1981).

Other considerations in ocular MG include decreased corneal sensitivity and exposure keratitis. If corneal sensitivity is affected, special attention should be given to those wearing contact lenses or those at risk for injury or infection. If exposure keratitis results from fatigue of the orbicularis oculi and incomplete lid closure, appropriate treatment with lubricating ointment and/or taping the lids should be considered.

CONCLUSION

Myasthenia gravis is an autoimmune disease that affects the neuromuscular junction, resulting in weakness and fatigue of voluntary muscles. A better understanding of the pathophysiology of MG has resulted in improved management. Ocular manifestations commonly occur during the course of the disease, often as the presenting sign, underscoring the importance of the eyecare practitioner's role in the diagnosis and subsequent management of this disorder.

REFERENCES

Berrih-Aknin S, Morel E, Raimond F, et al. The role of the thymus in myasthenia gravis: Immunohistological and immunological studies in 115 cases. *Ann NY Acad Sci.* 1987;505:50–70.

Bever CT, Aquino AV, Penn S, et al. Prognosis of ocular myasthenia. *Ann Neurol.* 1983;14:516–519.

Bryant RC. Asymmetrical pupillary slowing and degree of severity in myasthenia gravis. *Ann Neurol.* 1980;7:288–289.

Castronuovo S, Krohel GB, Kristan RW. Blepharoptosis in myasthenia gravis. *Ann Ophthalmol.* 1983;15:751–754.

Cogan DG. Myasthenia gravis. *Arch Ophthalmol.* 1965; 74:217–221.

Cogan DG, Yee RD, Gittinger J. Rapid eye movements in myasthenia gravis, 1. Clinical observations. *Arch Ophthalmol.* 1976;94:1083–1085.

Cohen MS. Epidemiology of myasthenia gravis. *Monogr Allergy.* 1987;21:246–251.

Compston DAS, Newsom-Davis VJ, Batchelor JR. Clinical, pathological, HLA antigen and immunological evidence for disease heterogeneity in myasthenia gravis. *Brain.* 1980; 103:579–601.

Consensus Conference. The utility of therapeutic plasmapheresis in neurologic disorders. *JAMA.* 1986;256:1333–1337.

Coppeto JR. Timolol-associated myasthenia gravis. *Am J Ophthalmol.* 1984;98:244–245. Letter.

Cornelio F, Peluchetti D, Mantegazza R, et al. The course of myasthenia gravis in patients treated with corticosteroids, azathioprine, and plasmapheresis. *Ann NY Acad Sci.* 1987; 505:517–525.

Daroff R. The office Tensilon test for ocular myasthenia gravis. *Arch Neurol.* 1986;43:843–844.

Drachman DB, De Silva S, Ramsay D, Pestronk A. Humoral pathogenesis of myasthenia gravis. *Ann NY Acad Sci.* 1987;505:90–105.

Drachman DB, McIntosh KR, De Silva S, et al. Strategies for the treatment of myasthenia gravis. *Ann NY Acad Sci.* 1988;540:176–186.

Ellenhorn N, Lucchese N, Greenwald M. Juvenile myasthenia gravis and amblyopia. *Am J Ophthalmol.* 1986;101:214–217.

Engel AG. Myasthenia gravis and myasthenic syndromes. *Ann Neurol.* 1984;16:519–534.

Genkins G, Kornfeld P, Papatestas AE, et al. Clinical experience in more than 2000 patients with myasthenia gravis. *Ann NY Acad Sci.* 1987;505:500–513.

Giese AC. *Cell Physiology.* Philadelphia: Saunders; 1979: Chapter 21.

Gorelick PB. Office Tensilon test. *Arch Neurol.* 1987; 44:689–690.

Grob D, Arsura EL, Brunner NG, Namba T. The course of myasthenia gravis and therapies affecting outcome. *Ann NY Acad Sci.* 1987;505:472–499.

Havard CWH, Fonseca V. New treatment approaches to myasthenia gravis. *Drugs.* 1990;39:66–73.

Herishanu Y, Lavy S. Internal "ophthalmoplegia" in myasthenia gravis. *Ophthalmologica.* 1971;163:302–305.

Honeybourne D, Dyer PA, Mohr PD, et al. Familial myasthenia gravis. *J Neurol Neurosurg Psychiatr.* 1982;45:854–856.

Howard FM, Lennon VA, Finley J, et al. Clinical correlations of antibodies that bind, block or modulate human acetylcholine receptors in myasthenia gravis. *Ann NY Acad Sci.* 1987;505:526–537.

Jay WM, Nazarian SM, Underwood DW. Pseudo-internuclear ophthalmoplegia with downshoot in myasthenia gravis. *J Clin Neuro-ophthalmol.* 1987;7:74–76.

Johns TR. Long-term corticosteroid treatment of myasthenia gravis. *Ann NY Acad Sci.* 1987;505:568–583.

Kaminski HJ, Maas E, Spiegel P, Ruff L. Why are the eye muscles frequently involved in myasthenia gravis? *Neurology.* 1990;40:1663–1669.

Lanska DJ. Indications for thymectomy in myasthenia gravis. *Neurology.* 1990;40:1828–1829.

Lepore FE, Sanborn GE, Slevin JT. Pupillary dysfunction in myasthenia gravis. *Ann Neurol.* 1979;6:29–33.

Linton DM, Philcox D. Myasthenia gravis. *Disease-a-Month.* November 1990;595–637.

Matell G. Immunosuppressive drugs: Azathioprine in the treatment of myasthenia gravis. *Ann NY Acad Sci.* 1987;505: 589–594.

Meyer D, Hamilton RC, Gimbel HV. Myasthenia gravis-like syndrome induced by topical ophthalmic preparations. *J Clin Neuro-ophthalmol.* 1992;12:210–212.

Miller NR, Morris JE, Maquire M. Combined use of neostigmine and ocular motility measurements in the diagnosis of myasthenia gravis. *Arch Ophthalmol.* 1982;100:761–763.

Monden Y, Fujii Y, Masaoka A. Clinical characteristics of myasthenia gravis with other autoimmune diseases. *Ann NY Acad Sci.* 1987;505:876–878.

Morel E, Eymard B. Immunological and clinical aspects of neonatal myasthenia gravis. *Ann NY Acad Sci.* 1987;505:879–880.

Nazarian J, O'Leary DJ. Corneal sensitivity in myasthenia gravis. *Br J Ophthalmol.* 1985;69:519–521.

Oda K. Ocular myasthenia gravis: Antibodies to endplates of human extraocular muscle. *Ann NY Acad Sci.* 1987;505:861–863.

Odel JG, Winterkorn JMS, Behrens MM. The sleep test for myasthenia gravis. A safe alternative to Tensilon. *J Clin Neuro-ophthalmol.* 1991;11:288–292.

Olanow CW, Wechsler AS, Sirotkin-Roses M, et al. Thymectomy as primary therapy in myasthenia gravis. *Ann NY Acad Sci.* 1985;505:595–606.

Osher RH, Glaser JS. Myasthenic sustained gaze fatigue. *Am J Ophthalmol.* 1980;89:443–445.

Osher RH, Griggs RC. Orbicularis fatigue. The "peek" sign of myasthenia gravis. *Arch Ophthalmol.* 1979;97:677–679.

Osher RH, Smith JL. Ocular myasthenia gravis and Hashimoto's thyroiditis. *Am J Ophthalmol.* 1975;79:1038–1043.

Osserman KE. Ocular myasthenia gravis. *Invest Ophthalmol.* 1967;6:277–287.

Osterman PO. Current treatment of myasthenia gravis. *Prog Brain Res.* 1990;84:151–161.

Pascuzzi RM, Phillips LH, Johns TR, Lennon VA. The prevalence of eletrophysiological and immunological abnormalities in asymptomatic relatives of patients with myasthenia gravis. *Ann NY Acad Sci.* 1987;505:407–415.

Perlo VP, Poskanzer DC, Schwab RS, et al. Myasthenia gravis: Evaluation of treatment in 1355 patients. *Neurology.* 1966;16:431–439.

Phillips LH, Melnick PA. Diagnosis of myasthenia gravis in the 1990s. *Sem Neurol.* 1990;10:62–69.

Rodgin SG. Ocular and systemic myasthenia gravis. *Am Optom Assoc.* 1990;61:384–389.

Rodriguez M, Gomez MR, Howard FM, Taylor WF. Myasthenia gravis in children: Long-term follow-up. *Ann Neurol.* 1983;13:504–510.

Romano PE, Stark WJ. Pseudomyopia as a presenting sign in ocular myasthenia gravis. *Am J Ophthalmol.* 1973;75:872–875.

Rowland LP. General discussion on therapy in myasthenia gravis. *Ann NY Acad Sci.* 1987;505:607–609.

Rowland LP. Therapy in myasthenia gravis: Introduction. *Ann NY Acad Sci.* 1987;505:566–567.

Sanders DB. The electrodiagnosis of myasthenia gravis. *Ann NY Acad Sci.* 1987;505:539–556.

Sethi KD, Rivner MH, Swift TR. Ice pack test for myasthenia gravis. *Neurology.* 1987;37:1383–1385.

Seybold ME. Plasmapheresis in myasthenia gravis. *Ann NY Acad Sci.* 1987;505:584–587.

Seybold ME. The office Tensilon test for ocular myasthenia gravis. *Arch Neurol.* 1986;43:842–844.

Sobocinsky-Olsson B, Sandström I, Pirskanen R, Matell G. Evaluation of press-on prisms for diplopia correction in myasthenia gravis. *Ann NY Acad Sci.* 1987;505:836–837.

Vogel MS, Soden R. The functional management of ocular myasthenia gravis. *J Am Optom Assoc.* 1981;52:829–831.

Walsh FB, Hoyt WF. *Clinical Neuro-ophthalmology.* Baltimore: Williams & Wilkins; 1969:1277–1297.

Walsh TJ. *Neuro-ophthalmology: Clinical Signs and Symptoms.* Philadelphia: Lea & Febiger; 1985:77–88, 110–126.

Yamazaki A, Ishikawa S. Abnormal pupillary responses in myasthenia gravis, a pupillographic study. *Br J Ophthalmol.* 1976;60:575–580.

Yee RD, Cogan DG, Zee DS, et al. Rapid eye movements in myasthenia gravis, 2. Electro-oculographic analysis. *Arch Ophthalmol.* 1976;94:1465–1472.

Younger DS, Jaretzki A, Penn AS, et al. Maximum thymectomy for myasthenia gravis. *Ann NY Acad Sci.* 1987;505:832–835.

Zweiman B, Arnason BGW. Immunologic aspects of neurological and neuromuscular diseases. *JAMA.* 1987;258:2970–2973.

15
Chapter

Myotonic Dystrophy

Diane T. Adamczyk

Myotonic dystrophy (MD) is a disease characterized by myotonia (increased muscle contraction and slow relaxation), muscle weakness, and atrophy. It affects many systems, including the cardiac, endocrine, and respiratory systems. Ocular manifestations are numerous, including cataracts, hypotony, and retinal pigmentary changes. Although the gene for MD has been localized (*19q*), the exact pathophysiology has yet to be determined.

EPIDEMIOLOGY

■ Systemic
Myotonic dystrophy is a familial disease, inherited in an autosomal dominant fashion, with variable penetrance. It affects all races and sexes equally. Incidence has been reported to be approximately 1 in 8000 (Allen & Barer, 1940). MD may affect infants and children, but it occurs more commonly in those in their 20s and 30s.

■ Ocular
Ocular manifestations are relatively common in MD, with cataracts the most frequent. Cataracts or lenticular changes probably affect all MD patients, with one third showing clinically significant changes. Almost half the patients have pigmentary changes in the peripheral retina and 20% have macular changes. Fifty to eighty-four percent have ptosis (Burian et al, 1966).

NATURAL HISTORY

■ Systemic
The exact pathogenesis of MD is not known. Historically, it has been considered to be a muscular disorder. Electron microscopic findings support MD as a myopathy, with a mitochondrial disorder (Ginsberg et al, 1978). However, other

studies refute this theory, supporting a neurogenic component (Jamal et al, 1986). It has been suggested that the defect is at the level of the cell membrane, causing an altered membrane transmission, with resultant hyperirritability, and myotonic discharges (Kuhn & Fiehn, 1981; Sarks et al, 1985).

Multiple systems are affected in MD. These include the endocrine, respiratory, and cardiovascular systems (Table 15–1). The respiratory and cardiovascular manifestations reflect specific muscle involvement. The endocrine system may also be affected in a number of ways, which include pituitary, adrenal, and thyroid involvement. In addition, abnormal insulin secretion and increased fasting plasma insulin may be present in patients, but the role of insulin in MD is uncertain (Huff et al, 1967).

Myotonic dystrophy often presents insidiously, at any age. Although infants may show disturbances indicative of myotonic dystrophy, such as difficulty sucking, more commonly patients in their 20s and 30s are affected. Generations may pass with only subtle signs of MD (eg, a history of high infant mortality or cataracts), before it is explicitly expressed. It is usually after three or four generations that decreasing intelligence or mental retardation may manifest.

MD is classically characterized by specific muscle presentations. Myotonia almost always occurs sometime in the course of the disease, often as the initial symptom. This may be brought on by use of a particular muscle or by

TABLE 15–1. SYSTEMIC MANIFESTATIONS OF MD

MUSCULAR MANIFESTATIONS
- Myotonia
- Myopathic facies
- Affected muscles
  - Muscles of facial expression
  - Small muscles of the hand
  - Muscles of mastication (difficulty chewing)
  - Sternocleidomastoid (difficulty raising head)
  - Muscles of arms
  - Muscles of feet (affected gait)
  - Quadriceps
  - Deep muscles of the neck
  - Palatal muscle (nasal voice)
  - Tongue
  - Deep tendon reflex (may be weak or absent)

SYSTEMIC MANIFESTATIONS
- **Endocrine**
  - Pituitary, adrenal, thyroid involvement; insulin changes (high fasting serum insulin levels, hypersecretion of insulin), irregular menses, abnormal carbohydrate metabolism
- **Cardiovascular**
  - Conduction involvement, left and right ventricular blocks, premature beats, atrial fibrillation, prolapsed mitral valve, heart enlargement, hypotension, systolic murmurs, electrocardiographic abnormalities
- **Respiratory**
  - Weakness of respiratory muscles (chest and diaphragm), weak pharyngeal and laryngeal muscles, hypoventilation syndrome, pulmonary infection
- **Gastrointestinal**
  - Pharyngeal and esophageal abnormalities (contraction/paresis), dysphagia, constipation
- **Genitourinary**
  - Gonadal atrophy (sterility), incontinence, urinary retention
- **Skeletal**
  - High palate, cleft palate, scoliosis

OTHER MANIFESTATIONS
- Scanty body hair (with frontal baldness)
- Psychological disturbances (eg, depression)
- Skin dryness
- Loss of high-tone hearing
- Weight loss
- Mental retardation
- Deficient immunoglobulin IgG
- Increased creatine in plasma concentration and urinary

mechanical or electrical stimulation. Myotonia is often exacerbated by emotional excitement, cold, and menstruation. It is relieved with increased or repetitive use of the muscle.

Other muscle manifestations include weakness and atrophy. This generally affects the distal muscles of the limbs, face, and neck. Muscle atrophy may follow a slowly progressive course over years, or may take a rapidly declining course within a year, possibly resulting in paralysis. When the facial muscles atrophy, a characteristic myopathic facies is seen (Figure 15–1). The patient presents with an expressionless, lean, narrowed, lengthened face, and ptosis.

Later involvement of MD includes the larynx, vocal cords, and pharynx, with resultant nasal voice and difficulty swallowing. MD patients may have a shorter life expectancy, with death resulting from pulmonary or cardiac complications (Longstaff et al, 1991).

■ Ocular

Ocular involvement is integral to the disease process. Common manifestations include cataracts; external ocular

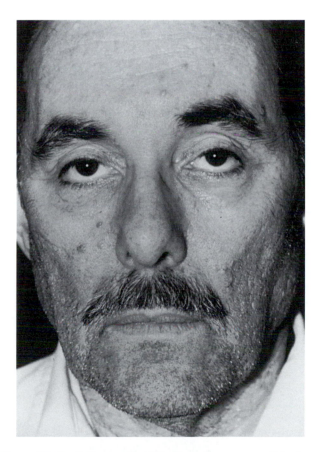

Figure 15–1. Patient with MD. Note lean, myopathic face. *(Reproduced with permission from Adamczyk DT, Oshinskie L. Oculopharyngeal muscular dystrophy.* The Journal of the American Optometric Association. *1987;58:408–412.)*

muscle involvement, particularly the orbicularis oculi and levator (ptosis); hypotony; and retinal changes (Table 15–2).

Cataracts occur in almost all patients with MD. The development and severity of MD are independent of the underlying disease process, and may occur before overt disease. The pathogenesis has yet to be established. Early generations that suffer from MD tend to develop cataracts at an older age, while later generations develop lens changes at a younger age. Bilateral lenticular changes occur in the anterior and posterior cortex. The opacities may concentrate at the suture lines, in the subcapsular area, or in a star formation at the poles of the lens (Figure 15–2). They are punctate, dust-like, iridescent, and white, red, green, or blue in color. The polychromatic lens changes are pathognomonic of MD and are probably due to the diffraction of light from the biomicroscope (Babel, 1981). When the cataracts advance, the opacities become denser and more globular (Walsh & Hoyt, 1969). The cataracts may remain stable, slowly progress, or less commonly, rapidly progress. Generally, vision is unaffected.

Retinal involvement in MD may vary in presentation and does not appear to be dependent on the overall progression

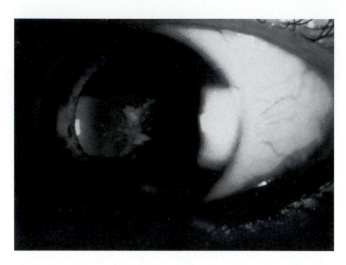

Figure 15–2. Myotonic cataract. Note the classic star formation. *(Courtesy of Optometry Service, FDR VA Hospital, Montrose, NY.)*

of the disease. The pathogenesis of the retinal changes is not known. These changes usually have little clinical or visual effect. Clusters of pigment in the peripheral retina may occur, along with yellow flecks. Rarely these pigmentary changes present with an appearance similar to retinitis pigmentosa (Sarks et al, 1985). In addition, affecting the deeper retina are bilateral, symmetric, macular changes. These include granular pigmentary changes that follow a streak or stellate pattern, with occasional gray-white or yellow spots. These sometimes resemble macular degeneration. In addition, a variant of retinal pigment epithelial patterned dystrophy may occur in MD as butterfly or reticular lesions (Hayasaka et al, 1984). Premature aging (possibly part of the disease course), quinine toxicity, or other etiology have all been attributed to the macular changes. Hayasaka and associates (1984) have also suggested that there is a widespread alteration in the pigment epithelial layer, with depigmentation of the ciliary processes and retinal changes.

Hypotony, another common manifestation of MD, may be the result of decreased aqueous secretion, possibly from degenerative or atrophic changes in the ciliary processes (Hayasaka et al, 1984) and/or increased outflow facility. Burian and co-workers (1967) found the intraocular pressure to range from 4 to 17 mm Hg in MD patients, with an overall average of 10 mm HG. The average pressure decreased with age, with 8.5 mm HG in patients aged 50 to 57 years. Burian and associates speculated that hypotony and cataracts may be the result of the same pathological process; however, they provide no substantiating evidence.

External ophthalmoplegia may also occur, with bilateral ocular motility disturbances, orbicularis oculi, and levator weakness. A common manifestation is ptosis, presenting with different degrees of severity. In addition, the orbicularis oculi weakens with infrequent blinking, and a myotonic response may be found with the Bell phenomenon.

TABLE 15–2. OCULAR MANIFESTATIONS OF MD

MORE COMMON
- Lens opacity
- Hypotony
- Extraocular muscle involvement
  Ptosis
  Orbicularis oculi: weakness (lagophthalmus, infrequent blink) and myotonia
  Motility disturbances
  Exotropia, exophoria, convergence insufficiency
  Poor Bell phenomenon
- Retinal changes: macular pigmentary changes, peripheral pigment changes, epiretinal membranes

LESS COMMON
- Enophthalmus
- Microphthalmos
- Low-amplitude ERG (abnormal)
- Abnormal dark adaptation curves
- Choroidal coloboma
- Cornea: exposure keratitis, keratopathy, decreased corneal sensation, vascularization, keratitis sicca/dry eye, filamentary keratitis
- Anterior segment: loss of iris pigment, pigment deposited on lens, angle, corneal endothelium
- Blepharoconjunctivitis/blepharitis
- Pupil dysfunction: miosis/weak pupil reflex (react sluggishly to light and near; with pupillograph)
- Optic atrophy
- Ectropion
- Loss of orbital fat

Here the eyes remain in the elevated position after forceful lid closure. Motility disturbances, which include decreased saccadic velocity and gaze restrictions, are uncommon but may occur. Rarely, the patient will have symptoms of diplopia. Studies on eye movement disorders have attempted to determine an underlying etiology (myopathy versus neuropathy); however, definitive conclusions have not been established.

DIAGNOSIS

■ Systemic
Diagnosis of MD is assisted by family history, clinical presentation, and electromyographic (EMG) findings in addition to the DNA probe (p5B1.4) used to detect the genetic mutation (Shelbourne et al, 1993). Diagnosis based on clinical presentation includes myopathy in the face, neck, and limbs; myotonia; testicular atrophy; lenticular changes; and baldness (Lessell et al, 1971). Percussion myotonia may assist in the diagnosis. Here, a prolonged contraction results from a blow, for example, to the thenar muscle, of the thumb (Kuhn & Fiehn, 1981). Another characteristic of myotonia is seen when the patient cannot release a hand grasp, such as after shaking hands. The warm-up phenomenon or training effect decreases the myotonia by repeated opening and closing of the hand, making the release of the hand grasp easier (Kuhn & Fiehn, 1981).

Characteristic EMG findings of myotonia were found in all clinically affected patients (Polgar et al, 1972). EMG results indicative of myotonia may be evident before clinical manifestation, particularly in apparently normal relatives.

■ Ocular
Ocular manifestations of MD are found through routine eye evaluation. Biomicroscopic examination will reveal lenticular changes, along with any anterior segment involvement.

Extraocular muscle involvement is determined through pursuits, observation of lid position for ptosis, and a myotonic response of the orbicularis oculi on forced lid closure. In addition, myotonia can be elicited from a flash of bright light that produces prolonged lid closure (Walsh & Hoyt, 1969).

Electrodiagnostic testing shows abnormal electroretinogram (ERG) and decreased dark adaptation findings. ERG findings are affected in almost all patients, even in the absence of ophthalmoscopic findings.

TREATMENT AND MANAGEMENT

■ Systemic
Treatment for MD is palliative (Table 15–3). This may include heat, cold avoidance, or quinine, which provides

TABLE 15–3. TREATMENT AND MANAGEMENT OF MD

- ■ **SYSTEMIC**
  - Palliative
  - Heat
  - Cold avoidance
  - Quinine
  - Antimyotonic drugs (eg, procainamide, diphenylhydantoin)
  - Comanagement with neurologist, and specialist per systemic involvement
  - Pharyngeal and esophageal testing if difficulty swallowing
  - Caution with general anesthesia
  - Genetic counseling

- ■ **OCULAR**
  - Lubricants
  - Surgery as needed: cataract removal, tarsorrhaphy (exposure keratitis), ptosis

relief from the myotonia but has its own side effects (eg, decreased vision). Rarely, antimyotonic drugs such as procainamide and diphenylhydantoin are used. (Kuhn & Fiehn, 1981).

A patient with MD should be co-managed with a neurologist. In addition, referral to the appropriate specialist may be necessary, dependent on the systemic manifestation of the disease. Pharyngeal and esophageal testing may be necessary if there is difficulty in swallowing. Any surgical procedure done with general anesthesia requires caution and testing for respiratory function, because of the potential for respiratory depression and exacerbation of myotonia.

Education and counseling are important aspects of patient management. This includes genetic counseling.

■ Ocular
Routine ocular care is necessary in the management of MD patients. Ocular manifestations are followed for progression and potential affect on visual function. Cataract extraction may be necessary in some cases, usually in the older patient. Visual prognosis is generally good after surgery. Occasionally surgical treatment is needed for exposure keratitis (tarsorrhaphy) and ptosis. In ptosis surgery, care must be taken not to raise the lids excessively, particularly because poor lid closure from orbicularis weakness usually already exists.

CONCLUSION

MD is a multisystemic disease, classically characterized by myotonia, ptosis, and facial weakness. Ocular manifestations are common, and may be a presenting sign in asymptomatic patients. Much still needs to be learned about the pathogenesis of the disease and its management. The role of the eye-care practitioner is integral in the care of these patients.

REFERENCES

Allen JH, Barer CG. Cataract of dystrophia myotonica. *Arch Ophthalmol.* 1940;24:867–884.

Babel J. Ophthalmological aspects of myotonic dystrophy. In: Huber A, Klein D, eds. *Neurogenetics and Neuro-ophthalmology.* New York: North-Holland Biomedical; 1981:19–30.

Betten MG, Bilchik RC, Smith ME. Pigmentary retinopathy of myotonic dystrophy. *Am J Ophthalmol.* 1971;72:720–723.

Bollen E, Den Heyer JC, Tolsma MHJ, et al. Eye movements in myotonic dystrophy. *Brain.* 1992;115:445–450.

Blanksma LJ, Kooijman AC, Sier Tsema JV, Roze JH. Fluorophotometry in myotonic dystrophy. *Documenta Ophthalmologica.* 1983;56:111–114.

Bruggen JP Ter, Bastiaensen LAK, Tyssen CC, Gielen G. Disorders of eye movement in myotonic dystrophy. *Brain.* 1990;113:463–473.

Burian HM, Burns CA. Ocular changes in myotonic dystrophy. *Am J Ophthalmol.* 1967;63:22–34.

Burian HM, Burns CA. Ocular changes in myotonic dystrophy. *Trans Am Ophthalmol Soc.* 1966;69:250–273.

Eustace P. Corneal lesions in myotonic dystrophy. *Br J Ophthalmol.* 969;53:633–637.

Garla PE. Cataracts in myotonic dystrophy. *J Am Optom Assoc.* 1983;54:1067–1068.

Ginsberg J, Hamblet J, Menefee M. Ocular abnormality in myotonic dystrophy. *Ann Ophthalmol.* 1978;10:1021–1028.

Hayasaka S, Kiyosawa M, Kastumata S, et al. Ciliary and retinal changes in myotonic dystrophy. *Arch Ophthalmol.* 1984;102:88–93.

Huff TA, Horton ES, Lebovitz HE. Abnormal insulin secretion in myotonic dystrophy. *N Engl J Med.* 1967;277:837–841.

Jamal GA, Weir AI, Hansen S, Ballantyne JP. Myotonic dystrophy. A reassessment by conventional and more recently introduced neurophysiological techniques. *Brain.* 1986;109:1279–1296.

Kuhn E, Fiehn W. Adult form of myotonic dystrophy. In: Huber A, Klein D, eds. *Neurogenetics and Neuro-ophthalmology.* New York: North-Holland Biomedical; 1981:31–43.

Lessell S, Coppeto J, Sanet S. Ophthalmoplegia in myotonic dystrophy. *Am J Ophthalmol.* 1971;71:1231–1235.

Longstaff S, Curtis D, Quick J, Talbot J. Genetic counselling for myotonic dystrophy: A comparison of lens examination and DNA linkage studies. *Eye.* 1991;5:93–98.

Mausolf FA, Burns CA, Burian HM. Morphologic and functional retinal changes in myotonic dystrophy unrelated to quinine therapy. *Am J Ophthalmol.* 1972;74:1141–1143.

Meyer E, Navon D, Auslender L, Zoni SS. Myotonic dystrophy: Pathological study of the eyes. *Ophthalmologica.* 1980; 181:215–220.

Polgar JG, Bradley WG, Upton ARM, et al. The early detection of dystrophia myotonica. *Brain.* 1972;95:761–776.

Raitta C, Karli P. Ocular findings in myotonic dystrophy. *Ann Ophthalmol.* 1982;14:647–650.

Sarks J, Penfold P, Liu H, et al. Retinal changes in myotonic dystrophy: A clinicomorphological study. *Aust NZJ Ophthalmol.* 1985;13:19–36.

Shelbourne P, Davies J, Buxton J, et al. Direct diagnosis of myotonic dystrophy with a disease-specific DNA marker. *N Engl J Med* 1993;328:471–475.

Thompson HS, Van Allen MW, von Noorden GK. The pupil in myotonic dystrophy. *Invest Ophthalmol.* 1964;3:325–338.

Walker SD, Brubaker RF, Nagataki S. Hypotony and aqueous humor dynamics in myotonic dystrophy. *Invest Ophthalmol Vis Sci.* 1982;22:744–751.

Walsh FB, Hoyt WF. *Clinical Neuro-ophthalmology.* Baltimore: Williams & Wilkins; 1969:1266–1277.

16
Chapter

Selected Muscle Disorders

Diane T. Adamczyk

There are a number of rare muscle disorders involving the extraocular muscles that fall under the all-encompassing term of chronic progressive external ophthalmoplegia (CPEO). These diseases have the underlying feature of external ophthalmoplegia, not involving the intrinsic muscles or the pupil; along with other characteristic features such as weakness of skeletal muscles, pigmentary retinopathy, or cardiac abnormalities. It is not known whether these conditions represent diverse expressions of the same disease process or different disease processes, with external ophthalmoplegia a common feature. Myopathic, neurogenic, and mitochondrial disorders have been considered to be possible etiologies.

The following disorders will be discussed: CPEO, and the specific entities of oculopharyngeal muscular dystrophy (ptosis and dysphagia), and Kearns–Sayre syndrome (progressive external ophthalmoplegia, retinal pigmentary changes and heart abnormalities).

■ CHRONIC PROGRESSIVE EXTERNAL OPHTHALMOPLEGIA

CPEO is a disorder of slowly progressive external ophthalmoplegia, often associated with other characteristic features specific to the presentation of the particular disease entity.

EPIDEMIOLOGY

■ Systemic

CPEO consists of a rare group of disease entities. Approximately half the cases occur in families, inherited in an autosomal dominant fashion, although recessive and sporadic cases also occur. Males and females are affected equally. The exact incidence is not known, because many cases are misdiagnosed. The age of onset is usually in the second decade; however, any age may be affected.

Petty and associates (1986) reported initial symptoms in mitochondrial myopathies to include fatigue (42.4%), limb weakness (27.3%), and dysphagia (6.1%), with normal intellegence in 80.3% of patients and dementia in 19.7%. Also reported was cerebellar ataxia in 40.9%. Other muscle involvement (facial and limb) occurs during the course of the disease in approximately 25% (Drachman, 1968).

■ Ocular

The most common ocular manifestation of CPEO is ptosis. Petty's study on mitochondrial myopathies in 1986 reported ptosis as the initial symptom in 59.1%. Ptosis and/or extraocular muscle involvement occur in 78.8%, and pigmentary retinopathy in 36% during the course of the disease.

NATURAL HISTORY

■ Systemic

The muscle disorders having external ophthalmoplegia as a common feature constitute a heterogenous group, both clinically and biochemically. The exact etiology of these disorders has yet to be determined. Myogenic, neurogenic, and

139

mitochondrial abnormalities have all been considered as possibilities. Electromyographic, histological, and clinical findings have supported a myogenic etiology; however, these findings are not always consistent, and at times lend support to a neurogenic or mitochondrial etiology. Mitochondria, the powerhouses of the muscle cell, have been found to be abnormal in many of these disorders, subsequently affecting muscle function and performance. On histologic stain these abnormal mitochondria appear as ragged red fibers. The exact cause of mitochondrial involvement has yet to be determined.

The characteristic feature of CPEO is slowly progressive muscle involvement (Table 16–1), with a familial tendency. In addition to the external ocular muscles, muscle weakness may affect the face, neck, and limbs. Manifestations may vary from mild to severe, some having the potential to lead to death (eg, heart block).

■ Ocular

CPEO is characterized by a slowly progressive ptosis and ophthalmoplegia, in the absence of pupillary involvement (Table 16–2). The external ocular muscles (EOMs) may be involved more frequently and earlier in CPEO because of

TABLE 16–1. SYSTEMIC MANIFESTATIONS

CHRONIC PROGRESSIVE EXTERNAL OPHTHALMOPLEGIA
- Weakness of muscles of the face, neck, limb (especially proximal), pharynx (causing dysphagia), larynx (causing nasal speech), skeleton
- Cardiac involvement (heart block)
- Central nervous system involvement: seizure, ataxia, deafness, dementia, cerebellum and corticospinal pathway disorders, increased CSF protein, dysmetria
- Endocrine dysfunction: growth and development, short stature
- Mental changes (lower IQ)

OCULOPHARYNGEAL MUSCULAR DYSTROPHY
- Dysphagia (pharyngeal muscle weakness): pharyngeal oral/nasal regurgitation, tracheal aspiration, pulmonary infection, weight loss, choking
- Rasping to nasal voice
- Other muscle weakness: facial, neck, shoulder, hip, limbs (especially proximal), masseter, tongue
- Esophageal carcinoma

KEARNS–SAYRE SYNDROME
- Cardiac involvement (heart block, bradycardia)
- Central nervous system involvement: cerebellar involvement (ataxia), deafness, mental retardation/dementia, elevated CSF protein, corticospinal dysfunction, vestibular system dysfunction
- Respiratory failure
- Endocrine involvement: diabetes, growth hormone deficiency, delayed puberty, amenorrhea, hypogonadism, hypoparathyroid, short stature

TABLE 16–2. OCULAR MANIFESTATIONS

CHRONIC PROGRESSIVE EXTERNAL OPHTHALMOPLEGIA
- Ptosis (Hutchinson facies)
- Ophthalmoplegia (restricted extraocular muscles, diplopia [rare], poor Bell phenomenon, proptosis—possibly from lax ocular muscles)
- Orbicularis oculi weakness (lagophthalmos, secondary corneal exposure)
- Pigmentary retinopathy
  Salt-and-pepper pigment, in equatorial region, bilateral, may have macular mottling; vision generally good unless associated optic atrophy
  Bone spicule pigment, optic atrophy, attenuated blood vessels, and macular pigment clumping, severe vision loss (to hand motion or light perception)
  RPE and choriocapillaris atrophy, vision good
- Reduced saccadic velocity
- Abnormal corneal endothelium (rare)

OCULOPHARYNGEAL MUSCULAR DYSTROPHY
- Ptosis (Hutchinson facies)
- Ophthalmoplegia (infrequent)

KEARNS–SAYRE SYNDROME
- Ptosis
- Ophthalmoplegia
- Salt-and-pepper retinopathy
- Visible choroidal vessels
- Peripapillary changes (metallic sheen, mottling)
- Corneal endothelium affected (corneal clouding)

morphologic differences from other muscles (eg, smaller fibers, richer blood supply; Scully et al, 1985), and/or EOMs' greater dependence on mitochondrial function, which result in a greater adverse affect from mitochondrial abnormalities than for other muscle groups (Mitsumoto et al, 1983).

Ptosis is often the presenting symptom, and is usually bilateral and relatively symmetric. In order to compensate for the ptosis, patients may raise their eyebrows and tilt their head back to see under the lids (Hutchinson facies).

Extraocular muscle involvement often presents insidiously, following the ptosis. Elevation of the eyes is usually affected initially, with progression to complete inability to move the eyes (Figure 16–1). Diplopia is rarely a symptom because of the symmetric, bilateral progression of the disease, in addition to the ptosis occasionally occluding one eye. The orbicularis oculi, along with other facial muscles, may also be involved.

In addition to extrinsic ocular muscle involvement, retinal changes often occur. Although the reason for retinal involvement is not known, disturbances in retinal mitochondria have been speculated. These changes include a pigmentary retinopathy, that may have three patterns of presentation (Mullie et al, 1985; Table 16–2). A bilateral

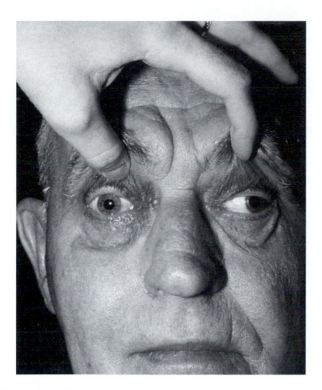

Figure 16–1. Patient with CPEO. Note the position of the eyes as lids are held open. *(Reprinted with permission from Adamczyk DT, Oshinskie L. Oculopharyngeal muscular dystrophy. The Journal of the American Optometric Association. 1987;58:408–412.)*

salt-and-pepper retinopathy located in the equatorial region may occur and usually is associated with good vision. A second presentation includes bone spicule pigmentation, optic atrophy, and attenuated blood vessels, with poor vision. A third type occurs with atrophy of the retinal pigment epithelium and choriocapillaris, and good vision. Salt-and-pepper retinopathy is the preferred terminology, and not atypical retinitis pigmentosa, because the classic features of retinitis pigmentosa do not occur.

DIAGNOSIS

■ Systemic
The diagnosis of CPEO is based on clinical presentation, family history, neurologic evaluation, and a negative Tensilon test. Associated systemic involvement and specific testing (eg, electromyography, blood workup) may also assist in the diagnosis. Systemic involvement is determined through a complete physical examination.

Differential diagnosis includes myasthenia gravis, thyroid disease, and cranial nerve pareses. Overall clinical presentation and neurologic evaluation, along with Tensilon, serum acetylcholine receptor antibody, and thyroid function tests, will help assist in the differential diagnosis.

■ Ocular
Chronic progressive external ophthalmoplegia is often misdiagnosed in the early stages of the disease. However, as the disease progresses, the classic presentation of ptosis, ophthalmoplegia, and lack of pupil involvement leaves little doubt about the correct diagnosis. Family history, complete physical and neurologic results, along with associated clinical manifestations (eg, dysphagia) may assist in the diagnosis. Ocular evaluation should include a cranial nerve workup, various testing procedures for extraocular muscle function (eg, sustained upgaze and forced duction) and fundus evaluation, which may include electrodiagnostic testing or fluorescein angiography. A careful evaluation of the retina may reveal pigmentary changes indicative of a specific muscle disorder syndrome, possibly assisting in the diagnosis. Ocular testing to rule out myasthenia may include sustained upgaze, Cogan lid twitch, and sleep test (see Chapter 14).

TREATMENT AND MANAGEMENT

Table 16–3 gives an overview of the treatment and management of CPEO.

■ Systemic
Treatment and management of the muscle disorders include neurological consultation, along with a complete physical evaluation to rule out any associated systemic involvement. The patient should be co-managed with the appropriate specialist for any subsequent systemic manifestations.

■ Ocular
Ocular manifestations of CPEO may initially be monitored. Advanced ptosis, which interferes with vision or is cosmetically unacceptable, may be treated with ptosis tape, lid crutches (Figure 16–2), or surgery. When surgery is the treatment choice, the patient should be educated on the potential of continued ptosis progression after surgery. Levator resection or brow suspension may be the surgery of choice, dependent on the function of the levator and frontalis muscles. Another important consideration in ptosis surgery is weakness of the orbicularis oculi muscle. Weak orbicularis function may contraindicate ptosis surgery because of poor lid closure. Lagophthalmos, particularly after ptosis surgery, may require lubricant therapy.

■ OCULOPHARYNGEAL MUSCULAR DYSTROPHY

Oculopharyngeal muscular dystrophy (OPMD) is a disease characterized by ptosis and dysphagia.

TABLE 16–3. TREATMENT AND MANAGEMENT

■ **SYSTEMIC**

CHRONIC PROGRESSIVE EXTERNAL OPHTHALMOPLEGIA
- Complete physical exam
- Neurologic workup
- Co-management with specialist dependent on systemic involvement

OCULOPHARYNGEAL MUSCULAR DYSTROPHY
- Include above for CPEO
- Co-management with ENT
- Cricopharyngeal myotomy
- Sphincter dilation
- Esophagram

KEARNS–SAYRE SYNDROME
- Include above for CPEO
- Co-management with cardiologist
- Pacemaker
- Vitamins
- Special considerations for potential respiratory involvement (eg, use of steroids, general anesthesia, high-altitude travel)

■ **OCULAR**

CHRONIC PROGRESSIVE EXTERNAL OPHTHALMOPLEGIA
OCULOPHARYNGEAL MUSCULAR DYSTROPHY
- Ptosis: tape, crutch, surgery
- Lagophthalmos: lubricants

KEARNS-SAYRE SYNDROME
- Include above for CPEO
- Special consideration for contact lens wear
- Special consideration for glaucoma treatment with β-blocker or adrenergic agents

EPIDEMIOLOGY

■ Systemic

OPMD occurs most commonly in French Canadians. The disease has been traced back to a couple that migrated from France to Canada in the 1600s, with subsequent generations affected. OPMD may also occur in other ethnic groups. OPMD differs from the classic presentation of CPEO in that the age of onset is usually in the 40s or 50s. Inheritance is often autosomal dominant, although autosomal recessive along with sporadic cases may occur. Males and females are equally affected.

The pharyngeal muscles are the second most commonly affected muscle group, with pulmonary infection reported in 25% of cases (Duranceau et al, 1983). Other muscles, such as facial, limb, and neck, are involved in 25% of the cases (Dayal & Freeman, 1976).

Ocular

The levator is the most commonly affected muscle in OPMD. Johnson and Kuwabara(1974) found 33% of patients they studied with ptosis had OPMD. This extremely high percentage was probably due to the large French-Canadian population that lived in the survey area.

NATURAL HISTORY

■ Systemic

OPMD is a slowly progressive disease (see Table 16–1) with the manifestations of ptosis and dysphagia. As with the other myopathies, the etiology has yet to be determined. Controversy has been centered around a myogenic, neurogenic, or mitochondrial cause, with favor toward a myopathic etiology.

Ptosis is usually the presenting symptom, with dysphagia following; however, the dysphagia may occur at the same

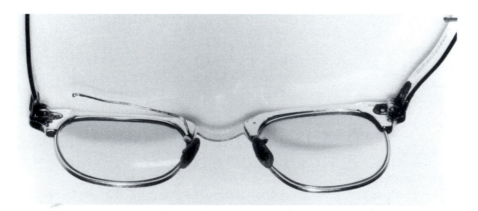

Figure 16–2. Ptosis crutch used by patient shown in Figure 16–1.

time or prior to the ptosis. Difficulty first begins in swallowing solid foods, later progressing to liquids. This is particularly pronounced when the patient is anxious or drinks cold fluids. The dysphagia is a result of the food not moving into the esophagus, secondary to poorly functioning pharyngeal muscles and lack of relaxation of the cricopharyngeal muscle. The dysphagia may vary from mild to severe, with regurgitation, aspiration pneumonia, and loss of weight potentially occurring. Although unlikely today, starvation and death have resulted.

Other muscle groups (those of the neck, shoulder, hip, and limbs) are inconsistently involved in OPMD. A nasal voice often accompanies the other symptoms. In addition, esophageal cancer is found more frequently with these patients.

■ Ocular

The levator is the most commonly affected muscle in OPMD. Patients characteristically present with a bilateral ptosis; however, one eye may be affected first. Progression is slow, with mild to severe manifestations (Figure 16–3). Ophthalmoplegia or extraocular muscle dysfunction usually does not occur in OPMD; and if it does, it has minimal involvement.

DIAGNOSIS

■ Systemic

Diagnosis of OPMD is based on family history and clinical presentation; specifically, a later age of onset and slow pro-

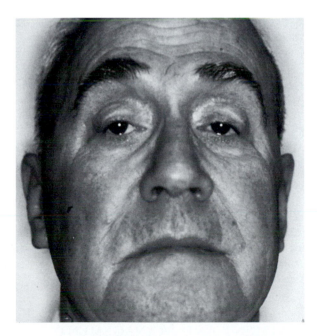

Figure 16–3. Patient with OPMD. Note Hutchinson facies. *(Reprinted with permission from Adamczyk DT, Oshinskie L. Oculopharyngeal muscular dystrophy. The Journal of the American Optometric Association. 1987;58:408–412.)*

gressive presentation of ptosis and dysphagia. Barium swallow testing may be necessary to diagnose and assess the swallowing mechanism. A complete workup to rule out other etiologies is as delineated under diagnosis for CPEO.

■ Ocular

The ocular diagnosis of OPMD is made by the characteristic features of the disease, as described in the systemic section, along with the general absence of other extraocular muscle involvement and lack of pupillary involvement. A complete workup for ocular involvement is delineated under ocular diagnosis for CPEO.

TREATMENT AND MANAGEMENT

See Table 16–3 for an overview of the treatment and management of OPMD.

■ Systemic

Co-management of OPMD with an ear, nose, and throat specialist is important to monitor the dysphagia. If dysphagia becomes severe, a cricopharyngeal myotomy or sphincter dilatation may be necessary to allow improved passage of food. These often provide relief. In addition, esophagrams should be done to rule out esophageal carcinoma.

■ Ocular

Ocular treatment of OPMD consists of initially monitoring the patient. As the ptosis advances, use of ptosis tape, lid crutches, or surgery should be considered. Molgat and Rodrigue (1993) reported ptosis to recur after surgery in 13% with OPMD. In addition, the patient should be followed closely for lagophthalmos and incomplete lid closure after ptosis surgery, with appropriate lubricant therapy used (Figure 16–4).

■ KEARNS–SAYRE SYNDROME

Kearns–Sayre syndrome (oculocraniosomatic neuromuscular disease) is a rare disease that afflicts the young. It consists of external ophthalmoplegia, pigmentary retinopathy (salt-and-pepper fundus), and cardiac involvement (heart block or conduction defects). The initial presentation is usually ptosis or ophthalmoplegia, generally followed by retinal and cardiac involvement.

EPIDEMIOLOGY

■ Systemic

Kearns–Sayre syndrome usually affects those under 20 years of age. It usually occurs sporadically. Systemic

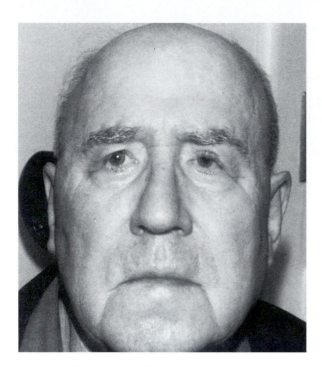

Figure 16–4. Patient in Figure 16–3 after ptosis surgery.

manifestations in addition to cardiac involvement in Kearns–Sayre syndrome include short stature (63%), cerebellar signs (69%), hearing loss (54%), mental retardation (40%), and vestibular dysfunction (33%), with a 20% mortality secondary to heart block reported (Berenberg et al, 1977).

■ Ocular
Ptosis or ophthalmoplegia initially presents in 88.6% of patients. Pigmentary degeneration may occur either alone or with ophthalmoplegia in 23% (Berenberg et al, 1977).

NATURAL HISTORY

■ Systemic
Kearns–Sayre syndrome has been attributed to an infectious/viral, genetic, autoimmune, or mitochondrial etiology. Although mitochondrial involvement is present, its exact role has yet to be determined (Moraes et al, 1989).

Kearns–Sayre syndrome may occur in infantile, juvenile, and adult forms, each progressive, but varied in severity. Age of onset appears related to severity, with the infantile form being the most severe (McKechnie et al, 1985). Ptosis or ophthalmoplegia is usually the presenting sign, with retinal and cardiac involvement often not present until 5 years after the ophthalmoplegia. The patient may remain symptom free for up to 33 years (Berenberg et al, 1977). Systemic manifestations (see Table 16–1) may involve neurologic abnormali-

ties (eg, deafness, ataxia, vestibular dysfunction, and less frequently, mental retardation), as well as endocrine abnormalities (eg, short stature, delayed puberty). When cerebrospinal fluid protein is increased in patients with ophthalmoplegia and retinal changes, the potential for heart block is increased (Berenberg et al, 1977). Vital functions may be affected, such as those of the heart and breathing, which may ultimately result in death.

■ Ocular
Kearns–Sayre syndrome is characterized by extraocular muscle and retinal involvement, generally with preservation of vision (see Table 16–2). Ptosis and ophthalmoplegia are frequently the initial presentation, with ptosis more commonly occurring first. Retinal abnormalities may be related to disturbances in the mitochondria and its affect on the photoreceptors (McKechnie et al, 1985). Eagle and co-workers (1982) suggests the defect is in the retinal pigment epithelium. Retinal manifestations usually occur in the posterior pole, with a salt-and-pepper retinopathy, visible choroidal vessels, and in advanced cases, peripapillary changes. The corneal endothelium may also be affected. These areas may be preferentially involved because of their increased number of mitochondria, and potential susceptibility to dysfunction.

DIAGNOSIS

■ Systemic
The diagnosis of Kearns–Sayre syndrome is based upon its clinical presentation with cardiac involvement. A complete physical and a cardiac evaluation with electrocardiogram is necessary for the diagnosis. Differential diagnosis is made based on the workup described under diagnosis for CPEO.

■ Ocular
The association of ocular symptoms with heart block provides a straight forward diagnosis. If pigmentary changes occur with a questionable diagnosis, differential diagnosis includes retinitis pigmentosa. Electrodiagnostic testing, along with difference in retinal pigment presentations (location and appearance), will assist in the diagnosis. Visual field testing can be done; however, results may vary from normal to having defects. Diagnosis of the external ophthalmoplegia is made based on that delineated under CPEO.

TREATMENT AND MANAGEMENT

See Table 16–3 for an overview of the treatment and management of Kearns–Sayre syndrome.

■ Systemic

Co-management with a cardiologist is necessary in Kearns–Sayre to monitor cardiac involvement. Cardiac conduction defects are usually successfully treated with a pacemaker, often extending life. Because of potential respiratory involvement, special considerations should be made with use of certain drugs (eg, sedatives and steroids), general anesthesia, and high-altitude travel. Certain vitamins may play a potential role in managing this disease, although more research is needed.

■ Ocular

Ocular manifestations of Kearns–Sayre are managed with routine eyecare and as delineated under CPEO. Special consideration is necessary for contact lens and glaucoma patients. Contact lenses wear should either be deferred or closely monitored because of the effect corneal endothelial abnormalities may have on corneal integrity. In treatment of glaucoma patients, the potential effect of β-blockers or adrenergic agents may have on cardiac involvement in Kearns–Sayre patients should be considered.

CONCLUSION

CPEO represents a general grouping of rare ocular myopathies, which include specific entities with associated clinical features, such as oculopharyngeal muscular dystrophy and Kearns–Sayre syndrome. A slowly progressive ptosis and ophthalmoplegia are characteristic of these diseases. Diagnosis may be initially difficult, because these disorders often mimic myasthenia gravis. The correct diagnosis is important not only for the potential of ocular intervention but also for appropriate referral and co-management of systemic involvement, which may be lifesaving.

REFERENCES

Chronic Progressive External Ophthalmopathy

Danta G, Hilton RC, Lynch PG. Chronic progressive external ophthalmoplegia. *Brain*. 1975;98:473–492.

Daroff RB. Chronic progressive external ophthalmoplegia. A critical review. *Arch Ophthalmol*. 1969;82:845–850.

Eshaghian J, Anderson RL, Weingeist TA, et al. Orbicularis oculi muscle in chronic progressive external ophthalmoplegia. *Arch Ophthalmol*. 1980;98:1070–1073.

Lane CM, Collin JRO. Treatment of ptosis in chronic progressive external ophthalmoplegia. *Br J Ophthalmol*. 1987;71:290–294.

Lowes M. Chronic progressive external ophthalmoplegia, pigmentary retinopathy and heart block (Kearns–Sayre syndrome). *Acta Ophthalmol*. 1975;53:610–619.

Metz HS, Meshel L. Ocular saccades in progressive external ophthalmoplegia. *Ann Ophthalmol*. 1974;6:623–628.

Mills PV, Bowen DI, Thompson DS. Chronic progressive external ophthalmoplegia and pigmentary degeneration of the retina. *Br J Ophthalmol*. 1971;55:302–311.

Mitsumoto H, Aprille JR, Wray SH, et al. Chronic progressive external ophthalmoplegia: Clinical, morphologic, and biochemical studies. *Neurology*. 1983;33:452–461.

Mullie MA, Harding AE, Petty RKH, et al. The retinal manifestations of mitochondrial myopathy. *Arch Ophthalmol*. 1985;103:1825–1830.

Petty RK, Harding AE, Morgan-Hughes JA. The clinical features of mitochondrial myopathy. *Brain*. 1986;109:915–938.

Scully RE, Mark EJ, McNeely BV. Case records of the Massachusetts general hospital. *N Engl J Med*. 1985;312:171–177.

Stanescu B, Ferriere G. Electroretinographic alterations in progressive external ophthalmoplegia, Kearns Sayres syndrome. In: Huber A, Klein K, eds. *Neurogenetics and Neuro-ophthalmology*. New York: Elsevier/North-Holland Biomedical; 1981:215–221.

Walsh FB (ed), Hoyt WR. *Clinical Neuro-ophthalmology*. Baltimore: Williams & Wilkins; 1969;2:1254–1265.

Oculopharyngeal Muscular Dystrophy

Adamczyk DT, Oshinskie L. Oculopharyngeal muscular dystrophy. *J Am Optom Assoc*. 1987;58:408–412.

Dayal VS, Freeman J. Cricopharyngeal myotomy for dysphagia in oculopharyngeal muscular dystrophy. *Arch Otolaryngol*. 1976;102:115–116.

Duranceau AC, Beauchamp G, Jamieson GG, Barbeau A. Oropharyngeal dysphagia and oculopharyngeal muscular dystrophy. *Surg Clin North Am*. 1983;63:825–832.

Duranceau A, Forand MD, Fauteux JP. Surgery in oculopharyngeal muscular dystrophy. *Am J Surg*. 1980;139:33–39.

Ford LH, Holinger PH. Hereditary dysphagia: The oculopharyngeal syndrome. *Laryngoscope*. 1971;81:373–378.

Fried K, et al. Autosomal recessive oculopharyngeal muscular dystrophy. *J Med Genet*. 1975;12:416–418.

Hardiman O, Halperin JJ, Farrell MA, et al. Neuropathic findings in oculopharyngeal muscular dystrophy. *Arch Neurol*. 1993;50:481–488.

Johnson CC, Kuwabara T. Oculopharyngeal muscular dystrophy. *Am J Ophthalmol*. 1974;77:872–879.

Molgat YM, Rodrigue D. Correction of blepharoptosis in oculopharyngeal muscular dystrophy: Review of 91 cases. *Can J Ophthalmol*. 1993;28:11–14.

Probst A, Tackmann W, Stoeckli HR, et al. Evidence for chronic axonal atrophy in oculopharyngeal "muscular dystrophy." *Acta Neuropathologica*. 1982;57:209–216.

Rare muscular dystrophy: Tracking disease through 300 years. *JAMA*. 1967;199:40–41.

Victor M, Hayes R, Adams RD. Oculopharyngeal muscular dystrophy. *N Engl J Med*. 1962;267:1267–1272.

Kearns–Sayre Syndrome

Bachynski BN, Flynn JT, Rodrigues MM, et al. Hyperglycemic acidotic coma and death in Kearns–Sayre syndrome. *Ophthalmology*. 1986;93:391–396.

‎

Bastiaensen I, Stadhovders A, Trijbels J, et al. Kearns syndrome. Concept of a disease. In: Huber A, Klein K, eds. *Neurogenetics and Neuro-ophthalmology*. New York: Elsevier/North-Holland Biomedical; 1981;205–210.

Berenberg RA, Pellock JM, DiMauro S, et al. Lumping or splitting? "Ophthalmoplegia-plus" or Kearns–Sayre syndrome. *Ann Neurol*. 1977;1:37–54.

Drachman DA. Ophthalmoplegia plus. *Arch Neurol*. 1968;18: 654–674.

Eagle RC, Hedges TR, Yanoff M. The atypical pigmentary retinopathy of Kearns–Sayre syndrome. A light and electron microscopic study. *Ophthalmology*. 1982;89:1433–1440.

Kalenak JW, Kolker AE. Kearns–Sayre syndrome and primary open-angle glaucoma. *Am J Ophthalmol*. 1989;108:335–336.

Kosmorsky GS, Meister DM, Sheeler LR, et al. Familial ophthalmoplegia-plus syndrome with corneal endothelial disorder. *Neuro-ophthalmology*. 1989;9:271–277.

McKechnie NM, King M, Lee WR. Retinal pathology in the Kearns–Sayre syndrome. *Br J Ophthalmol*. 1985;69:63–75.

Moraes CT, DiMauro S, Zeviani M, et al. Mitochondrial DNA deletions in progressive external ophthalmoplegia and Kearns–Sayre syndrome. *N Engl J Med*. 1989;320:1293–1299.

Ohkoshi K, Ishida N, Yamaguchi T, Kani K. Corneal endothelium in a case of mitochondrial encephalomyopathy (Kearns–Sayre syndrome). *Cornea*. 1989;8:210–214.

Phillips CI, Gosden CM. Leber's hereditary optic neuropathy and Kearns–Sayre syndrome: Mitochondrial DNA mutations. *Surv Ophthalmol*. 1991;35:463–472.

SECTION V

ENDOCRINE DISORDERS

17
Chapter

Diabetes Mellitus: An Overview

Jerry Cavallerano

Diabetes mellitus (DM) has been recognized as a disease for thousands of years, but the pathogenesis of the condition is still only partially understood. The ancient Greeks named the disease "diabetes," meaning "to run through," reflecting common symptoms of diabetes—excessive thirst and frequent urination. In the 19th century it was noticed that the urine of diabetic persons was sweet, and the Latin adjective "mellitus" (sweet) was added to the disease name.

Today, diabetes mellitus is recognized as a chronic syndrome or group of disorders characterized by the inability of the body to metabolize glucose properly, resulting in hyperglycemia as a common clinical finding.

EPIDEMIOLOGY

■ Systemic

Diabetes is a worldwide medical problem. The disease afflicts approximately 14 million Americans, 50 percent of whom have not been diagnosed and are unaware of their condition. Of those with diabetes in the United States, approximately 5 to 10% have type I, insulin-dependent diabetes mellitus (IDDM), and 90% have type II, noninsulin-dependent diabetes mellitus (NIDDM).

The various types of diabetes encompass the most common endocrine disorder in the United States. Each year, there are over 725,000 new cases of diabetes, and the aging American population suggests that the incidence will continue to rise as the population ages. There is a higher prevalence of NIDDM in American Indians, African Americans, and Hispanics.

Diabetes is a significant cause of morbidity and mortality in the United States and worldwide. The disease is the seventh leading cause of death in the United States, and the American Diabetes Association (1993) estimates that the total cost of diabetes in the United States is over $20 billion per year. Furthermore, despite advances in the treatment of diabetic retinopathy and diabetic macular edema, diabetes remains the leading cause of new blindness for working-aged Americans, and the leading cause of peripheral neuropathy in the world. Diabetes is also a significant risk factor for coronary artery disease, stroke, and renal failure, and a leading cause of nontraumatic amputation.

■ Ocular

Diabetes is a leading cause of blindness and visual impairment in the United States. A person with diabetes has 25 times the risk of blindness compared to a nondiabetic person, and diabetic retinopathy is the leading cause of new blindness in Americans of working age. Diabetes results in 8000 new cases of blindness annually representing 12% of new cases. Approximately 25% of individuals with IDDM have some level of diabetic retinopathy within 5 years of diagnosis; after 10 years, 60% have some level of retinopathy, and after 15 years, 80%.

Proliferative diabetic retinopathy is present in 25% of the IDDM population within 15 years of diagnosis, and 70% of

Special thanks to Ramachandiran Cooppan, MD, and George S. Sharuk, MD, for reviewing this manuscript, and to Lora Potter for help in preparing this manuscript.

that population can expect to have proliferative retinopathy during a lifetime. Diabetic macular edema develops in 40% of the IDDM population during a lifetime.

Presently, there are 700,000 Americans with proliferative diabetic retinopathy and 130,000 with high-risk proliferative diabetic retinopathy. Furthermore, there are 500,000 Americans with diabetic macular edema, and 325,000 with clinically significant macular edema. There are 63,000 new cases of proliferative diabetic retinopathy each year, with 29,000 cases of high-risk proliferative diabetic retinopathy. The annual incidence of diabetic macular edema in the United States is 75,000, with 50,000 cases of clinically significant macular edema.

Natural History

Pathophysiology

In normal metabolism of food, the human body breaks down ingested carbohydrates into glucose, a simple sugar. This glucose then enters the blood circulation and is delivered to other cells as the most important source of energy for the human body. Excess glucose is changed either to glycogen and stored in the liver or skeletal muscles, or to fat and stored in fatty tissue. Although stored glycogen can be converted into glucose when the body requires extra energy, without insulin glucose cannot enter and be used by human cells. Insulin allows cells to use glucose for energy or to store it as fat.

Insulin is produced, stored, and released into the bloodstream by the beta cells of the islets of Langerhans of the pancreas. Glucose is the major stimulus for regulating insulin secretion. Once released into the bloodstream, insulin binds to peripheral and hepatic cell membrane insulin receptors. This binding enhances peripheral glucose uptake and inhibits hepatic glucose production, resulting in a reduction of plasma glucose.

In IDDM, beta cells of the pancreas are destroyed and little or no insulin is produced. In NIDDM, these beta cells produce an inadequate amount of insulin, or the target cells are unable to respond properly to the insulin that is produced.

Classification of Diabetes Mellitus

Four main categories of diabetes mellitus are defined by the National Diabetes Data Group (NDDG) classification of DM (Table 17–1).

Type I or *insulin-dependent diabetes mellitus* (IDDM) was formerly called juvenile-onset diabetes. Although IDDM can be diagnosed at any age, the age of onset is usually at or below 40 years. Only 5 to 10% of the diabetic population has IDDM. The condition is caused by reduced or absent insulin production, and insulin injections are

TABLE 17–1. CLASSIFICATION OF DM

Type	Characteristics
Type I : IDDM	Any age; usually thin; have abrupt onset of signs and symptoms; usually before age 40
	Strongly positive urine glucose and ketone tests
	Dependent upon exogenous insulin to prevent ketoacidosis and to sustain life
Type II: NIDDM	Usually older than 40 years at diagnosis; usually obese; few classic symptoms
	Not prone to ketoacidosis except during periods of stress
	Not dependent upon exogenous insulin for survival, but may require insulin for stress-induced hyperglycemia and hyperglycemia that persists in spite of other therapy
Gestational DM (GDM)	Onset or discovery of glucose intolerance during pregnancy
	May or may not require insulin
Impaired glucose tolerance (IGT)	Plasma glucose levels higher than normal but not diagnostic for DM
Other types of DM and IGT	Secondary to pancreatic disease (eg, pancreatectomy, cystic fibrosis, chronic pancreatitis, hemochromatosis)
	Secondary to endocrinopathies (eg, Cushing syndrome, acromegaly, pheochromocytoma, primary aldosteronism, glucogonoma)
	Secondary to drugs and chemical agents (eg, certain antihypertensive drugs, thiazide diuretics, glucocorticoids, estrogen-containing preparations, psychoactive agents, catecholamines)
	Associated with insulin-receptor abnormalities (eg, acanthosis nigricans)
	Associated with genetic syndromes (eg, hyperlipidemia, muscular dystrophies, Huntington chorea)
	Associated with miscellaneous conditions (eg, malnutrition)

required to sustain life. Autoimmune destruction of pancreas beta cells results in a high incidence of islet-cell antibodies at the time of diagnosis of IDDM. Persons with IDDM are usually moderately to severely ill at the time of diagnosis, manifesting the classic diabetic symptoms of polyuria, polyphagia, and polydipsia. Other symptoms may include nausea, vomiting, abdominal pain, lethargy, or coma. Onset is usually rapid, and treatment includes daily insulin injections, appropriate diet and meal planning, and exercise.

In general, persons with IDDM

- May be of any age, are usually thin, and usually have abrupt onset of signs and symptoms before age 40 years.

- Have strongly positive urine glucose and ketone tests.
- Are dependent upon exogenous insulin replacement to prevent ketoacidosis and to sustain life.

There are multiple factors involved in the development of IDDM. Environmental and genetic factors seem to be implicated, although no specific genetic marker has yet been identified. Acute stress and viral infection are often suspected in the development of IDDM in a genetically predisposed or susceptible person. There is also a clear HLA association with the risk of development of IDDM, but studies of identical twins strongly support the role of environmental and other factors in the onset of the disease. Also, environmental factors may control the expression of any diabetic gene. Furthermore, it is not clear whether one or multiple etiologies are responsible for the various types of diabetes. Autoimmunity is a suspected etiologic factor, because 90% of patients with new-onset IDDM have islet cell antibodies in their plasma.

The risk of developing IDDM is approximately 5% if a person has a sibling with the condition. If two siblings have DM, the risk of IDDM rises to 10%. The risk of IDDM before the age of 20 years is 5 to 10% if a person's father has DM, and 3 to 5% if the mother has DM. If an aunt or uncle has DM, the risk of IDDM is approximately 1 to 2%.

In Type II or *noninsulin-dependent diabetes mellitus* (NIDDM), patients are usually over 40 years of age at onset; hence Type II DM was formerly called adult-onset diabetes. NIDDM is by far the most prevalent form of DM. Onset is frequently insidious, and the classic diabetic symptoms are usually absent. The risk of NIDDM increases with age and obesity. At the time of diagnosis a person may experience only minor symptoms or none at all. The cause of NIDDM is insulin resistance or relative or absolute insulin deficiency. Three factors seem to contribute to the development of NIDDM:

1. A defect in the insulin-producing beta cells of the pancreas, preventing the cells from adequately responding to glucose levels in the blood.
2. A reduced number of beta cells, preventing the pancreas from controlling elevated levels of blood glucose.
3. Insulin resistance, whereby insulin is unable to bind to receptor sites on the surfaces of cells.

This insulin resistance occurs due to either a reduced number of receptor sites on cell surfaces, or defects in the chemical reaction initiated by the binding of insulin to cell-receptor sites reducing signal transduction after binding has occurred.

Patients with NIDDM are frequently overweight, and proper diet and exercise are often sufficient to control NIDDM. Medical treatment when indicated includes oral hypoglycemic agents, insulin, or both insulin and oral agents. These patients are not prone to ketoacidosis and are not dependent upon exogenous insulin for survival, although they may require insulin for stress-induced hyperglycemia and hyperglycemia that persists in spite of other therapy. The risk of NIDDM increases with age and obesity. The etiology of NIDDM is poorly understood, and seems to be related to both environmental and genetic factors, although no specific HLA associations have been recognized.

Persons with NIDDM have both insulin deficiency and insulin resistance. Multiple factors are involved in the development of NIDDM. If both parents have NIDDM, the risk of a person developing NIDDM ranges as high as 75%. The risk is reduced to 25 to 30% if only one parent has NIDDM. Obesity is present in 60 to 80% of the NIDDM population. Studies of identical twins suggest a strong genetic factor in the development of NIDDM, and over 30% of the siblings of patients with NIDDM show abnormal glucose tolerance, although the exact genetic deficiency has not been delineated.

Gestational diabetes mellitus (GDM) has its onset or discovery of glucose intolerance during pregnancy. GDM does *not* include diabetic women who become pregnant, and patients with GDM may or may not require insulin. Elevated blood glucose levels or GDM are present in 2 to 3% of pregnant women, and diagnostic criteria specific for pregnancy have been developed (Table 17–2). The American Diabetes Association recommends that all pregnant women be screened for GDM during the 24th to 28th weeks of pregnancy. Women with GDM have a 25 to 30% risk of developing DM within 5 years postpartum.

Other types of diabetes mellitus are listed in Table 17–1 for completeness but are not discussed further in this chap-

TABLE 17–2. DIAGNOSIS OF DM

Type	Characteristics
Nonpregnant Adults	Classic symptoms[a] + unequivocal elevated plasma glucose
	Fasting plasma glucose (FPG) $\geq$ 140 mg/dL on more than one occasion
	Positive results on more than one oral glucose tolerance test
Children	Classic symptoms[a] + plasma glucose $\geq$ 200 mg/dL.
	FPG $\geq$ 140 mg/dL + sustained elevated glucose concentration on oral glucose tolerance test on more than one occasion
Pregnant women	Elevated glucose concentrations in two of the four samples below:
	Fasting plasma glucose $\geq$ 105 mg/dL
	1-hour sample $\geq$ 190 mg/dL[b]
	2-hour sample $\geq$ 165 mg/dL[b]
	3-hour sample $\geq$ 145 mg/dL[b]

[a]Polyuria, polydipsia, polyphagia, ketonuria, and rapid weight loss.
[b]Following 100-g glucose on oral glucose tolerance test.

ter. These types include diabetes secondary to pancreatic disease, endocrinopathies, or drugs and chemical agents; diabetes associated with insulin-receptor abnormalities or genetic syndromes; and miscellaneous conditions.

Impaired glucose tolerance (IGT) refers to patients with plasma glucose that are higher than normal but are not diagnostic for DM on oral glucose tolerance testing. Patients with IGT have less than a 5% risk of developing DM within a year. The category comprises normal patients, patients in transition to a diabetic state, and patients who have diabetes but who do not fulfill the diagnostic criteria.

Designating the type of diabetes in a patient is not always a straightforward task. The clinical stages of each category are similar, and determining whether or not a person is ketosis prone has inherent risks and is frequently not practical.

DIAGNOSIS

Screening tests for DM are indicated if a person has a strong family history of DM, is markedly obese, has a morbid obstetrical history or history of babies over 9 pounds at birth, or is pregnant (usually between the 24th and 28th weeks of pregnancy). The National Diabetes Data Group has established specific criteria for diagnosis of diabetes in adults, children, and pregnant women (see Table 17–2). For nonpregnant adults, a fasting plasma glucose level of 115 mg/dL or greater is an indication for diagnostic testing. A level of 130 mg/dL or greater in children is an indication for diagnostic testing. In pregnant women, an oral glucose tolerance test (OGTT) with a 50-g glucose load is suggested for screening. A fasting plasma glucose level of 150 mg/dL or greater 1 hour later is an indication for diagnostic testing.

A random plasma glucose test greater than 200 mg/dL in the presence of classic diabetic symptoms of polyuria, polyphagia, and polydipsia is diagnostic of diabetes in children. In children without diabetic symptoms, a plasma glucose concentration greater than 140 mg/dL and repeated readings greater than 200 mg/dL on an OGTT on more than one occasion are also diagnostic of DM.

TREATMENT AND MANAGEMENT

Insulin-dependent Diabetes Mellitus (IDDM)

Insulin is an endogenous hormone secreted by the pancreas directly into the blood circulation. When this hormone is absent, exogenous insulin must be injected to sustain human life. Patients with IDDM require exogenous insulin

in order to survive. The treatment of IDDM, however, is more complicated than merely injecting insulin once a day, and requires a careful balance of meal planning (diet), exercise, blood glucose monitoring, and medical management.

Insulin was first used to manage diabetes by Banting and Best in 1921. The goal of insulin therapy is to provide the body with the proper dose so circulating glucose can either be used as energy or stored. Insulin overdose lowers blood glucose levels, causing hypoglycemic reactions. Insufficient insulin dosage results in hyperglycemia, which can result in ketoacidosis or diabetic coma. Consequently, insulin dosage needs to be tailored to the specific metabolic needs of each individual, considering not only dietary habits, but personal activity and life style. In the nondiabetic person, this autoregulation is controlled by release of insulin from the pancreas in response to the level of blood glucose.

Four characteristics of commercially available insulin have clinical significance: the concentration, type, purity, and species of the insulin.

Insulin *concentration* is measured in units, and this measurement is consistent for all commercially available insulin worldwide. These units are labeled on the insulin bottles, with a number following the abbreviation for unit (U). The number following the U indicates the concentration of units in 1 cc of solution. For example, insulin marked U-100 has 100 units of insulin in 1 cc; this concentration must be drawn in a U-100 syringe. U-100 insulin is increasingly becoming the standard in the United States and worldwide, and this higher concentration of insulin (compared to U-40 and U-80, for example) permits the injection of a smaller amount of fluid.

Another important characteristic of insulin is its *type*, which reflects the speed of onset of insulin action, its period of peak action and the duration of action (Table 17–3; Figure 17–1). Short-acting insulins include regular and semilente insulin, whose onset of action varies from one-half to 2 hours after injection. The peak action is within several hours, and the duration of action is relatively brief, lasting an average of 6 to 8 hours. The intermediate-acting insulins include NPH (neutral protamine Hagedorn) and lente insulin, with an onset of action after injection of 1 to 3 hours. Peak action is 6 to 12 hours after injection, and the duration of action ranges from 18 to 26 hours. The long-acting insulins include ultralente and protamine zinc (PZI). These insulins act 4 to 6 hours after injection, and

TABLE 17–3. INSULIN PREPARATION

Preparation	Onset (hr)	Duration (hr)
Rapid acting	1/2–4	5–16
Intermediate acting	1–4	16–28
Long acting	4–6	36+

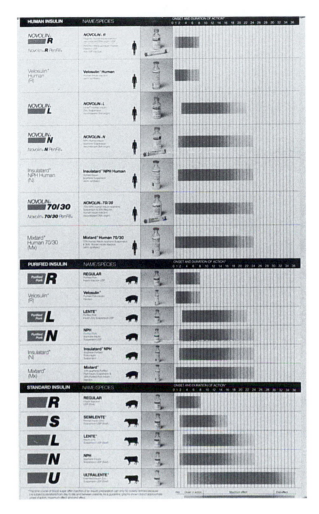

Figure 17–1. Chart showing various species of insulin and time of onset and duration of action of various types of insulin. *(Courtesy of Novo Nordisk Pharmaceuticals.)*

their peak action is 14 to 24 hours after injection. Their duration of action may last up to 36 hours.

The choice of insulin or combination of insulin types, and the mode of delivery (single daily injection, multiple daily injections, or insulin pump), need to be regulated and adjusted by the patient and primary physician, depending on the patient's life style, dietary habits, mode of glucose monitoring, compliance, social needs, and numerous other factors. Insulin types are frequently mixed for injection to take advantage of the peak action time of each type of insulin (see Figure 17–1). NPH and regular insulins make for more stable mixtures.

A third characteristic of insulin describes its *purity*. For many years insulin was available only from the pancreases of animals, particularly cattle and pigs. Because the pancreases used to produce insulin contain elements in addition to insulin, such as other hormones and cell fragments, these impurities were present in the insulin. Methods have been developed to extract these impurities from the final insulin

product because antibodies can develop in response to their presence. Today's animal extract insulins are 99.99% pure (proinsulin contaminants less than 10 parts per million). Side effects from impurities include redness or swelling at injection sites, tissue hypertrophy at injection sites, or resistance to the action of the injected insulin.

To overcome the problems of insulin impurities and to insure against shortages of animal pancreases needed to produce insulin, a biosynthetic "human" insulin has been developed. The source of insulin (biosynthetic or pork, beef, or other animal) defines the insulin's *species.* Insulins from different sources have amino acids linked in slightly different sequences. The insulin most similar to human insulin is derived from pigs. Although insulin from most animals is effective in humans, the differences can cause antibodies to the insulin to form, making the injected insulin less effective. The advent and use of synthetic insulin reduces the risk of this complication.

The goal of insulin therapy is to maintain circulating blood glucose levels as close to normal as possible; however, the autoregulation of the healthy human system to circulating levels of blood glucose cannot be duplicated by insulin injections. Strategies, therefore, have been devised to mimic the natural autoregulation of blood glucose levels. Multiple daily injections of insulin are the norm for most patients with IDDM, and the use of an artificial pancreas or the insulin pump reflects attempts to keep normal glycemic levels in a diabetic person. Frequency of insulin injection depends on a person's motivation and the severity of the diabetic condition, among other factors.

Regular exercise and appropriate meal planning to adjust the daily caloric intake and types of food are significant factors in diabetes control. Patients with diabetes need to work closely with their doctors, dieticians, and other members of their health care team to care for their diabetes. Dietary considerations are not limited merely to the total daily caloric intake. The temporal distribution of caloric intake and the food sources of the calories are also significant factors.

The Diabetes Control and Complications Trial (DCCT; 1993), a ten-year study sponsored by the National Institutes of Health, enrolled 1441 patients with type I, insulin-dependent diabetes mellitus, and investigated two questions:

1. *Primary prevention.* Does intensive therapy of diabetes prevent development of retinopathy and other long-term complications compared with conventional therapy?
2. *Secondary intervention.* Does intensive therapy affect the progression of diabetic retinopathy and other chronic complications compared with conventional therapy?

The DCCT study showed that intensive therapy reduced clinically meaningful diabetic retinopathy by 35 to 74%. Intensive therapy also reduced severe nonproliferative diabetic retinopathy, proliferative diabetic retinopathy, and a need for laser treatment by 45%. First appearance of any retinopathy was reduced by 27%. Furthermore, intensive therapy reduced the development of microalbuminuria by 35%, clinical proteinuria by 56%, and clinical neuropathy by 60%. Adverse effects of intensive therapy included hypoglycemia, catheter complications, weight gain, and ketoacidosis. Although these findings do not apply specifically to those with noninsulin-dependent diabetes mellitus, it is considered prudent to maintain as good control as possible of any diabetic condition based on the findings of the DCCT.

Noninsulin-dependent Diabetes Mellitus (NIDDM)

Diet, exercise, and weight loss in obese persons frequently may be sufficient to control NIDDM; however, in some cases pharmacological treatment is needed. Approximately 15% of persons with NIDDM control their condition by diet alone, and 25% are essentially on "no therapy." Patients with NIDDM may medically control their diabetic condition with oral hypoglycemic agents (OHGA) (35%), insulin (25%), or in some cases, both insulin and OHGA. Many patients with NIDDM require insulin for their control if oral agents fail to achieve proper blood glucose control. Also, high doses of injected insulin sometimes may not be effective without oral agents; conversely, oral agents may not be effective without injected insulin. These individuals are still considered to have NIDDM, because they can sustain life without insulin injections; but the insulin is crucial to maintain good health.

The oral hypoglycemic agents include sulfonylureas and biguanides. The biguanides presently are not available commercially in the United States, but are used in other areas of the world. These will not be discussed further in this chapter, but are mentioned for purposes of completeness.

The sulfonylureas are the oral agents presently available in the United States. These agents do not cure diabetes, and patients taking oral agents should recognize the continued importance of exercise and care in their diet and meal plan to control their diabetes. The action of these agents is to facilitate the release of insulin from the pancreas, enhance the sensitivity of insulin receptors on the target cells, decrease insulin resistance in the target cells, and regulate gluconeogenesis in the liver.

The sulfonylureas available in the United States fall into two classes, first-generation and second-generation oral hypoglycemic agents (Table 17–4). Both first- and second-generation oral hypoglycemic agents require functioning beta cells in the pancreas to be effective, and therefore oral agents cannot be used to treat IDDM. Furthermore, both generations of drugs control blood glucose levels by increasing insulin secretion and decreasing insulin resistance in the target cells. There are relatively few side effects from both classes.

TABLE 17–4. ORAL HYPOGLYCEMIC AGENTS–SULFONYLUREAS

Drug	Precautions	Duration (hr)
First Generation		
Acetohexamide (Dymelor)	Caution in elderly and patients with renal impairment	12–18
Chlorpropamide (Diabinese)	Caution in elderly and patients with renal impairment; higher frequency of alcohol flushing	24–72
Tolazamide (Tolinase)	Caution in elderly and patients with renal impairment	
Second Generation		
Glyburide (DiaBeta, Micronase)	Few side effects and drug interactions	24
Glipizide (Glucotrol)	Taken on empty stomach (before meals)	10–24

The major difference between the first- and second-generation agents concerns drug potency. In general, the second-generation agents are more potent per dose than the first-generation agents. Consequently, they are frequently effective in a once-daily dose, allowing for greater patient convenience and compliance. These second-generation agents are also more effective in decreasing insulin resistance, although they remain in the body for shorter periods and have rapid metabolic breakdown. Second-generation OHGA are less likely to react with other medications. The main drawback of second-generation oral agents, however, is a risk of hypoglycemic reaction because of their greater effectiveness.

The choice of medical therapy for those with NIDDM must be made carefully by the patient's primary physician. Consideration is given to a person's dietary habits, weight, exercise regime, and the consistency of day-to-day eating habits and dietary control. An oral hypoglycemic agent that may be effective when a person is controlling dietary intake and exercising regularly may cause serious hypoglycemia for a person who cuts back on meals, increases physical activity, or otherwise modifies his or her life style.

■ ASSOCIATED ACUTE COMPLICATIONS OF DIABETES MELLITUS

■ Systemic

Three major acute complications of DM are diabetic ketoacidosis, nonketotic hyperosmolar syndrome, and hypoglycemia. Each of these conditions is a medical emergency.

Diabetic Ketoacidosis

Diabetic ketoacidosis (DKA) is a potentially life-threatening condition that results from insulin deficiency. DKA is unlikely in NIDDM except during periods of significant stress such as those induced by trauma and intercurrent infection or disease. Despite modern treatment strategies and insulin availability, DKA is still relatively common, resulting in nearly 10% of hospital admissions for which diabetes is listed as the primary cause of hospitalization. Although DKA may be a presenting sign of DM, only 20% of cases of DKA occur in new-onset DM. The diagnosis of DKA may be difficult. Typically, polyuria and polydipsia are present for several days prior to onset. Gastric stasis and distension, nausea, vomiting, and anorexia are frequently present. Dehydration may result in tachycardia, disorientation, and tremulousness.

DKA results from a deficiency of insulin and an excess of counterregulatory hormones such as glucagon, catecholamines, cortisol, and growth hormone. The glucagon directly stimulates gluconeogenesis and ketogenesis in the absence of insulin. The degree of ketone body production correlates with the plasma glucagon concentration. Hepatic glucose production is further increased by excess catecholamine, cortisol, and growth hormone. These agents inhibit peripheral glucose utilization, resulting in increased fat conversion to free fatty acids and consequent production of ketone bodies.

Stress-induced release of counterregulatory factors is felt to play a significant role in the development of DKA. Infection and coexistent illness are the most common precipitating factors for DKA. Malfunction of insulin pumps and omission of insulin injections may also lead to DKA.

Prompt treatment of DKA is essential, with the goal being to increase glucose utilization, correct acidosis and ketonemia, and return normal hydration and electrolyte composition. However, there are serious complications due to treatment, including hypokalemia, hypoglycemia, and central nervous system deterioration. Meticulous diabetes management reduces the risk of complications, but DKA has been shown to cause nearly 10% of deaths associated with diabetes.

Alcoholic ketoacidosis is considered in the differential diagnosis of diabetic ketoacidosis. This condition is characterized by hyperketonemia, acidosis, and dehydration, although hyperglycemia is uncommon. The condition follows heavy and prolonged drinking, and may be marked by anorexia, nausea, vomiting, and abstinence from alcohol in the previous day.

Nonketotic Hyperosmolar Syndrome

Nonketotic hyperosmolar syndrome is an acute diabetic complication that most commonly affects the elderly with NIDDM who suffer from insidious hyperglycemia. Diuresis and subsequent dehydration leading to marked elevation in osmolarity result. Extreme hyperglycemia without ketoacidosis is the benchmark of this condition. Undiagnosed NIDDM or NIDDM stressed by infection, stroke, or steroid or diuretic therapy may precipitate nonketotic hyperosmolar syndrome. Treatment includes fluid replacement, insulin and electrolyte replacement, and identification of precipitating factors such as infection or cerebral vascular accident. The disorder can be fatal, and early recognition is essential in successful management. Treatment includes fluid replacement, and insulin and electrolyte administration. Identification of precipitating factors is important.

Hypoglycemia

Hypoglycemia is the most common and potentially the most serious acute complication of DM. Insulin, oral hypoglycemic agents, and alcohol are the most frequent causes of exogenous hypoglycemia. Insulin therapy results in monthly episodes of mild hypoglycemia in over 50% of patients. Attempts at tight metabolic control, such as in systems of continuous subcutaneous insulin infusion or with multiple daily injections, can result in profound hypoglycemia and a threefold increased risk of severe hypoglycemia, as was found in the Diabetes Control and Complications Trial (DCCT).

Several commonly used drugs can increase the hypoglycemia effect of insulin and oral hypoglycemic agents. These drugs include alcohol, sulfonylureas, biguanides, nonselective β–blockers, monoamine oxidase inhibitors, salicylates, and tetracyclines. Certain agents such as chloramphenicol, antibiotic sulfonamides, and doxycycline increase the risk of hypoglycemia by inhibiting the excretion or metabolism of sulfonylureas. This same effect is also seen with ethanol, phenylbutazone, coumadin, allopurinol, and phenyramidol. Competition for albumin-binding sites increases sulfonylurea action when used in combination with salicylates, antibiotic sulfonamides, and phenylbutazone. Beta-adrenergic receptor blocking agents, including some antiglaucoma drops, increase the risk of hypoglycemia by reducing gluconeogenesis.

■ ASSOCIATED CHRONIC COMPLICATIONS OF DIABETES MELLITUS

Persons with IDDM and NIDDM alike are susceptible to the chronic and acute complications of diabetes (Table 17–5).

■ Systemic

Microvascular Disease

Vascular diseases represent the major long-term complications of DM. Vascular diseases result from basement mem-

TABLE 17–5. COMPLICATIONS OF DM

Acute complications	Diabetic ketoacidosis (DKA)
	Nonketotic hyperosmolar syndrome
	Hypoglycemia
Chronic complications	Microvascular Disease
	Retinopathy
	Nephropathy
	Neuropathy
	Macrovascular disease
	Cardiovascular disease

brane disorders in the vessels, disorders of blood flow, and abnormalities of blood platelets. Diabetic microvascular disease usually is demonstrated in retinopathy, nephropathy, and neuropathies.

Functional loss of pericytes, endothelial cell proliferation, and thickening of the basement membrane of small vessels are frequently the earliest signs of diabetic changes in the body. These changes are reflected in the retina, kidneys, conjunctiva, skin, and elsewhere in the body. Such changes are frequently the earliest visible diabetic change, especially in the retina. There is some evidence that the degree of basement membrane damage reflects overall metabolic control. Blood flow disorders also result in vascular damage. Increased aggregation of red blood cells, secondary to abnormalities of blood platelets, causes endothelial cell injury, resulting in increased vascular permeability and, consequently, microangiopathy. Atherosclerotic plaques and signs develop in areas of altered blood flow.

Antiplatelet agents such as aspirin have been tested to determine their value in reducing diabetic vascular complications. Studies to date have been equivocal, although the Early Treatment Diabetic Retinopathy Study (ETDRS) demonstrated neither any advantage nor disadvantage to the daily use of 650 mg of aspirin in relation to diabetic retinopathy.

Nephropathy. The risk of renal disease for a person with DM is 20 times greater than in the general population. Approximately 4000 new cases of end-stage renal disease result from DM in the United States each year, and renal disease is the cause of death for one-half the deaths of all persons with IDDM under the age of 40 years. Approximately 40% with IDDM eventually become uremic, and 25 to 30% with NIDDM become uremic.

Glycemic control and blood pressure levels are closely related to renal disease. Renal disease may be asymptomatic for many years, although a person may have elevated levels of proteinuria. Early clinical signs include increased kidney size and increased glomerular filtration rate, which in turn leads to microalbuminuria. Diffuse thickening of the glomerular basement membrane results, leading to glomerular occlusion and renal insufficiency. Diet modifi-

cation and reduction of dietary protein are important management tools. Dialysis or transplantation become necessary in end-stage renal disease.

Neuropathy. Diabetic neuropathy is a common microvascular complication of diabetes. Diabetic neuropathies are generally considered in three categories: (1) symmetric distal polyneuropathy; (2) asymmetric neuropathies, such as cranial mononeuropathies and peripheral neuropathies; and (3) autonomic neuropathies.

There is evidence of demyelination and remyelination of nerve fibers, loss of endothelial cell tight junctions, and basement membrane thickening in patients with distal, symmetric, and autonomic neuropathy. The underlying etiology for symmetric distal neuropathies is a general metabolic abnormality involving neurons and Schwann cells. Symmetric distal neuropathy can be either painful or asymptomatic. The asymptomatic type is characterized by a numbness or tingling in the extremities, and the pain can result in either dull aches or severe pain.

Vascular occlusion or ischemia is considered the underlying problem for the asymmetrical or focal neuropathies, such as cranial mononeuropathies and peripheral neuropathies. Focal neuropathies are more common among older patients with NIDDM, while the incidence of symmetric neuropathies is approximately equal for those with NIDDM and IDDM.

Asymmetric mononeuropathy usually involves cranial nerves III, IV, or VI. The sixth and third nerves are most frequently affected, and there is pupillary sparing in approximately 80% of the cases of third-nerve palsy. Mononeuropathies of peripheral nerves usually involve nerves predisposed to pressure or entrapment, such as carpal tunnel syndrome. Neuropathic ulcers are frequent, especially in the foot, and are the result of decreased sensation and abnormal pressure distribution because of the weakness of intrinsic muscles of the foot from neuropathy.

Visceral (autonomic) neuropathy can result in gastroparesis, diabetic diarrhea, neurogenic bladder, impotence in men, and impaired cardiovascular reflexes. Mixed vascular and neuropathic disease can lead to leg ulcers and foot ulcers.

Treatment for diabetic neuropathy and its complications varies. Aldose reductase inhibitors have been suggested as a means to prevent diabetic neuropathy. Many complications of neuropathy can be prevented by prudent and judicious care, such as foot self-examination and appropriate choice of shoes. In some cases of diabetic neuropathy, medication, or vascular surgery is indicated.

Macrovascular Disease
Cardiovascular disease is the most frequent cause of death in diabetic patients. Coronary artery disease (CAD) is four to six times more prevalent in a diabetic population than in

a nondiabetic population. Risk factors for the development of CAD include age, smoking, hypertension, hyperlipoproteinemia, cholesterolemia, and elevated triglycerides. Duration of DM does not seem to be an independent risk factor for CAD in NIDDM patients, but the risk of CAD for IDDM patients rises from less than 10% after 25 years duration to over 60% after 40 years of IDDM.

Patients with DM also have a higher incidence of congestive heart failure, cardiomyopathy, cardiogenic shock, and recurrent myocardial infarction. The risk of stroke is two to four times greater for a diabetic person than for a nondiabetic person. Diabetes is a recognized independent risk factor for accelerated coronary vascular atherosclerosis, accelerated cerebrovascular atherosclerosis, and accelerated peripheral vascular disease.

■ Ocular

Ocular complications of DM are common, and all structures of the eye are susceptible to the deleterious effects of DM (Table 17–6.) Diabetic retinopathy is the leading cause of new blindness in Americans of working age. Vision loss from diabetes results from nonresolving vitreous hemorrhage, fibrovascular tissue growth leading to traction retinal detachment, and diabetic macular edema and macular nonperfusion (Table 17–7; Figures 17–2 to 17–5). Presently, there is no preventive means or cure for either diabetic retinopathy or diabetic macular edema, although the management of these conditions and their complications has been dictated by the findings of the Diabetic Retinopathy Study (DRS), Early Treatment Diabetic Retinopathy Study (ETDRS), and Diabetic Retinopathy Vitrectomy Study (DRVS)* Briefly, these studies show that:

- Appropriate and properly timed scatter (panretinal) laser photocoagulation surgery can reduce the risk of severe visual loss (best corrected acuity of 5/200 or worse) from proliferative diabetic retinopathy to 5% or less.
- Appropriate and properly timed focal laser photocoagulation surgery can reduce the risk of moderate visual loss (a doubling of the visual angle, such as a reduction from 20/40 to 20/80) from diabetic macular edema by 50% or more.
- Early vitrectomy may be valuable in restoring useful vision in patients with severe vitreous hemorrhage, particularly in those with IDDM, compared to delaying vitrectomy.

Diabetic retinopathy is a highly specific vascular complication that affects persons with either Type I or Type II

*A full discussion of diabetic eye disease is beyond the scope of this chapter, and the reader is referred to the reports of the DRS, ETDRS, and DRVS.

TABLE 17–6. OCULAR COMPLICATIONS OF DM

Visual function
  Reduced accommodation
  Fluctuating vision and refraction
  Tritan color defect
Increased incidence of primary open-angle glaucoma
Extraocular muscle palsy (III, IV, VI cranial nerve mononeuropathy)
Decreased tear production
Periorbital edema
Cornea
  Reduced corneal sensitivity
  Corneal abrasions and recurrent corneal erosions
  Slow, defective corneal re-epithelialization
Iris
  Rubeosis iridis (neovascularization of the iris)
  Ectropion uveae
  Neovascular glaucoma
Lens
  Premature cataract
  Diabetic cataract
Retina
  Nonproliferative diabetic retinopathy (NPDR)
  Proliferative diabetic retinopathy (PDR)
  Diabetic macular edema (DME)

DM. Almost all patients with IDDM after 20 years have at least some degree of retinopathy. Although laser surgery and other surgical modalities help minimize the risk of *moderate and severe visual loss* from DM, and in some cases restore useful vision for those who have suffered visual loss, there is no known method to prevent the development of diabetic retinopathy. These surgical modalities, particularly laser treatments, are most effective if initiated when a person *approaches* or just reaches *high-risk proliferative diabetic retinopathy* (PDR), or before a person has lost visual acuity from diabetic macular edema.

The 5-year risk of severe visual loss from high-risk PDR may be as high as 60%, and the risk of moderate visual loss from clinically significant macular edema (CSME) may be as high as 25 to 30%. Because proliferative retinopathy and macular edema may cause no ocular or visual symptoms when the retinal lesions are most amenable to treatment, the responsibility is to identify eyes at risk of visual loss and insure that patients receive referral for laser surgery at the most appropriate time. Diabetic macular disease may be present at any level of retinopathy.

Although retinopathy is the diabetic ocular complication most frequently recognized, diabetes can affect all structures of the eye. Appropriate examination and patient education can prevent or reduce the risk of some of these complications, and at times proper diagnosis, particularly in the presence of cranial nerve palsies, presents a significant diagnostic challenge.

TABLE 17–7. LEVELS OF RETINOPATHY

Nonproliferative Diabetic Retinopathy (NPDR)
A. Mild NPDR

At least one microaneurysm

Definition not met for B–F

B. Moderate NPDR

Moderate hemorrhages and/or microaneurysms (H/MA)

OR

Soft exudates, venous beading, and IRMA
   definitely present

Definition not met for C–F

C. Severe NPDR

Moderate H/MA in all four retinal quadrants

OR

Venous beading in two or more quadrants

OR

Moderate IRMA in at least one quadrant

Definition not met for D–F

D. Very Severe NPDR

Any two or more of C, above

Definition not met for E or F

Proliferative Diabetic Retinopathy (PDR)

Composed of
   Neovascularization on the disc or elsewhere
   Preretinal or vitreous hemorrhage
   Fibrous tissue proliferation

E. Early PDR

New vessels

Definition not met for F

F. High-risk PDR

NVD ≥ 1/3–1/2 disc area

OR

NVD and vitreous or preretinal hemorrhage

OR

NVE ≥ 1/2 disc area and preretinal or vitreous hemorrhage

Clinically Significant Diabetic Macular Edema

Thickening of the retina located less than or equal to 500 μm from
   the center of the macula

OR

Hard exudates with thickening of the adjacent retina located less
   than or equal to 500 μm from the center of the macula

OR

A zone of retinal thickening one disc area or larger in size located
   less than or equal to one disc diameter from the center of the
   macula

IRMA, intratretinal microvascular anomalies; NVD, neovascularization of the disc.
Based on ETDRS report 8.

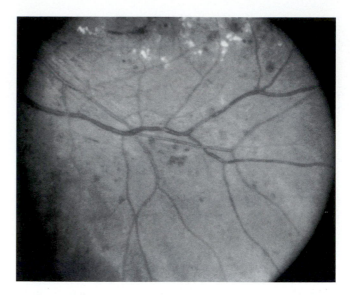

Figure 17–2. Severe nonproliferative diabetic retinopathy (NPDR). The various lesions of NPDR are represented, including cotton-wool spots, venous caliber abnormality, and hemorrhage and microaneurysms.

Proper ocular examination of the diabetic patient requires careful attention to visual acuity measurements and refraction, pupillary responses, extraocular muscle movements, the presence or absence of rubeosis iridis and cataracts, and careful fundus evaluation through dilated pupils annually. The presence of ocular or other medical abnormalities requires more frequent examination (Table 17–8).

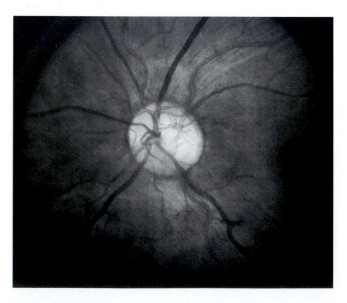

Figure 17–3. Proliferative diabetic retinopathy (PDR). There are new vessels on the optic nervehead greater than 1/4 disc area. This person has high-risk PDR and should be referred for prompt scatter (panretinal) laser photocoagulation surgery.

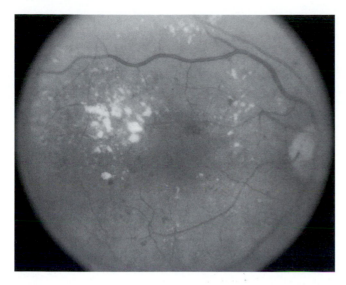

Figure 17–4. Diabetic macular edema. The retina shows clinically significant diabetic macular edema with hard exudates < 500 μm from the center of the macula with an adjacent area of retinal thickening (thickening not appreciated without stereoscopic viewing).

CONCLUSION

Diabetes mellitus is a complex disease with the potential for devastating systemic and ocular complications. Eyecare providers and other healthcare providers caring for diabetic patients need to pay constant attention to all potential ocular complications from diabetes. Furthermore, diabetes requires constant care by the patient, internist or diabetologist, and healthcare team. A patient's internist or diabetologist should be apprised of all eye examination findings, and

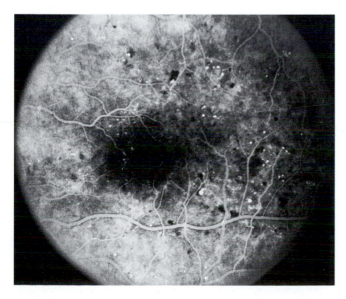

Figure 17–5. Fluorescein angiogram showing nonperfusion in the macular area.

TABLE 17–8. EYE EXAMINATION SCHEDULE

Type of DM	Recommended Time of First Exam	Routine Follow-up[a]
Type I IDDM	5 years after onset or during puberty	Yearly
Type II NIDDM	At time of diagnosis	Yearly

[a] Abnormal findings will dictate more frequent follow-up examinations.

patients should be encouraged to maintain an active role in the care of their diabetes in conjunction with their internist and other members of the healthcare team.

REFERENCES

American Diabetes Association. Position statement: Gestational diabetes mellitus. *Diabetes Care.* 1990;13(suppl):5–6.

American Diabetes Association. *Diabetes: 1991 Vital Statistics.* Alexandria, VA: American Diabetes Association, 1993.

Committee on Statistics, American Diabetes Association. Standardization of the oral glucose tolerance test. *Diabetes.* 1969;18:299.

Kahn R, Weir GC, eds. *Joslin's Diabetes Mellitus.* 13th ed. Philadelphia: Lea & Febiger; 1994.

Klein R, Klein BEK, Moss SE, et al. The Wisconsin Epidemiologic Study of Diabetic Retinopathy, 2. Prevalence and risk of diabetic retinopathy when age at diagnosis is less than 30 years. *Arch Ophthalmol.* 1984;102:520–526.

Klein R, Klein BEK, Moss SE, et al. The Wisconsin Epidemiologic Study of Diabetic Retinopathy, 3. Prevalence and risk of diabetic retinopathy when age at diagnosis is 30 or more years. *Arch Ophthalmol.* 1984;102:527–532.

Krall LP, Beaser RS. *Joslin Diabetes Manual.* 12th ed. Philadelphia: Lea & Febiger; 1989.

Moy CS, ed. *Diabetes: 1991 Vital Statistics.* Alexandria, VA: American Diabetes Association; 1991.

National Diabetes Data Group. Classification and diagnosis of diabetes mellitus and other categories of glucose intolerance. *Diabetes.* 1979;28:1039–1057.

Rifkin H, Porte D, eds. *Ellenberg and Rifkin's Diabetes Mellitus: Theory and Practice.* 4th ed. New York: Elsevier; 1990.

Diabetic Retinopathy Study

Diabetic Retinopathy Study report 1: Preliminary report on effects of photocoagulation therapy. *Am J Ophthalmol.* 1976;81:1–14.

Diabetic Retinopathy Study report 2: Photocoagulation of proliferative diabetic retinopathy. *Ophthalmology.* 1978;85:82.

Diabetic Retinopathy Study report 3: Four risk factors for severe visual loss in diabetic retinopathy. *Arch Ophthalmol.* 1979;97:658.

Diabetic Retinopathy Study report 4: A short report of long range results. Proceedings of the 10th Congress of International Diabetes Federation. *Excerpta Medica.* 1980;789–794.

Diabetic Retinopathy Study report 5: Photocoagulation treatment of proliferative diabetic retinopathy. Relationship of adverse treatment effects to retinopathy severity. *Dev Ophthal* (S Karger, Basel). 1981;2:1–15.

Diabetic Retinopathy Study report 6: Design, methods, and baseline results. *Invest Ophthalmol.* 1981;21:149–209.

Diabetic Retinopathy Study report 7: A modification of the Airlie House Classification of Diabetic Retinopathy. *Invest Ophthalmol.* 1981;21:210–226.

Diabetic Retinopathy Study report 8: Photocoagulation treatment of proliferative diabetic retinopathy. Clinical application of Diabetic Retinopathy Study (DRS) findings. *Ophthalmology.* 1981;88:583–600.

Diabetic Retinopathy Study report 9: Assessing possible late treatment effects in stopping clinical trials early: A case study by F. Ederer, MJ Podgor. *Controlled Clin Trials.* 1984;5:373–381.

Diabetic Retinopathy Study report 10: Factors influencing the development of visual loss in advanced diabetic retinopathy. *Invest Ophthalmol.* 1985;26:983–991.

Diabetic Retinopathy Study report 11: Intraocular pressure following panretinal photocoagulation for diabetic retinopathy. *Arch Ophthalmol.* 1987;105:807–809.

Diabetic Retinopathy Study report 12: Macular edema in Diabetic Retinopathy Study patients. *Ophthalmology.* 1987;94:754–760.

Diabetic Retinopathy Study report 13: Factors associated with visual outcome after photocoagulation for diabetic retinopathy. *Invest Ophthalmol.* 1989;30:23–28.

Diabetic Retinopathy Study report 14: Indications for photocoagulation treatment of diabetic retinopathy. *Int Ophthalmol Clin.* 1987;27:239–253.

Early Treatment Diabetic Retinopathy Study

Early Treatment Diabetic Retinopathy Study report 1: Photocoagulation for diabetic macular edema. *Arch Ophthalmol.* 1985;103:1796–1806.

Early Treatment Diabetic Retinopathy Study report 2: Treatment techniques and clinical guidelines for photocoagulation of diabetic macular edema. *Ophthalmology.* 1987;94:761–774.

Early Treatment Diabetic Retinopathy Study report 3: Techniques for scatter and local photocoagulation treatment of diabetic retinopathy. *Int Ophthalmol Clin.* 1987;27:254–264.

Early Treatment Diabetic Retinopathy Study report 4: Photocoagulation for diabetic macular edema. *Int Ophthalmol Clin.* 1987;27:265–272.

Early Treatment Diabetic Retinopathy Study Case reports 3 and 4: Case reports to accompany Early Treatment Diabetic Retinopathy Study Reports Numbers 3 and 4. *Int Ophthalmol Clin.* 1987;27:273–333.

Early Treatment Diabetic Retinopathy Study report 5: Detection of diabetic macular edema. Ophthalmoscopy versus photography. *Ophthalmology.* 1989;96:746–751.

Early Treatment Diabetic Retinopathy Study report 7: Early Treatment Diabetic Retinopathy Study design and baseline patient characteristics. *Ophthalmology.* 1991;98:741–756.

Early Treatment Diabetic Retinopathy Study report 8: Effects of aspirin treatment on diabetic retinopathy. *Ophthalmology.* 1991;98:757–765.

Early Treatment Diabetic Retinopathy Study report 9: Early photocoagulation for diabetic retinopathy. *Ophthalmology.* 1991;98:766–785.

Early Treatment Diabetic Retinopathy Study report 10: Grading diabetic retinopathy from stereoscopic color fundus photographs—an extension of the modified Airlie House Classification. *Ophthalmology.* 1991;98:786–806.

Early Treatment Diabetic Retinopathy Study report 11: Classification of diabetic retinopathy from fluorescein angiograms. *Ophthalmology.* 1991;98:807–822.

Early Treatment Diabetic Retinopathy Study report 12: Fundus photographic risk factors for progression of diabetic retinopathy. *Ophthalmology.* 1991;98:823.

Early Treatment Diabetic Retinopathy Study report 13: Fluorescein angiographic risk factors for progression of diabetic retinopathy. *Ophthalmology.* 1991;98:834–840.

Diabetic Retinopathy Vitrectomy Study

Diabetic Retinopathy Vitrectomy Study report 1: Two-year course of visual acuity in severe proliferative diabetic retinopathy with conventional management. *Ophthalmology.* 1985;92:492–502.

Diabetic Retinopathy Vitrectomy Study report 2: Early vitrectomy for severe vitreous hemorrhage in diabetic retinopathy. Two-year results of a randomized trial. *Arch Ophthalmol.* 1985;103:1644–1652.

Diabetic Retinopathy Vitrectomy Study report 3: Early vitrectomy for severe proliferative diabetic retinopathy in eyes with useful vision. Results of a randomized trial. *Ophthalmology.* 1988;95:1307–1320.

Diabetic Retinopathy Vitrectomy Study report 4: Early vitrectomy for severe proliferative diabetic retinopathy in eyes with useful vision. Clinical application of results of a randomized trial. *Ophthalmology.* 1988;95:1331–1334.

Diabetic Retinopathy Vitrectomy Study report 5: Early vitrectomy for severe vitreous hemorrhage in diabetic retinopathy. Four-year results of a randomized trial. *Arch Ophthalmol.* 1990;108:958–964.

The Diabetes Control and Complications Trial (DCCT)

DCCT Research Group. The effect of intensive treatment of diabetes on the development and progression of long-term complications in insulin-dependent diabetes mellitus. *New Engl J Med.* 1993;329:977–986.

DCCT Research Group. Baseline analysis of renal function in the diabetes control and complications trial. *Kidney Int.* 1993;5:668–674.

DCCT Research Group. Plasma lipid and HDL cholesterol levels in patients with Type I diabetes recruited for the Diabetes Control and Complications Trial. *Diabetes Care.* 1992;15:885–894.

DCCT Research Group. Epidemiology of severe hypoglycemia in the DCCT. *Am J Med.* 1991;90:450–459.

DCCT Research Group. The Diabetes Control and Complications Trial: An update. *Diabetes Care.* 1990;13:427–33.

DCCT Research Group. Are continuing studies of metabolic control and microvascular complications in IDDM justified? The Diabetes Control and Complications Trial. *N Engl J Med.* 1988;318:246–250.

DCCT Research Group. Assessment of hemoglobin A_{1c} in the Diabetes Control and Complications Trial. *Clin Chemistry.* 1987;33:2267–2271.

DCCT Research Group. Comparison of stereo fundus photography and fluorescein angiography in detecting early diabetic retinopathy: The Diabetes Control and Complications Trial experience. *Arch Ophthalmol.* 1987;105:1344–1351.

DCCT Research Group. The Diabetes Control and Complications Trial: Results of the feasibility study (phase II). *Diabetes Care.* 1987;10:1–9.

DCCT Research Group. Effects of age, duration and treatment of IDDM on residual b-cell function: Observations during eligibility testing for the Diabetes Control and Complications Trial. *J Clin Endocrinol Metab.* 1987;65:30–36.

DCCT Research Group. The Diabetes Control and Complications Trial: Design and methodologic considerations for the feasibility phase. *Diabetes.* 1986;35:530–544.

Schumer M, Burton G, Burton C, Crum D, Pfeifer MA, DCCT Research Group. Diabetic autonomic neuropathy, 1. autonomic nervous system data analysis by a computerized central unit in a multicenter trial. *Am J Med.* 1988;85(suppl 5A):137–143.

18
Chapter

Thyroid Dysfunction

Bernard J. Dolan

The thyroid gland secretes hormones that maintain the normal metabolic function of the body. The production and release of excess thyroid hormones results in increased metabolic activity, and is referred to as hyperthyroidism. The most common form of hyperthyroidism is Graves disease. A decrease in the production and release of thyroid hormones results in decreased metabolic activity and is called hypothyroidism. The most common cause of noniatrogenic thyroid failure in the United States is chronic autoimmune thyroiditis (Hashimoto disease). Normal production and release of thyroid hormones is called the euthyroid state. Goiter is a diffuse or nodular enlargement of the thyroid that can occur in the hyperthyroid, hypothyroid, or euthyroid states. The most common thyroid disorder is iodine deficiency, which leads to goiter and hypothryoidism. This discussion will emphasize those thyroid disorders that are associated with the ocular findings of thyroid related orbitopathy.

EPIDEMIOLOGY

■ Systemic

Hyperthyroidism
Graves disease most commonly presents in the second to third decade, although it is often seen in the fourth and fifth decades. It occurs about six times more often in females than males. It is much less common in the elderly and is unusual in children under 10 years of age. In the United States, a prevalence of 0.4% is estimated.

Hypothyroidism
There are a variety of causes for hypothyroidism; therefore, the epidemiology varies with the specific cause. Hypothyroidism is more common than hyperthyroidism, affecting approximately 2% of females and 1% of males in population studies. The presence of thyroid autoantibodies, which correlates with chronic autoimmune thyroiditis, can be detected in 10% of the population, with this presence four times more frequent in older women than men.

However, only half of these individuals have raised thyroid stimulating hormone (TSH) levels. Only 5% per year with both antibodies and elevated TSH levels will develop hypothryoidism. Sporadic congenital hypothyroidism arrests normal development and results in physical and mental retardation. It occurs in about one in every 4000 live births. Many states require screening for hypothyroidism in newborns to allow for prompt treatment of these individuals.

■ Ocular

Hyperthyroidism
Thyroid-related orbitopathy most commonly presents in 30- to 50-year-old females. The female-to-male ratio is 2.5 to 1. Elderly patients who develop Graves disease are less likely to develop eye findings. However, when elderly men develop eye findings, severe orbitopathy occurs more often than in younger individuals. Thyroid eye disease is less common in children and adolescents. When it occurs in children it is usually very mild. Smoking has been identified as a risk factor for developing ocular signs and is associated with increased severity of ocular findings.

Approximately 50% of cases have some component of clinically evident infiltrative orbitopathy.

Hypothyroidism

No information is available in the literature concerning the epidemiology of the ocular involvement, which is more an ocular manifestation of systemic hypothyroidism.

NATURAL HISTORY

Anatomy and Physiology

The thyroid is the largest endocrine gland in the normal adult. Located in the anterior portion of the lower neck, it consists of a right and left lobe that are lateral to the trachea and connected by a small isthmus. An embryologic remnant of the thyroglossal duct is sometimes present in the form of a pyramidal lobe. Due to the migration of the thyroglossal duct from the second pharyngeal pouch during embryonic development, thyroid tissue may be found throughout the neck region.

The thyroid is composed of numerous microscopic closed vesicles, called follicles, lined by a simple cuboidal epithelium and filled with a proteinaceous colloidal material. This colloidal material is composed of thyroglobulin, a high-molecular-weight iodinated glycoprotein that stores the thyroid hormones.

Iodine, an essential component of thyroid hormones, is a somewhat rare element. Therefore, proper dietary intake is necessary to ensure an adequate iodine supply. Iodized salt, sea fish, milk, and eggs are good dietary sources of this element. The epithelial cells lining the thyroid follicle act as a very efficient trap to concentrate the iodide available in the body. The presence of TSH, or thyrotropin, from the pituitary acts to stimulate thyroid iodide transport, while its absence results in markedly decreased iodide transport.

Iodide trapped by the thyroid is rapidly oxidized to iodine and through a series of complex reactions is incorporated into the tyrosine molecule to form the basic building blocks of the thyroid hormones triiodothyronine (T_3) and thyroxine (T_4). Thyroglobulin acts as a substrate for the iodination and coupling of the tyrosines. The T_3 and T_4 hormones are stored in the follicular lumen attached to thyroglobulin until they are released.

Both the production and release of the thyroid hormones are stimulated by TSH. The secretion of TSH is under control of thyroid-releasing hormone (TRH), which is synthesized in the hypothalamus. TRH binds to the thyrotrope cells of the anterior pituitary and stimulates the release of TSH. This hormone then binds to specific receptors of the thyroid follicular cell, stimulating the production and release of thyroid hormones (Figure 18–1).

The normal thyroid gland does not produce equal amounts of the thyroid hormones. The extrathyroidal pool

of T_4 is approximately 20 times greater than the pool of T_3 and the half-life of T_4 is 7 days versus 1 day for T_3. Although T_3 is the more potent thyroid hormone, only a small amount of the peripheral concentration comes from direct thyroidal secretion. The major component of thyroid secretion is T_4, which is converted by iodination in the peripheral tissues to produce active T_3. The effects of T_4 in the peripheral tissues may rely on its conversion to T_3. This has lead to the suggestion that T_4 is a T_3 prohormone. In addition, the conversion of T_4 to T_3 is controlled by different enzymes of various tissue types, which may provide additional regulation of thyroid hormone function.

Thyroid hormones in the blood are bound to specific serum proteins, thyroxine- binding globulins (TBG), thyroxine-binding prealbumin (TBPA), and albumin. These proteins have a higher affinity for T_4, which normally has only 0.03% of the hormone circulating in the free unbound state. T_3 is less tightly bound, with about 0.3% of the hormone in the unbound state. Serum-binding proteins act as a metabolic storage compartment for the thyroid hormones, protecting this reservoir from excretion and metabolic degradation. The metabolic effects of the thyroid hormones appear to be related to the amount of hormone circulating in the free state.

In order to prevent the excess production and secretion of thyroid hormones, a negative feedback loop is required. An increase in the serum concentration of the thyroid hormones is effective in inhibiting the pituitary secretion of TSH. In addition, thyroid hormones influence the inhibition of TSH when injected into the hypothalamus; however, the role they play in affecting TRH concentration is uncertain.

Thyroid hormones act to stimulate the cellular metabolic reactions of tissues throughout the body. By enhancing oxygen consumption, stimulating protein synthesis,

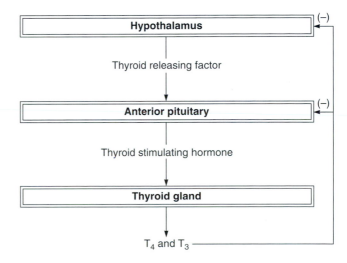

Figure 18–1. Feedback loop for thyroid hormones. The major site of the inhibition is at the pituitary level, with the inhibitory effect of T_4 primarily mediated through its conversion to T_3 within the gland.

stimulating lipolysis, and activating hepatic glyconeogenesis, the thyroid hormones enhance the generation of body heat. It has been estimated that thyroid hormones regulate 40% of the body's resting oxygen consumption. Normal growth and sexual development of the body will not occur in the absence of thyroid hormones. Skin and connective tissue depend on these hormones for the integrity of normal collagen and hair growth. Myocardial proteins regulating cardiac contractibility are affected by thyroid hormones. The nervous system requires these hormones for the normal production of neurons, dendrite and myelin formation, and normal nerve conduction. In addition, the thyroid hormones affect gastrointestinal motility, endocrine gland functions, and red blood cell production.

■ Systemic

Table 18–1 summarizes the systemic manifestations of thyroid disorders.

Thyrotoxicosis

Thyrotoxicosis refers to a clinical syndrome comprising many physiologic and biochemical changes. These are produced by the alterations in cellular metabolism due to increased amounts of thyroid hormones. The signs and symptoms of thyrotoxicosis involve many organ systems, because thyroid hormone receptors are present on all cells of the body. Thyrotoxicosis has a number of etiologies, including primary hyperthyroidism (Graves disease), excess thyroid medication in the treatment of hypothyroidism or goiter, a toxic multinodular goiter, toxic adenoma, excess iodine, inflammatory induced leakage of thyroid hormones, excess hormone produced by ectopic thyroid tissue, and thyroid carcinoma or choriocarcinoma. Thus, *thyrotoxicosis* refers to disorders of elevated thyroid hormones without regard for the source, while *hyperthyroidism* is reserved for those cases where excess thyroid hormones are a product of thyroid hypersecretion. The clinical presentation of thyrotoxicosis in these various disorders has many similar components; however, these will vary with the age of the patient, severity of the disorder, and pathophysiology of the specific syndrome.

Thyrotoxicosis affects the metabolism and removal of numerous drugs from the body. This usually results in requiring an increased medication dosage to maintain the

TABLE 18–1. SYSTEMIC MANIFESTATIONS OF THYROID DISORDERS

HYPERTHYROIDISM	HYPOTHYROIDISM
• **Symptoms**	• **Symptoms**
Nervousness	Cold intolerance
Heat intolerance	Weakness
Sweating	Reduced energy
Fatigue	Lethargy
Palpitation	Muscle cramps
Insomnia	Constipation
Early waking	Increased sleeping
Alopecia	Weight gain
Vitiligo	Reduced appetite
Brittle nails	Joint stiffness
• **Signs**	• **Signs**
Sweating	Cool, scaling skin
Proximal muscle weakness	Puffy hands and face
Emotionally labile	Deep voice
Tremor	Myotonia
Tachycardia	Delirium
Arrhythmia (atrial fibrillation)	Bradycardia
Hypertension (systolic)	Slow reflexes
Brisk deep-tendon reflexes	Obesity
Diabetes	Hypothermia
Increased triglycerides and calcium	Myxedema
Decreased cholesterol	• **Signs in children**
Microcytic anemia	**(cretinism)**
	Growth failure
	Delayed puberty
	Mental retardation
	Sparse hair
	Large abdomen
	Flat nose
	Poor muscle tone

therapeutic effect. However, the therapeutic activity of some drugs, including the anticoagulants heparin and coumadin, are enhanced by increased thyroid hormone levels.

Thyrotoxicosis varies in its clinical presentation from a syndrome with few clinical features to a life-threatening alteration of metabolic functions called thyroid storm. This is a rapidly progressing decompensation of hyperthyroidism. If not promptly identified and properly treated, it can result in death due to cardiovascular collapse. Thyroid storm is most commonly seen in patients with untreated chronic thyrotoxicosis and in patients with additional stress from surgery or illness.

Hyperthyroidism

Graves disease is an autoimmune induced thyrotoxicosis characterized by a diffuse goiter. About one half of cases have some clinically evident component of the associated infiltrative orbitopathy. This is due to cellular infiltration and mucopolysaccharide deposition in the extraocular muscle and cellular infiltration of the orbit. The associated dermopathy is an uncommon manifestation characterized by a localized nonpitting edema (myxedema) occurring in 0.5 to 4%. Also less commonly associated is clubbing of the fingers, called thyroid acropathy (1%). Stress or hormone change have been implicated as contributing to the onset.

In Graves disease, thyroid receptor antibodies of the IgG class are produced by lymphocytes and attach to the thyroid follicular cells at the site of TSH membrane receptors. The binding of thyroid receptor antibodies activates adenyl cyclase and initiates metabolic steps leading to increased production and release of thyroid hormones. The resulting higher serum concentration of thyroid hormones acts on the pituitary to inhibit the release of TSH and the thyrotopes response to TRH. Because there is no negative feedback to the lymphocytes producing the thyroid receptor antibodies, excess secretion of the thyroid hormones continues. This leads to thyroid growth, increased vascularity, and excess thyroid function, which are manifested clinically as goiter and thyrotoxicosis.

With constant stimulation by thyroid receptor antibodies, the production of thyroid hormones increases many times the normal rate. This excess stimulation of the thyroid hormones biosynthetic pathway results in a relative increase in the production of T_3 as compared to T_4. The amount of T_3 in the blood derived from thryoidal secretion has been estimated to increase from less than 20% in normals to more than 40% in hyperthyroidism.

The presence of excess thyroid hormones produces abnormalities in the biochemical pathways and has a marked effect on almost every tissue of the body. Numerous enzymes and proteins are synthesized, while others are broken down. The complex interaction of these tissues and their metabolic response cannot be explained by a single mechanism.

The natural history of Graves disease is unclear. It is evident that some patients can recover normal thyroid function spontaneously without treatment, sometimes even becoming hypothyroid. However, other untreated patients will remain chronically hyperthyroid, with cyclic periods of exacerbation and remission, and only after months or years will the thyrotoxic component burn itself out; still other patients will progress and die from the complications of thyroid storm. It has been estimated that one third of the patients with Graves disease would fall into each category; however, other forms of hyperthyroidism could not easily be distinguished at the time these observations were made (Michie et al, 1978). Although it is clear that some patients can improve without therapy, presently there is no reliable way to identify them. Therefore, until the clinical or laboratory testing characteristics of these patients who spontaneously return to normal are clearly identified, treatment is recommended for all symptomatic patients.

The signs and symptoms of Graves disease are a gradual onset of thyrotoxicosis, with or without the signs of thyroid-related ophthalmopathy. Symptoms of thyrotoxicosis can include heat intolerance, weight loss, increased appetite, palpitation, fatigue, muscular weakness, nervousness, irritability, depression, and increased bowel motility. Difficulty sleeping and early-morning wakening are common findings. The apparent need to be constantly active contrasts with the concurrent symptoms of fatigue and muscle weakness. Difficulty concentrating on tasks and a decreased tolerance to emotional stress may also be present. Increased bowel motility often results in more frequent and softer bowel movements, but rarely in frank diarrhea. Skin may be smooth, soft, warm, oily, and moist. Hair may also be oily. Alteration of libido or menstrual cycle may also be noted.

Often the symptoms may be vague, or the significance of an isolated complaint may be difficult to recognize. Heat intolerance may contribute to strain on the living situation, as the patient is constantly lowering the thermostat, opening windows, or removing covers from the bed. Climbing stairs leads to weakness, fatigue, and shortness of breath. Chronic muscular fatigue results in the need to be constantly active. Although weight loss with increased appetite is most common, a few patients may gain weight. Loss of ability to concentrate or to withstand emotional stress, or increased irritability, emotional lability, or depression may underlie complaints of difficulty with interpersonal relationships.

An increased basal metabolic rate and moderately elevated respiratory rate are also evident. Microcytic anemia and weak contraction of skeletal muscle may be seen in some cases. Changes in the skin include alopecia, vitiligo, and brittle nails. Thyrotoxicosis alters the carbohydrate, lipid, and calcium metabolism. This can result in abnormal glucose tolerance curves, diabetes, or the exacerbation of existing diabetes. Serum calcium, fasting free fatty acids, and triglyceride levels can increase, while cholesterol is reduced. In addition, there are brisk deep-tendon reflexes.

The cardiovascular signs can be among the most prominent, with increased demand due to elevated metabolic rate and the need to dissipate excess heat. Tachycardia is often present, with a pulse rate of greater than 90, even at rest. The increased force of contraction can be felt as palpitation. Some 10% of thyrotoxic patients may develop an arrhythmia, most often atrial fibrillation. The increased demand does not commonly lead to cardiac disorders unless underlying heart disease is present. Elevation of the systolic, but not the diastolic, blood pressure is common.

Thus, the classic thyrotoxicosis patient is a sweaty, tremulous, fidgety individual with a short attention span. Most often this complex of symptoms develops slowly over a period of months or years; however, it can occur within a few weeks or less. More acute development may be associated with emotional stress at the time symptoms appeared.

Hypothyroidism
Hypothyroidism is the clinical syndrome characterized by the deficiency of thyroid hormones and the resultant cellular responses. It is classified as primary hypothyroidism when alteration in the thyroid gland is responsible for the decrease in thyroid hormones. This occurs due to chronic autoimmune thyroiditis (Hashimoto disease), surgical or radioiodine treatment for Graves disease, irradiation of neck neoplasm, subacute thyroiditis, dietary deficiency of iodine (endemic goiter), drugs (eg, lithium), or congenital biosynthetic defect. Secondary hypothyroidism is the deficiency of thyroid hormones due to pituitary TSH deficit, which can occur in pituitary adenoma or ablative therapy. Tertiary hypothyroidism is due to deficiency of hypothalamic TRH, and is rare. Finally, hypothyroidism can be due to peripheral tissue resistance to the action of the thyroid hormones, an extremely rare condition.

Chronic autoimmune thyroiditis (Hashimoto disease) is the most common type of hypothyroidism in this country. This disorder frequently occurs in individuals with a positive family history or with family members but no clinical manifestations, who have antithyroidal antibodies. It may be associated with a goiter in younger patients, but the gland is often destroyed by the immune processes in the adult. It is characterized by the high titers of thyroid microsomal antibodies. Infrequently, patients with this disorder will develop thyroid-related orbitopathy.

Because the thyroid hormones are necessary for normal development, the clinical manifestations of hypothyroidism depend more on the age of onset than the specific cause of the disorder. Hypothyroidism in infants (cretinism) leads to interruption of bone growth, sparse hair, large abdomen, flat nose, poor muscle tone, and mental retardation. In children, the interruption of bone growth is seen, with retarded

sexual development. In adults, hypothyroidism is characterized by myxedema.

In addition to myxedema, adult hypothyroidism is characterized by symptoms that include lethargy, chronic fatigue, weakness, muscle cramps, inability to concentrate, cold intolerance, decreased sweating, weight gain, amenorrhea, and chronic constipation. Clinical signs include bradycardia, with cardiac enlargement, occasionally hypertension, shallow respirations, cool skin, dry skin and hair, puffy hands and face, and slow reflexes.

■ Ocular
Table 18–2 summarizes the ocular manifestations of thyroid disorders.

Hyperthyroidism
Thyroid-related orbitopathy is an autoimmune disorder that is often, but not exclusively, associated with Graves disease (Figure 18–2). There is no proven relationship between Graves disease and thyroid-related orbitopathy; however, numerous studies provide a firm basis for a strong association between these two disorders. Although some investigators consider thyroid-related orbitopathy and systemic

TABLE 18–2. OCULAR MANIFESTATIONS OF THYROID DISORDERS

HYPERTHYROIDISM
- Lids
  - Lid retraction
  - Lid lag
  - Lagophthalmus
- Cornea
  - Exposure
  - Photophobia
- Conjunctiva
  - Conjunctival or periorbital edema
- Extraocular muscles
  - Restriction
  - Diplopia
  - Increased IOP
  - Proptosis
  - Wide-eyed stare
- Optic nerve
  - Decreased vision
  - Visual field loss
  - Afferent pupillary defect
  - Decreased color vision
  - Blurred disc margins

HYPOTHYROIDISM
- Madarosis
- Periorbital myxedema
- Loss of lateral third of eyebrow
- Thyroid orbitopathy (rare)

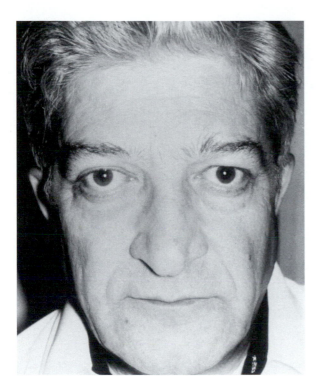

Figure 18–2. Patient with Graves disease. Note proptosis and position of lower lids. *(Photo courtesy of Dr. Diane T. Adamczyk.)*

hyperthyroidism to be components of a single disease, others suggest that ocular infiltration and hyperthyroidism may be distinct, organ-specific autoimmune disorders that are very closely related. Presently, the nature of the relationship between these disorders is unknown, but may be related to the complexity of the immune response. Various mechanisms have been proposed as the initiating event responsible for the development of the ocular findings. Despite the controversy as to the mechanism or antigen that is responsible for the development of thyroid orbitopathy, the autoimmune basis for this disorder is well established.

The majority of patients develop systemic hyperthyroidism prior to ocular findings. In some cases, eye findings present prior to the development of systemic hyperthyroidism; however, they both develop within 18 months of each other in 80% of cases with severe eye disorders. Occasionally, the separation between the diagnoses can be years. Therefore, a patient who first appears to have euthyroid orbitopathy may eventually develop systemic hyperthyroidism. Furthermore, ultrasound studies have demonstrated enlarged extraocular muscles in most Graves disease patients without clinically detectable ocular dysfunction. A more detailed analysis of patients with apparent euthyroid orbitopathy often reveals evidence of thyroid autoimmune disease when evaluated for presence of thyroid membrane antibodies or thyroiditis by biopsy. However, the course and severity of the ocular and systemic disorders do not necessarily correlate. The eye signs

associated with Graves disease are generally self-limited and mild, yet in some cases become severe and threaten vision.

Lids. Retraction of the upper or lower lid, and upper lid lag, are the ocular signs of thyrotoxicosis without regard to the specific cause. The normal position of the upper eyelid is 2 mm below the limbus, and the lower eyelid is at the limbus. Lid retraction is noted when the upper lid is positioned at the limbus or above with visible scleral tissue (Dalrymple sign) or the lower lid is 1 to 2 mm below the limbus. Widening of the palpebral fissure causes a characteristic stare. Closer observation is required to notice the upper lid lagging behind the globe as the eye is depressed (von Graffe sign). Elimination of thyrotoxicosis leads to the resolution of lid retraction and stare in one half to two thirds of patients.

The eye signs of infiltrative orbitopathy are due to the increased volume of the extraocular muscles or orbital tissue. These can include puffy, swollen lids; unilateral or bilateral proptosis; restriction of extraocular muscle; increased IOP upon up gaze; conjunctival injection; corneal exposure; decreased vision; blurred optic disc margins; or chorioretinal striae.

Conjunctiva/Periorbital Edema. Conjunctival or periorbital edema is a common early sign of thyroid eye disease. The swelling is most noticeable in the morning and decreases throughout the day. Inflammation of subcutaneous connective tissue and anterior displacement of orbital fat due to orbitopathy can lead to periorbital edema.

Extraocular Muscle Involvement/Proptosis. Enlargement of the extraocular muscles (EOM) is the prominent anatomical abnormality in infiltrative orbitopathy, which causes proptosis (Figure 18–3). Histologic studies have indicated lymphocytic infiltration, proliferation of fibroblasts, and edema within the interstitial tissue of the muscles. The muscle fibers appear normal. It is clear that both the extraocular muscle cells and the fibroblast play important roles in the pathogenesis of this disorder, and that the autoimmune basis for thyroid-related orbitopathy is directed against one or both of these tissues. Orbital fibroblasts have also been implicated in the production of glycoaminoglycans and collagenous connective tissue to replace orbital fat. This may occur by direct fibroblast stimulation, by antibodies, or due to interaction with lymphocytes within the inflammatory response. Despite the large body of clinical and experimental evidence regarding the role EOM cells and fibroblasts play in this disorder, the relationship between the orbital infiltration and hyperthyroidism remains unclear.

Approximately one fourth of Graves patients develop proptosis. The proptosis may be unilateral or bilateral, with about 50% of patients having a difference of less than 5

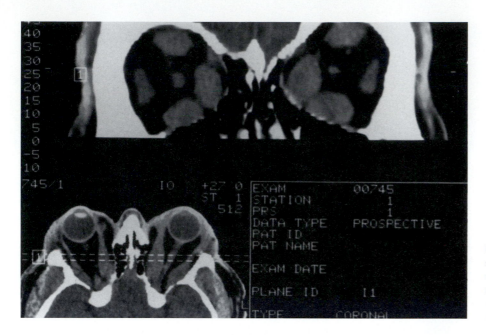

Figure 18–3. CT scan of the orbit demonstrating the enlargement of the extraocular muscles. Note that the inferior rectus and medial rectus are the two muscles most involved, with minimal involvement of the lateral rectus.

mm between eyes, 89% having less than 7 mm of difference, and none with over 11 mm. A complaint of lashes touching the back of spectacle lenses may occur in advanced proptosis. Proptosis most often remains stable after reaching its maximum, usually within the first 2 years.

Abnormalities in extraocular muscle function can lead to restriction of movements. Initial complaints are of diplopia in upgaze, because the inferior rectus muscle is most commonly involved, followed by the medial, superior, and lateral recti muscles. These complaints are most common upon wakening, when very tired, or after one alcoholic beverage. An abnormal head position with an elevated chin may be necessary for driving to relieve the diplopia in upgaze. However, symmetric restriction from enlarged muscles does not always cause symptoms. Increased vascularity over the medial or lateral rectus insertion is found both with thyroid eye disease and myositis.

Cornea. When proptosis is·severe enough to prevent lid closure, chronic corneal exposure can result. Ocular symptoms due to exposure keratopathy include gritty, irritable eyes and tearing. Proptosis can lead to complaints of corneal foreign body or reduced contact lens tolerance. This can be further complicated by the common loss of a Bell phenomenon due to significant involvement of the inferior rectus. Corneal scarring and ulceration can result with associated loss of vision. Occasionally this results in corneal perforation.

Optic Nerve Involvement. Only 2 to 7% develop severe, vision-threatening orbitopathy from optic nerve involvement. Patients with compressive optic neuropathy have gradual onset of visual loss, or visual field loss. The sco-

tomas can be central, arcuate, altitudinal, paracentral, or a generalized constriction. Decreased vision associated with reduced brightness of colors is suggestive of optic nerve compression. Associated signs include afferent pupillary defect, color vision loss, disc edema, chorioretinal striae, and visual evoked potential abnormalities. The vast majority have an extraocular muscle disorder. Recently imaging studies have revealed apical compression of the optic nerve by enlarged muscle bodies as the underlying cause of this finding. Unilateral compression occurs in approximately 30% of cases.

Although many patients with extraocular myopathy may have only transient problems, the course of compressive neuropathy is difficult to predict. The majority of patients that develop eye findings associated with Graves disease have mild disorders that are subject to exacerbations and remissions during the course of the disease.

NOSPECS. Historically, a detailed classification of the eye signs associated with Graves disease was devised, abbreviated NOSPECS. NOSPECS stands for class 0, *N*o signs or symptoms; class 1, *O*nly signs; class 2, *S*oft tissue involvement; class 3, *P*roptosis; class 4, *E*OM involvement; class 5, *C*orneal involvement; and class 6, *S*ight loss from optic nerve involvement. It is of little use in the clinical setting because it provides no prognostic value, contributes little assistance in management decisions, and does not present a logical progressive sequence of the disorder, with patients skipping over several steps in the progression.

Hypothyroidism

Ocular findings in hypothyroidism are usually the systemic manifestations of the disease expressed within the ocular tissues and adnexa. The ocular tissues most commonly involved are the skin of the eyelid and the eyebrows. Myxedema is sometimes especially prominent in the eyelids as a boggy, nonpitted edema. Another ocular sign is loss of the outer third of the eyebrow. In addition, a few patients with chronic autoimmune thyroiditis may develop thyroid-related orbitopathy and keratitis sicca.

DIAGNOSIS

■ Systemic

Hyperthyroidism

Laboratory investigation of hyperthyroidism is critically linked to the history and findings on physical examination. Therefore, the patient presenting with findings of thyrotoxicosis is best served by referral to an endocrinologist who can evaluate the laboratory findings within the context of the overall systemic health. With suspected Graves disease, the initial step would be to demonstrate the hyperthyroid state, with an elevated free T_4 level and a decreased thyrotropin (TSH) level with a newer and more sensitive immunometric assay, if available. If the free T_4 level is normal and the TSH level is reduced, a T_3 level or free T_3 will usually be elevated. Sensitive TSH tests have eliminated the need for TRH stimulation test or thyroid-suppression test in most cases. This occurs more often early in the disorder. Serum TSH receptor antibodies can be useful in the differentiation of euthyroid orbitopathy and orbital tumor.

Hypothyroidism

The diagnosis of hypothyroidism is based on the history and physical examination, along with laboratory studies used to differentiate between disorders with similar or confusing presentations. The classic presentation of myxedema leaves little doubt about the diagnosis. A history of radioiodine or surgical treatment of hyperthyroidism is also significant. Elevated TSH levels confirm the diagnosis of primary hypothyroidism with the appropriate clinical findings. Eventually T_4 levels and free T_4 will be depressed, and this will occur prior to decrease in T_3 levels. Serum antimicrosomal and antithyroglobulin tests are useful to confirm the presence of autoimmune disease.

■ Ocular

Hyperthyroidism

The diagnosis of thyroid-related eye disease may or may not coincide with systemic thyroid disease. Differentiation from other orbital disorders may include history and physical findings, laboratory evaluation, ultrasonography, and

imaging studies of the orbit. The ocular examination places emphasis on observation of lid position and function, corneal and conjunctival signs, position of the globe, and function of the extraocular muscles and optic nerve.

Lid lag may be an uncommon first presentation. It is best evaluated by instructing the patient to follow a target that is slowly moved downward while carefully observing the position of the lid relative to the globe. Lid movements may be spasmodic or jerky, and a fine tremor may be detected in a lightly closed lid. Increased adrenergic activity is presumed to be the basis for these findings. In addition, position of the lids should be evaluated and any retraction noted.

Proptosis of more than 22 mm, or a difference of more than 2 mm as measured by exophthalmometry between eyes, is considered suspicious for orbital disease. When proptosis is seen in combination with lid retraction and lid lag, diagnostic possibilities other than thyroid-related orbitopathy are limited. However, proptosis greater than 23 mm is unusual as an isolated presenting sign for thyroid-related orbitopathy, and other orbital disorders must be considered. The proptosis of thyroid-related orbitopathy is straight out and protrusion of the eye in any other direction suggests another diagnosis. Thyroid-related orbitopathy can present with unilateral proptosis; however, imaging studies often show subtle abnormalities in the other orbit. The most common cause of both bilateral and unilateral proptosis in the adult is thyroid-related orbitopathy.

The normal eye should be able to elevate and depress 5.5 mm or the approximate distance from limbus to pupil. Horizontal limitation secondary to extraocular muscle involvement is best noted as an inability to "bury the limbus" on full abduction or adduction and the amount of sclera showing can be measured. Due to EOM restriction, especially of the inferior rectus muscle, vertical diplopia and/or increased IOP may be elicited on attempted upgaze. Binocular fields of fusion and diplopia measured on a Goldmann perimeter are helpful in evaluation and following the EOM dysfunction. Forced duction tests can distinguish nonrestrictive ophthalmoplegias.

Special attention should be given to the evaluation of optic nerve function every time a patient with thyroid-related eye disease is examined. This should include pupils, brightness comparison, and color vision screening. Baseline threshold visual fields should be obtained and repeated if there is any symptom or sign that indicates an optic neuropathy may be present.

Because orbitopathy is occasionally the presenting sign of Graves disease, it must be considered as a diagnosis in patients presenting with proptosis, lid retraction, or impaired eye movement. When it presents with goiter and thyrotoxicosis, there is no difficulty making the diagnosis. Differentiating thyroid-related orbitopathy in an otherwise asymptomatic patient may require laboratory testing. A depressed TSH level by a very sensitive immunometric assay is highly suggestive of hyperthyroidism. Obtaining thyroid receptor antibody levels can be helpful. High antibody levels can be supportive but not conclusive in making a diagnosis. Orbital ultrasound studies can detect muscle enlargement and demonstrate it in patients with minimal thyroid orbitopathy. With unilateral proptosis or an atypical presentation, a CT scan of the orbit is indicated due to the possibility of orbital tumor.

Hypothyroidism

The ocular disorders in association with hypothyroidism are part of the systemic condition; therefore, the diagnosis is made on the systemic basis. External evaluation may reveal periorbital edema and loss of the lateral one third of the eyebrow.

TREATMENT AND MANAGEMENT

Table 18–3 summarizes the treatment and management of thyroid disorders.

■ Systemic

Hyperthyroidism

The treatment of Graves disease can involve medical drug therapy, radioactive iodine treatment, surgical treatment, or

TABLE 18–3. SYSTEMIC TREATMENT AND MANAGEMENT OF THYROID DISORDERS

HYPERTHYROIDISM
- **Medical**
  Radioactive iodine
     PLUS
  Propylthiouracil. Initial dosage: 200–300 mg, Q8h–Q12h, until normal metabolic state; monitor circulating levels of thyroid hormones, then decrease dosage 1/3 to 1/2, until maintenance dose, 50–150 mg, TID, continued for year or more
     OR
  Methimazole. Initial dosage: 10–20mg, Q12h, until normal metabolic state; monitor circulating levels of thyroid hormones, then decrease dosage 1/3 to 1/2, until maintenance dose, 5–15mg, qd, continued for year or more
     PLUS
  β-blocker
     OR
  Surgical: Subtotal thyroidectomy

HYPOTHYROIDISM
- **Medical**
  Levothyroxine 0.05–0.2 mg/d; average,0.125 mg/d

a combination of these modalities. Because the initial treatment with thionamides is often inadequate to control the thyrotoxicosis, a combination of drug therapy and radioactive iodine therapy or surgical intervention is often necessary. In the selection of treatment, consider the age of the patient, severity of the disease, and whether the patient is pregnant or desires to become pregnant.

Radioactive iodine therapy is the primary definitive treatment of hyperthyroidism in adults. Iodine 131 is the most commonly used isotope. Concentration of the radioactive iodine in the thyroidal tissues leads to local damage to the thyroid without involvement of the surrounding tissues of the neck. Alteration in thyroid function is slow to occur, and is usually seen 1 to 2 months after therapy, although full effect may not be seen for months or years. Therefore, patients must be medically treated in the interim. Any consideration of retreatment should be delayed 6 to 12 months after initial treatment.

Radioactive iodine therapy is very effective in establishing and maintaining control of hyperthyroidism. Relapse is rare. However, there is a high incidence of secondary hypothyroidism. Approximately 30% of those treated with radioactive iodine have been reported to develop hypothyroidism 5 years after therapy, with the incidence increasing to between 40 and 70% 10 years after treatment.

Concern regarding possible carcinogenic effects and uncertainty about the long-term effects of the hypothyroid state have frightened patients away from this treatment and led to recommendations against using radioactive therapy in children. Studies have documented the lack of evidence for carcinogenic or leukemogenic effects, and have led to lowering the age limit for this treatment. It should not be used in a pregnant or potentially pregnant woman. A recent report suggests that this form of therapy may exacerbate thyroid-related eye disease (Bartalena et al, 1989).

Thionamides are the primary drugs used in the treatment of Graves disease. These agents act to block the production of the thyroid hormones (T_3 and T_4) by preventing the iodide oxidation and inhibiting its organic binding. The thyroid has approximately a 3-month store of thyroid hormones; because thionamides do not interfere with the release of thyroid hormones, a delay of days to months occurs between the initiation of therapy and clinical evidence of drug efficacy. The length of this latent period depends on the amount of thyroid hormones stored, rate of secretion, severity of hyperthyroidism, and degree of inhibition by the pharmaceutical agent. Some improvement in symptoms is usually noted within a few weeks, and metabolic parameters are usually restored to normal within 6 weeks.

Propylthiouracil (PTU) and methimazole (Tapazole) are thionamides used in the treatment of hyperthyroidism. PTU acts to further reduce the circulation levels of T_3 by interfering with the peripheral conversion of T_4 to T_3. Methimazole has been reported to have a number of immunoregulatory effects that may enhance its action. Despite these minor differences in action, the clinical response time of these agents is approximately the same. When normal metabolic parameters are obtained after about 6 to 8 weeks of therapy, the circulating levels of thyroid hormones should be monitored. At this stage, patients with a normal metabolic state should have a one-third to one-half reduction in dosage, with future reductions every 4 to 8 weeks until arriving at a reasonable maintenance dosage, which is continued for a year or more. The total treatment time is approximately 18 to 24 months.

Complete remission of hyperthyroidism is obtained in one third to one half of patients on antithyroid medication. The best response has been seen in patients with less than 1 year of hyperthyroidism and a decrease in thyroid size during drug therapy. These agents are used as a primary treatment, mostly in younger patients, as a means of achieving the euthyroid state prior to surgical treatment, and as an adjunct to radioactive iodine treatment.

Other drugs are used to supplement medical, surgical, or radioactive iodine therapy. Propranolol is used with the thioamides or radioactive iodine as an agent to block sympathetic stimulation that may be contributing to thyrotoxic manifestations, as well as to protect the heart. Inorganic iodine or high-dose corticosteroids may be given intravenously in certain emergency circumstances when prompt control of thyrotoxicosis is necessary. Inorganic iodine acts to inhibit thyroid hormone release. Corticosteroids act to reduce circulating levels of T_3 by altering the peripheral conversion of T_4, and may act to lower T_4 levels by direct action on the thyroid. Use of inorganic iodine as a primary agent to control thyrotoxicosis is limited to situations where there has been previous treatment with radioactive iodine. Corticosteroid use is limited due to the high risk of numerous significant side effects with these agents. Lithium may also be used to block hormone release in patients allergic to both thionamide and iodide.

Subtotal thyroidectomy is an effective treatment for relieving hyperthyroidism in Graves disease. It is not an ideal treatment due to frequent complications of hypothyroidism (4 to 30%) and other surgical complications. The mortality and morbidity associated with surgery must be weighed against the complications of the disease process. Surgery is usually recommended in cases of noncompliance or complications with medical therapy; patients refusing radioactive iodine therapy; pregnancy; large goiter; and in children. There may be less secondary hypothyroidism associated with surgery than radioiodine treatment. Recurrence of thyrotoxicosis is uncommon.

Preoperative management usually includes the use of antithyroid therapy to restore the normal metabolic state. When this is achieved, iodine therapy is added to reduce the vascularity and establish a normal follicular cell layer. The goal is to deplete the gland of hormone stores and return the metabolic function to normal prior to the operation.

Hypothyroidism

Levothyroxine (T_4; Synthyroid) is used in the treatment of hypothyroidism. Levothyroxine is converted to T_3 peripherally in the body; thus both thyroid hormones are available to the tissues despite only one being administered.

■ Ocular

Table 18–4 summarizes the treatment of ocular findings of thyroid disorders.

Hyperthyroidism

Because this ocular disorder is often self-limiting and without severe ocular complications, most patients can be treated in the primary care setting with an endocrinologist managing the systemic aspects of the underlying thyroid disorder. However, some patients will require referral to experienced ophthalmic surgeons for treatment of severe exposure, proptosis, and optic nerve compression. Each examination of the patient with thyroid-related orbitopathy should be directed toward ensuring that these complications, which can profoundly affect vision, are not present. Special emphasis should be placed on ruling out optic nerve involvement each time a patient is examined. The goals are to preserve vision, maintain patient comfort, and address oculomotor disorders.

Treatment of the underlying thyrotoxicosis returns the lid retraction to normal in the majority of patients. However,

TABLE 18–4. TREATMENT OF OCULAR FINDINGS OF THYROID DISORDERS

HYPERTHYROIDISM	
● **Nonsurgical**	
Lid retraction	Guanethidine 2%
Corneal exposure	Artificial tears (Q1h) ointment
Lagophthalmus	Tape lids
Photophobia	Tints
Periorbital edema	Elevate head hs
Diplopia	Head position, prisms, occlusion
Advanced proptosis	Corticosteroids (40–80 mg/d)
	Immunosuppressive therapy
	Radiation therapy
● **Surgical**	
Optic neuropathy	Orbital decompression
Diplopia	Muscle surgery
Lid retraction	Eyelid surgery
HYPOTHYROIDISM	
● Systemic treatment	

during and prior to treatment some patients are symptomatic, with gritty eyes, tearing, or photophobia, which can be treated with artificial tears and tinted lenses. Nonpreserved artificial tears are recommended to reduce reactions to preservatives. Exposure should be treated aggressively with bland ointment and taping lids at night if closure is incomplete. Elevation of the head when sleeping is recommended for patients with periorbital edema. With recent onset of lid retraction and no increased IOP on upward gaze, a trial of 2% topical guanethedine eyedrops can be helpful in reducing the lid retraction. This drug acts to deplete sympathetic storage sites. However, corneal irritation and the temporary nature of the effects limit the use of this therapy.

Medical treatment of the complications that threaten vision in infiltrative orbitopathy include progressive proptosis, corneal exposure, and optic nerve compression. It is unclear if treating the thyrotoxicosis has any influence on any of the findings associated with infiltrative ophthalmopathy.

Oral corticosteroids have been used to reduce the inflammatory component that leads to proptosis, causing significant corneal symptoms. Patients are treated for 4 weeks and then slowly tapered. Unfortunately, exacerbations are often experienced when doses drop below 30 mg daily. The problem of complications with long-term steroid use must be considered. Generally patients with inflammation as the basis of the disease occurring during the first 3 to 12 months do better with steroids or radiation. Steroids are effective in stabilizing a recent-onset ophthalmoplegia or optic neuropathy until radiation or surgery is performed. Various immunosuppressive therapies have been attempted. However, the potential complications of carcinogenesis do not justify their use, given the comparable effectiveness of corticosteroids.

Radiotherapy continues to be used in some centers as a means of treating the infiltrative component of thyroid-related orbitopathy. The success of this therapy has been mixed in uncontrolled reports.

Orbital decompression is the treatment of choice when vision is threatened by optic nerve compression or severe exposure keratopathy has progressed to ulceration. Removal of the orbital walls relieves the pressure by allowing the orbital fat and EOMs to enter the sinuses.

Management of the diplopia associated with this disorder can be difficult. Discussing appropriate head position can be helpful, as is the use of Fresnel prisms. Surgical correction should be delayed until after orbital decompression or when the measurements of motility and deviation have been stable for 6 months.

Only after the optic nerve compression is controlled and the diplopia has been addressed should surgical correction of upper or lower lid retraction be attempted. Indication for surgery includes protection of the cornea and the improvement of appearance.

Hypothyroidism

Because the eye findings in hypothyroidism are manifestations of the systemic disease, most clear with the treatment of the systemic disease.

CONCLUSION

Thyroid disease is a challenging disorder for the clinician to treat and manage. Uncertainty regarding the pathogenesis of these autoimmune disorders, coupled with a clinical course of Graves disease that is characterized by exacerbations and remissions of varying duration, leads to difficulty in evaluating the effectiveness of therapy. In addition, thyroid-related orbitopathy often does not correlate with systemic severity or course, and it is difficult to predict which patients will develop sight-threatening complications. Nevertheless, ocular signs such as lid retraction and proptosis may lead to the diagnosis of this complex disorder.

REFERENCES

Bartalena L, Marcocci C, Bogazzi F, et al. Use of corticosteroids to prevent progression of Graves' ophthalmopathy after radio iodine therapy for hyperthyroidism. *N Engl J Med.* 1989;321:1349–1359.

Bernal J, Refetoff S. The action of thyroid hormones. *Clin Endocrinol.* 1977;6:227–249.

Char DH. The ophthalmopathy of Graves' disease. *Med Clin North Am.* 1991;75:97–119.

DeGroot LJ, Quintans J. The causes of autoimmune thyroid disease. *Endocrin Rev.* 1989;10:537–62.

Feliciano DV. Everything you wanted to know about Graves' disease. *Am J Surg.* 1992;164:404–411.

Fells P. Thyroid-associated eye disease: Clinical management. *Lancet.* 1991;388:29–32.

Hall R, Scanlon MF. Hypothyroidism: Clinical features and complications. *Clin Endocrin Metab.* 1979;8:29–38.

Kendler DL, Lippa J, Rootman J. The initial clinical characteristics of Graves' orbitopathy vary with age and sex. *Arch Ophthalmol.* 1993;111:197–201.

LaFranchi SH. Hypothyroidism. *Pediatr Clin North Am.* 1979;26:33–51.

Lamkin JC, Raizman MB. Update on laboratory tests for diagnosis of orbital disease. *Int Ophthalmol Clin.* 1992;32:27–44.

McDougall IR. Graves' disease: Current concepts. *Med Clin North Am.* 1991;75:79–95.

McGregor AM. Antibodies to the TSH receptor in patients with autoimmune thyroid disease. *Clin Endocrinol* (Oxf). 1990;33:683–685.

Michie W, Beck JS, Pollet JE. Prevention and management of hypothyroidism after thyroidectomy for thyrotoxicosis. *World J Surg.* 1978;2:307–319.

Perros P, Kendall-Taylor P. Antibodies to orbital tissues in thyroid-associated ophthalmopathy. *Acta Endocrinol.* 1992; 126:137–142.

Perros P, Kendall-Taylor P. Pathogenetic mechanisms in thyroid-associated ophthalmopathy. *J Int Med.* 1992;231:205–211.

Tallstedt L, Lundell G, Torring O, et al. Occurrence of ophthalmopathy after treatment for Graves' hyperthyroidism. *N Engl J Med.* 1992;326:1733–1738.

Weetman AP. Thyroid-associated eye disease: Pathophysiology. *Lancet.* 1991;338:25–28.

19
Chapter

Disorders of the Parathyroid Glands

Bernard J. Dolan

The parathyroid glands usually consist of four separate glands located on the posterior aspect of the thyroid gland, but may vary in number and position. The major secretion of the parathyroid glands is parathyroid hormone (PTH), a polypeptide that plays an important role in maintaining serum calcium levels within a normal range. Disorders of the parathyroid glands lead to the disruption of calcium regulation. The resulting clinical syndromes can be broadly classified into hyperparathyroidism (primary and secondary) and hypoparathyroidism, with pseudohypoparathyroidism a rare disorder of PTH resistance.

Ocular findings in parathyroid disorders are associated with physiological responses of the ocular tissues to the long term alteration of calcium levels in the body. Chronic hyperparathyroidism can result in calcium deposition in the cornea and conjunctiva. Chronic hypoparathyroidism can cause ocular surface disease, cataracts, and, rarely, papilledema. Pseudohypoparathyroidism can display lens opacities and is also occasionally associated with papilledema.

EPIDEMIOLOGY

The incidence of hyperparathyroidism has been estimated as high as 1 per 1000, making it one of the most common endocrine disorders. It is more common in women over 45, with estimates as high as 1 in 500 in this population.

Hypoparathyroidism is most commonly associated with postoperative thyroidectomy. It occurs in approximately 5% of these surgical cases. Primary idiopathic hypoparathyroidism is a rare disorder.

NATURAL HISTORY

Pathophysiology

Calcium is important in the regulation of nervous and muscle conduction. Nerve and muscle cells are sensitive to alterations in calcium levels. When calcium levels drop too low, depolarization of nerve and muscle cells is greatly enhanced, resulting in tetany, convulsions, and dysfunction of the central nervous system. Hypercalcemia leads to weakness, drowsiness, disorientation, and eventually coma. Therefore, calcium levels must be regulated within a narrow range. A variety of homeostatic mechanisms exist to regulate the serum calcium levels so as to maintain normal neuromuscular function.

The parathyroid glands serve as the primary regulator of serum calcium levels in the body. A decrease in serum calcium concentration stimulates parathyroid hormone secretion. PTH acts directly on bone tissue and the kidney, and indirectly on the intestine to increase serum calcium concentration. At each of these sites, PTH activates adenylate cyclase, which increases cyclic adenosine monophosphate (cAMP) production in the cells of the target organ.

Bone, a reservoir of calcium for the body, is the major target organ of PTH. Bone is not a static structure. The matrix, composed of a hypoxyapatite crystal containing calcium and phosphate, is constantly remodeled by ongoing resorption and replacement. PTH activates the osteoclast, the cell responsible for resorption of bone, promoting the breakdown of the organic and inorganic matrix of bone. This increases serum calcium levels. This activity appears to be potentiated by the active metabolite of vitamin D and blocked by calcitonin. The response of bone tissue to the interaction of these hormones plays a central role in calcium balance.

Parathyroid glands do not act alone in the maintenance of calcium levels in the body. Calcitonin, produced by the C-cells of the thyroid, is released in response to increased blood calcium concentration, and acts to decrease serum calcium by inhibiting bone resorption. Vitamin D production and metabolism involving the liver and kidney also act to regulate calcium levels by increasing calcium and phosphate absorption in the small intestine. PTH increases the synthesis of a vitamin D metabolite that indirectly acts upon the intestine to increase calcium absorption.

The collective response of the intestine, kidney, and bone determines the calcium serum level, which provides negative feedback to the parathyroid gland to regulate the release of PTH and also modifies the production of vitamin D. Calcium homeostasis can be disrupted by a number of factors. Excess quantities or increased sensitivity to PTH or vitamin D can lead to hypercalcemia. Insufficient quantities or interruption of the action of PTH or vitamin D on target organs can lead to hypocalcemia.

■ Systemic

Hyperparathyroidism
Primary hyperparathyroidism is a condition characterized by excess secretion of PTH, resulting in dysfunction of calcium, phosphate, and bone metabolism, which leads to hypercalcemia and hypophosphatemia. In the past, this disorder was considered rare; however, with the increased use of routine screening of serum calcium levels, the diagnosis is often made prior to the onset of symptoms or clinical signs. Familial primary hyperparathyroidism is an inherited disorder that is transmitted in an autosomal dominant pattern. In addition, there are several distinct syndromes, classified as multiple endocrine neoplasia (MEN), in which parathyroid tumors are associated with other endocrine tumors. A defect in the neural crest cell that gives rise to the parathyroid as well as other endocrine glands is thought to be responsible for these inherited disorders.

Primary hyperparathyroidism is caused by the neoplastic transformation of cells of the parathyroid gland. In 80 to 85% of cases, patients with primary hyperparathyroidism have a single hypersecreting gland, a solitary adenoma. All four glands are hyperfunctioning in chief cell parathyroid hyperplasia, representing about 12% of cases. Parathyroid cancer is present in about 1% of cases. In the remaining 3%

of cases, one but not all glands are involved in hyperplasia or simultaneous multiple adenomas have developed.

The clinical manifestations of primary hyperparathyroidism are often subtle, with most cases having a benign course for many years. Frequently, the diagnosis is made in patients with no symptoms and minimal signs of the disease. Clinical presentation varies greatly, but may include vague abdominal complaints, mental changes, or mild to moderate weakness (Table 19–1). Polyuria and polydipsia may occur due to urinary electrolyte depletion. Long-term complications from hypercalcemia can lead to kidney stones, chronic urinary tract infections, extensive bone resorption, peptic ulcer, chronic pancreatitis, pseudo-gout, and hypertension. Rarely, there is an acute onset of symptoms that may be severe in nature, including marked dehydration and coma. With routine blood screening leading to early detection and treatment of this disorder, many of the long-term complications are not seen as frequently as in the past.

There have been no prospective studies to document the natural history of hyperparathyroidism. Furthermore, due to the early diagnosis and treatment of patients with minimal clinical signs and symptoms, the natural history is less clear. However, studies of conservative medical therapy indicate that 26% of patients required surgical intervention

TABLE 19–1. SYSTEMIC MANIFESTATIONS OF PARATHYROID DISORDERS

HYPERPARATHYROIDISM
- Proximal muscle weakness
- Fatigue
- Headache
- Weight loss
- Mild depression
- Hypercalcemia
- Renal calculi
- Pseudo-gout (calcium-crystal-induced arthropathy)
- Peptic ulcer
- Hyperactive reflexes
- Osteoporosis
- Weak, easily fractured bones

HYPOPARATHYROIDISM
- Mild paresthesias
- Muscle cramps
- Carpopedal spasms
- Convulsions
- Mental status changes
- Irritability
- Hypocalcemia
- Hyperphosphatemia
- Normal renal function
- Dental problems
- Basal ganglia calcifications
- Brittle nails
- Cardiac arrhythmias

within 10 years of the diagnosis while 58% remained in the nonoperated group after 5 years (Sholtz & Purnella, 1981).

Secondary hyperparathyroidism refers to increased PTH secretion in response to chronically low serum calcium levels, and is most commonly associated with chronic renal failure. There is no specific abnormality of the parathyroid glands. In most cases, correction of the cause of hypocalcemia results in the normalization of PTH levels within 6 months. Occasionally, the elevated PTH levels persist. This is called tertiary hyperparathyroidism.

Hypoparathyroidism

Hypoparathyroidism is an uncommon disorder that can be subdivided into hereditary or acquired types. It is characterized by the decreased production of PTH or decreased sensitivity of the target organs to PTH. All patterns of inheritance have been identified. The acquired type most often occurs when too much parathyroid tissue is removed in the surgical treatment of primary hyperparathyroidism. Function of the parathyroid glands can also be compromised by thyroidectomy and rarely by radioiodine therapy for hyperthyroidism.

Hypoparathyroidism presents with the acute and chronic manifestations of untreated hypocalcemia (see Table 19–1). Complications of muscle contraction can include facial grimacing, cardiac arrythmia, and intestinal cramps with chronic malabsorption. Extreme cases may include laryngeal spasms, convulsions, and respiratory arrest. Behavioral changes include irritability, depression, paranoia, and psychosis. Typically, the hereditary type has a more gradual onset of symptoms that may go unrecognized for years.

Little is known of the natural history of hypoparathyroidism. It may be associated with other endocrine abnormalities such as those involving the thymus, thyroid gland, adrenal gland, or ovary. Many with thymus involvement die in early childhood. The acquired type occurs in a population with a known risk after parathyroid or thyroid surgery, although there may be considerable delay in presentation with the latter. Transient hypocalcemia following these procedures usually resolves without intervention. Reoperation is necessary in some cases of parathyroid disease, which greatly increases the risk of developing hypoparathyroidism.

■ Ocular

Table 19–2 summarizes the ocular manifestations in parathyroid disorders.

Hyperparathyroidism

Hyperparathyroidism is associated with the local deposition of calcium in the conjunctiva and the cornea. The corneal deposition of calcium is called band keratopathy (Figure 19–1). It has been suggested that it occurs at this location due to CO_2 diffusion creating an alkaline environment that

TABLE 19–2. OCULAR MANIFESTATIONS IN PARATHYROID DISORDERS

HYPERPARATHYROIDISM

● Disorder	● Manifestation
Band keratopathy	Decreased vision, surface irritation
Pannus formation Conjunctival calcification	Asymptomatic

HYPOPARATHYROIDISM

● Disorder	● Manifestation
Keratoconjunctivitis	Foreign body sensation, photophobia
Cataract (polychromatic)	Normal to decreased vision
Papilledema	Normal to transient vision loss (seconds)

would facilitate the precipitation of calcium. This deposition can progress into the corneal pupillary axis resulting in decreased vision or progress to epithelial disruption causing irritation and pain. Occasionally, pannus will develop.

Hypoparathyroidism

Hypoparathyroidism is associated with ocular surface disease, cataract, and occasionally papilledema due to long-term disease. The ocular surface disease is due to keratoconjunctivitis, and when associated with superficial candidiasis or adrenal insufficiency can lead to severe corneal involvement with blepharospasm and complaints of photophobia. Lens opacities that develop as bilateral discrete polychromatic opacities are found in the cortical and subcapsular portions of the lens. Visually significant cataracts may develop if the systemic disorder goes unrecognized; however, progression of lenticular changes is arrested with appropriate systemic therapy. Rarely, papilledema due to reduction in the absorption of cerebrospinal fluid (CSF) may be seen with hypoparathyroidism. Correction of the hypocalcemia has been reported to result in a return to normal CSF absorption with resolution of the papilledema.

DIAGNOSIS

■ Systemic

Hyperparathyroidism

The diagnosis of primary hyperparathyroidism is made primarily on the basis of clinical findings. Hypercalcemia in the presence of an unremarkable history and normal comprehensive physical examination is very suggestive of this diagnosis. Other causes of hypercalcemia must be excluded

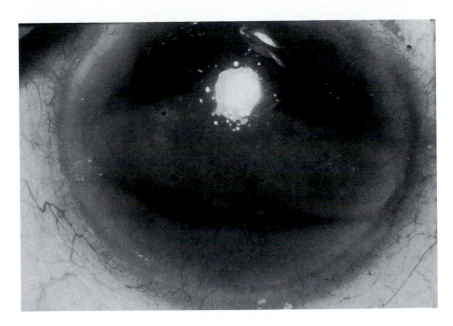

Figure 19–1. Band keratopathy.

prior to making the diagnosis of primary hypercalcemia. These may include malignancy (eg, breast cancer, leukemia); endocrine disorders, (eg, adrenal insufficiency, hyperthyroidism); excess ingestion of calcium or vitamin A or D; granulomatous disease (eg, sarcoidosis, tuberculosis); medications (eg, thiazide diuretics, lithium); renal failure; and laboratory error. A careful history for symptoms related to PTH hypersecretion and duration of hypercalcemia is of value, because an isolated duration of greater than 1 year eliminates most other causes of hypercalcemia. Familial hypocalciuric hypercalcemia is also consistent with chronic hypercalcemia, and is characterized by only moderately elevated PTH levels, with most patients exceeding 99% renal calcium absorption. Malignancy-related hypercalcemia is usually discovered in patients with known malignancy, but may occur as the presenting sign of an occult tumor. It is associated with a more acute presentation and seldom associated with the long-term complications of hypercalcemia. PTH levels are undetectable or extremely low in malignancy-related hypercalcemia. This diagnosis is often made in association with the clinical symptoms of the tumor. Other diagnostic possibilities that must be considered are hypercalcemia associated with vitamin D disorders, kidney failure, lithium therapy, hyperthyroidism, thiazides, excess vitamin A, and granulomatous diseases such as sarcoidosis and tuberculosis.

It is important to establish that hypercalcemia is truly present by several serum calcium measurements prior to further evaluation. Normal values of 8.5 to 10.5 mg/dL will vary with different laboratories, age, and sex. Generally, symptoms are present when calcium levels are above 11.5 mg/dL; renal insufficiency and calcification of tissues occurs when levels exceed 13 mg/dL; and severe

hypercalcemia is defined as 14.5 mg/dL or greater, a medical emergency that can lead to coma or cardiac arrest. Once the presence of persistent hypercalcemia is established, immunoassay for PTH levels is appropriate. An elevated PTH level in the presence of persistent hypercalcemia and without clinical evidence for other causes is the best guide to diagnosis. Other tests that can be helpful in the diagnosis include blood phosphorus, serum proteins, alkaline phosphate, chloride, and measurement of urinary cAMP.

Hypoparathyroidism

Hypoparathyroidism is characterized by hypocalcemia, hyperphosphatemia, and normal renal function. A careful history should attempt to determine the duration of the illness and associated clinical signs and symptoms. The inherited type usually presents early in life. Onset of symptoms in the adult may be due to nutritional deficiencies, renal failure, or disorders of vitamin D metabolism. A history of neck surgery, even many years ago, raises the possibility of postsurgical hypoparathyroidism. After comprehensive physical examination, diagnostic workup includes establishing chronic hypocalcemia, determination of PTH levels by radioimmunoassay, test of vitamin D metabolism, urinary cAMP levels, and urinary phosphate response to exogenous PTH.

■ Ocular

Hyperparathyroidism

Band keratopathy associated with hyperparathyroidism is diagnosed by the clinical appearance. A white, opaque material in the superficial corneal stroma having the appearance of frosted or ground glass is characteristically located at the 3- and 9-o'clock positions within the palpebral fissure. The peripheral edge is separated from the limbus by a sharp clear margin, while the central edge is diffuse and gradually fades into the corneal tissue. Conjunctival deposits of calcium appear as small, hard, white flecks or glass-like crystals in the palpebral conjunctiva.

Hypoparathyroidism

Ocular complications of hypoparathyroidism are diagnosed by the clinical appearance. Complaints of photophobia and blepharospasm can be associated with keratoconjunctivitis. More commonly, lens opacities associated with polychromatic crystals are found. The recognition of these lens opacities may lead to the systemic diagnosis. Papilledema is due to intracranial hypertension and sometimes associated with convulsions. This may be confused with a suspected intracranial mass.

TREATMENT AND MANAGEMENT

Any patient with ocular signs, systemic signs or symptoms, or a history consistent with hyperparathyroidism or hypoparathyroidism should be referred to an internist or endocrinologist for evaluation, systemic workup, definitive diagnosis, and treatment (Table 19–3).

■ Systemic

Hyperparathyroidism

Although there is no specific medical treatment for primary hyperparathyroidism, following the asymptomatic patient with periodic monitoring of renal, gastrointestinal, and bone

TABLE 19–3. TREATMENT AND MANAGEMENT OF PARATHYROID DISORDERS

■ **SYSTEMIC**
HYPERPARATHYROIDISM
- Observation versus parathyroidectomy

HYPOPARATHYROIDISM
- Calcium (1–2 g/d) and vitamin D (50,000–100,000 U/d) supplements

■ **OCULAR**
HYPERPARATHYROIDISM
- Band keratopathy: observation, EDTA

HYPOPARATHYROIDISM
- Cataract: observation, surgical removal
- Keratoconjunctivitis: topical lubricants
- Papilledema: correction of hypocalcemia

functions is indicated. Often a period of observation may be suggested for patients with no complications and a serum calcium level of less than 11.5 mg/dL. This may be the preferred treatment for older individuals without complications. However, there is evidence that asymptomatic patients who had surgery showed improved renal function and increased bone density. Therefore, it might be prudent to recommend parathyroidectomy to young asymptomatic patients prior to the development of symptoms or complications.

Parathyroidectomy is recommended as definitive treatment for all patients with a firm diagnosis and no contraindication to the operation. Recurrent hyperparathyroidism develops in less than 5% of cases with a single adenoma and in about 11% of cases with one or more glands involved. With successful surgical treatment, systemic symptoms due to hypercalcemia disappear.

Hypoparathyroidism

Hypoparathyroidism treatment consists of medical therapy with vitamin D and calcium supplements. Dosage will vary with each patient.

■ Ocular

Hyperparathyroidism

Band keratopathy can be removed by irrigating the chelating agent ethylenediaminetetraacetate (EDTA) onto the Bowman membrane after the corneal epithelium has been removed. Indications for removal include decreased vision and symptomatic irritation (see Table 19–3).

Hypoparathyroidism

Keratoconjunctivitis associated with hypoparathyroidism is treated with supportive therapy (eg, ocular lubricants). Consultation with a corneal specialist is advised in cases that are complicated by superficial stromal and extensive peripheral vascularization. Early lens opacities will not cause visual loss, but a visually significant cataract from long-term disease should be referred for surgical removal. Papilledema due to hypoparathyroidism should resolve as the systemic condition is treated (see Table 19–3). Neuro-ophthalmologic consultation is advised, because this uncommon complication can mimic an intracranial mass.

CONCLUSION

The disruption of the normal function of the parathyroid glands leads to alterations in calcium and phosphate blood levels, which manifest systemically as a disruption of the normal function of nerve, muscle, and gastrointestinal systems.

The ocular manifestations of parathyroid disease may include corneal and conjunctival changes, along with cataracts. The ocular disorders usually present in patients with established parathyroid dysfunction. However, the detection of the classic ocular signs, such as polychromatic lenticular opacities in hypoparathyroidism, may lead to its diagnosis.

REFERENCES

Blake J. Eye signs in idiopathic hypoparathyroidism. *Trans Ophthalmol Soc UK*. 1976;46:488–451.

Brown RC, Aston JP, Weeks I, et al. Circulating intact parathyroid hormone measured by a two-site immunochemiluminometric assay. *J Clin Endocrinol Metab*. 1987;65:407–414.

Cogan DG, Albright F, Bartter FC. Hypercalcemia and band keratopathy. Report of nineteen cases. *Arch Ophthalmol*. 1948;40:624–638.

Davies M. Primary hyperparathyroidism: Aggressive or conservative treatment? *Clin Endocrinol*. 1992;36:325–332.

Grant WM. New treatment for calcific corneal opacities. *Arch Ophthalmol*. 1974;1257–1261.

Hanley DA, Sherwood LM. Secondary hyperparathyroidism in chronic renal failure: Pathophysiology and treatment. *Med Clin North Am*. 1978;62:1319–1339.

Heath H III. Primary hyperparathyroidism: Recent advances in pathogenesis, diagnosis, and treatment. *Adv Intern Med*. 1992;37:275–293.

Lafferty FW, Hubay CA. Primary hyperparathyroidism: A review of the long-term surgical and nonsurgical morbidities as a basis for a rational approach to treatment. *Arch Intern Med*. 1989;149:789–796.

Mallete LE, Bilizikian JP, Heath DA, et al. Primary hyperparathyroidism: Clinical features and biochemical features. *Medicine*. 1974;53:127–146.

Mundy GR, Cove DH, Fisken R. Primary Hyperparathyroidism: Changes in the pattern of clinical presentation. *Lancet*. 1980;1:1317–1320.

Paloyan E, Lawrence AM. Primary hyperparathyroidism: Pathology and therapy. *JAMA*. 1981;246:1334.

Sambrook MA, Hill LF. Cerebrospinal fluid absorption in primary hypoparathyroidism. *J Neurol Neurosurg Psychiatr*. 1977;1015–1017.

Schneider AB, Sherwood LM. Pathogenesis and management of hypoparathyroidism and other hypocalcemic disorders. *Metabolism*. 1975;24:871–898.

Scholz DA, Purnell DC. Asymptomatic primary hyperparathyroidism. 10-year prospective study. *Mayo Clin Proc*. 1981;56:473–478.

Dysfunction of the Pituitary Gland

Bernard J. Dolan

The pituitary gland, or hypophysis cerebri, is composed of the anterior pituitary (adenohypophysis), derived from ectoderm, and the posterior pituitary (neurohypophysis), derived from neural ectoderm. It plays a central role in the endocrine system by releasing a number of hormones that regulate other endocrine glands and nonendocrine tissue. Dysfunction of the pituitary gland may be evidenced in both its systemic and ocular manifestations. Recognition of these are therefore important.

Disorders of the pituitary gland associated with ocular findings are primarily the result of expanding anterior pituitary lesions. Due to its proximity to the optic chiasm, a pituitary gland tumor may lead to compression of the optic pathway, with resultant visual loss. Because disturbances of the visual system are associated with anterior pituitary lesions, the following discussion will be limited to this area.

EPIDEMIOLOGY

■ Systemic

Adenomas are the most common pituitary tumors and can occur at any age. It is difficult to estimate true incidence of these disorders, but they accounted for 6 to 23% of intracranial tumors in an autopsy series of unselected adults (Kovacs & Horvath, 1987). Because the distinction between small areas of hyperplasia and neoplasia is difficult to make histologically, there is a wide range in the rate of lesion detection. Thus, reports on the incidence of pituitary adenomas vary from 2 to 27%.

Prolactin-secreting adenomas are the most common, with a frequency of about 40%. Nonsecretory adenomas compose 25 to 30% of pituitary adenomas. Growth-hormone-secreting adenomas are found in 14 to 17% of patients with pituitary tumors. Corticotrope adenomas probably present in about 10% of cases.

Gonadotropin-secreting adenomas are less common, with a prevalence in surgical specimen studies of 3.5 to 4.1%. Thyroid stimulating hormone (TSH) secreting adenomas are rare, representing 1% or less of pituitary adenomas.

■ Ocular

The prevalence of visual symptoms and signs associated with pituitary adenoma are decreasing because of earlier diagnosis due to endocrine complaints and imaging studies for unrelated causes. Decreased visual acuity was noted in 4% and visual field loss in 9% of pituitary tumor patients admitted to a neuroendocrine service between 1976 and 1981 (Anderson et al, 1983).

NATURAL HISTORY

The pituitary gland extends from the median eminence at the base of the hypothalamus into a bony projection of the sphenoid bone, the sella turcica. Dura mater lining the sella surrounds the gland, separating it laterally from the cavernous sinus and superiorly from the brain with a dural fold called the diaphragma sellae. Important anatomical relationships to the pituitary gland include the internal carotid arteries and cavernous sinus laterally, the sphenoid air sinus inferiorly and anteriorly, and the optic chiasm and the optic tracts.

Six major hormones have been identified as being produced and secreted in the anterior pituitary gland. These include glycoproteins and polypeptides. The polypeptides are adrenocorticotropin hormone (ACTH), which is derived from pro-opiomelanocortin (POMC); growth hormone (GH); and prolactin. The glycoproteins are thyrotropin or thyroid-stimulating hormone (TSH); luteinizing hormone (LH); and follicle-stimulating hormone (FSH). The glycoprotein hormones are made up of an identical alpha subunit and a slightly different beta subunit that appears to delineate the specific hormone function. Table 20–1 delineates each hormone's function.

All anterior pituitary hormones are secreted in bursts that result in sharp peaks in the systemic blood levels of the hormone. Between these bursts of hormone release, the blood levels may be low or undetectable by present assays. Therefore, a single random measurement of hormonal levels may not provide a clear indication of hormonal secretion.

Pituitary secretions are regulated by the hypothalamus, which is influenced by input from the nervous system (Figure 20–1). The hypothalamus produces specific peptides that act on the corresponding cells of the anterior pituitary to control hormone secretion. Although most releasing factors are stimulatory, dopamine inhibits prolactin secretion. Growth hormone has individual factors that stimulate

TABLE 20–1. HORMONE FUNCTIONS OF THE ANTERIOR PITUITARY GLAND

Polypeptides

Adrenocorticotropin hormone (ACTH)
  Synthesis and secretion of glucocorticoids
  Release of mineralocorticoids and adrenal androgens (minor
    influence)
Growth hormone (GH)
  Promote metabolism and growth
Prolactin
  Development of mammary gland and lactation
  Physiological function of liver, ovary, testes, and prostate

Glycoproteins

Thyroid-stimulating hormone (TSH)
  Production and release of thyroxine (T_4) and triiodothyronine (T_3),
    which increases metabolic activity
Follicle-stimulating hormone (FSH)
  Gonadotropin
  Gametogenesis; with LH produces sex hormones
  Follicular maturation
  Production of mature sperm
Luteinizing hormone (LH)
  Gonadotropin
  With FSH produces sex hormones
  Ovulation
  Maintains corpus luteum; production of estrogen and progesterone
  Testosterone production

and inhibit the release of this hormone. The hypothalamus also receives negative feedback via the hormones secreted by target organs or other metabolic products. Disruption of this balance may result in the selective overstimulation of one target gland or tissue, or deficiency of one or more of the pituitary hormones.

In addition to regulation by the hypothalamus, the anterior pituitary is influenced by the circulating levels of hormone from the target organ (see Figure 20–1). This provides a negative feedback loop for regulation in the levels of pituitary hormones. The thyroid hormones, cortisol, peptide growth factors, and sex hormones all act to inhibit the release of the corresponding pituitary hormone. Furthermore, the hormones from the target organs provide a feedback control upon the secretion of the hypothalamic-releasing hormones by influencing neuroregulators and other central neurotransmitters. These additional neural and endocrine influences act to maintain a homeostatic balance for each individual hormone.

■ Systemic

Pituitary Adenomas

Pituitary adenomas are classified as microadenomas or macroadenomas based on size of the lesion. When the tumor is an encapsulated lesion, 10 mm or less in diameter, and yet readily distinguished from the gland, it is a microadenoma. Tumors greater than 10 mm in diameter are macroadenomas. Most commonly, these tumors expand superiorly through the diaphragma sellae, which offers the least resistance. These larger tumors can grow down through the thin layer of bone into the sphenoid sinus, laterally into the cavernous sinus, or into the orbital surface of the frontal bone. Rarely does the tumor grow posteriorly and compress the basilar artery and brainstem.

The shape of the tumor is dependent on the resistance of the diaphragma sellae and the size of the pituitary stalk opening. Some tumors may pass easily through the opening; others take a dumbbell shape due to more resistance in the opening, and still others may expand within the diaphragma. All suprasellar extensions have the potential for the tumor to impinge on the optic chiasm, optic tracts, or optic nerves. Macroadenomas may also compress the hypothalamus.

Pituitary adenomas were originally classified based on the characteristic dye that the proliferating cells took up on light-microscopic examination. Acidophilic adenomas were associated with clinical syndromes implicating excess growth hormone, basophilic adenomas with clinical syndromes implicating excess ACTH, and chromophobe adenomas with clinical signs suggesting hypopituitarism. This classification began to break down when microscopic examination showed that chromophobes had secretory granules and clinical symptoms of endocrine activity were

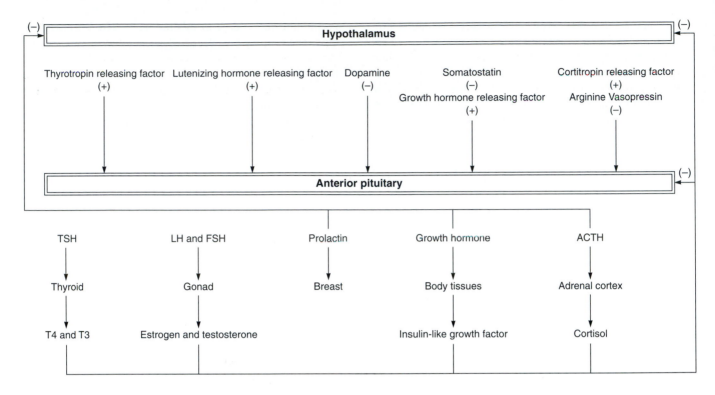

Figure 20–1. Diagram of the releasing factors and feedback loops for the pituitary hormones.

associated with more than half the chromophobe adenomas. Present classification of pituitary adenomas uses a functional morphological system where clinical and laboratory findings are correlated with histological, immunohistochemical, and electron-microscopic characteristics of normal and adenomatous cell types.

The signs and symptoms of pituitary adenoma are secondary to either the mass effects of the expanding gland or to excess production of hormone. The clinical manifestations of a pituitary adenoma vary with age, gender, cell type, and the extent of compression on the gland and surrounding structures (Table 20–2). The most common presenting symptom for pituitary tumors has changed from visual loss to endocrine dysfunction. This is related to the development of radioimmunoassays to measure the hormones of the anterior pituitary and the development of computed tomography (CT) scanning and magnetic resonance imaging (MRI). Mass effects include headache, hypopituitarism, and disturbance of the optic nerves. Headache from pituitary adenomas can vary in location, but may be localized to retro-orbital or bitemporal areas.

The three most common endocrine disorders due to excess hormone secretion with pituitary adenoma are amenorrhea and galactorrhea with hyperprolactinemia, acromegaly with hypersecretion of growth hormone, and Cushing disease with hypersecretion of ACTH and resultant excess cortisol. Other endocrine abnormalities include impotence, decreased libido, gigantism, dysthyroidism, and

hypogonadism. Some of these endocrine manifestations result from anterior pituitary hormone deficiency due to the mass effect causing destruction of the normal pituitary cells. The mass effect can also compress the pituitary stalk or hypothalamus, resulting in endocrine dysfunction of the anterior or posterior pituitary.

Initially, adenomas are classified as secretory or nonsecretory. Most pituitary adenomas are secreting. The secreting adenoma may be composed of any secretory cell type in the anterior pituitary. The majority of cases are classified based on the systemic manifestations they produce. This can be assisted by measuring the serum concentrations of specific anterior pituitary hormone levels or immunohistochemical study of tumor tissue. However, depending on the hormone being secreted, size and shape of the tumor, and age and sex of the patient, the adenoma may not produce clinical symptoms. In some cases, the adenoma may secrete more than one hormone and still produce no clinical signs and symptoms. Other tumors secreting more than one hormone may be associated with the clinical manifestations of only one hormone. Despite this variation, most tumors can be classified as a specific secretory type using clinical manifestations, serum hormone levels, and tumor tissue immunohistochemistry. These include prolactin-producing adenomas, growth-hormone-producing adenomas, ACTH-producing adenomas, TSH-producing adenomas, LH- and FSH-producing adenomas, mixed or multiple hormone-producing adenomas, and null-cell adenomas, which are

TABLE 20–2. SYSTEMIC MANIFESTATIONS OF PITUITARY DYSFUNCTION

PROLACTINOMAS
- Females: Galactorrhea, amenorrhea
- Males: Impotence, decreased libido
- Both: Infertility, headache, weight gain

GROWTH-HORMONE-SECRETING ADENOMAS
- Gigantism (child)
- Acromegaly (adult)
  Large jaw/nose, growth hands/feet, thickened skin, increased metabolic rate, enlargement of body organs, impaired glucose tolerance, headache, peripheral neuropathy, fibrous thickening joint capsule, fatigue, recurrent sinusitis, deepening of voice, increased spacing of teeth, menstrual disturbance

ACTH-SECRETING ADENOMAS (CUSHING DISEASE)
- "Moon face"
- Centripital obesity
- "Buffalo hump"
- Bruising easily

GONADOTROPIN-SECRETING ADENOMAS
- Female: Rare
- Male: Decreased libido, impotence

TSH-SECRETING ADENOMAS
- Heat intolerance
- Weight loss
- Nervousness
- Tremor
- Increased appetite

NONSECRETORY ADENOMAS
- Headache
- Hypopituitarism
- Visual loss

HYPOPITUITARISM
- Hypogonadism, hypothyroidism, adrenal insufficiency

PITUITARY APOPLEXY
- Sudden decrease in visual acuity, ophthalmoplegia, headache, sensory perception changes, nausea/vomiting, seizures, hemiplegia

devoid of clinical, biochemical, or immunohistochemical evidence of endocrine activity.

Prolactinomas

The most common secreting pituitary adenomas are prolactinomas. Common presenting symptoms in women of childbearing age are galactorrhea, amenorrhea, or infertility. Men may have decreased libido, impotence, infertility, and in some cases galactorrhea. The presence of endocrine

symptoms varies with gender and age, as well as the duration and size of the tumor. Postmenopausal women and men commonly complain of only headache. Hypogonadism is probably mediated by prolactin inhibiting the release of the hypothalamic LH-releasing factor and the resulting decreased gonadotropin production.

Prolactinomas are most commonly found in women 20 to 50 years old. Other symptoms include weight gain, decreased libido, fatigue, acne, oily skin, vaginal dryness, and constipation. The presence of these additional symptoms does not appear to change the probability of finding a pituitary tumor.

Men with hyperprolactinemia do not often present with galactorrhea, due to the poor development of acini in the breast. However, vigorous manipulation may demonstrate the presence of this finding. Partial or complete impotence, decreased libido, and infertility may be ignored for years and only recognized after successful treatment. Hypogonadism can also manifest as decreased body hair or beard. Increased appetite with resultant obesity, apathy, and headache may be present. Thus, prolactinomas in men are more likely to be diagnosed at 60 to 70 years of age.

Although the natural history of prolactinomas is not completely understood, it appears that there is slow growth of the tumor in most cases. In microadenoma autopsy studies where the majority of patients had no evidence of endocrine dysfunction, 40% of the tumors tested positive for prolactin with immunohistochemical stain. Studies following untreated prolactin-secreting microadenomas reveal that most tumors are unchanged over the 3- to 6-year observation period while a minority show a significant increase in tumor size. Factors responsible for tumor enlargement in these cases have not been identified. However, DNA analysis indicates that prolactinomas are monoclonal in origin.

Growth-hormone-secreting Adenomas

The hypersecretion of growth hormone is most often due to a pituitary adenoma. Rarely, the cause is excess production of GH-releasing factor by the hypothalamus or ectopic secretion of GH-releasing factor from a peripheral area such as a tumor of the pancreas. The normal circadian pattern in the secretion of GH is replaced with a pattern of variable bursts. This results in gigantism in a child or young adolescent where the epiphyseal plates have not closed. Growth of the long bones is stimulated and an individual can reach the height of 8 to 9 feet if untreated. In the adult, GH hypersecretion results in acromegaly. It most commonly presents between 20 and 40 years of age. The well developed case of acromegaly may be easily identified; however, early signs are often not recognized.

Acromegalics have characteristic growth changes in the soft tissues and bones of the face, hands, and feet. These patients may complain of increased shoe, glove, or ring size. Growth occurs in the mandible, nasal, malar, and frontal bones, changing facial appearance. Marked jaw projection and exaggerated nasolabial folds develop slowly over the years and may elicit no complaint from the patient; however, those who do not see the patient frequently may comment on the changes. Proliferation of the connective tissue leads to increased subcutaneous tissue and thickened oily skin. This can contribute to nerve entrapment as in carpel tunnel syndrome. Enlargement of body organs may occur, including the viscera, heart, kidney, pancreas, and liver. Metabolic rate may increase with normal thyroid hormone levels. Impaired glucose tolerance is common due to insulin resistance actions of GH, and may put the patient at risk for development of diabetes mellitus. Long-standing disease can lead to fatigue, weakness, and muscle abnormalities with electromyogram (EMG) changes. Peripheral neuropathy with paresthesias of the hand and feet may develop. Fibrous thickening of the joint capsule with joint pain may be confused with arthritis. Other manifestations include headache, increased spacing of teeth, recurrent sinusitis, otitis media, deepening of voice, and hyperhydrosis of the skin. Women may complain of menstrual disturbances, while men may experience decreased libido and impotence.

Adrenocorticotropin-secreting Adenomas

Hypercortisolism results in a distinctive clinical presentation of increased cortisol and associated systemic findings that is called Cushing syndrome. The cause of hypercortisolism may be excessive autonomous secretion of cortisol by an adrenal tumor (17%), an ectopic nonpituitary tumor producing ACTH (15%), or pituitary hypersecretion of ACTH (68%). Cushing syndrome due to pituitary hypersecretion of ACTH is almost always due to a pituitary tumor, and is called Cushing disease.

Clinical recognition is relatively easy when the disease is fully developed; however, the early presentation may present difficulty in establishing the clinical diagnosis. Cushing disease has been described most frequently in women between 20 and 40 years of age, but it can occur at any age, in both sexes, and any race. There is loss of the diurnal rhythm of ACTH secretion by the pituitary gland; however, many patients who are ill, under stress, or hospitalized demonstrate this loss of diurnal rhythm.

Cushing syndrome is characterized by increased weight due to adipose tissue deposition in the face, back of the neck, and trunk, with thin arms and legs. Prominent cheek fat pads produce a "moon face" appearance, and deposition of fat pads in the supraclavicular fossae and back of the neck ("buffalo hump") occur frequently. Sexual dysfunction is a common complaint with amenorrhea or oligomenorrhea in women and decreased libido or impotence in men. Protein loss leads to abnormalities of the skin, and muscle wasting. Common skin findings include thinning of the epidermis, purple striae from subcutaneous vasculature, slow repair, and easy bruising. Other skin changes include acne,

skin pigmentation, or rash. Generalized osteoporosis due to loss of bone matrix can lead to vertebral compression fractures and resultant back pain. Occasionally pathological fractures of the extremities may occur. Headache, increased body hair, and ankle edema may also be found. Impaired glucose tolerance without overt diabetes mellitus and hypertension associated with left ventricular hypertrophy are common associated findings. Mental disturbances range from mild anxiety to severe depression.

Gonadotropin and TSH-secreting Adenomas

Gonadotropin-secreting adenomas and TSH-secreting adenomas are uncommon. Therefore, these will not be further discussed in this chapter, but are summarized in Table 20–2.

Nonsecretory Pituitary Adenomas

Nonsecretory pituitary adenomas are pituitary tumors that do not produce any apparent endocrine abnormality. The absence of excess hormone production from these tumors may be due to abnormal transition of these cells or poor development of the hormonal-producing components of the cells.

Nonsecretory pituitary tumors can produce symptoms and signs associated with the mass effect of space-occupying lesions such as headaches or vision loss. In addition, they may produce symptoms of hypopituitarism, which include hypogonadism, hypothyroidism, and adrenal insufficiency. Large tumors may compress the pituitary stalk and interfere with the delivery of dopamine, the hypothalamic prolactin-inhibitory factor, to the lactotrophs of the anterior pituitary resulting in mild hyperprolactinemia. Suprasellar meningiomas, aneurysms, craniopharyngiomas, or granulomatous disease such as sarcoidosis can produce a hyperprolactinemia by this mechanism.

Hypopituitarism

Hypopituitarism is the loss of or reduction in function of the anterior pituitary. Total or selective loss may occur with pituitary adenomas due to the compromise of the normal cells from the tumor expansion. This occurs more commonly with macroadenomas such as prolactin-secreting, GH-secreting, or nonsecretory adenomas.

The clinical features of hypopituitarism will depend on the age, gender, and number and types of hormones that lose function. One or more hormone functions may be affected as the adenoma expands. The symptoms of loss of function due to tumor compression may be masked by the signs and symptoms of the pituitary tumor hypersecretion. Hypopituitarism is also seen in patients with head injury or parasellar disease, or who have undergone a surgical procedure or radiation treatment for pituitary adenomas.

The most common symptom of hypopituitarism is gonadal dysfunction in both men and women. Loss of pituitary hormonal secretion with systemic deficiency of the hormone is progressive and often occurs initially with gonadotropins, followed by GH, TSH, and ACTH. Variations occur so that adrenal dysfunction and hypothyroidism may be the initial presentation. Deficiency of the gonadotropins causes delayed or arrested puberty in adolescents, infertility, amenorrhea or menstrual disorders in women, and slow reduction of libido and impotence in men that may be attributed to aging. GH hyposecretion leads to interruption of normal growth and delayed puberty in children; however, there is no recognized pathologic syndrome in adults.

Secondary hypothyroidism usually occurs late in the development of hypopituitarism and is usually more mild than primary hypothyroidism. ACTH deficiency leads to a secondary adrenal deficiency with malaise, loss of energy, and postural hypotension. Adrenal insufficiency can lead to a medical emergency.

Pituitary Apoplexy

Pituitary apoplexy was originally used to describe a life-threatening, acute infarction of the pituitary gland; however, the present use of the term includes infarction and necrosis associated with a hemorrhage into a pituitary tumor. Clinical signs include sudden changes in visual function, ophthalmoplegia, headache, or sensory perception, often associated with nausea and vomiting. These signs result from sudden compression due to the rapid expansion of the lesion. Occasionally, compression of the carotid artery against the anterior clinoid process can result in cerebral hemispheric disorders including seizures and hemiplegia.

■ Ocular

The ocular disorders associated with pituitary adenomas are secondary to the expansion of the tumor and the compression of nerves that serve the ocular structures (Table 20–3). Due to the proximity of the optic chiasm, pituitary tumors can lead to compression of the optic pathway and result in visual loss. In addition, expansion laterally into the cavernous sinus may compress the oculomotor nerve (III), trochlear nerve (IV), abducens nerve (VI), and the ophthalmic and maxillary divisions of the trigeminal nerve (V). With the advancement of neuroimaging techniques, visual loss as the presenting sign of a pituitary tumor is less common.

Ocular findings are absent in microadenomas, because the tumor is too small to compress the adjacent nerves. Macroadenomas most commonly expand superiorly, and this often results in the compression of the optic chiasm. The type of visual field defect produced is dependent on the anatomic relationship between the chiasm and the pituitary gland. The chiasm is normally directly above the pituitary; however, the chiasm is anterior in about 15% of persons (prefixed chiasm) and posterior in about 5% of cases (post-

TABLE 20–3. OCULAR MANIFESTATIONS OF DYSFUNCTIONS OF THE PITUITARY GLAND

COMPRESSION OF OPTIC NERVE, CHIASM, OR PATHWAY
- Visual field loss: central and/or peripheral (classically bitemporal)
- Decreased visual acuity
- Decreased color vision
- Optic atrophy

COMPRESSION OF CRANIAL NERVES III, IV, OR VI
- Ophthalmoplegia
- Diplopia
- Ptosis

COMPRESSION OF CRANIAL NERVES V₁ OR V₂
- Facial pain

RETRO-ORBITAL VENOUS CONGESTION
- Proptosis (rare)

fixed chiasm). Lateral expansion of the tumor into the cavernous sinus occurs less frequently, but can result in complaints of diplopia, ptosis, and alteration of facial sensation.

The bitemporal hemianopic field defect is the classic sign of chiasmal disorder and the visual abnormality most commonly observed in a patient with a pituitary adenoma (Figure 20–2). The superior temporal quadrants are usually the first to be affected, with the inferior temporal quadrants following. The inferior nasal quadrants are the next to become involved, followed by the superior nasal quadrants and blindness. This correlates with the compression coming from directly below the chiasm and causing damage to the crossed fibers first and later involving the uncrossed fibers.

Visual field defects other than the classic bitemporal distribution are possible due to alterations in the relationship between the chiasm and the sella. Rarely, the compression is anterior on the intracranial portion of an optic nerve, with unilateral decreased vision and central or arcuate scotoma. With a postfixed chiasm, compression of one optic nerve just anterior to the chiasm can result in an ipsilateral visual loss, relative afferent pupillary defect, decreased color vision, and a visual field defect that may have a suggestion of temporal loss. The contralateral eye has a superior temporal defect that may be missed unless careful perimetry is performed. This is due to compression of inferior nasal fibers of the contralateral eye that project forward into the optic nerve of the ipsilateral eye just anterior to the chiasm (Wilbrand knee). With a prefixed chiasm, the field defect can be a bitemporal scotomatous pattern with normal vision from pressure on the posterior aspect of the chiasm. Incongruous homonymous hemianoptic defects are possible if the adenoma compresses the optic tract on one side. Rarely, growth of the tumor between the optic nerves may

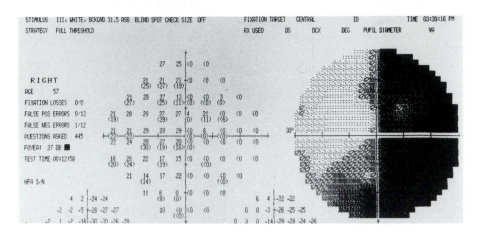

A

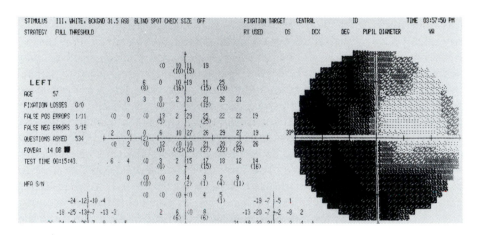

B

Figure 20–2. Visual fields examination (right eye [**A**] and left eye [**B**]) demonstrating a bitemporal hemianopsia in a patient with a pituitary adenoma. Note the slight assymetry with more involvement of the left inferior nasal quadrant.

produce binasal defects as the nerve is pushed laterally against the internal carotid arteries.

The visual field defects may be relative or absolute. The use of a red target may elicit a defect in a field that appears normal to a white target. The visual acuity may be normal in patients with early bitemporal field defects; therefore, these patients may be visually asymptomatic. However, a number of patients develop decreased visual acuity in one or both eyes as the bitemporal defects progress. This may be associated with other clinical signs of optic neuropathy such as color vision defects. Thus, the symptomatic patient may complain of central vision loss or peripheral field loss.

The visual loss associated with pituitary tumors is slowly progressive and gradual so that it can be well established prior to its detection. Continued expansion of the tumor leads to progressive visual field loss and can result in blindness if no treatment is instituted. Damage from compression of the pituitary adenoma eventually produces optic atrophy. This may be appreciated after 6 weeks of nerve compression. The atrophy due to pituitary adenomas is usually diffuse.

Paresis of the nerves controlling the extraocular muscles is associated with the complaint of diplopia. This finding can be caused by compression on the cavernous sinus wall or by invasion of the sinus. This occurs in about 15% of patients, usually without signs or symptoms. Both large tumors with lateral extension, possibly due to a small diaphragma opening, and smaller tumors, often associated with Cushing disease, may grow laterally into the cavernous sinus. With significant invasion of the cavernous sinus, the trigeminal nerve may also be affected, and venous stasis may rarely produce moderate proptosis.

A few patients with complete bitemporal hemianopsia may complain of horizontal or vertical diplopia and difficulty reading in the absence of extraocular muscle nerve paresis. This may result from loss of the normal overlap of ganglion-receptive fields in the nasotemporal fusional areas, causing the breakdown of preexisting phoria. The remaining nasal fields may overlap or separate, causing diplopia and reading disturbances.

DIAGNOSIS

■ Systemic

The clinical characteristics of a patient with a pituitary adenoma will vary with the size and cell type of the tumor. Microadenomas are associated with complaints suggesting an endocrine disorder, or they may be detected with imaging studies for an unrelated disorder. Young women with galactorrhea–amenorrhea syndrome, patients with acromegaly, and patients with Cushing disease are usually diagnosed due to complaints regarding their endocrine disorders. The presenting sign can be macroadenomas with associated visual system abnormalities as the tumor compresses the surrounding nerves. However, many patients with nonsecretory adenomas are diagnosed due to CT or MRI studies performed for reasons unrelated to the tumor. In addition, these large tumors can be associated with hypopituitarism as the function of the other secreting cells is compromised by the tumor expansion. The sequence of the diagnostic workup in pituitary adenomas will vary depending on the presenting signs or symptoms.

History and physical examination of the patient with a suspected or documented pituitary adenoma should include evaluation of growth curve, sexual development or dysfunction, presence of galactorrhea, diabetes insipidus, acromegaly, thyroid function, and adrenal function. Clinical evidence of acromegaly, hyperprolactinemia, or Cushing syndrome should focus the type of investigation. Because detecting the hypersecretion of one or more anterior pituitary hormones and documenting the normal function of other pituitary systems can lead to extensive and expensive testing, laboratory investigation should always be directed by the clinical findings and interpreted within the context of the physical examination and patient history. In addition, interpretation of the laboratory investigation relies upon understanding the limitations of each type of assay, the relationship between the levels of pituitary and target hormones, and the pulsatile hormonal secretion of the anterior pituitary. Other factors influencing hormone levels can include the time of day, developmental stage, stress level, fasting state, and level of patient activity. This evaluation is best performed by an endocrinologist or experienced internist.

In patients with suspected prolactinoma, serum prolactin levels should be repeated prior to the diagnosis of hyperprolactinemia due to the pulsatile secretion of this hormone and its response to breast manipulation. However, a single value of 200 µg/L or greater in a patient with a documented macroadenoma is likely to be due to a prolactinoma. A serum prolactin level of less than 150 to 200 µg/L in the presence of a macroadenoma most likely represents a secondary hyperprolactinemia. This is due to pituitary stalk compression from a nonprolactin-secreting tumor and the interruption of dopamine delivery from the hypothalamus. Serum levels of 20 to 60 µg/L represent mild elevations of prolactin and are more difficult to interpret. They must be repeated several times prior to concluding that pathologic hyperprolactinemia is present.

Postmenopausal women and men with prolactinomas are commonly identified on radiologic imaging for an unrelated problem or complaint of headache. In addition, a history of combined galactorrhea and amenorrhea with elevated prolactin levels increases the probability of a pituitary adenoma being found with high-resolution imaging techniques.

The measurement of growth hormone levels is not practical for the clinical setting in the evaluation of a suspected acromegalic due to the fluctuations in the pulse secretion. Measurement of serum IGF I concentration, a somatomedin which reflects growth hormone levels over the past 24 hours, is a valuable screening test. Elevated IGF I levels indicate excess GH secretion except during pregnancy and puberty, when IGF I levels are increased. An oral glucose tolerance test with monitoring of GH levels is the definitive test for acromegaly. After ingestion of glucose, GH levels will normally decrease to less than 2 µg/L. In acromegaly, serum GH fails to drop below this level.

Macroadenomas are rare in Cushing disease, and only about 50% of the microadenomas are detectable with imaging studies. This adds to the complexity of distinguishing between primary tumors of the adrenal glands, ectopic ACTH-secreting tumors, and ACTH-secreting pituitary tumors. After ruling out an iatrogenic source of cortisol, biochemical testing in the diagnosis of Cushing syndrome includes the dexamethasone suppression test and mytyrapone test, and occasionally a corticotropin-releasing factor test may be of assistance. A negative low-dose dexamethasone-suppression test confirms the diagnosis of Cushing syndrome. A high-dose dexamethasone-suppression test assists in distinguishing the cause of Cushing syndrome, or Cushing disease and when positive suggests a pituitary etiology. Mytyrapone acts to inhibit cortisol synthesis and is used to distinguish between the unresponsiveness of ectopic production of ACTH and pituitary-based dysfunction that remains responsive to short-term changes in plasma cortisol levels.

The diagnosis of nonsecreting adenomas is often based on visual disturbances, headache evaluation, particularly significant changes in headache pattern, or symptoms of hypopituitarism. Hypopituitarism should be evaluated by investigating the hormonal levels of the anterior and posterior pituitary. History and physical findings may suggest deficient hormones.

Appropriate imaging studies are essential for the diagnosis of pituitary tumor. CT and MRI (Figures 20–3 and 20–4) have replaced plain skull x-rays, cerebral angiography, and pneumoencephalography in the evaluation of pituitary adenoma. These earlier techniques provided poor visualization of the gland and the surrounding structures.

CT will provide direct imaging of the gland, identify large tumors, and delineate early hemorrhage. High-resolution and contrast CT, with 1.5-mm cuts, is recommended for detection of pituitary tumors. MRI provides the best method for direct imaging of the gland and its surrounding structures (optic chiasm, diaphragma sellae, and vascular structures), along with identifying large and small tumors. However, many microadenomas, particularly in Cushing disease, will not be resolved on MRI or CT. When intratumoral hemorrhage (pituitary apoplexy) is suspected, prompt evaluation with CT or MRI is required. Within the first few days CT is more sensitive in visualizing the hemorrhage; however, MRI is superior in the subacute stage. In addition, primary empty sella syndrome, a herniation of the subarachnoid space into the sella, once presented a confusing suggestion of pituitary tumor on x-ray, yet is now readily recognized and differentiated on CT or MRI.

■ Ocular

Although it is true that pituitary adenomas without endocrine symptoms were traditionally diagnosed due to dysfunction of the visual system, the frequency of this method of detection has been reduced by the common use of high-quality imaging studies. However, patients still present to eyecare practitioners with and without complaints of visual loss who harbor pituitary tumors compressing the optic pathway. A patient without endocrine or visual symptoms may have early visual signs that are missed due to lack of testing visual fields or poor technique in testing visual fields. When visual field defects are detected, the recognition of a bitemporal defect may lead to the proper diagnosis. However, if central arcuate, centrocecal, or nasal defects are revealed, the proper diagnosis may be missed. Some rare cases may mimic a retrobulbar neuritis. Therefore, any suggestion of a temporal defect that respects the vertical meridian or an asymptomatic defect in the other eye should raise the suspicion that the cause of visual loss is in the region of the chiasm. The eyecare practitioner should consider a pituitary mass as a potential etiology of unexplained visual loss.

Disorders of eye movements are less common than visual loss. In most cases, eye movement findings are associated with visual loss, field defect, or trigeminal deficit suggesting the presence of a tumor; nevertheless, these are sometimes isolated findings. Most commonly, the oculomotor nerve is partially affected with or without pupillary involvement. This normally occurs without pain; however, painful recurrent oculomotor palsy has been reported with

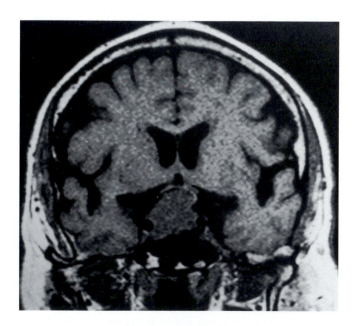

A

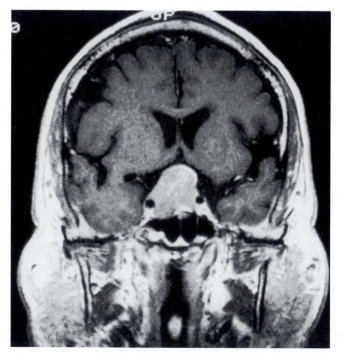

B

Figure 20–3. MRI of pituitary adenoma with **(A)** and without **(B)** contrast. Note the compression of the chiasm just above the adenoma.

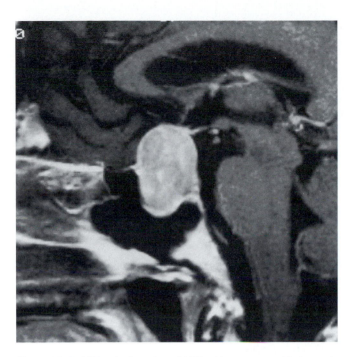

Figure 20–4. Midsagittal section of MRI with contrast, with the optic chiasm stretched over the pituitary adenoma.

TABLE 20–4. SYSTEMIC AND OCULAR TREATMENT AND MANAGEMENT OF PITUITARY ADENOMAS

PROLACTIN-SECRETING ADENOMAS
- Bromocriptine (2.5 mg TID; chronic treatment 2.5 mg BID)
- CT or MRI 1–2 years
- Transsphenoidal excision
- Adjunctive radiation therapy

GROWTH-HORMONE-SECRETING ADENOMAS
- Transsphenoidal excision
- Adjunctive bromocriptine (10–20 mg/d)
- Radiation

ACTH-SECRETING ADENOMAS
- Transsphenoidal excision
- Radiation therapy
- Adjunctive medical therapy

NONSECRETORY TUMORS
- Transsphenoidal excision
- Adjunctive radiation therapy
- Replacement therapy

OCULAR
- Systemic management
- Visual fields examination

prolactin-secreting adenoma. Damage to the oculosympathetic pathway may occur resulting in a smaller, less reactive pupil. The trochlear and abducens nerves are less frequently involved and seldom in isolation. Complete ophthalmoplegia occurs most often with pituitary apoplexy but is extremely rare.

TREATMENT AND MANAGEMENT

▪ Systemic

Pituitary Adenomas
The management of pituitary adenomas (Table 20–4) varies with the size of the tumor, cell type, age and health of the patient, and in women, any future desire for pregnancy. Present management may include observation, medical therapy, surgical excision, radiation, or a combination of these modalities. The goals of treatment are to return the hormonal hypersecretion to normal, decrease tumor size, return the pituitary to normal function, recover any visual loss (Figure 20–5), and resolve any cranial nerve impairment. Ideally this is achieved without chronic hormonal replacement therapy. Only partial achievement of these goals is often possible with very large tumors.

Prolactin-secreting Adenomas
When hyperprolactinemia is present in an asymptomatic woman of childbearing years, with no visible lesion on CT or

MRI, appropriate management may simply be monitoring the patient, which is based on the potential of long-term stability.

Medical therapy includes bromocriptine (Parlodel), a dopamine agonist, which is very effective in hyperprolactinemic women. Treatment results in 80 to 90% normalized prolactin levels, during therapy, with the return to menses and improved galactorrhea. Bromocriptine therapy in men results in increased testosterone levels with improvement of libido and potency. Effectiveness of bromocriptine therapy is correlated with the number and binding affinity of dopamine receptors on the tumor. Side effects of nausea, orthostatic hypotension, and headache cause 10% to discontinue therapy. Medical therapy for macroadenomas may involve a longer treatment period to get prolactin levels within the normal range. As this medical therapy is not tumoricidal, withdrawal of the medication usually leads to increased prolactin levels, reexpansion of the tumor, and return of symptoms. Continued therapy is required even after normal prolactin levels are achieved. Medically treated patients are followed with CT or MRI every 1 to 2 years. Patients with fewer receptors may respond partially or not at all to medical therapy. Surgical resection of the tumor should be considered when medical therapy fails.

Surgical removal of the tumor by the transsphenoidal approach was the most effective treatment prior to develop-

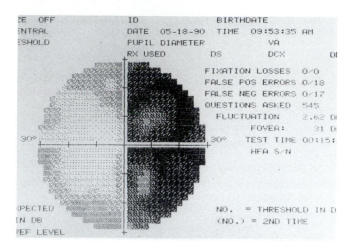
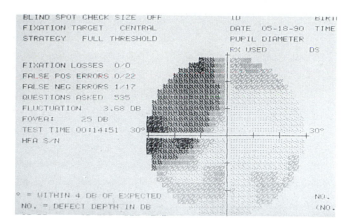

Figure 20–5. Visual fields examination of the patient in Figure 20–2 (right eye [A] and left eye [B]) 3 days after transsphenoidal resection of the tumor. Note the rapid recovery of the left eye.

ment of medical therapy. Surgical results vary with the skill and experience of the surgeon, size of the tumor, and the presurgical prolactin levels. Surgery is effective in resecting microadenomas, with a reversal of symptoms in 80 to 85% of cases and 60 to 80% achieving normal prolactin levels. However, due to recurrence, about 30% will return to preoperative metabolic conditions after 5 years. Surgical results in achieving normal prolactin levels with macroadenomas are less successful. However, surgical resection is effective in reducing the size of macroadenomas. Residual therapy is often required with large tumors, due to partial resection.

Radiotherapy is effective in arresting tumor growth but less effective in reducing serum prolactin levels. It is not the treatment of choice in prolactinoma, but is used in combination with bromocriptine in more rapidly growing tumors. Hypopituitarism and damage to optic pathways are complications seen with pituitary radiation therapy.

Growth-hormone-secreting Adenomas

Surgical removal is the preferred initial treatment for GH-secreting adenomas. Results depend on the skill of the surgeon and the size of the tumor, with tumor extension beyond the sella decreasing the chances of a surgical cure. However, immediate reduction in visual symptoms, other mass effects of the tumor, and hypersecretion of GH is often obtained. Postoperative radiotherapy is useful with persistent tumor to prevent tumor growth and control hormonal hypersecretion. Radiotherapy alone is less useful, because the time interval to reach normal levels is often 10 years. Bromocriptine is effective in only about 20% of GH tumors. It may be used in patients with persistent disease after surgery or radiation. Octreotide, a somatostatin analogue, has been used in clinical trials in patients not responsive to other therapy.

ACTH-secreting Adenomas

Transsphenoidal surgical excision is the preferred treatment in removing ACTH tumors that are identified on imaging and hemihypophysectomy or total hypophysectomy in cases where the tumor is not localized. The cure rate is approximately 80% with an identified microadenoma and experienced surgical team. Radiation is an option, with 80% of children responding to therapy; but disappointing in adults, with only about 20% being successful. The potential development of pituitary dysfunction and other long term-effects of radiation must be considered. Medical treatment includes metyrapone and aminoglutemide, which blocks or inhibits cortisol synthesis. These medications have limited usefulness due to side effects and ineffectiveness. Their main role is adjunctive use in preparing extremely ill patients for surgery or while waiting for the full effects to occur after radiation treatment.

Nonsecretory Tumors

Surgical excision, via transsphenoidal approach, is the recommended therapy for nonsecretory tumors. Radiation therapy may be required for residual tumors. Postoperative management includes evaluation for replacement therapy.

■ Ocular

Pituitary Adenomas

When successful, surgical recession, radiation therapy, or medical therapy results in reduction in the size of an adenoma with decompression of the chiasm and optic nerves. This results in improvement of visual acuity and the visual field. Eyes with preoperative visual acuity of at least 20/100 almost always improve postsurgically, as do 60% of eyes with less than 20/100 preoperative acuity. Surgical removal has resulted in improvement of visual function in 75 to 95% of patients. Improvement may start hours after the surgery and continue for months and occasionally years. Improvement in visual field defects with medical therapy can occur prior to detection of tumor regression on imaging studies. However, 4 to 10% of those treated with surgical removal have deterioration of the visual loss. Complications of radiation therapy include damage to the optic chiasm or optic nerves.

Ocular examination prior to and after surgical or medical treatment, including visual fields examination, is needed to document effectiveness of therapy and monitor tumor recurrence. This should be done in conjunction with imaging studies. In some cases, changes in visual field or visual acuity may indicate tumor recurrence that is not seen on imaging studies.

Conclusion

A pituitary adenoma can present with either systemic manifestations such as those attributed to hormonal involvement, or ocular disturbances, which may be the only sign prior to diagnosis. Bitemporal hemianopsia, a classic sign, is highly suggestive of a pituitary tumor. However, other ocular presentations may provide diagnostic difficulty, as evidenced by decreased vision that has been attributed to another cause. This emphasizes the need to consider a pituitary adenoma as a differential when unexplained vision loss occurs. Consequently, an understanding of both the ocular and systemic manifestations of pituitary dysfunction may lead the eyecare practitioner to the appropriate diagnosis and subsequent management.

References

Alexander JM, Biller BMK, Bikkal H, et al. Clinically nonfunctioning pituitary tumors are monoclonal in origin. *J Clin Invest.* 1990;86:336–340.

Anderson D, Faber P, Marrovitz S, et al. Pituitary tumors and the ophthalmologist. *Ophthalmology.* 1983;90:1265–1270.

Boggan JE, Tyrrell JB, Wilson CB. Transsphenoidal microsurgical management of Cushing's disease. Report of 100 cases. *J Neurosurg.* 1983;59:195–200.

Cohn AR, Cooper PR, Kupersmith MJ, et al. Visual recovery after transsphenoidal removal of pituitary adenomas. *Neurosurgery.* 1985;17:446–452.

Demura R, Jibiki K, Kubo O, et al. The significance of alpha-subunit as tumor marker for gonadotrophin-producing pituitary adenomas. *J Clin Endrocrinol Metab.* 1986;63:564–569.

Ebersold MJ, Quast LM, Laws ER Jr, et al. Long-term results in transsphenoidal removal of non-functioning pituitary tumors. *J Neurosurg.* 1986;64:712–719.

Fahlbusch R, Buchfelder M, Schrell U. Short-term preoperative treatment of macroprolactinomas by dopamine agonists. *J Neurosurg.* 1987;67:807–815.

Grisoli F, Leclircq T, Winteler JP, et al. Thyroid stimulating hormone pituitary adenomas and hyperthyroidism. *Surg Neurol.* 1986;25:361–368.

Kovacs K, Horvath E. Pathology of pituitary tumors. *Endocrinol Metab Clin North Am.* 1987;16:529–551.

Kovacs K, Lloyd R, Horvath E, et al. Silent somatotroph adenomas of the human pituitary. A morphologic study of three cases including immunocytochemistry, electron microscopy, in vitro examination, and in situ hybridization. *Am J Pathol.* 1989;134:345–353.

Laws ER Jr, Trautmann JC, Hollenhorst RW Jr. Transsphenoidal decompression of the optic nerve and chiasm. Visual results in 62 patients. *J Neurosurg.* 1977;46:717–722.

Molitch ME, Elton RL, Blackwell RE, et al. Bromocriptine as primary therapy for prolactin-secreting macroadenomas: Results in a multicenter study. *J Clin Endocrinol Metab.* 1985;60:698–705.

Ortiz JM, Stein SC, Nelson P, et al. Pituitary adenoma presenting as unilateral proptosis. *Arch Ophthalmol.* 1992;10:282–283.

Snyder PJ. Gonadotroph cell adenomas of the pituitary. *Endocrinol Rev.* 1985;6:552–563.

Snyder PJ, Fowble BF, Schatz NJ, et al. Hypopituitarism following radiation therapy of pituitary adenomas. *Am J Med.* 1986;81:457–462.

Tucker HS, Grubb SR, Wigand JP, et al. Treatment of acromegaly by transsphenoidal surgery. *Arch Intern Med.* 1980;140:795–802.

Yamada S, Kovacs K, Horvath E, et al. Morphological study of clinical nonsecreting pituitary adenomas in patients under 40 years of age. *J Neurosurg.* 1991;75:902–905.

21
Chapter

Dysfunction of the Adrenal Glands

Bernard J. Dolan

The adrenal glands, located on the superior pole of the kidney, are paired structures composed of two embryologically and functionally diverse components, the adrenal cortex and medulla. The adrenal cortex, derived from mesoderm, secretes glucocorticoids, mineralocorticoids, and androgen hormones. The glucocorticoids, cortisol being the most significant, act to influence sugar metabolism, activate lipolysis in adipose tissue, modulate the immune system, and mediate inflammatory reaction, along with other important functions. Mineralocorticoids, aldosterone being the most significant, act to regulate sodium, potassium, and electrolyte balance of extracellular tissues. Androgens secreted by the adrenal cortex are converted in the peripheral tissues to more potent androgens such as testosterone and act to promote normal growth. The adrenal medulla, derived from neural crest ectoderm, produces epinephrine and smaller amounts of norepinephrine, which act to increase overall sympathetic functions throughout the body.

There are a variety of adrenal cortex disorders, yet they can be broadly classified as disorders of hypersecretion or hyposecretion of adrenal cortical hormones. Chronic excess cortisol secretion is called Cushing syndrome. Chronic excess aldosterone secretion is called Conn syndrome or primary aldosteronism. Primary adrenal cortical insufficiency (Addison disease) can result in deficiency of glucocorticoids, mineralocorticoids, and androgen hormones. Secondary and tertiary adrenal cortical insufficiency is due to inadequate pituitary adrenocorticotropin hormone (ACTH) secretion and a defect in corticotropin-releasing hormone (CRH) secretion, respectively.

Adrenal medullary disorders seldom come to the attention of the eyecare practitioner. Tumors associated with cells of neural crest origin are the exception. Pheochromocytomas are uncommon tumors of the chromaffin tissue of the adrenal medulla, with resultant excess secretion of norepinephrine in most cases. Neuroblastomas are tumors of embryonic sympathoblasts, with an associated excess production of catecholamines and a tendency for aggressive malignant behavior.

The ocular findings associated with adrenal cortical and medullary disorders are commonly a result of a systemic manifestation of the adrenal disorder. As an isolated finding these are seldom of value in making the diagnosis of an adrenal disease. However, within the context of a unique clinical syndrome, it can assist in the diagnosis of the underlying systemic disease.

EPIDEMIOLOGY

■ Systemic

Cortex Hyperfunction
The incidence of Cushing syndrome varies with the cause. The most common form is thought to be iatrogenic, with an estimated 10 million people in this country taking glucocorticoids in pharmacological doses each year. The second most common form is probably ectopic ACTH syndrome, with an estimated incidence of about 660 per million per year. Cushing disease, due to pituitary dysfunction has an incidence of about 5 to 25 per million per year, and adrenal carcinoma has an estimated incidence of 2 per million per

year. Cushing disease is 3 to 8 times more common in females than in males.

Primary aldosteronism (Conn syndrome) has its peak incidence during the fourth to fifth decades. It is the cause of hypertension in less than 1% of cases.

Cortex Hypofunction

Primary adrenal insufficiency (Addison disease) has an incidence of approximately 50 cases per million adults. It is more common in females than males, at a ratio of 2.6 to 1.

Secondary and tertiary adrenal insufficiency has no specific epidemiology.

Medulla Disorders

Medulla neuroblastoma is the most common malignant tumor in children, representing about 15% of metastatic disease in this population. Pheochromocytoma is an uncommon tumor.

■ Ocular

Hypertension occurs in approximately 80% of Cushing syndrome cases; however, the incidence of hypertensive retinopathy is unknown. Exophthalmos has been reported in about 7% of cases, and raised intraocular pressure in about 25% of cases.

Ocular findings are uncommon in Cushing disease and rare in primary adrenal insufficiency. The frequency of ocular findings in primary aldosteronism and secondary and tertiary adrenal insufficiency is unknown.

NATURAL HISTORY

Table 21–1 gives an overview of the adrenal hormones. Adrenal hormone production and secretion is under the regulation of various systems. The pituitary hormone ACTH is the major regulator of glucocorticoids, playing a significant role in androgen secretion and a minor role in aldosterone secretion. ACTH production is under the control CRF secreted by the hypothalamus. The glucocorticoids provide negative feedback to the hypothalamus and anterior pituitary to inhibit the secretion of CRF and ACTH (Figure 21–1). Aldosterone secretion is primarily regulated by the renin–angiotensin system. Epinephrine from the adrenal medulla is directly influenced by the preganglionic sympathetic innervation.

■ Systemic

Table 21–2 summarizes systemic manifestations of adrenal disorders.

Cortex Hyperfunction

Cushing syndrome is the clinical manifestation resulting from chronic glucocorticoid hypersecretion. The cause may

TABLE 21–1. ADRENAL HORMONES

Adrenal Cortex

Glucocorticoid
    Cortisol (survival, sugar metabolism, activates lipolysis in adipose tissue, modulates immune system, mediates inflammatory reaction)
    Excess: Cushing syndrome
        ACTH dependent: primary microadenomas of the anterior pituitary (Cushing disease), nonpituitary tumor (ectopic ACTH), nonhypothalamic tumor (ectopic CRH)
        ACTH independent: iatrogenic and primary adrenocortical adenomas or carcinomas
    Insufficiency (primary): Addison disease
Mineralocorticoids
    Aldosterone (regulates sodium, potassium, electrolyte balance of extracellular tissues)
    Excess: Aldosteronism (primary: Conn syndrome)
    Insufficiency: (primary: Addison disease)
Androgen
    Testosterone (promotes normal growth)

Adrenal Medulla

Catecholamines, epinephrine, and norepinephrine (sympathetic function)
    Excess: Pheochromocytomas or neuroblastomas

be due to ACTH hypersecretion (ACTH dependent) or may be ACTH independent. The ACTH-dependent type most commonly occurs with primary ACTH secretion of the pituitary (Cushing disease). In addition, nonpituitary tumors (ectopic ACTH syndrome), which are often associated with malignant tumors, such as small-cell lung carcinoma, and nonhypothalamic tumors, which secrete CRH (ectopic CRH), may be responsible. Independent ACTH Cushing syndrome may result from iatrogenic administration of excessive glucocorticoids, primary adrenocortical adenoma, or carcinoma.

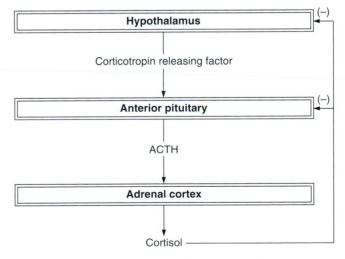

Figure 21–1. Feedback loop for cortisol.

TABLE 21-2. SYSTEMIC MANIFESTATIONS OF ADRENAL DISORDERS

CORTEX HYPERFUNCTION
- **Cushing Syndrome**
  Centripetal obesity
  Oily skin
  Easy bruisability
  Polyuria, polydipsia
  Weakness
  Headache
  Impotence
  Increased cholesterol
  Edema
  Renal calculi
  Vertebral compression fracture
  Backache
  Glucose intolerance
  Proximal myopathy
  Hypertension
  Increased low-density lipoproteins
  Congestive heart failure
  Oligomenorrhea or amenorrhea
  Acne
- **Primary Aldosteronism (Conn Syndrome)**
  Frontal headache
  Muscular weakness
  Nocturia
  Hypertension
  Hypokalemia
  Polyuria, polydypsia
  Glucose intolerance

CORTEX HYPOFUNCTION
- **Primary Adrenal Insufficiency (Addison Disease)**
  Hyperpigmentation
  Weakness
  Fatigue
  Nausea/vomiting
  Weight loss
  Hypotension
  Hypoglycemia
  Dehydration
  Hyponatremia
  Hypokalemia
  Decreased axillary hair (females)
  Decreased libido (females)
- **Secondary and Tertiary Adrenal Insufficiency**
  Weakness
  Fatigue
  Signs of chiasmal compression

MEDULLA DISORDERS
- **Neuroblastomas**
  Hypertension
  Bone pain
  Weight loss
  Fever, vomiting, diarrhea
- **Pheochromocytomas**
  Tremor
  Tachycardia
  Sweat
  Palpitation
  Headache
  Flush or blanch

Cushing syndrome is characterized by progressive obesity, prominent cheek fat pads ("moon face"), deposition of fat in the supraclavicular and dorsocervical fat pads ("buffalo hump"), weakness associated with proximal muscle wasting, and moderate hypertension. Easy bruising, poor wound healing, and visibility of subcutaneous vessels are the result of loss of subcutaneous fat and connective tissue in the skin. Oily skin, acne, and mild facial hirsutism in women are due to excess androgens. Osteoporosis with rib fractures, and lower back pain due to vertebral compression fractures, are common. Hypercalcuria or glucosuria leads to polydipsia and polyuria. Mild depression, emotional lability, irritability, anxiety, panic attacks, and loss of energy and libido are common psychiatric complications. Thromboembolic events occur with increased frequency.

In an older series, a 50% mortality in 5 years from the onset of symptoms was reported without treatment (Plotz et al, 1952). Mortality was due to the complications of chronic hypercorticolism, including cardiovascular, thromboembolic, and hypertensive complications. Inability to control bacterial infections may also lead to death. Death from malignant disease associated with ectopic-ACTH producing tumors usually occurs within 1 year.

ACTH-independent adrenocortical adenoma have an excellent prognosis with treatment, while the prognosis for adrenal carcinomas is poor due to lack of effective treatment for distant micrometastases.

Primary aldosteronism (Conn syndrome) presents with the symptoms of frontal headaches and hypokalemia, muscular weakness, loss of stamina, polyuria, polydypsia, nocturia, flaccid paralysis, and glucose intolerance. Signs include blood pressure that can vary from borderline to severe; however, malignant hypertension is rare.

Cortex Hypofunction

Primary adrenal insufficiency (Addison disease) presents with symptoms of weakness, weight loss, postural syncope, fatigue, nausea, and vomiting. Clinical signs may include hypotension, hypoglycemia, hyponatremia (decreased sodium), and hyperkalemia (decreased potassium). The earliest sign is often the classic hyperpigmentation of skin and mucous membranes, which is thought to be due to increased ACTH and other pro-opiomelanocortin (POMC) peptide levels. Weakness, fatigue, myalgias, and arthalgias occur with complete glucocorticoid deficiency. Decreased intravascular volume, hypotension, dehydration, and gastrointestinal disturbances present with complete mineralocorticoid deficiency. Androgen deficiency in women leads to decreased libido and axillary and pubic hair. Men retain the androgen supply from the testes.

Signs and symptoms are usually delayed until 90% of the adrenal cortex is destroyed. Chronic adrenal insufficiency develops in the majority of cases with gradual destruction of the gland. Untreated Addison disease may be fatal within 2 years of the diagnosis in more than 80% of cases. Major physiological stress can induce an acute adrenal crisis with shock, abdominal pain, fever, lethargy, confusion, or coma. This can rapidly lead to death if untreated.

Secondary adrenal insufficiency has many of the same features as chronic primary adrenal insufficiency. However, because mineralocorticoid secretion is usually normal, hypotension, shock, dehydration, and adrenal crisis are rarely encountered. With ACTH secretion being decreased rather than increased, hyperpigmentation is not seen.

Medulla-associated Disorders

The metastases of neuroblastomas, malignant tumors of the embryonic neural crest cells, occur in infants and children. Neuroblastomas originate from cells that normally differentiate into the paravertebral sympathetic ganglia and adrenal medulla. These tumors often secrete epinephrine and are associated with hypertension. Additional signs and symptoms will be determined by the site of metastasis, and may include fever, vomiting, diarrhea, progressive weight loss, and bone pain.

Pheochromocytomas, rare tumors of the chromaffin cells of the sympathetic nervous system, cause excess catecholamine secretion. This condition most often presents in the fourth to sixth decades. Signs and symptoms include hypertension, sudden, recurrent bouts of sweating, tremors, palpitations, tachycardia, headache, and flushing or blanching.

■ Ocular

Table 21–3 summarizes the ocular manifestations of adrenal disorders.

Cortex Hyperfunction

The ocular complications of Cushing syndrome can include hypertensive retinopathy, exophthalmos, and increased intraocular pressure. It has been suggested that this increased intraocular pressure is an expression of the genetic tendency of ocular steroid responders rather than a complication of Cushing syndrome. Posterior subcapsular cataracts have not been observed as a complication of hypercortisol secretion.

Primary aldosterone results in hypertension that produces a mild hypertensive retinopathy that rarely includes hemorrhages.

Cortex Hypofunction

The common presentation of hyperpigmentation with primary adrenal insufficiency seldom involves the lids or conjunctiva.

TABLE 21–3. OCULAR MANIFESTATIONS OF ADRENAL DISORDERS

CORTEX HYPERFUNCTION
- **Cushing Disease**
  Signs of chiasmal compression
- **Cushing Syndrome**
  Hypertensive retinopathy
  Exophthalmos
  Increased IOP
- **Primary Aldosteronism (Conn Disease)**
  Hypertensive retinopathy

CORTEX HYPOFUNCTION
- **Primary Adrenal Insufficiency (Addison Disease)**
  Pigmentation of lid or conjunctiva
- **Secondary Adrenal Insufficiency**
  Signs of chiasmal and cavernous sinus compression

MEDULLA DISORDERS
- **Pheochromocytomas**
  Hypertensive retinopathy
- **Neuroblastomas**
  Proptosis with ecchymosis
  Horner syndrome (under age 2)
  Papilledema

When secondary and tertiary adrenal insufficiency is due to a tumor, compression of the optic chiasm and cranial nerves in the cavernous sinus is possible. This results in loss of visual field, visual acuity, color vision, or oculomotor function.

Medulla Disorders

Neuroblastomas commonly involve the orbit, leading to the ocular finding of proptosis, which in about half the cases is associated with eyelid ecchymosis. Orbital metastases are frequent (35 to 55% of cases). Neuroblastomas of the upper thoracic or cervical ganglia may present as Horner syndrome prior to age 2. Metastasis to the skull can give rise to papilledema or optic atrophy.

In some cases pheochromocytoma causes sustained hypertension that gives rise to hypertensive retinopathy. This may include nerve fiber layer hemorrhages, cotton-wool spots, narrowed tortuous arterioles, engorged irregular veins, and swollen disc margins. Removal of the tumor leads to resolution of the hypertension and its ocular manifestations.

DIAGNOSIS

■ Systemic

Cortex Hyperfunction

The diagnosis of Cushing syndrome/disease is based on clinical findings in concert with laboratory analysis of adrenal cortex function. Twenty-four hour urinary cortisol testing, dexamethasone suppression testing, metyrapone, CRH testing and sampling, and imaging of the adrenal or pituitary are obtained as indicated by the history and physical examination to differentiate the cause of the disorder. The low-dose dexamethasone suppression test can confirm the diagnosis of Cushing syndrome when negative, with a high-dose dexamethasone suppression test distinguishing the cause, suggesting a pituitary etiology when positive. Metyrapone distinguishes ectopic ACTH production from a pituitary etiology by inhibiting cortisol synthesis. Pituitary dysfunction responds to plasma cortisol level changes, whereas ectopic ACTH production does not.

Hypertension, resulting from primary aldosteronism, is diagnosed by hyperaldosteronemia with suppressed plasma renin activity. Twenty-four hour aldosterone testing may also be done. It is also important to differentiate between adenomas and hyperplasia of the adrenal glands as the cause for therapeutic reasons.

Cortex Hypofunction

Rapid ACTH stimulation test is the initial step in the laboratory assessment of adrenal insufficiency. Plasma levels of ACTH are then used to distinguish primary, secondary, and tertiary forms. Prolonged ACTH stimulation can also aid in this differentiation. CRH stimulation testing can distinguish between secondary or tertiary forms, but there is no therapeutic advantage in making this distinction.

Medulla Disorders

Diagnosis of neuroblastomas and pheochromocytomas may be assisted with 24-hour urinary studies, which will show increased catecholamine and catecholamine metabolites. Particular to neuroblastomas are the main catecholamine catabolite, vanilyllmandelic acid. Appropriate imaging studies can follow positive urinary analysis.

■ Ocular

The ocular findings in all of these disorders are detected by appropriate clinical observation and correlation with the systemic signs and symptoms or diagnosis.

TREATMENT AND MANAGEMENT

Table 21–4 summarizes the treatment and management of adrenal disorders.

■ Systemic

Cortex Hyperfunction

The signs and symptoms of hypercortisolism, with proper treatment, resolve over a 2-to 12-month period. Treatment

TABLE 21–4. SYSTEMIC AND OCULAR TREATMENT AND MANAGEMENT OF ADRENAL DISORDERS

■ **SYSTEMIC**
CORTEX HYPERFUNCTION
- **Cushing Syndrome**
  Pituitary adenomas
    Transsphenoidal resection
    Adjunctive radiation or medical therapy
  Ectopic tumors
    Surgical resection
    Adjunctive radiation or chemotherapy
  Adrenal adenomas or carcinomas
    Surgical resection
    Supplemental medical therapy
  Iatrogenic
    Steroid withdrawal
- **Primary Aldosteronism**
  Antihypertensive medication
  Adenomas: Unilateral adrenalectomy
  Hyperplasia: Spironolactone (200–400 mg/d)

CORTEX HYPOFUNCTION
- **Primary Adrenal Insufficiency**
  Dexamethasone (maintenance 0.5 mg or 5 mg prednisone hs) and flurocortisone (0.1 mg/d)
  Acute: glucocorticoid replacement, IV saline and dextrose
  Chronic: steroid maintenance
- **Secondary and Tertiary Adrenal Insufficiency**
  Dexamethasone and replacement therapy for other pituitary hormones as necessary

MEDULLA DISORDERS
- Neuroblastomas: surgical removal, radiation, chemotherapy
- Pheochromocytomas: surgical removal, supportive medical therapy

■ **OCULAR**
- Treat underlying systemic disorder
- Topical antiglaucoma medication for increased IOP

of Cushing disease consists of surgical removal of the pituitary tumor (transsphenoidal microadenoectomy) with supplemental radiation and mitotane (adrenocorticolytic drug) medical therapy in resistant cases. Ectopic ACTH syndrome may be treated with surgical resection of the tumor, chemotherapy, or radiation therapy. Adrenal enzyme inhibitors are often required to suppress hypercortisolism. Bilateral adrenalectomy is reserved for patients who failed other treatments and require rapid cure of hypercortisolism. When adrenal tumor is the cause, surgical resection of the tumor is indicated with supplemental mitotane and adrenal enzyme inhibitors.

Treatment in primary aldosteronism varies with the underlying cause. Because adenomas are rarely bilateral, total unilateral adrenalectomy is recommended. In cases of bilateral hyperplasia or when surgery is contraindicated, medical therapy of spironolactone often controls the hypokalemia. Additional antihypertensive medical therapy is usually required.

Cortex Hypofunction

Acute adrenal crisis of primary adrenal insufficiency is treated with glucocorticoid replacement and by prompt action using intravenous saline and dextrose to eliminate dehydration, hypovolemia, and electrolyte abnormalities. Chronic primary adrenal insufficiency is treated with steroid maintenance therapy.

Chronic secondary and tertiary adrenal insufficiency is treated in the same manner as chronic primary adrenal insufficiency, but mineralocorticoid therapy is seldom required. Additional replacement therapy for other pituitary hormones may be necessary.

Medulla Disorders

Neuroblastomas are best managed by a pediatric oncologist, usually with surgical removal, along with radiation or chemotherapy. Pheochromocytomas are treated by surgical removal, with supportive medical therapy as needed.

■ Ocular

Generally, there is no specific treatment for the ocular manifestations of adrenal cortex disorders, because they reflect the systemic manifestation of the disease process. Treatment of the underlying systemic disorder may lead to resolution of any hypertensive retinopathy and exophthalmos. Some cases of raised intraocular pressure may require topical antiglaucoma agents until endogenous steroid levels are reduced by treatment of Cushing syndrome.

CONCLUSION

Adrenal disorders of the cortex and medulla may present in a variety of ways. Systemic manifestations are the most salient features of adrenal dysfunction. Although ocular presentations are not common, awareness of their manifestations can assist and lead to the diagnosis and treatment of the adrenal dysfunction.

REFERENCES

Burke CW. Adrenocortical insufficiency. *Clin Endocrinol Metab.* 1985;14:947–976.

Carey RM, Varma SK, Drake DR Jr, et al. Ectopic secretion of corticotropin-releasing factor as a cause of Cushing's disease. *N Engl J Med.* 1984;311:13–20.

Carpenter PC. Diagnostic evaluation of Cushing's syndrome. *Endocrinol Metab Clin North Am.* 1988;17:445–472.

Haas JS, Nootens RH. Glaucoma secondary to benign adrenal adenoma. *Am J Ophthalmol.* 1974;78:497–500.

Krieger DT. Physiopathology of Cushing's disease. *Endocrinol Rev.* 1983;4:22–43.

Mampalam TJ, Tyrell JB, Wilson CB. Transsphenoidal microsurgery for Cushing's disease. A report of 216 cases. *Ann Intern Med.* 1988;109:487–493.

Norton HJ. Photographic analysis of the retinopathy accompanying adrenal pheochromocytoma. *Am J Ophthalmol.* 1964;57:967–973.

Plotz CM, Knowlton AI, Ragan C. The natural history of Cushing's syndrome. *Am J Med.* 1952;13:597–614.

Young WF, Hogan MJ, Klee GG, et al. Primary aldosteronism: Diagnosis and treatment. *Mayo Clin Proc.* 1990;65:96–110.

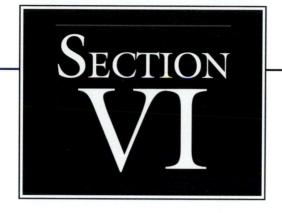

SECTION VI

RHEUMATOLOGIC AND INFLAMMATORY DISORDERS

22
Chapter

Rheumatoid Arthritis

Brian Patrick Mahoney

Rheumatoid arthritis (RA), a collagen vascular disorder, is the most common form of inflammatory joint disease. The degree of functional and physical limitation is so great that RA is the most common cause of physical disability in the United States. Ocular involvement includes anterior and posterior segment inflammation, which is related to poorly regulated immune mechanisms.

EPIDEMIOLOGY

■ Systemic

RA afflicts 5 million people in the United States, with the average age of onset between 35 and 50. There is a familial predisposition, and women are affected three times more frequently than men. Caucasians are also at higher risk than other races for developing RA.

■ Ocular

Dry eye leading to keratitis sicca is the most common ocular manifestation, affecting about 10 to 25% of RA patients (Lamberts, 1983). Episcleritis and scleritis occur less frequently, with Watson and Hayreh (1976) reporting the incidence of episcleritis in 5% of patients with collagen vascular disease. Nonrheumatoid episcleritis affects females and males equally; however, McGavin and associates (1976) found that all RA patients with episcleritis were female. The incidence of RA in the scleritis population may be as high as 33%; however, the incidence of scleritis in the RA population is less than 1%. Nonrheumatoid scleritis affects females five times more frequently than males. McGavin and co-workers (1976) found a similar sex distribution of RA-associated scleritis and episcleritis. Rao and associates (1985) reported that 28% of patients with necrotizing scleritis had RA. Twenty-one percent of patients with necrotizing scleritis associated with a systemic connective tissue disease die within 8 years.

NATURAL HISTORY

■ Systemic

Table 22–1 summarizes the features of RA. A single pathogenic mechanism is not responsible for all of the manifestations. An individual may be predisposed to RA development by altered immunologic mechanisms that are hereditary. Poorly controlled cellular infiltration and inflammation from immune deficiencies contribute to tissue destruction. Rheumatoid factors, antibodies to host tissues of the IgG and IgM classes, develop. Identification of host tissues as being foreign occurs and an inflammatory response is initiated, particularly in articular (joint) tissues. Cellular immunologic deficiencies, particularly in T-cell activity, contribute to inadequate control of inflammation and ultimate joint destruction.

The primary sites of RA inflammation are centered around musculoskeletal tissues. Small joints with synovial linings are affected most commonly (ie, small joints of the hands and feet) early in the disease, and with increasing severity as RA progresses. The rheumatoid joint is characterized by hypertrophic, inflamed synovial tissue with inflammatory fluid accumulation and adjacent soft tissue swelling. This is responsible for the hot, swollen, tender joints that are the hallmark of RA joint inflammation. RA joint stiffness normally resolves with activity after about 60 minutes.

TABLE 22–1. SYSTEMIC MANIFESTATIONS OF RA

ARTICULAR
- Early
    Affects small joints of the hands and feet
    Hot, swollen, tender joints
    Joint stiffness decreases with activitiy
- Progressive
    Bilateral, peripheral joints
    Extends to the trunk (hands, elbows, shoulders)
- Joint deformity
    Swan neck, boutonniere deformity, ulnar deviation

EXTRA-ARTICULAR
- Nodular formation most commonly in cutaneous/subcutaneous tissues but also in deep body tissues
- Infarction and/or hemorrhage of the nails, folds of the feet, and hands
- Anemia
- Pneumonitis/pulmonary nodules
- Pericarditis
- Vasculitis (eg, skin and bowel ulcerations, myocardial infarct)

RA has a bilateral predilection for the peripheral joints extending towards the trunk (hands, elbows, and ultimately the shoulders) after 20 years of progression. Chronic inflammation leads to erosion of the bony surfaces and cartilaginous destruction, which causes joint deformity (swan neck and boutonniere deformities of the fingers, and ulnar deviation of the hands; Figure 22–1). Progressive joint disease results in significant physical impairment of the extremities, which impacts on the quality of life for most patients. RA is a very debilitating disease, although patient mortality is not associated with the arthritis.

Large nodules of the cutaneous and subcutaneous tissues are seen in 25% of RA patients, but visceral organ nodules occur less frequently. An increase in the number and size of the nodules is associated with progression of the disease. The nodules have a necrotic center encapsulated with fibroblastic tissue and surrounded by inflammatory cells. These usually accompany exacerbations of the arthritis, yet the exact mechanism for their development is unknown.

Other extra-articular (outside the joint) features of RA are observed to varying degrees. Two or more extra-articular features occur in 75% of RA patients. Systemic vasculitis is rarely seen with RA, although focal areas of vasculitis are observed clinically. This vasculitis is not initiated by circulating levels of rheumatoid factors (RF) but appears related to deposition of anomalous immune complexes in the vessel wall, which triggers the inflammation. The inflammation may involve large and/or small vessels. Other symptoms manifest as tissues of various organs become involved by the vasculitis, such as neurologic deficits, skin and bowel ulceration, and myocardial infarcts. These manifestations are related to focal and systemic vasculitic inflammation. The presence of systemic vasculitis in a RA patient serves as a poor prognostic indicator.

The clinical features of RA differ from osteoarthritis in various ways. The etiology of joint involvement of RA is primarily inflammatory and improves with activity, in contrast to osteoarthritis, whose etiology is primarily mechanical and worsens with physical activity. Joint inflammation is secondary to mechanical insult in osteoarthritis, yet occurs without previous insult in rheumatoid arthritis. Joint cartilage is the primary site of articular involvement in osteoarthritis, whereas the bony surfaces of the joints are primarily involved in rheumatoid arthritis. Osteoarthritis has a monoarticular predilection with development of focal erosions, cartilage destruction, and osteophyte development in the joints, in contrast to the surface erosions and destruction that occur in RA.

■ Ocular

Table 22–2 summarizes the ocular manifestations of RA. The most commonly encountered ocular manifestation of RA is dry eye. The symptomatology is typically foreign body sensation and epiphora. The dry eye condition follows a chronic course, and its severity increases with disease progression but not directly with activity. Keratitis sicca can progress to filamentary keratitis on occasion for some RA patients, but not as a rule for all RA patients. Secondary keratopathies such as bacterial keratitis (ulceration) and toxic staphylococcal infiltration (from coincident blepharitis) occur in patients with moderately to severely compromised tear quality. Many patients may have dry eye or associated keratopathy when RA is first diagnosed.

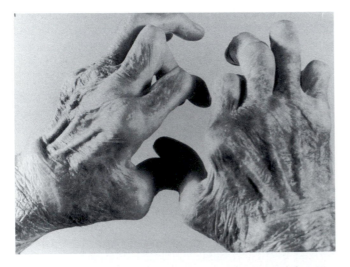

Figure 22–1. Hands of an RA patient. Note the finger deformities bilaterally. The metacarpal and interphalangeal joints are affected most severely. Significant functional impairment results from this level of deformity. (*Reprinted with permission from Mahoney BP. Rheumatologic disease and associated ocular manifestations. J Am Optom Assoc. 1993;64:403–415.*)

TABLE 22–2. OCULAR MANIFESTATIONS OF RA

- Dry eye
    Keratitis sicca
    Filamentary keratitis
    Secondary bacterial keratitis
- Furrowing of the peripheral cornea
- Episcleritis
- Scleritis
    Non-necrotizing
    Necrotizing

Furrowing of the peripheral cornea also occurs as RA progresses (Figure 22–2). This may result from an immune-mediated response in the perilimbal blood vessels, which subsequently affects the adjacent cornea, resulting in stromal thinning. This represents a relatively benign condition unless associated with episcleritis or scleritis. A marginal corneal ulceration may be observed without an infection by a pathogenic organism. An immune mechanism is proposed in these cases.

Episcleritis (Figure 22–3) can be a presenting sign for RA patients, and is usually observed in one eye only. Bilateral involvement may be observed, but simultaneous presentation is rare. Recurrent episodes of episcleritis usually manifest prior to active periods of the arthritis and for that reason correlate better with disease activity than keratitis sicca. Episcleritis does not progress to scleritis in RA

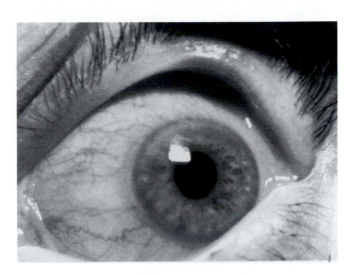

Figure 22–3. Episcleritis in an RA patient. This patient had recurrent episodes of episcleritis that responded well to topical steroid use. Note the deep injection that did not blanch with topical vasoconstrictors. No corneal involvement manifested during any of the active episodes.

patients and rarely progresses to involve any adjacent tissue. Episcleritis will recur despite systemic treatment. Scleritis associated with RA takes many forms, including the diffuse or nodular forms seen most frequently, and necrotizing scleritis (with or without inflammation) observed less frequently. The necrotizing forms have the most serious systemic implications, particularly scleromalacia perforans (without inflammation). Scleral thinning and scleral ectasias—loss of scleral and episcleral tissue layers—occur with progression of the disease, possibly leading to globe perforation. Necrotizing scleritis usually occurs in the advanced stages of RA, with implications for increased patient mortality, therefore requiring aggressive medical treatment. Corneal involvement from inflammatory extension occurs in 50 to 70% of scleritis patients; therefore, secondary corneal furrowing or keratolysis suggests an associated scleritis.

Diagnosis

■ Systemic

Many patients have symptoms that are not exclusive to RA, making the diagnosis difficult in some cases. Table 22–3 lists the diagnostic criteria for RA. Laboratory tests and radiographic studies are necessary for initial diagnosis and are helpful in monitoring progression.

Serologic testing for the presence of RF, including IgG and IgM autoantibodies and other immunoglobulins, should be ordered. RF are present in 75% of RA patients as opposed to less than 5% of the general population.

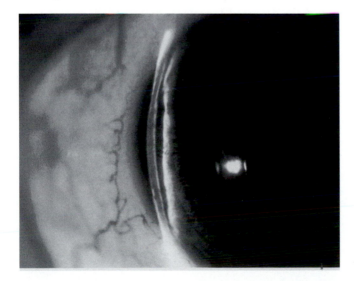

Figure 22–2. Peripheral corneal thinning in an RA patient. Note the stromal loss in a circumferential pattern near the limbus of the cornea. This was present bilaterally and was not accompanied by corneal perforation. No dry eye was present and no ocular treatment was necessary. (*Reprinted with permission from Mahoney BP. Rheumatologic disease and associated ocular manifestations. J Am Optom Assoc. 1993;64:403–415.*)

TABLE 22–3. CRITERIA FOR DIAGNOSIS OF RA

Four Criteria Must Be Met
1. AM joint stiffness lasting 1 hour
2. Joint swelling of three or more joints
3. Proximal interphalangeal, metacarpophalangeal, or wrist joint inflammation
4. Symmetric joint involvement
5. Positive RF
6. Joint erosion of involved joints of hand or wrist

Enzyme-linked immunosorbent assay (ELISA) testing is more accurate for the detection of immunoglobulin antibodies and may be ordered if the RF results are equivocal. A mild normochromic normocytic anemia is present in about 50% of patients, with a hemoglobin level under 10 gm/100 mL in rare cases. Fine-needle aspiration of synovial fluid reveals elevated levels of complement proteins and white blood cells (2000 to 50,000 cells with 70 to 85% polymorphonuclear neutrophil leukocytes). A drop in serum complement levels (particularly C_3) and elevated serum white blood cell count (above 15,000/mm³) may be seen with advanced extra-articular disease activity but not with joint disease only. Joint aspirations may be needed when clinical suspicion is high and other test results are equivocal.

Joint x-ray and radionuclide evaluation of suspected inflamed joints are also indicated. Radiographic evidence of joint damage may precede any patient symptoms. X-rays of affected joints (hands or feet) reveal surface erosion and degeneration resulting from inflammation. Radionuclide scanning is more sensitive in detecting joint involvement and inflammation than conventional x-ray evaluation.

■ Ocular

Detection of RA associated ocular involvement can be done following a thorough anterior and posterior segment evaluation. The use of B-scan ultrasonography should be considered if posterior scleritis is suspected.

TREATMENT AND MANAGEMENT

■ Systemic

There is no curative treatment for RA known at this time. The goal of treatment is to minimize inflammation and its sequelae while maximizing patient functioning. Nonpharmacologic modalities such as exercise and physical therapy are encouraged. Pharmaceutical agents used to inhibit the inflammatory responses include salicylates, nonsteroidal antiinflammatory drugs (NSAIDs), steroids, antimalarial agents (quinolines), gold salts, and cytotoxic and immunosuppressive agents. The appropriate treatment regi-

men is determined by the severity of patient symptoms and systemic involvement. Pharmacologic agents were traditionally employed using a step approach from weakest to strongest, although some rheumatologists ascribe to a newer philosophy of aggressive treatment utilizing stronger medications at an earlier stage. Most practitioners, however, determine the appropriate therapeutic regimen on an individual basis (Table 22–4).

Salicylates and NSAIDs are of little value in long-term treatment, because they inadequately inhibit the level of inflammation throughout the disease progression. Steroids and plaquenil (or chloroquine less frequently) are the primary treatment in RA. These drugs are effective in inhibiting inflammation while maintaining a high level of patient functioning. Penicillamine is an effective drug alternative, but it may be 2 to 3 months until the patient appreciates any subjective improvement, and up to 6 months until a reduction in the amount of synovitis is observed; therefore it is not an optimal treatment choice for acute exacerbations. Gold salt treatment has a limited role in RA therapy because of the high frequency of relapses with only partial remission and frequent toxic reactions. Methotrexate, a folic acid agonist, is used in patients who do not respond well or fail to sustain a favorable response to NSAIDs or gold treatment. Other immunosuppressive agents are used in RA therapy (eg, azathioprine, 5-fluoroucil, hydroxyurea, dapsone) when significant clinical improvement is not achieved with other, less toxic medications. They are usually reserved for refractory cases of RA and cases involving necrotizing scleritis. Detrimental side effects may preclude long-term use of these drugs. However, many can be used safely for sustained periods of time with the proper management by a rheumatologist. Changes in the combinations of these medications will be necessary for long-term management of RA patients. RA is a chronic, progressive disease with extra-articular involvement that will occur despite aggressive systemic management.

■ Ocular

Table 22–5 gives an overview of treatment of the ocular sequelae of RA. The use of ocular lubrication remains the

TABLE 22–4. SYSTEMIC TREATMENT OF RA

1. Physical therapy
2. Aspirin
3. NSAIDs
4. Steroids
5. Antimalarial medications (quinolines)
6. Gold salts
7. Cytotoxic agents
8. Immunosuppressive agents
9. Orthopedic and surgical intervention

TABLE 22–5. TREATMENT OF OCULAR SEQUELAE OF RA

DRY EYE
- Ocular lubricants (unpreserved)
- Solutions as needed and ointments at bedtime
- Punctal occlusion (temporary or permanent)

FILAMENTARY KERATITIS
- Filament removal
- Heavy lubrication
- Topical steroids (Pred Forte qid)
- Bandage contact lens or pressure patch (may worsen keratitis)

CORNEAL ULCERATION
- Appropriate antibiotic as determined by corneal scraping

EPISCLERITIS
- Topical steroids
- NSAIDs (indomethacin)

SCLERITIS
- Non-necrotizing
  NSAIDs (indomethacin)
  Subtenons steroid injection
  Systemic steroids
- Necrotizing
  Immunosuppressive or cytotoxic agents
  Steroids contraindicated

primary treatment for patients with compromised corneal integrity from poor tear quality. Moderate to severe keratitis sicca associated with epithelial compromise is best managed with unpreserved ocular lubricating agents, particularly with high-viscosity tear supplements (eg, carboxymethylcellulose). Lubricant treatment does not eliminate all epithelial staining. Improved symptomatology and decreased staining is considered a therapeutic success. Punctal plugs, either temporary or permanent, and punctal ablative procedures (cauterization) may offer symptomatic relief, but fall short of a curative treatment.

The treatment of episcleritis associated with RA is dependent on its severity and chronicity. Resolution may occur without intervention if very mild inflammation is present. More severe or chronic forms require topical vasoconstrictors or steroids (fluoromethalone, prednisone phosphate, or prednisone acetate). Short-term use is optimal to obtain symptomatic relief, but long-term use may be needed if structural damage is observed (eg, proximal corneal inflammation). Oral NSAIDs may be an effective adjunctive therapy in recurrent cases of episcleritis.

Treatment of scleritis depends on both the type and severity present. It requires more aggressive treatment than episcleritis because of the propensity for structural damage. Topical steroids are used but are not effective by themselves. NSAIDs have been an effective therapeutic modality for some scleritis patients. Subtenons injections of steroids (Kenalog) may be needed to sufficiently control the inflammation and limit any structural damage. Steroid use is contraindicated when scleral thinning is present because of the potential for scleral perforation. Aggressive medical therapy by the rheumatologist is required when necrotizing scleritis is detected, particularly without inflammation. These patients have a better prognosis when systemic immunosuppressive therapy is instituted.

Co-management with a rheumatologist for RA patients with ocular inflammation is essential. Short-term modifica-

tions of systemic medications (usually increased strength or dosage) are particularly important when ocular inflammation persists. Ocular side effects of systemic medications may require discontinuation or modification of the systemic medications to prevent irreversible vision loss (Table 22–6).

Close monitoring of the ocular side effects of systemic therapy is necessary. Most medications used to treat RA have ocular side effects that may be of significance to the eyecare practitioner. NSAIDs are associated with whorl keratopathy and photosensitivity, but these effects do not require discontinuation of the drug; however, optic neuropathy, nystagmus, and retinal hemorrhages do necessitate drug removal. Quinoline medications induce pigmentary retinopathy after reaching cumulative doses of 5000 g. These levels are normally achieved after a few years; however, electroretinogram (ERG) abnormalities can be

TABLE 22–6. OCULAR TOXICITY OF COMMONLY USED MEDICATIONS IN THE MANAGEMENT OF RA

Medication	Side Effect
NSAIDs	Whorl keratopathy (eg, Indomethacin)
	Optic neuropathy
	Photosensitivity
	Nystagmus
	Retinal or subconjunctival hemorrhages
Steroids	Posterior subcapsular cataracts
	Glaucoma
Gold salts	Corneal deposits
	Lens deposits
Chloroquine/Plaquenil	Whorl keratopathy
	Pigmentary retinopathy
	Toxic maculopathy
	Toxic neuropathy
Methotrexate	Punctate keratitis

detected earlier than the development of pigmentary retinopathy. High-quality serial color photographs may be the most sensitive method for detecting toxic maculopathy. Serial focal ERGs and color vision testing are helpful but not practical in clinical practice. Color vision testing with the D15 and Ishihara plates are of little value because both miss subtle color deficiencies. A 100 Hue test appears to be the best for detecting color abnormalities associated with early toxic maculopathy. Vision loss resulting from toxic accumulation of the drugs in the retinal pigment epithelium (RPE) layer of the retina may be permanent. This toxic effect lessens with time after the drug is discontinued; however, complete reversal of these effects does not occur. If macular toxicity is not detected at an early stage, the patient may experience additional vision loss despite cessation of the drug.

It may be difficult to discern toxic macular pigmentary disruption in patients on quinoline therapy from early age-related macular degeneration (ARMD). The appearance of pigmentary disruption associated with the use of chloroquine (or plaquenil) is a bull's-eye/circular pattern, whereas ARMD pigment disruption appears more patchy or diffuse. Although not routinely performed, a fluorescein angiogram may distinguish between ARMD and chloroquine pigment disruption.

The relationship between the use of steroids and associated posterior subcapsular cataract (PSC) or secondary glaucoma is well established. PSC and glaucoma development are attributable to both topical and oral steroid use. Glaucoma therapy should be directed towards aqueous inhibition (β-blockers or carbonic anhydrase inhibitors). The appropriate selection of medication should be made on an individual basis. Cataract extraction should be considered if patient function is affected.

The use of gold salts is associated with few ocular sequelae other than the deposition of gold in tissues (chrysiasis), which requires discontinuation of the drug only if corneal ulceration is present. Methotrexate is found in the tears and acts as a direct irritant to the corneal epithelium, which requires aggressive lubricant therapy, but not discontinuation of the drug. Ocular health evaluations should be performed on a regular basis, varying from every 3 to 12 months, depending on the clinical severity.

CONCLUSION

Rheumatoid arthritis is a progressive polyarticular inflammatory arthropathy that most frequently affects women. The predilection for the extremities with progression towards the trunk is frequently responsible for significant physical and functional impairment in the advanced stages of RA. The majority of the ocular manifestations and their treatment require little intervention other than chronic pal-

liative treatment by the eyecare practitioner. Necrotizing scleritis, unlike most ocular manifestations, is consistent with serious underlying disease and patient mortality, therefore requiring aggressive systemic treatment. The vision-threatening side effects of medications used to treat RA underscore the importance of the role of the eyecare provider. Co-management with a rheumatologist or internist is very important for optimal patient care.

REFERENCES

Baker D, Rabinowitz JL. Current concepts in the treatment of rheumatoid arthritis. *J Clin Pharmacol.* 1986;26:2.

Benson WE. Posterior scleritis. *Surv Ophthalmol.* 1988;32:297.

Bluestein H. Cellular immunity. In: Uttsinger PD, Zvaifler NJ, Ehrlich GE, eds. *Rheumatoid Arthritis.* Philadelphia: Lippincott; 1985:71.

Boers M, Ramsden M. Long-acting drug combinations in rheumatoid arthritis: A formal overview. *J Rheumatol.* 1991;18:316.

Clements PJ, Paulus HE. Nonsteroidal anti-inflammatory drugs (NSAIDs). In: Kelley WN, Harris ED, Ruddy S, Sledge CB, eds. *Textbook of Rheumatology.* Philadelphia: Saunders; 1993:700.

Conn DL, McDuffie FC, Holley KE, Schroeter AL: Immunologic mechanisms in systemic vasculitis. *Mayo Clinic Proc.* 1976;51:511.

Cruess AF, Schachat AP, Nicholl JA, et al. Chloroquine retinopathy. Is fluorescein angiography necessary? *Ophthalmology.* 1985;92:1127.

Dieppe PA, Doherty M, MacFarlane D, Maddison P. Rheumatoid arthritis. In: Dieppe PA, ed. *Rheumatologic Medicine.* Edinburgh: Churchill Livingstone; 1985:41.

Fauci AS, Young KR. Immunoregulatory agents. In: Kelley WN, Harris ED, Ruddy S, Sledge CB, eds. *Textbook of Rheumatology.* Philadelphia: Saunders; 1993:797.

Foster CS. Immunosuppressive therapy for external ocular inflammatory disease. *Ophthalmol.* 1982;87:140.

Friedlaender M. Arthritic and connective tissue disorders. In: Friedlaender M, ed. *Allergy and Immunology of the Eye.* New York: Raven; 1993:223.

Grant S, Greenseid DZ, Leopold IH. Toxic retinopathies. In: Tasman W, Jaeger EA, eds. *Duane's Clinical Ophthalmology.* Philadelphia: Lippincott; 1989;3:chapter 33.

Hardin JG, Longenecker GL. *Handbook of Drug Therapy in Rheumatic Disease.* Boston: Little, Brown; 1992.

Lamberts DW. Dry eye and tear deficiency. *Int Ophthalmol Clinics.* 1983;23:123–130.

McGavin DD, Williamson J, Forrester JV, et al. Episcleritis and Scleritis. A study of their clinical manifestations and association with rheumatoid arthritis. *Br J Ophthalmol.* 1976;60:192.

Melvin JL. *Rheumatic Disease in the Adult and Child: Occupational Therapy and Rehabilitation.* Philadelphia: Davis; 1989.

Panush RS. *Principles of Rheumatic Disease.* New York: Wiley; 1982:15–23.

Pincus SH. Immunoregulation and experimental therapies. In: McCarthy DJ, Koopman WJ, eds. *Arthritis and Allied Conditions.* Philadelphia: Lea & Febiger; 1993:683.

Rao NA, Marak GE, Hidayat AA. Necrotizing scleritis. *Ophthalmol.* 1985;92:1542.

Rynes RL. Antimalarial Drugs. In: Kelley WN, Harris ED, Ruddy S, Sledge CB, eds. *Textbook of Rheumatology*. Philadelphia: Saunders; 1993:731.

Sanz I, Alboukrek D. Treatment of rheumatoid arthritis: Traditional and new approaches. In: Fischbach M, ed. *Rheumatoid Arthritis*. New York: Churchill Livingstone; 1991:99.

Tierney DW. Ocular chrysiasis. *J Am Optom Assoc.* 1988;59:960.

Tilkian SM, Conover MB, Tilkian AG. *Clinical Implications of Laboratory Tests*. St. Louis: Mosby; 1987.

Wakefield D, McCluskey P. Cyclosporin therapy for severe scleritis. *Br J Ophthalmol.* 1989;73:743.

Watson PG. Diseases of the sclera and episclera. In: Tasman W, Jaeger E, eds. *Duane's Clinical Ophthalmology*. Hagerstown, MD: Harper & Row; 1987;4:chapter 23.

Watson PG, Hayreh SS. Scleritis and episcleritis. *Br J Ophthalmol.* 1976;60:163.

23
Chapter

Juvenile Rheumatoid Arthritis

Brian Patrick Mahoney

Juvenile rheumatoid arthritis (JRA) is a group of arthritides that are responsible for significant functional loss in children. JRA is the most common chronic disease with a genetic predisposition in children. These disorders can be classified according to their clinical characteristics into oligoarthritic JRA, polyarthritic JRA, and systemic JRA (or Still disease). The ocular sequelae vary for each category of JRA, as do the systemic features. The major ocular manifestations of JRA—iridocyclitis, cataracts, and band keratopathy—cause more severe vision loss than other types of rheumatic diseases. The systemic and ocular prognosis for most JRA patients is good with early detection and treatment.

EPIDEMIOLOGY

■ Systemic

JRA remains the most frequently encountered collagen vascular disease in children. Towner and associates (1983) reported the incidence of JRA to be 13.9 per 100,000 children annually. Sullivan and co-workers (1975) also reported that 0.01% of children per year were at risk for developing JRA. Affecting females more frequently than males in a 2 to 1 ratio, JRA incidence peaks between ages 2 and 4, and again between ages 10 and 12. Polyarthritic JRA represents 50% of cases, followed by oligoarthritic JRA in 30% and systemic JRA in 20% of cases.

■ Ocular

Chronic anterior uveitis (iridocyclitis) is the major ocular complication of JRA. It is associated with severe vision loss, and is seen in approximately 20% of patients with oligoarthritic JRA, 5% of patients with polyarthritic JRA, and rarely with systemic JRA. The iridocyclitis occurs bilaterally in 66% of patients, with one eye usually preceding the other. The iridocyclitis is more likely to be seen in females with early-onset JRA and minimal joint disease. Recurrent nongranulomatous iridocyclitis occurs in over 20% of patients with oligoarthritic JRA.

NATURAL HISTORY

■ Systemic

The pathogenesis of JRA is unknown. Immune-mediated activity directed towards Type II collagen has been identified among other immunologic abnormalities. Rheumatoid factor (RF) mediated responses are rarely found. Unlike adult RA, joint inflammation primarily involves the weight-bearing joints of the lower extremities (knees and ankles) as well as the joints of the elbows and hands. There is little associated pain or tenderness observed with these patients. The clinical manifestations observed in the first 6 months of the disease determine the appropriate classification. The course of JRA is variable depending on the specific type. The average duration of the clinical course of JRA is $6\frac{1}{2}$ years for all categories. JRA may be classified as described below (Table 23–1 lists the characteristics of each category).

- Polyarthritic JRA: Five or more joints are inflamed at diagnosis.
- Oligoarthritic JRA: Four or fewer joints are inflamed at diagnosis.
- Systemic JRA: A variable number of joints are inflamed, but prominent systemic manifestations are present.

TABLE 23–1. SYSTEMIC MANIFESTATIONS OF JRA

	■ POLYARTHRITIS	■ OLIGOARTHRITIS	■ SYSTEMIC (STILL DISEASE)
ARTICULAR FEATURES OF JRA			
● Frequency	50%	30%	20%
● Characteristics of arthritis	5 or more joints	4 or fewer joints	Variable number of joints
		Preceded months by low-grade fever	Preceded weeks or months by high fever
	Symmetric	Asymmetric	Symmetric or asymmetric
● Joints involved	Knees	Knees	Knees/hips
● Progressive involvement	Lumbar and cervical vertebrae	Minimal	Lymph and liver enlargement with pericarditis
● Testing	(+)ANA	(+) ANA	(–) ANA
	(+)RF (late onset > 10)	(+) RF (if onset < 10; rare if > 10)	

EXTRA-ARTICULAR FEATURES OF JRA

- Fever
- Pericarditis
- Pulmonary fibrosis
- Renal glomerulitis
- Myositis
- Macular rash
- Lymphadenopathy
- Hepatosplenomegaly
- Growth retardation
- Ocular inflammation

Extra-articular features may occur in all types of JRA, but with greater frequency and severity in systemic or Still disease.

Polyarthritic JRA is seen initially following a low-grade fever with minimal systemic manifestations, often in an older girl. The child may be free from symptoms despite significant joint enlargement. Some discomfort may be experienced with joint movement. Cycles of fever and arthritis progress, involving the vertebral and cervical joints, which results in limited range of motion of the back and neck. If the duration of the disease is short (under 7 years), then the amount of functional loss from joint destruction is not severe. The cycles of activity cease, but the arthritis remains with the child into adulthood, but with minimal progression after the second decade. Mortality is not associated with polyarticular JRA.

Oligoarthritic JRA often presents in a young boy with monoarthritis following a low-grade fever. The arthritis typically presents months after the fever resolves. Asymmetric joint involvement affecting the knees occurs in 75% of cases, unlike the symmetric involvement associated with polyarthritic JRA. Cycles of articular inflammation rarely persist beyond the early teens, with persistent arthritis evident in adulthood without significant progression. Patient mortality is rarely associated with this form of JRA.

Although systemic JRA (Still disease) represents the smallest percentage of cases, it has the most striking extra-articular (nonjoint) features. The arthritis development is preceded by high fever (102° F) by weeks or months. The fever frequently accompanies other extra-articular features (eg, macular rash of the skin, hepatosplenomegaly, lymphadenopathy, pericarditis), which require treatment. Over 90% of these patients manifest arthritis by the end of the first year. Severe polyarticular disease commonly results,

and progressive inflammation of the carpal joints continues for up to 20 years, despite remission of the other articular features. Arthritis persists as the child ages, but the cycles of arthritis activity rarely recur beyond the early to midteen years. Patients with systemic JRA are at highest risk for death, resulting from the systemic disease. Death occurs in 2 to 4% of all JRA patients, with systemic JRA identified in almost all cases. Death during childhood is associated with pericarditis (seen in 36% of patients), aortic valve regurgitation, and cardiac tamponade. Death in adulthood is frequently associated with cardiac involvement from amyloidosis, which can develop 1 to 20 years after the onset of arthritis. Despite the high frequency of systemic involvement, ocular involvement is rarely seen with these patients.

The articular responses of JRA are similar to adult RA; however, joint destruction is delayed or not appreciated despite disease progression. Rheumatoid nodules are rarely seen and are not a predominant feature of JRA. Small-vessel vasculitis of the skin is responsible for the pathognomonic rash commonly seen in polyarthritic and systemic JRA but rarely seen with oligoarthritic JRA. The discrete cutaneous lesions are 2 to 5 mm in size and are found most frequently on the back and proximal extremities during or following the fever. These lesions clear as the fever resolves.

■ Ocular

Table 23–2 lists the ocular manifestations of JRA. The classic triad of iridocyclitis, cataract, and band keratopathy is associated most frequently with oligoarthritic JRA; less frequently with polyarthritic JRA; and rarely with systemic

TABLE 23–2. OCULAR MANIFESTATIONS OF JRA

UVEITIS
- Overall incidence of 20%; most frequent with oligoarthritis; least frequent with Still disease

CATARACT
- Seen in 50% of chronic iridocyclitis patients

BAND KERATOPATHY
- Seen in 50% of chronic iridocyclitis patients

GLAUCOMA
- Common with chronic iridocyclitis

JRA. Overall incidence of iridocyclitis is approximately 20% for JRA patients. Cataract, glaucoma, and band keratopathy are seen in 50% of patients who develop persistent iridocyclitis. Severe vision loss results predominantly from cataract formation and less frequently from band keratopathy. Ocular involvement is insidious, with the mean age of onset of iridocyclitis at $5^1/_2$ years. The iridocyclitis commonly follows, but may precede the onset of arthritis. Patients with active iridocyclitis are asymptomatic in 50% of cases and require ocular evaluation for detection. Evidence of chronic iridocyclitis or associated findings (posterior synechiae or glaucoma) may be the presenting sign leading to the diagnosis of JRA. Posterior segment involvement from chronic iridocyclitis is not commonly seen despite the significant anterior segment sequelae.

Band keratopathy observed in children under 16 is pathognomonic for JRA. The band keratopathy results from aggressive ocular inflammation, not abnormal calcium metabolism, and does not reflect the severity of articular disease. Vision loss results when the visual axis becomes involved. Dry eye and keratitis sicca are not manifestations of JRA, in contrast to their high prevalence in adult RA. Poor epithelial wetting may reflect epithelial disruption associated with band keratopathy and not compromised tear quality.

DIAGNOSIS

■ Systemic

The diagnosis of JRA is based on clinical presentation and history. A fever or rash may have subsided at the time of the evaluation, but joint inflammation persists and will be evident, leading to the diagnosis of JRA. Hematologic and radiographic studies are beneficial in the diagnosis and classification of JRA. Routine hematologic testing for JRA includes antinuclear antibody (ANA), RF, erythrocyte sedimentation rate (SED rate), serum complement, and com-

plete blood count (CBC) tests. Fewer than 20% of JRA patients test positive for RF, in contrast to 75% of adult-onset RA patients. A positive ANA occurs in 40% of polyarticular JRA, 75% of oligoarticular JRA, and 10% of systemic JRA patients. A positive ANA, as well as some HLA haplotypes, are implicated as risk factors for the development of chronic iridocyclitis in JRA patients. Elevation of the SED rate, serum complement, and IgG occur in conjunction with acute systemic activity. Leukocytosis is found in 95% of patients with active systemic JRA, with white blood counts in the range of 25,000 per mm^3.

Radiographic evaluations of the inflamed joint reveal soft tissue swelling and peri-articular osteoporosis with possible new bone formation. Loss of the cartilaginous space with erosions occur after a long duration of JRA activity. Synovial fluid aspiration shows inflammatory debris, but an elevated white blood cell count may not be present. Radiographic attention should be directed toward any suspected joints, with consideration of synovial fluid aspiration if radiographic results are insufficient for diagnosis.

■ Ocular

The ocular manifestations of JRA (which include the triad of iridocyclitis, cataract, and band keratopathy) are diagnosed most accurately by biomicroscopic evaluation. Patients with a positive ANA, HLA-DR5, and DR8 are at highest risk for development of chronic iridocyclitis. Because the iridocyclitis may be present without symptoms, these high-risk patients should be thoroughly evaluated for its presence. JRA-associated iridocyclitis remains active despite apparent control of the articular disease, and persists long after systemic therapy is initiated.

The biomicroscopic appearance of band keratopathy is consistent with other etiologies. Dense lenticular opacities at the level of the anterior cortex of the lens are characteristic of JRA. A complicated cataract may develop when posterior subcapsular cataracts result from steroid therapy for the iridocyclitis. Glaucoma may result from impaired outflow mechanisms resulting from inflammatory debris obstructing the trabecular meshwork or posterior synechia causing an iris bombé.

TREATMENT AND MANAGEMENT

Table 23–3 describes the treatment of JRA.

■ Systemic

The goal of treatment with JRA is to control the pathologic changes primarily in articular tissues. All systemic therapy must be individualized depending on the type of JRA and the severity of joint involvement. Because JRA typically

TABLE 23–3. SYSTEMIC AND OCULAR TREATMENT OF JRA

- **SYSTEMIC**
  1. Aspirin plus exercise and physical therapy
  2. NSAIDs
  3. Gold salts/plaquenil/penicillamine
  4. Steroids
  5. Immunosuppressive agents
  6. Orthopedic surgery

  Extra-articular
  - Fever: monitor/acetominophen
  - Macular rash, lymphadenopathy, pulmonary fibrosis, hepatosplenomegaly: monitor
  - Growth retardation: growth hormone
  - Myositis: steroids
  - Pericarditis, renal glomerulitis: hospitalization

  Note: Extra-articular manifestations may influence overall treatment of the disease (eg, systemic medication changes, hospitalization)

- **OCULAR**

  UVEITIS
  - Topical cycloplegics (5% homatropine)
  - Topical steroids (Pred Forte)

  CATARACT
  - Surgery

  BAND KERATOPATHY
  - Chelating agents (EDTA)

runs a self-limiting course, medical therapy is needed only when the persistent arthritis warrants treatment.

Aspirin (ASA) plays a significant role in the treatment of articular inflammation in conjunction with exercise. Additional treatment to manage progressive joint involvement includes nonsteroidal antiinflammatory drugs (NSAIDs), particularly Tolmetin. Gold salts are used frequently for treating JRA patients when their arthritis has not responded to the use of ASA or NSAIDs after about 6 months. Antimalarial medications are not used as frequently in JRA as in adult RA, although the efficacy appears good. When they are used, they are usually limited to a 2-year course because of the potential for toxicity. The use of cytotoxic and immunosuppressive drugs is limited to those cases where life-threatening situations arise. Orthopedic surgical intervention is warranted in cases where joint destruction results in physical impairment. Proper diagnosis and treatment results in recovery in about 85% of JRA patients.

Ocular

Medical intervention may adequately control the articular inflammation but have minimal effect on ocular inflammation. Topical steroids and short-acting cycloplegics remain the primary treatment of JRA-associated iridocyclitis.

Long-term therapy (months to years) with cycloplegics is necessary for most patients to sufficiently control the persistent inflammation characteristic of JRA. Eyes with chronic iridocyclitis have a higher propensity for developing band keratopathy and cataracts, and therefore warrant aggressive therapy. Strong parasympatholytic agents for iridocyclitis should be used judiciously because of their high propensity for systemic toxicity. Topical steroids are used for acute and long-term management of ocular inflammation. Periocular injections of steroids are rarely needed to control the iridocyclitis—only when inadequate response to topical treatment is evident. Oral steroids (5 mg once daily) may be a necessary therapy when recalcitrant forms of iridocyclitis are encountered.

Cataract formation causing significant vision loss requires extraction to maximize visual function. Key and Kimura (1975) found that 30% of patients had vision of 20/200 or less secondary to cataracts. Postsurgically, 13% obtained a 20/30 acuity (Kanski, 1990).

Lubricant therapy with unpreserved ophthalmic solutions and ointments is needed in cases where epithelial disruption is present along with symptoms of foreign body sensation. Chelating agents (EDTA) have been used to treat band keratopathy successfully but do not prevent reformation. Patients with band keratopathy and cataracts require comanagement with a corneal/anterior segment specialist if surgical intervention is necessary.

Glaucoma in JRA patients is not easily managed, and may require topical or systemic aqueous inhibitors. The side effects of systemic carbonic anhydrase inhibitors preclude their use in children. Topical carbonic anhydrase inhibitors, if available, may be very effective for this type of glaucoma. Surgical trabeculectomy may be necessary to reduce the IOP if topical management alone is ineffective.

Patients with JRA should have regular examinations (every 3 to 6 months) to detect and monitor uveitis and other vision-threatening changes. Follow-up for active ocular involvement should be determined by its severity and specific therapeutic regimen. Supportive services for the patient and family should be considered in those patients with physical and visual impairment.

CONCLUSION

The hallmark clinical feature of JRA is the development of articular inflammation following a fever. Because JRA runs a less aggressive course than adult RA, the joint involvement is less debilitating. The potential for vision loss in JRA patients is much higher than for adult RA despite a less severe clinical course. The overall prognosis for JRA patients is good with early detection and adequate medical management. Unfortunately, patients with systemic JRA do not have as good a prognosis as other JRA patients due to the potential for developing life-threatening complications. Early diagnosis and treatment is imperative in order to preserve maximal physical and visual functioning.

REFERENCES

Calabro JJ, Holgerson WB, Sonpal GM, Khoury MI. Juvenile rheumatoid arthritis: A general review and report of 100 patients observed for 15 years. *Semin Arthritis Rheumatol*. 1976;5:257.

Cassidy JT. Juvenile rheumatoid arthritis. In: Kelley WD, Harris ED, Ruddy S, Sledge CB, eds. *Textbook of Rheumatology*. Philadelphia: Saunders; 1993;1189.

Friedlaender MH. Arthritic and connective tissue disorders. In: Friedlaender MH, ed. *Allergy and Immunology of the Eye.* New York: Raven; 1993.

Giles CL. Uveitis in childhood, 1. Anterior. *Ann Ophthalmol*. 1989;21:13.

Hardin JG, Longenecker GL. Drug therapy of specific rheumatic diseases. In: Hardin JG, Longenecker GL, eds. *Handbook of Drug Therapy in Rheumatic Disease*. Boston: Little, Brown; 1992:175.

Kanski JJ. Juvenile rheumatoid arthritis and uveitis. *Surv Ophthalmol*. 1990;34:253.

Key SN, Kimura SJ. Iridocyclitis associated with juvenile rheumatoid arthritis. *Am J Ophthalmol*. 1975;80:425.

Pachman LM, Poznanski AK. Juvenile rheumatoid arthritis. In: McCarty DJ, Koopman WJ, eds. *Arthritis and Allied Conditions*. Philadelphia: Lea & Febiger; 1992:1021.

Petty RE. Treatment of juvenile rheumatoid arthritis. In: McCarty DJ, Koopman WJ, eds. *Arthritis and Allied Conditions*. Philadelphia: Lea & Febiger; 1992:1039.

Rosenberg AM, Romanchuk KG. Antinuclear antibodies in arthritic and nonarthritic children with uveitis. *J Rheumatol*. 1990;17:60.

Sullivan DB, Cassidy JT, Petty RE. Pathogenic implications of age of onset of juvenile rheumatoid arthritis. *Arthritis Rheum*. 1975;18:251.

Towner SR, Michet C, O'Fallon WM, Nelson AM. The epidemiology of juvenile rheumatoid arthritis in Rochester, Minnesota. *Arthritis Rheum*. 1983;26:1208.

Wirostoko E, Johnson L, Wirostoko W. Juvenile rheumatoid arthritis inflammatory eye disease. Parasitization of ocular leukocytes by mollicute-like organisms. *J Rheumatol*. 1989;16:1446.

Ankylosing Spondylitis

Brian Patrick Mahoney

Ankylosing spondylitis (AS), also called Marie–Strümpell disease, is an inflammatory arthropathy most frequently seen in young men. Inflammation of the sacroiliac joints is the hallmark of AS, although the spinal column may also become involved. It is one of the first seronegative spondylarthropathies (a type of arthritic disease that tests negative for rheumatoid factor) to be associated with ocular inflammatory disease. The eyecare practitioner encounters few ocular sequelae in these patients other than an acute nongranulomatous iridocyclitis. This frequently manifests prior to any other symptoms, often leading to the diagnosis of AS.

EPIDEMIOLOGY

■ Systemic

AS is seen in approximately 1 to 2% of the Caucasian American population, with initial onset between the ages of 20 and 40. Men were once thought to be affected two to four times more frequently than women, but these numbers are misleading considering that AS is probably underdiagnosed in women, given the milder course of the disease in females. HLA-B27 is found in 90% of AS patients; however, less than 10% of HLA-B27 patients develop any spondyloarthropathy. Relatives of AS patients have a 20% greater chance of developing AS if they are HLA-B27 positive than do relatives of non-AS patients. This is related to the presence of HLA antigens, which are determined on a genetic basis. Calin (1975) reported 20% of patients with HLA-B27 antigens have symptomatic AS.

■ Ocular

AS is the most frequently identified systemic disease associated with recurrent iridocyclitis. Kimura and associates (1966) identified approximately 35% of uveitis patients as having probable or definite AS. Acute iridocyclitis occurs in approximately 25% of AS patients at some point during the course of their disease. Brewerton and co-workers (1973) found 29% of uveitis patients were HLA-B27 positive, without evidence of rheumatologic disease, and 33% of the patients in the same study did manifest rheumatologic-associated disease.

NATURAL HISTORY

Table 24–1 summarizes the systemic and ocular involvement of AS.

■ Systemic

AS is a progressive inflammatory arthropathy with a predilection for the axial skeleton, with the sacroiliac joint affected most severely and the vertebral column affected less extensively. The exact mechanism for AS development is unknown, although a postinfectious arthropathy is suspected. An immune reaction to the infectious organism appears to incite the arthropathy in a susceptible individual (HLA-B27 positive). *Klebsiella* has been implicated as one of the triggering organisms, and it is seen more frequently in AS patients. The joint inflammation is centered around the ligament to bone junction (entheses), which places many joints throughout the body at risk. The joints of the

TABLE 24–1. SYSTEMIC AND OCULAR INVOLVEMENT OF AS

EARLY
- **Articular**
  Axial skeleton, sacroiliac joint
- **Extra-articular**
  Iridocyclitis
  Anemia
  Prostatitis

LATE
- **Articular**
  Extensive vertebral involvement
  Peripheral joint involvement
  Tendinitis
- **Extra-articular**
  Pulmonary fibrosis
  Aortic valvular disease with reflux
  Cardiac conduction deficits
  Pericarditis
  Amyloidosis

axial skeleton and upper extremities are at highest risk for involvement.

The typical clinical presentation is of a young adult male with lower back or flank pain that is worse after periods of inactivity (eg, after sleep) and is associated with limited flexion of the back. The pain distribution may involve the lower back, buttock, hip, or leg (pseudo-sciatica). Other characteristics of AS-associated pain include an insidious onset, lasting 3 months, which is relieved by exercise. Milder symptoms are commonly experienced by women. Recurrent episodes of sacroiliitis leading to joint fusion is the most characteristic feature of AS. Patients with active sacroiliac joint inflammation are asymptomatic 50% of the time.

Calcification of the intervertebral spaces (capsules) results in the loss of joint space, giving rise to a bamboo appearance of the spine on radiography. The spinal arthritis progresses up the vertebral column without skipping regions. Although this feature is most characteristic of AS, it runs a variable course, and may not be seen despite a long duration of AS.

Extraspinal involvement occurs in 40% of AS patients. Progression of the arthritis to other joints of the upper extremities can involve the rib cage, leading to chest pain, decreased chest expansion, and associated breathing difficulties. Articular inflammation infrequently involves the elbows, hands, knees, or feet. The articular inflammation is self-limiting and results in less functional loss as the patient ages as compared to rheumatoid arthritis.

Aortic involvement affects 3 to 10% of patients and may manifest 15 or more years following the onset of AS. Valvular reflux may be related to amyloidosis (a rare feature of AS) and serves as a significant source of patient mortality. Conduction deficits of the heart including com-

plete block are observed (and may be associated with the presence of HLA-B27). Pericarditis and pulmonary fibrosis are rarer complications, which can potentially be fatal. Pulmonary fibrosis usually manifests after the fifth decade.

■ Ocular

Ocular involvement occurs in 20% of AS patients, with AS being the most commonly identified systemic disease in patients with recurrent iridocyclitis. The acute nature of the inflammation is the hallmark of AS iridocyclitis. Iridocyclitis may precede the symptoms associated with active sacroiliitis by months and serve as the sentinel for the diagnosis of AS. Simultaneous presentation of iridocyclitis is rare although recurrences may follow an alternating pattern with one eye predominantly affected. The ocular inflammation is usually confined to the anterior segment with few sequelae. Posterior synechiae develop frequently due to the acute onset of the iridocyclitis, although involvement of other tissues is not frequently encountered. Glaucoma and cataracts are more likely to result from therapy than from the inflammation itself. Posterior segment involvement is usually limited to macular edema, developing after multiple recurrences of iridocyclitis, and may affect vision when it is significant.

DIAGNOSIS

■ Systemic

Patient history and clinical presentation are instrumental to the diagnosis of AS (Table 24–2). There is no specific test for diagnosing AS, but certain findings on radiographic and serologic testing are consistent with AS. Diagnostic testing consists primarily of x-rays of the axial skeleton along with blood tests for the presence of HLA-B27 antigens and erythrocyte sedimentation (SED) rate. Radiographic studies are instrumental in the diagnosis of AS. Sacroiliac joint films are used to detect the presence of joint fusion or calcification

TABLE 24–2. DIAGNOSTIC CRITERIA FOR AS (MODIFIED NEW YORK CRITERIA)

1. Lower back pain not relieved by rest of at least 3 months duration
2. Lumbar restriction in the frontal and sagittal planes
3. Decreased chest expansion compared to normal age-matched values
4. Unilateral sacroiliitis (grades 3 or 4)
5. Bilateral sacroiliitis (grades 2 or 3)

Definite AS if number 4 or 5 above, along with any other criterion, is observed.

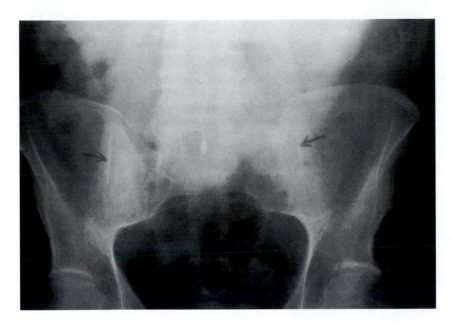

Figure 24–1. Sacroiliac joint film in AS patient. Note the loss of space of the sacroiliac joint on sides (*arrows*). This patient had buttock pain and recurrent episodes of iridocyclitis. (*Reprinted with permission from Mahoney BP. Rheumatologic disease and associated ocular manifestations.* J Am Optom Assoc. *1993;64:403–415.*)

bilaterally (Figure 24–1). A pelvic bone scan is more sensitive in detecting active sacroiliac joint inflammation, particularly if a patient is asymptomatic. X-rays of the vertebral column reveal intervertebral joint calcification, giving the characteristic bamboo appearance associated with AS.

A positive test for the presence of the HLA-B27 antigen is seen in over 90% of AS patients. AS has a higher association with HLA serotypes than any other disease. Normally only 8% of the Caucasian American and 4% of the African American population are HLA-B27 positive. The presence of the HLA-B27 haplotype is viewed as a predisposing factor for AS but does not imply eventual development of the disease. SED rates are elevated in 80% of AS patients with active articular disease.

■ Ocular

Ocular assessment of a patient with AS includes a complete eye evaluation. A mild to moderate amount of anterior chamber reaction is normally seen with AS-associated iridocyclitis. Posterior synechia develops rapidly given the acute nature of the iridocyclitis (Figure 24–2). Chronic uveitis may lead to the development of cataracts, increased IOP, and macular edema. Appropriate laboratory and radiological testing should be ordered if AS is suspected based on ocular examination.

TREATMENT AND MANAGEMENT

■ Systemic

Aggressive medical treatment is not necessary for most AS patients. Sustained therapy with nonsteroidal antiinflammatory drugs (NSAIDs), combined with an aggressive physi-

cal therapy program, remains the mainstay of AS treatment. The chronic use of NSAIDs is sufficient for delaying the vertebral calcification as well as minimizing sacroiliac joint fusion, thereby maximizing the patient's levels of activity and comfort. Indomethacin has replaced phenylbutazone as the NSAID of choice because of the toxicity associated with long-term use of phenylbutazone. Phenylbutazone is considered for short-term therapy when indomethacin is not sufficient to control disease activity. Salicylates have not been very effective in AS therapy. Stronger agents, like sulfasalazine, may help patient symptoms, but have little effect on delaying vertebral calcification. Changes in the dosage or type of medication may be necessary, but stronger antiinflammatory agents are rarely needed to manage most AS patients (Table 24–3).

TABLE 24–3. TREATMENT AND MANAGEMENT OF ANKYLOSING SPONDYLITIS

■ **SYSTEMIC**
- Physical therapy
- Antiinflammatories
   NSAIDS—indomethacin
   Rarely requires other stronger agents (eg, sulfasalazine)
- Orthopedic surgical intervention (rare)
- Pulmonary and cardiac manifestations managed by specialist

■ **OCULAR**
Iridocyclitis
- Topical cycloplegic and steroid preparations need be initiated quickly to prevent synechiae formation
- Antiglaucoma medication, if secondary glaucoma

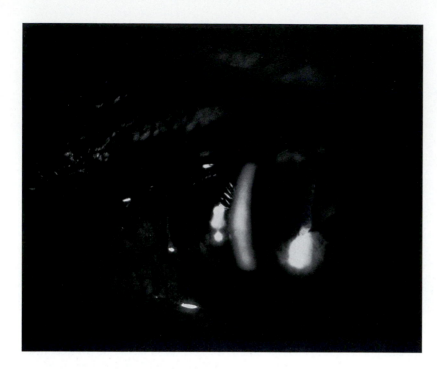

Figure 24–2. Iridocyclitis in AS patient. This is the same patient shown in Figure 24–1. Posterior synechia developed in addition to keratic precipitates within 1 day of symptoms. Topical steroids and cycloplegics quelled the inflammation and broke the synechia within 1 week.

Increased physical activity has a beneficial effect on the joint disease of AS. Joint inflammation and subsequent destruction are minimized with regular physical activity. Orthopedic surgical intervention is necessary if significant joint disease affects the hips or knees.

■ Ocular

Iridocyclitis associated with AS can frequently be managed by conventional therapy using topical steroids and cyclo-plegics. A stronger, longer-lasting cycloplegic agent (scopo-lamine versus homatropine) may be desired considering the propensity for development of posterior synechiae. The episodes usually resolve within a 2-week period, yet frequent recurrences warrant the use of long-term topical steroid use. The use of systemic NSAIDs may also be effective in con-trolling ocular inflammation; however, most patients have recurrences despite NSAID therapy. The use of periocular steroid injections is not warranted unless topical medications are insufficient or a chronic pattern develops. Patients with AS should be monitored on a regular basis—every 6 to 12 months—in conjunction with rheumatic evaluations, or as needed when acute exacerbations of iridocyclitis occur.

CONCLUSION

AS is the most frequently encountered seronegative spondyloarthropathy whose outstanding feature is its pro-gressive arthritis primarily involving the axial skeleton. Physical impairment is usually minor despite a long history of AS. AS is rarely associated with patient mortality, and does not require aggressive treatment and management. Extra-articular involvement is limited to the eye for many AS patients. Recurrent, nongranulomatous iridocyclitis is a hallmark of this disease, is usually mild to moderate, and responds well to conventional ocular therapy. Early detec-tion of ocular inflammation is necessary so therapy can be instituted to minimize complications that result from uncontrolled iridocyclitis. Eyecare practitioners play an integral role in the healthcare of AS patients because of the frequency of acute iridocyclitis in these patients.

REFERENCES

Abel GS, Terry JE. Ankylosing spondylitis and recurrent anterior uveitis. *J Am Optom Assoc.* 1991;62:844.

Beckingdale AB, Williams D, Gibson JM, et al. *Klebsiella* and acute anterior uveitis. *Br J Ophthalmol.* 1984;68:866.

Bergfeldt L, Vallin H, Edhag O. Complete heart block in HLA-B27 associated disease. Electrophysiological and clinical char-acteristics. *Br Heart J.* 1984;51:181.

Brewerton DA, Caffrey M, Nicholls A, et al. Acute anterior uveitis and HLA 27. *Lancet.* 1973;2:994.

Calin A. Striking prevalence of ankylosing spondylitis in "healthy" B27 positive males and females: A controlled study. *N Engl J Med.* 1975;293:835–839.

Catterall RD, Perkins ES. Uveitis and urogenital disease in the male. *Br J Ophthalmol.* 1961;45:109.

Clegg DO. Sulfasalazine. In: McCarty DJ, Koopman WJ, eds. *Arthritis and Allied Conditions.* Philadelphia: Lea & Febiger; 1993;637.

Dougados M, Boumier P, Amor B. Sulfasalazine in ankylosing spondylitis: A double-blind controlled study in 60 patients. *Br Med J.* 1986;293:911.

Goie The HS, Steven MM, Van der Linden SM, Cats A. Evaluation of the diagnostic criteria for ankylosing spondylitis: A comparison of the Rome, New York, and Modified New York Criteria in patients with a positive clinical history screening test for ankylosing spondylitis. *Br J Rheumatol.* 1985;24:242.

Hardin JG, Longenecker GL. Drug therapy of specific rheumatic diseases. In: Hardin JG, Longenecker GL, eds. *Handbook of Drug Therapy in Rheumatic Disease.* Boston, Little, Brown; 1992;175.

Kimura SJ, Hogan MJ, O'Connor GR, Epstein WV. Uveitis and joint disease: A review of 191 cases. *Trans Am Ophthalmol Soc.* 1966;64:301.

Russel AS, Lentle BC, Percy JS. Investigation of sacroiliac disease: Comparative evaluation of radiological and radionuclide techniques. *J Rheumatol.* 1975;2:45.

Scharf Y, Zonis S. Histocompatability antigens (HLA) and uveitis. *Surv Ophthalmol.* 1980;24:220.

Wollheim FA. Ankylosing spondylitis. In: Kelley WN, Harris ED, Ruddy S, Sledge CB, eds. *Textbook of Rheumatology.* Philadelphia: Saunders; 1993:943.

25
Chapter

Psoriatic Arthritis

John Elliott Conto

Psoriatic arthritis (PA) is an uncommon seronegative spondyloarthropathy (arthritis of the spine) that is distinguished from other inflammatory arthropathies by the presence of characteristic psoriatic skin and nail disease. The arthritis may be mild to severe, with single or multiple peripheral joints becoming affected. The degree of joint involvement is quite variable, and often several different patterns concurrently exist. Sacroiliitis and spondylitis may be seen in patients with PA, but are less commonly present than in patients with ankylosing spondylitis or Reiter syndrome. A genetic predisposition between psoriasis and seronegative arthritis has been supported by family and HLA studies (Marcusson, 1979). The inheritance pattern is thought to be a dominant inherited multifactorial trait with variable penetrance. Environmental factors are thought to play a role in the development of PA, including bacterial antigen induction, retrovirus antigen reaction, trauma, and immunologic agents.

Ocular involvement in PA ranges from a mild purulent conjunctivitis to a nongranulomatous iritis similar to that seen in Reiter syndrome or ankylosing spondylitis. Episcleritis may rarely develop. Unlike many other inflammatory arthropathies, keratoconjunctivitis sicca does not seem to occur in conjunction with PA.

EPIDEMIOLOGY

■ Systemic

Leczinsky (1948) suggested that the frequency of PA in patients with psoriasis is about 7%. The estimated incidence in the general population is thought to be 0.1 to 1%, which is similar to the prevalence of rheumatoid arthritis. It is generally accepted that psoriasis occurs three to six times more frequently in the arthritic population than in the general population. Males and females are affected equally as seen in uncomplicated psoriasis. The peak age of onset appears to be in the fourth or fifth decades, but there is a small subset of patients in whom the onset is under the age of 16.

■ Ocular

Generalized ocular inflammation occurs in about 30% of patients with PA. Conjunctivitis has been reported in approximately 20% of cases, while an anterior iritis appears in an estimated 7% of PA patients (Lambert & Wright, 1976).

NATURAL HISTORY

■ Systemic

PA usually has a slow onset, but is known to develop acutely in one third of patients. The psoriasis often precedes the arthritis by several years, although in 15 to 20% of cases the arthritis occurs before the development of the skin lesions. The skin disease consists of discrete erythematous lesions with flaking and scaling of the surrounding skin, which may elicit mild to moderate complaints of irritation and itching. The pattern varies from small hidden patches to broad exfoliation. The majority of patients with PA do not have severe skin disease.

Nail involvement is seen in the vast majority of PA patients, and may occur without overt skin changes. The severity of the arthritis appears to be related to the degree of nail changes. Common nail manifestations include discoloration, thickening of the distal nail, separation at the ungal bed, ridging, cracking, and nail pitting (Figure 25–1). A review by Gladmann (1991) suggested an increased association between nail disease and the likelihood of involvement of the distal joints.

PA is typified by a synovitis, which is indistinguishable from that seen in rheumatoid arthritis. The disease follows a course that includes periods of exacerbation and remission. Thickening of the synovial membrane and joint swelling are early arthritic changes, and usually involve the small finger joints. Patients will complain about joint pain and stiffness.

Progressive joint disease will demonstrate articular destruction, bone reabsorption, and marginal bony overgrowth at the insertion of the tendon. The knee, hip, ankle, and wrist can also be involved. Fibrous tissue development may cause the joints to fuse. The sacroiliac joint may be involved in 20 to 40% of HLA-B27 positive patients (Table 25–1).

Several arthritic patterns have been defined by Moll and Wright (1973), and can present in isolation or in combination (Table 25–2). The exact frequency is unknown, because many investigators use different criteria for each pattern.

The most common PA subtype is an asymmetric oligoarticular (involving few joints) form. This pattern is similar to the peripheral arthropathy seen in other spondyloarthropathies, such as ankylosing spondylitis or Reiter syndrome. One or more joints are involved, especially the small distal joints of the hands and feet. The toes or fingers

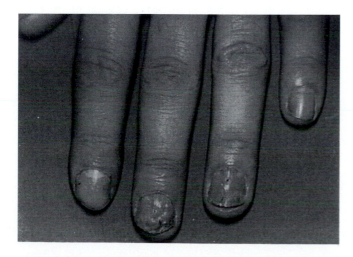

Figure 25–1. Psoriatic nail manifestations: discoloration, distal nail thickening, ridging, cracking, and nail pitting. *(Reprinted with permission from Gawkrodger DJ: An Illustrated Coulored Text of Dermatology. New York: Churchill Livingstone; 1992.)*

TABLE 25–1. SYSTEMIC MANIFESTATIONS OF PA

PSORIASIS
- **Symptoms**
  Mild to moderate itching
- **Signs**
  Discrete erythematous lesions
  Scaling and flaking of the skin

PSORIATIC NAIL DISEASE
- **Signs**
  Discoloration
  Ungal bed separation
  Cracking and ridging
  Nail pitting

PSORIATIC ARTHRITIS
- **Symptoms**
  Joint pain
  Joint stiffness
- **Signs**
  Synovial membrane thickening and joint swelling
  "Sausage swelling" of fingers and toes
  Sacroiliitis
  Asymmetric changes of the DIP joints
  Bony ankylosis
  "Pencil-in-cup" or "fishtail" deformities of phalanges

often have a "sausage swelling" look to them. The oligoarticular arthritis usually presents abruptly with mild or no systemic symptoms or signs. It may resolve rapidly or persist for several months.

Symmetrical polyarthritis is seen in about one quarter of PA patients. Women are more frequently affected than men. This form has a similar clinical presentation to rheumatoid arthritis, although the joint involvement is less extensive and deforming than rheumatoid arthritis. A small percentage of these patients are seropositive for rheumatoid factor (RF).

TABLE 25–2. JOINT INVOLVEMENT IN PA

PA Subtype	Involved Joints
Asymmetric oligoarticular	Distal and proximal interphalangeal joints of hands and feet Metatarsophalangeal joints Occasional involvement of wrists, hips, knees, ankles
Symmetrical polyarthritis	Wrist Proximal and distal interphalangeal joints
Predominant distal interphalangeal	Distal interphalangeal joints
Predominant axial	Spinal column Sacroiliac joint
Arthritis mutilans	Severe osteolysis of phalanges

Predominant distal interphalangeal joint (DIP) arthritis is characterized by isolated involvement of the fingers. It affects males more frequently than females, and is most often associated with the nail disease.

The two least common forms of PA are predominant axial arthritis and deforming erosive arthritis or arthritis mutilans. Predominant axial arthritis has a clinical picture that closely resembles ankylosing spondylitis, but with less severe symptoms. Deforming erosive arthritis causes progressive osteolysis and severe distortion of the involved digits (Figure 25–2). These patients seem to present in the second to third decade, and have widespread skin disease.

Patients with PA tend to have less functional loss, and they do not lose as much time from work, as patients with rheumatoid arthritis. Mortality due to PA is rare, and when death is associated with the disease, it is usually from complications related to medical therapy.

◼ Ocular

PA may cause ocular symptoms of minor irritation, redness, foreign body sensation, or photophobia. The conjunctivitis seen in PA is superficial, and is occasionally accompanied by a mucopurulent discharge. It is generally short in duration, but may follow a chronic course. The acute anterior uveitis is unilateral, and presents with the subjective complaints of pain and photophobia. It is most often seen in PA patients with sacroiliitis. Ciliary injection, a mild to marked anterior chamber reaction, and fine keratic precipitates are typical findings upon examination. The iritis may be recurrent and alternate between the eyes. Intraocular pressure may be lowered during iritis. The anterior vitreous is not usually involved, except in severe cases of iritis.

Posterior segment involvement is rare, and complications, such as cystoid macular edema or cataract, are uncommon if initial treatment of the anterior iritis is adequate. Episcleritis, not frequently found in PA, is usually self-limiting (Table 25–3).

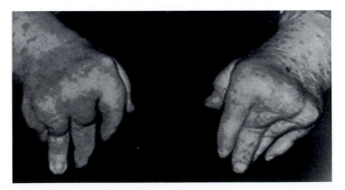

Figure 25–2. Deforming arthritis mutilans with severe distortion of the digits and hands. *(Reprinted with permission from Gawkrodger DJ: An Illustrated Coulored Text of Dermatology. New York: Churchill Livingstone; 1992.)*

TABLE 25–3. OCULAR MANIFESTATIONS OF PA

- **Symptoms**
  Irritation
  Redness
  Photophobia
  Foreign body sensation
  Decreased vision

- **Signs**
  Mucopurulent conjunctivitis
  Anterior iritis
  Episcleritis

DIAGNOSIS

◼ Systemic

The diagnosis of PA is made in the presence of psoriasis or psoriatic nail disease, along with the characteristic signs of the spondyloarthritis. The manifestations of the arthritis can be quite variable between patients. There are no characteristic laboratory abnormalities associated with PA. RF is negative in the vast majority of patients. Erythrocyte sedimentation rate may be elevated, but is nonspecific for PA. Anemia may be present. Analysis of the synovial fluid may show inflammatory components. There has been an increased linkage of psoriasis and PA with several HLA antigens, including HLA-B13, B17, B27, and Cw6 (Alonso et al, 1991). Radiographic findings may demonstrate asymmetric changes of the DIP joints, terminal phalanges, and sacroiliac joint. Other radiographic features, not characteristic of PA alone, are bony ankylosis or destruction of the joints of the hands and feet, and bony proliferation of the distal joints. Progressive erosion of the phalanges may appear as "pencil-in-cup" or "fishtail" deformities. In the most severe cases, extension of the phalanges may occur.

◼ Ocular

The conjunctivitis and anterior uveitis seen in PA are similar in clinical appearance to those seen in Reiter syndrome or ankylosing spondylitis, and are readily diagnosed with biomicroscopy. Differentiation of PA as the cause from other similar etiologies is based on the systemic findings.

TREATMENT AND MANAGEMENT

◼ Systemic

In most PA patients, the skin disease is relatively mild and requires no treatment. In patients with mildly active arthritis, NSAIDs are used. Indomethacin seems to be more effective than aspirin or ibuprofen. If necessary, the oligoarticular synovitis may be managed with local glucocorticoid injections. Oral steroids are rarely necessary. Parenteral or oral gold has been used with various degrees of success in severe erosive cases. However, about one third of patients will have a severe skin reaction from gold therapy. Other therapeutic agents reported to be effective are antimalarials, such as hydroxychloroquine; antimetabolites, such as methotrexate; or the retinoid, etretinate (Table 25–4). Many of these drugs have toxic side effects that limit their broad use. Some patients may benefit from photochemotherapy with methoxypsoralen and long-wave ultraviolet-A light (PUVA).

Physical therapy and exercise are helpful in preserving the range of motion of the involved joints. Hand and ankle splints may prevent contracture from developing. Surgical reconstruction of damaged joints can be considered when extreme functional loss occurs, but has a less favorable result than in rheumatoids.

■ Ocular

The conjunctivitis follows a benign course, resolving over a period of 7 to 10 days. Supportive therapy with cold compresses, vasoconstrictors, and ocular lubricants as needed may be helpful for subjective relief. Acute anterior uveitis can be managed with varying dosages of topical steroids depending on the severity of anterior chamber reaction, and cycloplegic agents (see Table 25–4).

CONCLUSION

PA is an arthropathy that is seen with psoriatic skin or nail disease. The clinical course is often benign, but can be quite variable in the overall effect on physical function. Many joints are affected, from the small distal joints of the digits, to the larger joints of the spine or hip. Like the other seronegative arthropathies, PA can have associated ocular findings, most commonly conjunctivitis or anterior iritis. The ocular complications are usually mild, without longstanding sequelae.

REFERENCES

Alonso JCT, Perez AR, Castrillo JMA, et al. Psoriatic arthritis (PA): A clinical immunological and radiological study of 180 patients. *Br J Rheum.* 1991;30:245–250.

Dieppe PA, Doherty M, Macfarlene D, Maddison P. Psoriatic arthropathy. In: Dieppe PA, Doherty M, Macfarlene D, Maddison P. *Rheumatology Medicine.* Edinburgh: Churchill Livingstone; 1985:86–90.

Gladman DD. Psoriatic arthritis: Review of current concepts. *Isr J Med Sci.* 1991;27:228–232.

Lambert JR, Wright V. Eye inflammation in psoriatic arthritis. *Ann Rheum Dis.* 1976;35:354–356.

Leczinsky CG. The incidence of arthropathy in a ten-year series of psoriasis cases. *Acta Dermatol Venereol.* 1948;28:483–485.

Marcussion J. Psoriasis and arthritic lesions in relation to the inheritance of HLA genotypes. *Acta Dermatol Venereol.* 1979; 59(suppl 82):1–48.

Melvin JL. Rheumatic disease in the adult and child. In: Melvin JL. *Occupational Therapy and Rehabilitation.* 3rd ed. Philadelphia, Davis; 1989:88–92.

Michet CJ, Conn DL. Psoriatic arthritis. In: Kelley WN, Harris ED, Ruddy S, Sledge CB, eds. *Textbook of Rheumatology.* 3rd ed. Philadelphia: Saunders; 1989:1053–1063.

Moll JMH, Wright V. Psoriatic arthritis. *Semin Arthritis Rheum.* 1973;3:55–78.

Wright V. Psoriatic arthritis. In: Kelley WN, Harris ED, Ruddy S, Sledge CB, eds. *Textbook of Rheumatology.* 2nd ed. Philadelphia: Saunders; 1985:1021–1031.

TABLE 25–4. TREATMENT AND MANAGEMENT OF PA

■ **SYSTEMIC**	
● Mildly active arthritis	NSAIDs
● Oligoarticular synovitis	Local glucocorticoid injections
● Severe erosions	Parenteral or oral gold
● Other therapeutic agents	Antimalarials, antimetabolites, retinoids, photochemotherapy
● Mobility preservation	Surgical joint reconstruction, physical therapy and exercise
■ **OCULAR**	
● Conjunctivitis/episcleritis	Vasoconstrictors, ocular lubricants
● Uveitis	Topical corticosteroids (1% prednisolone acetate Q2H to QID) Cycloplegics (0.25% scopolamine BID or 5% homatropine BID)

Reiter Syndrome

Brian Patrick Mahoney

Reiter syndrome (RS) is a disease of the joints of the spine. RS tests negative for rheumatoid factors (a seronegative spondyloarthropathy) and is characterized by urethritis, arthritis, and conjunctivitis (or iridocyclitis). Although a reactive etiology (eg, infection) is strongly supported for RS, it differs from other reactive arthritides in its association with ocular and urethral inflammation as its primary extra-articular (nonjoint) features. Sacroiliac inflammation and associated HLA-B27 are shared features of RS and ankylosing spondylitis (also a seronegative spondyloarthropathy); however, each is distinguished by a different clinical course. Active ocular involvement coincides with articular activity for many RS patients, requiring aggressive medical management.

EPIDEMIOLOGY

■ Systemic

RS is the most common cause of arthralgia in the 20- to 35-year-old age group. It affects men five times more frequently than women, with over 90% of RS patients being young adult males. The prevalence is about 3 in 100,000 in a male population only. RS occurs more commonly in Caucasians, coinciding with the higher prevalence of HLA-B27. RS develops in about 1 to 3% of patients with nonspecific urethritis. Progression of the disease results in severe physical disability in approximately 15% of RS patients.

■ Ocular

Ocular involvement is seen in about 66% of RS patients at the time of diagnosis. Recurrent iridocyclitis occurs more frequently in patients with chronic exacerbations, and conjunctivitis occurs more frequently in patients with self-limiting disease. Conjunctivitis occurs in approximately 33% of RS patients over the course of their disease, and acute iridocyclitis manifests in 8 to 40% of RS patients. There may be a higher association between RS and iridocyclitis than initially thought. Rosenbaum (1989) reported a higher frequency of associated uveitis in RS (7.2%) than in anky-losing spondylitis (5.5%) in a population of uveitis patients who had seronegative spondyloarthropathies.

NATURAL HISTORY

Table 26–1 summarizes both systemic and ocular manifestations of RS.

■ Systemic

The exact etiology for RS has yet to be determined, but significant evidence supports its classification as a reactive arthropathy. This inflammatory arthropathy often follows a venereal (particularly in males) or enteric/intestinal (particularly in females) infection. Infectious organisms associated with RS include *Shigella*, *Salmonella*, and *Chlamydia*. The pathogenic organism is not the cause of the arthropathy. An altered immune response to the infective pathogen directed toward the patient's own tissues (particularly articular or joint) initiates the disease in a susceptible individual. The presence of HLA-B27 identifies those patients most susceptible to developing this response. Antibodies to *Chlamydia* have shown cross-reactivity to HLA lymphocytes and can bind to various tissues, triggering an

TABLE 26–1. SYSTEMIC AND OCULAR MANIFESTATIONS OF RS

ARTICULAR
- Sacroiliitis
- Enthesitis: Achilles tendinitis most commonly
- Inflammation of the small peripheral joints of the lower extremities

EXTRA-ARTICULAR
- Prostatitis/urethritis
- Cervicitis
- Ocular
  Conjunctivitis
  Uveitis; unremitting, may lead to cataract, vitritis, increased IOP, macular edema
- Oral ulcers
- Keratoderma blenorrhagicum of palms of hands and soles of feet
- Balanitis
- Amyloidosis
- Cardiac
  Conduction deficits
  Pericarditis
  Aortic insufficiency
- Pulmonary fibrosis

inflammatory reaction. About 50% of RS patients have antibodies to *Chlamydia*, and about 10% of patients treated for chlamydial infections develop arthritis.

Other enteric and sexually transmitted infections are associated with a reactive arthritis. Patients with reactive arthritis may manifest joint involvement similar to RS, including achilles tendinitis. Extra-articular features, including ocular inflammation, are not observed and the complete syndrome does not develop. There is not a strong association with HLA-B27 when compared to RS and ankylosing spondylitis.

The clinical course for RS patients is not always predictable. There are no known clinical indicators to predict which patients will develop an unrelenting clinical course. Patients with the classic triad seem to run a milder course than those patients who manifest an incomplete triad at the time of diagnosis. The clinical course in women is less severe than in men for unknown reasons. The early clinical presentation includes asymmetric arthralgia of the knee, ankle, or toe developing about a month (or more) following infection. The initial episode of arthropathy lasts 2 to 3 months. The patient may be diagnosed only after recurrent episodes because of the mild degree of joint inflammation. The quiescent periods between active cycles shorten as the disease becomes more aggressive. Years may lapse between active arthritic cycles during the early stage of the disease, decreasing to only months between cycles as the disease develops into a chronic course.

Active sacroiliac joint inflammation manifests early in the course of the disease, although patients may be asymptomatic. Sacroiliac joint inflammation is seen in about 40 to 60% of patients with the chronic disease and less frequently in those with a remitting course. Sacroiliac inflammation is less severe in RS than in ankylosing spondylitis. Symptoms of lower back, buttock, and sciatic-like pain, as well as a limited range of motion of the lower back, are all consistent with active sacroiliitis. Axial skeletal involvement, including sacroiliitis, occurs in 20% with a remitting course and more frequently in patients with the chronic course. Inflammation of the ligament and tendon insertions on the bone (enthesitis) most frequently affect the Achilles tendon, but other joints may also be involved. Inflammation of these joints is associated with pain and restricted movement.

Recurrent cycles of arthritis affect the weight-bearing joints of the lower extremities. The joints in the hips, knees, ankles, and toes are the most frequently involved, resulting in some degree of decreased function for all RS patients and severe physical disability in 15 to 20%. Involvement of the upper extremities (shoulders, elbows, wrists, and fingers) occurs to a lesser degree as RS progresses. Exacerbations of articular inflammation commonly occur without any extra-articular activity.

Recurrent mucocutaneous membrane inflammation is a common feature, with episodes of noninfectious urethritis or cervicitis present in 33% of RS patients, which frequently signals the beginning of another cycle of activity. Mucopurulent discharge of the urethra may not be appreciated by the male patient due to its transient nature. The associated genitourinary inflammation frequently goes undetected in women because of the occult nature of these infections. Oral ulcerations develop along with a vesicular rash on the head of the penis (balanitis) or cervix (cervicitis) with little associated pain. Keratoderma blenorrhagicum, a papulosquamous eruption similar to psoriasis, frequently involves the hands and feet. This is the most common mucocutaneous manifestation of RS.

The recurrent cycles of arthritic activity in RS are centered around the weight-bearing joints of the lower extremities. The hips, knees, and ankles are involved most frequently, with gradual loss in function as joint damage occurs. Joint involvement of the lower extremities progresses and results in some degree of functional impairment for most patients. Severe functional impairment is seen in 15% of RS patients. Exacerbations of the arthralgia may occur without significant extra-articular inflammation, yet extra-articular inflammation is almost always accompanied by exacerbations of arthritis.

Approximately 20 to 50% of RS patients run a chronic course with significant systemic sequelae. In a study by Fox (1979), 83% of RS patients had active arthritis after 5.6 years of follow-up, 42% had active urethritis or cervicitis, and 50% had active back or heel pain. Severe joint disease in the lower extremities and axial skeleton accounts for functional impairment in RS patients by the seventh decade. RS rarely results in death, but when it occurs, it is usually attributed to cardiac complications, including amyloidosis.

■ Ocular

Exacerbations and remissions of the ocular involvement in RS follow a pattern similar to the arthritis. The exact triggering mechanism is unknown; however, antibodies, particularly to *Chlamydia*, have shown to cross-react with HLA lymphocytes and bind to conjunctival tissues, resulting in an inflammatory reaction. The cycles of ocular inflammation are self-limiting, lasting about 2 weeks without medical intervention. Nonspecific conjunctival inflammation is characterized by palpebral and bulbar injection. A mixed papillary and follicular response of the palpebral conjunctiva can be observed days after the onset of the urethritis or cervicitis. There may be a mild noninfectious mucoid discharge present. A mild superficial punctate staining of the cornea is commonly observed, without associated bacterial keratitis, and resolves with the conjunctivitis. A decreased tear breakup time is present. Tendinitis commonly occurs with the conjunctivitis or precedes it by days or weeks.

Acute iridocyclitis is a frequent manifestation of chronic RS. Patients present with symptoms typically associated with iridocyclitis (pain, photophobia, and lacrimation). These symptoms recur with each episode and worsen with the duration of ocular inflammation. The acute onset and aggressive nature of the inflammation places the patient at risk for developing posterior synechiae unless prompt treatment is instituted. Recalcitrant forms of uveitis may occur, resulting in posterior synechiae, cataract, elevated intraocular pressure (secondary to impaired outflow from inflammatory debris), vitritis or macular edema (Figure 26–1).

DIAGNOSIS

■ Systemic

Diagnosis of RS is based on a thorough history that includes previous enteric or venereal disease, mucocutaneous lesions, peripheral arthritis, lower back pain, and ocular inflammation. Diagnostic testing, although not specific for RS, may include HLA-B27, erythrocyte sedimentation rate (SED rate), and a complete blood count, along with x-ray (Figure 26–2), or bone scans. The most frequently ordered battery includes HLA-B27 test and a sacroiliac joint study (x-ray or bone scan). The definitive diagnosis of RS may be difficult to differentiate from other spondyloarthropathies or reactive arthropathies despite extensive evaluation. Sufficient clinical follow-up is necessary so the clinical course can be accurately assessed and specific diagnosis can ultimately be determined.

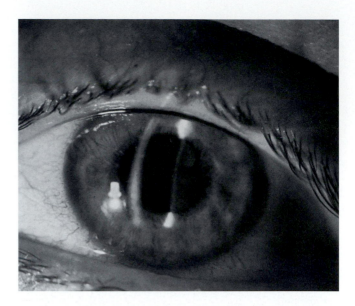

Figure 26–1. Uveitis in an RS patient. This patient required very aggressive systemic and ocular treatment to manage his chronic RS (20+ years). He had bilateral uveitis with both anterior and posterior segment sequelae in each eye. A mild anterior chamber reaction persisted in each eye despite the resolution of symptoms. (*Reprinted with permission from Mahoney BP. Rheumatologic disease and associated ocular manifestations.* J Am Optom Assoc. *1993;64:403–415.*)

There is a high association between RS and HLA-B27 (70 to 90%). Similar to ankylosing spondylitis, the presence of HLA-B27 appears to represent a predisposition for the development of RS, but it is not a determining factor for its development. Significant controversy exists regarding the exact relationship between the presence of HLA-B27 and its role in the development of seronegative spondyloarthropathies. Seronegative spondyloarthropathies do not have rheumatoid factors present, or serologic indicators of immunologic abnormalities (IgG and IgM proteins). Sufficient evidence exists to suggest the presence of HLA-B27 antigens with altered immunologic responses, although a causal relationship cannot be proven. Elevated SED rate and leukocytosis are commonly associated with disease activity. Keratoderma blenorrhagicum of the planar region of the feet, although rarely seen, is pathognomonic for RS. Cultures of the urethral or cervical surfaces are of no benefit in RS diagnosis because pathogen activity is not the cause of the inflammatory response.

Sacroiliac joint evaluation by x-ray or bone scan is needed to determine the amount of joint inflammation and fusion. Bone scans are more sensitive at detecting low-grade joint inflammation and may be preferred in cases where x-ray results are equivocal. Radiographic studies of the back are not necessary because extensive vertebral involvement is not a common feature. X-rays of any affected joints reveal areas of active osteoporosis at the

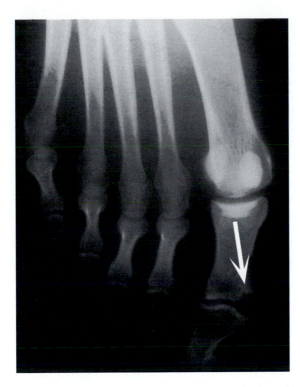

Figure 26–2. X-ray of the feet of an RS patient. Note the loss of bone at the lateral aspects of the joints of the toes (*arrow*). This patient had symptoms of tendinitis and had previously been treated for a chlamydial infection. He experienced nonspecific ocular irritation of both eyes on a recurrent basis following the chlamydial infection.

lateral aspects of the joints with adjacent areas of bony proliferation. Surrounding soft tissue swelling and bony proliferation near the inflamed entheses are evident on x-ray.

Other findings suggestive of the diagnosis of RS include fever, weight loss, fatigue, and malaise in the early stages. Cardiac involvement, including heart block and nonspecific S-T segment abnormalities, are seen in 10% of RS patients. Aortic regurgitation is a late manifestation, similar to ankylosing spondylitis. Amyloidosis, serositis, and pulmonary infiltrates are also rarely associated with RS usually as a manifestion of chronic disease.

■ Ocular

Ocular manifestations of RS are diagnosed with the use of biomicroscopy to appropriately evaluate for conjunctival (mixed papillary response), corneal, or anterior chamber (iridocyclitis) involvement. A tear breakup time should also be performed to help determine tear quality. A dilated fundus evaluation is necessary to rule out any vitreal or retinal involvement.

TREATMENT AND MANAGEMENT

Table 26–2 gives an overview of RS treatment and management.

TABLE 26–2. TREATMENT AND MANAGEMENT OF RS

■ SYSTEMIC
- Physical therapy
- NSAIDs (eg, indomethacin)
- Steroids[a]
- Cytotoxic agents[a]
- Immunosuppressive agents[a]

■ OCULAR
- Conjunctival inflammation
    - Lubricants
    - Vasoconstrictors
- Iridocyclitis
    - Topical cycloplegic
    - Topical steroid
    - Subtenon steroid injection
    - Systemic immunosuppressant agents
    - Antiglaucoma medications if needed

[a]These agents are indicated for recalcitrant forms of RS and are used infrequently.

■ Systemic

There is no known cure for RS. The mainstay of medical therapy consists of an aggressive physical therapy program combined with oral nonsteroidal antiinflammatory agents (NSAIDs), primarily indomethacin. Long-term management with NSAIDs is adequate to manage most RS patients with a remitting course. The relatively benign course and episodic nature of this disease do not warrant a more aggressive therapeutic approach. Intralesional steroid injections may be needed on an episodic basis to control local articular inflammation not responding to oral medications. Other treatment options include the use of systemic steroids, cytotoxic agents, and immunosuppressive agents for patients whose symptoms of arthritis are not adequately controlled with conservative measures.

■ Ocular

Palliative therapy is sufficient for most episodes of conjunctival inflammation associated with RS. Lubrication or mild vasoconstrictors can be used during exacerbations of the conjunctivitis. The conjunctivitis should resolve on its own in about 7 days if no medical intervention is instituted. Antibiotic use is not indicated because an infective pathogen is not responsible for the conjunctivitis. The iridocyclitis can be adequately controlled with the use of topical cycloplegic agents and corticosteroids. Chronic topical steroid use may be needed to manage the iridocyclitis in between episodes of significant activity. Subtenon steroid injection may be necessary if progressive ocular tissue damage occurs. Systemic immunosuppressive agents may be used for recalcitrant forms of iridocyclitis. Management of elevated intraocular pressure should be considered as needed on an individual basis. Treatment should be directed toward the anterior chamber reaction and inhibiting aqueous formation, because the etiology of the pressure elevation is related to impaired outflow by inflammatory debris.

When vision is affected, a more aggressive treatment is needed. Cataract extractions for patients with chronic inflammation may improve vision, but residual macular edema may preclude them from attaining a substantial visual improvement.

CONCLUSION

The most striking features of RS include the arthritic predilection for the lower spine, pelvis, and lower extremities in addition to the ocular and mucocutaneous manifestations. Patients with the more aggressive course of RS suffer from arthritis, physical impairment, and ocular inflammation to a greater degree than patients with a remitting course. Thorough patient education regarding the cyclical nature of both the articular and extra-articular features of RS is necessary to minimize patient frustration with this potentially unrelenting disease.

REFERENCES

Csonka GW. Recurrent attacks in Reiter's syndrome. *Arthritis Rheum.* 1960;3:164.

Cush JJ, Lipsky PE. Reiter's syndrome and reactive arthritis. In: McCarty DJ, Koopman WJ, eds. *Arthritis and Allied Conditions.* Philadelphia:Lea & Febiger; 1993:1061.

Fan PT, Yu DTY. Reiter's syndrome. In: Kelley WN, Harris ED, Ruddy S, Sledge CB, eds. *Textbook of Rheumatology.* Philadelphia: Saunders; 1993:961.

Ferry AP. The eye and rheumatic disease. In: Kelley WN, Harris ED, Ruddy S, Sledge CB, eds. *Textbook of Rheumatology* Philadelphia: Saunders; 1993:509.

Fox R, Calin A, Gerber RC, Gibson D. The chronicity of symptoms and disability in Reiter's Syndrome: An analysis of 131 consecutive patients. *Ann Int Med.* 1979;91:190.

Hardin JG, Longenecker GL. Drug therapy of specific rheumatic diseases. In: Hardin JG, Longenecker GL, eds. *Handbook of Drug Therapy in Rheumatic Disease.* Boston: Little, Brown; 1992:175.

Hemady R, Tauber J, Foster CS. Immunosuppressive drugs in immune and inflammatory ocular disease. *Surv Ophthalmol.* 1991;35:369.

Lally EV, Ho G. A review of methotrexate therapy in Reiter's syndrome. *Semin Arthritis Rheum.* 1985;15:139.

Lee DA, Barker SM, Su WPD, et al. The clinical diagnosis of Reiters syndrome: Ophthalmic and nonophthalmic aspects. *Ophthalmology.* 1986;93:350.

Noer HR. An "experimental" epidemic of Reiter's syndrome. *JAMA.* 1966;198:693.

Paronen I. Reiter's Disease: A study of 344 cases observed in Finland. *Acta Med Scandanavia.* 1948;131(suppl 212):1.

Rosenbaum JT. Characterization of uveitis associated with spondyloarthritis. *J Rheumatol.* 1989;16:792.

Wakefield D, Penny R. Cell-mediated immune response to chlamydia in anterior uveitis: Role of HLA-B27. *Clin Exp Immunol.* 1983;51:191.

27
Chapter

Systemic Lupus Erythematosus

Lloyd P. Haskes

Systemic lupus erythematosus (SLE) is an idiopathic, multisystemic inflammatory disorder characterized by hyperactivity of the immune system and prominent autoantibody production. Acute periods of disease activity followed by periods of remission are common, giving the disease an unpredictable course. A definite genetic predisposition has been demonstrated, although the full extent remains unknown. Environmental factors also play a role in inducing SLE in genetically predisposed individuals. Systemic manifestations of SLE include cutaneous lesions; arthritis; cardiac, renal, and other major organ disease; and central nervous system (CNS) involvement. Ocular manifestations include retinal involvement, vascular occlusion, neuro-ophthalmological signs, inflammation, and various other disorders.

In addition to classic SLE, several disorders exist that share it clinical features: drug-induced lupus and two cutaneous forms (discoid lupus and subacute cutaneous lupus).

EPIDEMIOLOGY

■ Systemic

The overall prevalence of SLE in the United States has been reported to be between 15 and 50 cases per 100,000 persons (Hahn, 1991). The average annual incidence is estimated to be 1.8 to 7.6 cases per 100,000 persons per year (Hochberg, 1990). Females constitute 80 to 90% of SLE patients. The average age of onset is 30 years, although SLE may occur at any age. African-Americans exhibit a threefold increased frequency and severity of SLE.

■ Ocular

Approximately 20% of SLE patients have ocular manifestations (Steinberg, 1988). Episcleritis/scleritis is seen in 10%, and retinal complications in approximately 5% of lupus patients (Hahn, 1991). Keratoconjunctivitis sicca occurs in approximately 10% of cases (Steinberg,1987).

NATURAL HISTORY

Autoimmune phenomena are the hallmark of SLE. Increased production of autoantibodies occurs. These antibodies react with "self" antigens such as nuclear constituents (eg, DNA, histones, ribonucleoproteins), cytoplasmic components, and cell membrane components (Steinberg, 1987). It is not known exactly what triggers production of these autoantibodies, but the following have been implicated: bacterial and viral infection, parasitic infection, UV light exposure, hormonal abnormalities, genetic predisposition to hyperimmunity, and drugs or food that increase immune activity or decrease suppressor function. The antibody–antigen complexes circulate in the blood and usually deposit on the walls of small vessels in most organ systems of the body.

Increased vascular permeability, smooth venular muscle contraction, and mast cell and basophil degranulation occur due to activation of the complement system. Polymorphonuclear leukocytes and macrophages are drawn to the complex

227

deposit site, resulting in the phagocytosis of the complex and the cells to which it is attached. Lysosomal enzymes, released due to phagocytosis and cell death, cause further inflammation and broad tissue damage. Stresses such as surgery, infections, pregnancy, abortions, and psychological pressures have been known to exacerbate SLE. Female patients with SLE who undergo hysterectomies exhibit improvement of symptoms. This implies that female hormones may play a role in SLE.

■ Systemic

The onset and course of SLE is highly variable. The particular organ system involved varies among patients as will the severity within each organ system. Classically, SLE will include periods of active disease followed by either periods of less intense disease or remissions. The classic presentation of SLE actually occurs in few patients and is characteristically described as affecting young women in their early 30s with a butterfly rash, sun sensitivity, arthritis, fever, fatigue, weight loss, alopecia, and some renal involvement.

The butterfly rash may appear as a mild blush or more severely as an edematous and erythematous rash of both cheeks including the bridge of the nose (Figure 27–1). This rash occurs in approximately 40% of patients and often precedes the other disease manifestations (Stevens, 1988). It may appear without sun exposure but will often be exacerbated by it.

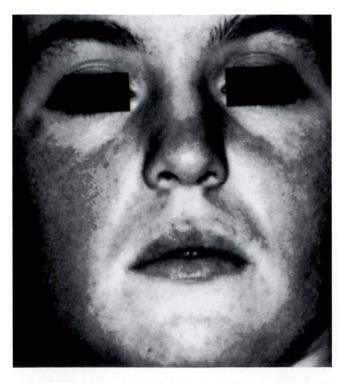

Figure 27–1. Erythematous, slightly edematous, "butterfly" rash typical of SLE. *(Photo courtesy of Machiel Polano, MD, Clinic of Dermatology, University Hospital, Leiden, Netherlands.)*

Behavioral disturbances, ranging from mild anxiety and memory deficits to major psychoses, have been observed in about 35% of cases as a result of CNS involvement (Stevens, 1988).

Renal disease is seen in approximately 40 to 50% of patients and may present clinically as an acute nephritis, nephrotic syndrome, or glomerulonephritis (Spalton, 1990). Patients with drug-induced lupus or lupus-like symptoms rarely exhibit renal or CNS involvement.

A systemic inflammatory disorder that satisfies the traditional criteria for SLE may be induced by a number of drugs. These include chlorpromazine, hydralazine, methyldopa, isoniazid, procainamide, and phenytoin. The manner in which these drugs induce SLE symptoms is poorly understood. The clinical features of drug-induced SLE are usually mild and include arthritis or arthralgia, myalgia, and fever. Lymphadenopathy, renal, and CNS involvement, rarely occur. The symptoms usually resolve once the offending agent is discontinued.

Discoid lupus includes skin lesions not commonly found in SLE patients. These lesions may recur or persist for many years in individuals who never develop multisystem disorders. Occasionally joint pains, mild anemia, and leukopenia may present in the absence of typical SLE findings. Approximately 10% of patients with discoid lesions will develop clinical and laboratory abnormalities characteristic of SLE later in their illness (Stevens, 1988).

Subacute cutaneous lupus differs from discoid lupus in all respects and has less systemic involvement than SLE. The dominant manifestation is intense photosensitivity. Arthritis is found in only 30%, and less than 20% have neurological involvement, nephritis, and hematologic abnormalities (Stevens, 1988).

The majority of SLE patients usually have only one or two signs or symptoms at initial presentation and develop additional symptoms later in the disease course. A myriad of clinical disorders may be encountered in SLE (Table 27–1). Therefore criteria have been developed to aid in establishing a diagnosis of SLE.

The 10-year survival rate now nears 90% (Stevens, 1988). Usually the various manifestations of SLE appear sequentially over a period of years. Remissions are spontaneous or in response to drug therapy. Nephritis with renal failure may occur despite adequate control of other manifestations. When the disease occurs solely in the skin or joints and no major organ involvement occurs, a favorable prognosis is made. In cases of severe involvement of the brain, lungs, heart, or kidney, a poor prognosis is made. Leading causes of death are infections and renal failure.

■ Ocular

SLE produces various ocular complications, which tend to manifest in more acutely ill patients (Table 27–2). SLE retinal vasculopathy is believed to be due to autoimmune

TABLE 27–1. SYSTEMIC MANIFESTATIONS OF SLE

- Constitutional (90%)
  Fatigue, fever, weight loss, anorexia
- Musculoskeletal (90%)
  Arthritis, arthralgia, myalgia
- Cutaneous (80%)
  Butterfly rash, alopecia, photosensitivity, oral ulcers, discoid lupus, Raynaud phenomenon
- Hematologic (80%)
  Anemia, hemolytic anemia, leukopenia, thrombocytopenia, vasculitis
- Central Nervous System (60%)
  Personality disorders, seizures, psychoses, stroke, migraine headaches, pseudotumor cerebri
- Cardiopulmonary (60%)
  Pleurisy, pericarditis, myocarditis, endocarditis
- Renal (50%)
  Proteinuria, nephrotic syndrome, renal failure
- Gastrointestinal (45%)
  Mild pain, diarrhea, abnormal liver enzymes, colitis
- Fetal loss (30%)
- Thrombosis (15%)
  Venous, arterial

TABLE 27–2. OCULAR MANIFESTATIONS OF SLE
(Most common to least common)

- Cornea
  Keratoconjunctivitis sicca, stromal infiltration, ulceration, vascularization, superficial punctate keratitis, marginal infiltrates, pannus formation
- Conjunctiva
  Nonspecific conjunctivitis affecting palpebral and bulbar regions
- Episclera/Sclera
  Scleritis (usually diffuse or nodular)
- Uvea
  Nongranulomatous uveitis
- Vitreous
  Hemorrhage
- Retina
  Vasculitis, including cotton-wool spots, hemorrhages, vascular occlusion (usually arterial), neovascularization, detachment
- Optic Nerve
  Optic neuritis, anterior optic neuropathy, atrophy
- Neuro-ophthalmic
  Cranial nerve palsies with possible diplopia, ptosis, pupil abnormalities; visual field loss, cortical blindness, internuclear ophthalmoplegia, nystagmus, papilledema secondary to pseudotumor cerebri

mechanisms with antigen–antibody complexes deposited in the retinal and choroidal vessel walls (Singerman & Jampol, 1991). Retinal manifestations most commonly found include cotton-wool spots and hemorrhages. Vascular occlusion is uncommon, but if it does occur the arteries are more frequently affected than the veins. Involved arteries will appear thin, sheathed, white, and nonperfused. The resultant retinal nonperfusion and hypoxia may cause neovascularization of the optic nerve head and retina. Vitreous hemorrhage and retinal detachment may also occur. Optic atrophy and blindness may result with severe occlusion.

Scleritis, usually diffuse or nodular, is fairly common and may be a presenting feature of SLE. A nongranulomatous uveitis is sometimes found and appears to be associated with immune reactants in the uveal blood vessels (Singerman & Jampol, 1991). Nonspecific conjunctivitis is another abnormality seen with SLE patients and may affect the bulbar and palpebral regions. Superficial punctate keratitis (SPK) is the most common corneal manifestation of SLE. Occasional corneal manifestations include stromal infiltration, ulceration, and vascularization. In patients with inadequately controlled systemic disease, sicca syndrome is common. Discoid lupus involves skin changes, especially of the face and lid margins. Secondary corneal irritation may result in marginal infiltrates and pannus formation. SPK may also be found in these patients.

CNS involvement can cause neuro-ophthalmic signs and symptoms. Cranial nerve palsies may manifest as diplopia, ptosis, or pupillary abnormalities. Homonymous visual field loss, cortical blindness, internuclear ophthalmoplegia, nystagmus, pseudotumor cerebri, and migraine headaches are other sequelae with CNS involvement (Singerman & Jampol, 1991). Optic nerve involvement may include optic neuritis, anterior ischemic optic neuropathy, and slowly progressive visual loss. Immune complex vasculitis, lupus anticoagulant, and other antiphospholipid antibodies may play a role in the pathogenesis of the neuro-ophthalmic complications (Singerman & Jampol, 1991).

DIAGNOSIS

■ Systemic

A diagnosis of SLE is based on the clinical presentation and laboratory results. In 1982 the American Rheumatological Association established eleven criteria, eight clinical manifestations, and three laboratory investigations in order to assist in the diagnosis of SLE. A minimum of four of the eleven established criteria is suggested to make the diagnosis of SLE (Table 27–3). The four criteria may be present serially or simultaneously during any interval of observation. The most common clinical manifestations include a

TABLE 27–3. DIAGNOSTIC CRITERIA FOR SLE

A minimum of 4 of the 11 criteria is suggested for diagnosis

1. Malar rash. Fixed erythema, flat or raised, over the malar eminences, tending to spare the nasolabial folds.
2. Discoid rash. Eythematous raised patches with adherent keratotic scaling and follicular plugging; atrophic scarring may occur in older lesions.
3. Photosensitivity. Skin rash as a result of unusual reaction to sunlight, by patient history or physician observation.
4. Oral ulcers. Painless oral or nasopharyngeal ulceration, observed by a physician.
5. Arthritis. Nonerosive arthritis involving two or more peripheral joints, characterized by tenderness, swelling, or effusion.
6. Serositis. Pleuritis with convincing history of pleuritic pain or rub heard by physician or evidence of pleural effusion, OR pericarditis documented by electrocardiogram or rub or evidence of pericardial effusion.
7. Renal disorder. Persistent proteinuria, OR cellular casts: may be red cell, hemoglobin, granular, tubular, or mixed.
8. Neurologic disorder. Seizures in the absence of offending drugs or known metabolic derangements, OR psychosis in the absence of offending drugs or known metabolic derangements.
9. Hematologic disorder. Hemolytic anemia, OR leukopenia on two or more occasions, OR lymphopenia on two or more occasions, OR thrombocytopenia in the absence of offending drugs.
10. Immunologic disorder. Positive lupus cell preparation, OR anti-DNA antibody to native DNA in abnormal titer, OR anti-*Sm* antibody to *Sm* nuclear antigen, OR false-positive serologic test for syphilis known to be positive for 6 months and confirmed by *Treponema pallidum* immobilization or fluorescent treponemal-antibody absorption test.
11. Antinuclear antibody. An abnormal titer of antinuclear antibody by immunofluorescence or an equivalent assay at any point in time and in the absence of drugs known to be associated with drug-induced lupus syndrome.

Adapted with permission from Steinberg AD. Systemic lupus erythematosus. In: Wyngaarden JB, Smith LH, eds. Cecil Textbook of Medicine. 18th ed. Philadelphia: Saunders, 1988, p 2011.

butterfly rash, arthritis, fever, fatigue, weight loss, and some renal involvement.

Laboratory investigations are specific for the autoimmune aspect of SLE. The immunofluorescent assay for antinuclear antibodies (ANAs) detects multiple autoantibodies to nuclear constituents (Stevens, 1988). A positive test for ANAs supports the diagnosis of SLE because ANAs are present in 99% of all SLE patients (Steinberg, 1988). This test is not specific because ANAs are present in other collagen vascular diseases. If the patient is ANA negative, SLE can virtually be eliminated. It has been found that 25% of women over the age of 65, about one third of patients with liver disease, and about 5% of the normal population are ANA positive (Rosenberg et al, 1988).

If a patient tests positive for ANAs then a test for serum antibodies to native DNA should be performed. Antibodies to native DNA are present in about 70 to 80% of SLE patients and are rarely seen in patients without SLE

(Roberts & Hughes, 1989; Rosenberg et al, 1988). High serum levels of ANA and anti-DNA usually reflect disease activity, especially in patients with nephritis.

Lupus erythromatosus (LE) cell preparation tests are no longer considered important in confirming the diagnosis of SLE. The test has a low sensitivity and variable specificity and is difficult to perform. The LE cell consists of a phagocytized nucleus. The phagocytosis requires antibodies reactive with DNA–histone and complement.

Hematologic abnormalities may be detected. A mild normochromic normocytic anemia is commonly found, and the patient should be evaluated for iron deficiency. Hemolytic anemia occurs in up to 10% of SLE patients who exhibit a positive Coombs test, which detects autoantibodies directed against red blood cells (Roberts & Hughes, 1989). Leukopenia, as indicated by a decrease in total lymphocytes, occurs in up to 50% of SLE patients, and thrombocytopenia occurs in about one third and may be detected by the presence of antiplatelet antibodies (Meyerhoff, 1983).

Antibodies to coagulation factors may be measured in coagulation abnormalities. Antiphospholipid antibodies are found in 10 to 15% of patients and are known as lupus anticoagulants (Meyerhoff, 1983). They cause a prolonged partial thromboplastin time (PTT) and an increased tendency toward coagulation, which results in recurrent arterial or venous thrombosis and recurrent spontaneous abortions.

Antibodies exist that react with various low-molecular-weight RNA species such as SS-A and SS-B. Anti-Ro (SSA) and Anti-La (SSB) antibodies also are associated with Sjögren syndrome, nephritis, and subacute cutaneous lupus.

A decreased serum complement C_3 level is 90% predictive for SLE, and the simultaneous presence of both a decreased serum C_3 level and native DNA antibodies has been reported to be virtually 100% predictive of SLE (Rosenberg et al, 1988). Decreased serum C_3 levels result from activation and consumption of complement components.

■ Ocular

Ocular examination, including a thorough history, visual acuity examination, external examination, and anterior and dilated posterior segment evaluations, are crucial for revealing any ocular involvement.

Fluorescein angiography may exhibit arterial and capillary nonperfusion in patients with retinal vasculopathy, with neovascular leakage and staining of the involved vessels. There also may be vascular incompetence and fluorescein leakage in patients with apparently normal funduscopic appearance.

TREATMENT AND MANAGEMENT

■ Systemic

A cure for SLE does not exist. Patients with SLE require much rest and should avoid stress in order to minimize exacerbation of the disease. Ultraviolet light should be avoided as it too is associated with disease flare-ups.

Medical management involves four major classes of drugs (Table 27–4). Salicylates and nonsteroidal antiinflammatory drugs (NSAIDs) are employed to treat the arthralgias, arthritis, myalgias, and fever in the 20 to 30% of patients who have mild disease with no life-threatening manifestations (Hahn, 1991).

Antimalarials, such as hydroxychloroquine (Plaquenil), are employed in an attempt to treat the discoid skin lesions and rheumatic sequelae (joint disease) of SLE.

High-dose, short-acting corticosteroids, such as prednisone or methylprednisolone, are used in life-threatening and severely disabling cases of SLE. These include active involvement of the kidneys, skeletal muscle, myocardium, and CNS, as well as hemolytic anemia, thrombocytopenia, and intravascular clotting (Stevens, 1988). Usually, prolonged maintenance at low dosages (less than 30 mg per day) is needed to prevent recurrence of symptoms.

Cytotoxic agents (azathioprine, chlorambucil, cyclophosphamide) are controversal in the treatment of SLE nephritis. These agents are employed when steroids are not effective or the dosage level cannot be tolerated in treating major organ inflammation.

■ Ocular

Patients receiving more than 200 mg/day of Plaquenil may develop a pigmentary retinal degeneration and/or corneal changes. This irreversible retinal disturbance is also known as bull's-eye retinopathy because it appears first in the macula. The retinopathy usually occurs after 2 to 3 years of therapy. The most common initial symptom is a decrease in visual acuity. Color vision defects and visual field defects may occur before loss of visual acuity. Visual field changes include central and paracentral scotomas and peripheral defects. These patients should be monitored every 6 months with visual acuity, color vision, and central (Amsler grid) and peripheral visual field testing

Reversible corneal changes, which include edema and a whorl-like pigmentary deposit in the epithelium, may occur after only 2 to 3 weeks of therapy with 200 mg or more of Plaquenil. The corneal changes may cause a complaint of halos around lights that cease with drug discontinuation.

Glaucoma and posterior subcapsular cataracts are ocular complications of steroidal therapy. The cataracts occur in patients taking 15 mg or more for 2 years or more. These patients should be monitored every 3 months, with careful attention to intraocular pressures and a dilated lenticular evaluation.

Retinal vascular occlusive disease and its consequences are treated using conventional therapy. Laser photocoagulation for retinal neovascularization, vitrectomies and scleral buckling for vitreal hemorrhages, and retinal detachment are employed. Topical steroidal drops may be employed along with cycloplegics for an SLE-related uveitis.

Lubricating ophthalmic drops and ointments may be used for any keratoconjunctivitis sicca symptoms.

CONCLUSION

SLE is a multisystemic disease with potentially devastating complications. The exact etiology has yet to be firmly established, but an autoimmune disruption or malfunction clearly exists. Despite the host of systemic signs and symptoms that may exist, diagnosis may initially be difficult or delayed, because the average new SLE patient presents with only a few symptoms. These symptoms may not occur at once but can present sequentially, further delaying the diagnosis of SLE.

The ocular manifestations are sometimes presenting features of the disease. Therefore, a knowledgeable eyecare provider may aid in the prompt diagnosis, treatment, and management of SLE. The continued involvement of an eyecare provider is crucial to guard against the potential for ocular side effects secondary to systemic treatment protocols,

TABLE 27–4. TREATMENT AND MANAGEMENT OF SLE

■ Systemic
LIFE STYLE ADJUSTMENTS
- Stress avoidance
- Rest
- Avoidance of ultraviolet light

MEDICAL MANAGEMENT
- **Salicylates and NSAIDs**
  For treatment of arthralgias, arthritis, myalgia, fever
- **Antimalarials (hydroxychloroquine [Plaquenil] 200–600 mg/d)**
  For treatment of discoid skin lesions and rheumatic sequelae
- **Corticosteroids (prednisone or methylprednisolone)**
  For treatment of life-threatening cases of renal involvement, myocardial involvement, CNS involvement
- **Cytotoxic agents (azathioprine, chlorambucil, cyclophosphamide)**
  Employed when corticosteroids are not indicated for treatment of nephritis

■ Ocular
- Laser photocoagulation for retinal neovascularization
- Vitrectomies for vitreous hemorrhage
- Scleral buckling for retinal detachment
- Dry eye therapy for keratitis sicca symptoms
- Topical corticosteroids and cycloplegic agents for uveitis

as well as to monitor the patient for further ocular manifestations of this disease.

REFERENCES

Hahn BH. Systemic lupus erythematosus. In: Wilson JD, Braunwald E, Isselbacher KJ, Petersdorf RG, et al, eds. *Harrison's Principles of Internal Medicine.* 12th ed. New York: McGraw-Hill; 1991:1432–1437.

Hochberg MC. Systemic lupus erythematosus. *Rheum Dis Clin North Am.* 1990;16:617–639.

Meyerhoff J. Systemic lupus erythematosus, 6. Hematologic and serologic abnormalities. *Md State Med J.* 1983;32:935–939.

Roberts DM, Hughes WM. Systemic lupus erythematosus: How to manage this chronic, complicated disorder. *Postgrad Med.* 1989;86:191–200.

Rosenberg SA, Blaiss MS, Springgate CF. Emerging therapies for autoimmune disease, such as systemic lupus erythematosus. *Modern Med.* 1988;56:44–47.

Singerman LJ, Jampol LM. *Retinal and Choroidal Manifestations of Systemic Disease.* Baltimore: Williams & Wilkins; 1991:6–15.

Spalton DJ. Systemic lupus erythematosus. In: Gold DH, Weingeist TA, eds. *The Eye in Systemic Disease.* Philadelphia: Lippincott; 1990:72–74.

Steinberg AD. Systemic lupus erythematosus. In: Wyngaarden JB, Smith LH, eds. *Cecil Textbook of Medicine.* 18th ed. Philadelphia: Saunders; 1988:2011–2018.

Steinberg AD. Systemic lupus erythematosus. *Hospital Med.* August 1987;24–46.

Stevens MB. Systemic lupus erythematosus. In: Harvey AM, Johns RJ, McKusick VA, Owens Jr AH, Ross RS, eds. *The Principles and Practice of Medicine.* 22nd ed. Norwalk, CT: Appleton & Lange; 1988:494–500.

28
Chapter

Polymyalgia Rheumatica

Lloyd P. Haskes

Polymyalgia rheumatica (PMR) is a syndrome characterized by pain and stiffness in the shoulders, pelvic girdle musculature, and torso. A poorly understood relationship exists between PMR and giant-cell arteritis (GCA), an inflammatory condition of medium and large arteries. Both disorders often occur together or at different times in the same population. It has been suggested that PMR and GCA represent a variable expression of the same disorder. In those with PMR and GCA, severe visual disturbance and blindness may occur.

EPIDEMIOLOGY

■ Systemic

PMR almost always occurs in patients over age 50, with the mean age of onset approximately 70 years. The prevalence in persons over age 50 is about 1 in 100, and the annual incidence is close to 1 in 2000 (Chuang et al, 1982). Women are affected 2.5 times more often than men (Healey, 1988). A genetic predisposition is suggested by the greater incidence among Caucasians, within families, and the association with HLA haplotypes.

When PMR initially occurs alone, 10 to 50% of patients will develop GCA. Forty-one to 44% of all polymyalgia cases will have a positive temporal artery biopsy whether or not arteritic signs or symptoms exist (Fauchald et al, 1972). In a population-based study in Sweden, positive biopsies ranged from 31% in PMR alone to 87% in PMR with GCA symptoms (Bengtsson & Malmvall, 1981).

■ Ocular

When associated with GCA, patients with PMR run the same risk of developing ocular manifestations as patients with GCA only (about 50% have ocular symptoms).

NATURAL HISTORY

■ Systemic

No infectious agent, environmental factor, toxin, or drug has been identified as the definitive cause of PMR. The disease usually presents gradually over a number of weeks but occasionally may be sudden in onset. Symptoms include pain and morning stiffness in the neck, shoulders, lumbar area, and thighs. The stiffness often subsides as the day progresses. The neck and shoulder muscles are initially affected, with the symptoms becoming bilateral and symmetric (Table 28–1).

Fatigue, anorexia, weight loss, and low-grade fever are common and may be presenting complaints. Despite the severity of complaints, physical examination reveals little and muscle strength is normal. The cause of the severe musculoskeletal pain is unclear but it has been attributed to muscular or arterial inflammation. Resolution of the disease may occur naturally over the course of several months but may extend up to 10 years.

Vision may be affected if this disease coexists with or is followed by GCA. It is not known whether PMR patients with a negative temporal artery biopsy represent an earlier or milder form of the same disease as biopsy-positive PMR patients. PMR may occur before or after the onset of GCA.

TABLE 28–1. SYSTEMIC MANIFESTATIONS OF PMR

- Muscle pain and stiffness in at least two of the following muscle groups: shoulders, neck, back, upper arms, thighs
- Normal muscle strength
- Erythrocyte sedimentation rate (Westergren) > 50 mm/hr
- Low-grade fever
- Malaise
- Weight loss
- Possible associated GCA

TABLE 28–2. OCULAR MANIFESTATIONS OF PMR

PURE PMR
- No ocular manifestations

PMR WITH GCA
- Transient visual loss
- Anterior ischemic optic neuropathy (AION) leading to vision loss
- Diplopia (usually transient due to ischemia of the extraocular muscles)

Some consider PMR and GCA to be a single entity termed polymyalgia arteritica.

In most cases PMR/GCA is a self-limited disease. The statistical survival rate for these patients is usually favorable. The overall mortality is no different than that of the general population.

■ Ocular

Ocular involvement with severe visual consequences results from anterior ischemic optic neuropathy (AION) secondary to the GCA. Ocular manifestations will not appear in PMR patients unless GCA is also present (Table 28–2).

DIAGNOSIS

■ Systemic

Currently there are no diagnostic tests to confirm the diagnosis of PMR. It is a diagnosis of exclusion because muscle pain, stiffness, and an elevated erythrocyte sedimentation rate (ESR) may occur with other disorders. The differential diagnosis includes polymyositis, systemic lupus erythematosis, dermatomyositis, rheumatoid arthritis, neoplasms, and infections (Stander, 1989).

The final diagnosis of PMR is based on the symptoms of aching and morning stiffness in at least two of the following muscle groups: neck, shoulder, and pelvic girdles. An elevated ESR is also present, usually greater than 50 mm/hr by the Westergren method, averaging 70 to 80 mm/hr (Chuang et al, 1982). Occasionally, the ESR may exceed 100 mm/hr. A good correlation exists between disease activity and ESR. Temporal artery biopsies should be obtained if coexisting GCA is suspected. In addition to the variable frequency of positive biopsy in PMR cases, a major hindrance in the evaluation of the PMR/GCA association has been the lack of uniformity in temporal artery biopsy technique.

■ Ocular

If PMR occurs without GCA then no ocular manifestations will be present. Ocular signs and symptoms emerge when

PMR occurs along with GCA. The most common ocular manifestation is an AION diagnosed by its clinical presentation of decreased visual acuity, afferent pupillary defect, altitudinal visual field loss, and edematous optic nerve head, with disc hemorrhages and cotton-wool spots.

TREATMENT AND MANAGEMENT

■ Systemic

PMR responds well and rapidly to low-dose corticosteroid therapy (Table 28–3). A higher dose may be required initially in those with arteritic involvement. Daily dosages of oral prednisone may provide dramatic relief of symptoms in pure PMR within 24 hours. If a 50% improvement in symptoms is not seen within 48 hours of initiation of steroid therapy, another diagnosis should be considered. The ESR usually returns to normal after about a month of therapy. A low daily maintenance dose of oral prednisone may be required for approximately 2 years.

Nonsteroidal antiinflammatory drugs (NSAIDs) have been used in early or mild PMR in an attempt to alleviate the musculoskeletal pain and systemic symptoms. However, the adequacy of NSAIDs alone is controversial. Antimalarial and cytotoxic agents have also been employed

TABLE 28–3. TREATMENT AND MANAGEMENT OF PMR

- Prednisone:
    10-15mg po daily (20-30 mg po daily if arteritic involvement suspected)
    Daily maintenance dose of 2.5-7.5 mg for 2 years after symptoms resolve
- NSAIDs
    Used in cases of early or mild PMR to alleviate systemic symptoms
    Usage of this drug class alone is controversial
- Antimalarial / cytotoxic agents:
    Exhibit some success where steroids are contra indicated and other therapy fails

with some success when steroids are contraindicated or when severe side effects occurred, as well as in cases of therapeutic failure.

■ Ocular

No ocular treatment is necessary in pure PMR as there is no ocular involvement. When PMR occurs with GCA, the systemic corticosteroid treatment (with slow tapering to prevent relapse) is all that is necessary to treat ocular manifestations.

CONCLUSION

PMR is a disorder that affects specific muscle groups. The diagnosis is one of exclusion, as its symptoms of muscle stiffness and aching are common to several other diseases. PMR is strongly associated with GCA. Therefore, any case of PMR must be further investigated for the possible presence of GCA, and vice versa. Thus, any patient with presumed PMR also must be examined for possible ocular complications secondary to GCA.

REFERENCES

Bengtsson BA, Malmvall BE. The epidemiology of giant cell arteritis including temporal arteritis and polymyalgia rheumatica. *Arthritis Rheum.* 1981;24:899.

Chuang TY, Hunder GG, Ilstruo DM, et al. Polymyalgia rheumatica: A 10-year epidemiologic and clinical study. *Ann Intern Med.* 1982;97:672–680.

Fauchald P, Rygvold O, Oystese B, et al. Temporal arteritis and polymyalgia rheumatica: Clinical and biopsy findings. *Ann Intern Med.* 1972;77:845.

Healey LA. Polymyalgia rheumatica and giant cell arteritis. In: Wyngaarden JB, Smith LH, eds. *Cecil Textbook of Medicine.* 18th ed. Philadelphia: Saunders; 1988:2033.

Stander PE. Polymyalgia rheumatica: Clinical features and management. *Postgrad Med.* 1989;86:131–138.

29
Chapter

Giant-cell Arteritis

Lloyd P. Haskes ■ William J. Tullo

Hutchinson, in 1890, described "thrombotic arteritis" in which a man with "painful red temples" was unable to wear his hat. Nearly 50 years later in 1938, Jennings described blindness and other visual complications associated with this disease, then called temporal arteritis.

Giant-cell arteritis (GCA), also known as temporal arteritis or cranial arteritis, is now known to be a multisystemic inflammatory condition of medium and large arteries common in older patients. Although arteries throughout the body may be affected, there is a predilection for the cranial arteries. If untreated, this disease may result in catastrophic vision loss due to involvement of the posterior ciliary arteries. Interestingly, over 50% of GCA patients develop a syndrome called polymyalgia rheumatica (PMR) characterized by pain and stiffness in the shoulders, pelvic girdle musculature, and torso. Conversely, 20 to 40% of patients with PMR also have GCA (Goodman, 1979).

EPIDEMIOLOGY

■ Systemic
GCA usually occurs between the ages of 50 and 85, with an average age of onset of 70 (Troost, 1992). As the average age of the population increases, so does the incidence of this disease. The incidence reported in the literature is quite variable. In Olmstead County, Minnesota between 1950 and 1985, the incidence of GCA was reported to be 17 per 100,000 in the population aged 50 years and older (Machado et al, 1988). The incidence increased from 2.6 per 100,000 aged 50 to 59 years, to 44.7 per 100,000 aged 80 and above. GCA is found predominately in Caucasians, and is more common in women than men.

■ Ocular
Visual symptoms occur in approximately 50% of cases, with the most common complaint being sudden complete monocular vision loss. Transient monocular blindness and scintillating scotomas are important prodromal symptoms in 2 to 19% of GCA patients (Goodman, 1979). The complete vision loss is a result of anterior ischemic optic neuropathy (AION) due to arteritic involvement of the posterior ciliary arteries. Inferior altitudinal visual field loss is present in 70 to 80% of these patients (Ishak et al, 1988).

One percent of vision loss is secondary to central retinal artery occlusion, and it has been noted that 10% of central retinal artery occlusions are secondary to GCA (Cullen, 1967; Wagener & Hollenhorst, 1958). Fifty to seventy-five percent of GCA patients with unilateral ocular involvement will proceed to bilateral involvement, usually in 1 to 10 days, if there is no therapeutic intervention (Crawford, 1990).

NATURAL HISTORY

■ Systemic
The exact etiology of GCA is unknown, but an immunologic mechanism may be involved. GCA is an inflammatory

condition of the medium and large arteries with a distinct elastica in which all layers of the blood vessel are involved. Electron microscopy shows very early damage to the smooth muscle cells. Persistent inflammation causes segmental fragmentation of the elastic lamina, swollen endothelium, smooth muscle necrosis, and cellular infiltration with lymphocytes, giant cells, and epithelioid cells. Fibrosis, hyalin thickening, and thrombosis are found with eventual vessel occlusion. The lack of an internal elastic lamina in small vessels is postulated to protect them from involvement in GCA. A similar histological mechanism is found in PMR.

GCA most often affects the temporal and occipital arteries. The ophthalmic artery, posterior ciliary arteries, and central retinal artery are also affected. Less commonly, the aorta, coronary, subclavian, femoral, radial, cerebral, coronary, hepatic, renal, mesenteric, and iliac arteries may be affected.

The most common initial symptoms of GCA are headache, jaw claudication, low-grade fever, and weight loss. The headache may be temporal, frontal, or occipital, and is pulseless. The onset of the headache is gradual and then becomes diffuse, more severe, and more insistent. The headache is often worse at night, and may be aggravated by cold temperature. The involved temporal artery is often tortuous, nodular, red, and tender (Figure 29–1). The temporal artery and scalp may be so tender that the patient is unable to comb his or her hair, wear a hat, or sleep using a pillow.

A classic systemic sign is a significant elevation in the erythrocyte sedimentation rate. Other systemic signs and symptoms are listed in Table 29–1. The systemic sequelae of the disease, if left untreated, include myocardial infarction, stroke, ruptured aortic aneurysm, PMR, and psychosis. Few deaths are reported secondary to GCA. Most are secondary to lack of treatment. GCA patients improve rapidly, both symptomatically and clinically, after initiation of treatment.

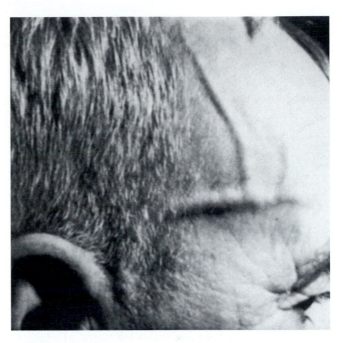

Figure 29–1. Temporal arteritis with typical appearance of the swollen, tender, inflamed temporal artery with involvement of both the anterior and posterior branches *(Reprinted with permission from Healey LA, Wilske KR:* The Systemic Manifestations of Temporal Arteritis. *New York: Grune & Stratton, 1978).*

■ Ocular

Ocular symptoms usually occur several weeks to months after the onset of systemic symptoms. The posterior ciliary arteries, ophthalmic artery, and central retinal artery may become involved, resulting in ischemia to the optic nerve, ciliary ganglion, and retina. The classic ocular manifestation is an acute AION, characterized by a pale swollen optic disc with disc and peripapillary retinal hemorrhages and cotton-wool spots, an afferent pupillary defect, and altitudinal visual field loss. Other, rarer findings may also occur (Table 29-2).

TABLE 29–1. SYSTEMIC MANIFESTATIONS OF GCA

- Elevated ESR
- Headache
- Jaw claudication
- Prominent and tender temporal artery
- Tender scalp
- Malaise
- Weakness
- Anorexia
- Fever
- Vertigo
- Deafness
- Nausea
- Abnormal sensation of taste and smell
- Abdominal pain
- Associated PMR

TABLE 29–2. OCULAR MANIFESTATIONS OF GCA

- Anterior ischemic optic neuropathy (AION)
    - Decreased visual acuity
    - Afferent pupillary defect
    - Altitudinal visual field defect
    - Reduced color vision
    - Disc edema
    - Peripapillary retinal hemorrhages
    - Cotton-wool spots
- Diplopia secondary to third and sixth cranial nerve palsies
- Central retinal artery occlusion
- Ocular pain
- Cortical blindness secondary to occipital lobe infarction
- Rubeosis irides and secondary glaucoma

Episodes of transient visual disturbance may precede vision loss. Sudden, persistent visual loss is most often secondary to severe AION (Figure 29–2). Total blindness may occur. The other eye may become involved one day to several weeks after the initial onset of visual symptoms. Visual disturbances are unusual in the absence of systemic signs of

GCA. After resolution of the AION, the affected nerve will retain temporal disc pallor along with a residual altitudinal field loss and afferent pupillary defect.

DIAGNOSIS

■ Systemic

The diagnosis of GCA is made primarily from the patient history, physical signs, and symptoms. Clinical diagnosis is usually established by the dramatic elevation of the erythrocyte sedimentation rate (ESR 80 to 100 mm/hr by the Westergren method), and a positive temporal artery biopsy. However, 2% of patients with positive temporal artery biopsies will have a normal ESR (Healey & Wilske, 1978).

The ESR is normally higher in females than in males, and increases with age. A general rule of thumb for normal ESR determination by the Westergren method is as follows: Normal male ESR $\leq$ (age in years) / 2; normal female ESR $\leq$ (age in years + 10) / 2 (Miller & Green, 1983).

Laboratory testing should also include a complete blood count with differential to rule out any other systemic diseases. The levels of alpha 2-globulin and fibrinogen are also commonly elevated, and there is an increased incidence of human leukocyte antigens (HLA) B8 and B10 in GCA.

Biopsy of the temporal artery provides the most reliable diagnostic information and valuable insight regarding treatment effectivity. A positive biopsy confirms the presence of GCA. However, a negative biopsy does not rule out the possibility of GCA. The biopsied artery should be 2.5 cm or greater in length in order to avoid the possibility of only biopsying a skip area. These skip lesions (areas of normal artery in between diseased artery) exist in 28% of GCA patients (Klein et al, 1976). According to Hall and associates (1983), a properly performed and analyzed temporal artery biopsy will result in a correct diagnosis in 94% of cases. If negative, many practitioners biopsy the contralateral artery. However, the presence of giant cells is not necessary to make the diagnosis.

■ Ocular

Optic nerve involvement secondary to an AION may be diagnosed by the presence of an afferent pupillary defect, altitudinal visual field loss, and decreased visual acuity. The optic nerve may be edematous, with peripapillary retinal hemorrhages and cotton-wool spots. Fluorescein angiography may also be useful in determining the extent of ischemia to the optic nerve head. Electroretinogram, although usually not performed, often exhibits an extremely large a-wave in both affected and normal eyes. Normal a-wave returns with therapy.

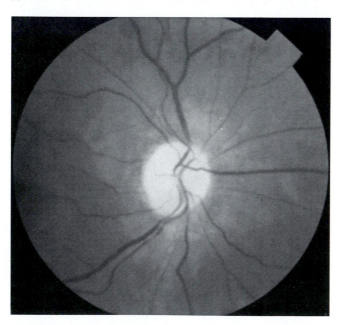

Figure 29–2. A. Acute anterior ischemic optic neuropathy secondary to GCA. Note the elevation of the nerve head with blurred disc margins and adjacent flame hemorrhages. **B.** Atrophic appearance of the same nerve head several months later. (*Courtesy of Jerome Sherman, OD.*)

TREATMENT AND MANAGEMENT

■ Systemic

Corticosteroids are the mainstay of GCA treatment (Table 29–3). A baseline ESR should be ordered, and if elevated, a temporal artery biopsy should be considered. If the patient is seen within 36 hours of onset of symptoms, steroid therapy involves intravenous methylprednisolone for several days. After 5 days, another ESR is obtained to determine the effectiveness of treatment. Other standard therapy involves oral prednisone. As the ESR declines, dosage is reduced daily. A low maintenance dose is usually continued for 9 to 12 months, after which the patient is regularly monitored. Common systemic side effects of steroid therapy are fluid retention, hypertension, peptic ulcer (with possible perforation and hemorrhage), facial erythema, diabetes, and cushingoid state. Immunosuppressive agents have little effect in this disease.

■ Ocular

Ocular therapy is simply systemic therapy. The primary goal of therapy is to prevent vision loss in the fellow eye. If the acute vision loss is less than 36 hours old, pulsed steroid therapy may significantly improve vision. The addition of a retrobulbar depot steroid injection may help resolve the acute ocular involvement. Usually, a negative response to steroid treatment suggests an incorrect diagnosis of GCA. However, some cases of GCA may unfortunately progress to total bilateral vision loss despite steroid therapy. Ocular side effects due to steroid therapy include glaucoma and posterior subcapsular cataracts.

CONCLUSION

GCA is a systemic disease characterized by an inflammatory obliterative arteritis. Any patient over the age of 50 years who presents with acute onset of anterior ischemic optic neuropathy, diplopia, or central retinal artery occlusion should have an ESR obtained to rule out GCA. Due to the dramatic effect of steroids in preventing involvement of the other eye, treatment with systemic steroids should begin immediately upon suspicion of GCA. Unfortunately, GCA is one of the most frequently misdiagnosed extraocular causes of preventable vision loss.

REFERENCES

Crawford JB. Cranial arteritis. In: Gold DH, Weingeist TA, eds. *The Eye in Systemic Disease*. Philadelphia: Lippincott; 1990:45–48.

Cullen JF. Occult temporal arteritis: A common cause of blindness in old age. *Br J Ophthalmol*. 1967;51:513–525.

Goodman BW. Temporal arteritis. *Am J Med*. 1979;67:839–852.

Hall S, Lie JT, Kurland LT, et al. The therapeutic impact of temporal artery biopsy. *Lancet*. 1983;2:1217–1220.

Healey LA, Wilske KR. *The Systemic Manifestations of Temporal Arteritis*. New York: Grune & Stratton; 1978:119–120.

Hutchinson J. Diseases of the arteries. *Arch Surg* (Lond). 1890;1: 323–329.

Ishak AW, Persak GC, Mitchell PC, Warwick S. Giant cell arteritis. *J Am Optom Assoc*. 1988;59:864–868.

Klein RG, Campbell RJ, Hunder GG, Carney JA. Skip lesions in temporal arteritis. *Mayo Clinic Proc*. 1976;51:504–510.

Machado EBV, Michet CJ, Ballard DJ, et al. Trends in incidence and clinical presentation of temporal arteritis in Olmstead County, Minnesota, 1950–1985. *Arthritis Rheum*. 1988;31:745–749.

Miller A, Green M. Simple rule for calculating normal erythrocyte sedimentation rate. *Br Med J*. 1983;286:266.

Troost BT. Migraine and other headaches. In: Tasman W, Jaeger EA, eds. *Duane's Clinical Ophthalmology*. Philadelphia: Lippincott; 1992;2:1–30.

Wagener HP, Hollenhorst RW. The ocular lesions of temporal arteritis. *Am J Ophthalmol*. 1958;45:617–630.

TABLE 29–3. TREATMENT AND MANAGEMENT OF GCA

- Baseline ESR and temporal artery biopsy if ESR is elevated
- Methylprednisolone (1 g IV bid × 5 days; if ESR declines, switch to 80 mg PO; taper by 10–20 mg daily as ESR continues to decline)

  OR

- Prednisone (100 mg PO; taper by 10 mg daily as ESR declines)

  THEN

- Low maintenance dose for 9–12 months

30
Chapter

Polyarteritis Nodosa

Michael A. Chaglasian

Polyarteritis nodosa (PAN) is a systemic condition characterized by inflammation of small- and medium-sized arteries. Although the specific cause of this disease is unknown, it is likely to have both immunologic and allergic origins.

Polyarteritis is classified as a systemic necrotizing vasculitis with greatest similarity to allergic angiitis and granulomatosis (Churg–Strauss syndrome), and polyangiitis syndrome. All these vasculitic syndromes are characterized by inflammation and damage to blood vessels. Classic immune-complex-mediated mechanisms are the primary pathogenesis. Single or multiple organ systems may be involved.

Rheumatoid arthritis, Sjögren syndrome, mixed cryoglobulinemia, and hairy-cell leukemia are associated with PAN. More significantly, approximately 10% of patients with PAN will be hepatitis-B-antigen positive. This is the only good link between PAN and specific antigen–antibody complexes (Michalak,1978). Vasculitis may precede, occur simultaneously with, or follow clinical hepatitis.

This immune-complex vasculitis may affect the medium to small arteries of any organ system. Most significantly affected are the kidney, heart, skin, liver, and gastrointestinal tract. Because patient symptoms are often vague, nonspecific, and may involve several organ systems, initial diagnosis is often difficult or delayed.

Ocular complications are a direct consequence of the vasculitis, and thus will vary depending on which ocular vessels become involved. In general, ocular manifestations are rare.

EPIDEMIOLOGY

■ Systemic
PAN is an uncommon disease with an incidence of only 0.9 per 100,000 and a prevalence of 6.3 per 100,000, as detected in a study in Rochester, Minnesota. The onset is usually by the fourth or fifth decades. Males have been noted to have twice the incidence of females (Kurland et al, 1984).

■ Ocular
A 1951 study reported ocular involvement in 10 to 20% of patients (Stillerman). No later study has demonstrated a higher incidence, but ocular signs may frequently go unde-

tected because of the widespread systemic manifestations. Almost every tissue can become involved (Gold, 1980).

NATURAL HISTORY

■ Systemic
Pathological examination of patients affected with PAN demonstrate focal, panmural necrotizing inflammatory lesions in the small- to medium-sized arteries. Inflammation is characterized by fibrinous necrosis and pleomorphic cellular infiltration, generally with polymorphonuclear leukocytes. The lesion site may show aneurysm dilation with thrombosis. Occlusion of the arterial lumen may occur after

the lesion has healed, due to proliferation of fibrous tissue and endothelial cells.

In 1975, Sams and co-workers first demonstrated the presence of immunoglobulin deposits in blood vessels of patients with polyarteritis. This established a potential immune–allergic mechanism for polyarteritis and related vasculitic diseases. More recently, Purcell and associates (1984) identified IgM, IgG, and complement within the arterioles of conjunctival and skin lesions of a patient with iritis secondary to polyarteritis.

Although there is no specific set of symptoms for all patients, fever, malaise, and weight loss are generally among the presenting complaints. Progressive organ involvement leads to the more dramatic clinical manifestations of skin rash, peripheral neuropathy, abdominal pain, renal disease, and polyarteritis (Table 30–1).

Oster nodules are painful, purple (hemorrhagic) cutaneous nodules that appear throughout the body in association with vasculitis (Figure 30–1). Other cutaneous lesions include painful, ecchymotic digital tip infarctions and palpable purpura. As many as 50% of patients will have an asymmetric, episodic polyarteritis (Cohen et al, 1980). Between 70 and 80% of patients will manifest kidney involvement with proteinuria and renal sediment (Ralston & Kvale, 1949). Segmental necrotizing glomerulonephritis is responsible for progressive renal insufficiency. Hypertension develops in 25% of patients and may lead to congestive heart failure or death. Gastrointestinal disturbances include abdominal pain correlating with the involved organ. Patients with cardiac complications are usually asymptomatic. Congestive heart failure may develop as a result of coronary insufficiency and hypertension.

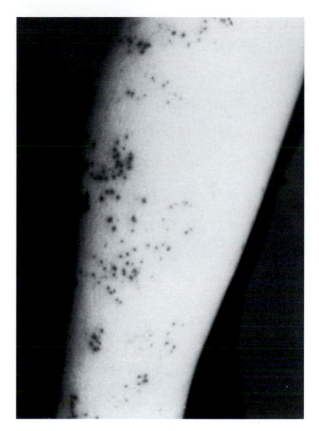

Figure 30–1. Cutaneous inflammatory nodules secondary to necrotizing vasculitis. *(Courtesy of Scott I.M. Lim, DO.)*

Untreated cases of PAN have a very poor prognosis, with a survival rate of approximately 13%. With corticosteroid therapy, the 4-year survival rate increases to 50%. Many of the deaths from this disease occur within the first year of diagnosis.

■ Ocular

As stated previously, ocular involvement in PAN will vary, depending on the specific location of involved vessels. There are no published data as to which tissue is most frequently affected, although posterior segment disease is most commonly reported in the literature. Anterior segment complications include conjunctival chemosis and hemorrhages, iridocyclitis, episcleritis, and scleritis (Table 30–2).

Retinopathy associated with PAN may be characterized as "ischemic" in appearance (Figure 30–2). Typically there is a mixture of cotton-wool spots, marked irregular caliber of vessels, arterial occlusion, retinal and subhyaloid hemorrhage, and exudates. The etiology of this retinal picture may be a direct manifestation of vasculitis, secondary to severe hypertension, or both (Wise, 1952). The most frequently affected posterior structures are the posterior ciliary arteries and choroidal vessels. Choroidal vasculitis is very common (Morgan et al, 1986). Central retinal artery occlu-

TABLE 30–1. SYSTEMIC MANIFESTATIONS OF PAN

SIGNS AND SYMPTOMS
- Fever
- Weight loss
- Malaise
- Headache
- Abdominal pain
- Myalgia
- Hypertension
- Rash, digital-tip infarction
- Oster nodules

ORGAN SYSTEMS AFFECTED
- Kidneys
- Heart
- Skin
- CNS
- Liver
- Peripheral nerves
- Gastrointestinal
- Skeletal muscle

TABLE 30–2. OCULAR MANIFESTATIONS OF PAN

- Photophobia
- Conjunctival hyperemia
- Conjunctival inflammation
- Extraocular muscle palsy
- Diplopia
- Exophthalmos
- Iridocycilitis
- Scleritis
- Intraocular pain
- Decreased visual acuity
- Papilledema
- Ischemic optic neuropathy
- Ischemic retinopathy
- Choroidal vasculitis

sion is not uncommon. Arteritis and phlebitis are well-demonstrated with fluorescein angiography.

Isolated cases of optic nerve involvement and fibrinous iridocyclitis have been reported and may precipitate ischemic optic neuropathy, disc edema, and hemorrhages. Exophthalmos may be noted as a consequence of orbital vessel inflammation (Van Wein & Merz, 1963). When scleral vessels become involved, patients may demonstrate a necrotizing scleritis and/or a sclerokeratitis (Moore & Sevel, 1966). It is also important to be aware of the possibility of a PAN-like vasculitis in patients with Cogan syndrome (nonsyphilitic keratitis and nerve deafness).

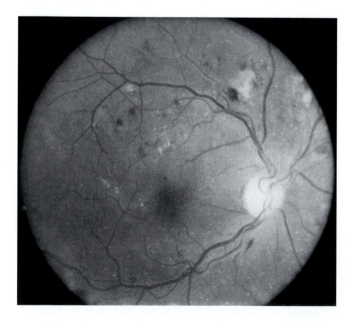

Figure 30–2. Ischemic retinopathy typical of polyarteritis nodosa. *(Courtesy of Scott I.M. Lim, DO.)*

DIAGNOSIS

■ Systemic

The results of laboratory tests for a suspected case of PAN are generally nonspecific, reflecting diffuse systemic inflammation. Abnormal findings may include an elevated erythrocyte sedimentation rate, normochromic anemia, decreased serum albumin, and thrombocytosis. Neutrophilic leukocytosis and increased globulins may also be found. Mild to moderate eosinophilia may be encountered. Urinalysis shows protein and red-cell casts. Diminished serum complement should also be screened for in patients with a cutaneous vasculitis.

Biopsy of involved tissue will more definitively prove vascular inflammation and should be considered whenever possible. Abdominal arteriography will demonstrate characteristic small and large aneurysms with focal constrictions between dilated segments along arterioles.

■ Ocular

Ocular diagnosis is made based on clinical examination, generally following a systemic diagnosis. Thorough slit lamp and dilated fundoscopic examination is obviously recommended for patients presenting with any of the symptoms of PAN. Intravenous fluorescein angiography is useful for clarifying the amount of retinal ischemia by identifying areas of capillary nonperfusion, although this is not specifically diagnostic of PAN. Angiography may also show staining and hyperflouorescence of the walls of inflamed arterial and venule segments. Delayed choroidal filling can also be seen. For patients presenting with decreased vision or any of the ocular symptoms associated with PAN, a careful medical history and workup is required. Temporal artery biopsy can also be diagnostic of PAN by demonstrating fibrinoid necrosis and granulomatous arteritis. In contrast to patients with giant-cell arteritis (temporal arteritis), the biopsy in PAN will not demonstrate any giant cells.

TREATMENT AND MANAGEMENT

■ Systemic

The majority of patients with PAN will be treated with corticosteroids. Prednisone may bring active inflammation under control. If more aggressive therapy is needed, intravenous methylprednisolone may be given. Dosages should be tapered as the patient's condition improves. Cyclophosphamide, a cytotoxic antineoplastic agent, has been found to be quite effective in several diseases associated with abnormal immune function. In patients with PAN the use of this agent may result in an improved survival rate and in long-

TABLE 30–3. TREATMENT AND MANAGEMENT OF PAN

- ■ **SYSTEMIC**
  - Oral corticosteroids (prednisone 60–100 mg/d)
  - IV corticosteroids (methylprednisolone: 1 g qd × 3–4 days)
  - Cyclophosphamide

- ■ **OCULAR**
  - Treatment of underlying systemic condition
  - Iridocyclitis
    Topical steroids (prednisolone acetate 1.0% qid)
    Cycloplegia (eg, atropine, homatropine)
  - Scleritis
    Oral steroids (prednisone 40–60 mg/d)

term remission even after the termination of treatment. The use of this agent also may allow the reduction of corticosteroids used in therapy (Fauci, 1979). Continued therapy for a year or more is often required.

■ Ocular

All ocular complications in PAN are initially managed by treating the underlying systemic condition. Localized ocular therapy has a role when iridocyclitis or scleral keratitis is present. These patients may be placed on topical steroids in conjunction with a long-acting cycloplegic. For patients with scleritis, oral prednisone is prescribed (Table 30–3).

CONCLUSION

PAN is a systemic necrotizing vasculitis involving multiple organ systems. It is a rare disease that may be classified with other vasculitic syndromes. The specific etiology is unknown, but an immune–allergic mechanism may contribute to the clinical picture. The disease may follow an acute, subacute, or chronic course. Untreated patients with PAN have a poor prognosis, and even treated patients do not fare well. There is high mortality from renal failure, GI complications, myocardial infarction, congestive heart failure, and cerebral infarction.

Although ocular complications are thought to be few, they may often go undetected due to the severity of other involved systems. Some patients have ocular symptoms that develop early in the course of the disease; appropriate awareness of the clinical features of PAN is thus prudent to all primary eyecare practitioners. Treatment needs to be directed toward controlling the diffuse systemic vascular inflammation.

REFERENCES

Cohen RD, Conn DL, Ilstrup DM. Clinical features, prognosis and response to treatment in polyarteritis nodosa. *Mayo Clin Proc.* 1980;55:146–150.

Fauci AS, Katz P, Haynes BF, Wolff SM. Cyclophosphamide therapy of severe systemic necrotizing vasculitis. *New Engl J Med.* 1979;301:235–238.

Gold DH. Ocular manifestations of connective tissue diseases. In: Tasman W, Jaeger EA, eds. *Duane's Clinical Ophthalmology.* Philadelphia: Lippincott; 1980;5:17–19.

Kimbrill OC Jr, Wheliss JA. Polyarteritis nodosa complicated by bilateral optic neuropathy. *JAMA.* 1967;201:139–140.

Kurland LT, Chuang TY, Hunder GG. The epidemiology of systemic arteritis, In: Lawrence RC, Shulman LE, eds. *Epidemiology of the Rheumatic Diseases.* New York: Gower; 1984:196–206.

Michalak T. Immune complexes of hepatitis B surface antigen in the pathogenesis of periarteritis nodosa: A study of seven necropsy cases. *Am J Pathol.* 1978;90:619–632.

Moore JG, Sevel D. Corneal–scleral ulceration in periarteritis nodosa. *Br J Ophthalmol.* 1966;50:651–655.

Morgan CM, Foster CS, D'Amico DJ, Gragoudas ES. Retinal vasculitis in polyarteritis nodosa. *Retina.* 1986;6:205–209.

Purcell JJ Jr, Birkenkamp R, Tsai CC. Conjunctival lesions in periarteritis nodosa: A clinical immunopathologic study. *Arch Ophthalmol.* 1984;102:736–738.

Ralston DE, Kvale WF. The renal lesions of periarteritis nodosa. *Proc Staff Meet Mayo Clin.* 1949;24:28.

Sams WM Jr, Clayrian HN, Kohler PF. Human necrotizing vasculitis: Immunoglobulins and complement in vessel walls of cutaneous lesions and normal skin. *J Invest Dermatol.* 1975;64:441.

Stillerman ML. Ocular manifestations of diffuse collagen disease. *Arch Ophthalmol.* 1951;45:239–250.

Van Wein S, Merz EH. Exophthalmos secondary to periarteritis nodosa. *Am J Ophthalmol.* 1963;56:204–208.

Wise GN. Ocular periarteritis nodosa. Report of two cases. *Arch Ophthalmol.* 1952;48:1–11.

31
Chapter

Wegener Granulomatosis

Michael A. Chaglasian

Wegener granulomatosis is a systemic necrotizing granulomatous vasculitic disease of unknown etiology. It is perhaps initiated by an allergic hypersensitivity to airborne allergens.

Three major anatomic sites are affected: the upper respiratory tract, lower respiratory tract, and kidneys. This triad defines the "classic" (complete) form of the disease. In the "limited" form of the disease, all three criteria are not present simultaneously or renal disease is absent. A fourth predominant characteristic is a disseminated vasculitis that affects the arteries and veins of numerous other organ systems.

Ocular manifestations reflect the rapid course of the systemic disease and are visually threatening due to dramatic and severe inflammation throughout the globe. In the limited form of the disease and, less commonly, in the classic form, ocular manifestations may be the initial presenting sign. Wegener granulomatosis is typically classified with other respiratory vasculitic syndromes that affect medium- to small-sized arteries. These include allergic angiitis and granulomatosis (Churg–Strauss syndrome) and lymphomatoid granulomatosis.

The prognosis for patients with Wegener granulomatosis is guarded, and in the past there was a significant mortality rate. Fortunately, systemic corticosteroids and immunosuppressive/cytotoxic drugs are effective in controlling this devastating disease.

EPIDEMIOLOGY

■ Systemic

Wegener granulomatosis is an uncommon disease, but it is not rare. There are very few data regarding its prevalence. A total of 140 patients were diagnosed with the disease between 1966 and 1982 at the Mayo Clinic (Bullen et al, 1983). The average age of onset of initial symptoms was 48 years (range, 7 to 73 years). Definitive diagnosis was made approximately 6 years later.

There is no racial or sexual predilection, although more females are noted to have the limited form of the disease. Untreated, the classic form is rapidly fatal, with a mean survival rate of 50% at 5 months and an 82% morbidity at 1 year. The limited form has a much better prognosis.

■ Ocular

The incidence of ocular involvement in Wegener granulomatosis ranges from 28 to 58% in the classic form. The numerous ocular manifestations also appear in the limited form, and are often among the major signs in the early stages of the disease.

NATURAL HISTORY

■ Systemic

The necrotizing vasculitis characteristic of Wegener granulomatosis (and other vasculitic syndromes) involves granulomatosis (Table 31–1). A granuloma is a histological man-

TABLE 31–1. SYSTEMIC MANIFESTATIONS OF WEGENER GRANULOMATOSIS

SYMPTOMS
- Rhinitis
- Sinusitis
- Cough
- Otitis media
- Fever
- Malaise
- Weight loss
- Purpuric rash
- Arthralgia

SIGNS
- Necrotizing granulomatous inflammation of upper respiratory tract
- Necrotizing granulomatous inflammation of lower respiratory tract
- Glomerulonephritis
- Diffuse focal vasculitis affecting other organ systems: heart, skin, nervous system

ifestation of inflammation. It is an aggregation of mononuclear, epithelial, and multinucleated giant cells. The specific etiology of Wegener granulomatosis is still unknown. Due to its concentration in the respiratory system, a hypersensitivity to an inhaled antigen is hypothesized. Abnormalities of the T-cell system and immune complex formation are then responsible for triggering the pathological findings.

Initial systemic manifestations are primarily otorhinolaryngolic, pulmonary, and rheumatologic. The patient will have a lasting cough, sinusitis, or secretions that do not respond to antibiotics. Weight loss, fever, and malaise soon follow. Chronic otitis media may occur, leading to sensorineural hearing loss. Nasal obstruction and ulceration may develop.

Pulmonary features besides a productive cough and hemoptysis (expectoration of blood) include chronic dyspnea, reflecting lower respiratory tract inflammation, and bronchiolar spasm. Glomerulonephritis, proteinuria, and red-blood casts are the typical renal complications. They are never an initial manifestation, and severe hypertension is rarely seen.

A manifestation of skin involvement (Figure 31–1) that can develop is a palpable purpura, an erythematous papule that does not blanch when the skin is pressed. Ulcers, nodules, or hemorrhagic vesicles are also scattered over the lower extremities. Individual lesions spontaneously resolve within 4 weeks, although they leave an atrophic scar behind. Overall, cutaneous involvement continues indefinitely in recurrent episodes (Hu et al, 1977). Many patients (50%) go on to develop nonspecific arthralgias, but this is transient and not a true arthritis.

Fewer patients develop neurological involvement, which may include polyneuropathy, peripheral neuritis, paresthesias, and cranial nerve palsies.

Patients with this disease are also at risk for developing a lethal midline granuloma. This destructive process involves the paranasal sinuses, palate, orbit, and central facial bones. The course of Wegener granulomatosis is insidious and rapidly progressive. Left undiagnosed and untreated, it is most certainly fatal.

■ Ocular

Ocular findings in Wegener granulomatosis are numerous and common (Table 31–2). They are found in about 50% of patients, with virtually all vascularized ocular tissues potentially affected, including the orbit. Ocular disease is classified as either focal (primary) or contiguous. Focal disease occurs independently of respiratory tract involvement; contiguous disease is caused by spreading from affected paranasal sinuses (Robin et al, 1985). Ocular involvement may often be the presenting sign. It may be unilateral or bilateral. Left untreated, ocular complications can lead to permanent visual loss.

Orbital Disease

Orbital disease is the most common ophthalmic complication in Wegener granulomatosis, occurring in 50% of patients with ocular manifestations. Orbital granulomatosis is caused by spreading from contiguous paranasal sinuses and not a primary or focal vasculitis. Diffuse orbital inflammation (eg, scleral/episcleral vascular engorgement) is the most frequent presenting sign and symptom. Pain, tender-

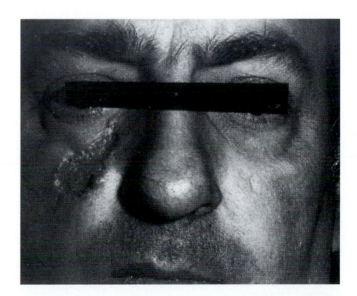

Figure 31–1. A cutaneous lesion in which a diagnosis of Wegener granulomatosis was established by biopsy *(Reprinted with permission from Mandel ER, Wagoner MD:* Atlas of Corneal Disease. *Philadelphia: Saunders; 1989.)*

TABLE 31–2. OCULAR MANIFESTATIONS OF WEGENER GRANULOMATOSIS

ORBITAL
- Granulomatosis and vasculitis
- Proptosis
- Eye movement restrictions
- Ulceration
- Optic nerve compression

SCLERAL/CONJUNCTIVAL/UVEAL
- Conjunctival injection
- Episcleritis
- Scleritis
- Uveitis

CORNEAL
- Subepithelial infiltrates
- Marginal infiltration
- Circumlimbal ulceration/furrowing
- Exposure keratitis

RETINAL/CHOROIDAL
- Diffuse vasculitis
- Disseminated retinitis (ischemic)
- Venous congestion
- Retinal and choroidal detachments

ADNEXAL
- Dacryoadenitis
- Dacryocystitis
- Nasolacrimal duct obstruction
- Eyelid edema and erythema

ness, chemosis, and limitation of extraocular movement increase as proptosis rapidly develops. Continued orbital vasculitis and granulomatosis lead to severe proptosis, painful ophthalmoplegia, tissue loss, skin ulceration, and optic nerve compression, causing vision loss (Robin et al, 1985).

Presentation of orbital disease in Wegener granulomatosis may resemble idiopathic pseudotumor. However, in Wegener granulomatosis, orbital disease is bilateral and will recur without complete treatment of the systemic disease.

Scleral Disease
A diffuse mild scleritis that parallels the systemic disease is another common finding. Less commonly, it may be quite severe with painful nodules and necrosis, as is seen in rheumatoid arthritis and other collagen vascular diseases (Bullen, 1983).

Corneal Disease
Marginal corneal thinning and ulceration are seen in association with adjacent scleritis. Beginning with focal perilimbal infiltrates there is circumferential extension and

furrowing (Figure 31–2). Ring ulcers may develop and can extend into the central cornea with devastating visual consequences. Multifocal stromal infiltrates may extend centrally during periods of disease exacerbation. Exposure keratitis may result from orbital disease and proptosis.

Anterior Segment Disease
Conjunctival disease manifests as a recurrent nonspecific conjunctival injection. It is never seen as an isolated finding. Nasolacrimal duct obstruction has been detected in 25% of patients with Wegener granulomatosis. It appears to be a late manifestation of the disease and may become more widely detected as better treatment strategies prolong patient survival (Hardwig et al, 1991). Other anterior segment complications include periorbital lid edema, dacryocystitis, dacryoadenitis, and uveitis.

Posterior Segment Disease
Retinal and choroidal complications in Wegener granulomatosis are rare, with only 7 to 20% of patients demonstrating any significant involvement (Bullen et al, 1983; Robin et al, 1985). Most commonly, a retinal vasculitis will be detected. Other patients may have retinal venous congestion and optic nerve edema associated with a retrobulbar mass. Disseminated retinitis with cotton-wool spots, hemorrhage, and edema may develop secondary to renal failure. Kinyoun and associates (1987) observed a choroidal vasculitis in two patients with Wegener granulomatosis. Choroidal and retinal detachments can potentially develop in patients with severe overlying scleritis and uveitis.

DIAGNOSIS

■ Systemic
Workup for Wegener granulomatosis begins with a thorough history and otorhinolaryngological and systemic

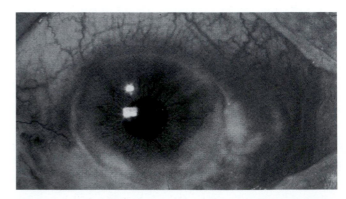

Figure 31–2. Peripheral ulcerative keratitis with associated scleritis. *(Reprinted with permission from Mandel ER, Wagoner MD: Atlas of Corneal Disease. Philadelphia: Saunders; 1989.)*

examination looking for signs of diffuse inflammatory disease.

Diagnostic criteria for Wegener granulomatosis were established by Godman and Churg in 1954. Diagnosis requires (1) respiratory granulomatosis lesions, (2) diffuse focal vasculitis, and (3) granulomatous lesions of renal glomeruli. Clinical diagnosis is often made in patients with symptomatology of a systemic vasculitis affecting the upper (nasal sinus mucosa) and lower (lungs) respiratory tracts and glomerulonephritis. It is important to remember that in the limited form of the disease, renal disease may be absent; and even in the classic form it will be asymptomatic. In addition to this clinical triad, focal vasculitis affecting other systems must be investigated. This would include the smaller arteries of the spleen, heart, pancreas, and adrenal glands.

Thus, patients with a combination of rhinitis, sinusitis, a lasting cough, arthralgias, erythematous cutaneous lesions, and renal failure may be suspected of having Wegener granulomatosis.

The differential diagnosis for these patients would include other granulomatous and/or vasculitic diseases. Lymphomatoid granulomatosis, allergic angiitis, and granulomatosis (Churg–Strauss syndrome) have both granulomatous and vasculitic characteristics but affect different organ systems. Sarcoidosis is a granulomatous disease but there is no vasculitis. Polyarteritis is a vasculitis without granulomatous inflammation, as are other collagen vascular diseases.

Infectious causes of granulomatosis should also be ruled out, including tuberculosis, syphilis, histoplasmosis, blastomycosis, and coccidiomycosis. Nasopharyngeal neoplasma, such as Hodgkin disease, can also have similar initial presentations (Bullen et al, 1983).

Additional tests to help confirm diagnosis include x-rays, biopsy, and specific laboratory tests. Sinus x-rays demonstrate mucosal thickening or sinus opacification. Pulmonary x-rays show cavitation (formation of cavities) and infiltration. Nasal mucosal biopsy is the best location for histological confirmation of vasculitis and granuloma formation (Charles et al, 1991). Renal impairment from glomerulonephritis causes significant proteinuria and reduced creatinine clearance. Other abnormal blood tests include an elevated erythrocyte sedimentation rate, elevated C-reactive protein, anemia, leukocytosis, and increased immunoglobulins.

Another important serologic test for Wegener granulomatosis is the antineutrophil cytoplasmic antibody test (ANCA). This test, which detects the presence of antibodies for components of primary granules of neutrophils and monocytes, has been a very useful diagnostic adjunct for diagnostic confirmation of the disease (Nolle et al, 1989). The ANCA titer is increased at presentation in almost every patient with the disease.

■ Ocular

As previously stated, ocular complications in Wegener granulomatosis are very common and may often be the presenting sign. Patients with periorbital pain, scleritis, marginal corneal infiltrates (corneoscleral disease), and/or proptosis may be suspected of having the disease. Ocular diagnosis is most frequently made following a definitive systemic diagnosis. However, recent research has investigated making a diagnosis based on ophthalmic signs. Soukiasian and associates (1992) obtained serum ANCA on seven patients in whom scleritis alone was the presenting sign. All patients tested positive, and systemic diagnosis of Wegener was further corroborated with physical and histological examination. Their study demonstrates high sensitivity and specificity for ANCA testing.

The usefulness of orbital biopsy was investigated by Kalina and associates in 1992. They found only 54% of their patients (n=13) showed the classic histopathological triad of granulomatous inflammation, tissue necrosis, and vasculitis. Due to their lack of sensitivity they recommend a definitive clinical correlation in patients with orbital disease who are suspected of having Wegener granulomatosis.

Leavitt and Butrus (1991) were able to correctly diagnose a patient via lacrimal gland biopsy. Their patient presented with a dacryoadenitis, and later developed a glomerulonephritis and classical necrotizing granulomatosis.

TREATMENT AND MANAGEMENT

■ Systemic

Until the early 1970s when cyclophosamide (Cytoxan) was introduced into a therapeutic regimen, Wegener granulomatosis was considered to be a fatal disease. The use of corticosteroids alone was only moderately beneficial and did not produce a lasting remission. Cyclophosphamide now has a well-established place in the management of Wegener granulomatosis as the disease is now much less likely to be fatal. It can still, however, lead to significant functional loss.

Cyclophosphamide given in an approximate dosage of 2 mg/kg/day orally is the most frequent first-line therapy. Oral prednisone (1 mg/kg) is often given simultaneously with the cyclophosphamide for greater effectiveness. Intravenous dosages are a second highly successful option for advanced presentations. This "pulsed immunosuppressive therapy" is a series of injections of methylprednisolone and cyclophosphamide at 3-day intervals over a short period of time (Meyer et al, 1987).

Treatment with cyclophosphamide often needs to be continued for a year or more after the disappearance of symptoms. Permanent remission is never guaranteed and reactivations have been documented 20 years after initial therapy. There are numerous significant side effects with cyclophosphamide, which include: severe leukopenia, alopecia, hemorrhagic cystitis, cytomegalovirus retinitis, and teratogenesis. The side effects of oral steroids are also to be considered. Blood cell counts should be checked as often as twice weekly (Charles et al, 1991; Robin et al, 1985).

Other treatment modalities that have been employed with some success include azathioprine (an immunosuppressive for patients who cannot tolerate cyclophosphamide) and plasma exchange (for severe renal disease). Other investigators have been successful maintaining disease inactivity with the adjunctive use of the antibiotic trimethoprim–sulfamethoxazole; however, the complete role of this medication is not fully understood (DeRemee et al, 1985; West et al, 1987).

The therapeutic management of patients with Wegener granulomatosis is difficult, complicated, and variable from patient to patient. It is best managed by specialists with expertise in the use of these medications.

■ Ocular

Because ophthalmic involvement in Wegener granulomatosis is a reflection of systemic disease, ocular therapy is primarily based on complete systemic management (Table 31–3). Jampol and associates (1978) demonstrated the effectiveness of cytotoxic agents in the treatment of scleritis. This has been corroborated by many other studies. Topical steroidal therapy for patients with conjunctivitis, episcleritis, and scleritis may supplement systemic medications. Advancing corneal disease and ulceration are poorly controlled with topical therapy and will generally only respond to oral treatment, though prophylactic lubrication and antimicrobial agents should be used when necessary.

TABLE 31–3. TREATMENT AND MANAGEMENT OF WEGENER GRANULOMATOSIS

■ Systemic
- Systemic oral prednisone 1mg/kg/d
- Oral cyclophosphamide 1–4 mg/kg/d
- Pulsed immunosuppressive therapy: IV methylprednisolone and cyclophosphamide
- Plasma exchange
- Azathioprine
- Trimethoprim–sulfamethoxazole

■ Ocular
- Initiate appropriate systemic therapy
- Topical steroids
- Topical lubricants and antibiotics
- Optic nerve decompression
- Penetrating keratoplasty
- Dacryocystorhinostomy

With increased longevity of patients, surgical management may be required in certain patients with specific ocular complications. Most importantly, surgical optic nerve decompression (removal of the roof or medial wall of the optic canal) is necessary in those patients with expulsive proptosis. Corneal perforation from significant ulceration can be managed with penetrating keratoplasty or cyanoacrylate adhesive. Although controversial, dacryocystorhinostomy is effective in cases of nasolacrimal duct obstruction, and can be employed when the disease is quiescent (Hardwig et al, 1992).

CONCLUSION

Wegener granulomatosis is a complicated granulomatous vasculitis primarily affecting the upper and lower respiratory tracts and kidneys. There can be extensive ophthalmic complications leading to permanent visual loss. The specific etiology is unknown. Significant strides have been made in management, with the use of systemic steroids and immunosuppressive/cytotoxic agents. Long-term remission of the disease is now possible. Ocular inflammatory complications are primarily managed through systemic treatment regimes. The eyecare practitioner should be aware that scleritis and/or proptosis may be the presenting sign of Wegener granulomatosis.

REFERENCES

Bullen CL, Liesegang TJ, McDonald TJ, DeRemee RA. Ocular complications of Wegener's granulomatosis. *Ophthalmology.* 1983;90:279–290.

Charles SJ, Meyer PA, Watson PG. Diagnosis and management of systemic Wegener's granulomatosis presenting with anterior ocular inflammatory disease. *Br J Ophthalmol.* 1991;75:201–207.

DeRemee RA, McDonald TJ, Weiland LH. Wegener's granulomatosis: Observations on treatment with antimicrobial agents. *Mayo Clinic Proc.* 1985;60:27–32.

Godman GC, Churg J. Wegener's granulomatosis. Pathology and review of the literature. *Arch Ophthalmol.* 1954;58:533–553.

Hardwig PW, Bartley GB, Garrity JA. Surgical management of nasolacrimal duct obstruction in patients with Wegener's granulomatosis. *Ophthalmology.* 1992;99:133–139.

Hu CH, O'Loughlin S, Winkelman RK. Cutaneous manifestations of Wegener's granulomatosis. *Arch Dermatol.* 1977;113:175–182.

Jampol LM, West C, Goldberg MF. Therapy of scleritis with cytotoxic agents. *Am J Ophthalmol.* 1978;86:266–271.

Kalina PH, Lie JT, Campbell RJ, Garrity JA. Diagnostic value and limitations of orbital biopsy in Wegener's granulomatosis. *Ophthalmology.* 1992;99:120–124.

Kinyoun JL, Kalina RE, Klein ML. Choroidal involvement in systemic necrotizing vasculitis. *Arch Ophthalmol.* 1987; 105:939–942.

Koyama T, Matsuo N, Watanabe Y, et al. Wegener's granulomatosis with destructive ocular manifestations. *Am J Ophthalmol.* 1984;98:736–740.

Leavitt JA, Butrus SI. Wegener's granulomatosis presenting as dacryoadenitis. *Cornea.* 1991;10:542–545.

Meyer PAR, Watson PG, Franks W, Dubord P. "Pulsed" immunosuppressive therapy in the treatment of immunologically induced corneal and scleral disease. *Eye.* 1987;1:487–495.

Nölle B, Specks U, Rohrbach MS, DeRemee RA, Gross WL. Anticytoplasmic autoantibodies: Their immunodiagnostic value in Wegener granulomatosis. *Ann Int Med.* 1989;3:28–40.

Robin JB, Schanzlin DJ, Meisler DM, DeLuise VP, et al. Ocular involvement in the respiratory vasculitides. *Surv Ophthalmol.* 1985;30:127–140.

Sorter NA, Wolff SM. Necrotizing vasculitis. In: Fitzpatrick TB, Eizen AZ, Wolf K, et al, eds. *Dermatology in General Medicine.* 3rd ed. New York: McGraw-Hill; 1986:1300–1306.

Soukiasian SH, Foster CS, Niles JL, Raizman MB. Diagnostic value of anti-neutrophil cytoplasmic antibodies in scleritis associated with Wegener's granulomatosis. *Ophthalmology.* 1992; 99:125–132.

West BC, Todd JR, King JW. Wegener's granulomatosis and trimethoprim–sulfamethoxazole: Complete remission after a twenty year course. *Ann Intern Med.* 1987;106:840–842.

32
Chapter

Sjögren Syndrome

Brian Patrick Mahoney

Sjögren syndrome is an autoimmune disease that involves diffuse exocrine gland dysfunction throughout the body. Decreased lacrimal gland secretion (resulting in keratitis sicca) together with decreased salivary gland secretion, causing dry mouth (xerostomia), are referred to as the sicca complex. Primary Sjögren syndrome occurs when the sicca complex manifests by itself; secondary Sjögren syndrome occurs in association with a collagen vascular disease such as rheumatoid arthritis or systemic lupus erythematosus. The ocular and systemic manifestations are a source of significant patient discomfort because of the progressive nature of the disease. The identification of patients with Sjögren syndrome is important not only to provide palliative treatment, but also because of the potential development of malignant lymphoma.

EPIDEMIOLOGY

The incidence of Sjögren syndrome in the general population is not well known. Over 90% of Sjögren patients are women, with the age of onset between 40 and 60. The age of onset correlates well with the high incidence of other autoimmune syndromes in women of this age group. Approximately 25% of patients with Sjögren syndrome have rheumatoid arthritis. Approximately 90% of Sjögren syndrome patients have keratitis sicca as their primary ocular manifestation.

NATURAL HISTORY

Table 32–1 summarizes the manifestations of Sjögren syndrome. The etiology of Sjögren syndrome is poorly understood, yet the infiltration of exocrine glands by lymphocytes and plasma cells is well documented. Autoimmune-mediated responses targeting exocrine glands occur, resulting in glandular insufficiency.

The clinical course can follow one of two patterns, either slowly progressive and chronic, or acutely progressive and less chronic. Patients with the acutely progressive type have more severe ocular and oral presentations. Because tears and saliva both have lubricating and immunologic properties, a decrease in these functions results in mucous membrane drying and discomfort as well as the potential for secondary infection. These patients present with keratitis sicca and xerostomia of varying degrees. Other oral features include fissures at the corner of the mouth, tongue, and buccal surfaces, and an increased incidence of dental caries. Impaired ability to taste also occurs. Dysphagia results from inadequate lubrication of food transport down the esophagus. Patients with Sjögren syndrome develop these symptoms at a young age, with greater severity, along with other systemic manifestations.

The classic symptoms of keratitis sicca are associated with Sjögren syndrome. These may range from a mild burning sensation to severe pain, depending on the level of ocular surface drying and epithelial compromise. Emotional tearing is not commonly affected unless extensive involvement of the lacrimal gland occurs, which may be observed by gross examination. A papillary response of

TABLE 32–1. SYSTEMIC AND OCULAR MANIFESTATIONS OF SJÖGREN SYNDROME

ORAL
- Xerostomia
- Dysphagia
- Dry lips, mouth fissures
- Dental caries

SALIVARY GLANDS
- Enlarged parotid glands

GASTROINTESTINAL
- Achlorhydria
- Gastritis

IMMUNOLOGIC/HEMATOLOGIC
- Lymphoma
- Pernicious anemia
- Elevated SED rate
- Antinuclear antibodies
- Thyroglobulin antibodies
- Rheumatoid factor
- Hypergammaglobulinemia
- Malignant lymphoproliferation
- Other rheumatic disease

ARTICULAR
- Inflammatory arthritis

GENITOURINARY
- Vaginal dryness
- Discomfort with intercourse
- Discomfort with urination

DERMATOLOGIC
- Dry skin
- Intermittent purpura
- Allergic drug reactions

NASOPHARYNGEAL
- Dry nose
- Decreased smell
- Epistaxis
- Difficulty speaking
- Dry pharynx

PULMONARY
- Subjective labored breathing
- Lower respiratory infections

RENAL
- Tubular acidosis

NEUROLOGIC
- Multiple-sclerosis-like syndrome
- Cranial nerve palsies
- Altered cognitive abilities
- Peripheral neuropathies

OCULAR
- Keratitis sicca
- Filamentary sicca
- Bacterial keratitis/blepharitis
- Nongranulomatous orbital pseudotumor (rare)

the palpebral conjunctiva along with a bulbar conjunctival injection may develop. A noninfectious, ropey discharge results from irritation of the ocular surface and disruption of normal tear physiology. A staphylococcal infection of the ocular surface or eyelids (blepharitis) occurs in about 75% of patients with keratitis sicca. Ulcerative bacterial keratitis can result in corneal scar formation or perforation. Progression in the severity of keratitis sicca leads to filamentary keratitis from anomalous regrowth of the corneal epithelium after significant insult.

Development of filamentary keratitis (Figure 32–1) can occur on an acute basis despite treatment for keratitis sicca. Severe pain is commonly associated with filamentary keratitis. Corneal opacification and pannus from chronic insult is observed in the later stages of ocular involvement. These ocular manifestations are progressive and serve as a source of chronic symptoms for Sjögren syndrome patients.

Parotid gland enlargement occurs in 50% of Sjögren syndrome cases, with bilateral involvement more common. A "chipmunk" appearance to the face occurs as the parotid gland enlargement progresses. Palpation of the glands frequently reveals a firm consistency, but this does not occur in all cases. Acute parotid and other glandular infiltration is frequently accompanied by fever; therefore, these patients can be acutely ill. Infiltration and enlargement of other lymph glands is of a mild degree but can be severe if life-threatening malignant lymphoma develops.

Abnormalities of the nasopharynx and respiratory tract occur in about 50% of Sjögren syndrome patients. Drying of the mucous membranes of the nasopharynx is associated with many symptoms, including epistaxis (nosebleeds), decreased sensation of smell, subjective labored breathing, difficulty speaking, and lower respiratory infections. Drying of the vaginal membranes and vulvar area is associated with discomfort during sexual intercourse as well as during urination. Drying of the skin, purpura with ulcerations, and allergic dermatitis are all dermatologic manifestations seen with increasing frequency with disease progression.

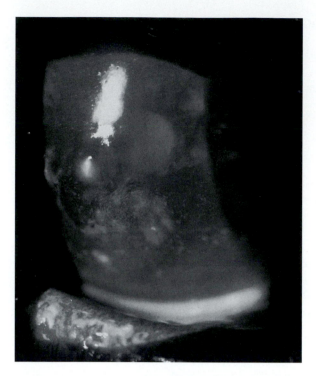

Figure 32–1. Filamentary keratitis in a Sjögren syndrome patient. This 61-year-old patient has rheumatoid arthritis. Note the diffuse epithelial staining with fluorescein. Heavy dye uptake by the filament is observed. Filament stripping and heavy lubrication was sufficient to control this episode of keratitis.

Other extraglandular features of Sjögren syndrome include renal tubular acidosis, with electrolyte imbalance that can exacerbate symptoms of weakness associated with polymyopathy. Extraglandular manifestations of Sjögren syndrome also occur including an inflammatory arthritis. Vasculitis of the skin, although rare, may present as a focal or diffuse rash or ulceration of the legs. Neurologic abnormalities from central nervous system involvement are seen in 66% of patients with cutaneous vasculitic involvement. Cranial nerve palsy, diminished cognitive abilities, and peripheral sensory and motor neuropathies that may imitate multiple sclerosis are all neurologic manifestations of Sjögren syndrome.

Associations with other hematologic and immunologic diseases includes Hashimoto thyroiditis, polymyositis, rheumatoid arthritis, systemic lupus erythematosus, anemia, and hypergammaglobulinemia. Of significant importance is a 44 times greater incidence of non-Hodgkin lymphoma, which may develop in a Sjögren syndrome patient anywhere from 6 months to 29 years following initial onset of the syndrome. Rheumatoid arthritis is present in about 50% of Sjögren patients, and in these cases, the arthritis follows the course consistent with rheumatoid arthritis. If arthritis does not develop within the first year following the onset of the sicca complex, then there is only a 10% chance that it will develop after that time.

DIAGNOSIS

Patient presentation and history consistent with the clinical manifestations of Sjögren syndrome aid in the diagnosis. These include dry eye, dry mouth, and parotid gland enlargement. The diagnosis of Sjögren syndrome is made when the patient meets two or more of the following criteria:

1. Drying mucous membranes (oral, ocular, and nasopharyngeal)
2. Enlarged parotid or salivary gland
3. A connective tissue disorder

Dental and otolaryngological evaluation of the oral and nasopharyngeal tissues respectively will reveal mucous membrane drying or ulceration of these tissues. Tissue biopsies of the parotid, salivary, or lacrimal glands reveal the typical infiltrative cells and debris with loss of exocrine glandular structure.

Dynamic evaluation assessing the parotid glands production and secretory abilities is accomplished by secretory sialiography, and the salivary gland is assessed by sequential salivary scintography. The technique of secretory sialiography involves injection of a radiopaque medium into the parotid duct with visualization of the duct by radiographs. Sequential salivary scintography also evaluates parotid gland function. The results of these procedures parallel each other and correlate directly with the degree of xerostomia.

Hematologic studies such as serum protein electrophoresis, rheumatoid factor (RF), antinuclear antibodies (ANA), and complete blood count (CBC) are used in monitoring the progression of the disease. Hypergammaglobulinemia, found in 30% of Sjögren patients, and cryoglobulinemia, found in 20%, will be detected by serum protein electrophoresis. Elevated immune complexes frequently occur. An increase in serum B_2-microglobulin levels usually precedes renal and lymphoproliferative disorders. The CBC with differential will confirm the presence of lymphoproliferative disease, lymphoma, or anemia. Rheumatoid factor is present in 90% of Sjögren patients, with 70% ANA positive. Antithyroglobulin antibodies are also found in 35% of these patients.

The ocular diagnosis of keratitis sicca is based on the patient symptoms of foreign body sensation, photophobia, and burning and irritability of the eye and eyelid. Decreased vision results from significant corneal drying. Conjunctival and lacrimal gland biopsies assist in the diagnosis and reveal infiltrative cells with glandular loss. Decreased Schirmer strip wetting is indicative of severe tear production deficiency. A combination of fluorescein and rose bengal staining is present. Areas of epithelial nonwetting with fluorescein stain accompany the staining pattern. A dramatic clinical picture is appreciated when corneal filaments readily take up both fluorescein and rose bengal dye. Tear lysozyme deficiencies are present; however, this test is not necessary considering the clinically obvious ocular manifestations in Sjögren syndrome patients. Corneal opacification and pannus, both long-term sequelae of corneal and conjunctival desiccation, are easily seen.

TREATMENT AND MANAGEMENT

Management of Sjögren syndrome remains palliative at this time (Table 32–2). The concurrent treatment for associated collagen vascular disease has little impact on reversing or stabilizing the mucocutaneous processes involved with Sjögren syndrome. Increased fluid intake and increased humidity in the home and work environments help maximize patient comfort level. Mucomimetic agents to the affected mucous membranes are used as often as needed by the patient.

Deficiencies in salivary secretions are more difficult to compensate for than tear deficiencies. Frequent fluid intake, particularly water, help keep the oral mucosa moist. Bromhexine is a salivary substitute that patients may find beneficial. It is imperative that patients with Sjögren syndrome receive regular dental care (every 3 to 4 months) and maintain impeccable oral hygiene. The use of sugar-free lozenges may stimulate release of residual amounts of salivary secretions and keep patients comfortable.

Systemic treatment for associated arthritic conditions has little effect on the progression of exocrine gland dysfunction. Treatment with oral nonsteroidal antiinflammatory drugs (NSAIDs) is beneficial for many cases of arthralgia.

TABLE 32–2. TREATMENT AND MANAGEMENT OF SJÖGREN SYNDROME

- **SYSTEMIC**
  - Treatment aimed at associated connective tissue disease
  - Artificial mucomimetic agents for oral cavity
    Bromhexine
    Sugar-free lozenges
    Increased water intake
    Dental hygiene
    Saline nasal sprays
    Increased humidity in home and work environments

- **OCULAR**
  - Artificial tear supplements—unpreserved solutions and ointments (dosage determined by patient presentation)
  - Punctal occlusion by plug or ablation
  - Management of filaments if present
  - Management of associated bacterial keratitis/blepharitis

Low-dose steroids may be needed for cases refractory to NSAID therapy. Oral steroids are used when allergic vasculitis presents with cutaneous lesions, and are discontinued after the lesions resolve. Central nervous system manifestations, particularly pseudo-multiple sclerosis, require oral steroid use for extended periods. Necrotizing vasculitis and lymphoproliferative disease have been treated with cyclophosphamide with success, but this treatment does not improve the glandular involvement of Sjögren syndrome.

Ocular treatment includes unpreserved ophthalmic lubricant solutions and ointments. Unpreserved solutions are preferred because they do not contribute to epithelial insult nor are they associated with patient sensitivities. Treatment regimen must be individualized, and some patients may require hourly instillations of topical drops. The use of ophthalmic ointments is usually restricted to bedtime due to associated blurred vision. This side effect may be tolerable during the day for patients whose symptoms become severe. Chronic therapy is necessary and patient compliance is instrumental in any therapeutic success.

Collagen punctal implants, punctal plugs, and punctal ablative procedures can be successful and warrant consideration on an individual basis. Unrealistic expectations of therapy should be avoided, because complete elimination of ocular surface staining will not be achieved. A decrease in corneal staining and patient symptoms are the therapeutic goal.

Appropriate antimicrobial medications should be used concurrent with ophthalmic lubrication when bacterial keratitis presents. Rapid healing of the corneal tissues does not occur due to the loss of adequate tear quality and quantity necessary for epithelial healing. It may take an extended period of time to heal (greater than 4 weeks) compared to that expected in a patient with adequate tear quality.

Filament stripping, topical steroids, and Mucomyst are all treatment modalities to consider with filamentary keratitis. Pressure patching may aggravate filamentary keratitis, and therefore should be avoided. Bandage contact lenses have been helpful in managing patient discomfort following filament stripping, but their use should be limited considering their propensity to dry out on the eye, placing the patient at increased risk for secondary bacterial keratitis. Patients with Sjögren syndrome should receive regular eye examinations as often as every 3 to 4 months. This allows for early detection of vision-threatening changes, and subsequent treatment to prevent permanent vision loss.

CONCLUSION

Sjögren syndrome is a disease not only of exocrine gland dysfunction but also with significant and potentially life-threatening extraglandular manifestations. The progressive nature of glandular destruction causes Sjögren syndrome to be one of the most frustrating diseases for both patient and healthcare provider. Ocular involvement is a predominant feature of this syndrome, and can be associated with permanent vision loss despite aggressive medical therapy. Thorough patient education regarding the chronicity and progressive nature of Sjögren syndrome is necessary, because compliance plays an integral role in the successful management of this disease.

REFERENCES

Bloch KJ, Buchanan WW, Wohl MJ, Bunim JJ. Sjögren's syndrome. A clinical, pathological and serological study of sixty two cases. *Medicine.* 1965;44:187.

Chisholm DM, Waterhouse JP, Mason DK. Lymphocytic sialadenitis in major and minor glands: A correlation in post mortem studies. *J Clin Pathol.* 1970;23:690.

Fox RI, Kang HI. Sjögren's syndrome. In: Kelley WN, Harris ED, Ruddy S, Sledge CB, eds. *Textbook of Rheumatology.* Philadelphia: Saunders; 1993:931.

Freidlaender MH. Arthritic and connective tissue disorders. In: Freidlaender MH, ed. *Allergy and Immunology of the Eye.* New York: Raven; 1993:223.

Hardin JG, Longenecker GL. Drug therapy of specific rheumatic diseases. In: Hardin JG, Longenecker GL, eds. *Handbook of Drug Therapy in Rheumatic Disease.* Boston: Little, Brown; 1992:175.

Krachmer JH, Laibson PR. Corneal thinning and perforation in Sjögren's syndrome. *Am J Ophthalmol.* 1974;78:917.

Maddison PJ. Dry Eyes: Autoimmunity and relationship to other systemic disease. *Trans Ophthalmol Soc UK.* 1985;104:458.

Mikulicz JJ. Concerning peculiar symmetrical disease of the lacrimal and salivary glands. *Med Classics.* 1937;2:165.

Miyasaka N, Seaman W, Bakshi A, et al. Natural killing activity in Sjögren's syndrome: An analysis of defective mechanisms. *Arthritis Rheum.* 1983;72:52.

Preston SJ, Buchanan WW. Rheumatic manifestations of immune deficiency. *Clin Exp Rheumatol.* 1989;7:547.

Shearn MA. Sjögren's syndrome. *Sem Arthritis Rheumatol.* 1972;2:165.

Strand V, Talal N. Advances in the diagnosis and concept of Sjögrens syndrome (autoimmune exocrinopathy). *Bull Rheum Dis.* 1980;30:1046.

Talal N. Sjögrens syndrome and connective tissue disease with other immunologic disorders. In: McCarty DJ, ed. *Arthritis and Allied Conditions.* Philadelphia: Lea & Febiger; 1989:810.

33
Chapter

Sarcoidosis

Esther S. Marks

Sarcoidosis is a multisystemic granulomatous disease of unknown etiology. It was first described by the British physician Jonathon Hutchinson in 1898 as a dermatologic disorder termed Mortimer's malady (named for one of his patients). The current name was derived from the term "sarkoid," coined by the Norwegian dermatologist Caesar Boeck in 1899, who felt the granulomatous skin lesion resembled a sarcoma. In 1909, Schumacher, a German physician, was the first to describe ocular involvement in sarcoidosis, in the form of an anterior uveitis.

Sarcoidosis is characterized most commonly by bilateral hilar lymphadenopathy, pulmonary infiltration, and dermatologic and ocular manifestations. In the nearly 100 years since it was first described, advances in diagnostic technology have significantly furthered the understanding of the pathogenesis of sarcoidosis, although medical researchers still remain puzzled as to the inciting agent.

EPIDEMIOLOGY

■ Systemic

The epidemiology of sarcoidosis varies around the world. In the United States, sarcoidosis occurs in approximately 5 per 100,000 Caucasians and in 40 per 100,000 African-Americans. Although there is no overall sex predilection, in African-Americans, females are affected almost twice as often as males. The disease also appears to be more virulent in African-Americans. Peak incidence occurs in the third and fourth decades of life, although there appears to be another peak in the fifth to seventh decades, particularly in females. Reports of seasonal outbreaks have lent credence to an infectious or environmental etiologic agent (Badrinas et al, 1989). A weak genetic susceptibility has been reported.

Sarcoidosis involves many systems. Close to 95% of patients have pulmonary involvement. Muscle involvement is present in at least 50% of patients with little symptomatology. Although renal granulomas are common (demonstrated in up to 40% of patients), kidney dysfunction is unusual. Other manifestations include bone and joint involvement (up to 35%), dermatologic manifestations (20 to 35%), splenomegaly (up to 15%), hepatomegaly (up to 20%), bone marrow involvement (17%), neurological manifestations (5 to 10%), clinically significant cardiac involvement (5%), clinically evident salivary gland involvement (5%), and mucous membrane manifestations (5%). The gastrointestinal system, pancreas, and endocrine system are rarely affected.

■ Ocular

Ocular manifestations may occur in 17 to 64% of patients, although a frequency of 20 to 25% is most often cited. The most common abnormality is an anterior granulomatous uveitis, occurring in 50 to 85% of patients with ocular involvement. Posterior segment lesions of the choroid and retina may occur in 25%, and optic nerve involvement in as few as 5% of patients. Sarcoidosis of the skin of the eyelid has been reported in 12 to 27%, and conjunctival granulomas in 44 to 56%. Keratoconjunctivitis sicca secondary to lacrimal gland involvement has been reported in 4 to 66% of patients.

NATURAL HISTORY

The etiology of sarcoidosis has been variably ascribed to infectious agents (viruses, mycobacteria, fungi), environmental factors (pine pollens, peanut dust, clay eating, hairsprays), drugs, chemicals, and autoimmune dysfunction. Despite continuing controversy regarding etiology, the pathogenesis of sarcoidosis has become clearer.

Sarcoidosis is characterized by noncaseating granuloma formation in multiple systems. These granulomas are composed mainly of epithelioid cells, as well as some giant cells. Activated T lymphocytes interact with monocytes, macrophages, and other inflammatory cells, encouraging the formation of granulomas and eventual fibrosis and hyalinization. Heightened cell-mediated immune processes (in particular, elevated T-lymphocyte helper/suppressor ratios) occur at disease sites, and are depressed in the blood and at unaffected sites. Humoral immunity is elevated, with increases in many serum immunoglobulins.

■ Systemic

Sarcoidosis falls into two general groups: subacute/acute and chronic. The subacute/acute patient tends to have an abrupt onset of asymptomatic bilateral hilar lymphadenopathy, sometimes with parenchymal infiltration, and occasional erythema nodosum. The majority of these patients experience spontaneous resolution of the disorder without treatment within 2 years. The chronic sarcoidosis patient has usually had 2 or more years of symptoms. Onset is more insidious, consisting of pulmonary infiltrates, progressive dermatologic lesions, hepatosplenomegaly, and chronic ocular and other system involvement. The prognosis is generally poorer in chronic sarcoidosis. Treatment is usually required to relieve symptoms and signs.

Clinical presentation depends on the organ system or tissues affected, and the degree of resulting dysfunction (Table 33–1). The vast majority of patients demonstrate pulmonary involvement (Figure 33–1). This usually begins as an alveolitis, and proceeds to granuloma and fibrosis formation. The most common pulmonary symptoms are cough (mild to severe), dyspnea (mild to severe), wheezing, frequent chest pain, and occasional hemoptysis. Pleural effusion may occasionally occur, although pneumothorax is rare. Constitutional symptoms—malaise, weight loss, fever, fatigue—occur in approximately 20 to 30% of patients. Hilar, cervical, axillary, epitrochlear, inguinal, and supraclavicular lymphadenopathy are exceedingly common. The nodes are firm and nontender.

Dermatologic lesions, representing granulomatous infiltration, occur in about one third of patients. Erythema nodosum may erupt quite suddenly and severely in acute sarcoidosis, with tender red nodules often on the legs, accompanied by joint pain. Despite the severity of symptoms, this manifestation confers a favorable prognosis for spontaneous resolution of both the skin lesions and other concurrent sarcoidosis symptoms. Löfgren syndrome is a symptom complex characterized by erythema nodosum and bilateral hilar lymphadenopathy, with or without arthritis. It too has a very favorable prognosis.

Other cutaneous manifestations may occur, often associated with chronic disease, requiring treatment or sometimes regressing on their own. The lesions may be plaque-like, papular, nodular, or infiltrative. The most common sites of involvement are the face (especially around the mouth, nose, and eyes), neck, and extensor surfaces of the extremities. These lesions may cause serious disfigurement such as in lupus pernio involving the face and nose. Even scars may become infiltrated by granulomas. Dermatologic lesions are usually accompanied by mucous membrane, joint, and bone lesions.

Bone lesions in sarcoidosis may include cysts, punched-out lesions, or lattice-like lesions. Most commonly the hands and feet are involved, followed by the nasal bones, skull, axial skeleton, and ends of long bones. It may be asymptomatic, or present as painful, sausage swelling, with resulting bone deformity. Acute arthritis, particularly a migratory polyarthritis involving the joints of the ankles, knees, wrists, elbows, and proximal interphalanges, is more common in females with sarcoidosis. Joints are red, inflamed, and tender. Pain and limitation of motion are characteristic. The arthritis may last a couple of weeks to several months without permanent joint changes. Chronic arthritis is usually mono- or oligoarticular, involving the knees or ankles.

Mucous membrane involvement includes the nasal cavity, sinuses, and larynx. Patients may complain of sinus headaches, nasal congestion, and hoarseness. If nasal septum perforation from granulomatous infiltration occurs, the patient develops a saddle nose deformity. Salivary gland involvement may also occur with nontender bilateral parotid gland enlargement. This usually indicates chronic sarcoidosis. Parotid gland involvement is often accompanied by lacrimal gland infiltration resulting in a sicca complex of dry mouth and eyes.

Neurological manifestations commonly involve the cranial nerves and meninges. Facial nerve palsy is the most common sign of neurosarcoidosis, occurring in greater than 50%, and usually is due to lower motor neuron dysfunction. It may be unilateral or bilateral, and may appear alone or along with other cranial nerve palsies. Most often it is transient. Various theories have been suggested to explain the pathogenesis of this palsy including compression by a swollen parotid gland, and demyelinization. None have been substantiated. Other commonly involved cranial nerves are the optic nerves, glossopharyngeal and vagus nerves (resulting in hoarseness), and the auditory nerves (resulting in deafness). These manifestations carry a poorer

TABLE 33–1. SYSTEMIC MANIFESTATIONS OF SARCOIDOSIS

PULMONARY INVOLVEMENT
- Alveolitis, followed by granulomatous infiltration, and fibrosis
- Occasional pleural effusion, rare pneumothorax
- Symptoms include cough, dyspnea, wheezing, chest pain, hemoptysis

LYMPH NODE INVOLVEMENT
- Firm and nontender enlargement of various nodes, especially hilar and mediastinal
- Others include cervical, axillary, epitrochlear, inguinal, and supraclavicular

CONSTITUTIONAL SYMPTOMS
- Weight loss, anorexia
- Fatigue, general malaise

DERMATOLOGIC INVOLVEMENT
- Erythema nodosum (Löfgren syndrome: erythema nodosum, bilateral hilar lymphadenopathy, with or without arthritis)
- Plaque-like, nodular, papular or infiltrative lesions of the face (especially around the nose, mouth, and eyes), neck, and extensor surfaces of the extremities.
- Lupus pernio—disfiguring lesions of the face and nose
- Scar infiltration

MUCOUS MEMBRANE AND SALIVARY GLAND INVOLVEMENT
- Nasal cavity, sinuses, and larynx, enlarged parotid glands
- Symptoms include nasal congestion, sinus headache, and hoarseness
- Nasal septum perforation results in saddle nose deformity

BONE AND JOINT INVOLVEMENT
- Most commonly affects hands and feet with painful sausage swelling
- Nasal bones, skull, axial skeleton, and long bones may also be affected
- Bone cysts, lattice-like lesions, or punched-out lesions may occur
- Acute migratory polyarthritis (ankles, knees, wrists, elbows, proximal interphalanges)
- Chronic mono- or oligoarticular arthritis (knees or ankles)
- Arthritic symptoms: painful, red, inflamed joints with limitation of motion

NEUROLOGICAL AND MUSCULAR INVOLVEMENT
- Cranial nerve palsies, most commonly nerve VII, followed by IX, X, VIII, and others
- All types of peripheral neuropathies with paresthesias, neuralgias, muscle weakness, and atrophy
- Tendon reflexes may be decreased or absent
- Asymptomatic muscle infiltration more common than myopathy
- Aseptic meningitis with headache, fever, and neck rigidity
- Space-occupying granulomatous lesions throughout CNS (predilection for the base of the brain) with headaches, papilledema, lethargy, visual acuity and field loss, and seizures

RETICULOENDOTHELIAL INVOLVEMENT
- Hepatosplenomegaly
- Occasional serious liver dysfunction: hepatitis, cirrhosis, portal hypertension
- Hypercalcemia and hypercalciuria may lead to nephrolithiasis and/or nephrocalcinosis

CARDIAC INVOLVEMENT
- Cardiomyopathy, congestive heart failure, angina, valvular incompetence, arrhythmias
- Cor pulmonale and sudden death

OTHER INVOLVEMENT
- Gastrointestinal, pancreatic, and reproductive system involvement (rare)
- Endocrine involvement may lead to diabetes insipidus and panhypopituitarism

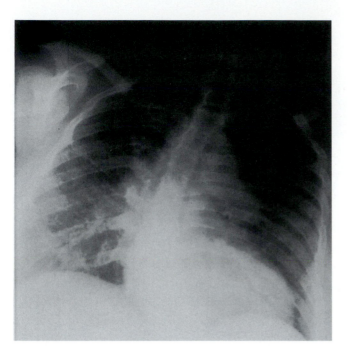

Figure 33–1. Chest x-ray demonstrating stage 2 sarcoidosis with bilateral hilar lymphadenopathy and pulmonary infiltrates.

prognosis. The remaining cranial nerves are less commonly involved. Peripheral neuropathy may occur with paresthesias, neuralgias, and weakness or atrophy of muscles. Tendon reflexes may be depressed or absent. Several types of neuropathy have been described with sarcoidosis, including Guillain–Barré syndrome. Muscular involvement is most commonly asymptomatic although myopathy has been observed.

Aseptic meningitis due to granulomatous infiltration of the meninges has been reported in up to one quarter of neurosarcoidosis patients. Fever, headache, and neck rigidity are common symptoms in both the acute and chronic forms. Seizures have also been reported in up to one quarter of patients with neurologic involvement, and generally indicate a poor prognosis. Although uncommon, space-occupying granulomatous lesions have been reported throughout the central nervous system, with a predilection for the base of the brain. Symptoms, common to most space-occupying masses, include headaches, seizures, decreased visual acuity, papilledema, and lethargy.

Both the liver and spleen may be enlarged asymptomatically. Occasionally serious liver dysfunction may result in hepatitis, cirrhosis, or portal hypertension. Bone marrow and kidney involvement are also usually asymptomatic. However, hypercalcemia and the associated hypercalciuria may lead to nephrolithiasis (kidney stones) or nephrocalcinosis (diffuse kidney calcification). Hypercalcemia results from the production of 1,25-dihydroxy vitamin D by sarcoidosis granulomas. This increases the resorption of calcium from the gastrointestinal tract.

Although cardiac granulomatous infiltration may occur in up to one third of patients, it is clinically significant in only 5%. It may lead to cardiomyopathy, congestive heart failure, angina, valvular incompetence, arrhythmias, or sudden death. The most common cardiac manifestation of sarcoidosis is cor pulmonale. This results from pulmonary hypertension due to extensive pulmonary disease. Prognosis is quite poor.

Although granulomatous involvement of the gastrointestinal tract, pancreas, reproductive system, and endocrine system are rare, two disorders deserve mention. Diabetes insipidus should be suspected in a sarcoidosis patient presenting with polydipsia and polyuria. It is the result of involvement of the hypothalamic–pituitary axis. Panhypopituitarism is also reported secondary to sarcoidosis.

The mortality rate in sarcoidosis is primarily due to the complications of pulmonary insufficiency and cardiac involvement. Overall, the rate reported is up to 5%.

■ Ocular

Ocular manifestations may involve almost any ocular structure or tissue, and may be the first sign of sarcoidosis (Table 33–2). Uveitis, particularly anterior, is the most common ocular manifestation. It may present as subacute or chronic (as an incidental discovery on routine examination). If symptomatic, the patient may complain of a red, watery, photophobic, and blurry eye(s). The uveitis may be unilateral or bilateral, and is characterized by cells and flare, mutton-fat keratic precipitates, and occasionally, iris nodules. Patients may not develop symptoms until complications occur, such as anterior and posterior synechiae (Figure 33–2), secondary glaucoma, secondary cataract, band keratopathy, or cystoid macular edema. Recurrent or chronic uveitis is usually associated with chronic sarcoidosis.

Posterior segment involvement most commonly presents as a periphlebitis or posterior uveitis (chorioretinitis). The vitreous may demonstrate spillover of inflammatory cells from an anterior uveitis, or present with fluffy snowballs or "string-of-pearls" opacities. Retinal veins may demonstrate yellow-white perivascular exudates ("candle-wax drippings"). Sheathing of the vessels may occur anywhere in the fundus. Retinal and optic nerve neovascularization, believed to be due to capillary nonperfusion, may lead to vitreous hemorrhage and tractional retinal detachment. Initially, patients may be asymptomatic or present with blurry vision. Frank occlusion of the central retinal vein or one of its branches is rare. Choroidal granulomas may occur, appearing as yellow-gray lesions with or without an overlying vitritis, or accompanying vasculitis.

Keratoconjunctivitis sicca may develop secondary to lacrimal gland infiltration. Patients may present with dry, gritty, burning eyes. Conjunctival involvement in sarcoidosis results in the formation of granulomas described as yellow nodules. These are most often found in the fornices and

TABLE 33–2. OCULAR MANIFESTATIONS OF SARCOIDOSIS

LID/ADNEXAL INVOLVEMENT
- Granulomatous lid lesions—papular, nodular, ulcerative, or plaque-like
- Lacrimal gland enlargement with displacement of globe and distension of lid

ANTERIOR SEGMENT INVOLVEMENT
- Conjunctival (palpebral and fornix) granulomatous nodules—symptoms of irritation
- Keratoconjunctivitis sicca—symptoms of sore, gritty, burning eyes
- Anterior uveitis
  - May be asymptomatic
  - Symptoms include red, watery, photophobic, blurry eye(s)
  - Signs include cells, flare mutton-fat KPs, vitreal spillover
  - If long-standing may have posterior and/or anterior synechiae, secondary glaucoma, secondary cataracts, cystoid macular edema, and band keratopathy
  - Uveoparotid fever (Heerfordt syndrome): fever, parotid enlargement, and uveitis

POSTERIOR SEGMENT INVOLVEMENT
- Vitreal opacities—snowballs, string-of-pearls
- Periphlebitis or posterior uveitis with retinal perivenous sheathing and yellow-white exudates (candle-wax drippings)
- Rare occlusion of retinal veins
- Neovascularization of disc or retina
- Yellow-gray choroidal granulomas with or without overlying vitritis and vasculitis

NEURO-OCULAR INVOLVEMENT
- Cranial nerve palsy (restricted motilities, diplopia, ectropion, and lagophthalmos possible)
- Papilledema secondary to intracranial lesions (headache, visual field defects, and visual acuity loss possible)
- Direct optic nerve infiltration (disc edema, visual acuity loss, dyschromatopsia, visual field defects)
- Optic atrophy (visual acuity loss, relative afferent pupillary defect)

TOXIC DRUG EFFECTS
- Steroids
  - Cataract formation
  - Glaucoma
- Chloroquine
  - Corneal deposits
  - Bull's-eye retinopathy

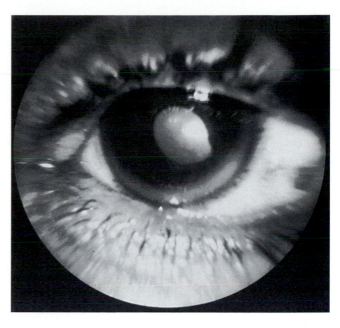

Figure 33–2. Chronic granulomatous uveitis resulting in posterior synechiae.

on the palpebral conjunctiva. Large nodules may produce irritation. Progressive cicatricial conjunctivitis has also been reported, with symptoms of chronic conjunctivitis—sore, red, itchy eyes. Granulomas of the skin of the eyelid may also occur. These may be nodular, papular, ulcerative, or plaque-like.

Neuro-ocular manifestations include extraocular muscle dysfunction secondary to cranial nerve palsies, papilledema secondary to intracranial sarcoid mass lesions, disc edema secondary to intraocular inflammation, and granulomatous involvement of the optic nerve at its head, intraorbital, or intracranial locations. Patients may report diplopia in the case of cranial nerve palsies, visual field defects from optic nerve involvement due to an intracranial mass lesion, along with painless loss of visual acuity and color vision, particularly with direct optic nerve infiltration. Optic atrophy may result when the optic nerve is compromised.

Ocular manifestations may occur in isolation, or may precede or occur concurrently with other manifestations. Certain symptom complexes may occur. Heerfordt syndrome, also known as uveoparotid fever, is characterized by fever, parotid gland enlargement, facial nerve palsy, and uveitis.

DIAGNOSIS

■ Systemic

Diagnosis requires a clinical and radiographic picture compatible with sarcoidosis, histologic confirmation of non-caseating granulomas via biopsy, and the elimination of other granulomatous diseases (eg, tuberculosis). Initial examination must include a thorough history and physical examination to reveal past or current signs and symptoms consistent with sarcoidosis. This should be followed by routine nonspecific hematologic tests (including erythrocyte sedimentation rate, or ESR), serum chemistries (including calcium and liver function tests), urinalysis, and chest x-rays.

Further tests used to determine the presence of sarcoidosis include serum angiotensin-converting enzyme, serum lysozyme, tissue biopsy, tuberculin skin testing (PPD) and anergy panel, Kveim–Siltzbach skin test, and when indicated, pulmonary function tests (PFTs), bronchoalveolar lavage (BAL), cerebrospinal fluid (CSF) examination, gallium scans, computed tomography (CT), magnetic resonance imaging (MRI), and electrocardiograms (ECG) to reveal possible cardiac involvement. Many of these laboratory and imaging tests are nonspecific, and therefore must be interpreted in the context of the clinical picture.

Routine laboratory tests may reveal a leukopenia (specifically lymphopenia and decreased T-lymphocyte helper/suppressor ratios), thrombocytopenia, and occasional anemia, eosinophilia, monocytosis, and elevated ESR. Hypercalcemia, hypercalciuria, proteinuria, and abnormal liver function tests may also occur.

Elevated ACE levels have been observed in 34 to 90% of patients with active sarcoidosis. The sarcoid granulomas produce ACE, an enzyme that catalyzes the conversion of angiotensin I to the vasoconstrictor angiotensin II. However, ACE levels are elevated in a number of other diseases (eg, lymphoma, tuberculosis, cirrhosis, diabetes mellitus, Gaucher disease, and leprosy). The same is true of serum lysozyme levels. This enzyme is produced by the sarcoid granulomas, and therefore is usually elevated in active disease. However, it may also be elevated in other disease processes.

Chest radiography in sarcoidosis, although nonspecific, has been widely studied. Many diseases may present similarly (eg, tuberculosis, lymphoma, carcinoma). Therefore, diagnostic tests to exclude other diseases must also be considered, such as the culturing of sputum, blood, and CSF to eliminate the possibility of an infectious etiology (eg, tuberculosis).

A widely used staging (or typing) method has been devised for interpreting chest x-ray results, despite controversy concerning whether or not patients pass through the stages in a sequential fashion. Stage 0 denotes a clear chest x-ray, even though the patient may have abnormal pulmonary function. This stage may occur either early or late in the disease. Stage 1 is characterized by bilateral hilar lymphadenopathy, usually a manifestation of early disease that resolves within 1 to 2 years. Stage 2 represents bilateral hilar lymphadenopathy plus parenchymal infiltration, which does not carry as good a prognosis, although symptoms usually resolve. Stage 3 presents as pulmonary infiltration only, whereas stage 4 is characterized by fulminant

infiltration and fibrosis. Patients with stage 4 sarcoidosis have the least favorable prognosis, as they may develop respiratory failure, pneumothorax, and cor pulmonale. In addition to chest x-rays, radiography of suspected bone and/or joint involvement may be performed looking for punched-out lesions, cysts, and lattice-like lesions.

Patients suspected of having restrictive pulmonary disease should undergo pulmonary function tests. Although nonspecific in nature, these tests may provide information concerning the presence of infiltrative lung disease, even prior to being visible on radiography. Forced vital capacity and forced expiratory volume are often reduced.

Characteristic immune changes in sarcoidosis include increased humoral immunity (elevations in serum complement, circulating immune complexes, and autoantibodies); depressed peripheral cell-mediated immunity (lymphopenia and cutaneous anergy on PPD skin testing and anergy panels); and increased cell-mediated immunity at disease sites as seen with bronchoalveolar lavage (BAL). BAL uses a fiberoptic bronchoscope in the distal airway. Saline is instilled and then removed by suction. Elevated levels of T-lymphocytes are recovered in active pulmonary sarcoidosis.

The Kveim–Siltzbach skin test, another immunologic test for sarcoidosis, is believed to be a delayed hypersensitivity reaction to some unknown antigen. A saline suspension of human sarcoidal tissue is injected intradermally in the flexor surface of the forearm. Approximately 4 to 6 weeks later, a positive result will demonstrate the appearance of a nodule that may be biopsied to reveal noncaseating granuloma formation. Positive results are found in 59 to 94% (75% being the most commonly stated figure) of sarcoidosis patients, with a very low false-positive rate. Although less invasive than lung biopsy or bronchoalveolar lavage, the skin test has several disadvantages. It is limited by the excessive length of time necessary to obtain positive results, requires the avoidance of systemic steroids for the duration of the test, and most importantly, the Kveim antigen is not commercially available.

Examination of CSF is usually reserved for aiding in the diagnosis of meningitis. Meningeal involvement in neurosarcoidosis may reveal elevated protein levels, normal or decreased glucose levels, and pleocytosis. The CSF may also be cultured to rule out an infectious etiology.

Tissue biopsy provides histologic confirmation of noncaseating granulomas. Tissue samples should first be obtained from easily accessible sites (eg, skin, mucous membranes, conjunctiva, or lacrimal gland) if available. If not, transbronchial lung biopsy, or biopsies of lymph nodes, liver, or skeletal muscle may be considered.

Imaging techniques other than chest radiography may be used for diagnosis of intra-or extrathoracic sarcoidosis. The routine use of chest CT scans for the diagnosis of pulmonary sarcoidosis is often advocated because of reported higher sensitivity (Hansell & Kerr, 1991). CT and MRI scans are especially useful in the diagnosis of neurosarcoidosis. Gallium scans are also useful because gallium 67 has been found to accumulate in active sarcoidal tissue. It is particularly helpful in delineating lacrimal gland, parotid gland, and intrathoracic involvement. However, its use is limited in abdominal and skeletal evaluation, because normal bone and abdominal viscera will absorb gallium.

■ Ocular

Ocular manifestations may be readily diagnosed with comprehensive eye examination. Evaluation may reveal decreased visual acuity, dyschromatopsia, pupil abnormalities, or restricted motilities secondary to neuro-ocular involvement or intraocular inflammation. Slit-lamp biomicroscopy may reveal an apparently prolapsed lacrimal gland, lid swelling and erythema, a displaced globe, a dry eye, superficial punctate keratitis, symblepharon formation, or conjunctival or lid nodules. Intraocular inflammation will manifest characteristically with cells, flare, keratic precipitates (usually mutton fat), along with potential complications such as posterior or anterior synechiae, increased intraocular pressure (secondary glaucoma), secondary cataract, band keratopathy, and cystoid macular edema in long-standing cases.

Posterior segment involvement may be visualized with dilated fundus examination. Vitreal opacities, perivenous retinal yellow exudates and sheathing, choroidal granulomas, neovascularization of the optic nerve or retina, papilledema, or optic nerve pallor may be revealed. Fluorescein angiography may assist in the evaluation of chorioretinal involvement and neovascularization.

Intraocular inflammation suspected to be secondary to sarcoidosis, should be investigated with routine laboratory tests as well as a serum ACE level, chest x-ray, PPD with anergy panel, syphilis serology, toxoplasmosis titers (for posterior uveitis), and antinuclear antibody testing to rule out an autoimmune etiology. A lacrimal gland mass, optic nerve involvement, or cranial nerve palsy requires imaging techniques—CT, MRI, or gallium scans of the head and orbits to rule out tumors, demyelinating diseases, vascular lesions, and so forth. Conjunctival or lacrimal gland biopsy should be considered to demonstrate noncaseating granulomas. Patients suspected to have sarcoidosis should be evaluated by an internist for medical management, and further evaluation by a dermatologist, neurologist, or pulmonary specialist may be indicated.

TREATMENT AND MANAGEMENT

■ Systemic

Patients with asymptomatic hilar lymphadenopathy do not require treatment. Routine chest x-rays every 6 months should be performed until the adenopathy disappears (usually within 1 to 2 years). However, patients with symptomatic or progressive intrathoracic disease, persistent constitutional symptoms, or sarcoidosis involving other organ systems require systemic medical therapy (Table 33–3). Corticosteroids are the mainstay of sarcoid treatment. A 2-week loading dose, followed by a 6-week taper, and then a minimum 6-month maintenance dose followed by another taper (as long as a relapse does not occur), are usually recommended. Local administration of corticosteroids may be useful. Steroid inhalers or nasal sprays may alleviate local symptoms. Intralesional injections of steroids may resolve certain cutaneous lesions. Complications due to steroid therapy may result, such as weight gain, diabetes mellitus, hypertension, cataracts, and glaucoma. The patient on systemic corticosteroid therapy must, therefore, be closely monitored. Despite immune suppression from steroid therapy, there have been reports of sarcoid patients concurrently infected with the human immunodeficiency virus (HIV) who have been effectively treated with corticosteroids (Lowery et al, 1990).

Chloroquine is used to treat cutaneous sarcoidosis. A daily loading dose for 2 weeks followed by a 6-month maintenance dose has been particularly efficacious in disfiguring skin involvement. Hydroxychloroquine (Plaquenil) is reportedly not as effective. Should chloroquine treatment be instituted, a preliminary ocular examination and follow-up examinations every 6 months must be performed to rule out the development of toxic ocular side effects. Methotrexate has also been found to be effective in the treatment of disfiguring cutaneous sarcoidosis. Other immunosuppressive/cytotoxic medications (eg, azathioprine, chlorambucil, cyclophosphamide, cyclosporine A) have been used, particularly in cases refractory to steroids; however, controlled studies are needed to determine their true efficacy.

Surgical intervention may be required in certain cases. Cardiac involvement may necessitate the placement of pacemakers or defibrillators. Expanding intracranial masses or increased intracranial pressure in neurosarcoidosis may demand surgical intervention.

■ Ocular

The treatment of ocular sarcoidosis varies according to the ocular tissue(s) involved (see Table 33–3). The presence of other organ involvement also determines treatment protocol. Many ocular manifestations may be managed with topical, local, and/or systemic steroids.

Anterior uveitis is treated with the standard protocol of topical steroids and cycloplegic agents. Antiglaucoma medications may be required in cases of secondary glaucoma. Recalcitrant anterior uveitis, as well as cicatricial conjunctivitis, may be relieved with subconjunctival or sub-Tenon steroid injections. Lid lesions may respond to intralesional injections of steroids. Systemic steroids are required with

TABLE 33–3. TREATMENT AND MANAGEMENT OF SARCOIDOSIS

■ **SYSTEMIC**
- Asymptomatic bilateral hilar lymphadenopathy monitored every 6 months with chest x-ray without treatment
- Symptomatic or progressive pulmonary disease, persistent constitutional symptoms, or involvement of other organ systems requires corticosteroid medical therapy
    - Oral corticosteroids
        Oral prednisone loading dose 40 mg qd × 2 wk
        Taper to 30 mg qd × 2 wk, 25 mg × 2 wk, 20 mg × 2 wk
        Then maintenance dose 15 mg qd × minimum 6 mo
        If stable, taper 2.5 mg every 2–4 wk
    - Local corticosteroids
        Steroid inhalers or nasal sprays may be used for pulmonary involvement
        Intralesional injections for cutaneous lesions
    - Chloroquine
        Used to treat cutaneous sarcoidosis
        Loading dose 250–500 mg qd × 2 wk
        Maintenance dose 250 mg qd × 6 mo
        Hydroxychloroquine not as effective
    - Methotrexate
        Used to treat cutaneous sarcoidosis, particularly disfiguring lesions
        5 mg once weekly × 3 mo, repeated if relapse occurs
    - Others
        In cases refractory to steroids
        Immunosuppressive/cytotoxic drugs
        Chlorambucil, cyclophosphamide, cyclosporine A, azathioprine
    - Surgical treatment
        Cardiac pacemakers or defibrillators
        Intervention for expanding intracranial masses or increased intracranial pressure

■ **OCULAR**
- Co-management with the healthcare team
- Recalcitrant anterior uveitis, and posterior segment and orbital involvement, require standard systemic treatment with oral prednisone, although additional local ocular therapy may be necessary
- Eyelid lesions
    Intralesional injection of steroids
- Cicatricial conjunctivitis
    Subconjunctival or sub-Tenon steroid injection
- Keratoconjunctivitis sicca
    Artificial tears sol PRN
    Artificial tears ung qhs if indicated
    Punctal occlusion if necessary
- Anterior uveitis
    Topical prednisolone acetate 1% q 1–6 h
    Topical cycloplegia (eg, scopolamine 0.25% bid to tid)
    Periocular steroid injections if recalcitrant
    Antiglaucoma medications if necessary
- Chorioretinal involvement
    Systemic steroids required but in higher doses (eg, 60–100 mg prednisone qd with taper)
    If cystoid macular edema exists consider acetazolamide 250 mg qd or a NSAID (eg, indomethacin 25 tid mg × 6 wk)
    Retinal capillary nonperfusion and neovascularization may require panretinal photocoagulation
    Vitrectomy and retinal detachment repair if necessary
- Toxic drug effects
    Monitor patients on prednisone for cataract formation and glaucoma development
    Monitor patients on chloroquine for corneal deposits, decreased visual acuity, and bull's-eye retinopathy

an anterior uveitis, which is unresponsive to topical and injected steroids, posterior segment manifestations, and orbital involvement (eg, lacrimal gland enlargement).

Patients on topical or systemic steroids, as well as patients on antimalarials such as chloroquine, must be monitored for potential toxic effects. Although steroids may cause the development of cataracts or glaucoma, both these complications may be treated successfully (cataract extraction or medical glaucoma therapy) without necessarily discontinuing the medication. However, should a patient develop toxic ocular complications from chloroquine, a prompt decrease in dose or total withdrawal may be required to avoid irreversible vision loss from a dose-related pigmentary retinopathy (bull's-eye retinopathy). Patients on chloroquine should be examined every 6 months for changes in visual acuity, color vision, Amsler grid, retinal changes, and corneal deposits. Amsler grid monitoring at home should be encouraged.

Prophylactic panretinal photocoagulation may be considered for retinal capillary nonperfusion. The goal is to prevent proliferative retinopathy. However, retinal and/or optic nerve neovascularization often occurs despite prophylaxis, requiring further photocoagulation. Vitrectomy and retinal detachment surgery may be required.

Keratoconjunctivitis sicca symptoms should be relieved with topical lubricants. The severity will determine the appropriate treatment regimen. Occasionally, punctal occlusion may be required.

Conclusion

Sarcoidosis is a granulomatous disease characterized by pulmonary, cutaneous, ocular, and other organ system involvement. Although the pathogenesis of the disease has been elucidated, the etiology still remains unknown despite intensive research. Frequent ocular involvement, often presenting as the initial manifestation of the disease, may lead to the correct systemic diagnosis. Therefore, the eyecare provider is an integral member of the healthcare team managing the patient with sarcoidosis.

References

Alexander LJ. Ocular manifestations of sarcoidosis. In: *Primary Care of the Posterior Segment.* Norwalk, CT: Appleton & Lange; 1989:194–196.

Arnold WJ. Sarcoidosis. In: Kelley WN, Harris ED, Ruddy S, Sledge CB, eds. *Textbook of Rheumatology.* Philadelphia: Saunders; 1993.

Austin JHM. Pulmonary sarcoidosis: What are we learning from CT? *Radiology.* 1989;171:603–604.

Badrinas F, Morera H, Fite E, Plasencia A. Seasonal clustering of sarcoidosis (letter). *Lancet.* 1989;2:455–456.

Bascom R, Johns CJ. The natural history and management of sarcoidosis. *Adv Intern Med.* 1986;31:213–241.

Bell NH. Endocrine complications of sarcoidosis. *Endocrin Metab Clin North Am.* 1991;20:645–654.

Brownstein S, Liszauer AD, Carey WD, Nicolle DA. Sarcoidosis of the eyelid skin. *Can J Ophthalmol.* 1990;20:645–654.

Chapelon C, Ziza JM, Piette JC, et al. Neurosarcoidosis: Signs, course and treatment in 35 confirmed cases. *Medicine.* 1990;69:261–276.

Collison JMT, Miller NR, Green WR. Involvement of orbital tissues by sarcoid. *Am J Ophthalmol.* 1986;102:302–307.

Drosos AA, Constantopoulos SH, Psychos D, et al. The forgotten cause of sicca complex: Sarcoidosis. *J Rheum.* 1989;16: 1548–1551.

Duker JS, Brown GC, McNamara JA. Proliferative sarcoidosis retinopathy. *Ophthalmology.* 1988;95:1680–1686.

Ferry AP. The eye and rheumatic diseases. In: Kelley WN, Harris ED, Ruddy S, Sledge DB, eds. *Textbook of Rheumatology.* Philadelphia: Saunders; 1993:516–517.

Geggel HS, Mensher JH. Cicatricial conjunctivitis in sarcoidosis: Recognition and treatment. *Ann Ophthalmol.* 1989;21:92–94.

Hansell DM, Kerr IH. The role of high resolution computed tomography in the diagnosis of interstitial lung disease. *Thorax.* 1991;46:77–84.

Jabs DA, Johns CJ. Ocular involvement in chronic sarcoidosis. *Am J Ophthalmol.* 1986;102:297–301.

James DG, Williams WJ. Kveim–Siltzbach test revisited. *Sarcoidosis.* 1991;8:6–9.

Johns CJ, Scott PP, Schonfeld SA. Sarcoidosis. *Annu Rev Med.* 1989;40:353–371.

Jordan DR, Anderson RL, Nerad JA, Scrafford DB. The diagnosis of sarcoidosis. *Can J Ophthalmol.* 1988;23:203–207.

Jordan DR, Anderson RL, Nerad JA, et al. Optic nerve involvement as the initial manifestation of sarcoidosis. *Can J Ophthalmol.* 1988;23:232–237.

Karma A, Huhti E, Poukkula A. Course and outcome of ocular sarcoidosis. *Am J Ophthalmol.* 1988;106:467–472.

Kimmel AS, McCarthy MJ, Blodi CF, Folk JC. Branch retinal vein occlusion in sarcoidosis. *Am J Ophthalmol.* 1989; 107:561–562.

Lieberman J. Enzymes in sarcoidosis: Angiotensin-converting-enzyme (ACE). *Clin Lab Med.* 1989;9:745–755.

Lightman S, Chan CC. Immune mechanisms in chorio-retinal inflammation in man. *Eye.* 1990;4:345–353.

Lowery WS, Whitlock WL, Dietrich RA, Fine JM. Sarcoidosis complicated by HIV infection: Three case reports and a review of the literature. *Am Rev Respir Dis.* 1990;142:887–889.

Mayers M. Ocular sarcoidosis. *Int Ophthalmol Clin.* 1990;30: 257–263.

Rothova A, Alberts C, Glasius E, et al. Risk factors for sarcoidosis. *Documenta Ophthalmologica.* 1989;72:287–296.

Sharma OP. *Sarcoidosis: Clinical Management.* London: Butterworths; 1984.

Sharma OP, Sharma AM. Sarcoidosis of the nervous system: A clinical approach. *Arch Intern Med.* 1991;151:1317–1321.

Siltzbach LE, James DG, Neville E, et al. Course and prognosis of sarcoidosis around the world. *Am J Med.* 1974;57:847–852.

Spaide RF, Ward DL. Conjunctival biopsy in the diagnosis of sarcoidosis. *Br J Ophthalmol.* 1990;74:469–471.

Stampfl DA, Grimm IS, Barbot DJ. Sarcoidosis causing duodenal obstruction: Case report and review of gastrointestinal manifestations. *Digestive Diseases and Sci.* 1990;35: 526–532.

Stanford MR, Graham EM. Systemic associations of retinal vasculitis. *Int Ophthalmol Clin.* 1991;31:23–33.

Thomas PD, Hunninghake GW. Current concepts of the pathogenesis of sarcoidosis. *Am Rev Respir Dis.* 1987;135: 747–760.

Tingey DP, Gonder JR. Ocular sarcoidosis presenting as a solitary choroidal mass. *Can J Ophthalmol.* 1992;27:25–29.

Toews GB, Lynch JP. Editorial commentary: Methotrexate in sarcoidosis. *Am J Med Sci.* 1990;300:33–36.

Toner GC, Bosl GJ. Sarcoidosis, "sarcoid-like lymphadenopathy," and testicular germ cell tumors. *Am J Med.* 1990;89:651–656.

Weinreb RN, Tessler H. Laboratory diagnosis of ophthalmic sarcoidosis. *Surv Ophthalmol.* 1984;28:653–664.

Zic JA, Horowitz DH, Arzubiaga C, King LE. Treatment of cutaneous sarcoidosis with chloroquine: Review of the literature. *Arch Dermatol.* 1991;127:1034–1040.

34
Chapter

Scleroderma

John Elliott Conto

Scleroderma is a progressive multisystemic disorder of connective tissue primarily involving the skin, joints, and visceral organs. Thickening and fibrosis of the skin are the classic clinical signs. The etiology and true pathogenesis of scleroderma remain unclear, but vascular, immunologic, and abnormal collagen synthesis mechanisms have been proposed. Scleroderma can present in several forms that have various degrees of morbidity and mortality. The two most often described types are limited (CREST—calcinosis, Raynaud phenomenon, esophageal dysmotility, sclerodactyly, telangiectases) and diffuse (systemic sclerosis). Scleroderma has been known to overlap with other connective tissue disorders such as systemic lupus erythematosus, mixed connective tissue disease, and sclerodermatomyositis.

Scleroderma is known to cause several ocular disorders that are either a direct result of local fibrosis or from the effects of systemic disease. The best-recognized ocular component of scleroderma is keratoconjunctivitis sicca associated with Sjögren syndrome.

EPIDEMIOLOGY

■ Systemic

The exact incidence of scleroderma is unknown, but has been reported to be between 4 and 12 cases per million of population per year (Medsger, 1985). In the United States, there are 50,000 to 100,000 cases. All age groups can be affected, but it is rarely seen in children or males under 30 years of age. Onset is highest between the ages of 30 and 50.

Scleroderma occurs in all geographic areas and racial groups, but African-Americans may be at a moderately increased risk. It has been reported to be three to four times more common in women than in men, with women of childbearing age at the highest risk. Familial occurrences of scleroderma are unusual. Diffuse scleroderma represents about 60% of the cases, while the limited form occurs in about 20%. The remaining 10 to 20% of cases are comprised of patients who exhibit overlap characteristics of both the limited and diffuse form of the disease. Rapid development of diffuse scleroderma with visceral involvement is seen in 10% of patients.

■ Ocular

The eyelid is the most frequent ocular structure involved in scleroderma, and is affected in about 65% of cases (Horan, 1969). Decreased tear production is found in 40 to 50% of the cases, with keratoconjunctivitis sicca seen in 30% of patients with the disease. Conjunctival involvement is variable with shallowing of the fornices in 20% of cases, and conjunctival microvascular changes in 70% of patients. Posterior segment changes associated with hypertension are eventually found in at least 50% of patients with late-stage scleroderma (Grennan & Forrester, 1977).

NATURAL HISTORY

■ Systemic

Although the etiology of scleroderma is unclear, current concepts include vascular, immunologic, and abnormal collagen synthesis mechanisms. Several exogenous agents have been described as causing scleroderma-like illnesses, including vinyl chloride, silica dust, various hydrocarbons, and amines. Drug-induced scleroderma-like illnesses have been linked to L-tryptophan, bleomycin, pentazocine, and silicon breast augmentation.

Patients with scleroderma clinically present with a wide range of symptoms depending on the stage of the disease (Table 34–1). Generalized fatigue, weight loss, intolerance to cold temperatures, or puffiness and stiffness of fingers in the morning are common complaints. Heartburn may also be an initial concern to the patient. Less frequently, a patient might present with signs and symptoms similar to rheumatoid arthritis, such as inflamed and painful joints, or with accelerated hypertension and papilledema.

Raynaud phenomenon is the initial sign in 70% of patients with systemic sclerosis and in almost every patient with the limited form. It may precede other clinical signs by several months to years. Exposure to a cold environment or emotional stress precipitate vasospasm in the fingers or toes. Pallor of the skin results, followed by cyanosis, and eventual redness as the cutaneous blood vessels vasodilate. The digital arteries demonstrate microscopically marked intimal hyperplasia and adventitial fibrosis with resultant severe narrowing of the arterial lumen. In severe instances of Raynaud disease, fingertip necrosis may occur.

Cutaneous disease typically follows the onset of Raynaud disease within 2 to 5 years. Early nonpitting edema and skin thickening usually occur first on the fingers and hands in nearly all cases, followed by the face and neck. The skin thickening is due to accumulation of excess collagen, glycosaminoglycan, and fibronectin. The skin appears to be shiny, taut, or erythematous in the early stages, and superficial landmarks of the skin will be obscured. Patients are often concerned about the swollen appearance. As the facial skin tightens, the lips thin and the opening of the mouth narrows. This may make dental hygiene difficult for the patient. The skin may develop a blotchy appearance due to areas of hyperpigmentation and hypopigmentation (Figure 34–1). Patients with the limited form of the disease will have skin involvement confined to the fingers, distal extremities, and face. Those individuals with diffuse disease will have progression of skin changes to the proximal extremities and trunk. Significant clinical findings that suggest development of the diffuse form rather than the limited form are capillary dropout of the nailbed and tendon adhesions.

Progressive cutaneous disease results in adhesion to deeper structures and decreased mobility of the involved joints. In the later stages of the skin disease, atrophy develops and the superficial dermis becomes fragile and loose. Ulceration of the skin overlying bony protuberances may occur. In the limited form, the progression to the later stages gradually occurs over a period of about 10 years, with the appearance of telangiectasias or calcinosis. With diffuse disease, the extent and severity of the skin changes stabilize in about 3 years. Complications include digital ischemia and gangrene of the digits. Amputation is often necessary. The patient may also experience dryness of the skin, loss of hair, and impaired sweating in the later cutaneous stage.

The risk of developing sclerodermal involvement of the musculoskeletal system and internal organs closely parallels the progression and extent of skin disease. The esophagus, lungs, and kidneys are the visceral organs most likely to become affected. Patients with the diffuse form of the

TABLE 34–1. SYSTEMIC MANIFESTATIONS OF SCLERODERMA

SYMPTOMS
- Intolerance to cold
- Generalized fatigue
- Weight loss
- Joint stiffness
- Joint pain
- Dysphagia
- Gastric bloating
- Heartburn
- Constipation
- Dypsnea

SIGNS
- Raynaud phenomenon
- Skin edema
- Thickening and tightness of skin
- Arthralgia
- Esophageal hypomotility
- Pulmonary fibrosis
- Renal insufficiency

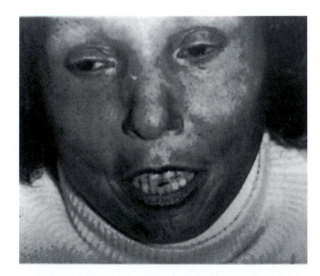

Figure 34–1. This patient with scleroderma demonstrates the characteristic swollen and tight facial appearance. The mouth is narrowed and skin hypopigmentation is evident. *(Reprinted with permission from Constantine V: Two week progression of subcapsular cataracts in scleroderma: General overview and case presentation. Clin Eye Vision Care. 1989;1:80–85.)*

disease will show systemic symptoms typically 5 years after the onset of the skin findings. The clinical course of limited scleroderma is longer, and usually will take 10 years for advancement of the disease to occur.

The esophagus is the most common visceral site of involvement in scleroderma. About 80 to 90% of patients will experience hypomotility of the lower two thirds of the esophagus. Symptoms include intermittent heartburn, dysphagia, and regurgitation. Peptic esophagitis and lower esophageal strictures may result. Other disturbances to the gastrointestinal tract can occur, such as gastric bloating, diarrhea, malabsorption, and constipation. These findings are more likely to be found in limited scleroderma.

Pulmonary interstitial fibrosis, pleurisy, and pulmonary arterial hypertension are common complications in scleroderma, and these conditions are the second leading cause of mortality and morbidity in scleroderma, especially in the limited form. Progressive dyspnea on exertion and coughing are common complaints.

Kidney involvement is found in about 35% of patients. Advancing disease may lead to sclerodermal renal crisis. This ominous complication is characterized by rapidly progressive renal insufficiency, hyper-reninemia, and the sudden onset of malignant hypertension. Kidney failure is the leading cause of death in scleroderma.

Generalized arthralgia and morning stiffness of the small joints, features of incipient musculoskeletal involvement, can be confused with early rheumatoid arthritis. However, clinically significant joint inflammation is uncommon. The hands lose mobility as fibrosis of the tendons occurs, causing entrapment neuropathy and carpal tunnel syndrome. The muscles may weaken due to disuse atrophy or primary myopathy. Subcutaneous calcinosis develops in 40% of cases with late-stage limited disease. The most common site of these deposits is the finger, which often becomes inflamed and uncomfortable. Spontaneous erosion through the skin may arise, with subsequent superinfection of the wound.

Less commonly affected visceral organs are the heart and liver. Heart disease is usually the result of visceral Raynaud disease producing focal myocardial infarction and necrosis. Arrhythmias may be present. Primary biliary cirrhosis is the most frequent hepatic complication.

Progression and outcome of scleroderma can be variable and dependent on the extent of visceral organ involvement. The 5-year survival rate is about 70%, with the majority of deaths due to kidney or lung complications (Tuffanelli, 1989).

■ Ocular

Patients with scleroderma may have ocular symptoms and complaints ranging from mild irritation to loss of vision. The majority of these complaints are from eyelid thickening or decreased tear production (Table 34–2). The onset of ocular findings is highly variable and often directly related to the degree of cutaneous and systemic involvement.

TABLE 34–2. OCULAR MANIFESTATIONS OF SCLERODERMA

SYMPTOMS
- Foreign body sensation
- Photophobia
- Vision loss

SIGNS
- Tightening of the eyelids
- Lagophthalmos
- Ptosis
- Conjunctival microvascular abnormalities
- Decreased tear production
- Keratoconjunctivitis sicca
- Anterior iritis
- Presenile cataracts
- Hypertensive retinopathy
- Papilledema
- Choroidopathy
- Optic neuropathy

Dermal lid sclerosis causes tightening of the eyelid and may lead to narrowing of the palpebral aperature, lagophthalmos, and ptosis. Upper tarsal scarring and shallowing of the fornix may also be present. Telangiectasias may be evident in the skin of the eyelid. Decreased tear production is the result of either inflammatory lesions or lacrimal gland fibrosis, causing keratoconjunctivitis sicca. Characteristic findings, identical to other causes of dry eye, are sodium fluorescein and rose bengal corneal and conjunctival epithelial staining, decreased Schirmer or tear breakup time (BUT), and mucous filaments. Severe dry eye cases may result in corneal scarring and subsequent vision loss. Exposure keratitis is rare. Venous dilation, telangiectasia, and varices of the conjunctival blood vessels are commonly seen. Serup and associates (1984) reported that unlike many other collagen tissue disorders, patients with scleroderma can have increased corneal thickness. Presenile anterior and posterior subcapsular cataracts have been documented to occur in the absence of the chronic use of corticosteroids (Constantine, 1989). Rush (1981) suggested that paralysis of the extraocular muscles, primarily the superior oblique, does infrequently occur. As in other connective tissue diseases, a nongranulomatous iritis may develop.

Vision is usually preserved, except in severe untreated cases of dry eye, cataracts, or retinopathy. Vision loss associated with scleroderma is usually from hypertensive retinopathy and choroidopathy or optic neuropathy. These findings are secondary to malignant hypertension due to advanced renal disease. Splinter hemorrhages of the retinal nerve fiber layer, cotton-wool spots, hard exudates and macular edema may be present. Elschnig spots, papilledema, and serous retinal detachment may also be found in severe cases.

DIAGNOSIS

■ Systemic

The diagnosis of scleroderma is usually based on the well-established clinical signs and symptoms. Classification into the limited or diffuse variant is helpful in predicting disease extent and prognosis for management, although separation may be difficult in the very early stages of the disease (Table 34–3). Limited disease is characterized by skin involvement that is confined to the digits, distal extremities, and face. Extension into the proximal extremities and trunk signifies the diffuse form of scleroderma. Biopsy of the skin should demonstrate cutaneous sclerosis. Diagnosis may become difficult if overlap occurs with other connective tissue disorders, most notably systemic lupus erthymatosus, or mixed connective tissue disease. Dysfunction of other target organs can be evaluated using standard diagnostic techniques.

Laboratory findings reflect connective tissue disease and are not specific for scleroderma. Immunologic testing reveals various nonspecific serologic abnormalities. Antinuclear antibodies (ANA) are present in 90% of cases. Anti-smooth muscle (ASM) antibody is lacking. About 30% of scleroderma patients have serum rheumatoid factor present. Serum anticentromere antibody (ACA) may be useful to make an early diagnosis between limited and diffuse disease; it is present in 50 to 95% of limited case and in less than 10% of diffuse cases (McCarty et al, 1983). Tan and co-workers (1980) demonstrated that the antibody to soluble nuclear antigen Scl-70 may be detected in 20 to 40% of patients with diffuse disease. At least 50% of patients will have hypergammaglobulinemia, and the erythrocyte sedimentation rate may be elevated.

■ Ocular

The ocular manifestations of scleroderma are usually discovered after the systemic disease has been diagnosed. Biopsy of the lacrimal gland is helpful in determining if tear dysfunction is due to inflammation or fibrosis. Measurement of decreased tear production can best be assessed with the Schirmer strip tear test. Examination with a biomicroscope should reveal any abnormalities of the anterior segment associated with scleroderma. Posterior segment findings are best demonstrated with the use of binocular indirect ophthalmoscopy, and closer inspection of the posterior segment vasculature can be aided with fluorescein angiography.

TREATMENT AND MANAGEMENT

■ Systemic

Because the etiology for scleroderma is unknown, there is no specific cure or management philosophy that encompasses all aspects of the disease. D-penicillamine, which interferes with the linkage of collagen, has been recently used to control the progression of the disease, but long-term beneficial results have been questionable (Medsger, 1989). Treatment is tailored towards the individual involvement of the various organ systems (Table 34–4).

Raynaud phenomenon is managed with a variety of sympathetic vasoconstrictor blocking drugs, such as guanethidine, prazosin, methyldopa, reserpine, or phenoxybenzamine. Verapamil, nifedipine, and diltiazem are calcium-channel blockers that may be useful in controlling the effects of Raynaud disease. Protection against exposure to cold, cessation of cigarette smoking, and avoidance of undue emotional stress may help reduce the number and severity of the vasospasm episodes and prevent fingertip ulceration.

Low-dose oral corticosteroids help reduce the inflammation of arthralgia and myalgia. No effective treatment for skin changes has been found, although salicylates and nonsteroidal antiinflammatory agents provide analgesic relief. General skin care to protect from exposure and drying is encouraged. Physical and occupational therapy can preserve joint mobility. Surgical debridement of calcinosis is indicated in severe cases.

Prevention of dysphagia, peptic esophagitis, and esophageal stricture secondary to esophageal hypomotility is accomplished by careful eating habits, antacids, and bethanechol. Histamine H_2-receptor blockers like cimetidine

---

TABLE 34–3. FEATURES OF DIFFUSE AND LIMITED SCLERODERMA

Feature	Diffuse	Limited
Cutaneous involvement	Extremities and trunk	Below elbow, telangiectasia
Rate of disease course	Rapid	Slow
Presenting sign	Skin thickening	Raynaud phenomenon
Raynaud phenomenon	Minor	Prominent and severe
Organ involvement	Lungs, heart, kidneys	Esophagus, lungs, liver
Musculoskeletal findings	Digit edema, arthritis, contractures, tendon adhesions	Mild contractures, calcinosis

TABLE 34–4. TREATMENT AND MANAGEMENT OF SCLERODERMA

- **SYSTEMIC**
  - General
    D-penicillamine
  - Raynaud phenomenon
    Calcium channel blockers, vasodilators, protection against cold exposure, cessation of cigarette smoking, avoidance of undue stress
  - Musculoskeletal
    Low dose corticosteroids
  - Skin
    Nonsteroidal antiinflammatory agents, salicylates, generalized skin care, mobility preservation exercise, surgical debridement of calcinosis
  - Esophagus
    Antacids, H$_2$ antagonists
  - Kidney
    Antihypertensives

- **OCULAR**
  - Dry eye
    Ocular lubricants (sol q1h–qid with ung qhs)
    Punctal occlusion (silicone plugs or electrocautery)
    Debridement of filaments
  - Ptosis
    Ptosis crutches or tape
  - Uveitis
    Topical corticosteroids (prednisolone acetate 1% q2h–qid)
    Cycloplegics (homatropine 5% or scopolamine 0.25% bid)

(Tagamet) can control gastric complications. Management of pulmonary disease is usually supportive and designed towards increasing function. Remaining renal function in renal scleroderma may be maintained by blockage of renin and angiotensin by various medications, including Captopril. Severe kidney disease may require dialysis or transplantation. Malignant hypertension needs immediate antihypertensive therapy. Management of coronary heart disease and congestive heart failure is controlled in scleroderma patients as in any other cardiac patients.

◼ Ocular

Keratoconjunctivitis sicca is managed according to the severity of the condition. Mild cases may be controlled with only artificial tear therapy during waking hours and ointment at bedtime. Severe cases may require punctal occlusion either by electrocautery of the puncta or by silicone plugs. Mucous filaments should be mechanically removed. Surgical correction of the eyelids to improve ptosis or exposure is difficult because of the fibrosis. Conservative measures like ptosis crutches or tape may provide relief.

Acute anterior iritis may be managed with topical steroids and cycloplegia. Hypertensive retinopathy and choroidopathy usually will resolve with adequate treatment of pulmonary arterial hypertension or malignant hypertension.

CONCLUSION

Scleroderma is a progressive disease of connective tissue that is characterized by Raynaud phenomenon, thickening and fibrosis of the skin, and sclerosis of the internal organs. Limited and diffuse scleroderma are the most common forms. Decreased joint mobility, esophageal hypomotility, pulmonary interstitial fibrosis, and renal insufficiency are common sequelae. No single treatment method is satisfactory, and management of the disease is focused towards controlling the complications. Common ocular complications are lagophthalmos, dry eye, and hypertensive retinopathy. Permanent vision impairment is unusual.

REFERENCES

Constantine V. Two-week progression of subcapsular cataracts in scleroderma: A general overview and case presentation. *Clin Eye Vision Care.* 1989;1:80–85.

Grennan DM, Forrester J. Involvement of the eye in SLE and scleroderma. *Ann Rheum Dis.* 1977;36:152–156.

Horan EC. Ophthalmic manifestations of progressive systemic sclerosis. *Br J Ophthalmol.* 1969;53:388–392.

McCarty GA, Rice JR, Bembi M, Barada FA. Anticentromere antibody. Clinical correlations and association with favorable prognosis in patients with scleroderma variants. *Arthritis Rheum.* 1983;26:1–7.

Medsger TA. Epidemiology of progressive systemic sclerosis. In: Black CM, Myers AR, eds. *Systemic Sclerosis (Scleroderma).* New York: Gowers; 1985:10–16.

Medsger TA. Treatment of systemic sclerosis. *Rheum Dis Clin North Am.* 1989;15:513–531.

Rush JA. Isolated superior oblique paralysis in progressive systemic sclerosis. *Ann Opthalmol.* 1981;29:217–231.

Seibold JR. Scleroderma. In: Kelley WN, Harris ED, Ruddy S, Sledge CB, eds. *Textbook of Rheumatology.* 3rd ed. Philadelphia: Saunders; 1989:1213–1238.

Serup L, Serup J, Hagdrup HK. Increased central corneal thickness in systemic sclerosis. *Acta Ophthalmol.* 1984;62:69–74.

Tan EM, Rodnan GP, Garcia I, et al. Diversity and antinuclear antibody in progressive systemic sclerosis: Anti-centromere antibody and it's relationship to CREST syndromes. *Arthritis Rheum.* 1980;23:617–625.

Tuffanelli DL. Systemic scleroderma. *Med Clin North Am.* 1989;73:1167–1180.

35

Chapter

Inflammatory Bowel Disease

Susan P. Schuettenberg

Inflammatory bowel disease (IBD) is a term used to describe a variety of chronic bowel afflictions ranging from mild to severe. Although ocular complications are not frequent, they may occur. Inflammatory bowel disease is usually divided into two categories: ulcerative colitis (UC) and Crohn disease. UC is an inflammatory disease of the colon characterized by diffuse inflammation of the colon's mucosal layer. Crohn disease, which is found throughout the gastrointestinal tract, involves full-thickness inflammation of the gut wall.

EPIDEMIOLOGY

■ Systemic

IBD is found to be more common among Caucasians than African-Americans. It affects an equal number of men and women. Although IBD is a disease of the young adult (peak occurrences between age 15 and 35), it can occur at any age. The incidence of IBD is higher in the Jewish population, especially those of Ashkenazi heritage. Two to five percent of IBD patients will have at least one affected relative.

Worldwide, the incidence of UC has been found to be 6 to 8 cases per 100,000, while its prevalence is numbered at 50 to 70 cases per 100,000. Although the incidence of Crohn disease is set at 2 cases per 100,000, with a prevalence of 20 to 40 cases per 100,000, many feel that this disease is on the rise.

■ Ocular

The overall frequency of extraintestinal manifestations of IBD is approximately 35%. On average, 10% of all patients with Crohn disease have ocular complications. With UC, ocular manifestations occur much less frequently and are much less severe. Posterior segment involvement has also been reported, but the incidence is less than 1% of patients with IBD.

NATURAL HISTORY

■ Systemic

The cause of IBD remains unknown. Although there is a possible genetic predisposition for the disease, environmental influences probably play a role. In addition, a higher than normal prevalence of haplotype HLA-B27 has been found among IBD patients. An autoimmune etiology is currently theorized, because immune complexes have been found circulating in patients' blood. These are thought to be the cause of the many extraintestinal manifestations. Alteration of the mucosal barrier of the intestine allows for microorganisms to act as antigens. This in turn elicits an immune response from the lymph tissue of the intestines. The resultant antigen–antibody complexes circulate systemically, and once deposited in distant tissue provoke an inflammatory response, causing tissue damage.

UC and Crohn disease are chronic conditions characterized in most patients by exacerbations and remissions that range from mild to severe, and even life-threatening (Table 35–1).

UC is restricted to the mucosal lining of the colon, and usually involves the rectum. The major symptoms are abdominal pain and bloody diarrhea. Fever, weight loss, anorexia, dehydration, and anemia can occur in those

TABLE 35–1. SYSTEMIC MANIFESTATIONS OF IBD

ULCERATIVE COLITIS
- Crampy lower abdominal pain, relieved with bowel movement
- Bloody diarrhea
- Fever, weight loss, anorexia
- Proctitis
- Pyoderma gangrenosum
- Kidney stones
- Bowel carcinoma
- Erythema nodosum

ENDOSCOPY REVEALS
- *Only* mucosal involvement
- Bowel foreshortening
- Blurred vascular pattern
- Deep ulcerations
- Pseudopolyps

CROHN DISEASE
- Constant abdominal pain, usually in the lower right quadrant, relieved with bowel movement
- Formed or diarrheal stool, usually *not* bloody
- Fever, weight loss > 5% body weight, malnutrition
- Intermittent bowel obstruction
- Aphthous ulcers
- Perianal/perirectal abscesses
- Bowel carcinoma
- Liver and kidney involvement
- Arthritis

ENDOSCOPY REVEALS
- Involvement of *all* layers of bowel wall
- Strictures
- Fistulas
- Skip lesions
- String signs

patients with severe colitis. Patients may present in a number of ways, ranging from proctitis alone (inflammation of the anus and rectum) to pancolitis (inflammation of the entire colon). The prognosis is good for those patients with proctitis as the sole manifestation, but for those presenting with pancolitis, hospitalization is required. For cases of mild colitis, remission can be achieved through medical or surgical treatment (colectomy).

An extreme case of acute UC can result in a condition termed toxic megacolon. This complication is marked by dilation of the colon (more than 6 cm in diameter) with extreme thinning of the bowel wall. The patient becomes critically ill and is at risk for perforation of the colon with resulting peritonitis. This is a life-threatening situation with a high rate of mortality.

Prolonged periods of spontaneous remission can occur in cases of UC, with a patient enduring only minimal symptoms. Clinically, the course of the disease may vary, with more than half of all UC patients suffering a relapse within 1 year of diagnosis. Most patients suffering from UC have a normal lifespan, with death occuring only as a result of a severe complication such as bowel perforation or the development of carcinoma of the colon.

The inflammatory lesions of Crohn disease may be found throughout the gastrointestinal tract, from the mouth to the anus and rectum. Unlike UC, bowel involvement in Crohn disease tends to be irregular and discontinuous.

Crohn disease can be subdivided by bowel distribution. In approximately 30% of patients, the inflammation involves the small intestine only (especially the terminal ileum). This is called regional enteritis. Another 30% suffer from inflammation of the colon alone, and this is termed either Crohn colitis, granulomatous colitis, or Crohn dis-

ease of the colon. The final 40% have ileocolitis, with involvement of the ileum and parts of the large intestine (usually the ascending colon).

The clinical course of this disease is marked by unpredictable flare-ups and spontaneous remissions. Diarrhea, abdominal pain (especially in the lower right quadrant), weight loss exceeding 5% of total body weight, vomiting, dehydration, and a low-grade fever signal the onset of a flare-up. If the small intestine is extensively involved, intermittent bowel obstruction is likely to occur. Perianal or perirectal abscesses may also be present. The mortality rate is found to increase with the duration of Crohn disease, with as many as 10% dying due to complications such as sepsis and peritonitis.

Extraintestinal manifestations of IBD are quite common. For example, UC is characterized by nephrolithiasis (kidney stones), erythema nodosum (an inflammatory reaction of subcutaneous fat resulting in tender red nodules of the skin), and an indolent necrotic skin lesion termed pyoderma gangrenosum. Patients with UC also have a high incidence of colonic cancer.

Crohn disease is marked by arthritis (both ankylosing and migratory), renal disorders, liver function abnormalities, and bowel carcinoma. In addition, stomatitis (inflammation of the mouth) with aphthous ulcers of the buccal mucosa (superficial ulcers of the mouth), are a frequent finding.

One serious complication that occurs in up to 30% of children and adolescents with IBD is delayed growth and development. Decreased nutritional intake due to malabsorption from the affected bowel is partially responsible for this problem. Therefore, an aggressive nutritional program is extremely important in preventing or reversing growth retardation and delayed sexual maturation.

The extraintestinal manifestations found in IBD may on occasion precede a bowel flare-up, and are often the most disabling part of the disease. Not only do these complications occur after the diagnosis of IBD has been made, but they can also be a presenting symptom. Most will be relieved by an improvement in the colitis or following treatment or surgery.

■ Ocular

The ocular manifestations found in both UC and Crohn disease may (1) precede the onset of the disease or an acute attack of either form of IBD; (2) follow the same pattern of exacerbation and remission as the systemic disease; or (3) present as a chronic condition with exacerbations and remissions of its own. The ocular complications may range from benign to blinding.

Ocular manifestations of UC are relatively rare, but when present, the most common is uveitis (Figure 35–1). For those patients suffering from Crohn disease, uveitis and episcleritis are among the most common findings. In addition, conjunctivitis and keratopathy as well as other ocular manifestations have been reported (Table 35–2).

In the IBD literature, keratopathy is the general term used to describe any corneal involvement ranging from stromal infiltrates to corneal ulcers. Conjunctival changes associated with Crohn disease have been divided into three patterns: granuloma formation, fibrovascular membrane proliferation, and blepharoconjunctivitis. Scleritis, although a less common ocular complication, is important because it is one of the most sight-threatening ocular manifestations of IBD (Figure 35–2).

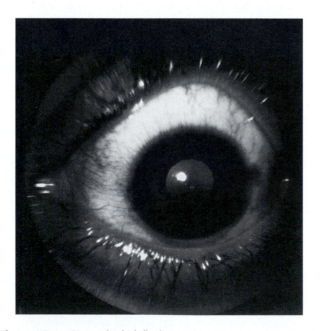

Figure 35–1. Circumlimbal flush is evident in this patient with anterior uveitis.

TABLE 35–2. OCULAR MANIFESTATIONS OF IBD

CROHN DISEASE
● Episcleritis	Common
● Uveitis	Common
● Blepharitis	Rare
● Conjunctivitis	Rare
● Keratitis	Rare
● Scleritis	Rare
● Scleromalacia perforans	Rare
● Xerophthalmia	Rare
● Cataracts	Rare
● Orbital myositis	Rare
● Proptosis	Rare
● Optic disc edema	Rare
● Central serous retinopathy	Rare
● Macular hemorrhage	Rare
● Macular edema	Rare
● Neuroretinitis	Rare
● Exudative retinal detachment	Rare
● Choroidal folds	Rare
● Retrobulbar neuritis	Rare
● Endophthalmitis	Rare
● Orbital cellulitis	Rare

ULCERATIVE COLITIS
● Uveitis	Rare
● Optic neuritis	Rare

DIAGNOSIS

■ Systemic

The diagnosis of IBD is based on the presenting signs and symptoms (see Table 35–1). Laboratory studies are *not* considered to be beneficial in the diagnosis of IBD, except to rule out other etiologies.

The diagnosis of UC requires a view of the sigmoid colon via endoscopy, revealing a red mucosa that bleeds easily, the absence of a normal mucosal blood vessel pattern, and possibly pseudopolyps. Radiographic findings may include a foreshortened colon with a narrowed lumen, strictures, deep ulcerations, and pseudopolyps (Figure 35–3). A biopsy of the rectal mucosa is necessary to rule out carcinoma or amebiasis (colitis caused by the *Entamoeba histolytica* parasite), and a stool sample is needed to exclude bacterial diarrhea.

The diagnosis of Crohn disease is also one of exclusion, and is based on endoscopy and radiologic studies including a barium enema. Biopsy of the bowel will reveal *full-thickness* inflammation of the bowel wall, with granulomas found in the serosa. This results in adhesions between adjacent loops of the intestine and to other abdominal organs. Major radiographic findings include intestinal strictures, longitudinal ulcers, and internal bowel fistulas (bowel to bowel, bladder, vagina, abdominal wall, or skin), which can contribute to

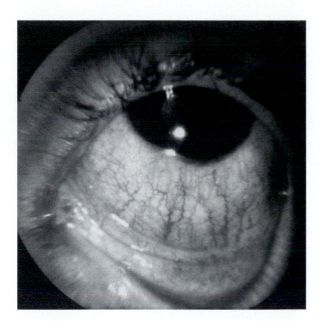

Figure 35–2. Nodular scleritis secondary to Crohn colitis. Nodule appears at the 7-o'clock position at the limbus. (*Reprinted with permission from Schuttenberg SP. Nodular scleritis, episcleritis, and anterior uveitis as ocular complications of Crohn's Disease. J Am Optom Assoc. 1991;62:377–381.*)

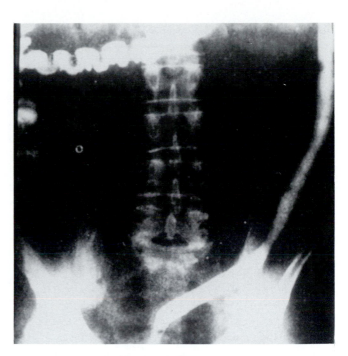

Figure 35–3. The marked colonic narrowing and strictures seen in this x-ray can be characteristic of chronic ulcerative colitis. (*©1990 reproduced from HOSPITAL MEDICINE September 1990, with the permission of Cahner's Publishing Co.*)

nutritional problems. In addition, "skip" areas—sections of normal intestine intervening between diseased bowel—can occur. A reduction in the size of the intestinal lumen of the small bowel is termed the "string sign," and is also characteristic of Crohn disease. Again, there is no truly reliable lab test to indicate the activity of the disease.

■ Ocular

The eyecare professional must be aware that ocular manifestations can occur prior to, during, or after a bout of IBD. Therefore, IBD should be considered in the systemic differential diagnosis of a patient who presents with recurrent episcleritis, recurrent uveitis, or scleritis.

TREATMENT AND MANAGEMENT

■ Systemic

The treatment of Crohn disease and UC are similar as both require the use of many of the same agents. In addition, general supportive and dietary measures will benefit patients with either ailment (Table 35–3).

In treating these disease entities, the goal of therapy is to control the disease activity by decreasing the bowel inflammation, reducing the abdominal pain, controlling the episodes of diarrhea, and optimizing nutrition.

Mild to moderate acute UC is treated with supportive measures (bed rest, change in eating habits such as remov-

ing roughage from the diet) and by treating with sulfasalazine. Sulfasalazine is absorbed systemically and then cleaved in the colon to form sulfapyridine, an antibiotic, and 5-aminosalicylic acid (5-ASA). An antiinflammatory agent, 5-ASA is the active ingredient that locally inhibits the synthesis of prostaglandins and leukotrienes (a group of compounds that act as mediators of the inflammatory reaction). If the sulfasalazine therapy is not sufficient, corticosteroid therapy may be helpful. Either oral prednisone or a hydrocortisone enema can be administered. When the acute attack of UC has subsided, sulfasalazine should be continued because it decreases the incidence of future flare-ups. Chronic prednisone therapy is sometimes required for those patients who cannot achieve a remission without it, or in those whose disease flares up whenever steroids are tapered.

Treatment of toxic megacolon (an extreme case of acute UC) consists of immediate hospitalization and initiation of high doses of corticosteroids and broad-spectrum antibiotics. If the dilation of the colon continues, emergency colectomy is the treatment.

Twenty to twenty-five percent of all UC patients will require surgical treatment. This consists of a total colectomy and is considered a "cure," because UC is confined to the colon. A colectomy is necessary when the colitis is either unremitting or unresponsive to therapy.

Medical and surgical treatment for Crohn disease is helpful in controlling the disease, but neither will cure it. The

TABLE 35–3. TREATMENT AND MANAGEMENT OF IBD

■ **SYSTEMIC**

ULCERATIVE COLITIS
- Supportive measures (bed rest, change in eating habits)
- Sulfasalazine (4–6 g PO daily)
- Prednisone (10–20 mg PO daily) or hydrocortisone enema (100 mg)
- Colectomy if unresponsive to medical treatment

CROHN DISEASE
- Supportive measures (bed rest, change in eating habits)
- Sulfasalazine (3–4 g PO daily)
- Prednisone (50–80 mg PO daily or IV if severe)
- Colectomy if unresponsive to medical treatment

■ **OCULAR**

CONJUNCTIVITIS
- Topical steroid therapy

EPISCLERITIS
- Warm/cold compresses prn
- Mild to moderate cases: add artificial tears or topical decongestant qid
- Severe cases: mild steroid (eg, prednisolone acetate 0.125%)

KERATOPATHY
- Topical antibiotic (eg, tobramycin, gentamicin) or topical steroid (eg, prednisolone acetate 1%) depending on type of corneal involvement

UVEITIS
- Topical steroid (eg, prednisolone acetate 1%) qid to q4h depending on severity
- Mydriatic/cycloplegic (eg, cyclopentolate 1%) bid or homatropine 5% bid

SCLERITIS
- Topical steroid (eg, prednisolone acetate 1% q4h) or more for patient comfort, rarely sufficient alone
- Indomethacin (75–100 mg PO daily) or flurbiprofen (300 mg PO daily)
- If unresponsive or severe, add prednisone (60–80 mg PO daily, taper once the pain has subsided, then discontinue after 2 weeks)
- Combined therapy using lower dosages of NSAID and corticosteroid if treatment fails or patient cannot tolerate required doses
- If unremitting use penicillamine or cyclophosphamide
- Scleral inlay grafts if scleral perforation occurs (rare)

NSAID, nonsteroidal antiinflammatory drug.

medical management of Crohn disease is similar to that of UC. In those patients whose active disease continues despite supportive measures, treatment consists of large-dose steroid therapy. Usually, oral prednisone is administered daily, with those that are severely ill requiring intravenous administration. Due to the many unacceptable side effects of long-term steroid therapy, the dose is gradually reduced to the minimum level needed to suppress inflammation.

Sulfasalazine therapy is also instituted in those patients who suffer from Crohn disease of the colon. Daily doses of sulfasalazine are required during the active phase of the disease. It should be noted, however, that neither prednisone nor sulfasalazine can effectively maintain remission in those patients with Crohn disease.

Surgical therapy (ie, bowel resection) is reserved for the complicated cases of Crohn disease. Those who suffer from bowel narrowing, fistula formation, abscesses, toxic megacolon (much less common in Crohn disease than UC), and bowel perforation require surgery. However, there is a 50 to 75% recurrence rate over a 5-year period; many physicians are therefore reluctant to advise surgery. Often, those patients who have suffered from Crohn disease for a number of years will have had much of their small intestine removed, because new lesions are always developing.

When a flare-up of Crohn disease persists and all other medical and surgical options have been attempted, patients are sometimes treated with more potent immunosuppressive agents, such as azathioprine or 6-mercaptopurine. However, both are toxic agents and cause many side effects, even with short-term use, and are therefore generally avoided.

The National Cooperative Crohn Disease Study was conducted to investigate the response of extraintestinal manifestations to therapy. According to Rankin and associates (1979), a significant difference in response between placebo and drug-treated patients was noted for perianal abscess in patients receiving high-dose sulfasalazine, and for anal fissure in patients receiving high-dose prednisone or azathioprine. Although the results are statistically significant in favor of treatment, Rankin and co-workers feel that further confirmation with a larger series of patients is necessary for proof of the treatment's effectiveness.

■ Ocular

In cases of both UC and Crohn disease, steroid therapy is particularly indicated in the treatment of extraintestinal manifestations, including ocular complications. The steroid therapy will help keep the bowel inflammation in check, thereby reducing the likelihood of other complications. Most ocular problems occur after a flare-up has begun, but they have been found to precede the bowel inflammation as well.

The most common ocular complications found in patients with IBD are anterior uveitis, episcleritis, keratopathy, and conjunctivitis.

Uveitis is treated with a course of topical steroids and mydriatic or cycloplegic agents. The frequency and duration of the medication depends on the presentation and severity of each case. Typically, the steroid is tapered to prevent a rebound of the inflammation.

Episcleritis is usually treated with supportive measures: warm/cold compresses several times a day, artificial tears, or topical decongestants. In severe cases, some have been known to use a mild steroid.

The treatment of the keratopathy varies from the use of topical antibiotics to topical steroid therapy, depending on the type of corneal involvement.

The conjunctival changes associated with Crohn disease have been successfully treated with topical steroid therapy (Wright, 1980).

The treatment of scleritis can begin with topical steroid therapy for patient comfort, but this is rarely sufficient to control the condition. Systemic nonsteroidal antiinflammatory agents such as indomethacin or flurbiprofen are then added to suppress the destructive process until remission occurs naturally. For unresponsive scleritis or severe inflammation such as necrotizing scleritis, systemic steroids are needed. Patients with IBD may already be on a course of steroids for the bowel inflammation, but if they are not, then daily doses of prednisone are initiated, tapered once the pain has subsided, and then discontinued after 2 weeks. If either of these treatments fails to control the inflammation, or if the patient cannot tolerate the dosage required, then combination therapy using lower dosages of both the corticosteroid and the nonsteroidal antiinflammatory agent can be initiated. In unremitting cases of scleritis, cytotoxic immunosuppressive agents such as penicillamine or cyclophosphamide may be used, but with extreme caution due to their severe systemic side effects. Subconjunctival injections of steroids are to be avoided, because this action may accelerate the deterioration of the sclera. Surgical treatment (scleral inlay grafts) is useful only in the *rare* case of perforation.

Because ocular involvement may occur during a bout of IBD, treatment of the bowel inflammation with steroids and antiinflammatory agents will have a beneficial effect on any ocular complications.

CONCLUSION

Inflammatory bowel disease primarily affects younger patients, and may range from mild to severely debilitating. Existing treatment protocols may be beneficial, although the side effects of long-term corticosteroid use may be problematic. Removal of the diseased colon will ultimately cure ulcerative colitis, but no known cure exists for Crohn disease. Ocular complications can occur at any point in the disease process (even prior to diagnosis); therefore, IBD should be considered in the systemic differential diagnosis of a patient with recurrent uveitis, recurrent episcleritis, or scleritis. Appropriate intervention early in the course of the disease is particularly beneficial.

REFERENCES

Crohn BB. Ocular lesions complicating ulcerative colitis. *Am J Med Sci.* 1925;169:261–267.

Ernst BB, Lowder CY, Meisler DM, et al. Posterior segment manifestations of inflammatory bowel disease. *Ophthalmology.* 1991;98:1272–1280.

Evans JP, Eustace P. Scleromalacia perforans associated with Crohn's disease. *Br J Ophthalmol.* 1973;57:330–335.

Greenstein AJ, Janowitz HD, Sachar DB. The extraintestinal complications of Crohn's disease and ulcerative colitis: A study of 700 patients. *Medicine.* 1976;55:401–412.

Hopkins DJ, Horan E, Burton IL, et al. Ocular disorders in a series of 332 patients with Crohn's disease. *Br J Ophthalmol.* 1974;58:732–737.

Knox DL, Schachat AD, Mustonen E. Primary, secondary and coincidental ocular complications of Crohn's disease. *Ophthalmology*. 1984;91:163–173.

Korelitz BI, Coles RS. Uveitis (iritis) associated with ulcerative and granulomatous colitis. *Gastroenterology*. 1967;52:78–82.

Macoul KL. Ocular changes in granulomatous ileocolitis. *Arch Ophthalmol*. 1970;84:95–97.

Mondino BJ, Phinney RB. Treatment of scleritis with combined oral prednisone and indomethacin therapy. *Am J Ophthalmol*. 1988;106:473–479.

O'Morain C. *Crohn's Disease: Treatment and Pathogenesis*. Boca Raton, FL: CRC; 1987.

Petrelli EA, McKinley M, Troncale FJ. Ocular manifestations of inflammatory bowel disease. *Ann Ophthalmol*. 1982;14:356–360.

Present DH. Inflammatory bowel disease: Extraintestinal manifestations. *Mt Sinai J Med*. 1983;50:126–132.

Rankin GB, Watts HD, Melnyk CS, Kelley ML. National cooperative Crohn's disease study: Extraintestinal manifestations and perianal complications. *Gastroenterology* 1979;77:914–920.

Rosenthal S, Snyder J, Hendricks K, et al. Growth failure and inflammatory bowel disease: Approach to treatment of a complicated adolescent problem. *Pediatrics*. 1983;72:481–490.

Schachter H, Kirsner J. *Crohn's Disease of the Gastrointestinal Tract*. New York: Wiley; 1980:12–124.

Schuettenberg SP. Nodular scleritis, episcleritis and anterior uveitis as ocular complications of Crohn's disease. *J Am Optom Assoc*. 1991;62:377–381.

Sedwick LA, Klingele TG, Burde RM, et al. Optic neuritis in inflammatory bowel disease. *J Clin Neuro-ophthalmol*. 1984;4:3–6.

Sleisenger MH, Fordtran JS. *Gastrointestinal Disease: Pathophysiology, Diagnosis and Management*. Philadelphia: Saunders; 1989:1327–1358.

Strauss RE. Ocular manifestations of Crohn's disease: Literature review. *Mt Sinai J Med*. 1988;55:353–356.

Watson P. Diseases of the sclera and episclera. In: Duane TD, ed. *Clinical Ophthalmology*. Philadelphia: Harper & Row; 1989;4:1–30.

Watson PG. The diagnosis and management of scleritis. *Ophthalmology*. 1980;87:716–720.

Wright P. Conjunctival changes associated with inflammatory disease of the bowel. *Trans Ophthal Soc UK*. 1980;100:96–97.

36
Chapter

Behçet Disease

William J. Tullo

Behçet disease is a chronic multisystemic disorder commonly associated with the triad of uveitis and recurrent ulcers of the mouth and genitalia. Although the etiology is poorly understood, this disease has been recognized since the time of Hippocrates. Behçet disease is characterized by chronic widespread and progressive obliterative perivasculitis. It involves multiple organ systems including the central nervous system. The ocular manifestations usually result in significant visual loss.

EPIDEMIOLOGY

■ Systemic

Behçet disease often presents in the third or fourth decades of life. It is most commonly found in Mediterranean, Middle Eastern, and Japanese populations. The prevalence is reported to be 1 per 10,000 in Japan and 2.1 per 100,000 in Kuwait. Rarely found in the United States, a prevalence of 1 per 300,000 has been reported in Minnesota.

■ Ocular

Ocular manifestations, usually bilateral, appear in 70 to 85% of Behçet disease patients. Ocular involvement is more common in male patients. In Japan, 15 to 25% of all uveitis patients have Behçet disease as a diagnosis. However, in San Francisco, only 0.4% of all cases of uveitis are caused by this disease.

NATURAL HISTORY

Behçet disease is of unknown etiology and is characterized by chronic exacerbations and remissions. The disease process is the result of multifocal vasculitis affecting many of the major organ systems of the body. Tissue destruction is due to local ischemia.

No clear hereditary component has been identified, although it is suspected to play a role. Studies implicating viral and autoimmunologic causes have proven inconclusive at this time. Recent studies implicate prior infection with uncommon serotypes of *Streptococcus sanguis*. A delayed hypersensitivity reaction to the bacteria with antigen–antibody-mediated cytotoxicity is theorized to cause the lesions found in Behçet disease. Actual tissue damage is due to neutrophil hyperfunction.

■ Systemic

Aphthous (small 2- to 10-mm round or oval mucous membrane lesions with yellow-white exudate) oral ulceration (Figure 36–1) is the most frequent (70 to 100%) initial manifestation, and resembles erythema nodosum or common canker sores. Often multiple and painful, the oral lesions last 1 to 4 weeks and heal without scarring. Recurrence is seen at irregular intervals lasting days to months.

Genital ulcers (Figure 36–2) occur in 89 to 93% and epididymitis (inflammation of a portion of the excretory duct of the testis) occurs in 6% of Behçet disease patients. Genital ulcers are also multiple and painful. Unlike the oral ulcers, genital ulcers tend to scar. They heal in 1 to 4 weeks, but recurrence is less common.

Recurrent episodes of cough, chest pain, dyspnea, and hemoptysis are the primary systemic clinical signs noted.

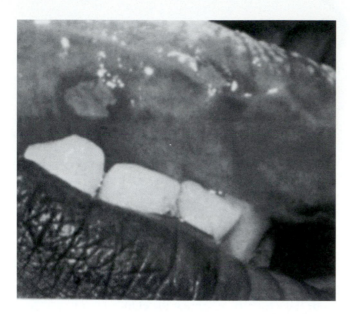

Figure 36–1. Ulcerating sublingual lesions. *(Reprinted with permission from Rahman A, et al: Behçet's disease in Kuwait, Arabia. Scand J Rheum. 1986;15.)*

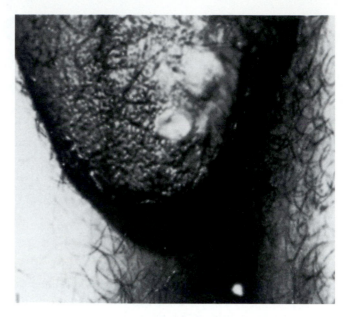

Figure 36–2. Healing genital ulcer. *(Reprinted with permission from Rahman A, et al: Behçet's disease in Kuwait, Arabia. Scand J Rheum. 1986:15.)*

Fever, anemia, and elevated erythrocyte sedimentation rate (ESR) are also noted.

Vascular complications are seen in 34% of patients. Arterial findings include occlusions and saccular aneurysms of the aorta, pulmonary, brachiocephalic, and visceral arteries. Cerebral arteries and veins may also be affected. Colitis is a common finding involving multiple ulcers of diverse size, depth, and appearance. Similar ulcers can affect any portion of the digestive tract.

Arthritis of both small and large joints is found in 50 to 60% of Behçet disease patients. The knees and the ankles are most commonly affected. The arthritis is intermittent, subacute, self-limiting, and nondestructive.

As many as 49% of patients with Behçet disease may have neurologic deficits. Vestibular lesions causing a sudden mild to complete deafness may represent one of the earliest signs of neurological involvement. Neuro-Behçet disease is characterized by central nervous system involvement including meningomyelitis (autoimmune inflammatory disorder) or local ischemia, often in the brainstem, resulting in a poor prognosis. Paralysis and paresis of extremities are common. Death from Behçet disease is rare, but usually secondary to neurological and vascular defects in the brainstem (Table 36–1).

■ Ocular

There are many ocular manifestations of Behçet disease (Table 36–2). Visual disability is the most common presenting symptom. Ocular symptoms tend to recur on an average of every 2 months. Anterior segment involvement most commonly presents with a bilateral nongranulomatous

uveitis with fine keratic precipitates. This often leads to a sterile hypopyon in 34% of patients.

Posterior segment involvement usually presents with vitreous inflammatory cells from an underlying retinal and choroidal vasculitis. Secondary complications may include central retinal vein occlusion (CRVO) or branch retinal vein occlusion (BRVO), retinal exudates, and retinal or vitreous hemorrhages. Local retinal infarcts can lead to fibrous scarring and retinal detachment.

Early and late ophthalmic signs are obvious during routine ocular examination. Long-term complications include

TABLE 36–1. SYSTEMIC MANIFESTATIONS OF BEHÇET DISEASE

- Recurrent aphthous stomatitis
- Genital aphthous ulcerations
- Epididymitis
- Arthropathy
- Gastrointestinal disease: Colitis
- Subcutaneous nodules
- Erythema nodosum-like eruptions
- Cutaneous vasculitis
- Thrombophlebitis
- Multifocal peripheral vasculitis
- CNS involvement: Vestibular lesions, meningomyelitis, ischemia
- Pulmonary signs: Chest pain, cough, dyspnea, hemoptysis
- Fever
- Anemia
- Increased erythrocyte sedimentation rate

TABLE 36–2. OCULAR MANIFESTATIONS OF BEHÇET DISEASE

EARLY
- Ulcerative eyelid lesions
- Conjunctivitis
- Episcleritis
- Scleritis
- Keratitis
- Bilateral granulomatous anterior uveitis
- Hypopyon
- Iris neovascularization
- Posterior synechiae
- Vitreous cells
- Vitreal hemorrhage
- Papillitis
- Papilledema
- Macular edema
- Macular hemorrhage
- Central/branch retinal vein occlusion
- Focal retinal lesions
- Peripheral retinal vasculitis
- Choroidal vasculitis
- Retinal detachments
- Cranial nerve palsies

LATE
- Secondary glaucoma
- Cataracts
- Optic nerve atrophy
- Retinal vascular sheathing
- Retinal pigment epithelial hypertrophy
- Retinal atrophy

TABLE 36–3. DIAGNOSTIC CRITERIA FOR BEHÇET DISEASE

Major Criteria

1. Recurrent aphthous mouth ulcerations
2. Genital ulcerations
3. Eye lesions
   Recurrent uveitis, hypopyon
   Chorioretinitis
4. Skin lesions
   Erythema nodosum-like eruptions
   Subcutaneous thrombophlebitis
   Hyperirritability of the skin

Minor Criteria

1. Arthritic signs and symptoms
2. Gastrointestinal lesions
3. Epididymitis
4. Vascular lesions
5. Central nervous system involvement

Adapted from Peplinski LS. Ocular involvement in Behçet's disease. J Am Optom Assoc. 1989;60:854–857.

cataract from long-standing inflammation and steroid use. Optic atrophy is also seen from chronic papilledema and microcapillary nonperfusion of the optic nerve resulting from untreated intracranial hypertension secondary to dural venous thrombosis. Severe visual impairment within 6 years of ocular involvement is seen in 50 to 80%, and 25 to 30% are blind. The typical period between onset of visual symptoms and blindness is 3.5 years.

DIAGNOSIS

There is no specific laboratory test to diagnose Behçet disease. Diagnosis is dependent upon the clinical signs and symptoms. Diagnostic criteria (Table 36–3) were established by the Ministry of Health and Welfare, Behçet's Disease Research Committee of Japan in 1972.

Two types of Behçet disease have been described. Complete Behçet disease exhibits all four of the major criteria. Incomplete disease exhibits three of the four major criteria, or one of the eye lesions plus one other major criterion.

A positive pathergy test is considered by some to be of value when diagnosing Behçet disease. The pathergy test looks for skin hypersensitivity to a needle prick. The positivity of the pathergy test seems to differ significantly between various countries around the world, possibly due to different test techniques (eg, needle diameter used). A positive test (sterile pustule 24 hours after trauma) has been found highly specific in Israel (97%), and in Japan, and Turkey (both 79 to 84%). In the United States and Britain, the pathergy test seems to be much less reliable.

Radiographs and computed tomography (CT) scans are of little diagnostic help in Behçet disease. Magnetic resonance imaging (MRI) has been valuable monitoring brainstem lesions in neuro-Behçet syndrome. In-111 (radioactive Indium) labeled leukocyte imaging is useful for detecting active bowel disease.

There is a close association between HLA-B5 and HLA-Bw51 antigens and Behçet disease. The ocular disease is more closely related to HLA-B5. Other weaker associations have been noted. The association of major histocompatibility class II antigens is less significant in the United States.

■ Ocular

Ocular findings are the most common signs that lead to the proper diagnosis of Behçet disease. Fluorescein angiography is useful in detecting and monitoring retinal vascular changes in Behçet disease, even when no ocular symptoms are reported by the patient. Anterior segment flourophotometry indicates that fluorescein dye leakage from uveal vasculature is significantly higher in posterior uveitis type Behçet disease as compared to anterior uveitis type and normal patients. Fluorescein iris angiography is used to indicate the extent of the damage to the systemic vascular system while the patient was in the remission stages of the disease. Fluorescein angiography is essential for early diagnosis.

Active ocular inflammation in Behçet disease is reflected in the visual evoked potentials (VEP), flash electroretinography (FERG), and pattern visually evoked cortical potential (PVECP). Electrodiagnostic testing results alone are of no diagnostic value, but can be very valuable in monitoring posterior segment changes and visual prognosis.

Ocular differential diagnosis must include the ocular manifestations of cytomegalovirus, herpes simplex virus, reticulum cell sarcoma, inflammatory bowel disease, and sarcoidosis. A careful history, and collection of clinical and laboratory data, are necessary to form the correct diagnosis. Due to similarity of clinical signs and symptoms, some investigators believe that Behçet disease and inflammatory bowel disease are part of the spectrum of the same syndrome.

TREATMENT AND MANAGEMENT

■ Systemic

There is no current effective treatment (Table 36–4) for the systemic manifestations of Behçet disease. Systemic corticosteroid therapy is not effective for long-term therapy. Although temporary reduction of inflammatory signs and symptoms is often seen, recurrences and increased frequency of attacks usually occur. Standard therapy can be oral or pulsed intravenous dosages.

Immunosuppressive agents are effective alternatives or adjuncts to systemic steroids. Cyclosporine-A has been found to rapidly improve most ocular and some auditory findings within 1 week, along with decreasing the severity and frequency of attacks. Its mechanism of action is thought to be its anti-T-cell effects. Due to nephrotoxicity and lymphoproliferative disease, dosage and length of treatment must be carefully monitored. Azathioprine is also effective in severe oral and genital ulcerations. Unfortunately, when immunosuppressive agents are discontinued, symptoms tend to return.

Topical recombinant interferon-alpha-2c hydrogel (IFN alpha 2c) and superoxide dismutase (SOD) cream applied to oral aphthous and skin lesions for 4 weeks seem to be very effective. No serious side effects have been noted to date. Topical steroid (hydrocortisone) ointments have also been shown to reduce healing time of mucocutaneous lesions. Oral indomethacin is effective therapy for Behçet patients with joint disease.

When standard systemic therapy fails, some temporary reduction in symptoms and inflammation is observed with anticoagulant or antithrombotic therapy. Fibrinolytic therapy is thought to reduce the adhesiveness of blood platelets,

TABLE 36–4. TREATMENT AND MANAGEMENT OF BEHÇET DISEASE[a]

SYSTEMIC THERAPY
- Systemic immunosuppressives
  Cyclosporine-A (7–16 mg/kg/d po)
  Azathioprine (1.0–2.5 mg/kg/d po)
  Cyclophosphamide (2–3 mg/kg/d po)
  Chlorambucil (0.1–8.0 mg/kg/d po)
  Levamisole (50 mg tid 2 days each week po)
  Colchicine (0.5–1.0 mg/d po)
  Mizoribine (2–4 mg/kg/d po)
  Thalidomide (25 mg/d po)[b]
- Systemic antiinflammatory
  Methylprednisolone (1000 mg tid IV alt. days)
  Prednisone (100 mg po)
  Indomethacin (100–200 mg/d po)
- Systemic antibiotics
  Dapsone (100 mg/d po)
- Antithrombotic/coagulants and plasma exchange
  Fibrinolytic therapy (ethylestrenol or phenformin)
  Plasmapheresis
  Isovolemic hemodilution

TOPICAL THERAPY
- Topical antiinflammatory
  5-aminosalicylic acid (5-ASA) ung
  5% hydrocortisone ung
- Topical immunosuppressive
  Interferon-alpha-2c ung
  Superoxide dismutase (SOD) cream (0.6 mg/mL)

OCULAR ORAL THERAPY
- Immunosuppressives
  Cyclosporine-A (7–16 mg/kg/d po)
  Azathioprine (1.0–2.5 mg/kg/d po)
  Colchicine (0.5–1.0 mg/d po)
  Chlorambucil (0.1–8.0 mg/kg/d po)
  Cyclophosphamide (2–3 mg/kg/d po)
  Levamisole (50 mg tid 2 days each week po)
  Mizoribine (2–4 mg/kg/d po)
  Thalidomide (25 mg/d po)[b]
- Antiinflammatory
  Prednisone (100 mg po)
  Indomethacin (100–200 mg/d po)

OCULAR TOPICAL THERAPY
- Cyclopentolate/homatropine (1.0%/5.0% bid)
- Prednisolone acetate (1.0% q2h)

[a] Listed in prescribing order.
[b] Not currently available in the United States.

thereby preventing extension of thromboses. Plasmapheresis and isovolemic hemodilution therapy effectively removes the immune complexes from the circulation.

■ Ocular

Topical prednisone and subconjunctival, sub-Tenon, and retrobulbar prednisone can be effective for ocular manifestations, but results are inconsistent. Oral doses of systemic steroids are often only palliative. Topical mydriatics or cycloplegics are useful in preventing posterior synechiae.

Chlorambucil has been the treatment of choice for sight-threatening chorioretinitis for many years. Favorable results are found as compared to systemic corticosteroids. Serious side effects, including suppressed bone marrow function (leukopenia, thrombocytopenia), infertility (amenorrhea), and carcinogenesis, limit the use of such immunosuppressive agents.

Currently, immunosuppressive therapy utilizing cyclosporine-A has replaced standard chlorambucil therapy for better control and suppression of ocular signs and symptoms. Improvement in visual acuity, color vision, and anterior and posterior segment inflammation was noted by Caspers-Velu and colleagues (1989). The severity of recurrent attacks also decreased with cyclosporine-A therapy. As mentioned previously, serious side effects such as nephrotoxicity require careful monitoring of patients.

Azathioprine has also been shown (Yazici et al, 1990) to be effective in maintaining visual acuity and preventing new eye disease. Other agents under investigation include colchicine, levamisole cyclophosphamide, mizoribine, dapsone, and fusidic acid. Although no longer available in the United States due to its teratogenic effects, thalidomide has been shown to reduce the severity and healing rates of oral and genital ulceration. Combination antiinflammatory, antibiotic, and immunosuppressive therapy has also met with some success.

Pars plana vitrectomy in patients with vitreous hemorrhage is not indicated, because it usually results in hypotony and ocular phthisis in less than 2 years. Retinal photocoagulation has been shown to be effective in eyes with retinal capillary nonperfusion, branch retinal vein occlusion, or retinal or disc neovascularization, to prevent vitreous hemorrhage and the development of secondary glaucoma.

Treatment of ocular inflammation is continued as long as useful vision remains. It is generally agreed that once inflammatory eye signs are quiet for 2 years, treatment should be discontinued.

CONCLUSION

Behçet disease is a multifaceted syndrome characterized by oral and genital ulcerations and ocular abnormalities due to a chronic progressive perivasculitis. Multiple relapses and remissions are common. The etiology is unknown, but an immunologic reaction caused by prior streptococcal infection is highly suspected. The utilization of immunosuppressive agents rather than corticosteroids is the mainstay of modern treatment. Early diagnosis and initiation of treatment is the key to maximizing favorable long-term prognosis.

REFERENCES

Arbesfeld SJ, Kurban AK. Behçet's disease. *J Am Acad Dermatol.* 1988;191:767–779.

Aronsson A, Tegnar E. Behçet's syndrome in two brothers. *Acta Dermato-Venereologica.* 1983;63:73–74.

Atmaca LS. Experience with photocoagulation in Behçet's disease. *Ophthal Surg.* 1990;21:571–576.

Atmaca LS. Fundus changes associated with Behçet's disease. *Graef Arch Clin Exp Ophthalmol.* 1989;227:340–344.

Caspers-Velu LE, Decaux G, Libert J. Cyclosporine in Behçet's disease resistant to conventional therapy. *Ann Ophthalmol.* 1989;21:111–116.

Cruz RD, Adachi-Usami E, Kakisu Y. Flash electroretinograms and pattern visually evoked potentials in Behçet's disease. *Jpn J Ophthalmol.* 1990;34:142–148.

Davies PG, Fordham JN, Kirwan JR, et al. The pathergy test and Behçet's syndrome in Britain. *Ann Rheum Dis.* 1984;43:70–73.

Efthimiou J, Addison IE, Johnson BV. In vivo leucocyte migration in Behçet's syndrome. *Ann Rheum Dis.* 1989;48:206–210.

Friedman-Birnbaum R, Bergman R, Aizen E. Sensitivity and specificity of pathergy test results in Israeli patients with Behçet's disease. *Cutis.* 1990;45:261–264.

Fukuyama H, Kameyama M, Nabatame H, et al. Magnetic resonance images of neuro-Behçet syndrome show precise brain stem lesions. *Acta Neurol Scand.* 1987;75:70–73.

Gemignani G, Berrettini S, Bruschini P, et al. Hearing and vestibular disturbances in Behçet's syndrome. *Ann Otol Rhinol Larynol.* 1991;100:459–463.

Godfrey WA. Acute anterior uveitis. In: Tasman W, Jaeger EA, eds. *Duane's Clinical Ophthalmology.* Hagerstown, MD: Harper & Row; 1990;4:40:7–9.

Hamuyudan V, Yurdakul S, Serdaroglu S, et al. Topical alpha inerferon in the treatment of oral ulcers in Behçet's syndrome. *Clin Exp Rheum.* 1990;8:51–54.

Harre RG, Conrad GR, Seabold JE. Colonic localization of Indium-111 labeled leukocytes in active Behçet's disease. *Clin Nuc Med.* 1988;13:459–462.

Hashimoto T, Takeuchi A. Treatment of Behçet's disease. *Curr Opin Rheum.* 1992;4910;31–34.

Hirohata S, Oka H, Mizushima Y. Streptococcal-related antigens stimulate production of IL6 and interferon-gamma by T-cells from patients with Behçet's disease. *Cell Immun.* 1992;140:410–419.

Jorizzo JL. Behçet's disease. *Neurol Clin.* 1987;5:427–440.

Kaneko F, Takahashi Y, Muramatsu Y, Miura Y. Immunological studies on aphthous ulcer and erythema nodosum-like eruptions in Behçet's disease. *Br J Dermatol.* 1985;113:303–312.

Kirkali Z, Yigitbasi O, Sasmaz R. Urological aspects of Behçet's disease. *Br J Urol.* 1991;67:638–639.

Lim SD, Haw CR, Kim NI, Fusaro RM. Abnormalities of T-cell subsets in Behçet's syndrome. *Arch Dermalol.* 1983;119:307–310.

Masuda K, Mishima S. Behçet's disease. In: Fraunfelder FT, Roy FH, eds. *Current Ocular Therapy.* 2nd ed. Philadelphia: Saunders; 1985:258–259.

Mizushima Y. Behçet's disease. *Curr Opin Rheum.* 1991;3:32–35.

Mizushima Y. Hoshi K, Yanagawa A, Takano K. Topical application of superoxide dismutase cream. *Drugs Exp Clin Res.* 1991;17:127–131.

Moore SB, O'Duffy JD. Lack of association between Behçet's disease and major histocompatibility complex class II antigens in an ethnically diverse North American Caucasoid patient group. *J Rheumatol.* 1986;13:771–773.

Mousa AR, Marafie AA, Rifai KM, et al. Behçet's disease in Kuwait, Arabia. *Scand J Rheum.* 1986;15:310–332.

Muftuoglu AU, Pazarli H, Yurdakul S, et al. Short term cyclosporin A treatment of Behçet's disease. *Br J Ophthalmol.* 1987;71:387–390.

Nakajima A, Kanai A, Minami S, Kogure M. Application of mizoribine after keratoplasty and in the treatment of uveitis. *Am J Ophthalmol.* 1983;100:161–163.

O'Duffy JD, Lehner T, Barnes CG. Summary of the third international conference on Behçet's disease. *J Rheumatol.* 1983;10:154–158.

O'Duffy JD, Robertson DM, Goldstein NP. Chlorambucil in the treatment of uveitis and meningoencephalitis of Behçet's disease. *Am J Med.* 1984;76:75–84.

Özarmagan G, Saylan T, Azizlerli G, Övül C, et al. Re-evaluation of the pathergy test in Behçet's disease. *Acta Dermato-Venereologica.* 1991;71:75–76.

Ozdemir O, Erkam N, Bakkaloglu A. Results of pars plana vitrectomy in Behçet's disease. *Ann Ophthalmol.* 1988;20:35–38.

Peplinski LS. Ocular involvement in Behçet's disease. *J Am Optom Assoc.* 1989;60:854–857.

Raizman MB, Foster CS. Plasma exchange in the therapy of Behçet's disease. *Graef Arch Clin Exp Ophthalmol.* 1989;227:360–363.

Ramselaar CG, Boone RM, Kluin-Nelemans HC. Thalidomide in the treatment of neuro-Behçet's syndrome. *Br J Dermatol.* 1986;115:367–370.

Raz I, Okon E, Chajek-Shaul T. Pulmonary manifestations in Behçet's syndrome. *Chest.* 1989;95:585–589.

Rizzo PA, Valle E, Mollica A, et al. Multimodal evoked potentials in neuro-Behçet. *Acta Neurol Scand.* 1989;79:18–22.

Serdaroglu P, Yazici H, Ozdemir C, et al. Neurologic involvement in Behçet's syndrome. *Arch Neurol.* 1989;46:265–269.

Wizemann AJ, Wizemann V. Therapeutic effects of short-term plasma exchange in endogenous uveitis. *Am J Ophthalmol.* 1984;97:353–357.

Yazici H, Barnes CG. Practical treatment recommendations for pharmacotherapy of Behçet's syndrome. *Drugs.* 1991;42:796–804.

Yazici H, Pazarli H, Barnes CG, et al. A controlled trial of azathiopine in Behçet's syndrome. *N Engl J Med.* 1990;322:281–285.

Yoshikawa K, Takahashi Y, Ohsone T, et al. Fluorescein iris angiography and anterior segment fluorophotometry in patients with Behçet's disease. *Jpn J Ophthalmol.* 1987;31:425–432.

37
Chapter

Vogt–Koyanagi–Harada Syndrome

William J. Tullo

Vogt–Koyanagi–Harada (VKH) syndrome is a multisystemic inflammatory condition that represents a spectrum of disorders, including bilateral panuveitis, meningismus (meningeal irritation), dysacousia (especially high-frequency sounds), poliosis, and vitiligo. The immune system attacks the melanocytes throughout the body, resulting in inflammation of the retina, uvea, meninges, and the skin. VKH syndrome is observed most frequently in Asian and darkly pigmented populations.

EPIDEMIOLOGY

Asian descendants are more frequently affected by VKH syndrome than other races. In Japan, where the incidence of VKH syndrome is very high, 54% of patients are male. The average age of onset is 36.3 years for men and 39.3 years for women. Most affected men are between 20 and 39 years of age, and women are between 30 and 59 years. Both eyes are affected simultaneously in 63% of patients. Of all the uveitis patients seen in Japan, 8% are diagnosed with VKH syndrome.

In the United States, a study at the National Eye Institute (Nussenblatt, 1988) found 78% of patients to be female, 50% Caucasian, 35% African-American, and 13% Hispanic. A large number of the patients reported American Indian antecedents.

NATURAL HISTORY

The exact etiology of VKH syndrome is unknown. There is a strong tendency for symptoms to occur in the spring and the late autumn. Due to its seasonal occurrence, infectious agents such as a virus, bacterium, or fungus have been theorized to cause VKH syndrome. However, extensive serological studies have failed to isolate any single agent as a causative factor in VKH syndrome.

Destruction of the melanocyte seems to be the underlying cause of both vitiligo (Figure 37–1) and VKH syndrome. The disappearance of choroidal melanocytes, and the appearance of epithelioid cells containing pigment granules at lesion sites, indicate the existence of an autoimmune response. The exact cause or predilection for the events to occur has yet to be understood. VKH syndrome may be part of the systemic autoimmune disease, vitiligo.

Most recent studies also seem to implicate an autoimmune reaction. Immunopathologic study of the uvea of VKH patients reveals nongranulomatous inflammation of mainly T lymphocytes, B lymphocytes, and macrophages, indicating both a humoral and cell-mediated response. Hypersensitivity to uveal pigment and antiganglioside antibodies is seen in 71% of VKH patients. Circulating antibodies to the outer segments of the photoreceptors and Müller cells of the retina have been isolated. It is therefore postulated that VKH syndrome is an autoimmune response against various neuronal elements and/or melanocytes.

VKH syndrome is associated with many systemic and ocular manifestations (Tables 37–1 and 37–2). It progresses in three distinct stages. Stage 1 is the prodromal stage and usually lasts a few days. It is characterized by headaches, deep orbital pain, vitiligo, nausea, low-grade fever, photophobia, and lacrimation. Other common signs and symptoms include vertigo, tinnitus, general malaise, skin rashes, arthralgia, and neck rigidity.

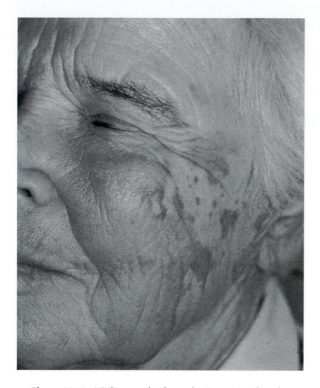

Figure 37–1. Vitiligo on the face of a Caucasian female.

Stage 2 is the ophthalmic stage and may last weeks to months. Common signs and symptoms include iris posterior synechiae, vitreous cells, bilateral serous nonrhegmatogenous retinal detachments (usually starting at the macula and proceeding inferiorly), chorioretinal scarring, papilledema, bilateral uveitis, retinal vascular sheathing,

TABLE 37–1. SYSTEMIC MANIFESTATIONS OF VKH SYNDROME

- Poliosis (VC)
- Pleocytosis of cerebrospinal fluid (VC)
- Dysacousis (VC)
- Scalp supersensitivity (VC)
- Headaches (VC)
- Tinnitus (C)
- Fever (C)
- Vomiting/nausea (C)
- General malaise (C)
- Vitiligo (C)
- Alopecia (C)
- Vertigo (LC)
- Skin hyperesthesia (LC)
- Meningismus (ND)
- Neck stiffness (ND)
- Arthralgia (ND)
- Skin rashes (ND)

VC, very common (100–60%); C, common (59–33%); LC, less common (<33%); ND, no data.

TABLE 37–2. OCULAR MANIFESTATIONS OF VKH SYNDROME

- Poliosis (VC)
- Sugiura sign (perilimbal vitiligo) (VC)
- Blurry vision (ND, considered VC)
- Photophobia (ND, considered VC)
- Bilateral uveitis (VC)
- Posterior synechiae (VC)
- Vitreous cells (VC)
- Bilateral serous nonrhegmatogenous retinal detachments (VC)
- Chorioretinal scarring (VC)
- Sunset glow fundus (diffuse RPE depigmentation) (VC)
- Papilledema (VC)
- Keratic precipitates (C)
- Subcapsular cataracts (C)
- Macular edema (ND, considered C)
- Macular scarring (ND, considered C)
- Retinal vascular sheathing (ND, considered C)
- Subretinal neovascularization (ND, considered C)
- Lacrimation (ND, considered C)
- Ocular pain (C)
- Secondary glaucoma (LC)
- Iris nodules (LC)
- Iris rubeosis (ND, considered LC)

VC, very common (100–63%); C, common (62–30%); LC, less common (< 30%); ND, no data.

keratic precipitates, ocular pain, blurred vision, photophobia; as well as nonocular manifestations such as dysacousis, meningismus, and skin hyperesthesia. Less common signs and symptoms are listed in Table 37–2.

Stage 3 is the convalescent stage, and may also last weeks to months. During this period ocular and neurological symptoms subside. Dysacousis, deafness, poliosis (Figure 37–2), vitiligo, and alopecia continue. Sugiura sign (perilimbal vitiligo) and sunset-glow fundus (widespread retinal pigment epithelium dropout) become evident.

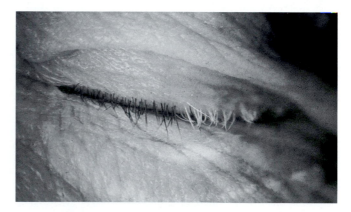

Figure 37–2. Poliosis adjacent to normal lashes.

Classically, this inflammatory syndrome was divided into two types. The Harada type was described as having no anterior chamber reaction, in contrast to the Vogt–Koyanagi type, which was described as having a severe anterior chamber reaction. All patients were shown to have bilateral asymmetric ocular disease.

More recently, Chan and associates (1989) describe three clinical types. Type 1 VKH syndrome (25%) manifests typical ocular features but no skin or ear involvement. Type 2 (50%) has ocular manifestations, and at least one manifestation of skin or ear involvement. Type 3 (25%) has ocular involvement and two or more skin or ear manifestations. The duration of illness in 70% of Types 1 and 2 is less than 1 year, while 67% of Type 3 are found to have active disease for more than 1 year. Types 1 and 2 have been described as an incomplete form of VKH syndrome.

The ocular manifestations occur primarily in the posterior segment of the eye. Anterior segment involvement alone has not been reported. Disease recurrence has been found in 43% of patients within the first 3 months, often associated with rapid tapering of steroid dosage. If no recurrence is seen in the first 6 months, the visual prognosis is significantly improved.

Prompt treatment in VKH syndrome has a good visual prognosis; however, if left untreated the prognosis is very poor. The best predictive factor of final visual acuity is the entering visual acuity. With treatment most patients (81%) have final visual acuity greater than 20/40, while only 11% have visual acuity less than 20/200. Other factors such as severe ocular complications and age of onset can also influence final visual acuity. No correlation has been found between sex, race, disease type, type or number of extraocular manifestations, and final visual acuity.

DIAGNOSIS

No laboratory or serological test is diagnostic of VKH syndrome. Diagnosis is made primarily by the clinical presentation of bilateral panuveitis, meningismus, dysacousis, poliosis, and vitiligo. The combined results of clinical and laboratory tests, ocular examination, and thorough case history are needed to obtain a diagnosis of VKH syndrome. Tests include fluorescein angiography, ultrasonography, human leukocyte antigen (HLA) haplotype, cerebrospinal fluid analysis (lumbar puncture), computed tomography (CT) scan, and magnetic resonance imaging (MRI) studies.

Anterior and posterior segment evaluation reveals the characteristic ocular findings: bilateral panuveitis, iris synechiae, serous retinal detachments, chorioretinal scarring, papilledema, and retinal vascular sheathing. Fluorescein angiography reveals patchy areas of delayed choroidal filling with leakage at the level of the retinal pigment epithelium and the optic nervehead in the early phases. In later phases, pooling of dye behind abnormal retinal pigment epithelium is seen. Fluorescein angiography also assists in clearly delineating choriocapillary dropout, retinal vasculitis, and subretinal neovascular nets.

Ultrasound may reveal diffuse low to medium reflective thickening of the choroid posteriorly, serous retinal detachment, mild vitreous opacities, and thickening of the sclera and episclera in the posterior pole. Resolution of these findings can be monitored with ultrasound as treatment progresses.

Lumbar puncture reveals cerebrospinal fluid that has elevated protein and mononuclear pleocytosis. CT scan of the brain may reveal areas of low density (active inflammation). MRI studies often reveal brain atrophy secondary to infarction in patients with neurologic signs and symptoms.

Most patients exhibit the presence of many HLA haplotypes, in particular, HLA-DRw53 (100%) and HLA-DQwa (73.9%). Although the presence of an HLA haplotype is not the cause of the disease, these specific genotypes yield a susceptibility to VKH syndrome via an altered immune response.

Differential diagnosis includes sympathetic ophthalmia, acute multifocal placoid pigment epitheliopathy (AMPPE), uveal effusion syndrome, geographic choroidopathy, and posterior scleritis. The above conditions often exhibit signs such as iridocyclitis and retinal pigmentary disruption.

TREATMENT AND MANAGEMENT

It is necessary to treat both the systemic and ocular effects of VKH syndrome (Table 37–3) in a timely manner to avoid permanent and severe complications. Currently, VKH syndrome is treated with systemic steroids and/or other immunosuppressive agents. Steroid treatment protocol may be either oral steroids alone, or oral and intravenous pulse steroids. When this fails, systemic cyclosporine A, chlorambucil, and other immunosuppressive agents may be successful alone or in combination with steroids. Disease relapse may occur after cyclosporine is discontinued.

Prompt treatment of ocular manifestations is necessary to prevent severe visual impairment. Final visual acuity is significantly better in patients treated with high-dose systemic steroids. Topical steroids and periocular injections of dexamethasone or methylprednisolone may also be used.

Secondary glaucoma, the result of severe intraocular inflammation or neovascularization of the anterior chamber angle, is very difficult to treat. Treatment of the intraocular inflammation with increased intraocular pressure requires topical steroids, cycloplegia, topical β-blockers, and oral carbonic anhydrase inhibitors (see Table 37–3). This combination can often reduce the inflammation and intraocular

TABLE 37–3. TREATMENT AND MANAGEMENT OF VKH SYNDROME

SYSTEMIC THERAPY
- Methylprednisolone 500–1000 mg (IV) × 3 days; then prednisone 40 mg PO taper × 4–6 weeks
OR
- Prednisone 100–200 mg PO at breakfast × 1 week, then taper × 4–6 weeks
OR
- Cyclosporine-A 7–10 mg/kg taper × 3 months

OCULAR THERAPY
- Systemic therapy PLUS treatment for:
- **Uveitis**
  Topical steroid: Prednisolone acetate 1.0% q1h OU 7–10 days, then taper
  Cycloplegia: Homatropine 5% bid
- **Secondary Glaucoma**
  Topical β-blocker: Timolol maleate 0.5% bid
  Carbonic anhydrase inhibitor: Acetazolamide 500 mg PO bid
- **Neovascular Glaucoma**
  Panretinal/goniophotocoagulation

pressure to acceptable levels. Argon laser panretinal photocoagulation and goniophotocoagulation is necessary when iris neovascularization is present.

CONCLUSION

VKH syndrome is a rare multisystem disease often presenting initially to the primary eyecare provider. Proper diagnosis and early treatment usually result in remission of symptoms and preservation of vision. Aggressive use of systemic corticosteroids and slow gradual tapering will usually minimize damage to organ systems and prevent recurrence.

REFERENCES

Barnes L. Vitiligo and Vogt–Koyanagi–Harada syndrome. *Dermatol Clin.* 1988;6:229–239.

Belfort JR, Nishi M, Hayashi S, et al. Vogt–Koyanagi–Harada's disease in Brazil. *Jpn J Ophthalmol.* 1988;32:344–347.

Chan CC, Palestine AG, Nussenblatt RB. Vogt–Koyanagi–Harada syndrome. In: Tasman W, Jaeger EA, eds. *Duane's Clinical Ophthalmology.* Philadelphia: Lippincott; 1993, 4:5–10.

Chan CC, Palestine AG, Nussenblatt RB, et al. Antiretinal autoantibodies in Vogt–Koyanagi–Harada's disease, Behçet's disease, and sympathetic ophthalmia. *Ophthalmology.* 1985;92: 1025–1028.

Chan CC, Palestine AG, Kuwabara T, Nussenblatt RB. Immunopathologic study of Vogt–Koyanagi–Harada syndrome. *Am J Ophthalmol.* 1988;105:607–611.

Forster DJ, Cano MR, Green RL, Rao NA. Echographic features of the Vogt–Koyanagi–Harada syndrome. *Arch Ophthalmol.* 1990;108:1421–1426.

Nussenblatt RB. Clinical studies of Vogt–Koyanagi–Harada's disease at the National Eye Institute, NIH, USA. *Jpn J Ophthalmol.* 1988;32:330–333.

Nussenblatt RB, Palestine AG, Chan CC. Cyclosporin A therapy in the treatment of intraocular inflammatory disease resistant to systemic corticosteroids and cytotoxic agents. *Am J Ophthalmol.* 1983;96:275–282.

Ohno S. Vogt–Koyanagi–Harada's disease. In: Saari KM, ed. Uveitis update. *Excepta Medica* (Amsterdam). 1984:401–405.

Ohno S. Immunological aspects of Behçet's and Vogt–Koyanagi–Harada's disease. *Trans Ophthalmol Soc UK.* 1981;101:335–341.

Ohno S, Char DH, Kimura SJ, O'Connor GR. Vogt–Koyanagi–Harada syndrome. *Am J Ophthalmol.* 1977;83: 735–740.

Ohno S, Minakawa R, Matsuda H. Clinical studies of Vogt–Koyanagi–Harada's disease. *Jpn J Ophthalmol.* 1988; 32:334–343.

Rubsamen PE, Gass JD. Vogt–Koyanagi–Harada syndrome. Clinical course, therapy, and long-term visual outcome. *Arch Ophthalmol.* 1991;109:682–687.

Sakamoto T, Murata T, Inomata H. Class II major histocompatibility complex on melanocytes of Vogt–Koyanagi–Harada disease. *Arch Ophthalmol.* 1991;109:1270–1274.

Sasamoto Y, Ohno S, Matsuda H. Studies on corticosteroid therapy in Vogt–Koyanagi–Harada disease. *Ophthalmologica.* 1990;201:162–167.

Wakatsuki Y, Kogure M, Takahashi Y, Oguro Y. Combination therapy with cyclosporin A and steroid in severe case of Vogt–Koyanagi–Harada's disease. *Jpn J Ophthalmol.* 1988; 32:358–360.

Wakefield D, McCluskey P, Reece G. Cyclosporin therapy in Vogt–Koyanagi–Harada disease. *Aust NZ J Ophthalmol.* 1990;18:137–142.

Zhao M, Jiang Y, Abrahams IW. Association of HLA antigens with Vogt–Koyanagi–Harada syndrome in a Han Chinese population. *Arch Ophthalmol.* 1991;109:368–370.

38
Chapter

Kawasaki Disease

Michael A. Chaglasian

Kawasaki disease, or mucocutaneous lymph node syndrome, is an acute febrile illness occurring predominantly in infants and young children. Bilateral conjunctival injection is one of its main diagnostic features, although multisystem involvement is always present. The disease was first described by Kawasaki in 1967. Although it initially appeared to be limited to Japan, it has since been recognized worldwide. The disease is usually self-limiting without significant complications, although a small number of fatalities occur due to coronary artery aneurysm formation. Severe visual complications are very rare.

EPIDEMIOLOGY

The majority of patients diagnosed with Kawasaki disease are children and infants; 80% of patients are under 5 years of age. The peak age of onset is 12 months. Numerous cases have been diagnosed in Japan, with 84,000 reported between 1967 and 1986. Periodic outbreaks are now recognized worldwide, with several occurring in major U.S. cities at 2- to 4-year intervals. For uncertain reasons, these outbreaks have a seasonal predilection, being most common in winter and spring. This information lends some support to an unidentified infectious origin. The incidence in males is twice that of females. Sibling occurrences represent 2% of all cases. Conjunctival injection is found in approximately 90% of cases.

NATURAL HISTORY

■ Systemic

The onset of Kawasaki disease begins with an acutely high fever (104°F), which will generally last 7 to 10 days. Two to five days following the onset of fever, several characteristic systemic manifestations will begin to appear. The lips,

tongue, and oral cavity become markedly red. There is swelling and induration of the hands and feet, while the palms and soles become erythematous. Concurrent bilateral conjunctival injection is almost always noted (Figure 38–1). This injection is often dramatic enough to be the presenting sign or complaint of the parent. Other concurrent systemic signs at this time include an erythematous, polymorphous rash over the trunk, and possibly a nonpurulent cervical lymphadenopathy (Kawasaki, 1988).

At approximately 2 weeks, when the fever begins to subside, these systemic manifestations will also begin to abate. This subacute phase, occuring between days 10 through 30, is characterized by a membranous desquamation of the fingertips (see Figure 38–1). Arthritis and coronary complications may also begin to appear.

Pericarditis is frequently detected (50%) during the acute stages of the disease. Coronary aneurysms may develop 3 to 4 weeks after fever onset. Aneurysms are best, and most safely, detected with two-dimensional echocardiography. Aneurysms reach a peak incidence of 40% in the 3- to 4-week time period, with a gradual regression of aneurysm size and incidence thereafter. One year after the disease only 3 to 5% of infants will have a clinically detectable aneurysm (Nakano et al, 1985).

Aneurysms of 8 mm or more are of much more clinical significance. They generally do not show regression over

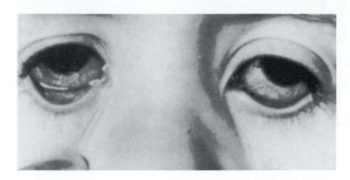

A

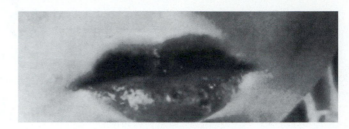

B

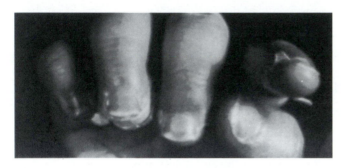

C

Figure 38–1. Nonexudative conjunctivitis (**A**), fissured lips (**B**), and fingertip desquamation (**C**) in Kawasaki disease. *(Reprinted with permission from Jacob JL, et al. Ocular manifestations of Kawasaki disease (mucocutaneous lymph node syndrome). Can J Ophthalmol. 1982;17:200.)*

time, and are more likely to develop stenotic occlusions leading to myocardial infarction. Aneurysms of 4 mm or less demonstrate the most favorable prognosis (Kato et al, 1986). Sudden death due to acute cardiac failure may occur in 2% of patients with Kawaski disease. Males (up to 1 year of age) with fever lasting 16 days or more and other cardiac abnormalities have a higher mortality rate. In addition to myocardial infarction, arrhythmia and aneurysm rupture are life-threatening complications for these children.

Other significant findings that may be observed are diarrhea, arthralgia, abdominal pain, and gall bladder hydrops (Table 38–1). Kawasaki disease naturally progresses into a convalescent phase 6 to 8 weeks after onset in which all symptoms disappear spontaneously.

■ Ocular

Nonexudative conjunctivitis (see Figure 38–1) is one of the early presenting signs in Kawasaki disease. In most cases, the conjunctiva will be significantly injected 360 degrees around the limbus. The hyperemia is primarily limited to the entire bulbar conjunctiva and does not progress to pseudomembrane formation. The palpebral conjunctiva shows minimal change; no hyperemia, follicles, or papillae are noted. In most cases conjunctival hyperemia spontaneously resolves without any sequelae. Conjunctival scarring has been demonstrated in one patient with Kawasaki disease (Ryan & Walton, 1983).

Bilateral iridocyclitis is seen in 78% of patients; it is rare, however, in patients under 2 years of age. The inflammation typically lasts several days to weeks and responds well to topical medications. The iridocyclitis is neither recurrent nor is it of a particularly severe nature (Ohno et al, 1982).

Other less common ocular complications include superficial punctate keratitis, subconjunctival hemorrhage, papilledema, vitreal opacities, and chorioretinal inflammation (Jacob et al, 1982; Table 38–2).

TABLE 38–1. SYSTEMIC MANIFESTATIONS OF KAWASAKI DISEASE

- Acute, high fever
- Erythema of lips, tongue, oral cavity
- Swelling of hands, feet
- Desquamation of fingertips and toetips
- Cervical lymphadenopathy
- Truncal rash
- Arthralgia
- Diarrhea
- Abdominal pain
- Arthritis
- Pericarditis
- Coronary aneurysms
- Gall bladder hydrops

TABLE 38–2. OCULAR MANIFESTATIONS OF
KAWASAKI DISEASE

- Bilateral conjunctival hyperemia
- Bilateral iridocyclitis
- Less common findings
    - Superficial punctate keratitis
    - Subconjunctival hemorrhage
    - Vitreal opacities
    - Papilledema
    - Chorioretinal inflammation

DIAGNOSIS

■ Systemic and Ocular

Kawasaki disease is diagnosed via clinical findings. These findings should satisfy the criteria initially established by the Japan MCLS Research Committee in 1974 (Table 38–3). The disease should be highly suspected in acute febrile children with red hands, strawberry tongue, and swollen hands and feet. Bilateral conjunctival hyperemia aids in calling attention to the possibility of Kawasaki disease.

Laboratory studies taken during the acute phase reveal leukocytosis with left shift differential (more immature forms of leukocytes), thrombocytosis, increased ESR, anemia, increased levels in C-reactive protein (a vitamin-K-dependent protein that stops fibrin formation and stimulates fibrinolysis) and alpha-2-globulin (a serum plasma protein). Urinalysis shows proteinuria. An electrocardiogram may show numerous nonspecific changes. The differential diag-

TABLE 38–3. KAWASAKI DISEASE: CLINICAL CRITERIA FOR DIAGNOSIS

Five of the six criteria below are required in order to make the diagnosis. One or more of the findings listed under 3 and 4 will fullfill that particular criterion.
1. Fever lasting 5 days or more, not responding to antibiotics
2. Bilateral bulbar conjunctival injection
3. Changes of lips and oral cavity
    A. Dryness, redness and fissuring of lips
    B. Strawberry tongue
    C. Reddening of oral mucosa
4. Changes of peripheral extremity
    A. Induration of hands and feet
    B. Erythema of palms and soles
    C. Desquamation of finger and toe tips
    D. Transverse grooves across fingernails and toenails
5. Erythematous truncal rash
6. Cervical lymphadenopathy

Adapted from Kawasaki T, Kosaki V, Okawa S, et al. A new infantile acute febrile mucocutaneous lymph node syndrome (MLNS) prevailing in Japan. Pediatrics. 1974;54:271–276, and Japan MCLS Research Committee. Diagnostic Guideline of Infantile Acute Febrile Mucocutaneous Lymph Node Syndrome. 3rd ed. Tokyo: Japan Red Cross Medical Center, 1978.

nosis of Kawasaki disease includes erythema multiforme, Stevens–Johnson syndrome, and juvenile arthritis.

TREATMENT AND MANAGEMENT

■ Systemic

During the acute phase, Kawasaki disease is best managed with aspirin. It is universally recommended as its antiplatelet and antiinflammatory effects help both symptomatically and may prevent coronary artery thrombosis. Aspirin may also promote aneurysm regression (Hicks, 1977). Dosages range from 30 to 180 mg/kg/day in four divided doses. The dosage may be reduced (3–5 mg/kg/day) following resolution of fever and inflammatory signs (Gersony, 1991). The goal of therapy is control of the acute inflammatory phase and prevention of coronary artery complications.

Infants during the acute phases should be hospitalized for close observation and management of a dangerously high fever. In addition, echocardiography may be performed regularly to monitor aneurysm development. Corticosteroids have been used in the past with poor success, and have perhaps even led to a predisposition for aneurysm formation. Recently, intravenous gamma globulin has been found to be preventative for coronary artery aneurysm formation. Its use may be considered in high-risk cases (Newberger et al, 1986). Gamma globulin is more beneficial in reducing the coronary vasculitis in Kawasaki disease as compared to aspirin alone. Its mechanism of action may be prevention of immune activation. A large prospective study indicates that a single, large dose of gamma globulin (2 g/kg) is effective in symptom reduction and can shorten hospitalization of the infant (Newberger, 1990).

Any child with significant residual coronary artery disease will require regular long-term follow-up. Among the many recommendations for these patients are the following: (1) antiplatelet therapy for patients with small aneurysms; (2) yearly cardiac examinations with electrocardiogram; (3) anticoagulant therapy for patients with multiple aneurysms; and (4) stress testing to determine any necessary physical restrictions. Coronary artery bypass surgery has been performed in rare cases to help symptomatic patients with significant residual disease (Table 38–4).

■ Ocular

The ocular manifestations in Kawaski disease are generally mild, self-limiting, and resolve without visual or physiological complications; treatment is therefore delivered on a supportive-only basis (Puglise et al, 1982). Conjunctival injection does not require any therapy. Iridocyclitis may require traditional antiinflammatory and cycloplegia therapy (see Table 38–4).

TABLE 38–4. TREATMENT AND MANAGEMENT OF KAWASAKI DISEASE

■ **SYSTEMIC**

ACUTE
- High-dose aspirin therapy
- Hospitalization to monitor cardiac complications
- IV gamma globulin

CHRONIC
- Low-dose antiplatelet agents
- Coronary artery bypass in severe cases
- Regular cardiac evaluations

■ **OCULAR**
- None, or supportive therapy, for conjunctival hyperemia
- Topical steroid (prednisolone acetate 1%) and cycloplegia for iridocyclitis.

CONCLUSION

Kawasaki disease is an acute febrile illness occurring primarily in infants and young children. The disease is recognized by bilateral conjunctival hyperemia, erythema of the tongue and mouth, and swelling of the palms and feet in conjunction with a high fever. Cardiac abnormalities are common but rarely develop into significant complications. The mainstay of systemic therapy is high-dose aspirin and intravenous gamma globulin. Ocular findings are primarily limited to conjunctival injection and iridocyclitis. A low incidence of superficial punctate keratitis, vitreal opacities, and subconjunctival hemorrhage have been reported. Because the disease is self-limiting, ocular treatment is often supportive and limited to close observation.

REFERENCES

Gersony WM. Diagnosis and management of Kawasaki disease. *JAMA.* 1991;265:2699–2703.

Hicks RM. Mucocutaneous lymph node syndrome in Hawaii. *Arthritis Rheum.* 1977;20:389.

Jacob JL, Polomeno RC, Chad Z, Lapointe N. Ocular manifestations of Kawasaki disease (mucocutaneous lymph node syndrome). *Can J Ophthalmol.* 1982;17:199–202.

Japan MCLS Research Committee. *Diagnostic Guideline of Infantile Acute Febrile Mucocutaneous Lymph Node Syndrome.* 3rd rev ed. Tokyo: Japan Red Cross Medical Center; 1978.

Kato H, Ichinose E, Kawasaki T. Myocardial infarction in Kawasaki disease: Clinical analysis in 195 cases. *J Pediatr.* 1986;108;923–927.

Kawasaki T. Kawasaki disease. In: *Primer on the Rheumatic Diseases.* 9th ed. Atlanta: Arthritis Foundation; 1988:130–131.

Kawasaki T, Kosaki V, Okawa S, et al. A new infantile acute febrile mucocutaneous lymph node syndrome (MLNS) prevailing in Japan. *Pediatrics.* 1974;54:271–276.

Nakano H, Ueda K, Saito A, et al. Repeated quantitative angiograms in young children with acute febrile mucocutaneous lymph node syndrome. *J Pediatr.* 1975;86:892–898.

Newberger JW. Preliminary results of multicenter trial of IVGG treatment of Kawasaki disease with single-infusion vs. four-infusion regimen. *Pediatr Res.* 1990:27:22A.

Newberger JW, Takahshi M, Burns JC, et al. The treatment of Kawasaki syndrome with intravenous gammaglobulin. *N Engl J Med.* 1986;315:341–347.

Ohno S, Miyajima T Higuchi M, et al. Ocular manifestations of Kawasaki's disease (mucocutaneous lymph node syndrome). *Am J Ophthalmol.* 1982;93:713–717.

Puglise JF, Rao NA, Weiss RA, et al. Ocular features of Kawasaki's disease. *Arch Ophthalmol.* 1982;100:1101–1103.

Ryan EH, Walton DS. Conjunctival scarring in Kawaski disease: A new finding? *J Pediatr Ophthalmol.* 1983;20:106–108.

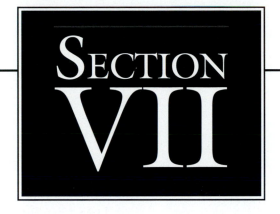

SECTION VII

SKELETAL AND CONNECTIVE TISSUE DISORDERS

39
Chapter

Paget Disease

Margaret McNelis

Paget disease, also known as osteitis deformans, is a chronic, progressive disorder of bone characterized by abnormal osteoclastic activity. Abnormal and accelerated bone formation and resorption can cause prominent skeletal deformities as well as vascular and nervous systems manifestations. Ocular involvement can occur as a result of local bone deformity causing compression of the optic nerve, globe, or lacrimal duct. Angioid streaks are also found in patients with Paget disease.

EPIDEMIOLOGY

■ Systemic
Paget disease affects between 0.1 and 3.0% of the population by the fifth decade, and 11% in their ninth decade. It shows no gender predilection and is most prevalent in persons from the United Kingdom and their descendants.

■ Ocular
Angioid streaks are found in 8 to 15% of patients with Paget disease. In addition, there is a clear association of optic neuropathy; however, the incidence is not known.

NATURAL HISTORY

■ Systemic
The etiology of Paget disease is unknown, but there appears to be a hereditary predisposition. A viral etiology has also been proposed. The pathophysiologic mechanism is one of excessive bone resorption followed by the production of abnormal new bone, leading to structural and functional alterations of the skeleton and adjacent tissues.

The disease takes place in three phases, and each may occur simultaneously in one or more bones. The osteolytic phase is characterized by excessive osteoclastic bone

resorption and increased vascularity of the affected bone. The osteoclasts in Paget disease are especially large, sometimes containing up to 100 nuclei. This stage is followed by the mixed phase, in which simultaneous osteolytic and osteoblastic activity occurs, with the deposition of lamellar (also called pagetic) bone. Lastly, in the osteoclastic phase, dense, less vascular bone is laid down in a mosaic pattern. The most commonly affected bones are the cranium (osteoporosis circumscripta), clavicles, and long bones, especially in the lower extremities. When there is vertebral involvement, it usually occurs in the thoracic and lumbar region.

Skeletal findings include deformity and pathologic "chalkstick" (the bone breaks cleanly) fractures, which can occur as a result of the abnormal bone activity. Symptoms may include deep bone pain and warmth over the affected areas. Other systems can be affected, depending upon the site(s) of bone malformation (Table 39–1). When the cranium is involved, the superficial temporal artery may become more prominent. Basilar invagination may develop as the skull base softens and weight of the cranium increases (Figure 39–1). As this occurs, the basilar arteries may become compressed, leading to severe brainstem and cerebellar dysfunction. Neurological symptoms may suggest compression of the brain, spinal cord, and peripheral and cranial nerves. These include headaches with valsalva maneuver or straining, trigeminal neuralgia, hemifacial spasm, and numbness or weakness of the extremities. Later,

TABLE 39–1. SYSTEMIC MANIFESTATIONS OF PAGET DISEASE

SKELETAL SYSTEM
- Skeletal deformities of cranium, clavicles, long bones (especially lower extremities), vertebrae (thoracic and lumbar region) (C)
- Chalkstick fractures (C)
- Basilar invagination of the skull, compressing basilar artery and leading to severe brainstem and cerebellar dysfunction, hydrocephalus (M)
- Bone tumors: osteogenic sarcoma; fibrosarcoma; multiple myeloma; lymphatic leukemia (R)

HEARING LOSS
- Secondary to (1) bone changes and vascular ischemic damage to 8th cranial nerve and (2) conduction loss from ossicle sclerosis and otitis media from chronic eustachian tube obstruction (M)

VASCULAR ABNORMALITIES SECONDARY TO PAGETIC BONE CHANGES
- Arterial calcification (C)
- Congestive heart failure (M)
- Vascular ischemia of neural structures secondary to shunting of blood through hypervascular pagetic bone (pagetic steal) (M)
- Temporal artery prominence (M)
- Heart block from intracardiac calcification (R)

C, common; M, more frequently than rarely; R, rare.

flexor spasms and sphincter difficulties may develop. Similar complications arise from hydrocephalus, when communication between the ventricular–aqueductal system is impaired.

Several serious vascular abnormalities may develop secondary to the pagetic bone changes. These include congestive heart failure, heart block from intracardiac calcification, and arterial calcification. Shunting of blood through hypervascular pagetic bone also leads to vascular ischemia of neural structures. This phenomenon is known as "pagetic steal."

Hearing loss is extremely variable and occurs in 30 to 50% of patients with skull involvement. Sensory neural loss is due primarily to temporal bone and petrous ridge changes with resultant vascular ischemic damage to the eighth cranial nerve. These patients may also report tinnitus and vertigo. Conductive hearing loss can also occur as a result of ossicle sclerosis and chronic otitis media from constriction of the eustachian tube.

The most serious complication of Paget disease is the development of primary bone tumors. These tumors almost always arise in pagetic bone. The most frequent tumor is the osteogenic sarcoma. Less than 1% of Paget patients develop this tumor; however, in patients who have multiple Pagetic sites (or polyostotic disease), it may occur in as many as

10% of patients. The second most common tumor is the fibrosarcoma. Occasional occurrence of hematopoietic tumors, such as multiple myeloma and lymphatic leukemia, have also been reported. All of these tumors are aggressive and lethal.

■ Ocular

Ocular compromise in Paget patients may occur due to local bone deformity, angioid streaks, and metabolic and/or vascular disturbances (Table 39–2). Angioid streaks are the most common ocular manifestation. Clarkson and Altman (1982) reviewed active cases of Paget disease. They found that those patients with angioid streaks had been diagnosed for a longer period of time and had more sites of the disease than those with normal eye findings. This implies a correlation between disease duration and amount of ocular involvement. This study also indicated that approximately 20% of patients with active skull involvement developed angioid streaks. These may become complicated by subretinal neovascularization and disciform macular scars. Ocular symptoms may include metamorphopsia or scotomas if subretinal neovascularization occurs.

Optic neuropathy may be caused by local bone compression to the optic nerve. Interestingly, Eretto and colleagues (1984) found that only 2 of 9 patients with Paget disease exhibiting visual field defects associated with optic neuropathy had optic canal encroachment, indicating another cause for the neuropathy, possibly a result of pagetic "steal." Elevation of intraocular pressure and glaucoma have also been reported.

Local bone compression of the globe or cranial nerves can cause exophthalmos or extraocular muscle involvement with subsequent diplopia. Patients may complain of epiphora if the lacrimal duct is compressed.

DIAGNOSIS

■ Systemic

Paget disease is rarely diagnosed before the age of 35, and is often a spurious finding when x-ray or blood examinations are performed for another disorder. Diagnosis is based on clinical signs and symptoms, as well as laboratory testing. Elevation of the serum alkaline phosphatase (an index of osteoblastic activity) and urine total peptide hydroxyproline (an index of bone matrix resorption) to more than twice the upper normal limit are used to diagnose Paget disease. Characteristic radiographic findings will confirm the diagnosis. Technetium-99 diphosphonate bone scans are used to determine the extent of bony involvement, and are the most sensitive means to detect active lesions of Paget disease, although this is not a specific test for the disease (Figure 39–2). In this test, the scanning agent is adsorbed (attached)

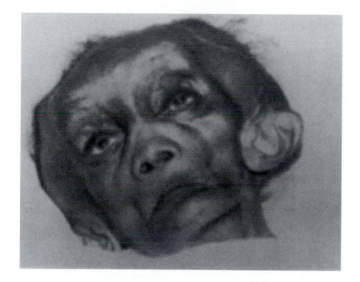

A

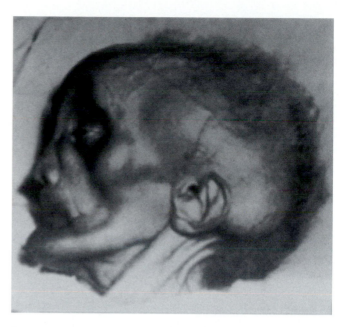

B

Figure 39–1. Increased cranium size due to bony malformation. *(Reprinted with permission from Renie WA. Goldberg's Genetic and Metabolic Eye Disease. 2nd ed. Boston: Little, Brown; 1986, p 484.)*

onto "hot" areas, indicating regions of increased bone vascularity and mineralization. Confirmational x-rays are then taken of the positive regions of the scans. Bone biopsy is rarely necessary, but may occasionally be used when differentiating "burned out" Paget sites from primary hyperparathyroidism, osteomyelitis, and osteomalacia.

Some patients have elevated serum metabolites of vitamin D. Serum concentration of calcium and inorganic phosphorous is normal, but urinary calcium may be elevated and may lead to renal calculi. If serum calcium or inorganic phosphorous are abnormal, other disease entities must be ruled out, such as malignancy or primary hyperparathyroidism.

TABLE 39–2. OCULAR MANIFESTATIONS OF PAGET DISEASE

ANGIOID STREAKS IN RETINA
- Can cause subretinal neovascularization and disciform macular scar

LOCAL BONE DEFORMITY
- Optic neuropathy
- Extraocular muscle palsy
- Exophthalmos
- Epiphora secondary to lacrimal duct obstruction

VASCULAR DISTURBANCES
- Optic neuropathy

OTHER
- Increased intraocular pressure and glaucoma

■ Ocular

Diagnosis of angioid streaks is made by fundoscopy and fluorescein angiography. They appear in the peripapillary area and radiate outward, roughly in the directions of the extraocular muscles. They may appear reddish to gray, depending on the amount of fundus pigmentation present (see Chapter 41 for more detailed discussion of the fluorescein pattern associated with angioid streaks).

Clinical signs of optic neuropathy will be evident on fundus and visual field examinations as well as through patient history. Forced ductions can be used to differentiate muscle entrapment versus cranial nerve palsy in cases of extraocular muscle paralysis. Exophthalmos secondary to bone deformity can be measured through exophthalmometry. If the lacrimal duct is obstructed, symptoms of epiphora along with clinical signs of blockage (Jones dye test) will help make the diagnosis. X-ray and CT scan of the involved areas can be used to confirm the diagnosis.

TREATMENT AND MANAGEMENT

■ Systemic

Most patients with Paget disease require no therapy or only mild analgesic agents such as aspirin or indomethacin for pain in affected areas. Table 39–3 includes a summary of treatment and management of Paget disease. Orthopedic surgery, including total hip replacement, can aid in ambulation when needed. These patients also respond well to

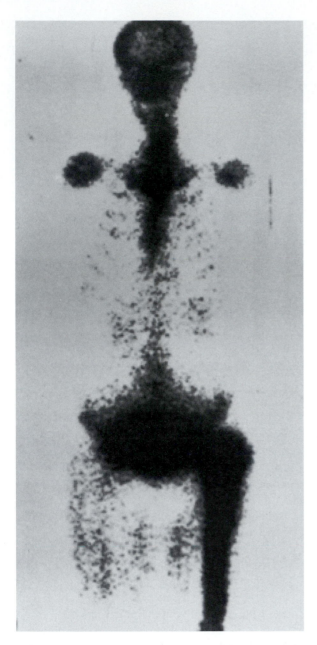

Figure 39–2. Technetium-99 diphosphonate bone scan shows increased areas of vascularity and mineralization, particularly in the left femur. *(Reprinted with permission from Singer FR.* Paget's Disease of Bone. *New York: Plenum; 1977, p 108.)*

TABLE 39–3. TREATMENT AND MANAGEMENT OF PAGET DISEASE

SKELETAL INVOLVEMENT
- No treatment if bone involvement is minor
- Analgesics for pain in affected areas
- Salmon calcitonin injections in courses, or human calcitonin, as alternative therapy
- Orthopedic surgery
- Cytotoxic agents
- Occipital craniotomy in cases with basilar compression
- Chemotherapy or radical resection with bone tumors

HEARING LOSS
- Calcitonin and disodium etidronate

OCULAR INVOLVEMENT
- **Angioid Streaks**
  Routine fundus examination and visual field examination
  Home Amsler grid monitor
  Fluorescein angiography
  Laser surgery, when indicated
- **Bone Deformity Causing Muscle Paralysis, Exophthalmos**
  No specific treatment, follow only with supportive measures
  Debulking of bones
- **Optic Neuropathy Caused By Pagetic "Steal"**
  Surgical debulking
  Systemic salmon calcitonin, sodium etidronate, or mithramycin
- **Lacrimal Obstruction**
  Monitor, supportive measures
  Local debulking of bones

salmon calcitonin injections of 40 μg daily or on alternate days. Salmon calcitonin causes an inhibition of the ongoing bone resorptive process by decreasing the number of osteoclasts. It has been shown to relieve bone pain and help heal osteolytic lesions. It also reduces increased cardiac output and may cause the reversal of some neurological damage. Due to the formation of antibodies to salmon calcitonin, its long-term efficacy tends to diminish with time. Some of these patients do well when switched to human calcitonin. Patients tend to respond best when they receive intermittant courses of therapy, rather than remaining on it chronically. Recent advances have been made in the administration of calcitonin in the form of a nasal spray for patients with milder disease. This has good acceptance in geriatric cases where subcutaneous injection is less convenient.

Both sensorineural and conductive hearing loss have been reported to stabilize and occasionally reverse with combination therapy of calcitonin and disodium etidronate. Disodium etidronate is the only FDA-approved biphosphonate. It can be taken orally at 5 mg/kg of body weight with similar results to calcitonin. Cytotoxic agents such as mithramycin have been used to suppress several manifestations of the disease by inhibiting bone resorption and reducing hypercalcemia. They offer dramatic relief from bone pain but they are also highly toxic to hepatic, renal, and platelet tissue and are reserved for patients unresponsive to other therapy.

Patients with basilar compression may require occipital craniotomy for decompression of neurologic structures. In cases of sarcoma, chemotherapy has been largely ineffective, and radical resection of the affected limb has the best outcome for survival.

■ Ocular

Complete dilated fundus ophthalmoscopic examination and visual fields are indicated in Paget patients. Ocular management consists of laser therapy to subretinal neovascularization when serous detachment of the macula is a possible threat. Prophylactic photocoagulation of angioid streaks is contraindicated, as it may stimulate new vessel growth. Angioid streaks without neovascularization should be followed at least every 6 months by stereo fundus photography and fluorescein angiography, when indicated. The patient should also self-monitor for any changes with a home Amsler grid. If optic neuropathy or lacrimal duct obstruction results from a compressive lesion, surgical debulking is an option. However, this is of limited aid due to excessive bleeding and regrowth of the surgical site. Optic neuropathy is thought to be caused by bony compression and Pagetic "steal" of vascular supply secondary to hypervascular bone lesions. Although it is difficult to restore neural function, treatment is the systemic administration of salmon calcitonin, sodium etidronate, or mithramycin.

CONCLUSION

Paget disease is a common disorder of bone, which can lead to many systemic manifestations. In addition to skeletal deformities, advanced disease affects the vascular and nervous system, including the eyes. Its manifestations can occur in various forms and degrees in the affected sites. Although a specific etiology remains elusive, recent developments in medicine have proven helpful in reducing its severity. The eyecare practitioner can play an important role in management of the patient with Paget disease through education, follow-up, and timely referral when indicated.

REFERENCES

Ballin M. Parathyroidism in reference to orthopedic surgery. *J Bone Jt Surg.* 1933;15:120.

Berman L. The endocrine treatment of Paget's disease. *Endocrinology.* 1932;16:109.

Clarkson JG, Altman RD. Angioid streaks. *Surv Ophthalmol.* 1982;26:235.

D'Agostino HR, Barnett CA, Zielinski XJ, Gordan GS. Intranasal salmon calcitonin treatment of Paget's disease of bone. Results in nine patients. *Clin Orthop.* 1988;230:223–228.

Davis AE Jr. Simultaneous occurrence of osteitis deformans and Hodgkin's disease. *JAMA.* 1960;173:153.

Eretto P, Krohel GB, Shihab ZM, et al. Optic neuropathy in Paget's disease. *Am J Ophthalmol.* 1984;97:505.

Federman JL, Shields JA, Tomer TL. Angioid streaks. Fluorescein angiographic features. *Arch Ophthalmol.* 1975;93:951.

Foldes J, Shamir S, Brautbar C, et al. HLA-D antigens and Paget's disease of bone. *Clin Orthop.* 1991;266:301–303.

Foldes J, Shamir S, Kidroni G, Menczel J. Vitamin D in Paget disease of bone. *Clin Orthop.* 1989;243:275–279.

Gagel RF, Logan C, Mallette LE. Treatment of Paget's disease of bone with salmon calcitonin nasal spray. *J Am Geriatr Soc.* 1988;36:1010–1014.

Gass JDM, Clarkson JG. Angioid streaks and disciform macular detachment in Paget's disease (osteitis deformans). *Am J Ophthalmol.* 1973;75:576.

Haddad JG. Paget's disease of bone. In: Stein J, ed. *Internal Medicine.* 3rd ed. Boston: Little, Brown; 1990:2361–2364.

Healey JH, Buss D. Radiation and pagetic osteogenic sarcomas. *Clin Orthop Sep.* 1991;270:128–134.

Krane SM. Paget's disease of bone. *Clin Orthop.* 1977;127:24.

Kukita A, Chenu C, McManus LM, et al. Atypical multinucleated cells form in long-term marrow cultures from patients with Paget's disease. *J Clin Invest.* 1990;85:1280–1286.

Lando M, Hoover LA, Finerman G. Stabilization of hearing loss in Paget's disease with calcitonin and etidronate. *Arch Otolaryngol Head Neck Surg.* 1988;114:891–894.

McKusick VA. *Heritable Disorders of Connective Tissue.* 4th ed. St. Louis: Mosby; 1960:718–723.

Mills BG, Singer FR. Nuclear inclusions in Paget's disease of bone. *Science.* 1976;194:201.

Muff R, Dambach MA, Perrenaud A, et al. Efficacy of human calcitonin in patients with Paget's disease refractory to salmon calcitonin. *Am J Med.* 1990;89:181–184.

O'Doherty DP, Dickerstaff DR, McCloskey EZ, et al. A comparison of the acute effects of subcutaneous and intranasal calcitonin. *Clin Sci.* 1990;78:215–219.

Paton D. *The Relation of Angioid Streaks to Systemic Disease.* Springfield: Thomas; 1972:38–46.

Potter HG, Schneider R, Ghelman B, et al. Multiple giant cell tumors and Paget's disease of bone: Radiographic and clinical correlations. *Radiology.* 1991;180:261–264.

Proops D, Bayley D, Hawke M. Paget's disease and the temporal bone—A clinical and histopathological review of six temporal bones. *J Otolaryngol.* 1985;14:20–29.

Rassmussen H, Bordier P. *The Physiologic and Cellular Basis of Metabolic Bone Disease.* Baltimore: Williams & Wilkins; 1974:272–304.

Rebel A, Malkani K, Basle M, Bregeon C. Osteoclast ultrastructure in Paget's disease. *Clin Orthop.* 1987;217:4.

Rosenkrantz JA, Gluckman EC. Co-existence of Paget's disease of bone and multiple myeloma: Case reports of two patients. *Am J Roentgenol Rad Ther Nuc Med.* 1957;78:30.

Shields JA, Federman JL, Tomer TL, et al. Angioid streaks. Ophthalmoscopic variations and diagnostic problems. *Br J Ophthalmol.* 1975;59:257.

Singer FR. Paget's disease of bone. In: Wyngaarden JB, Smith LH, eds. *Cecil's Textbook of Medicine.* 17th ed. Philadelphia: Saunders; 1985:1461–1463.

Singer FR. *Paget's Disease of Bone.* New York: Plenum; 1977:93–102, 121–158.

Verhoeff FH. Histological findings in a case of angioid streaks. *Br J Ophthalmol.* 1948;32:531.

40
Chapter

Marfan Syndrome

Margaret McNelis

Marfan syndrome is composed of a group of connective tissue disorders that exhibit characteristic skeletal, cardiovascular, and ocular abnormalities with a wide range of expressivity. The typical presentation of a Marfan syndrome patient is that of a tall individual with long, thin arms and legs, hypermobile joints, and a long face. It has been suggested that Abraham Lincoln may have had Marfan syndrome, as well as the composer Rachmaninov, who wrote piano music that is best played by very long, hyperextensible hands. Subluxation of the crystalline lens is the most common ocular manifestation of this disease.

EPIDEMIOLOGY

■ Systemic

Marfan syndrome occurs in 4 to 6 per 10,000 births. Between 5 and 35% of these cases are new mutations and are associated with an increased paternal age. Sporadic cases tend to be more severely affected than familial ones. The disease shows no racial or sexual predilection. Skeletal involvement is found in every patient with Marfan syndrome. Aortic involvement occurs in 80% of patients with the disease.

■ Ocular

Subluxation of the crystalline lens occurs in 50 to 58% of patients with Marfan syndrome, with little effect on acuity in most patients. Visual acuity is 20/40 or better in 60% of patients with lens subluxation. Glaucoma occurs in 8% of patients, secondary to lens dislocation or a congenital angle anomaly. Retinal detachment is found in 9% of patients with dislocated lenses. Iris transillumination is present in about 10% of patients, and approximately 20% of patients with Marfan syndrome are strabismic.

NATURAL HISTORY

■ Systemic

While once considered to be exclusively autosomal dominantly transmitted with variable penetrance, Marfan syndrome is now thought to be comprised of several molecular defects that cause a group of phenotypically similar disorders. It has been linked to a defect in the fibrillin gene on chromosome 15. A phenotypically similar but distinct disorder, congenital contractural arachnodactyly, has been linked to a defect in the fibrillin gene on chromosome 5, and it is probably this disorder that Antoine Marfan described in 1896.

Fibrillin is a major component of the microfibrils found in the connective tissue space of blood vessel walls and the suspensory ligaments of the crystalline lens. Fibrillin is probably a family of connective tissue proteins, rather than a single protein in itself, and Marfan-like changes may arise when mutations occur on other fibrillin genes. This may account for the variability in phenotypes of different Marfan patients.

Skeletal abnormalities of Marfan syndrome manifest as long, spiderlike fingers (arachnodactyly; Figure 40–1) and armspan equal to or greater than height. The Marfan patient

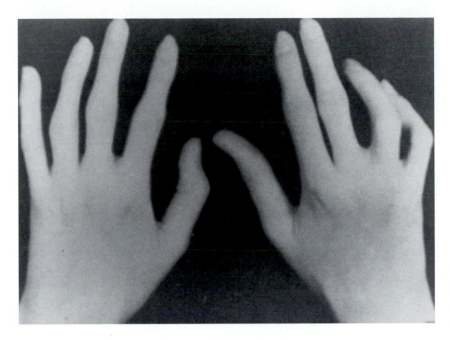

Figure 40–1. Long, spiderlike fingers in a patient with Marfan syndrome *(Reprinted with permission from McKusick VA. Heritable Disorders of Connective Tissue. 4th ed. St. Louis: Mosby; 1960, p 172.)*

is tall within his or her family, with the upper segment of the body (head to pubic bone) much shorter than the lower segment (pubic bone to floor). Scoliosis is frequent and is the most debilitating of the skeletal complications. Overgrowth of the ribs can cause sternal displacement inward (pectus excavatum) or outward (pectus carinatum or pigeon chest). The number and severity of skeletal abnormalities in Marfan syndrome increase during puberty.

The joints will be hyperextensible, and repeated dislocations of the hips, clavicles, patellas, and mandibles may occur. Patients usually have a high arched palate and an abnormal smallness of the jaw. Other variable physical signs include a broad nasal bridge, large floppy low-set ears, partially cleft palate, inguinal hernia, femoral fracture, overlapping toes, foot deformities, decreased muscle tone, diminished reflexes, and peripheral muscle wasting.

Mitral valve prolapse is common, characterized by midsystolic click and late systolic murmur on auscultation. An association has been made between mitral valve prolapse and cerebrovascular events such as transient ischemic attacks, retinal vascular emboli, and stroke. See Chapter 4 for a more complete discussion of valve disorders. Aortic involvement is the most common cause of death, with the average age 32 years. Histologic examination of Marfan aortas exhibit cystic medial necrosis with focal fragmentation of the elastic fibers in the media. Structurally altered cardiac valves may give rise to bacterial endocarditis, arrhythmias, rupture of the chordae tendineae, sudden mitral insufficiency, and sudden death.

Marfan patients may also exhibit skin folds and stretch marks in places where body fat has been neither gained nor lost. These patients are also more prone to inguinal hernias, as well as other hernia types. Spontaneous pneumothorax

and bullous emphysema have been reported, but the incidence is unknown. A high frequency of sleep apnea in these patients has also been noted, perhaps due to a floppy, easily collapsible pharynx.

Various central nervous system manifestations have been documented (Table 40–1), as well as an association with schizophrenia.

■ Ocular

The major ocular sign in Marfan syndrome is ectopia lentis, or bilateral displacement of the crystalline lenses (Figure 40–2). The lenses will almost always be displaced upward in a superotemporal direction, usually occurring in utero. This type of dislocation is incomplete, and nonprogressive, and accommodation is possible because the zonules remain attached to the lens. This is to be differentiated from the ectopia lentis found in homocystinuria (see Chapter 76), in which the zonules rupture and the lenses dislocate down and in. In these cases, accommodative function is impaired. Lenticular astigmatism may be induced with lens subluxation, depending on the degree of dislocation. Phakic eyes are more commonly myopic in the Marfan patient.

Increased axial length can cause moderate to severe myopia and the risk of spontaneous retinal detachment increases with increased axial length. The choroid in these patients may be thin, displaying various degrees of scleral crescents, but staphylomas are uncommon. Peripheral retinal degenerations may also occur, leading to retinal detachment. Other peripheral retinal manifestations include prominent areas of white without pressure, lattice degeneration, retinal holes, and less commonly, retinoschisis. Colobomas of the iris, lens, and optic nerve have been associated with Marfan syndrome.

TABLE 40–1. SYSTEMIC MANIFESTATIONS OF MARFAN SYNDROME

SKELETAL
- Arachnodactyly (C)
- Armspan that exceeds height (C)
- Hyperextensible joints (C)
- High, arched palate (C)
- Small jaw bones (C)
- Hernias (C)
- Flat feet and foot deformities (C)
- Scoliosis (C)
- Pectus excavatum/carinatum (C)
- Broad nasal bridge (M)
- Large, floppy, low-set ears (M)
- Partially cleft palate (M)
- Femoral fracture (M)
- Overlapping toes (M)

CARDIOVASCULAR
- Mitral valve prolapse (C)
- Arrhythmias (C)
- Dilated ascending aorta; rupture or aneurysm of aorta (C)
- Cerebrovascular accidents such as transient ischemic attacks, strokes (C)

- Structurally altered cardiac valves with resultant bacterial endocarditis, arrhythmia, rupture of chordae tendineae, sudden mitral insufficiency (C)

CUTANEOUS
- Skin folds and stretch marks (C)

MUSCULAR SYSTEM
- Decreased muscle tone (C)
- Diminished reflexes (C)
- Peripheral muscle wasting (M)

PULMONARY SYSTEM
- Spontaneous pneumothorax (R)
- Bullous emphysema (R)
- Sleep apnea (R)

CENTRAL NERVOUS SYSTEM
- Dural ectasia such as lumbosacral meningocele (a congenital hernia in which the meninges protrude through an opening in the skull or spinal column) (M)
- Dilated cisterna magna (M)
- Learning disability (M)
- Hyperactivity with or without attention deficit disorder (M)
- An association with schizophrenia has been suggested (R)

C, common; M, more frequently than rarely; R, rare.

Relatively flat corneas are typical in Marfan syndrome, but a few cases of keratoconus have also been reported. Corneal diameter may be increased up to 14 mm without an increase in intraocular pressure.

As is common in many other connective tissue disorders, the anterior chamber angle in Marfan syndrome is deep

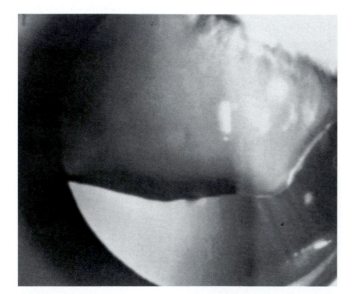

Figure 40–2. Ectopia lentis in a Marfan patient in which the lens is displaced in an upward direction *(Reprinted with permission from Renie WA, ed.* Goldberg's Genetic and Metabolic Eye Disease. *2nd ed. Boston: Little, Brown; 1986, p 395.)*

with structural abnormalities. Glaucoma may occur due to pupil block, congenital angle anomalies, or anterior lens subluxation. If glaucoma occurs, further stretching of the globe, which already may have an increased axial length, may cause retinal detachment.

Retinal arterial occlusions associated with emboli from inflamed mitral valve leaflets have been reported.

Due to the thinness of the sclera in Marfan syndrome, as well as other connective tissue disorders, it often appears blue. Upon careful observation, iridodonesis may be seen, as may heterochromic irides. The iris dilator muscle is often hypoplastic, causing miotic pupils that dilate poorly, and the pupils are occasionally eccentric. Iris topography is also reduced, giving it a smooth appearance. The iris transilluminates in about 10% of patients, more prominently at the iris base.

Cases of microspherophakia and cataracts have been reported in conjunction with Marfan syndrome. Coloboma of the fundus, and macula have also been reported.

Reiger anomaly, characterized by a prominent anteriorly displaced Schwalbe line, iris strands to Schwalbe line, and anterior iris–stromal hypoplasia, has been reported in three cases of Marfan syndrome. This is an autosomal dominant disorder, and presently there does not appear to be a common embryologic or metabolic factor associating the two disorders.

Acquired Brown syndrome, which is defined as an inflammation of the microfibrillar fibers of the superior oblique tendon, is accompanied by diplopia and pain in upgaze, and has also been associated with Marfan syndrome. Other binocular complications associated with Marfan syndrome include amblyopia, strabismus, anisometropia, and rarely, nystagmus. Table 40–2 gives a complete list of the ocular manifestations of Marfan syndrome.

TABLE 40–2. OCULAR MANIFESTATIONS OF MARFAN SYNDROME

SCLERA/CONJUNCTIVA
- Blue sclera (M)
- Flat or increased corneal diameter (R)
- Keratoconus (R)

IRIS, PUPIL, AND ANGLE ANOMALIES
- Iridodonesis (C)
- Reiger anomaly (C)
- Deep anterior chamber angle (C)
- Heterochromic irides (C)
- Miotic pupils that dilate poorly secondary to hypoplastic iris dilator (C)
- Reduced iris topography (giving a smooth appearance) or iris transillumination defects (more prominent at iris base) (C)

LENS
- Ectopia lentis (C)

GLAUCOMA
- Secondary glaucoma from pupil block, congenital angle anomalies, or anterior lens subluxation (M)

RETINA
- Retinal detachment (C)
- Peripheral retinal degenerations such as white without pressure, lattice degeneration, retinoschisis, and retinal holes (M)
- Retinal arterial occlusions (R)

BINOCULAR
- Strabismus (C)
- Amblyopia (C)
- Anisometropia (M)
- Nystagmus (R)

OTHER
- Enophthalmos (C)
- Down-slanting palpebral fissures (M)
- Colobomas (M)
- Brown tendon sheath syndrome (R)

C, common; M, more frequently than rarely; R, rare.

DIAGNOSIS

■ Systemic

Diagnosis of Marfan syndrome (Table 40–3) is made based primarily upon skeletal, ocular, and cardiovascular manifestations. Patients with arachnodactyly and armspan equal to or greater than height may be suspected to have the disease. Most of these patients' height is in the 95th percentile or greater for their age. Signs of hyperextensible joints, such as a history of repeated dislocations of the hips, clavicles, patellas, and mandible, or other systemic features, may lend further evidence to the diagnosis. On physical examination, a murmur or click on auscultation may be detected.

In the absence of a family history of Marfan syndrome, diagnosis is based upon skeletal involvement as well as manifestations in at least two other systems. If one (or more) first-degree relatives are affected, diagnosis requires the involvement of two systems, of which one manifestation should be major.

Diagnostic echocardiographic findings include a dilated ascending aorta, and late in the disease, left ventricular failure. Echocardiography also provides a more definitive diagnosis of mitral valve prolapse.

Tissue biopsies will indicate a disruption in the elastic fibers in the blood vessel walls. There will be increased collagen deposition overall, and proliferation of smooth muscle cells. Several Marfan cases have shown decreased synthesis of type I collagen. In some patients, urinary hydroxyproline levels are elevated, indicating increased collagen turnover.

■ Ocular

Marfan syndrome may be diagnosed after the discovery of bilateral lens subluxation on routine eye examination. Other causes of lens subluxation (eg, homocystinuria) must be ruled out. Very rarely, the less common manifes-

TABLE 40–3. MARFAN SYNDROME: CRITERIA FOR DIAGNOSIS[a]

Criteria	Hard Manifestations	Soft Manifestations
Ocular features	Subluxated lenses	Myopia
Cardiovascular features	Aortic dilatations	Mitral valve prolapse
Skeletal features	Severe scoliosis	Tall stature
	Deformity of anterior chest	Joint laxity
		Arachnodactyly

[a] In the presence of a family history of the disease, a minimum of two criteria must be present to make a diagnosis of Marfan syndrome. In the absence of family history, three criteria must be present.
Adapted with permission from Cohen PR, Schneiderman P: Clinical manifestations of Marfan syndrome. Int J Dermatol. 1983;23:292.

tations discussed in the ocular natural history section earlier in the chapter will be found on routine examination.

TREATMENT AND MANAGEMENT

■ Systemic

Currently there is no treatment for the fundamental defect that produces Marfan syndrome (Table 40–4). Severe scoliosis may warrant the use of a brace, or spinal fusion. There has been an attempt to prevent the severity of scoliosis in young girls by administering estrogen, thereby speeding up puberty and shortening the amount of time for scoliosis to progress. The effect of this therapy is unknown, but these young women have not grown to as great a height as would be expected with the disease. Orthotics are used in the treatment of foot deformities.

Annual echocardiograms should be performed in order to monitor the progression of aortic dilatation. When the diameter is greater than 50% normal size, echocardiograms are done every 6 months. Prophylactic repair is warranted when the diameter of the aortic root reaches 6 centimeters. A β-blocker is typically prescribed to prevent further aortic enlargement. Low-impact aerobic sports such as swimming and cycling are encouraged for patients to maintain good cardiovascular fitness, but contact sports and isometric exercises should be discouraged. In the

TABLE 40–4. TREATMENT AND MANAGEMENT OF MARFAN SYNDROME

CARDIOVASCULAR COMPLICATIONS
- Echocardiogram every 6 months or annually
- Surgical intervention for aortic dilatation, aneurysm, or rupture, when indicated
- Systemic β-blockers
- Low-impact aerobic sports

SKELETAL COMPLICATIONS
- Braces or spinal fusion for severe scoliosis
- Estrogen therapy in young females (efficacy has not yet been determined)
- Orthotics for foot deformities

OCULAR COMPLICATIONS
- Appropriate phakic/aphakic prescriptions as early as possible to prevent amblyopia
- Annual fundus evaluation to detect retinal complications; retinal consultation and repair of retinal detachment, as indicated
- Mydriatics and miotics to reposition subluxated lenses
- Treatment of secondary glaucoma with standard regimen
- Sub-Tenon steroid injections in Brown syndrome

cases of aortic aneurysm or rupture, surgical intervention is necessary.

■ Ocular

Reduced visual acuity may result from delayed or inadequate correction of refractive error. Therefore, it is important to fit children early with appropriate phakic/aphakic prescriptions to prevent amblyopia from developing. Because the lens maintains normal accommodative function, it is not removed unless it induces a secondary glaucoma or prevents adequate visualization of the retina. In cases where subluxation occurs into the anterior chamber and causes a secondary glaucoma, mydriatics are used to reposition the lens, sometimes followed by chronic miotic ophthalmic drops to maintain its position. Retinal detachments are treated with surgical repair. In the case of Brown syndrome, sub-Tenon steroid injections near the trochlea have relieved both symptoms and diplopia.

CONCLUSION

Marfan syndrome manifests as abnormalities in several tissue systems leading to skeletal, ocular, cardiovascular, and cutaneous manifestations. It is not uncommon for an eye-care provider to be the first to discover this disorder in a patient with bilaterally subluxated lenses. Management of these patients is interdisciplinary, and prompt referral to the appropriate healthcare provider is indicated.

REFERENCES

Allen RA, Straatsma BR, Apt L, Hall MO. Ocular manifestations of the Marfan syndrome. *Trans Am Acad Ophthalmol Otolaryngol*. 1967;71:18.

Barnett HJM, Boughner DR, Taylor DW, et al. Further evidence relating mitral valve prolapse to cerebral ischemic events. *N Engl J Med*. 1980;302:139.

Bergen RL, Cangemi FE, Glassman R. Bilateral arterial occlusion secondary to Barlow's syndrome. *Ann Ophthalmol*. 1982;14:673–675.

Cheitlin M. Thromboembolic studies in the patient with a prolapsed mitral valve. *Circulation*. 1979;60:46.

Cistulli PA, Sullivan CE. Sleep disorders in Marfan's syndrome. *Lancet*. 1991;337:1359–1360.

Collins M, Swann PG, See ML. Case report: Marfan's syndrome. *Clin Exp Optom*. 1988;71:58–59.

Good WV, Corbett TD. Acquired Brown's syndrome in association with Marfan's syndrome. *Binoc Visn Q*. 1991;6:101–102.

Gott VL, Pyeritz RE, MacGovern GJ, et al. Surgical treatment of aneurysms of the ascending aorta in the Marfan syndrome. *N Engl J Med*. 1986;314:1070–1074.

Grin TR, Nelson LB. Rieger's anomaly associated with Marfan's syndrome. *Ann Ophthalmol*. 1987;19:380–384.

Halme T, Savunen T, Aho H, et al. Elastin and collagen in the aortic wall: Changes in the Marfan syndrome and annuloaortic ectasia. *Exp Mol Pathol*. 1985;43:1–12.

Joseph KN, Kane HA, Milner RS, et al. Orthopedic aspects of the Marfan phenotype. *Clin Orth Rel Res*. 1992;277:251–261.

Kainulainen K, Pulkkinen L, Savolainen A, et al. Location on chromosome 15 of the gene defect causing the Marfan syndrome. *N Engl J Med*. 1990;323:935–939.

Kanski J. *Clinical Ophthalmology*. London: Butterworths; 1984: 8.17–8.18.

Lee B, Godfrey M, Vittale E, et al. Linkage of Marfan syndrome and a phenotypically related disorder to two different fibrillin genes. *Nature*. 1991;330–333.

Maddox BK, Sakai LY, Keene BR, Glanville RW. Connective tissue microfibrils. *J Biol Chem*. 1989;264:21381–21385.

Maslen CL, Corsen GM, Maddox BK, et al. Partial sequence of a candidate gene for the Marfan syndrome. *Nature*. 1991; 352:334–337.

Maumenee IH. The eye in the Marfan syndrome. *Trans Am Ophthalmol Soc*. 1981;79:684.

McKusick VA. The defect in Marfan syndrome. *Nature*. 1991;352:279–281.

Morse RP, Rockenmacher S, Pyeritz RE, et al. Diagnosis and management of infantile Marfan syndrome. *Pediatrics*. 1990;86:888–894.

Nelson LB, Maumenee IH. Ectopia lentis. In: Renie WA, ed. *Goldberg's Genetic and Metabolic Eye Disease*. 2nd ed. Boston: Little, Brown; 1986:389–395.

Pyeritz RE. The Marfan syndrome. *Am Fam Physician*. 1986;34:83–94.

Pyeritz RE. Marfan syndrome. In: Emery AEH, Rimoin DL, eds. *Principles and Practice of Medical Genetics*. New York: Churchill Livingstone; 1983;2:820–835.

Pyeritz RE, McKusick VA. The Marfan syndrome: Diagnosis and management. *N Engl J Med*. 1979;300:772–777.

Robert L. Inborn metabolic disorders of the eye. In: Peyman GA, Sanders DR, Goldberg MF, eds. *Principles and Practice of Ophthalmology*. Philadelphia: Saunders; 1980:1746–1749.

Sirota P, Frydman M, Sirota L. Schizophrenia and the Marfan syndrome. *Br J Psychiatry*. 1990;157:433–436.

Skovby F, McKusick VA. Estrogen treatment for tall stature in girls with the Marfan syndrome. *Birth Defects*. 1977;13:155.

Traboulsi EI, Aswas MI, Jalkh AE, Malouf JE. Ocular findings in mitral valve prolapse syndrome. *Ann Ophthalmol*. 1987; 19:354–359.

Tsipouras P, Del Mastro R, Sarfarazi M, et al. Genetic linkage of the Marfan Syndrome, ectopia lentis, and congenital contractural arachnodactyly to the fibrillin genes on chromosomes 15 and 5. *N Engl J Med*. 1992;326:905–909.

Woerner EM, Royalty K. Marfan syndrome: What you need to know. *Postgrad Med*. 1990;87:229–236.

Worobec-Victor SM, Bain MAB. Oculocutaneous genetic diseases. In: Renie WA, ed. *Goldberg's Genetic and Metabolic Eye Disease*. 2nd ed. Boston: Little, Brown; 1986:510–511.

Zito G. Neurological complications of mitral leaflet prolapse. *Lancet*. 1979;1:784.

41
Chapter

Pseudoxanthoma Elasticum

Margaret McNelis

Pseudoxanthoma elasticum (PXE) is a generalized, inherited disorder of elastin, a major component of connective tissues. The primary defect in this disease causes calcification of the elastic fiber component of connective tissue, primarily in the skin, blood vessels, and eyes. Its most prominent manifestations occur in these areas, and angioid streaks of the retina are considered pathognomonic for the disease.

EPIDEMIOLOGY

■ Systemic

Classic PXE is inherited through autosomal recessive transmission, but dominant forms exist as well. It occurs in one person per 160,000 and shows no racial predilection. Clinical manifestations are usually evident by age 30, but may also be encountered in the very old and very young. Mitral valve prolapse occurs in up to 70% of individuals affected with the disease, and hemorrhage (usually gastrointestinal) affects up to 15% of patients.

■ Ocular

Angioid streaks are found in 85% of patients with PXE, and loss of central vision occurs in 70% of patients with angioid streaks. About 50% of PXE patients with angioid streaks become legally blind in a follow-up period of 4 years. Optic disc drusen are inherited in an autosomal dominant pattern in PXE, with an incidence of 3.4 per 1000 patients.

NATURAL HISTORY

■ Systemic

PXE was divided into four types by Pope (1974b), and this is known as Pope's classification. Type I recessive is the most common form of the disease, in which only moderate changes in skin, blood vessels, and the eyes occur. It is this type that will be detailed in this chapter (Table 41–1).

Type II recessive PXE is rarely encountered in clinical practice. The manifestations are mild, with only skin changes evident. Ocular and blood vessel manifestations are absent.

The other two types of PXE are dominantly inherited. Type I dominant is characterized by peau d'orange (dimpled skin resembling that of an orange) and severe cardiovascular manifestations including angina, hypertension, and claudication, along with prominent angioid streak formation. Type II dominant is four times more common than type I dominant. It is characterized by focal areas of extremely stretchable skin, a high arched palate, loose joints, and blue sclera.

The cutaneous findings of PXE are very helpful in the diagnosis of the disease. The lesions are described as peau d'orange, as they resemble the texture of an orange peel. They are yellowish coalescent papules, most prominent in the skin folds of the neck, axillas, and inguinal and antecubital areas. Exaggeration of nasolabial folds can lead to a "hound-dog" appearance of the face.

Cardiovascular complications are common in PXE and can cause serious sequelae. Significant arterial calcification and thickening of the muscular walls of the vessels are present by age 30, leading to peripheral vascular disease. Peripheral vascular disease is usually accompanied by

TABLE 41–1. SYSTEMIC MANIFESTATIONS OF PXE

DERMATOLOGIC
- Peau d'orange skin, especially in the neck, axilla, inguinal, and antecubital areas
- Exaggeration of nasolabial folds

VASCULAR DISEASE:
- Hypertension secondary to narrowing of renal arteries (common)
- Peripheral vascular disease (common)
- *The following occur with approximately equal incidence:*
  - Premature coronary atherosclerosis and complications (myocardial infarction and angina)
  - Valvular heart disease
  - Restrictive cardiomyopathy
  - Mitral valve prolapse
  - Cerebrovascular disease and complications (lacunar infarcts, aneurysms, subarachnoid and intracerebral hemorrhage)
  - Gastrointestinal disease and complications (GI hemorrhage, ulcerative colitis, internal hemorrhoids, atrophic gastritis, duodenal ulcer)
  - Urinary tract hemorrhage
  - Uterine hemorrhage

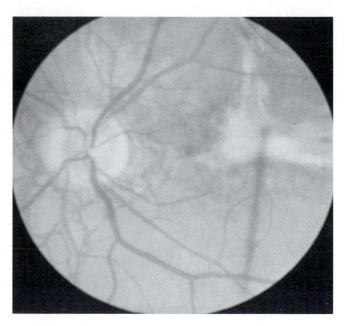

Figure 41–1. Angioid streaks emanating from disc and active neovascularization present at fovea. *(Courtesy of Stuart Richer, OD.)*

symptoms of cramping and intermittent claudication, more common in the lower extremities, because the upper extremities develop collateral circulation more readily. Peripheral pulses may be weak or absent in patients by age 30. Narrowing of the renal arteries often causes hypertension. Mitral valve prolapse is another cardiovascular complication in patients with PXE. Premature coronary atherosclerosis, angina, and myocardial infarction may occur in patients as young as age 20. Valvular heart disease and restrictive cardiomyopathy may also occur.

Neurological complications of cerebrovascular disease include lacunar infarcts and/or aneurysm with progressive intellectual deterioration and mental disturbances due to cortical atrophy. Subarachnoid and intracerebral hemorrhages are a common cause of death.

Gastrointestinal (GI) complications such as hemorrhage may occur as early as age 7, with an average age of about 26. Other GI complications include ulcerative colitis, internal hemorrhoids, atrophic gastritis, and duodenal ulcer. Acute GI hemorrhage can lead to death. Urinary tract and uterine hemorrhage have been reported with somewhat lesser frequency.

■ **Ocular**

Angioid streaks (Figure 41–1) are a common finding in PXE; when present, the association is known as Grönblad–Strandberg syndrome. Fundus peau d'orange (Figure 41–2) and salmon spots precede angioid streaks. Peau d'orange fundus is believed to be due to focal areas

of RPE thinning overlying the irregularly calcified but unbroken Bruch membrane. These are characterized by multiple small yellow dots against a red background, most prominently in the midperipheral temporal fundus. These dots are not drusen, but thinned and focally degenerated areas of Bruch membrane with secondary atrophy of the retinal pigment epithelium. This pigment mottling of the fundus is followed by the appearance of salmon spots.

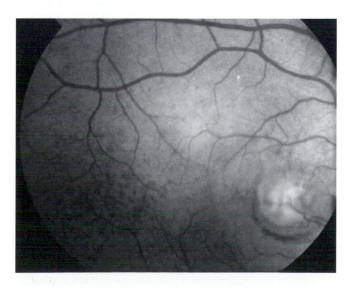

Figure 41–2. Fundus peau d'orange.

These are focal areas of Bruch membrane dehiscences. The spots are round, white-yellow, glistening lesions one-third disc diameter or less in size, which may represent calcified drusen of the retinal pigment epithelium. They can also occur at the posterior pole, temporal to the macula. Salmon spots may be accompanied by irregular atrophic spots in the periphery similar to those seen in presumed ocular histoplasmosis syndrome (POHS). This degeneration may progress to angioid streaks, which are found in most patients, usually between the ages of 20 and 50. The streaks are bilateral and asymmetric, reddish brown to gray in color, originating as an incomplete peripapillary ring with spokes radiating anteriorly toward the equator, three to five disc diameters in length. The spokes narrow as they extend forward. They are typically asymptomatic until they involve the macula area. Peripherally, they may be associated with white refractile drusen. The streaks may remain stationary, or they may progress periodically in length and number.

Progression is thought to occur as the cracks radiate from the optic nervehead in the direction of force of the extraocular muscles. These cracks may be bridged by a thin, hypopigmented pigment epithelium. Once they become full thickness, complications such as serous or hemorrhagic maculopathy and retinopathy associated with choroidal neovascularization may ensue. The neovascular changes most commonly affect the papillomacular bundle, but can occur elsewhere, not necessarily associated with a streak. Because the integrity of the blood–retinal barrier is impaired, hemorrhage from choroidal neovascularization may leak into the macula area, causing edema and distortion. When the macula is affected, it is usually after age 40, manifesting as either a disciform degeneration secondary to choroidal neovascularization or central areolar dystrophy of the RPE. The exudative form is more common than the atrophic form of macular degeneration in this condition. Subsequent scarring, choroidal atrophy, and sclerosis, with progressive retinal pigment epithelial atrophy, follow. Due to the fragile condition of these tissues, they are highly susceptible to even minor ocular trauma and the development of secondary hemorrhagic retinopathy. Symptoms of decreased visual acuity, impaired color vision, metamorphopsia, and scotomas can occur when angioid streaks lead to macular subretinal neovascular membranes.

Other posterior pole findings may include drusen, peripheral punched-out lesions, optic atrophy, and optic nerve drusen. Corneal manifestations include nonspecific opacities, keratoconus, and wrinkles in Descemet membrane. Subluxation of the crystalline lens, acquired cataracts, exophthalmos, and oculomotor paralysis have also been found to be associated with this disease. Table 41–2 gives the ocular manifestations of pseudoxanthoma elasticum.

TABLE 41–2. OCULAR MANIFESTATIONS OF PXE

POSTERIOR POLE
- Angioid streaks and complications
    Serous/hemorrhagic maculopathy and retinopathy associated with choroidal neovascularization
    Disciform macular scar or central areolar dystrophy of the RPE with possible hemorrhagic retinopathy
- Drusen of the fundus
- Peripheral punched-out lesions
- Optic nerve drusen
- Optic atrophy secondary to compression from optic nerve drusen

CORNEA
- Nonspecific opacities
- Keratoconus
- Wrinkles in Descemet membrane

OTHER
- Subluxation of the crystalline lens
- Cataract
- Exophthalmos
- Extraocular muscle paralysis

DIAGNOSIS

■ Systemic

The diagnosis of PXE is usually made based on the characteristic changes of the skin, and to a lesser extent, the vessel and ocular manifestations. The skin will appear loose and wrinkled, similar to the appearance of a plucked chicken. It may feel velvety, thickened, or atrophic. Skin biopsy is used when the disease is suspected and on biopsy these changes are very distinctive. Fragmentation and clumping of elastin fibers in the middle and lower dermis will be found. Biopsy of arteries will display fragmentation of the tissue causing swelling of the media and occlusion of the lumen. Calcification of the peripheral arteries may also be detected by x-ray.

Signs and symptoms of hypertension, GI or intracranial bleeding, peripheral vascular disease, or atherosclerosis may lead to or support the diagnosis of PXE.

■ Ocular

Angioid streaks may be seen on routine fundus examination in a patient with or without the diagnosis of PXE. However, since approximately 65% of patients presenting with angioid streaks have PXE, it is important for the eyecare practitioner to be aware of this disease in the differential diagnosis. If there is no diagnosis of coexistent systemic disease, referral should be made to an internist for evaluation. Important differential diagnoses include Paget and sickle cell disease (Table 41–3). A diagnostic workup should include serum alkaline phosphatase levels; calcium

TABLE 41–3. DIFFERENTIAL DIAGNOSIS OF ANGIOID STREAKS

Pseudoxanthoma elasticum[a]
Paget disease of bone[a]
Sickle-cell hemoglobinopathies[a]
Acromegaly
Ehlers–Danlos syndrome
Neurofibromatosis
Dwarfism
Pituitary tumor
Lead poisoning
Facial angiomatosis
Diffuse lipomatosis
Familial polyposis
Hyperphosphatemia
Senile elastosis

[a] Most common.

and phosphorous levels (Paget disease); hemoglobin electrophoreses (sickle-cell disease); skin biopsy (PXE); and x-ray of the skull, abdomen, and lower extremities (Paget disease).

Angioid streaks are more easily visualized during the retinal arterial phase of fluorescein angiography (FA) due to choroidal intravascular fluorescence and defects in Bruch membrane. A persistent late fluorescence will be visualized due to staining of collagen in Bruch membrane. Evidence of subretinal neovascularization will also be seen on FA, if present. Peripheral visual fields and electroretinogram will be normal in these patients. Color vision may be affected, manifesting as red-green or blue-yellow defects.

TREATMENT AND MANAGEMENT

■ Systemic

Treatment and management of PXE consists of controlling the secondary systemic diseases, cosmetic repair of the dermatologic manifestations, and often genetic counseling (Table 41–4). Standard medical control of hypertension in PXE is mandatory, but difficult. Encouraging results have been reported following coronary artery bypass surgery in young adults with coronary artery disease. Surgical repair of acute gastrointestinal hemorrhagic sites may be indicated. Due to problems with peripheral circulation, digits and extremities often may have to be amputated.

Cosmetically, the surgical removal of redundant skin folds may be desirable. This may be complicated by keloid formation with calcium particles extruding through the scar tissue, but the surgery generally meets with favorable results. Because of vascular impairment, slow wound healing and sepsis are surgical risks. Also, coronary artery

TABLE 41–4. TREATMENT AND MANAGEMENT OF PXE

- **■ SYSTEMIC**
  - Control of hypertension
  - Medical management of atherosclerosis, peripheral vascular disease, or other vascular complications
  - Surgical repair of hemorrhagic sites
  - Cosmetic surgery to remove redundant skin
  - Genetic counselling

- **■ OCULAR**
  - Patients with PXE and no ocular manifestations
    - Annual eye examination including retinal evaluation
    - Patient education regarding ocular complications of PXE
  - Patients with angioid streaks but no subretinal neovascularization and otherwise normal findings
    - Annual eye examination with retinal evaluation and FA, if indicated
    - Self-monitor with acuity chart and Amsler grid daily
    - Avoidance of ocular trauma and valsalva maneuvers
  - Patients with angioid streaks and evidence of subretinal leakage
    - Self-monitor with acuity chart and Amsler grid daily
    - Repeat FA every 1 to 2 months
    - Laser photocoagulation if symptomatic drop in acuity occurs with a neovascular membrane at least 300 μm from the fovea
    - DFE and repeat FA 5 to 7 days postlaser therapy and again at 3 weeks
    - Daily self-monitor of acuity and Amsler grid
    - Repeat laser as needed

insufficiency may predispose the patient to arrhythmias and sudden death; general anesthesia should therefore be used only when acutely necessary.

■ Ocular

Fluorescein angiography is indicated if there is a change in clinical status. If leakage is detected on FA, a retinal consultation is indicated. FA is then repeated every 1 to 2 months to aid in treatment. Currently there is no therapy for preventing angioid streak formation or progression. Laser photocoagulation may be performed on neovascular membranes, but appears to be of limited benefit, as recurrent neovascularization can be stimulated by photocoagulation. Therefore, this contraindicates performing prophylactic laser therapy. However, if a patient experiences a symptomatic drop in acuity with a neovascular membrane at least 300 μm (one-fourth disc diameter) from the fovea, laser therapy is indicated. Argon or red krypton is used in the papillomacular area, directly to the neovascular membranes, less than one-half disc diameter in extent. Subretinal neovascularization one-half disc diameter away from the fovea should also be photocoagulated. Follow-up is especially critical during the first 6 to 8 weeks after laser surgery, because recurrence of the membrane is most likely during this time. Patients should be given an Amsler grid and a home acuity chart to monitor any changes on a daily basis. Follow-up consists of a dilated fundus examination with repeat FA 5 to 7 days following laser therapy and again at 3 weeks. Once stabilized, patients should be examined every 3 months, and FA should be done every 6 months. Follow-up consists of visual acuity, Amsler grid testing, and dilated fundus examination. Repeat FA and reapplication of laser should be done as indicated. When successful, this treatment has been found to minimize the final scotoma size, as well as the amount of distortion experienced, while preventing further loss of vision.

Avoidance of ocular trauma, as well as valsalva maneuvers, is critical to preserve vision as long as possible, and protective eyewear is advised. Many of these patients become candidates for low-vision care and vision rehabilitation.

CONCLUSION

PXE is a rare disorder of connective tissue with serious systemic and ocular manifestations. It may be discovered upon routine fundus examination; therefore the eyecare practitioner may be the first to discover this disease. In these cases, timely referral is important, to an internist for management of systemic complications and to a retinologist when indicated for retinal complications. Patients should be counselled on the need for frequent eyecare follow-up, protective eyewear, and the avoidance of ocular trauma.

REFERENCES

Chumbley LC. *Ophthalmology in Internal Medicine.* Philadelphia: Saunders; 1981:203–206.

Clarkson JG, Altman RD. Angioid streaks. *Surv Ophthalmol.* 1982;26:235–246.

Connor PJ, Juergens JL, Perry HO, et al. Pseudoxanthoma elasticum and angioid streaks. A review of 106 cases. *Am J Med.* 1961;30:537.

Deutman AF, Kovacs B. Argon laser treatment in complications of angioid streaks. *Am J Ophthalmol.* 1979;88:12–17.

Fitzpatrick TB, Eisen AZ, Wolff K, et al, eds. *Dermatology in General Medicine.* 2nd ed. New York: McGraw-Hill; 1979:1144–1154.

Franceschetti A, Francois J, Babel J. *Chorioretinal Degenerations.* Springfield, IL: Thomas; 1974:275.

Fraunfelder FT, Roy FH, eds. *Current Ocular Therapy.* Philadelphia: Saunders; 1990:200–201.

Gelisken O, Hendriske F, Deutman AF. A long-term follow-up study of laser coagulation of neovascular membranes in angioid streaks. *Am J Ophthalmol.* 1988;105:299–303.

Goodman RM, Smith EW, Paton D, et al. Pseudoxanthoma elasticum: A clinical and histopathological study. *Medicine.* 1963;43:297.

Grand M, Isserman MJ, Miller CW. Angioid streaks associated with pseudoxanthoma elasticum in a 13-year-old patient. *Ophthalmology.* 1987;94:197–200.

Guiffre G. The pathogenesis of the fundus peau d'orange and salmon spots. *Metabol Ped Syst Ophthalmol.* 1987;10:95–98.

Johnson BW, Oshinski L. Diagnosis and management of angioid streaks. *J Am Opt Assoc.* 1988;59:704–711.

Kayazawa F. A successful argon laser treatment in macular complications of angioid streaks. *Ann Ophthalmol.* 1981;13:581–584.

Lebwohl MG, DiStefano D, Prioleau PG, et al. Pseudoxanthoma elasticum and mitral valve prolapse. *N Engl J Med.* 1982;307:228–231.

L'Esperance FA. Miscellaneous macular diseases. In: *Ophthalmic Lasers.* 3rd ed. St. Louis: Mosby; 1989:609–620.

Lorenzen SE. Drusen of the optic disc: A clinical and genetic study. *Acta Ophthalmol.* 1966;suppl:90.

Mausolf FA, ed. *The Eye and Systemic Disease.* St. Louis: Mosby; 1980:372–375.

McDonald HR, Schatz H, Aaberg TM. Reticular-like pigmentary patterns in pseudoxanthoma elasticum. *Ophthalmology.* 1988;95:306–311.

McKusick VA. *Heritable Disorders of Connective Tissue.* 4th ed. St. Louis: Mosby; 1960:474–520.

Newsome DA. Angioid streaks and Bruch's membrane degenerations. In: Newsome DA, ed. *Retinal Dystrophies and Degenerations.* New York: Raven; 1988.

Piro PA, Scheraga D, Fine SL. Angioid Streaks: Natural history and visual prognosis. In: Fine SL, Owens SL, eds. *Management of Retinal Vascular and Macular Disorders.* Baltimore: Williams & Wilkins; 1983:136–139.

Pope FM. Autosomal dominant pseudoxanthoma elasticum. *J Med Genet.* 1974a;11:152–157.

Pope FM. Two types of autosomal recessive pseudoxanthoma elasticum. *Arch Dermatol.* 1974b;110:209–212.

Rongioletti F, Bertamino R, Rebora A. Generalized pseudoxanthoma elasticum with deficiency of vitamin K-dependent clotting factors. *J Am Acad Dermatol.* 1989;21:1150–1152.

Rosen E. Fundus in pseudoxanthoma elasticum. *Am J Ophthalmol.* 1968;66:236–244.

Shields JA, Federman JL, Tomer TL, Annesley WH Jr. Angioid streaks: Ophthalmoscopic variations and diagnostic problems. *Br J Ophthalmol.* 1975;59:257–266.

Singerman L. Current management of choroidal neovascularization. *Ann Ophthalmol.* 1988;20:415–420.

Singerman LJ, Hatem G. Laser treatment of choroidal neovascular membranes in angioid streaks. *Retina.* 1981;1:75–83.

Verhoff FH. Histological findings in a case of angioid streaks. *Br J Ophthalmol.* 1948;32:531.

Viljoen DL, Bloch C, Beighton P. Plastic surgery in pseudoxanthoma elasticum: Experience in nine patients. *Plast Reconstr Surg.* 1990;85:233–238.

Wilkinson CP. Stimulation of subretinal neovascularization. *Am J Ophthalmol.* 1975;79:997.

42

Chapter

Ehlers–Danlos Syndrome

Margaret McNelis

Ehlers–Danlos syndrome is an inherited disorder of collagen synthesis whose manifestations may include skin abnormalities, joint hyperextensibility, and the tendency to bruise. The disease has typically been described as autosomal dominant, but more recent studies indicate recessive and x-linked transmission as well. The various subtypes of the disease result from different mutations of the gene that produces type III procollagen. These mutations appear to affect the synthesis, organization, and degradation of collagen fibrils.

Ehlers–Danlos syndrome is broken into 11 types, each expressing variable degrees of penetrance. Types I through IV make up the vast majority of all cases, and will be discussed in this chapter. Type VI is the purely ocular form, displaying the classic Ehlers–Danlos ocular abnormalities but rarely encountered in clinical practice. Ocular findings in Ehlers–Danlos syndrome include keratoconus, prominent epicanthal folds, angioid streaks, microcornea, and blue sclera.

EPIDEMIOLOGY

■ Systemic

Ehlers–Danlos syndrome occurs in approximately 1 per 200,000 persons. About 80% exhibit types I or II, 10% type III, 4% type IV, and 6% types V through XI.

■ Ocular

Prominent epicanthal folds are found in 25% of types I and II Ehlers–Danlos syndrome. Blue scleras are found in less than 10%, most commonly type VI. Eight percent exhibit moderate myopia, while 7% are strabismic. Loose, easily everted upper eyelids and widely spaced eyes are common in these patients, but epidemiologic data are not available.

NATURAL HISTORY

■ Systemic

The type of Ehlers–Danlos syndrome determines the natural history of the disease (Table 42–1). This can be predicted from familial and biochemical studies and can also be used to determine potential pregnancy and surgical risks. Type I Ehlers–Danlos syndrome is inherited in an autosomal dominant manner and clinical features include very soft, hyperextensible skin (Figure 42–1), extreme joint hypermobility, easy bruising, and poor wound healing and scarring. Hernias occur in 10 to 20% of patients, as well as premature birth in 50% due to weakness of fetal membranes. Mitral valve prolapse is common, usually manifesting by adolescence, and often in early childhood. Life expectancy of this type is normal.

Type II (Mitis) Ehlers–Danlos syndrome is also inherited in an autosomal dominant pattern. It presents with milder features than type I. Joint hypermobility is usually limited to the hands and feet. Skin changes are mild to absent, displaying the characteristic thin, atrophic "cigarette paper" scars of Ehlers–Danlos types I through III. Life expectancy is also normal in this type.

Type III (familial hypermobility) also has an autosomal dominant inheritance pattern and exhibits marked joint laxity and soft skin with minimal extensibility and bruisability. Recurrent dislocations and early degenerative

TABLE 42–1. SYSTEMIC MANIFESTATIONS OF EHLERS–DANLOS SYNDROME

- Soft, hyperextensible skin
- Thin, atrophic "cigarette-paper" scarring
- Joint hypermobility
- Easy bruising
- Poor wound healing
- Hernias secondary to weak tissues
- Premature birth secondary to weak fetal membranes
- Mitral valve prolapse, "floppy" mitral valve syndrome
- Recurrent joint dislocations
- Degenerative arthritic changes
- Scoliosis
- Arterial rupture
- Traumatic or spontaneous carotid cavernous sinus fistula
- Cardiovascular and GI complications secondary to fragile vessels rupturing, and/or intestinal rupture or perforation

arthritic changes due to unstable joints may require surgery. These patients also demonstrate signs of prolapsed mitral valve (also referred to as "floppy mitral valve" syndrome).

Both autosomal dominant and autosomal recessive forms of type IV (ecchymotic, Sach–Barabas) exist. This type has the worst prognosis for life because of such effects on the cardiovascular system as ruptured aorta or intracranial vessels. Gastrointestinal system afflictions such as intestinal perforation are often life threatening. One half of patients die before the age of 40.

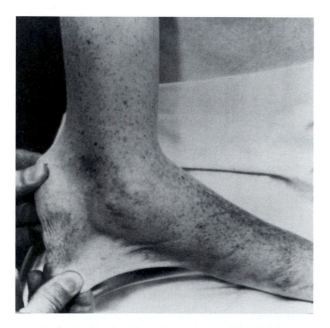

Figure 42–1. Hyperextensible skin in a patient with Ehlers–Danlos syndrome. *(Reprinted with permission from Perry HO, Bietti G. Ocular involvement in dermatologic disease. In: Mousoff F, ed. The Eye in Systemic Disease. St. Louis: Mosby, 1980, p 413.)*

■ Ocular

Myopia and strabismus are common findings in patients with Ehlers–Danlos syndrome (Table 42–2). Epicanthal folds and blue sclera are other less commonly encountered manifestations. Microcornea, retinal detachment, keratoconus, and angioid streaks have also been associated with this syndrome. Due to hyperextensibility of the skin, easy eversion of the upper eyelid is possible (Metenier sign).

Ocular signs of Ehlers–Danlos, unique to type VI, include keratoglobus and corneal haze at the level of Bowman layer. Glaucoma is often present by the third decade, and retinal detachment by the fourth. Vitreoretinal degeneration and angioid streaks with associated neovascularization and disciform scarring occur with minimal trauma. Corneas or globes may rupture upon minimal trauma. Rare cases of ectopia lentis have also been reported.

DIAGNOSIS

■ Systemic

Diagnosis and differentiation is primarily made through physical examination following signs of skin, joint, and bruising abnormalities, along with detailed family history to determine the mode of inheritance, as well as tissue biopsy. Prenatal diagnosis of type IV is possible via type III collagen analysis.

■ Ocular

Routine ocular examination may reveal any ocular manifestation of Ehlers–Danlos syndrome. External and anterior segment evaluation may reveal epicanthus, strabismus,

TABLE 42–2. OCULAR MANIFESTATIONS OF EHLERS–DANLOS SYNDROME

- Myopia
- Strabismus
- Prominent epicanthal folds
- Blue sclera
- Microcornea
- Retinal detachment
- Keratoconus
- Angioid streaks
    Neovascularization and disciform scarring with minimal trauma
- Keratoglobus
- Corneal haze at Bowman membrane
- Secondary glaucoma
- Vitreoretinal degeneration
- Rupture of cornea or globe with minimal trauma
- Ectopia lentis

myopia, blue sclera, microcornea, corneal haze, keratoconus, or keratoglobus. Angioid streaks, subsequent macular scarring, and retinal detachment may be found on dilated fundus examination.

TREATMENT AND MANAGEMENT

■ Systemic
Management of Ehlers–Danlos syndrome is mostly through supportive measures (Table 42–3). Some forms of Ehlers–Danlos syndrome have had beneficial results from 2 to 4 g of ascorbic acid per day. These patients should avoid trauma, but if it occurs, it is important to provide lacerations and wounds with good support, because it takes a longer period of time for these patients to heal. Physical therapy is important to maintain strength and stability of hypermobile joints.

These patients are challenging surgical candidates because of tissue weakness in suturing, excessive bleeding, and very slow wound healing. Surgery is generally avoided in the more severe cases except in emergency. When possible, genetic counseling may be helpful.

■ Ocular
Ocular treatment poses many risks to patients with Ehlers–Danlos syndrome (Table 42–3). In the case of strabismus, surgery may or may not be advised, depending on the degree of ocular tissue compromise. Contact lenses may be used to correct the corneal irregularities of keratoconus. This may be accomplished with rigid gas-permeable lenses, soft lenses, or a piggyback combination.

Special consideration needs to be given to those patients who develop retinal detachments, due to the fragility of the globe and the possibility of rupture under stress. This characteristic makes scleral buckling risky, and detachments are

TABLE 42–3. TREATMENT AND MANAGEMENT OF EHLERS–DANLOS SYNDROME

■ **SYSTEMIC**
- 2–4 g ascorbic acid daily to stimulate collagen synthesis, promote wound healing, and reduce vessel fragility
- Avoidance of trauma
- Appropriate supportive measures to promote healing of wounds
- Physical therapy
- Genetic counseling

■ **OCULAR**
- Contact lenses for corneal irregularities
- Extreme care during or avoidance of unnecessary surgery

usually repaired with laser photocoagulation or cryotherapy. In certain cases of macular degeneration, laser therapy may be indicated.

CONCLUSION

Ehlers–Danlos syndrome is a group of generalized collagen disorders. The organs most dramatically affected include the skin, joints, and skeletal system, gastrointestinal tract, and the cardiovascular system. Ocular manifestations are variable, and although they may not appear to be sight threatening, the fragility of the globe may make these patients risky candidates for ocular surgery.

REFERENCES

Arkin W. Blue scleras with keratoglobus. *Am J Opthalmol.* 1964; 58:678–672.

Bahn CF, Falls HF, Varley GA, et al. Classification of corneal endothelial disorders based on neural crest origin. *Ophthalmology.* 1984;91:558–563.

Beighton P. *The Ehlers–Danlos Syndrome.* London: Heinemann; 1970.

Beighton P. Serious ophthalmological complications in the Ehlers–Danlos syndrome. *Br J Ophthalmol.* 1970;54:263–268.

Biglan AW, Brown SI, Johnson BL. Keratoglobus and blue sclera. *Am J Ophthalmol.* 1979;83:225–233.

Byers PH. Type IV Ehlers–Danlos syndrome. In: Akeson W, Bornstein P, Glimcher MJ, eds. *Proceedings of the Workshop on Heritable Disorders of Connective Tissue.* St. Louis: Mosby; 1982:61–101.

Cole WG, Evans R, Sillence DO. The clinical features of Ehlers–Danlos type VII due to a deletion of 24 amino acids from the pro-alpha 1(I) chain of type I procollagen. *J Med Genet.* 1987;24:698–701.

Eyre DR, Shapiro FD, Aldridge JF. A heterozygous collagen defect in a variant of the Ehlers–Danlos syndrome type VII. *J Biol Chem.* 1985;260:11322–11329.

Fox R, Pope FM, Narcisi P, et al. Spontaneous carotid cavernous fistula in Ehlers–Danlos syndrome. *J Neurol Neurosurg Psychiatr.* 1988;51:984–986.

Gorlin RJ, Cohen MM. Craniofacial manifestations of Ehlers–Danlos syndromes, Cutis Laxa syndromes, and Cutis Laxa-like syndromes. In: Frias JL, Paul NW, eds. *Craniofacial Structures in Connective Tissue Disorders.* New York: Wiley-Liss; 1988:47–61.

Greenfield G, Romano A, Stein R, Goodman RM. Blue sclera and keratoconus: Key features of a distinct disorder of connective tissue. *Clin Genet.* 1973;4:8–16.

Gregoratos N, Bartsocas CS, Papas K. Blue sclera with keratoglobus and brittle cornea. *Br J Ophthalmol.* 1971;55: 424–426.

Hollister DW. Ehlers–Danlos type VIII. *Clin Res.* 1980;28:99A.

Hood OJ, Horton WA, Duvic M. Ehlers–Danlos syndrome caused by an apparent structural mutation in the carboxy portion of pro-alpha 2(I). *Am J Hum Genet.* 1987;41:A100.

Hyams SW, Dar H, Neumann E. Blue sclera and keratoglobus. Ocular signs of a systemic connective tissue disorder. *Br J Ophthalmol.* 1969;53:53–58.

Kaplan JA, LaFranco FP, Garoon I. Hereditary retinal detachment and vitreoretinal dysplasias. In: Renie WA, ed. *Goldberg's Genetic and Metabolic Eye Disease.* 2nd ed. Boston: Little, Brown; 1986:411–422.

May MA, Beauchamp GR. Collagen maturation defects in Ehlers–Danlos keratopathy. *J Ped Ophthalmol Strab.* 1987;24:78–82.

McKusick VA. The Ehlers–Danlos syndrome. In: McKusick VA: *Heritable Disorders of Connective Tissue.* 4th ed. St. Louis: Mosby; 1972:292–360.

Meyer E, Ludatscher RM, Zonis S. Collagen fibril abnormalities in the extraocular muscles in Ehlers–Danlos syndrome. *J Ped Ophthalmol Strab.* 1988;25:67–72.

Miura S, Shirakama A, Ohara A, et al. Fibronectin receptor on polymorphonuclear leukocytes in families of Ehlers–Danlos syndrome and other hereditary connective tissue diseases. *J Lab Clin Med.* 1990;116:363–368.

Nelson LB, Maumenee IH. Ectopia Lentis. *Surv Ophthalmol.* 1982;27:143–160.

Paton D. *The Relation of Angioid Streaks to Systemic Disease.* Springfield, IL: Thomas; 1972:62–63.

Perry HO, Bietti G. Ocular involvement in dermatologic disease. In: Mausolf FA, ed. *The Eye in Systemic Disease.* 2nd ed. St. Louis: Mosby; 1980:413–415.

Pinnell SR, Krane SM, Kenzora JE, Glimachen MJ. A heritable disorder of connective tissue, hydroxylysine-deficient collagen disease. *N Engl J Med.* 1972;286:1013–1020.

Pope FM, Narcisi P, Nicholls AC, Lieberman M. Clinical presentation of Ehlers–Danlos syndrome type IV. *Arch Dis Child.* 1988;63:1016–1025.

Robertson I. Keratoconus and the Ehlers–Danlos syndrome. A new aspect of keratoconus. *Med J Aust.* 1975;1:571–573.

Schievink WI, Piepgras DG, Earnest F, Gordon H. Spontaneous carotid cavernous fistula in Ehlers–Danlos syndrome type IV. Case report. *J Neurosurg.* 1991;74:991–998.

Siegel RC, Black CM, Baily AJ. Cross-linking of collagen in the x-linked Ehlers–Danlos type V. *Biochem Biophys Res Commun.* 1979;88:281–287.

Steinmann B, Tuderman L, Peltonen L, et al. Evidence for a structural mutation of procollagen type I in the Ehlers–Danlos syndrome VII. *J Biol Chem.* 1980;255:8887–8893.

Stewart RE, Hollister DW, Rimoin DL. A new variant of the Ehlers–Danlos syndrome: An autosomal disorder of fragile skin, abnormal scarring, and generalized periodontitis. *Birth Defects.* 1977;13:85–93.

Thomas IT, Frias JL. The cardiovascular manifestations of genetic disorders of collagen metabolism. *Ann Clin Lab Sci.* 1987;17:377–382.

Vissing H, D'Alessio M, Lee B, et al. Multiexon deletion in the procollagen III gene is associated with mild Ehlers–Danlos syndrome Type IV. *J Biol Chem.* 1991;266: 5244–5248.

Wenstrup RJ, Murad S, Pinnell SR. Ehlers–Danlos syndrome type VI: Clinical manifestations of collagen lysyl hydroxylase deficiency. *J Pediatr.* 1989;115:405–409.

Wirtz MK, Keene DR, Hori H, et al. In vivo and in vitro noncovalent association of excised alpha 1 (I) amino-terminal propeptides with mutant pN alpha 2(I) collagen chains in native mutant collagen in a case of Ehlers–Danlos syndrome, type VII. *J Biol Chem.* 1990;265:6312–6317.

43
Chapter

Osteogenesis Imperfecta

Margaret McNelis

Osteogenesis imperfecta (OI), also known as fragilitas ossium and maladie de Lobstein, is an inherited disorder of connective tissue. It affects bone, joints and ligaments, skin, eyes, and ears. The classic clinical triad of OI includes blue sclera, deafness, and bone fracture.

EPIDEMIOLOGY

■ Systemic
OI has a frequency of greater than 1 in every 20,000 births. There is no sex or racial predilection.

■ Ocular
Blue scleras are most frequent in type I OI. No further epidemiological data are available regarding the ocular manifestations of OI.

NATURAL HISTORY

■ Systemic
There are four varieties of OI. All four types exhibit a disorder of type I collagen synthesis in all affected tissues. Type I collagen is the major structural protein of bone, skin, and vessels. It also provides tensile strength and sites for anchoring cells and platelet aggregation. Unaffected family members may be carriers of an abnormal gene of connective tissue. Table 43–1 contains a summary of the systemic manifestations of OI. Dentin protein analysis shows that although OI teeth may appear clinically normal, the majority of collagen in all types of OI dentin is abnormal.

OI type I is the mildest and most common form. It is inherited as autosomal dominant in two varieties, with and without dental abnormalities. When dental abnormalities are present, decreased production of pulp and dentin produce irregular yellowish-blue teeth. Brittleness of bone and multiple fractures may be present at birth. Nonunion of fractures occurs in all forms of OI much more frequently than normals. This can lead to repeated fractures at a progressively deformed site. This improves after puberty, but returns with pregnancy and menopause. Deafness occurs in about one third of patients due to otosclerosis beginning in the second to third decades, along with a progressive sensorineural hearing loss that develops independently. Loose joint and tendons result in flat feet, kyphosis (hunchback), and frequent dislocations.

OI type II, the most severe type of the disease, is the perinatal lethal form. It is a result of a sporadic dominant mutation, or can be inherited recessively. Almost all bones break in utero, leading to marked deformity of limbs. Dismemberment can also occur during birth. If the infant survives delivery, he or she rarely lives longer than a few days.

OI type III, less severe than type II, is inherited in a heterogeneous autosomal recessive manner. There are numerous fractures at birth; however, bones are better developed than type II, with the infant's condition nearly normal. These children develop short stature and severe bone deformities, which are often independent of fracture. Kyphoscoliosis is dramatic, and can ultimately lead to respiratory failure. There is moderate looseness of joints, and variable dental and hearing changes.

TABLE 43–1. SYSTEMIC MANIFESTATIONS OF OI

BONE
- Bony fragility and brittleness causing multiple fractures (type I,II,III)
- Bone deformity secondary to repeated fractures (types I,II,III)
- Compressive fractures (types I,II,III)
    Leading to an increased susceptibility to large hematomas or intracranial hemorrhages
- Short stature (types I,III)

JOINTS AND LIGAMENTS
- Loose joints and tendons may cause flat feet, kyphosis, frequent joint dislocations (types I,III)
- Severe kyphoscoliosis can lead to respiratory failure

SKIN
- Thin and translucent skin (type IV)
- Tears at the corners of the mouth and groin (type IV)
- Easy bruising and hemorrhaging (type IV)

EARS
- Otosclerosis leading to hearing loss (types I,III)
- Sensorineural hearing loss (types I,III)

TEETH
- Abnormal dentin and pulp leading to irregular teeth (types I,III,IV)

CARDIOVASCULAR
- Aortic regurgitation, floppy mitral valve, fragile vessels (type IV)

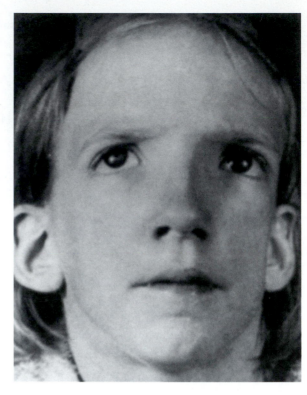

Figure 43–1. Blue sclera. *(Reprinted with permission from McKusick VA. Heritable Disorders of Connective Tissue. 4th ed. St. Louis: Mosby, 1972, p 417.)*

OI type IV has the most variable presentation of the four, and is transmitted both recessively and in a dominant form. Joint and hearing involvement are less frequent than in other types. The skin appears thin and translucent. Skin tears at the corners of the mouth and groin areas may occur. This type can be almost indistinguishable from Ehlers–Danlos syndrome when joints are involved. Some patients show significant cardiovascular alterations such as aortic regurgitation, floppy mitral valves, and fragile blood vessels. These may all lead to an increased susceptibility to large hematomas, compressive skull fractures, and intracranial hemorrhages.

■ Ocular

Electron microscopy of the scleral tissue of all OI patients reveals fibrils that resemble immature collagen. These fibrils are more translucent and uniformly arranged than normal, allowing uveal blood and pigment to become clinically visible as a blue cast. Blue sclera (Figure 43–1) are most frequent in type I. The degree of blueness is dependent upon the severity of collagen defect, and there is significant variability in color, due to the high heterogeneity of the disease. OI is associated with reduced ocular rigidity, although there

does not seem to be a correlation between the degree of blueness of the sclera and amount of reduction in rigidity.

Corneal fibril arrangements are similar to those found in the sclera. This may manifest as reduced central corneal thickness, keratoconus, megalocornea, or anterior embryotoxin.

Congenital glaucoma, crystalline lens dislocation, zonular cataract formation, partial color blindness, and choroidal sclerosis have been described in association with OI, as well as a report of subhyaloid hemorrhage (Table 43–2). Optic neuropathy and atrophy may occur in the more severe forms in which skull fractures cause optic nerve compression.

DIAGNOSIS

■ Systemic

Diagnosis of OI types I and II can be made in utero by ultrasound early in the second trimester. At birth, multiple fractures in an infant without a history of abuse may lead to diagnosis of any type; however, it may be more difficult to distinguish until later in life, when the diagnosis is aided

TABLE 43–2. OCULAR MANIFESTATIONS OF OI

BLUE SCLERA
- Associated with reduced ocular rigidity

CORNEAL COLLAGEN IRREGULARITIES
- Can lead to decreased central corneal thickness, keratoconus, megalocornea, anterior embryotoxin

OTHER
- Congenital glaucoma
- Crystalline lens dislocation
- Zonular cataract formation
- Partial color blindness
- Choroidal sclerosis
- Subhyaloid hemorrhage
- Optic neuropathy/atrophy secondary to skull fractures causing optic nerve compression

TABLE 43–3. TREATMENT AND MANAGEMENT OF OI

ORTHOPEDIC MEASURES
- Braces
- Molded seating
- Surgical straightening with long-bone rodding

PHYSICAL THERAPY
- Swimming and exercise to maintain muscle tone and range of motion

HEARING
- Hearing aids
- Surgical management

GENETIC COUNSELING

OCULAR
- Standard management (contact lenses) for keratoconus
- Standard glaucoma management
- Low-vision devices if visual impairment present

by family history, pedigree, and x-rays. Hypercalcuria occurs in OI children and can be detected through blood testing. Its magnitude reflects the severity of the skeletal disease. This may predict the stature of the child when he or she is older. Bone biopsy is of limited use in OI. Differential diagnosis includes juvenile osteoporosis, osteomalacia, and rickets, and is distinguished through biochemical measures of calcium, phosphorous, parathyroid hormone, and vitamin D.

■ Ocular

Blue sclera is the most obvious ocular finding in OI and may be helpful in the diagnosis of this disease. In addition, lens subluxation, choroidal sclerosis, and retinal and subhyaloid hemorrhages may be found following birth trauma.

TREATMENT AND MANAGEMENT

■ Systemic

Systemic therapy for all types of OI (Table 43–3) is primarily through orthopedic measures such as using lightweight external bracing, molded seating, and surgical straightening with long-bone rodding. Physical therapy and swimming to maintain muscle tone and range of motion are crucial. Progressive hearing loss has been treated surgically with stapes operations, but results have been disappointing. Genetic counseling is recommended in families of patients with OI.

■ Ocular

Management of the ocular manifestations of OI is limited (Table 43–3). No treatment exists or is necessary for blue sclera, and it does not appear that these eyes are more prone to rupture than normal eyes. Keratoconus is managed in a standard manner, with appropriate contact lenses. Glaucoma is also managed with standard medical treatment. If vision becomes severely impaired, low-vision devices may become necessary; however, it is important to keep in mind limitations in mobility due to bone deformities (eg, kyphoscoliosis). Yoked base-up prisms may be helpful for reading in a case of severe kyphoscoliosis or impaired head and neck movement.

CONCLUSION

OI is a generalized disorder of connective tissue that manifests itself specifically in the bones and eyes, as well as other tissues and systems. It can occur sporadically, or can be inherited either dominantly or recessively, displaying a wide variety of penetrance. There is limited therapy available; however, many advances have been made in understanding its mechanism and genetics. The eyecare practitioner may play an important role in the diagnosis or management of this disorder.

REFERENCES

Beighton P, Winship I, Behari D. The ocular form of osteogenesis imperfecta: A new autosomal recessive syndrome. *Clin Genet.* 1985;28:69–75.

Brons JT, van der Harten HJ, Wladmiroff JW, et al. Prenatal ultrasonographic diagnosis of osteogenesis imperfecta. *Am J Obstet Gynecol.* 1988;159:176–181.

Byers PH, Bonadio JF. Osteogenesis imperfecta: Clinical heterogeneity. In: Brown KS, Salinas CS, Paul NW, eds. *Craniofacial*

Mesenchyme in Morphogenesis and Malformation. New York: Liss; 1983:65–75.

Chan CC, Green WR, de la Cruz ZC, et al. Ocular findings in osteogenesis imperfecta congenita. *Arch Ophthalmol.* 1982;100:1459–1463.

Chines A, Petersen DJ, Schranck FW, Whyte MP. Hypercalcuria in children severely affected with osteogenesis imperfecta. *J Pediatr.* 1991;119:51–57.

Gage JP, Francis MJ, Smith R. Abnormal amino acid analyses obtained from osteogenesis imperfecta dentin. *J Dent Res.* 1988;67:1097–1102.

Gamble JG, Rinsky LA, Strudwick J, Bleck EE. Non-union of fractures in children who have osteogenesis imperfecta. *J Bone Joint Surg.* 1988;70:439–443.

Garretsen TJ, Cremers CW. Stapes surgery in osteogenesis imperfecta: analysis of postoperative hearing loss. *Ann Otol Rhinol Laryngol.* 1991;100:120–130.

Gerber LH, Binder H, Weintrob J, et al. Rehabilitation of children and infants with osteogenesis imperfecta. A program for ambulation. *Clin Orthop.* 1990;251:254–262.

Kaiser-Kupfer MI, McCain L, Shapiro JR, et al. Low ocular rigidity in patients with osteogenesis imperfecta. *Invest Ophthalmol Vis Sci.* 1981;20:807–809.

Khalil M. Subhyaloid hemorrhage in osteogenesis imperfecta tarda. *Can J Ophthalmol.* 1983;18:251–252.

Krane SM. Heritable and developmental disorders of connective tissue. In: Stein IJ. *Internal Medicine.* 3rd ed. Boston: Little, Brown; 1990:1818–1820.

McKusick VA. *Heritable Disorders of Connective Tissue.* 4th ed. St. Louis: Mosby; 1972:390–454.

Miura S, Shirakami A, Ohara A, et al. Fibronectin receptor on polymorphonuclear leukocytes in families of Ehlers–Danlos syndrome and other hereditary connective tissue diseases. *J Lab Clin Med.* 1990;116:363–368.

Nager GT. Osteogenesis imperfecta of the temporal bone and its relation to otosclerosis. *Ann Otol Rhinol Laryngol.* 1988;97:585–593.

Nogami H, Oohira A. Defective association between collagen fibrils and proteoglycans in fragile bone of osteogenesis imperfecta. *Clin Orthop.* 1988;232:284–291.

Opheim O. Loss of hearing following the syndrome of van der Hoeve–de Kleyn. *Acta Otolaryngol.* 1968;65:337.

Pedersen U, Bramsen T. Central corneal thickness in osteogenesis imperfecta and otosclerosis. *J Otorhinolaryngol Relat Spec.* 1984;46:38–41.

Rowe DW. Osteogenesis imperfecta. In: Wyngaarden JB, Smith LH, eds. *Cecil Textbook of Medicine.* 17th ed. Philadelphia: Saunders; 1985:1151–1152.

Smith R, Francis MJO, Sykes B. The eye and collagen in osteogenesis imperfecta. In: *The Eye and Inborn Errors of Metabolism.* Oxford: National Foundation–March of Dimes at the Radcliff Infirmary; 1975:563–568.

Starman BJ, Eyre D, Charbonneau H, et al. Osteogenesis imperfecta. The position for substitution for glycine by cysteine in the triple helical domain of the pro alpha 1(I) chains of type I collagen determines the clinical phenotype. *J Clin Invest.* 1989;84:1206–1214.

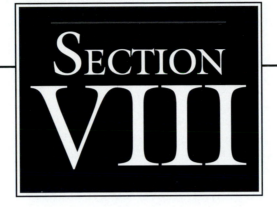

SECTION VIII

PHAKOMATOSES

44
Chapter

Neurofibromatosis

Joan Katherine Portello

Neurofibromatosis (NF) is a member of the group of diseases called the phako-matoses. These hereditary disorders are characterized by the appearance of multiple benign tumors called hamartomas involving various body tissues. Hamartomas are not true neoplasms, but consist of disorganized overgrowth of cells appropriate for that organ. NF is characterized by small pigmented skin lesions (café-au-lait spots), fol-lowed by the development of multiple peripheral nerve tumors (neurofibromas and schwannomas). Several different forms of NF have been identified. The most common are referred to as NF-1 and NF-2.

The systemic and ocular manifestations of NF can be extremely variable in severity due to the incomplete penetrance of this autosomal dominant condition, as well as its variable age-dependent expression. Familial expressivity does not contribute to the severity of the disease in future generations.

NF may have been first recognized as early as the mid-1600s. In 1882, the German pathologist Frederick Daniel von Recklinghausen described in his classic treatise a dis-order comprised of multiple fibromas of the skin and their relationship to multiple neuromas. He is credited for giving the disease the eponym von Recklinghausen dis-ease.

Possibly the most famous victim of NF was Joseph Carey Merrick, born August 5, 1862. He was known as the Elephant Man because his forehead was distinctly grooved towards the middle, with enlarged swellings on either side resembling that of an Indian elephant. Although Merrick died at the age of 27, photographs, casts of his head and limbs, and reconstruction of his skeletal bones have provided information about his disorder. Although it is believed that Merrick probably suffered from NF (Seward, 1990), the possibility exists that he may have suffered from other diseases involving bone and skin malformations (Tibbles & Cohen, 1986).

EPIDEMIOLOGY

■ Systemic

NF-1, an autosomal dominant disorder, affects approxi-mately 1 of every 4000 live births. There is a prevalence of 30 cases of NF-1 per 10,000 of the total population in a given year. In the United States alone over 100,000 patients have been diagnosed with NF-1. Spontaneous mutations are accountable for about 50% of all new cases reported.

Riccardi (1989) provided substantiating data that sporadic mutations may be correlated with advanced paternal age. NF-2, also autosomal dominant, has a frequency of 1 in 50,000 individuals, with just under 1000 cases reported in the United States. There is no race or sex predilection for NF-1 or NF-2.

Approximately 94% of NF-1 patients have one or more dermal café-au-lait spot and approximately 75% have six or more. One or more café-au-lait spots are present in approxi-mately 42% of patients with NF-2, and virtually no cases have six or more spots. Plexiform neurofibromas (involving a proliferation of Schwann cells from the inner aspect of nerve sheaths that follow the nerve pathway to possibly involve the spinal roots and spinal cord) occur in over 50% of patients diagnosed with NF. Riccardi (1989), observed that at least 85% of women with NF developed areolar neurofibromas after puberty. Bilateral acoustic neuromas are present in 95% of NF-2 patients, and approximately 5% of NF-1 patients.

■ Ocular

Over 50% of the patients with NF-1 have ocular features. Iris hamartomas, called Lisch nodules, are the most common ocular finding, occurring in approximately 90% of patients. Choroidal hamartomas, the second most common ocular finding, are present in 35% of patients. Optic nerve gliomas occur in 12 to 38% of patients. A significant number of NF-2 patients have cataracts as the sole ocular manifestation.

NATURAL HISTORY

■ Systemic

In order to clarify any preexisting inconsistencies in the terminology of different types of NF, the Panel for the National Institutes of Health Consensus Development on Neurofibromatosis in 1987 classified this disease. The Panel acknowledged that two distinctive forms of NF exist, but that variability of these forms may also be found. These forms are quite difficult to classify at this time due to insufficient clinical and/or genetic criteria.

NF-1 is most common, involving peripheral nervous system manifestations, specifically neurofibromas, as described by von Recklinghausen. NF-2 primarily has central nervous system manifestations, specifically bilateral acoustic neuromas. Frequently, patients with bilateral acoustic neuromas suffer from hearing loss. A specific allele has been identified on different chromosomes for these two distinct categories. In some cases the clinical and pathological criteria for NF-1 and NF-2 overlap. When this occurs, the syndrome is referred to as NF-3. Other variants of NF (NF-4 through NF-8) have also been reported (Riccardi, 1989).

Genetic linkage studies have recently shown the NF-1 gene to be linked to the nerve growth factor receptor on the long distal arm of chromosome 17. The mapping of the NF-2 allele has been localized to chromosome 22. Current research shows that this information can be used in DNA analysis to permit molecular prenatal or presymptomatic diagnosis. It has not been determined whether distinct genetic loci or variable expressions of the NF gene is responsible for the variant forms.

It is very difficult to describe a singular natural history of NF given its tremendous diversity (Figure 44–1). Pigmented skin lesions called café-au-lait spots are often present at birth or within the first 5 years of life. These dermal spots usually increase in number and size by adulthood but do not cause any adverse effects. Multiple freckling within skin folds, usually in the axillary region and/or the groin area, is another attribute found in NF-1 patients. Hamartomas involving neural tissue are termed neurofibromas. It is not known what causes neurofibromas to be present initially, to progress, or to recur. The higher levels of sex hormones present during puberty and during pregnancy may stimulate growth of the tumors. A circulating nerve growth factor, which stimulates growth in the peripheral nervous system, has been implicated in the systemic and orbital tumors. Further research is needed in this area before a definitive answer will emerge.

Neurofibromas that arise from Schwann cells and perineural cells, fibroblasts, endothelial cells, pericytes, and mast cells occur in the central and peripheral nervous system. At least three types of neurofibromas have been reported to occur in either NF-1 or NF-2, cutaneous, subcutaneous, and plexiform. Cutaneous and subcutaneous neurofibromas are usually first noticeable at the time of puberty and increase in number throughout adulthood. Cutaneous neurofibromas are present in the integument and can be found on the face, trunk, and proximal limbs, usually sparing the shins. These flesh-colored, soft, vascular lesions vary in size from several millimeters to approximately 65 centimeters in diameter (Figure 44–2). They can number from one to thousands, and typically are not associated with pain or tenderness. The tumors are mobile and as the dermis is moved the tumor moves simultaneously. Cutaneous neurofibromas are not as prominent in size or number in NF-2 or other forms of the disease as they are in NF-1.

Subcutaneous neurofibromas are very solid tumors ranging anywhere in size from a few millimeters to 4 centimeters (Figure 44–3). They are associated with pain and tenderness. These tumors are located under the dermis, therefore if the skin moves, the tumor does not move with it. Subcutaneous neurofibromas are primarily present in NF-1, although Riccardi (1989) reported paraspinal subcutaneous neurofibromas in both NF-1 and in NF-2.

The onset of plexiform neurofibromas is either before or after puberty. Plexiform neurofibromas may be further categorized into two subtypes, diffuse and nodular (Riccardi, 1989). The diffuse plexiform neurofibroma is a soft, rubbery tumor with occasional overlying hyperpigmentation of the dermis. These tumors are usually localized and are due to dysplasia of skin, muscles, and afferent blood vessels with subsequent overgrowth in that region. Nodular plexiform neurofibromas involve the superficial and deep major and minor nerves. These painful and tender nodules tend to be dense and grow in an array or undulated strings along the nerves.

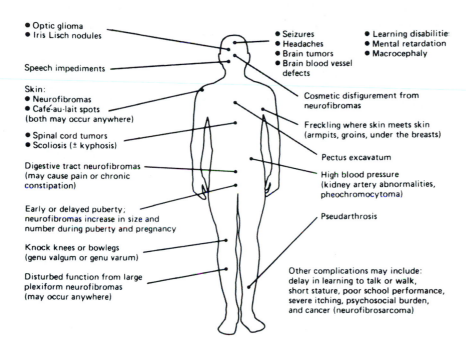

- Optic glioma
- Iris Lisch nodules

Speech impediments

Skin:
- Neurofibromas
- Café-au-lait spots
(both may occur anywhere)

- Spinal cord tumors
- Scoliosis (± kyphosis)

Digestive tract neurofibromas
(may cause pain or chronic
constipation)

Early or delayed puberty;
neurofibromas increase in size and
number during puberty and pregnancy

Knock knees or bowlegs
(genu valgum or genu varum)

Disturbed function from large
plexiform neurofibromas
(may occur anywhere)

- Seizures
- Headaches
- Brain tumors
- Brain blood vessel
defects

- Learning disabilitie
- Mental retardation
- Macrocephaly

Cosmetic disfigurement from
neurofibromas

Freckling where skin meets skin
(armpits, groins, under the breasts)

Pectus excavatum

High blood pressure
(kidney artery abnormalities,
pheochromocytoma)

Pseudarthrosis

Other complications may include:
delay in learning to talk or walk,
short stature, poor school performance,
severe itching, psychosocial burden,
and cancer (neurofibrosarcoma)

Figure 44–1. A schematic diagram of the clinical features of NF-1. *(Reprinted with permission from Powell PP, Schematic representation of von Recklinghausen neurofibromatosis (NF-1): An aid for patient and family education.* Neurofibromatosis. 1988;1:164–165.)

Other than being cosmetically unappealing and causing pruritus, cutaneous neurofibromas do not cause any serious threat to the patient's life. Involvement of either a paraspinal and/or nodular plexiform neurofibroma may lead to paraplegia or quadriplegia, and premature death has occurred due to these serious paralytic disorders (Riccardi, 1989). Diffuse plexiform neurofibromas not only have moderate to severe cosmetic abnormalities but, depending on location of the tumor, surgery may be necessary to prolong the patient's life. For instance, a diffuse plexiform neurofibroma found encompassing the trachea will require excision and occasionally tracheostomy.

Schwannomas rarely occur in NF-1, but will primarily affect the fifth and eighth cranial nerves in NF-2. Malignant schwannomas, although uncommon, decrease survival rate. Six percent or more of patients with NF-1 are likely to develop neurofibrosarcomas, usually from a preexisting benign neurofibroma. This malignancy also contributes to premature death. Other invasive tumors associated with neurofibromatosis are meningiomas, ependymomas, and pheochromocytomas (tumors of the adrenal glands that lead to secondary hypertension). Neurofibromas of the gastrointestinal tract are found in approximately 10% of patients and can cause constipation.

Nontumorous characteristic features common to NF-1 are learning disabilities (diagnosed in 60% of NF-1 patients), speech impediments, seizures, headache, hydrocephalus, macrocephaly (seen in 16% of NF-1 patients), and premature

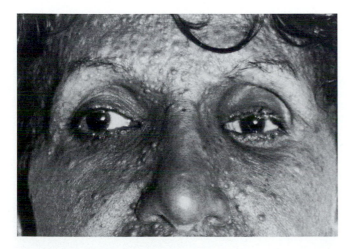

Figure 44–2. A 55-year-old Caucasian female with NF-1 and cutaneous neurofibromas of the face and left upper lid margin.

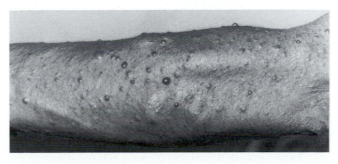

Figure 44–3. The same 55-year-old Caucasian patient from Figure 44–2 with NF-1 and subcutaneous neurofibromas of the arm.

or delayed puberty. Skeletal abnormalities include short stature, kyphoscoliosis (curvature of the lower and upper thoracic spine accompanying acute anteroposterior angulation), pseudarthrosis (a condition that mimics arthritis), sphenoid wing dysplasia, pectus excavatum (the sternum is abnormally concave), genu valgum/varum (knock-knee/bowleggedness), and pes planus (flat footedness). Vascular disorders (involvement of the afferent blood vessels) can affect the cerebral, gastrointestinal, and renal systems. Spinal and cerebral arachnoid cysts have also been reported (Table 44–1).

■ Ocular

Ocular involvement, especially in NF-1, may affect any part of the eye (Table 44–2). It can present during infancy before any systemic signs appear. One of the earliest signs and most common ophthalmic findings is the presence of iris Lisch nodules. These are found almost exclusively in NF-1, and may aid in the early diagnosis of neurofibromatosis (Figure 44–4). These tumors are usually bilateral, small, well-defined elevated masses arising from the iris

TABLE 44–1. SYSTEMIC MANIFESTATIONS OF NF

SKIN LESIONS
- Café-au-lait spots
- Freckling on skin folds

PERIPHERAL NERVE HAMARTOMAS
- Neurofibromas: cutaneous, subcutaneous, plexiform (diffuse and nodular)
- Schwannomas primarily affecting cranial nerves 5 and 8
- Neurofibrosarcomas
- Meningiomas
- Ependymomas
- Pheochromocytomas

CENTRAL NERVE TUMORS
- Bilateral/unilateral acoustic neuromas (vestibular schwannomas)
- Schwann cell tumors of the lining of the brain
- Meningiomas
- Ependymomas

NONTUMOROUS FEATURES
- Learning disabilities
- Speech impediments
- Seizures
- Headaches
- Hydrocephalus
- Macrocephaly
- Premature/delayed puberty
- Skeletal abnormalities: short stature, kyphoscoliosis, pseudoarthritis, sphenoid wing dysplasia, pectus excavatum, genu vulgum/varnum, pes planus
- Vascular disorders affecting cerebral, GI, and renal systems

TABLE 44–2. OCULAR MANIFESTATIONS OF NF

ANTERIOR SEGMENT AND ADNEXA
- Iris Lisch nodules
- Nodular plexiform neurofibromas of upper or lower lids
- Café-au-lait spots on eyelids
- Neurofibromas or schwannomas of conjunctiva, cornea, and/or orbit
- Corneal nerve thickening
- Decreased corneal sensitivity
- Exposure keratitis secondary to 5th- or 7th-nerve paralysis
- Hamartomas of anterior chamber

GLAUCOMA
- Congenital glaucoma
- Neovascular glaucoma

CATARACTS
- Posterior subcapsular, anterior cortical, nuclear sclerotic

RETINA AND CHOROID
- Choroidal hamartomas
- Retinal astrocytic hamartomas

OPTIC NERVE TUMORS
- Optic nerve gliomas
- Chiasmal gliomas

ORBITAL TUMORS
- Intraorbital/intracranial meningiomas
- Diffuse neurofibromas
- Orbital plexiform neurofibromas
- Orbital schwannomas (neurilemmomas)

surface. They can appear as clear to yellow or brown in color. Lisch nodules become increasingly prevalent with age. The severity of the disease is independent of the number as well as the age of onset of these nodules.

During the progression of the disease, nodular plexiform neurofibromas may be found on the upper or lower lids.

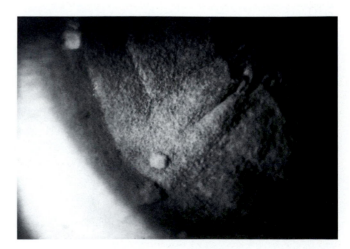

Figure 44–4. Iris Lisch nodules.

When they occur on the upper lid they can create pseudoptosis; if they occur on the lower lid, lagophthalmos may result. When palpated, they feel like a "bag of worms." If the lesions are large, they can be surgically removed, or if smaller, they can be debulked for cosmetic purposes. Café-au-lait spots may also exist on the eyelids. Neurofibromas and neurilemmomas (schwannomas) may be found on the conjunctiva, cornea, and/or orbit. Conjunctival hamartomas may be found rarely. These lesions consist of small tumors found on the bulbar and/or palpebral conjunctiva.

Corneal nerve thickening is seen with NF-1. In NF-2, reduced corneal sensitivity due to fifth-nerve involvement has been reported. Exposure keratitis from dry eye or Bell palsy secondary to seventh-nerve compromise have also been reported.

Other ophthalmic signs may include hamartomas in the anterior chamber angle causing a decrease in aqueous outflow. Fifty percent of patients with lid neurofibromas also develop ipsilateral buphthalmos secondary to congenital glaucoma. Grant and Walton (1968) showed that congenital abnormal tissue growth, presumably a hamartoma, covers most of the anterior chamber angle. This obstruction blocks aqueous outflow and results in glaucoma. Other studies suggest glaucoma could also be caused by a tumor thickening the choroid and ciliary body, thus closing the angle.

In adults with NF, neovascular glaucoma may be caused by the development of a fibrovascular membrane over the surface of the iris and trabecular meshwork. It is thought that the same mechanism that causes fibrovascular membrane formation in other systemic conditions is responsible for the neovascular membrane formation in NF. However, it is not known what precipitates this process.

Posterior subcapsular cataracts are known to occur in NF-2 patients (at any age), but several reports have demonstrated that the disease can also be accompanied by anterior cortical and/or nuclear opacities.

Choroidal hamartomas are the second most common ocular finding in NF. They appear clinically as choroidal nevi, flat or slightly elevated, and yellow, light, dark brown, or black in color. Histologically they are a proliferation of Schwann cells rather than a proliferation of choroidal melanocytes. The lesions can be 1 to 2 disc diameters in size and as many as 2 to 20 in number.

Optic nerve gliomas (of astrocytic origin) and the less common chiasmal gliomas are the most common intraorbital tumors in NF. The highest incidence of optic nerve gliomas is within the first decade of life, with peak incidence from 2 to 6 years (Chutorian et al, 1964). Proptosis, an early ocular sign of an optic nerve glioma, may be followed by visual loss and motility restriction with severity depending upon the degree of the proptosis and the size of the tumor. In the early stages, the optic nerve becomes atrophic but has distinct borders. Disc elevation, swelling, or gliosis of the optic nerve will not be present. Optic nerve gliomas have never

been reported to have infiltrated the muscle cone nor any orbital nerves. Evidence of an optic nerve glioma in a young child may become apparent before any other neurofibroma manifestations. Chiasmal pathway invasion by a growing intraorbital tumor is a rare occurrence. Chiasmal tumors often present with strabismus or nystagmus (especially in children), followed by hypothalamic disturbances and increased intracranial pressure.

Due to the variability of the natural history of optic nerve and chiasmal gliomas, it is difficult to predict visual prognosis in these patients. Optic nerve gliomas may recur after excision, may never progress with or without treatment, or may even improve with or without treatment. Long-term survival with optic gliomas is more favorable than with chiasmal tumors. The initial presentation of increased intracranial pressure associated with chiasmal tumors usually leads to hydrocephalus. In these cases cerebrospinal fluid bypass surgery has not been shown to increase the survival rate.

Intraorbital and intracranial meningiomas, typical of NF-2, occur less frequently than optic gliomas. Meningiomas that grow along the optic nerve or just behind the globe eventually result in a proptotic eye with vision loss. Meningiomas that infiltrate within the optic nerve will demonstrate signs of disc swelling and/or optic atrophy. Optic nerve optociliary shunt vessels, venous stasis retinopathy, and intraretinal hemorrhages tend to appear as the tumor progresses. Generally, intraorbital and intracranial meningiomas occur in the first decade of life, but they may present at any age. Early diagnosis and treatment is essential to preserve any functional vision. The survival rate is very good because meningiomas do not metastasize.

Retinal astrocytic hamartomas of the retinal nerve fiber layer or optic nerve (which are typical of tuberous sclerosis) have also been rarely reported.

Orbital plexiform neurofibromas are usually accompanied by sphenooccipital bony deformities and defects in other parts of the skull. These bony defects may cause the patient's pulse to be transmitted to the cerebrospinal fluid, and result in pulsatile exophthalmos. Temporal lobe herniation through the bony deformities may also create a pulsatile exophthalmos (Jakobiec & Jones, 1991). Pulsating exophthalmos due to neurofibromas occurs mostly in adulthood and should not be confused with carotid–cavernous sinus fistulas, arteriovenous malformations, large frontal mucoceles, or orbital varices. If left untreated, these benign, slow-growing tumors can cause enormous craniofacial disfigurement.

DIAGNOSIS

■ Systemic

The National Institute of Health Consensus Development Conference on Neurofibromatosis in 1987 proposed diagnostic criteria for NF-1 and NF-2 (Table 44–3). Although, these guidelines greatly aid the healthcare practitioner in diagnosing this disease, *there can be overlap between the two categories.*

NF may be suspected on routine physical examination when dermal hamartomas are present. They may appear anywhere on the body. Another characteristic finding during routine physical examination is café-au-lait lesions, which may also occur anywhere on the body. Freckling in the skin folds, such as the axillary and inguinal regions, is diagnosed on clinical examination especially at puberty. A first-degree relative with NF-1 is helpful in establishing the diagnosis, although one should be aware that no set patterns differentiate hereditary from sporadic mutations.

A complaint of hearing impairment in an individual with a first-degree relative positive for NF-2 calls for diagnostic testing, including an audiogram, brainstem auditory-evoked responses, and magnetic resonance imaging (MRI) procedure to aid in the potential diagnosis of NF-2.

■ Ocular

In an undiagnosed individual, Lisch nodules, found on biomicroscopy, may be the most common initial sign of NF. Optic nerve gliomas or meningiomas may be the first evidence of NF in undiagnosed children. Optic nerve gliomas are best detected by MRI, although computed tomography (CT) is utilized in some cases. Indirect ophthalmoscopy may reveal astrocytic tumors of the retina or choroidal lesions in a patient with no previous visual symptoms. If a

young child has been diagnosed with a posterior subcapsular cataract and no evidence of prior trauma, then a differential diagnosis should include NF, particularly NF-2.

TREATMENT AND MANAGEMENT

■ Systemic

The treatment of NF (Table 44–4) varies depending on the organs affected and to what degree. Although there is no cure, early intervention in some cases may result in preservation of the organ. Modalities of treatment include surgical excision of tumors, radiation therapy, and chemotherapy. Surgical treatment is sometimes warranted for purely cosmetic reasons. Patients diagnosed with NF require physical examinations at least once a year. This is essential because the tumors can progress at any time.

Genetic counseling is imperative and should be suggested to patients as well as their families. Molecular prenatal diagnosis of NF-1 is now possible, and should be considered, because a child born to an affected parent has a 50% chance of having NF-1. Emphasis on the variability of the disorder should be stressed to each family member; one child may have a mild case of neurofibromatosis, but this does not always imply that another child will manifest the same pattern. Psychosocial issues should be addressed such as cosmetic concerns and parental feelings of guilt. Patient/family educational information may be provided by the National Neurofibromatosis Foundation and the Acoustic Neuroma Association.

■ Ocular

Ocular treatment varies depending upon the extent and location of the ocular manifestations. Once again, surgical intervention and/or radiotherapy may be indicated to preserve the functional components of the organ or to address cosmetic concerns.

Lid neurofibromas that cause a secondary ptosis, entropion, or ectropion are surgically resected for both functional and cosmetic reasons. Optic nerve and chiasmal gliomas are either totally or partially excised, or radiotherapy is applied.

Surgical excision is the treatment of choice when dealing with orbital tumors because neurofibromas are radioinsensitive. Rarely is enucleation performed, and only if the orbital tumors are progressive or recurrent.

Congenital glaucoma is sometimes intractable, resulting in a blind, painful eye that may require enucleation. Otherwise, glaucoma secondary to NF is treated with standard therapy.

The majority of tumor findings in the eye are localized; however, all ocular findings such as Lisch nodules, choroidal hamartomas, retinal astrocytomas, and posterior lenticular changes should be carefully monitored over time for any change or growth (Table 44–4).

TABLE 44–3. DIAGNOSTIC CRITERIA FOR NF-1 AND NF-2

The clinical pathological entities to establish the diagnosis for NF-1 include two or more of the following:

1. Six or more café-au-lait macules of over 5 mm in greatest diameter in prepubertal persons and 15 mm or over in greatest diameter in postpubertal persons.
2. Two or more neurofibromas of any type or one plexiform neurofibroma (systemic and/or ocular).
3. Freckling in the axillary, inguinal, or other inguinal regions.
4. Optic glioma unilateral or bilateral, best detected with MRI techniques.
5. Two or more iris Lisch nodules as seen with a biomicroscope.
6. A distinctive osseous lesion such as sphenoid dysplasia or thinning of long-bone cortices, with or without pseudarthrosis.
7. A first-degree relative (a parent, sibling, or offspring) with NF-1 by any of the above criteria.

The diagnostic criteria for NF-2 are met if a person has either of the following:

1. Bilateral 8th-nerve masses seen with appropriate imaging techniques such as MRI or CT.
2. A first-degree relative with NF-2 and either unilateral 8th-nerve mass or two of the following: neurofibroma(s), meningioma(s), glioma(s), schwannoma(s), or posterior subcapsular cataracts developing at any age.

TABLE 44–4. TREATMENT AND MANAGEMENT OF NF

■ **SYSTEMIC**

SKIN LESIONS
- Cosmetic surgical removal of the lesions

PERIPHERAL NERVE HAMARTOMAS
- Monitor for any progression; if malignancy of the tumor ensues then surgical intervention, radiation therapy, or chemotherapy is necessary

CENTRAL NERVE TUMORS
- Monitor for any change in shape, size, or extension; if the tumor progresses, surgical treatment is necessary

■ **OCULAR**

ANTERIOR SEGMENT AND ADNEXA
- Iris Lisch nodules: No treatment necessary
- Nodular plexiform neurofibromas of upper or lower lids: Cosmetic surgical removal
- Exposure keratitis secondary to 5th or 7th-nerve paralysis: Standard dry eye treatment
- Hamartomas of anterior chamber: Monitor for any progression; if severe, surgical intervention may be necessary

GLAUCOMA
- Congenital glaucoma: If intractable, enucleation is required
- Neovascular glaucoma: Standard therapy

OPTIC NERVE TUMORS
- Monitor using MRI and CT to document any progression of the tumor; if severe, surgical resection, radiotherapy, or chemotherapy may be warranted

ORBITAL TUMORS
- Monitor utilizing MRI and CT to document any progression of the tumor or malignancy; if severe, surgical resection, radiation therapy, or chemotherapy is warranted

CONCLUSION

NF has a wide range of clinical expression. It can be so mild that it goes undiagnosed until adulthood, or it can be evident at birth and include severe deformities with subsequent lifelong complications. Once diagnosed, multidisciplinary management (neurologist, dermatologist, orthopedist, internist, and eyecare provider) should provide follow-up care regularly. At present, research has permitted extensive genetic insight into this disease. Further genetic studies and investigation of the pathogenesis of NF are needed to attempt to prevent the complications of this disorder in the future.

REFERENCES

Binitie OP, Obikili AG. Pulsating orbital plexiform neurofibroma and optic nerve glioma. *East African Med J.* 1989;66:362–364.

Bolshauser E, Stocker H, Machler M. Neurofibromatosis type 1 in a child of a parent with segmental neurofibromatosis (NF-5). *Neurofibromatosis.* 1989;2:244–245.

Burke JP, Bowell R, O'Doherty N. Proteus syndrome: Ocular complications. *J Pediatr Ophthalmol Strabismus.* 1988;25:99–102.

Cawthon RM, Andersen LB, Buchberg AM, Xu GF. DNA sequence and genomic structure of EV12B, a gene lying within an intron of the neurofibromatosis type 1 gene. *Genomics.* 1991;9:446–460.

Chutorian AM, Schwartz SF, Evans RA, Carter S. Optic gliomas in children. *Neurology.* 1964;14:83–95.

Clementi M, Alessandra M, Franca A, et al. Linkage analysis of neurofibromatosis type 1. *Hum Genet.* 1991;87:91–94.

Eggers H, Jakobiec FA, Jones IA. Optic nerve gliomas. In: Tasman W, Jaeger EA, eds. *Duane's Clinical Ophthalmology.* Philadelphia: Lippincott; 1991;2:1–17.

Garretto NS, Ameriso S, Molina HA, et al. Type 2 neurofibromatosis with Lisch nodules. *Neurofibromatosis.* 1989;2:315–321.

Good WV, Brodsky MC, Edwards MS, Hoyt WF. Bilateral retinal hamartomas in neurofibromatosis type 2. *Br J Ophthalmol.* 1991;75:190.

Grant WM, Walton DS. Distinctive gonioscopic findings in glaucoma due to neurofibromatosis. *Arch Ophthalmol.* 1968;79:127–134.

Huson S, Dylan J, Beck L. Ophthalmic manifestations of neurofibromatosis. *Br J Ophthalmol.* 1987;71:235–238.

Jakobiec FA, Jones IS. Neurogenic tumors. In: Tasman W, Jaeger EA, eds. *Duane's Clinical Ophthalmology.* Philadelphia: Lippincott; 1991;2:1–45.

Kobrin JL, Blodi FC, Weingeist TA. Ocular and orbital manifestations of neurofibromatosis. *Sur Ophthalmol.* 1979;24:45–51.

Martyn LJ, Knox DL. Glial hamartoma of the retina in generalized neurofibromatosis. *Br J Ophthalmol.* 1972;56:487–491.

Michels VV, Whisnant JP, Garrity JA, Miller GM. Neurofibromatosis type 1 with bilateral acoustic neuromas. *Neurofibromatosis.* 1989;2:213–217.

Mulvihill JJ. Neurofibromatosis: History, nomenclature, and natural history. *Neurofibromatosis.* 1988;1:124–131.

National Institutes of Health. *Neurofibromatosis: National Institutes of Health Consensus Development Conference Statement.* Bethesda: National Institutes of Health; July 1987.

National Institute of Health Conference. Neurofibromatosis 1 (Recklinghausen disease) and neurofibromatosis 2 (bilateral acoustic neurofibromatosis). *Ann Intern Med.* 1990;113:39–52.

Neurofibromatosis Conference statement. National Institutes of Health Consensus Development conference. *Arch Neurol.* 1988:45:575–578.

Obringer AC, Meadows AT, Elaine MD, Zackai MD. The diagnosis of neurofibromatosis-1 in the child under the age of 6 years. *AJDC.* 1989;143:717–719.

Pou-Serradell A, Ugarte-Elola AC. Optic pathway gliomas in neurofibromatosis. *Neurofibromatosis.*1989;2:227–232.

Powell PP. Schematic representation of von Recklinghausen neurofibromatosis (NF-1): An aid for patient and family education. *Neurofibromatosis.* 1988;1:164–165.

Pulst SM. Prenatal diagnosis of the neurofibromatoses. *Clin Perinatol.* 1990;17:829–843.

Riccardi VM. Neurofibromatosis update. *Neurofibromatosis.* 1989;2:284–291.

Riccardi VM. Is NF-1 always distinct from NF-2? *Neurofibromatosis.* 1989;2:193–194. Editorial.

Rosner J. Clinical review of neurofibromatosis. *J Am Optom Assoc.* 1990;61:613–618.

Seiff SR, Brodsky MC, MacDonald G, et al. Orbital optic glioma in neurofibromatosis: Magnetic resonance diagnosis of perineural arachnoidal gliomatosis. *Arch Ophthalmol.* 1987;105:1689–1692.

Seward GR. The elephant man, parts 1 to 3. *Br Dental J.* 1990;169:173–175, 210–216, 252–255.

Tibbles JA, Cohen MM. The proteus syndrome: The elephant man diagnosed. *Br Med J.* 1986;293:683–685.

45

Chapter

Tuberous Sclerosis

Elizabeth B. Aksionoff

Tuberous sclerosis was first described by Bourneville in 1880, and in 1908 Vogt associated the triad of epileptic seizures, mental retardation, and facial angiofibromas (adenoma sebaceum). Van der Hoeve was the first to associate retinal involvement with tuberous sclerosis in 1920. Tuberous sclerosis (Bourneville disease) is now recognized as a multisystem, hamartomatous disorder. It belongs to the class of neurocutaneous syndromes called the phakomatoses, which are characterized by disseminated hamartomas (tumor-like nodules) of the eye, skin, central nervous system, and viscera.

EPIDEMIOLOGY

■ Systemic

Signs of tuberous sclerosis may be present at birth; however, patients usually present during the third decade of life. Tuberous sclerosis is diagnosed in 25% of patients by age 2, 60% by age 10, and 80% by age 20. Because the gene for tuberous sclerosis is pleiotrophic and variable in expression, the estimates of incidence in the literature are quite variable.

Seizure disorders are found in 82 to 90% of the patient population. The incidence of mental retardation is reported between 41 and 60%. Benign brain nodules may be detected in 14% of tuberous sclerosis patients by age 1 and in almost 60% by age 10. Giant-cell astrocytomas will develop in 2% of patients. An abnormal electroencephalograph (EEG) reading is found in 87% of those affected with tuberous sclerosis.

The incidence of skin lesions in tuberous sclerosis is 96%; by age 35, almost all patients will have the characteristic skin lesion, adenoma sebaceum. There is an 86% incidence of hypomelanotic macules and 20% present with Shagreen patches. The skeletal system is affected in 40% of patients. Phalangeal cysts are found in the hands or feet of 66%.

Cardiac rhabdomyomas, as evidenced by echocardiogram, are found in 43% of tuberous sclerosis patients. Renal angiolipomas occur in 50 to 80% of patients.

■ Ocular

Ocular involvement occurs in at least 50% of tuberous sclerosis patients. Benign astrocytic hamartomas of the retina or optic nerve occur in 50 to 87% of tuberous sclerosis patients.

NATURAL HISTORY

■ Systemic

Tuberous sclerosis is a multisystem, hamartomatous disorder involving the brain, skin, viscera, and the eye (see Table 45–1). Hamartomas are congenital anomalies of tissue formation arising from tissue normally present at the involved site. They typically contain large blood vessels and areas of calcification. Most hamartomas, although congenital, are usually inconspicuous at birth and become clinically apparent during the first two decades of life.

Inheritance of tuberous sclerosis is autosomal dominant, with low penetrance and variable expressivity. The disease has a high new mutation rate and may therefore appear as a

327

sporadic condition in up to 80% of affected patients. The defective gene has been isolated to the long arm of chromosome 9, locus 9q34. Tuberous sclerosis is a result of dysplasia of the neuroectodermal embryologic layer.

It is difficult to predict the course of tuberous sclerosis in any patient. Depending on the manifestations, a patient may lead a normal life or show rapid systemic or neurological deterioration from the disease.

Central Nervous System

The neurological features of tuberous sclerosis are mental retardation and seizure disorder. "Tuber-shaped" cerebral cortical malformations are responsible for the effects of tuberous sclerosis on the central nervous system. Fibrillary gliosis is often associated with these cortical malformations.

Cortical tubers are large astrocytic hamartomas most commonly found in the cerebral cortex, but which occasionally may appear in the cerebellum, basal ganglia, and rarely in the brainstem and spinal cord. They may cause alterations in the normal convolutional pattern of the gyri.

Subependymal giant-cell astrocytomas are usually benign. These are most commonly found in the region of the basal ganglia and protrude into the lateral and third ventricles. They may grow to obstruct the foramen of Munro and cause hydrocephalus and increased intracranial pressure. The presenting symptoms of an expanding cranial mass may include headache, decreased vision, and/or vomiting.

The most common, and often first, manifestation of tuberous sclerosis is a seizure disorder. The seizures are a result of cerebral cortical malformations. The seizures, or infantile spasms, usually begin in infancy or childhood, with repetitive myoclonic spasms of the head, neck, and limbs. These attacks are also known as "salaam attacks." They last for only a few seconds, but occur in groups of 10 to 50. These seizures may present as early as 4 months of age. With increasing age the infantile spasms become grand mal seizures. According to Pampliglione and Pugh (1975), 25% of children with seizures will develop other signs of tuberous sclerosis within 4 years. After the seizures present, the child may demonstrate a slowing in subsequent development. Although the seizures may arise from anywhere in the brain, they are usually concentrated in the periventricular distribution, where most of the tubers are found. There is a high correlation between seizures and irregularity on EEG.

Another manifestation of cerebral cortical malformations is mental retardation. Mental retardation is a common but not inevitable association with tuberous sclerosis.

There is a great deal of variability of the severity of seizures and mental retardation. Approximately one third of tuberous sclerosis patients will be of normal intelligence, with no significant health problems, while others may have severe mental retardation and/or seizures that are difficult

to control. Developmental delays may also be evident from birth. Borberg (1951) found that 15% of mentally retarded patients develop normally until between the ages of 8 and 14, when they began to show signs of intellectual deterioration. This may be due to frequent uncontrolled seizures or increased intracranial pressure due to an obstruction of the foramen of Munro.

Cutaneous

The earliest visible skin lesion associated with tuberous sclerosis is the hypomelanotic macule (Figure 45–1). This depigmented area, 1 to 2 cm in diameter, usually presents at birth. Hypomelanotic macules are a very common occurrence and are pathognomonic for tuberous sclerosis. They may be found on the trunk, limbs, or scalp and can range in number from 4 to 100. These lesions are called the "ash leaf" sign because they may resemble the shape of an ash tree leaf, oval at one end and tapered at the other, although they are quite variable in shape. These diagnostic lesions are often the first clinical sign of tuberous sclerosis.

Facial angiofibromas or adenoma sebaceum are also common, and may be the only cutaneous sign of tuberous sclerosis. These are small, red-brown, raised nodules distributed in a butterfly pattern of the nasolabial fold, malar area, and on the chin. The angiofibromas are composed of an overgrowth of sebaceous glands, connective tissue, and small blood vessels. They are first visible at ages 2 to 5 and may be progressive to young adulthood. This condition is usually present in all affected individuals over age 35.

Shagreen patches, another cutaneous presentation, are fibrous plaques in the skin presenting with a waxy, yellow-brown, or flesh-colored appearance. These raised, irregular, rough areas of skin are most commonly found on the forehead, eyelids, back, or legs. Other less common cutaneous manifestations are listed in Table 45–1.

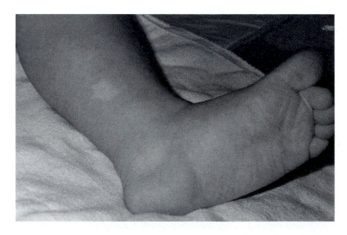

Figure 45–1. Hypomelanotic macule (ash-leaf spot) on the leg of a 1-year-old with tuberous sclerosis.

TABLE 45–1. SYSTEMIC MANIFESTATIONS OF TUBEROUS SCLEROSIS

CENTRAL NERVOUS SYSTEM
- Cerebral cortical malformations
- Astrocytic hamartomas
- Subependymal giant-cell astrocytomas

- The above can all lead to
    Seizures
    Mental retardation
    Increased intracranial pressure
    Hydrocephalus

CUTANEOUS
- Hypomelanotic macules (ash-leaf spots)
- Adenoma sebaceum
- Shagreen patches
- Subungual fibromas of fingers and toes
- Pitted hypoplasia of the teeth
- Café-au-lait spots
- Poliosis
- Vascular nevi

VISCERAL
- Renal angiomyolipomas may cause hematuria, uremia, hypertension
- Cardiac rhabdomyomas may cause cardiac arrhythmia
- Sclerotic areas of the calvarium and spine
- Phalangeal cysts
- Pleural cysts may cause emphysema, hemoptysis, recurrent pneumothorax

OTHER (LESS COMMON) HAMARTOMAS
- Liver
- Gastrointestinal tract
- Thymus
- Adrenal gland
- Pancreas

Visceral

The most commonly affected organ in tuberous sclerosis is the kidney. Polycystic renal disease is very common. Renal angiomyolipomas, usually benign multiple hamartomas of the kidneys, are common. They do not typically metastasize to other sites. They appear as nodules usually less than 2 cm in diameter. They may be solid or cystic, solitary or multiple, and unilateral or bilateral. The kidney tumors and cysts are usually asymptomatic. If symptoms do arise they may include pain, uremia, and other signs of renal failure as well as hypertension.

Cardiac rhabdomyomas are usually benign, asymptomatic, whitish tumors less than a centimeter in size. They may appear as a solitary tumor, usually at the apex of the left ventricle, as multiple nodules throughout the heart, or as diffuse infiltration of the myocardium. Cardiac rhabdomyomas may be responsible for pulmonic or aortic stenosis. Possible presenting signs include cardiac arrhythmias, heart failure, or ECG changes.

Other less common visceral manifestations of tuberous sclerosis are listed in Table 45–1.

The lifespan is normal in those patients with tuberous sclerosis who show minimal manifestations of the disease. However, with severe epilepsy and mental retardation, the prognosis for life beyond the third decade is poor. The cause of death is usually due to seizures, associated tumors, or concurrent disease.

■ Ocular

The primary ocular manifestations of tuberous sclerosis are hamartomas of the retina and optic nerve. These benign lesions can develop as early as a few months of life. Solitary astrocytic hamartomas may be seen in normal individuals. However, in tuberous sclerosis, the astrocytomas may be bilateral and multifocal. The hamartomas have been classified into three different morphological types.

Type 1 is the most common, usually appearing in the early stage of the disease, and located in the superficial retinal layers overlying the retinal blood vessels. They most commonly occur at or near the posterior pole, but may affect any part of the fundus. The hamartomas often arise in the retinal ganglion layer but may later involve all layers of the retina. The tumor is smooth and circular or oval in shape. It is relatively flat, although it might be slightly raised above the retina. It appears semitransparent and can range from grayish white to salmon in color, often with ill-defined margins. The lesion varies in size from one-half to three disc diameters in width. Its appearance may be very subtle and difficult to detect except for an abnormal light reflex or blurred underlying blood vessel. The lesion has little effect on the neighboring retina or choroid.

Type 2 is a well-circumscribed, calcified, white, opaque lesion that may be elevated and multinodular. This is considered the classic "mulberry"-type lesion (Figure 45–2). These astrocytic hamartomas are usually found at or around the optic disc and posterior pole. They range in size from one-half to three disc diameters in size. Some of these lesions have been known to dislodge and float freely in the vitreous and then possibly reattach and grow in other areas of the retina.

Type 3 is a combination of the first two varieties. The central core is calcified and nodular while the perimeter is smooth, semitranslucent, and salmon in color.

The hamartomas may be richly vascularized but present with varying degrees of vascularization. They usually do not grow over time; however, their appearance may change as they become calcified. The tumors are usually extramacular, arising in the inner retina, with little damage or vision loss. Hamartomas of the optic disc generally arise in the superficial layers of the papilla and interfere little with its structure or function. It is less common for the tumors to

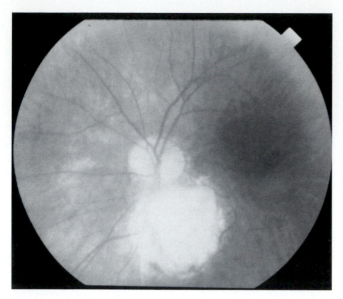

Figure 45–2. Solitary, multinodular retinal astrocytoma (type 2 or classic "mulberry" lesion).

involve all layers of the retina or optic nerve, but the choroid and vitreous may be affected secondarily. Retinal detachments are rarely associated with the hamartomas.

Vascular malformations may occur at or adjacent to a large hamartoma. These malformations may lead to preretinal or vitreous hemorrhage. Papilledema and/or optic atrophy may occur and are signs of associated intracranial lesions.

Other retinal findings are less common, and include pigment epithelial defects such as peripheral retinal hypopigmentation and atypical colobomas. Although rare, localized areas of choroidal atrophy have been reported to occur at or adjacent to retinal astrocytomas.

Visual loss is more commonly due to intracranial lesions, especially paraventricular tumors resulting in raised intracranial pressure, papilledema, and subsequent optic atrophy. Intracranial tumors may also be responsible for diplopia and extraocular muscle paresis.

The main nonretinal manifestation of tuberous sclerosis is adenoma sebaceum of the eyelids. Other rare ocular manifestations are listed in Table 45–2.

DIAGNOSIS

■ Systemic

Although the original criteria for diagnosis of tuberous sclerosis included the triad of seizures, mental retardation, and adenoma sebaceum, this no longer holds true because of the variable presentation of this disease. A scheme for the diagnosis of tuberous sclerosis (Table 45–3) is based on the criteria set by Gomez (1979). To make the diagnosis, one of the major requirements, or two of the minor requirements, must be met.

TABLE 45–2. OCULAR MANIFESTATIONS OF TUBEROUS SCLEROSIS

- Adenoma sebaceum of the eyelids
- Retinal astrocytic hamartoma
- Optic nerve astrocytic hamartoma
- Papilledema secondary to increased intracranial pressure, which can lead to:
    - Optic atrophy secondary to chronic papilledema
    - Extracranial nerve paresis
- Pigment epithelial defects
- Atypical coloboma
- Poliosis
- Iris hypopigmentation

The hypomelanotic macules are easily identified by reflecting ultraviolet light onto the skin from a Wood lamp in a darkened room. This helps to identify lesions in an infant. The other cutaneous signs are easily identified by physical and dermatologic examination. A careful search for depigmented nevi is of particular diagnostic importance in early life. A skin biopsy of the hypopigmented macules will show melanocytes with decreased tyrosinase activity characteristic of tuberous sclerosis. This is in contrast to areas of vitiligo where there is an absence of melanocytes.

The diagnostic tests used for the central nervous system manifestations include the EEG, CT scan, or MRI. The EEG is abnormal in most patients and may show a grossly abnormal hypsarrhythmic pattern in one third of tuberous sclerosis patients. Hypsarrhythmia is characterized by high-voltage arrhythmic slow waves mixed with spike discharges showing a multifocal distribution.

TABLE 45–3. CRITERIA FOR DIAGNOSIS OF TUBEROUS SCLEROSIS[a]

Major Requirements

Facial angiofibromas (adenoma sebaceum)
Ungual fibromas
Cortical tubers
Subependymal hamartomas
Multiple retinal hamartomas
Fibrous plaque of the forehead

Minor Requirements

Infantile spasms
Hypopigmented macules
Shagreen patch
Single retinal hamartoma
Calcified subependymal or cortical lesion
Bilateral renal angiomyolipoma or cysts
Cardiac rhabdomyoma
First-degree relative with a primary diagnosis of tuberous sclerosis

[a] One major or two minor requirements are necessary for diagnosis.

MRI will show high signal lesions most commonly of the cerebral cortex, but also of the posterior fossa and brainstem (Figure 45–3). The MRI may also show hamartomas and gliotic areas of the brain. More severely affected patients tend to have a higher number of cerebral cortical lesions detected by MRI. In this manner, MRI is useful in predicting the clinical severity of tuberous sclerosis in younger children and those newly diagnosed.

Calcified lesions in the subependymal region or deeper can be identified by CT scan and will confirm the diagnosis of tuberous sclerosis. This imaging study will demonstrate multiple scattered calcium deposits located close to the wall of the lateral and third ventricle in the proximity of the foramen of Munro. A CT scan also best resolves periventricular calcific lesions. Fifty percent of patients with tuberous sclerosis will show evidence of intracranial calcified hamartomas. Cerebral cortical atrophy and mild to moderate ventricular dilatation may also be evident. Less commonly, lesions have been seen in the superficial brain parenchyma or the cerebellum.

Other useful diagnostic tests include positron emission tomography (PET) to study the seizure activity, and skull x-rays for intracranial calcifications. Nonimaging tests include blood work with a CBC and electrolyte analysis, urinalysis, blood pressure measurements, chest x-rays, abdominal CT scan, ultrasound of the kidney, echocardiogram, ECG, and EEG.

Most of the visceral manifestations of tuberous sclerosis are asymptomatic and will be identified through diagnostic testing. Larger kidney tumors may present with hematuria and can be identified with intravenous pyelography. Cardiac rhabdomyomas are also usually asymptomatic; however, they may produce cardiac arrhythmias or obstruction of blood flow. Prenatal diagnosis by fetal echocardiogram and ultrasound may be possible in certain instances.

■ Ocular

Comprehensive ocular evaluation may reveal retinal or optic disc astrocytic hamartomas. Visual fields and visual acuity are normal in the absence of retinal hamartoma involving the macula or a central nervous system lesion affecting the visual pathways.

Fluorescein angiography can be used in the diagnosis of retinal hamartomas. The hamartomas will exhibit mild autofluorescence and late-phase staining. The mulberry lesions in particular are highly reflectile, and exhibit a marked autofluorescence that is obvious prior to injection of the dye or during the retinal arterial phase before the dye reaches the tumor circulation. During the venous phase, the tumors will appear hypofluorescent in comparison to the retinal and choroidal circulations. During the late venous stage, however, the phakomas fluoresce intensely. The type 1 lesions will also remain hypofluorescent up to the venous phase,

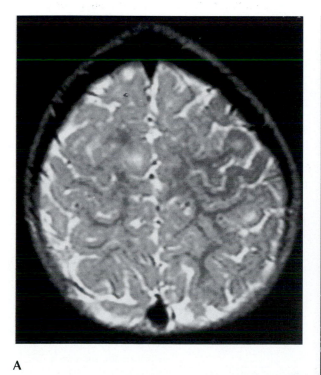

A

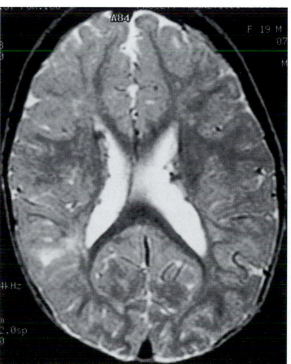

B

Figure 45–3. MRI showing high signal lesions (tubers) along the central sulcus and lateral ventricles.

and then a faint, diffuse hyperfluorescence occurs during the late venous phase. Small phakomas not noted ophthalmoscopically can be identified with angiography because of this hyperfluorescence. In this way, fluorescein angiography may be used as a screening tool to identify cases of suspected tuberous sclerosis.

Ultrasound B scan will show a strong echo with bright spots in the areas of calcified lesions.

An important differential diagnosis for the hamartomas of tuberous sclerosis is retinoblastoma of the optic nerve and retina. Other signs of tuberous sclerosis will help to make the diagnosis. Also, in tuberous sclerosis, the lesions will show little or no increase in size, while the retinoblastoma will increase dramatically.

The early-stage ocular lesions are characterized by opaque, white lesions that resemble myelinated nerve fibers. These are differentiated by bright fluorescence on angiography and are slightly raised above the surface of the retina in comparison to myelinated nerve fibers. These are also less discrete and lack the striate configuration of myelinated nerve fibers.

Inflammatory lesions such as early-stage toxocara or toxoplasmosis may cause a pale whitening of a focal region of retina and must be included in the differential diagnosis.

Optic disc astrocytic hamartomas may be confused with optic disc drusen. The differentiating factor is that disc drusen lie within the disc while the hamartomas protrude above it and obscure the disc and retinal vasculature. Also to be considered in the differential diagnosis is optic disc glioma, which may present with disc swelling, or the disc may be obscured by a mass protruding above its surface.

TREATMENT AND MANAGEMENT

■ Systemic

Treatment of tuberous sclerosis is directed toward the alleviation of symptoms (Table 45–4). Tumors are not generally treated because growth and change of these lesions are rare. Anticonvulsant medication is used in the control of seizures. The seizures are often difficult to control with medication; however, long periods of remission may develop spontaneously. There is some controversy regarding the role of pertussis immunizations provoking the onset of infantile spasms in patients predisposed to seizures. In the past, pertussis immunization had been linked with seizure onset. Currently, many feel this not to be true; however, many physicians still may want to withhold this immunization in order to avoid any possible cause for seizure onset. The decision to administer this immunization may have to be made after discussion between the patient's neurologist, pediatrician, and parents.

Administration of ACTH or steroids may lead to an improvement in the EEG pattern and a cessation of the seizure attacks. However, clinical relapse with a deterioration of the EEG is not infrequent. Occasionally surgical procedures are indicated in patients with severe seizures or expanding intracranial lesions. In some cases radiation therapy has been useful. Depending on the level of severity, patients with mental retardation may benefit from specialized schooling or vocational training.

Elimination of cutaneous and systemic lesions by dermabrasion and surgery is considered for cosmetic purposes. The adenoma sebaceum nodules can be treated but often result in regrowth and scarring. The tumors occurring in the visceral organs, kidney, and heart are usually benign and treated when complications arise. However, careful monitoring of pulmonary, renal, and cardiac function is warranted.

Although cases do arise from spontaneous mutations, genetic counseling is important for the patient, his or her parents, and siblings. CT or MRI scans of asymptomatic relatives to detect a carrier is a component of genetic counseling and is essential to those directly at risk. The finding of intracranial calcification in a parent of an affected child is helpful to confirm that the disease was inherited in an autosomal dominant manner rather than through spontaneous mutation. Parents of affected individuals should undergo a thorough examination of the skin, ophthalmoscopic evaluation through a dilated pupil for phakomata, and cranial imaging such as x-ray, MRI, or CT scan. An echocardiogram, ultrasound, or CT study of the kidneys and a physical examination of skin and nails are indicated. With the major advances in isolating the location of the gene to locus 9q34 of the long arm of chromosome 9, a prenatal test for tuberous sclerosis may be very close.

■ Ocular

Treatment of the ocular tumors is not indicated because the growth and change of these lesions are rare. Sequelae such as papilledema, vitreous hemorrhage, and retinal detachment

TABLE 45–4. TREATMENT AND MANAGEMENT OF TUBEROUS SCLEROSIS

● Seizures	Anticonvulsant medication
	Adrenocorticotrophic hormone or steroids
● Mental retardation	Specialized schooling, if necessary
● Visceral tumors	Careful monitoring and symptomatic treatment
● Cutaneous tumors	Cosmetic treatment
● Ocular tumors	Monitor Photodocumentation

are treated accordingly. Photodocumentation is indicated to ensure that a malignant lesion is not overlooked.

CONCLUSION

Tuberous sclerosis is a disorder associated with a variable presentation of central nervous system, cutaneous, ocular, and visceral manifestations. Although the retinal hamartomas common in tuberous sclerosis are generally benign, the eyecare practitioner has a responsibility to refer patients presenting with ocular signs for neurological and systemic evaluations.

REFERENCES

Bansley D, Wolter JR. The retinal lesion in tuberous sclerosis. *J Pediatr Ophthalmol.* 1971;8:261–265.

Borberg A. Clinical and genetic investigations into tuberous sclerosis and Recklinghausen's neurofibromatosis. *Acta Psychiatr. Neurol.* 1951;71(suppl):2–239.

Brett EM. Neurocutaneous syndromes. In: Brett EM, ed. *Paediatric Neurology.* Edinburgh: Churchill Livingstone, 1991:571–576.

Cruess AF. Tuberous sclerosis and the eye. In: Ryan SJ, ed. *Retina.* St. Louis: Mosby; 1989;1:571–578.

Gomez MR. Neurocutaneous diseases. In: Bradley WG, Daroff RB, Fenichel GM, Marsden CD, eds. *Neurology in Clinical Practice.* Boston: Butterworth-Heinemann; 1991.

Gomez MR. *Tuberous Sclerosis.* New York: Raven; 1979.

Krill AE. Tuberous sclerosis. In Krill AE, ed: *Krill's Hereditary Retinal and Choroidal Diseases.* Vol 2, *Clinical Characteristics.* Hagerstown, Md: Harper & Row; 1977: 1219–1248.

Miller NR. Phakomatoses. In Miller NR, ed: *Walsh and Hoyt's Clinical Neuro-ophthalmology.* Baltimore: Williams & Wilkins; 1988:1765–1788.

Pampiglione G, Moynahan EJ. The tuberous sclerosis syndrome, and clinical and EEG studies in 100 children. *J Neurol Neurosurg Psychiatr.* 1976;39:666–673.

Pampiglione G, Pugh E. Infantile spasms and subsequent appearance of tuberous sclerosis syndrome. *Lancet.* 1975;2:1046.

Roach ES, Williams DP, Laster DW. Magnetic resonance imaging in tuberous sclerosis. *Arch Neurol.* 1987;44:301–304.

Robertson DM. Ophthalmic manifestations of tuberous sclerosis. *Ann NY Acad Sci.* 1991;615:17–25.

Williams R, Taylor D. Tuberous sclerosis. *Surv Ophthalmol.* 1985;30:143.

Zion, V. M. Phakomatoses. In: Tasman W, Jaeger EA, eds. *Duane's Clinical Ophthalmology,* Philadelphia: Lippincott; 1992;5:6–7.

46
Chapter

Sturge–Weber Syndrome

Elizabeth B. Aksionoff

Sturge–Weber syndrome, also called encephalotrigeminal angiomatosis, is one of a group of congenital neurocutaneous syndromes called the phakomatoses. These syndromes are characterized by disseminated hamartomas (tumor-like nodules) of the eye, skin, and central nervous system.

Schirmer, in 1860, first associated buphthalmos with an ipsilateral facial nevus flammeus. In 1879, Sturge correlated unilateral buphthalmos, ipsilateral facial hemangioma, and contralateral epileptic seizures. It was not until 1922 that Weber established the triad of facial hemangioma, glaucoma, and cerebral dysfunction as the clinical entity, Sturge–Weber syndrome. Alexander and Norman (1960) believed that both facial and leptomeningeal angiomas must be present for the diagnosis of Sturge–Weber syndrome.

EPIDEMIOLOGY

■ Systemic

Sturge–Weber syndrome shows no racial or sex predilection. Focal or generalized seizures are found in 80% of patients, with 50% occurring before the age of 1 year. Mental retardation occurs in 54 to 60%. Hemiplegia contralateral to the angiomas occurs in 31%.

■ Ocular

The most common ocular manifestations of Sturge–Weber syndrome are choroidal hemangiomas and glaucoma. Choroidal hemangiomas are found in 40% of patients, and of these, 88% will develop glaucoma. Exudative retinal detachments will occur in 50% of patients with choroidal hemangioma. There is a 30% incidence of glaucoma in Sturge–Weber syndrome, of which 60% of cases are congenital. The remaining 40% develop glaucoma before early adulthood. Iris heterochromia is found in 8% of these individuals.

NATURAL HISTORY

■ Systemic

Sturge–Weber syndrome is believed to arise from a developmental error in a portion of the cephalic neural crest resulting in abnormal vasculature in the mesodermal derivatives of the supraocular dermis, choroid, and pia mater. Irregularity in the distribution and structure of small vessels results in abnormal proliferation of perivascular cells. Because these tumors are composed of cells normally present in this tissue, they are classified as hamartomas.

Sturge–Weber syndrome has no established genetic pattern. Its appearance is usually sporadic with variable expressivity.

Dermatologic

A common presenting feature of the disease is the nevus flammeus or port wine stain (Figure 46–1). This is a facial hemangioma within, but not always limited to, the distribution of the trigeminal nerve. The hemangioma primarily involves the ophthalmic and maxillary divisions, and rarely

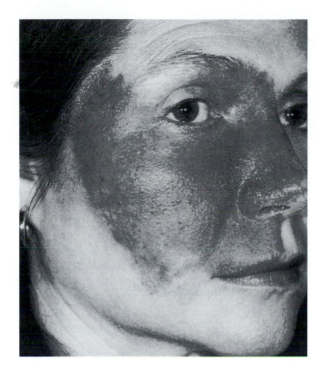

Figure 46-1. Nevus flammeus (port wine stain) of the face. *(Reprinted with permission from Habif TP.* Clinical Dermatology: A Color Guide to Diagnosis and Therapy. *2nd ed. St. Louis: Mosby, 1990, p 585.)*

the mandibular division. The supraorbital region is almost always affected.

The hemangioma consists of large, dilated capillaries in the dermis and subcutaneous tissues, and is usually present at birth. It presents as irregular, flat, dull, red patches. The nevus may darken with age and become more nodular, but will not increase in size. The nevus flammeus is usually unilateral but may extend past the midline. Hypertrophy of the face may occur ipsilateral to the hemangioma. The globe on the affected side may become enlarged even in the absence of glaucoma. Hemangiomas of the oral or nasal cavity are also possible.

Central Nervous System
Angiomatosis of the cerebral leptomeninges, the layer overlying the cerebral cortex, occurs on the same side as the facial hemangioma and results in altered circulation of the underlying cerebral cortex. These areas show degenerative changes with subsequent calcification. Once the calcium is deposited, the lesions can be evaluated radiographically. Calcification is usually seen before the age of 1 year. These lesions increase in size up to the second decade of life and then stabilize. Usually the occipital or occipital–parietal regions of one of the cerebral hemispheres are affected, but the lesions may extend over an entire hemisphere. It is a rare exception if the brain lesions are not on the same side as the skin lesions.

Epileptic seizures are a frequent occurrence in Sturge–Weber syndrome. The seizures present early in life,

with one half of patients developing them between the ages of 2 and 7 months. After seizure onset, development may be dramatically set back. When Sturge–Weber syndrome manifests with seizures in infancy, they may become intractable, with progressive hemiparesis, motor weakness, and mental retardation. The manifestations of seizure activity occur contralateral to the skin lesion. They usually begin as partial seizures but become more generalized with time. Patients with seizures unresponsive to medical therapy may develop slowly progressive neurological deficits and ultimately become moderately or severely disabled.

Unilateral cerebral cortical angiomatoses and associated atrophy and calcification can lead to cerebral dysfunction. If present, mental retardation ranges from mild to profound deficiencies. Bilateral involvement of the brain is associated with earlier onset of seizures and a poorer prognosis for mental development.

Almost one third of patients will have some degree of transient hemiplegia or visual field defect contralateral to the facial angioma.

Visceral tumors have been associated with a wide range of organ systems. Visceral involvement is less common in Sturge–Weber syndrome than in the other phakomatoses (Table 46–1).

Many patients with Sturge–Weber syndrome die in their second or third decades from the progressive central nervous system manifestations.

■ **Ocular**
The first visible ocular manifestation of Sturge–Weber syndrome is usually the nevus flammeus of the eyelid. When the upper eyelid is involved, there is a greater correlation with glaucoma and intracranial angiomatosis. The nevus flammeus may cause the lid to become ptotic.

Choroidal hemangioma, the most common ocular manifestation, is a diffuse, flat, vascularized cavernous hemangioma usually located at the posterior pole, often temporal to the optic disc. It is usually unilateral, but may be bilateral if the facial angioma is bilateral. Histologically, the hemangioma is composed of dilated vascular channels lined by attenuated endothelial cells or fibrocytes. The

TABLE 46–1. SYSTEMIC MANIFESTATIONS OF STURGE–WEBER SYNDROME

- Nevus flammeus (Port wine stain) along the distribution of the trigeminal nerve
- Seizure disorder
- Mental retardation
- Hemiparesis or hemiplegia contralateral to the nerves
- Angiomatosis of the cerebral leptomeninges ipsilateral to the nevus
- Visceral tumors of the lung, thymus, spleen, testes, ovaries, GI tract, pituitary, thyroid, pancreas

tumor gives a diffuse red appearance to the retina, especially in contrast to the fellow eye. It is referred to as "tomato catsup" fundus.

Localized hemangiomas are less common but are associated with serous retinal detachments. These lesions are circular or oval, slightly elevated, and reddish-orange in color. The overlying retina may exhibit tortuosity and dilatation of the retinal vasculature. The retinal pigment epithelium above the choroidal hemangioma may exhibit drusen, areas of calcification, or atrophy. At this stage, visual function may not be affected. With time, cystoid degeneration of the overlying retina may occur, leading to exudation and retinal pigment alterations, as well as to exudative retinal detachments, subsequent iris neovascularization, and secondary glaucoma. Subretinal hemorrhage from the choroidal hemangioma may result in retinal detachment with forward displacement of the iris and angle closure secondary to peripheral anterior synechiae formation.

There are several theories on the pathogenesis of the glaucoma in Sturge–Weber syndrome. Some associate the disease with an angle anomaly in which there is an anterior insertion of the ciliary muscle and uveal tissue in the angle. The thick uveal meshwork, poorly developed scleral spur, and anteriorly inserted iris root lead to outflow obstruction. Another theory involves the presence of limbal and episcleral vascular malformations that increase the episcleral venous pressure and thus impede aqueous outflow, subsequently raising intraocular pressure.

Glaucoma may develop in infancy, childhood, or adulthood. Buphthalmos occurs if IOP is elevated in an infant less than 3 years of age, causing the cornea and sclera to enlarge. The glaucoma usually occurs on the same side as the facial hemangioma, especially if it involves the skin of the upper eyelid, tarsus, and conjunctiva. Patients with bilateral facial lesions may have glaucoma in either or both eyes. Visual acuity and field loss is variable depending on the severity of the glaucoma.

TABLE 46–2. OCULAR MANIFESTATIONS OF STURGE–WEBER SYNDROME

- Choroidal hemangioma
- Glaucoma
- Buphthalmos, if glaucoma occurs prior to 3 years of age
- Nevus flammeus of the eyelid; may also cause ptosis
- Iris heterochromia, caused by small iris hamartomas
- Serous or exudative retinal detachment
- Anomalous vessels of the episclera and conjunctiva
- Intracranial malformations may cause homonymous hemianopias and papilledema
- Retinal pigmentary atrophy/retinitis pigmentosa
- Choroidal coloboma
- Atrophic chorioretinitis
- Retinoblastoma

Large, anomalous blood vessels may be present in the conjunctiva, episcleral tissue, choroid, and retina. Episcleral hemangiomas are found in all Sturge–Weber patients with glaucoma (Phelps, 1978). An episcleral hemangioma may appear as a faint blue or purplish blush lying under the Tenon capsule and conjunctiva.

Iris heterochromia may occur, with the iris darker on the side of the facial nevus, because melanocytes are grouped into small hamartomas on the anterior surface of the iris.

Contralateral homonymous hemianopias with or without macular sparing may occur secondary to occipital intracranial lesions. The hemianopia probably occurs from a thrombosis of the vessels of the malformation that penetrate the cortex.

The retinal pigment epithelium above the choroidal hemangioma may also exhibit changes. Drusen, areas of calcification, and RPE atrophy have been reported. Papilledema may result from increased intracranial pressure secondary to intracranial lesions. Other less commonly associated ocular manifestations of Sturge–Weber syndrome are included in Table 46–2.

DIAGNOSIS

■ Systemic

Nevus flammeus, present at birth, is the first presenting sign of Sturge–Weber syndrome, and is diagnosed by clinical appearance. Occurrence of the nevus flammeus alone, without additional involvement of the eye or central nervous system, does not constitute a diagnosis of Sturge–Weber syndrome. However, if glaucoma also exists, the diagnosis of Sturge–Weber syndrome can be made. Neurologic abnormalities are seldom evident at birth. Although seizures may not be initially present, neuroimaging and ocular evaluation is indicated if a nevus flammeus and/or glaucoma is diagnosed.

CT scans, especially axial and coronal views, are useful for the evaluation of the angiomatosis of the cerebral leptomeninges. They are more sensitive than x-rays to identify calcification and vascular lesions. The pathognomonic feature on radiographic studies is intracranial calcification arranged in parallel lines or "railroad tracks" showing a gyriform distribution. This is most commonly seen in the occipital or parietal lobes. MRI is the method of choice to detect intracranial involvement, but abnormal calcifications are not appreciated as well as with CT scan. Enhancement with gadolinium-DTPA improves the diagnostic value of MRI, before neurological symptoms arise. Cerebral angiography may also serve to identify and determine the extent of the angiomatous malformation. It will show a lack of superficial veins, tortuosity, enlargement of the deep subependymal and medullary veins, and nonfilling of the superior sagittal sinus.

Seizures may be evaluated with electroencephalography. Patients with unilateral involvement will show ipsilateral signal attenuation on EEG.

■ Ocular

External examination may reveal facial hemangioma, episcleral or conjunctival hemangioma, and iris heterochromia. Fundus examination may reveal hemangioma, glaucomatous optic nerve cupping, papilledema, retinal pigmentary atrophy, or retinal detachment.

Fluorescein angiography is a useful tool to diagnose choroidal hemangioma. A rapidly appearing, diffusely speckled background choroidal fluorescence beginning in the early transit phase with late staining is characteristic. In the absence of a retinal detachment, there is no leakage of the dye from the choroidal hemangioma into the retina. In isolated hemangiomas, the lesions fluoresce brightly during the early phases of angiography. An irregular lacy pattern may occur, probably due to the rapid filling of the cavernous channels of the hemangioma. Late hyperfluorescence of the tumor may result from the leakage of dye into the overlying subretinal space.

A- and B-scan ultrasonography can be useful to assess choroidal thickening found with choroidal hemangioma. A-scan sonography will exhibit high internal reflectivity. The B scan will show a solid echogenic mass.

A complete glaucoma workup is mandatory for any patient with a nevus flammeus. Gonioscopy may reveal malformations of the anterior chamber and prominent iris processes adhering to the trabeculum, especially in those with the congenital form.

Visual fields are not only important to follow glaucoma patients but also to detect field defects associated with visual pathway lesions. Visual field defects may include contralateral homonymous hemianopsias associated with occipital leptomeningeal angiomas, or sectorial defects associated with hemangiomas of the choroid.

TREATMENT

■ Systemic

Epileptic seizures may be treated medically or surgically (Table 46–3). Anticonvulsant medications are effective in about one half of patients with seizures due to Sturge–Weber syndrome. Surgery, such as cerebral resections and hemispherectomy, is indicated only for patients with severe progressive disease unresponsive to medical management to avoid continued deterioration. Patients who develop intractable seizures in the first 6 months of life and unilateral hemispheric involvement should be considered

TABLE 46–3. TREATMENT AND MANAGEMENT OF STURGE–WEBER SYNDROME

- Seizures
  Anticonvulsant medications
  Surgical procedures: cerebral resection or hemispherectomy
- Mental retardation
  Specialized schooling or vocational rehabilitation
- Facial nevus
  Cosmetics
  Laser surgery
- Glaucoma
  Medical management
  Surgical management: goniotomy, trabeculotomy, trabeculectomy, cyclocryotherapy
- Retinal detachment
  Surgical management

for early resection of the involved hemisphere. There is evidence that with earlier intervention, less intellectual deterioration will occur.

Visceral tumors are rare and are only treated when symptoms arise from them. Cutaneous angiomas are usually asymptomatic and not treated. Facial cosmetics can be used to conceal the lesions. Laser therapy is an option for the cosmetic management of the facial nevus flammeus.

■ Ocular

Follow-up eye care is important for Sturge–Weber patients, particularly if glaucoma or serous retinal detachment are present. Glaucoma in Sturge–Weber syndrome is variable in severity and subsequent treatment modalities (see Table 46–3). It often responds poorly to medical management. If medical treatment fails or if the glaucoma is congenital, surgical intervention is necessary. Buphthalmos requires immediate treatment. Goniotomy is a common procedure in infants with congenital glaucoma. Trabeculotomy is performed if corneal clouding prevents visualization of the angle or previous goniotomy has failed. In adults, after medical management fails, argon laser trabeculoplasty may be attempted first. However, if the pressure reduction is insufficient, conventional surgery is the next alternative. Trabeculectomy bypasses any component of the glaucoma caused by elevated episcleral venous pressure, whereas goniotomy does not. If external filtration fails, cyclocryotherapy may be attempted as a last resort. Various other surgical techniques are employed including combined trabeculectomy and cyclocryotherapy. Surgical glaucoma treatment may have complications such as intraoperative expulsive choroidal hemorrhage and choroidal effusion. It may be necessary to perform a posterior sclerotomy before opening the eye to prevent choroidal effusion.

Retinal detachment in Sturge–Weber patients is difficult to treat. When the retina is reattached, fibrous metaplasia of the RPE and cystoid degeneration of the retina overlying the choroidal hemangioma can cause poor visual prognosis.

Conclusion

Sturge–Weber syndrome is a congenital disorder involving hamartomas of the skin, central nervous system, and eye. It is characterized by facial hemangioma, glaucoma, and cerebral dysfunctions such as seizures and mental retardation. Although these entities may occur in isolation, Sturge–Weber syndrome is diagnosed when two or more systems are affected. Any patient presenting with a facial hemangioma in the trigeminal distribution or with idiopathic seizures must have comprehensive ocular and neurological evaluation to rule out other manifestations of this disease.

References

Alexander GL, Norman RM. *The Sturge–Weber Syndrome.* Bristol, England: Wright: Stonebridge Press; 1960.

Brett EM. Neurocutaneous syndromes. In: Brett EM, ed. *Paediatric Neurology.* Edinburgh: Churchill Livingstone, 1991:580–583.

Krill AE. *Sturge–Weber Syndrome Hereditary Retinal and Choroidal Diseases.* Vol 2, *Clinical Characteristics.* Hagerstown, Md: Harper & Row; 1977:1275–1290.

Miller NR. Phakomatoses. In: *Walsh and Hoyt's Clinical Neuro-ophthalmology.* Baltimore: Williams & Wilkins; 1988:1800–1816.

Phelps CD. The pathogenesis of glaucoma in Sturge–Weber syndrome. *Ophthalmology.* 1978;85:276–286.

Susac JO, Smith JL, Scelfo RJ. The "tomato-catsup" fundus in Sturge–Weber syndrome. *Arch Ophthalmol.* 1974;92:69.

Tripatini B, Inpathi RC, Cibis GW. Sturge–Weber syndrome. In: Ryan SJ, ed. *Retina.* St. Louis: Mosby; 1991;1:443–447.

Weiss JS, Ritch R. Glaucoma in the phakomatoses. In: Ritch R, Shields MB, eds. *The Secondary Glaucomas.* St. Louis: Mosby; 1982.

Zion VM. Phakomatoses. In: Tasman W, Jaeger EA, eds. *Duane's Clinical Ophthalmology.* Philadelphia: Lippincott; 1992;5:7–9.

47
Chapter

Von Hippel–Lindau Disease

Elizabeth B. Aksionoff

Von Hippel–Lindau disease, also called retinocerebellar capillary hemangiomatosis, is one of a group of congenital syndromes called the phakomatoses. These syndromes are characterized by disseminated hamartomas (tumor-like nodules) of the eye, skin, and central nervous system. However, von Hippel–Lindau disease is the only phakomatosis without an associated skin lesion. It is a rare, hereditary disorder whose complete complex consists of angiomatosis of the retina, capillary hemangioblastomas of the central nervous system, and cysts or vascular tumors of the viscera. Retinal angiomatoses were first described by von Hippel in 1904. The correlation with hemangiomatous tumors of the cerebellum was made by Lindau in 1926.

EPIDEMIOLOGY

Von Hippel–Lindau disease shows no sexual or racial predilection. It usually presents in the second to fourth decades of life, later than most of the other phakomatoses.

Headache is the presenting symptom in 90% of von Hippel–Lindau patients. Cerebellar hemangioblastomas may occur in 35 to 75% of patients. Renal cell carcinoma has an incidence of 33% in those with von Hippel–Lindau disease and pheochromocytoma occurs in 17%. Half of the patients with cerebellar tumors also present with polycythemia. Cysts present in various visceral organs, with the pancreas (72%), kidney (59%), liver (17%), and epididymis (7%) the most common locations. The complete symptom complex is found in 20% of those with the cerebellar hemangioblastomas, and only 25% of patients with retinal angiomas develop neurological symptoms.

NATURAL HISTORY

■ Systemic

Von Hippel–Lindau disease is characterized by angiomatosis of the retina, capillary hemangioblastomas of the central nervous system, and cysts or tumors of the viscera. It exhibits autosomal dominant inheritance with variable expression and incomplete penetrance. However, almost 80% are due to sporadic mutations. The gene has been isolated to chromosome 3.

Generalized developmental dysgenesis of the neuroectoderm and mesoderm cause hemangioblastomas of the cerebellum (Figure 47–1), medulla, and spinal cord, which are the characteristic central nervous system lesions in von Hippel–Lindau disease. The hemangioblastomas are single or multiple cysts, fed and drained by large vessels. The cyst is fluid filled and contains a nodule of tumor cells in its wall. Hemangioblastomas are usually found in the posterior fossa, and they become symptomatic when they increase intracranial pressure or cause cerebellar dysfunction. Headache is the most common symptom occurring during the course of the disease, and may occur as a result of increased intracranial pressure or the direct affect of the hamartomas on the meninges. Signs of cerebellar dysfunction may include vomiting, ataxic gait, dysdiadochokinesia (the inability to perform rapidly alternating movements), vertigo, and dysmetria (movements overshooting their intended targets). Intracranial hemorrhage or compression of vital brainstem centers are the major causes of death in von Hippel–Lindau disease,

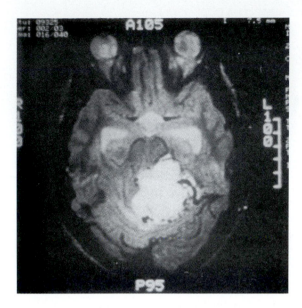

Figure 47–1. MRI with contrast shows cerebellar hemangioblastoma. *(Reprinted with permission from Burk RR: Von Hippel–Lindau disease (angiomatosis of the retina and cerebellum).* J Am Optom Assoc. *1991;62:384.)*

secondary to cerebellar hemangioblastomas and less commonly to medullary hemangioblastomas.

Less common systemic manifestations of von Hippel–Lindau disease are listed in Table 47–1. Spinal cord hemangioblastomas can cause pain, bilateral weakness of the extremities, and sensory disturbances. Renal cell carcinoma may present with hematuria, obstructive nephropathy, or an abdominal mass. This can be fatal secondary to metastasis or uremia. Pheochromocytoma, a tumor of the adrenal medulla, is often bilateral and results in vasoconstrictive hypertension. Polycythemia, an increase in red cell count, may be found in patients with cerebellar tumors related to the erythropoietic activity of the CNS cyst fluid.

■ **Ocular**

Half the patients diagnosed with von Hippel–Lindau disease will eventually suffer visual loss. Angiomatosis retinae is often the first observed manifestation of von

TABLE 47–1. SYSTEMIC MANIFESTATIONS OF VON HIPPEL–LINDAU DISEASE

- Hemangioblastomas of the cerebellum, medulla oblongata, spinal cord
- Hemangioblastomas of the pancreas
- Renal cell carcinomas
- Pheochromocytomas of the adrenal medulla
- Paragangliomas of the sympathetic chain
- Cysts and tumors of miscellaneous visceral organs: meninges, lung, liver, spleen, ovary, bladder, bones, skin, epididymis

Hippel–Lindau disease, and usually is asymptomatic when it is discovered in the second or third decades. Although the angioma may occur anywhere in the retina, it is often found in the midperiphery (Figure 47–2). Angiomas often present bilaterally and may be multiple.

Welch (1970) divided the natural history of the retinal angioma into several stages (Table 47–2). Angiomas of the disc or peripapillary region usually do not have dilated feeder vessels and are the capillary type. There are two varieties, endophytic and exophytic. The endophytic type are circular, reddish, slightly elevated masses internal to the vasculature of the optic disc. The earliest sign of the disc angioma is a small group of dilated capillaries usually on the temporal side. As it enlarges, this mass begins to resemble a nodule. These tumors give rise to surface neovascularization similar to the peripheral capillary hemangioma. The exophytic type is not seen as a distinct mass but as a blurring and elevation of the margin of the optic disc without prominent vascular channels.

Papillary, juxtapapillary, and peripheral angiomas may cause macular edema, the major cause of vision loss in von Hippel–Lindau disease. Even peripheral angiomas, especially those in the temporal fundus, may cause macular edema despite the presence of normal intervening retina. The maculopathy first presents as early edema or as discrete exudates in a star-shaped pattern. Further progression will result in a circular, elevated mass of subretinal exudate. This may lead to macular gliosis, extensive cystoid

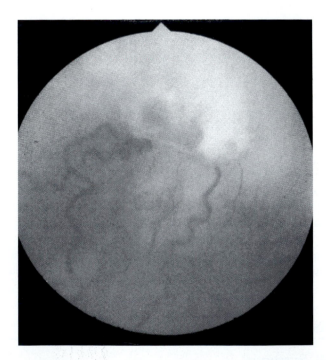

Figure 47–2. Retinal angioma with dilated, tortuous feeder vessels. *(Reprinted with permission from Burk RR: Von Hippel–Lindau disease (angiomatosis of the retina and cerebellum).* J Am Optom Assoc. *1991;62:385.)*

TABLE 47–2. STAGES OF RETINAL ANGIOMA DEVELOPMENT

Stage I: Preclassical

Microaneurysm-sized lesion consisting of a small capillary cluster

Endothelial cells of lesion are fenestrated, unlike a true capillary

Lack of tight junctions leads to leakage of plasma and blood components into the retina and subretinal space

Stage II: Classical

Larger lesion appearing as a small pink nodule or as a cluster of capillaries with associated dilated feeder vessels

Stage III: Exudation

Tumor enlarges, and secondary to incompetent capillary wall, lipid exudation into the retina and subretinal space occurs

Stage IV: Retinal Detachment

Internal limiting membrane is breached by a proliferation of fibrovascular tissue, causing vitreal traction and nonrhegmatogenous exudative retinal detachment

Stage V: End Stage

May include retinal hemorrhage, gliosis, neovascularization, rubeotic glaucoma, chronic uveitis, phthisis bulbi

TABLE 47–3. OCULAR MANIFESTATIONS OF VON HIPPEL–LINDAU DISEASE

- Angiomatosis retinae
- Optic disc or peripapillary angioma
- The above may cause
    Exudation
    Vitreous traction
    Macular edema
    Macular gliosis
    Exudative retinal detachment
    Neovascularization
    Secondary glaucoma
    Phthisis bulbi
- Cerebellar or central nervous system angiomas may cause
    Papilledema
    Cranial nerve dysfunctions
    Nystagmus

degeneration, and hole formation, resulting in a significant loss of central vision. These hemangiomas can lead to serous detachments of the peripapillary sensory retina and a ring of intraretinal lipid exudate. The angiomas may extend through a break in the internal limiting membrane and attach to the vitreous. If the vitreous produces traction on the tumor vessels, vitreous hemorrhage or retinal detachment may occur. This may lead to secondary glaucoma, chronic uveitis, and eventually a phthisical eye.

Increased intracranial pressure may lead to papilledema and subsequent optic atrophy as well as cranial nerve dysfunction, such as abducens nerve paresis. Nystagmus is a possible manifestation of cerebellar dysfunction resulting from cerebellar hemangioblastomas (Table 47–3).

DIAGNOSIS

■ Systemic

To make the diagnosis of von Hippel–Lindau disease, evidence of multisystem involvement must be present rather than isolated retinal, intracranial, or visceral lesions. Diagnosis is made when a patient has a hemangioblastoma of the central nervous system or retina and one or more of the following: first-degree relative with the disease; renal carcinoma; or renal, pancreatic, or epididymal cysts. Diagnosis is often difficult because of the variability in presentation. The first manifestation to become symptomatic is

usually the retinal lesion, followed by CNS hemangioblastomas and visceral lesions.

Von Hippel–Lindau disease is usually diagnosed during routine physical or ocular examination. Intracranial or visceral lesions may be discovered upon investigating the subjective symptoms or signs correlating with the involved areas. In these patients, complete blood chemistry (CBC) and urine analysis, which includes catecholamine, epinephrine, and norepinephrine levels, are recommended. Norepinephrine and epinephrine levels will help detect such manifestations as pheochromocytoma. If urine catecholamine levels are normal but blood pressure is elevated, plasma catecholamine levels should be taken. Any biochemical abnormalities warrant an abdominal CT scan. An MRI of the abdomen will highlight renal carcinoma and other visceral lesions.

Subjective complaint of headache is very common, and other symptoms indicating cerebellar or spinal cord involvement may occur, as described in the natural history section. In the presence of these symptoms, CT of the head and upper cervical spinal cord are indicated, along with MRI of the brain.

■ Ocular

Von Hippel–Lindau disease may be diagnosed in an asymptomatic individual during routine ocular examination. These patients warrant a complete systemic workup as outlined in the systemic natural history section. Ocular diagnosis of von Hippel–Lindau disease is based upon the presence of retinal angioma. Fluorescein angiography is a valuable tool in this diagnosis, and may be the only way to detect subclinical lesions. The enlarged capillaries act hemodynamically as shunts, with resultant enlargement of the afferent and efferent vessels. Because of the shunting mechanism, fluorescein travels through the tumor rapidly.

The arterial phase shows a single, rapid-filling artery feeding each angioma, which also quickly fills with dye. The angioma will show varying amounts of dye leakage throughout the late phases. Also, due to the rapid flow of fluorescein, the lamellar flow of the vein may be disrupted. Without stereoscopic fluorescein angiography, retinal angiomas may be confused with papilledema, papillitis, choroiditis, choroidal neovascularization, or choroidal hemangioma.

Differential diagnosis includes Wyburn–Mason syndrome, Coats disease, and sickle-cell disease. In Wyburn–Mason syndrome and Coats disease, no tumor is present. Sea fans found in sickle-cell disease may simulate a capillary hemangioma; however, the sea fans do not have feeder vessel enlargement or produce the high-flow shunt seen in von Hippel–Lindau disease.

If symptomatic, the ocular lesions may cause disturbances of vision, headache, papilledema, ocular motor dysfunction, or nystagmus.

TREATMENT

■ Systemic
The systemic therapy of CNS hemangioblastomas is often directed toward the alleviation of symptoms. However, asymptomatic cerebellar hemangioblastomas may be surgically removed to prevent complications of enlarging lesions. Hemangioblastomas of the spinal cord and brainstem are not treated if asymptomatic. Radiation therapy is warranted when symptoms arise (Table 47–4).

Cysts of the kidney, liver, and pancreas are usually asymptomatic and do not require treatment. However, early surgical removal of pheochromocytomas and renal cell carcinomas is indicated, because these are the most life-threatening lesions in von Hippel–Lindau disease.

Annual physical, kidney ultrasound, and neurological examinations are indicated in any patient at risk. This includes patients with a characteristic retina, CNS or visceral lesion, or a direct relative having the disease. The physical examination should include CBC and urine analysis. The neurological examination may include baseline CT scan of the head and upper cervical spinal cord. MRI of the brain, with particular attention to the posterior fossa, provides more information regarding the presence of cerebellar hemangioblastomas, and should be done when indicated.

Patients with any systemic manifestation of von Hippel–Lindau disease must have a comprehensive ocular examination to rule out the ocular manifestations of the disease.

By examining family members and/or through family history, an effort should be made to determine if the affected individual inherited the disease by autosomal dom-

TABLE 47–4. TREATMENT AND MANAGEMENT OF VON HIPPEL–LINDAU DISEASE

- ■ **SYSTEMIC**
  - Cerebellar dysfunction
    Surgical removal
  - Hemangioblastomas of the spinal cord and medulla
    Radiation therapy
  - Pheochromocytomas
    Surgical removal
  - Renal cell carcinomas
    Surgical removal
  - Visceral lesions
    Symptomatic treatment

- ■ **OCULAR**
  - Preclassical angiomas
    Photodocumentation, 6-month follow-up
  - Classical retinal angiomas
    Fluorescein angiography
    Argon photocoagulation, cryotherapy
  - Retinal detachment
    Reattachment procedures
  - Optic nerve angiomas
    Photocoagulation at first sign of exudation

inant transmission or as a result of spontaneous mutation. This information is useful for genetic counseling.

■ Ocular
The majority of tumors in von Hippel–Lindau disease progress and lead to serious visual loss. Therefore, indirect ophthalmoscopy is advised annually for family members of von Hippel–Lindau patients and every 6 months for those affected.

Retinal angiomas that are small, stable, and asymptomatic may be followed by photodocumentation (see Table 47–4). Follow-up is important because of the great variability in tumor growth rate. When the tumors are small, photocoagulation may obliterate them with little complication. The tumor itself and not the abnormal vessels is treated in order to prevent tumor growth and its sequelae. Treatment destroys the angioma, leaving a pigmented scar and involuted feeder vessels. Treatment of the peripheral angioma will often resolve any macula edema produced by the angioma. Complications of photocoagulation include hemorrhage, exudative retinal detachment, and an increase in intraretinal lipid deposits.

For tumors larger than 0.8 disc diameter and those with subretinal fluid, cryotherapy is recommended. Several treatments may be necessary. Less posttreatment exudative detachment occurs after cryotherapy of large angiomas than after photocoagulation. For tumors greater than one disc diameter in size, a combination of cryotherapy followed by photocoagulation of the tumor itself is indicated. In instances of large tumors, multiple tumors, or vitreous membranes, vitrectomy should be considered. Penetrating diathermy and eye wall resection are other techniques used to treat large peripheral capillary hemangiomas.

After treatment, patients should be followed with fluorescein angiography. Retreatment is indicated if the tumor persists in the pigmented scar or if fluorescein angiography shows the persistence of hyperfluorescence.

Intraretinal juxtapapillary capillary hemangiomas are difficult to treat because they are diffusely situated in the retina. Laser burns needed to destroy the abnormal vascular tissue must also penetrate the retinal tissue including the nerve fiber layer. When treated, there is a potential for full-thickness damage to the retina and disc, with resultant visual loss. If untreated, however, exudation, retinal detachment, and neovascular glaucoma may result from lesion growth. Treatment is usually indicated at the first sign of exudation.

For traction detachment or surface-wrinkling retinopathy, pars plana vitrectomy and membrane peeling may be used. Retinal detachments may require reattachment procedures such as scleral buckling.

Follow-up is recommended every 3 to 6 months depending on the extent of retinal findings. If a retinal or optic disc angioma is observed, a systemic workup with urinary catecholamine and CT or MRI of the head, upper cervical spinal cord, and abdomen are indicated.

CONCLUSION

Von Hippel–Lindau disease is a multisystem disease characterized by angiomatoses of the retina, hemangioblastomas of the central nervous system, and cysts or tumors of the viscera. This disease is of particular importance to the eyecare practitioner, because its first presenting signs are often ocular. Any retinal angioma should alert the practi-tioner to the need for a complete physical and neurological evaluation, because the associated renal cell carcinoma, pheochromocytoma, and cerebellar hemangioblastoma are potentially lethal lesions. Because the disease is autosomal dominant in nature, genetic counseling is advised.

REFERENCES

Annesley WH, Leonard BC, Shields JA, Tasman WS. Fifteen-year review of treated cases of retinal angiomatosis. *Ophthalmology.* 1977;83:446.

Goldberg MF, Duke JR. Von Hippel–Lindau disease. *Am J Ophthalmol.* 1968;66:693–705.

Gomez MR. Neurocutaneous diseases. In: Bradley WG, Daroff RB, Fenichel GM, Marsden CD, eds. *Neurology in Clinical Practice.* Boston: Butterworth-Heinemann; 1991.

Hardwig PW, Robertson DM. Von Hippel–Lindau disease: A familial, often lethal, multi-system phakomatosis. *Ophthalmology.* 1984;91:263–270.

Krill AE. Von Hippel–Lindau disease. In: Krill AE, ed: *Krill's Hereditary Retinal and Choroidal Diseases.* Vol 2, *Clinical Characteristics.* Hagerstown, Md: Harper & Row; 1977: 1249–1274.

Miller NR. Phakomatoses. In: Miller NR, ed: *Walsh and Hoyt's Clinical Neuro-ophthalmology.* Baltimore: Williams & Wilkins; 1988:1788–1800.

Nicholson DH. Capillary hemangioma of the retina and von Hippel–Lindau disease. In: Ryan SJ, ed. *Retina.* St. Louis: Mosby; 1989;1:563–570.

Ridley M, Green J, Johnson G. Retinal angiomatosis: The ocular manifestations of Von Hippel–Lindau disease. *Can J Ophthalmol.* 1986;21:276–283.

Welch RB. Von Hippel–Lindau disease: The recognition and treatment of early anastomosis retinae and the use of cryosurgery as an adjunct to therapy. *Trans Am Ophthalmol Soc.* 1970;68:367–424.

Zion, V.M. Phakomatoses. In: Tasman W, Jaeger EA, eds. *Duane's Clinical Ophthalmology.* Philadelphia: Lippincott; 1992;5:3–4.

48
Chapter

Wyburn–Mason Syndrome

Elizabeth B. Aksionoff

Wyburn–Mason syndrome, also known as racemose hemangiomatosis or Bonnet–Dechaume–Blanc syndrome, belongs to a group of disorders known as the phakomatoses, which are characterized by hamartomas (tumor-like nodules) of the eye, skin, and central nervous system. This disorder is characterized by retinal and systemic arteriovenous malformations (AVMs). AVMs, direct communications between the arterial and venous circulations without an intervening capillary bed, were first described in the retina by Magnus in 1874. In 1930, Yates and Paine noted the correlation of vascular malformation in the ipsilateral cerebral hemisphere and retina. Although an isolated AVM of the retina can occur, there is an association with ipsilateral AVMs of the brain and face.

EPIDEMIOLOGY

■ Systemic
AVMs of the central nervous system are found in 59% of patients with Wyburn–Mason syndrome. The majority of the malformations are found in the midbrain. AVM of the nasopharynx occurs in 16% of patients with this disease.

■ Ocular
Intracranial malformation will also be found in 90% of patients with large, racemose retinal arteriovenous malformation. Retinal malformation also occurs in 70% of patients with an AVM of the midbrain. Decreased vision in the affected eye occurs in 80%, and homonymous hemianopic visual field defects occur in 30% of these patients. AVMs within the orbit occur in 19% of affected patients and 5% are found within the eyelid.

NATURAL HISTORY

■ Systemic
There is no hereditary pattern associated with Wyburn–Mason syndrome. It has variable clinical manifes-

tations, with ocular or neurologic symptoms usually occurring before the fourth decade of life.

AVMs are the most common form of intracranial vascular hamartoma (Table 48–1). Malformation results from abnormal persistence of the embryonic vascular stage that precedes the differentiation of arteries, veins, and capillaries. Embryologically, the vascular mesoderm is shared by the optic cup and the anterior portion of the neural tube, which develops into the hyaloid vascular system of the eye and the vascular supply of the mesencephalon. Due to this proximity, a disturbance prior to 7 weeks gestation can produce arteriovenous malformations of both the visual structures and of the mesencephalon. If abnormalities occur after 7 weeks gestation, it is less likely for both systems to be affected. In these cases, AVMs may occur in either the eye or mesencephalon, but usually not both. Therefore these would not be classified as Wyburn–Mason syndrome.

The intracranial arteriovenous malformations are usually fed by branches from the ipsilateral carotid and vertebral–basilar arteries. They have a predilection for the midbrain and posterior fossa. Neurologic symptoms of AVMs are related either to direct compression from the intracranial AVM or to secondary changes such as infarction or hemorrhage (cerebral or subarachnoid). Hemorrhage is more likely to result from a larger AVM.

TABLE 48–1. SYSTEMIC MANIFESTATIONS OF WYBURN–MASON SYNDROME

- **AVMs of the midbrain may cause**
  Headaches
  Seizures
  Hemiparesis
  Cerebral or subarachnoid hemorrhages
  Mental retardation
  Hydrocephalus
- **Nasopharyngeal AVMs may cause**
  Epistaxis
  Oral hemorrhage
  Bruits

Central nervous system AVMs may produce varied symptoms. Headaches are often the first presenting feature. Other manifestations of central nervous system dysfunction include seizures, mental retardation, cranial nerve palsies, hemiparesis, and hydrocephalus secondary to blockage of the sylvian aqueduct.

Unlike the other phakomatoses, cutaneous manifestations are less common in Wyburn–Mason syndrome. Nevus flammeus, as seen in Sturge–Weber syndrome, may occur. Nasopharyngeal AVMs may also exist in Wyburn–Mason syndrome. They may cause epistaxis, oral hemorrhage, or bruits.

■ Ocular

Vascular malformations may occur anywhere along the visual pathway. A congenital, unilateral retinal arteriovenous malformation that is ipsilateral to the intracranial AVM is the most common finding (Figure 48–1). The retinal vascular

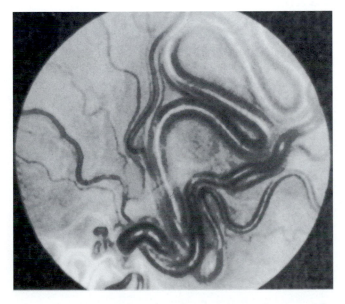

Figure 48–1. Congenital, unilateral retinal AVM. *(Courtesy of the Upjohn Company.)*

abnormality consists of one or more feeding arteries directly connecting with one or more draining veins with a predilection for the posterior pole and the superotemporal quadrant. This differentiates it from the retinal angioma of von Hippel–Lindau disease, which is usually seen in the peripheral retina. The majority of patients with a retinal AVM have poor vision in the affected eye. Reduced vision may occur if the AVM affects the macula or results in retinal hemorrhage.

Retinal vascular malformations range from very localized areas of arteriovenous communications to large, clustered, or racemose malformations involving the entire fundus. Three grades of anastomoses have been determined. Grade I is considered an anastomosis between an arteriole and a venule. Grade II is an anastomosis between a branch artery and a branch vein. Grades I and II present as dilatation and tortuosity in a sector of retina. Vision is usually good unless the lesion is in the posterior pole. Only a small percentage of these patients have associated systemic AVMs. Because these tend to be asymptomatic, the average presenting age for these patients is 42, at a routine eye examination. Grade III anastomoses show a diffuse, marked dilatation and tortuosity of the entire vascular system. This group has a high association with cerebral and facial arteriovenous anomalies. These patients exhibit vision loss or systemic symptoms. Therefore, the average age of presentation for grade III anastomoses is 25 years. If there are no symptoms associated with the intracranial malformation, the patient usually presents with vision loss due to a retinal AVM causing a steal phenomenon, resulting in retinal ischemia surrounding the AVM. The steal phenomenon results from low resistance in the direct communication between artery and vein. This causes higher blood flow through the AVM than the surrounding area. These vessels may become more tortuous and sclerotic over time due to the hemodynamic stress of this high-pressure vascular system.

AVMs of the CNS that impinge upon the visual pathway may lead to optic atrophy and visual field loss. Homonymous hemianopia or other visual field defects occur in one third of Wyburn–Mason syndrome patients.

Malformations in the optic nerve, optic chiasm, or optic tract can produce unilateral or bilateral decreased vision. Proptosis may occur due to an orbital AVM or from increased venous pressure from the cavernous sinus. Orbital AVMs may also produce bruits and dilitation of the conjunctival vessels. AVMs in the eyelid may produce ptosis. Table 48–2 includes other less common ocular manifestations of Wyburn–Mason syndrome.

DIAGNOSIS

■ Systemic

The diagnosis of Wyburn–Mason syndrome is based upon the presentation of signs and symptoms as well as imaging

TABLE 48–2. OCULAR MANIFESTATIONS OF WYBURN–MASON SYNDROME

- **Retinal AVMs may cause**
  Retinal ischemia
  Macular hemorrhage
  Central retinal vein occlusion
  Branch retinal vein occlusion
  Vitreous hemorrhage
  Neovascular glaucoma (rare)
- **Orbital or optic nerve AVMs may cause**
  Papilledema, subsequent optic atrophy
  Proptosis
  Cranial nerve 3,4, and 6 palsies
  Dilated conjunctival blood vessels
  Ptosis (if AVM present in lid)
  Parinaud syndrome
- **Increased intracranial pressure from intracranial AVMs may cause**
  Papilledema with subsequent optic atrophy
  Proptosis

studies. MRI is the diagnostic tool of choice to identify and follow the AVMs. Contrast-enhanced computed axial tomography is also used in the neuroradiographic evaluation of malformations. Investigation for bruits and carotid arteriogram provides important diagnostic information for the neurologically symptomatic patient. Cerebral angiography is reserved for patients with large retinal lesions or neurological symptoms. Electroencephalography is also useful, especially when a seizure disorder is present.

The presenting symptoms may be useful in determining the site of the AVM. Nasopharyngeal AVMs may produce epistaxis and oral hemorrhage, especially during or following dental surgery. AVMs in the ipsilateral basifrontal area and sylvian fissure may result in seizures, intracranial hemorrhages, hemiplegia, or hemianopia. Brainstem or cranial nerve damage may be evident with an AVM in the posterior fossa.

■ Ocular

Fundus evaluation will reveal an AVM in the posterior pole and superotemporal quadrant. Spontaneous venous pulsation is absent in the retinal vascular malformation. Grades I and II retinal AVMs are usually unilateral. They will appear as markedly dilated and tortuous retinal blood vessels. It is difficult to differentiate the arteries from the veins, especially by color. Because they are asymptomatic, the patients may be well into adulthood when first presenting for routine ophthalmoscopic evaluation. Patients with Grade III AVMs usually present at a younger age because of visual loss or related systemic or ocular symptoms. Grade III AVMs appear as a large mass of convoluted vessels. When a retinal AVM is found, a systemic workup is mandatory.

Unilateral or bilateral reduced visual acuity is a possible presenting symptom caused by malformations in the visual pathway. Increased intracranial pressure may present as papilledema or subsequent optic atrophy.

Proptosis may occur due to an orbital AVM or from increased venous pressure from the cavernous sinus. Exophthalmometry can quantify proptosis occurring secondary to an orbital AVM.

Von Hippel–Lindau disease, an autosomal dominant phakomatosis, is an important differential diagnosis. In von Hippel–Lindau disease, retinal lesions, with a distinct 2 to 3 disc diameter size, are usually located in the peripheral retina. These tumors can lead to subretinal exudate and retinal detachment. In Wyburn–Mason syndrome, there is a direct arteriovenous connection without any intervening angiomatous tumor formation. The retinal vascular abnormalities are usually stationary and seldom cause exudative retinal detachments.

Fluorescein angiography is a useful diagnostic technique in Wyburn–Mason syndrome. The characteristic appearance is a rapid transit of blood through the arteriovenous communication.

TREATMENT

■ Systemic

Arteriovenous malformations in Wyburn–Mason syndrome are usually situated deep in and around the mesencephalon. Therefore, surgical resection or embolization therapy is not suitable, and only the symptoms are treated through anticonvulsant medication if seizures are present (Table 48–3).

■ Ocular

Retinal vascular abnormalities are usually stationary and seldom cause the exudative retinal detachments seen with other phakomatoses. No treatment is indicated for these lesions, but photodocumentation is warranted because there is some evidence that the malformations may gradually

TABLE 48–3. TREATMENT AND MANAGEMENT OF WYBURN–MASON SYNDROME

- **Intracranial AVMs**
  Treat the symptoms (anticonvulsant medication)
  Surgery is not indicated
- **Retinal AVMs**
  Grades I and II
    Monitor yearly
    Photodocument
  Grade III
    Refer for systemic and neurological workup

enlarge over time while others may regress spontaneously. Yearly follow-up is indicated. The presence of grade III anastomoses mandates a systemic and neurologic workup. Appropriate treatment for any ocular sequelae is indicated. This may include vitrectomy, prism therapy for nerve palsies, photocoagulation, or glaucoma therapy.

CONCLUSION

Wyburn–Mason syndrome, classified as one of the phakomatoses, is characterized by unilateral vascular malformations of the retina and brain. This disease presents in a variable manner and it may be diagnosed in an asymptomatic patient presenting for routine eye care. The primary care practitioner should be aware of this disease and proper patient management. Careful follow-up and appropriate referral is indicated for these patients.

REFERENCES

Archer DB, Deutman A, Ernest JT, Krill AE. Arteriovenous communications of the retina. *Am J Ophthalmol.* 1973;75:224–241.

Lakhanpal V, Krishna Rao CVG, Schocket SS, Salcman M. Wyburn–Mason syndrome. *Ann Ophthalmol.* 1980;6:694–699.

Mansour AM, Walsh JB, Henkind P. Arteriovenous anastomoses of the retina. *Ophthalmology.* 1987;94:35–40.

Mansour AM, Wells CG, Jampol LM, et al. Ocular complications of arteriovenous communications of the retina. *Arch Ophthalmol.* 1989;107:232–236.

Miller NR. Phakomatoses. In: *Walsh and Hoyt's Clinical Neuroophthalmology.* Baltimore: Williams & Wilkins; 1988:1816–1820.

Wyburn–Mason R. Arteriovenous aneurysm of midbrain and retina, facial naevi and mental changes. *Brain.* 1943;66:163–203.

Zion VM. Phakomatoses. In: Tasman W, Jaeger EA, eds. *Duane's Clinical Ophthalmology.* Philadelphia: Lippincott; 1992;5:4–6.

SECTION IX

DERMATOLOGIC DISORDERS

49
Chapter

Atopic Dermatitis

Michael A. Chaglasian

Atopic dermatitis is a chronic, relapsing skin disease of unknown etiology. It is characterized by eczematous inflammation in patients with a family history of atopy. Atopy is a term that identifies persons who have an IgE-mediated hypersensitivity to environmental allergens, as in hay fever, asthma, eczema, or allergic rhinitis. In its most protracted course, the disease spans infancy, childhood, and adolescence, and may continue on into adulthood. It is also known as allergic eczema, infantile eczema, or allergic dermatitis. Ocular complications of atopic dermatitis were first noted in 1914 (Brunsting et al, 1955). Cataracts are very common and may appear at an early age. Other common ocular complications include keratoblepharoconjunctivitis, keratitis, and herpes simplex virus infection.

EPIDEMIOLOGY

■ Systemic

Surveys investigating the prevalence of atopic dermatitis vary as to the specific diagnostic criteria used. Most reports demonstrate that 2 to 5% of all children will exhibit some form of atopic dermatitis. In groups with a family history of atopy or asthma, the percentage may increase to 33%. The male-to-female ratio is about equal. Ninety percent of atopic dermatitis cases develop prior to age 5, most often within the first year of life. Atopic dermatitis rarely appears in adulthood (Leung et al, 1986).

■ Ocular

Ocular complications are present in approximately 42% of patients (Garrity & Liesegang, 1984), with atopic keratoconjunctivits the most common. Age and race characteristics of these patients are unknown. A slight male predominance may exist. Uehara (1981) studied 300 patients with atopic dermatitis and detected a prominant infraorbital fold of the lower eyelid in 25% of them, while finding it in only about 2% of the normal population. Anterior and posterior subcapsular cataracts are found in 13 to 25% of atopic der-

matitis patients. The frequency of keratoconus in patients with atopic dermatitis is most likely between 0.5% and 1.5%. (Brunsting et al, 1955; Garrity & Liesegang, 1984).

NATURAL HISTORY

■ Systemic

The systemic complications of atopic dermatitis will generally begin in early childhood, and will primarily be limited to the skin. The hallmark symptom is an intense pruritis (itching) that may be generalized or local and is intermittent throughout the day. Pruritis may be aggravated by several factors, including exposure to soaps, wool, acrylic, lotions, low humidity, heat, and sweat.

The cutaneous manifestations of atopic dermatitis are continually changing in severity and appearance. Various morphologic skin lesions will present through periods of exacerbation and remission. Included among these cutaneous lesions are xerosis, dermatitis, lichenification (a thickening and accentuation of skin markings), and ichthyosis (abnormal keratinization of the skin). Often an aggravating factor can be identified. Identification and removal of these factors may be the best therapy for the patient. Constant rubbing and scratching may cause or aggravate some of these cutaneous findings.

Common areas that show patchy dermatitis in the infant include the cheeks (Figure 49–1), forearms, legs, and diaper area. The dermatitis is a scaly, rough, reddish area of skin. In days or weeks, further crusting and weeping of the area is frequent. As the child learns to crawl and walk, the affected areas shift to elbows, knees, wrists, and ankles. Lichenification replaces the erythematous dermatitis. The itching remains severe at this stage.

In later childhood, the disease may improve, or continued manifestations may appear, including xerosis, lichenification, follicular eczema, fissuring and scaling of hands or feet, and skin hyper- or hypopigmentation. Some of these changes are aggravated by chronic scratching. Patients with atopic dermatitis have a tendency to develop generalized infections. The lengthy presence of weeping skin lesions is subject to secondary staphylococcal superinfection and thus requires careful monitoring. Cutaneous, nonocular viral infections from herpes simplex and vaccina are also common.

At around 2 years of age, half of the children with atopic dermatitis will demonstrate clear skin, while the other 50% will have continued recurrences up through ages 5 to 9. Those patients who have extended recurrences through adolescence are likely to have them continue into adulthood. The adult form of atopic dermatitis is usually more localized than the infantile or childhood forms. Areas of persistant eczematous irritation include the hands, face, neck, genitalia, and legs (Table 49–1).

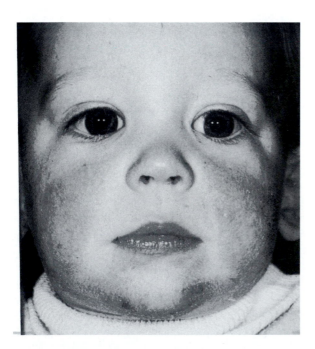

Figure 49–1. Atopic dermatitis of the cheeks. *(Reprinted with permission from Habif TP.* Clinical Dermatology: A Color Guide to Diagnosis and Therapy. *2nd ed. 1990;77.)*

TABLE 49–1. SYSTEMIC MANIFESTATIONS OF ATOPIC DERMATITIS

- Pruritis
- Eczematous inflammation of hands, face, and neck
- Lichenification
- Xerosis
- Ichthyosis
- Fissuring and scaling of hands and feet
- Hypo- or hyperpigmentation of skin
- Staphlyococcal superinfections
- Herpes simplex
- Herpes zoster

BODY AREA INVOLVED
- Infants: Cheeks, forearms, legs, diaper area
- Mobile infant: Elbows, knees, wrists, ankles
- Ault: Hands, face, neck, genitalia, legs

■ Ocular

The ocular manifestations of atopic dermatitis are numerous (Table 49–2). Although an association of the disease with cataracts was first made in 1914, it was not until 1952 that Hogan described an "atopic keratoconjunctivitis" as a clinical entity. Other significant ocular manifestations include keratoconus, herpes simplex, anterior uveitis, and retinal detachment.

Ocular disease in patients with atopic dermatitis usually begins in the late teens and may persist for 20 years or more. Patients have a predictable history of dermatitis in

TABLE 49–2. OCULAR MANIFESTATIONS OF ATOPIC DERMATITIS

- Prominent infraorbital fold of lower eyelid (Dennie–Morgan fold)
- Pruritis of the lids and periorbital skin
- Foreign body sensation
- Decreased VA secondary to cataract formation
- Blepharitis
- Thickening of lid margins
- Superficial punctate keratitis
- Keratoconjunctivitis
- Symblepharon
- Keratoconus
- Herpes simplex
- Cataracts

LESS FREQUENTLY REPORTED
- Uveitis
- Ocular hypertension
- Branch retinal vein occlusion
- Central serous choroidopathy
- Retinal detachment

early childhood, followed by occasional recurrences in adolescence. It has been noted that many of these patients will have a prominent fold of the lower eyelid, known as a Dennie–Morgan fold. The exact significance of this fold is uncertain, but is likely to indicate past or present inflammation and marked edema of the eyelid (Leung et al, 1986).

Atopic keratoconjunctivitis (Figure 49–2) is seen some time after localized cutaneous activity. It is bilateral and is characterized by pruritis, burning, and a slight mucus discharge. The eyelid will be mild to moderately erythematous and edematous. Blepharitis is a predominant finding (Tuft et al, 1991). Chronic eyelid inflammation and rubbing may leatopic dermatitis to excoriation (loss of skin), lichenification, and lid eversion with secondary epiphora. The bulbar conjunctiva will be hyperemic and edematous during the acute phase. Further changes may include shrinkage of the fornix, symblepharon formation, Trantas dots, and inclusion cysts at the limbus (Hogan, 1953).

Hogan (1953) noted that early corneal signs begin with a superficial punctate keratitis at the superior limbal area. Over several years, areas of pannus may develop (Figure 49–3). A haziness to the anterior stroma is subsequently noted. If the ocular disease persists, marginal ulceration and vascularization can progress and lead to severe vision loss.

The association between keratoconus and atopic disease has been noted and is well established. Keratoconus in atopic dermatitis patients follows the typical course of corneal thinning and ectasia with irregular astigmatism.

A high susceptibility to herpes simplex viral infection has been noted in several studies (Brunsting et al, 1955; Easty et al, 1975; Garrity & Liesegang, 1984). This corneal infection may be more difficult to manage in patients with atopic dermatitis.

The frequently-occurring anterior subcapsular cataracts are often described as white, polygonal, shield-like opacifi-

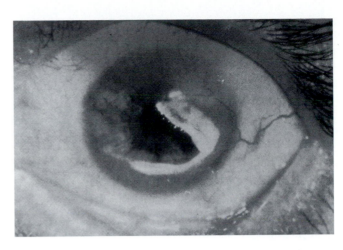

Figure 49–3. Peripheral corneal neovascularization and active pannus in a patient with recurrent atopic keratoconjunctivitis. (*Reprinted with permission from Foster CS, Calonge M. Atopic keratoconjunctivitis.* Ophthalmology. *1990;97:992–1000.*)

cations. Lens opacities usually first appear at age 20 and may either progress slowly or mature rapidly (Smolin & O'Conner, 1986). Because many atopic dermatitis patients may be treated with steroids, this etiology should be ruled out. Lens changes are most likely related to the severity of the disease.

Other ocular manifestations have been less frequently reported. These include retinal detachment, uveitis, ocular hypertension, branch retinal vein occlusion, and central serous chorioretinopathy. Retinal dialysis appears to be a common cause of retinal detachment in patients with atopic dermatitis (Katsura & Hida, 1984). The etiology of the dialysis is unknown.

DIAGNOSIS

■ Systemic

The multiple, varied, and ever-changing manifestations of atopic dermatitis have led to confusion in its diagnosis. The diagnosis is primarily clinical and should be made based on criteria suggested by Hannifin and Lobitz (Table 49–3). Thorough patient questioning usually reveals some prior family history of hay fever, asthma, allergic rhinitis, atopic dermatitis, or other atopic disease. A positive personal or family history of atopy and proper cutaneous features are principal criteria for diagnosis. Patch testing, although infrequently done, may be considered to rule out contact dermatitis.

Laboratory findings may be significant for increased serum IgE levels (6000 ng/mL versus 780 ng/mL in normal patients). Although many patients with the disease will have elevated serum IgE levels, some studies show 50% of atopic dermatitis patients have normal levels. Thus, this feature should be considered nonspecific. IgE values are also not related to the degree of ocular manifestations.

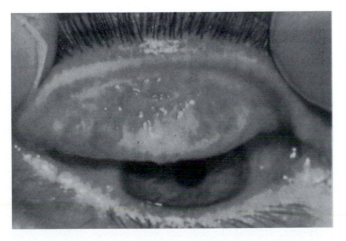

Figure 49–2. Prominant giant papillae with marked subepithelial sheets of fibrosis in a 42-year-old man with atopic keratoconjunctivitis. (*Reprinted with permission from Tuft et al, Clinical features of atopic keratoconjunctivitis.* Ophthalmology. *1991;98:150–158)*

TABLE 49–3. DIAGNOSTIC CRITERIA FOR ATOPIC DERMATITIS

Absolute Features

Pruritis

Typical morphology and distribution
  Flexural lichenification in atopic dermatitisults
  Facial and extensor involvement in infancy

Tendency towards relapses or chronicity

Plus Two or More of the Following

Personal/family history of atopy

Immediate skin test reactivity

White dermographism (skin swelling from scratching)

Anterior subcapsular cataracts

Or Plus Four or More of the Following

Xerosis/ichthyosis/hyperlinear palms (prominent palm creases)

Keratosis pilaris (keratotic papules of the hair follicles usually involving the extensor surfaces of the arms and thighs)

Facial pallor/infraorbital darkening

Dennie–Morgan infraorbital lid fold

Elevated serum IgE level

Keratoconus

Tendency towards nonspecific hand dermatitis

Tendency towards repeated cutaneous infections

Atopic dermatitisapted with permission from Hannifin and Lobitz, Newer concepts of atopic dermatitis. Arch Dermatol. 1977;113:663–670.

■ Ocular

Ocular diagnosis is made in patients with a history of atopic dermatitis and any of the ocular complications previously mentioned, most commonly atopic keratoconjunctivitis. Atopic keratoconjunctivitis can be more definitively diagnosed through conjunctival histopathologic studies that have demonstrated specific changes (Foster et al, 1991). Some of these changes include epithelial invasion by mast cells and eosinophils, goblet cell proliferation, and chronic mononuclear cell infiltration of the substantia propria (Hogan, 1952). Abnormal numbers of T cells, T-helper/inducer cells, macrophages, and Langerhans cells were found by Foster and associates (1991). These findings indicate that many cell types are involved in atopic keratoconjunctivitis and point out that successful long-term therapy cannot be solely aimed at mast cell stabilization. This is the rationale for systemic therapy in this topical disease.

TREATMENT AND MANAGEMENT

■ Systemic

Treatment is directed towards any acute manifestations as well as the removal of all potentially inciting agents or antigens (Table 49–4). Most important is educating the patient

TABLE 49–4. TREATMENT AND MANAGEMENT OF ATOPIC DERMATITIS

- ■ **SYSTEMIC**
  - Avoidance of scratching
  - Removal of inciting agent (soaps, clothing)
  - "Tap-water" bath with bath oils for damaged skin
  - Cold compresses
  - Topical steroids (eg, hydrocortisone acetate cream 0.5–1%; triamcinolone acetonide cream 0.025–0.5%)
  - Topical antipruritics
  - Bland emmolient creams and lotions
  - Oral antihistamines
  - Systemic steroids (rarely): prednisolone 5 mg qd; for short courses only
  - Systemic antibiotics (erythromycin) for staphylococcal control

- ■ **OCULAR**
  - Cold compresses
  - Artificial tear preparations
  - Decongestants
    Naphazoline 0.1% qid
    Phenylephrine 0.12% qid
  - Decongestant/antihistamine combinations
    Naphazoline/Pheneramine (Vasoclear A, Naphcon A, Albalon A)
  - Cromolyn sodium 4% (Optichrom)
  - Topical steroids
    FML 0.1% qid
    Pred Mild 0.125%
    Inflammase Mild 0.125%
  - Oral Antihistamines
    Seldane 60–120 mg bid
    Hismanal 10 mg qd

to avoid itching and scratching, because this will significantly hinder all treatment strategies. Damaged skin is treated aggressively, with an attempt to restore its normal condition and to control the pruritis. Treatment measures primarily include "tap-water" baths with water-trapping agents such as mineral oil and petrolatum USP. Creams and lotions should be avoided because they often contain fragrances, solubilizers, and preservatives. Cold compresses are used to relieve itching. Secondary bacterial superinfections are best treated with systemic antibiotics. Systemic antihistamines and oral cromolyn sodium have been used with mixed results in helping control and reduce acute flare-ups. Topical steroids are very helpful in controlling the dermatitis and pruritis found in the follicular eczema and lichenification stages. The best agents are low to mid potency, in a cream or ointment base. Systemic steroids are reserved for refractory cases.

■ Ocular

Ocular management (see Table 49–4) is also directed toward acute symptomatic relief. For keratoconjunctivitis, cold compresses and topical decongestants or decongestant/antihistamines will relieve most patients. For more symptomatic presentations, topical steroids will provide a more rapid resolution. Between the acute phases, artificial tear preparations are useful for corneal protection. Topical 4% cromolyn sodium has been used with some success for the relief of itching, inflammation, and lichenification. Its use can reduce the need for topical steroids.

Patients who develop chronic keratoconjunctivitis may require systemic therapy in addition to their topical medications. Foster and Calonge (1990) recommend maximizing systemic antihistamine therapy.

Due to increased corneal epithelial breakdown in keratoconic patients with atopic dermatitis, rigid gas-permeable contact lenses must be fit cautiously and patients followed closely, as corneal irritation is common in these patients. Frequent topical lubrication can improve patient success.

Cataract surgery is indicated for those patients with decreased acuity. Significant ocular complications are associated with cataract surgery in patients with atopic disease; thus there is a higher risk for poor visual outcome (< 20/100).

CONCLUSION

Atopic dermatitis is a relatively common, potentially chronic, superficial inflammation of the skin. Characterized by intense itching, it is commonly found in patients with a personal or family history of atopy. The skin is dry and pruritic; patchy lesions are distinguished by edema, erythema, excoriation, scaling, and resulting hyperpigmentation. There are numerous ocular complications, most commonly keratoconjunctivitis and subcapsular cataracts. Decreased vision is most commonly a result of anterior or posterior subcapsular cataracts, although corneal disease (marginal inflammation and vascularization, stromal haziness, and HSV keratitis) can cause permanent visual loss. Although various topical treatment modalities offer patients some symptomatic relief, it is difficult to avoid permanent cutaneous or ocular damage in the chronic forms of the disease.

REFERENCES

Brunsting LA, Red WB, Bair HL. Occurrence of cataracts and keratoconus with atopic dermatitis. *Arch Dermatol.* 1955; 72:237–241.

Easty D, Enstwistle C, Funk A, Witcher J. Herpes simplex keratitis and keratoconus in the atopic patient: A clinical and immunologic study. *Trans Ophthalmol Soc UK.* 1975;95:267–276.

Foster CS, Calonge M. Atopic keratoconjunctivitis. *Ophthalmology.* 1990;97:992–1000.

Foster CS, Rice BA, Dutt JE. Immunopathology of atopic keratoconjunctivitis. *Ophthalmology.* 1991;98:1190–1196.

Garrity JA, Liesegang TL. Ocular complications of atopic dermatitis. *Can J Ophthalmol.* 1984;19:21–24.

Hannifin JM, Lobitz WC Jr. Newer concepts of atopic dermatitis. *Arch Dermatol.* 1977;113:663–670.

Hogan MJ. Atopic keratoconjunctivitis. *Am J Ophthalmol.* 1953;36:937–947.

Hogan MJ. Atopic keratoconjunctivitis. *Trans Am Ophthalmol Soc.* 1952;50:265–281.

Katsura H, Hida T. Retinal detachment associated with atopic dermatitis. *Retina.* 1984;4:148–151.

Leung DYM, Rhodes AR, Geha RS. Atopic dermatitis. In: Fitzpatrick TB, Eisen AZ, Wolf K, et al, eds, *Dermatology in General Medicine.* 3rd ed. New York: McGraw-Hill; 1986: 1385–1411.

Smolin G, O'Connor GR. *Ocular Immunology.* Boston: Little, Brown; 1986:171–179.

Tuft SJ, Kemeny DM, Dart JKG, Buckley RJ. Clinical features of atopic keratoconjunctivitis. *Ophthalmology.* 1991;98:150–158.

Uehara M. Infraorbital fold in atopic dermatitis. *Arch Dermatol.* 1981;117:627.

50
Chapter

Rosacea

Michael A. Chaglasian

Rosacea dermatitis is a classic disorder affecting the cheeks, nose, forehead, chin, and eyes. Its characteristic rhinophyma (gross hypertrophy of the sebaceous glands of the nose) is a well-established hallmark, along with persistent erythema, telangiectasias, papules, and pustules. It is a syndrome of unknown etiology, although numerous associations and theories have been proposed.

The term "rosacea" is preferred over "acne rosacea" as the facial lesions are not similar to those found in acne vulgaris or cystic acne.

Ocular rosacea refers to patients with definitive ophthalmic manifestations. Ocular involvement in rosacea is common and typically includes blepharitis, meibomianitis, chalazia, and a mild to severe keratitis. Left untreated, permanent visual loss is possible. Unfortunately, both the ocular and cutaneous conditions are widely underdiagnosed by eyecare practitioners. Treatment with oral tetracycline is very effective for both disorders.

EPIDEMIOLOGY

Rosacea affects adults 30 to 60 years of age. Women are twice as likely as men to have rosacea without ocular signs. However, ocular rosacea is equally divided between the sexes. Patients with ocular rosacea tend to be slightly older than those patients with facial manifestations alone.

The specific distribution of rosacea among different races has not been well researched. The clinical impression is that it primarily affects fair-skinned Celtics and Northern Europeans. It was believed at one time that African-Americans were not affected, but it is now recognized that they also suffer from rosacea (Browning & Rosenwasser, 1986; Rosen & Stone, 1987).

Ocular involvement is present in upwards of 58% of patients. One third of all patients develop both ocular and facial manifestations simultaneously. Fifty percent develop skin lesions initially, while the remaining 20% will develop only ocular complications first (Borrie, 1953).

NATURAL HISTORY

■ Systemic

The cutaneous lesions of rosacea (Figure 50–1) have been well recognized for many centuries. Common patient complaints include facial flushing and warmth and painful pustules (small, circumscribed fluid-containing elevations that are usually purulent) around the central one third of the face. Patients may first notice an erythematous blush over the cheeks and nose. The onset is slow and insidious and initially the lesions may be intermittent, though slow to resolve. Acneform papules (small, solid raised skin lesions) 2 to 3 mm in size begin to appear in the same area. Telangiectatic vessels also cover the cheeks, nose, and forehead. Rhinophyma can progress to prominent vascularity, swelling, and disfigurement. It usually occurs after other cutaneous lesions have been present for some time, and may be more pronounced in males (Table 50–1).

The course of rosacea is prolonged with frequent recurrences. Transient skin papules and pustules resolve without

356

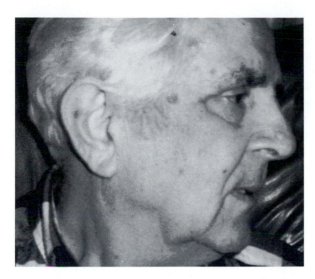

Figure 50–1. Cutaneous manifestations of rosacea. *(Courtesy of Diane T. Adamczyk, OD.)*

scarring. After a few years the disease may spontaneously disappear (Fitzpatrick et al, 1992).

Numerous pathophysiologic mechanisms have been suggested for rosacea. To date, none have been definitively established. Bacterial infection, specifically *Staphylococcus aureus*, has been linked to 60% of patients with rosacea; however cultures of many patients are sterile. Climatic exposure to sun, wind, heat, or cold might exacerbate lesions, but evidence is not absolutely convincing.

Extensive research has studied the hypertrophic sebaceous glands of patients with rosacea to determine an origin for the disease. No clear consensus has evolved as of yet; fatty acids in meibomian gland secretions are being studied as a possible route of irritation and tear disruption to the ocular surface (Browning & Proia, 1986).

The role of the follicle mite, *Demodex folliculorum*, in rosacea has also been investigated for many years. Initially, the mites were believed to be quite common in rosacea patients, but current literature purports that the mites have a relatively insignificant role, if any, in the pathogenesis of rosacea.

■ Ocular

The ocular manifestations in rosacea are numerous and nonspecific (Table 50–2). Except for a rare iritis, they all appear on the ocular surface or eyelids.

Commonly seen signs include blepharitis, meibomianitis, hordeola, chalazia, conjunctival hyperemia, punctate keratitis, epithelial erosions, and corneal vascularization leading to thinning or perforation.

Patients will typically present with complaints of foreign body sensation, pain, or burning. The symptoms may be constant or intermittent, but are generally bilateral. They may be more marked than clinical findings would suggest. Other initial complaints include red eyes, decreased vision, chalazia, and epiphora (Jenkins et al, 1979).

Blepharitis and meibomianitis are virtually universal findings in ocular rosacea patients. Inspissation of meibomian gland secretions will be noted during clinical examination.

Hordeola and chalazia are highly prevalent within the rosacea population. Lempert and colleagues (1979) found 64% of patients scheduled for chalazia excision to have clinically significant rosacea.

The tear film in rosacea patients has also been an area of study. Clinical examination reveals a significant disturbance to the ocular surface's protective layer. There is an excessive accumulation of debris, decreased tear breakup time, and an oily–foamy consistency to the tears similar to that seen with seborrheic blepharitis (McCulley & Sciallis, 1977).

TABLE 50–1. SYSTEMIC MANIFESTATIONS OF ROSACEA

- Erythema
- Flushing warmth
- Pustules
- Acneform papules
- Telangiectatic blood vessels
- Sebaceous gland hypertrophy
- Rhinophyma

TABLE 50–2. OCULAR MANIFESTATIONS OF ROSACEA

SYMPTOMS
- Foreign body sensation
- Pain, irritation
- Burning
- Photophobia
- Redness
- Epiphora
- Decreased vision

SIGNS
- Blepharitis
- Meibomianitis
- Disrupted tear film
- Hordeola
- Chalazia
- Conjunctival hyperemia
- Punctate keratitis
- Epithelial erosions
- Corneal vascularization
- Corneal thinning, ulceration, and perforation
- Iritis

Controversy still exists as to whether or not there is an alteration in the tear film pH. Abelson and co-workers (1980) found an alkaline shift; Jaros and Coles (1983) found an acidic shift, while Browning (1985) did not find any diagnostically useful difference between rosacea patients and normal controls. Different methods of determining the tear film pH may possibly explain these conflicting results.

Many patients with ocular rosacea may also have a coexisting keratoconjunctivitis sicca. Lemp and associates (1984) found almost 40% of rosacea patients with ocular manifestations to have a decreased Schirmer test. They concluded that this significantly contributed to patient symptomatology.

Corneal complications in ocular rosacea begin with a superficial punctate keratitis along the inferior two thirds of the cornea. The keratitis progresses with a dramatic peripheral vascularization, and subepithelial infiltrates central to the vessels may subsequently develop. Gross ulceration or infiltrate resolution causes further thinning of the cornea, which may ultimately lead to frank perforation of the cornea (Brown & Shahinan, 1978). Corneal erosions may develop at any time during active corneal disease. Other less common ocular findings include entropion, episcleritis, and iritis.

There are very few histologic or immunopathologic studies of ocular rosacea that help identify a pathophysiologic mechanism. Hoang-Xaun and associates (1990) studied the conjunctiva in patients with ocular rosacea. They found an overall increase of inflammatory cells, especially T-helper/inducer cells, macrophages, and antigen-presenting cells. This finding suggests a type IV hypersensitivity reaction that accounts for conjunctival inflammation. An unidentified antigen may be reaching the globe through the meibomian gland secretions via the tear film. Ocular manifestations therefore may be an exaggerated inflammatory response to this antigen and other toxic products.

Diagnosis

No strict criteria have been established for the diagnosis of rosacea or ocular rosacea. Diagnosis is based on a clinical impression following identification of characteristic cutaneous lesions.

For rosacea, this would include erythema, telangiectasia, papules, pustules, and rhinophyma. The ocular findings in rosacea are too nonspecific to make a definitive diagnosis; thus the facial features must be identified to confirm the diagnosis.

This presents a problem for the 20% of patients who develop ocular prior to facial manifestations. These patients often go undiagnosed, as specific testing for ocular rosacea

has not been formulated. As previously discussed, tear pH results remain controversial. Browning and Proia (1986) have suggested a point scale system for each clinical sign or symptom associated with ocular rosacea. Patients can be categorized as tentative, probable, or certain, depending on their total points.

Generally, if clinical suspicion is high, then initiation of proper therapy is warranted, as the side effects are minimal. It is helpful to remember that symptoms are often greater than the clinical appearance would suggest.

The differential diagnosis for rosacea includes seborrheic dermatitis, lupus erythematosus, cutaneous tuberous sclerosis (adenoma sebaceum), and acne vulgaris (teenage acne). Rosacea is differentiated from acne vulgaris by the lack of comedones (whiteheads), older age of the patient, and confinement of lesions to the face. In addition, the pustules of rosacea will resolve without scarring (Lempert et al, 1979).

Treatment and Management

■ Systemic

The treatment of choice for cutaneous lesions in rosacea is oral antibiotics. Tetracycline 250 mg/qid for 4 to 6 weeks, and then tapered to a level that controls active flareups, is the most widely prescribed medication. Within 3 to 6 weeks a dramatic improvement is noted in about 80% of patients. Some patients may be able to discontinue the drug, while others require a low maintenance dosage. Other prescribed antibiotics include ampicillin, erythromycin, and metronidazole. Tetracycline therapy does not improve the cutaneous erythema.

The long-acting tetracycline semisynthetic derivitives, doxycycline (Vibramycin) and minocycline (Minocin), have also proven effectiveness in the therapy of rosacea. They have the benefit of reduced administration and improved absorption with ingestion of dairy products. However, they are more costly for the patient. The contraindications and side effects of tetracycline therapy and its derivitives should be recognized by the practitioner.

An explanation for the therapeutic efficacy of tetracycline has been extensively researched. Current theories suggest a combination of bacterial eradication and decreased free fatty acid concentration in sebaceous gland secretions.

Metronidazole has been utilized both as an oral and more recently as a topical agent in the therapy of rosacea. It is a synthetic derivative of nitroimidazole and has antibacterial, antiprotozoal, antithelminthic, and even some inhibitory influences on the immune system (antiinflammatory). Oral dosages of 200 mg bid were found to be superior to placebo in the treatment of rosacea. In general this medication is reserved for those patients who do not respond to the tetracyclines. It may be more effective on the papules and pustules in patients with advanced cutaneous disease (Nielsen, 1988). Greater use of oral metronidazole is limited by concerns over toxicity with long-term use.

Topical metronidazole gel (Metro Gel 0.75%) has become a very popular medication in rosacea management. Its usefulness has been well documented in several clinical trials (Aronson et al, 1987; Lowe et al, 1989; Nielsen, 1988). This safe and effective drug has no serious side effects or allergic reactions. It is not to be used on or near the eyes. Applied twice daily, its greatest actions are against the papules, pustules, and erythema of rosacea. It is not helpful for the telangiectasia. Facial lesions will reappear upon discontinuation of the drug. Its mechanism of action is thought to be immunologic and antiinflammatory rather than antimicrobial (Schmadel & McEvoy, 1990).

Dietary restriction of alcohol, spicy foods, and hot beverages may help to improve skin lesions. These items are vasodilative and clinical experience has shown that eliminating them can help improve cosmetic appearance. Stress reduction has also been advocated. Topical antibiotics or benzoyl peroxide are not beneficial to the rosacea patient.

For severe rhinophyma, more aggressive surgical treatment may be warranted. Dermabrasion, surgical reduction, and carbon dioxide laser therapy for hypertrophic sebaceous glands have been implemented for rosacea patients with persistent lesions (Table 50–3). The CO_2 laser carbonizes superficial tissue, allowing it to be shaved off with a scalpel.

■ Ocular

Therapy for ocular manifestations of rosacea is not significantly different than treatment for its facial manifestations. Tetracycline at similar dosages (250 mg qid 4 to 6 weeks) has demonstrated its effectiveness throughout the literature.

TABLE 50–3. TREATMENT AND MANAGEMENT OF ROSACEA

- ■ **SYSTEMIC**
  - Tetracycline 250 mg/qid × 4–6 weeks, OR doxycyline 100 mg/qid × 4–6 weeks, OR topical metrodiazole gel 0.75% (for tetracycline nonresponders) bid
  - Dietary restriction of alcohol and spicy foods
  - For severe cases: Dermabrasion, CO_2 laser therapy

- ■ **OCULAR**
  - The above plus
    Eyelid hygiene
    Artificial tears
    Topical antibiotics
    Low-dose topical steroids
    Keratoplasty (in cases of severe corneal compromise)

Recently, Frucht-Perry and associates (1989) investigated the use of doxycycline in ocular rosacea. Fourteen of their 16 patients did very well with a dosage of 100 mg/qd × 4 to 6 weeks. One patient was switched to tetracycline because of ineffectiveness and one patient failed to improve with either medication.

Concomitant lid hygiene therapy is recommended for all patients with ocular rosacea. Conventional combinations of dilute shampoo lid scrubs, warm compresses, and lid massage can help eliminate blepharitis, return meibomian gland secretions to normal, and decrease the incidence of hordeola and chalazia. Topical metronidazole gel is not indicated for skin lesions near to the eyes as it may cause burning, tearing, or ocular irritation. It is very useful for treating the facial manifestations of rosacea.

Patients with corneal involvement require careful monitoring, due to the heightened risk for corneal ulceration and secondary infection. Systemic tetracycline is the primary therapeutic measure to thwart corneal complications. Patients should demonstrate improvement within 2 to 6 weeks of initiating therapy.

Topical antibiotics may be added prophylactically for patients with keratitis. Artificial tear preparations will provide symptomatic relief for patients as well as supplementing a deficient tear film in patients with coexisting dry eye. Topical steroids can be used for a short period of time (1 to 2 weeks) for iritis, peripheral keratitis, and episcleritis until the tetracycline takes affect. Low-dose steroids must be used, as high concentrations may result in corneal melting.

Patients who develop corneal ulcerations and perforations may require surgical management, either keratoplasty or conjunctival flaps.

CONCLUSION

Rosacea is a chronic dermatologic disease of unknown etiology. It is characterized by recurrent episodes of inflammatory papules, facial erythema, and telangiectasias. Potentially devastating visual complications may arise from the common ocular manifestations of this disease.

Oral antibiotics are the mainstay of treatment and work quite well for both the facial and ocular components of rosacea. Newer topical medications have also proven beneficial. Patients with significant cutaneous involvement warrant a dermatologic referral for more intensive therapy including surgical treatment options.

Eyecare practitioners should be aware that rosacea is underdiagnosed, because subtle facial features in patients who present with ocular signs and symptoms are often overlooked. Therefore, older patients who present with blepharitis, meibomianitis, and chalazia (especially if chronic or recurrent) should be carefully evaluated for rosacea.

REFERENCES

Abelson MB, Sadun AA, Udell IJ, Weston JH. Alkaline tear pH in ocular rosacea. *Am J Ophthalmol.* 1980;90:866–869.

Aronson IK, Rumsfield JA, West DP, et al. Evaluation of topical metronidazole gel in acne rosacea. *Drug Intell Clin Pharm.* 1987;21:346–351.

Borrie P. Rosacea with special reference to its ocular manifestations. *Br J Dermatol.* 1953;55:458–463.

Brown SI, Shahinian L Jr. Diagnosis and treatment of ocular rosacea. *Ophthalmology.* 1978;85:779–786.

Browning DJ. Tear studies in ocular rosacea. *Am J Ophthalmol.* 1985;99:530–533.

Browning DJ, Proia AD. Ocular rosacea. *Surv Ophthalmol.* 1986;31:145–158.

Browning DJ, Rosenwasser G, Lugo M. Ocular rosacea in blacks. *Am J Ophthalmol.* 1986;101:441–444.

Fitzpatrick TB, Johnson RA, Polano MK, et al. *Color Atlas and Synopsis of Clinical Dermatology.* 2nd ed. New York: McGraw-Hill; 1992:10–11.

Frucht-Perry J, Chayet AS, Feldman ST, et al. The effect of doxycycline on ocular rosacea. *Am J Ophthalmol.* 1989; 107:434–435.

Hoang-Xuan T, Rodrigyez A, Zalitas MM, et al. Ocular rosacea. *Ophthalmology.* 1990;97:1468–1475.

Jaros PA, Coles WH. Ocular surface pH in rosacea. *CLAO J* 1983;9:333.

Jenkins MS, Bown SI, Lempert SL, Weinberg RJ. Ocular rosacea. *Am J Ophthalmol.* 1979;88:618–622.

Lemp MA, Mahmood MM, Weiler HH. Association of rosacea and keratoconjunctivitis sicca. *Arch Ophthalmol.* 1984;102:556–557.

Lempert SL, Jenkins MS, Brown SI. Chalazia and rosacea. *Arch Ophthalmol.* 1979;97:1652–1653.

Loss RJ Jr. Common dermatoses. In: Noble J, ed. *Textbook of General Medicine and Primary Care.* Boston: Little, Brown; 1987:638.

Lowe NJ, Henderson T, Millikan LE, et al. Topical metronidazole for severe and recalcitrant rosacea: A prospective open trial. *Cutis.* 1989;43:283–286.

McCulley JP, Sciallis GF. Meibomian keratoconjunctivitis. *Am J Ophthalmol.* 1977;84:788–793.

Nielsen PG. Metronidazole treatment in rosacea. *Int J Dermatol.* 1988;27:1–5.

Nielsen PG. Treatment of rosacea with 1% metronidazole cream. A double blind study. *Br J Dermatol.* 1983;108:327–332.

Rosen T, Stone MS. Acne rosacea in blacks. *J Am Acad Dermatol.* 1987;17:70-73.

Salaman SSM. Tetracyclines in ophthalmology. *Surv Ophthalmol.* 1985;29:265–275.

Schmadel LK, McEvoy GK. Topical metronidazole: A new therapy for rosacea. *Clin Pharm.* 1990;9:94–101.

51
Chapter

Erythema Nodosum

Michael A. Chaglasian

Erythema nodosum is a cutaneous inflammation that presents as multiple nodular, erythematous lesions over the extensor surfaces of the lower extremities. The lesions are small, raised, tender nodules that are symmetrically distributed over the affected area. The condition will almost always be found in association with an underlying systemic disease; however, in 20 to 30% of patients, no instigating cause can be identified. Erythema nodosum has no specific, direct ocular complications. They are only found when the provoking systemic affliction has secondary ocular manifestations. In general, intraocular inflammation will be the most common ocular complication seen in connection with erythema nodosum.

EPIDEMIOLOLGY

Erythema nodosum is most prevalent in young adults (aged 20 to 40 years), although it can occur at any age. It is three times more common in females than in males. Both age and sex distribution will vary, depending on the particular underlying systemic affliction.

NATURAL HISTORY

■ Systemic

The cutaneous lesions of erythema nodosum rapidly appear over 1 to 2 days as tender red nodules on the anterior surfaces of the legs (Figure 51–1). The lesions may less frequently be observed on the forearms, face, and neck. Specifically, erythema nodosum is a septal panniculitis (an inflammation of the subcutaneous fat), without vasculitis. There may also be areas of raised erythematous plaques. There is no ulceration, crusting, or discharge associated with the nodules. Maximum size of the nodules is 0.5 to 2.0 cm, progressing in size within the first week. Preceding or

accompanying symptoms of erythema nodosum include fever, malaise, and arthralgia. The nodules remain for 1 to 3 weeks, undergoing a color change from red to dark purple. Complete cutaneous resolution, like a bruise fading, occurs in 3 to 6 weeks, leaving no scarring or pigmentary changes. Many patients may have a persistent mild arthritis long after dermatologic resolution (Bondi & Lazarus, 1986).

The specific etiology of erythema nodosum is unknown. Its pathogenesis is presumed to be an immunologic reaction to one or more circulating antigens (Bondi & Lazarus, 1986). Many systemic diseases have an etiologic association with erythema nodosum (Table 51–1). Pharmacologic agents, including sulfonamides and oral contraceptives, have been reported to cause erythema nodosum (Figure 51–2). Several infectious agents, principally streptococcus, also have an etiologic association with erythema nodosum. Upper respiratory infections with β-hemolytic streptococci may have erythematous nodules appearing within 3 weeks of infection (MacPherson, 1970).

Although cases of idiopathic erythema nodosum have been reported, any patient presenting with this inflammation must be appropriately evaluated. The most probable etiology will vary with geographical area and prevalent endemic diseases. It is useful to remember that in children with

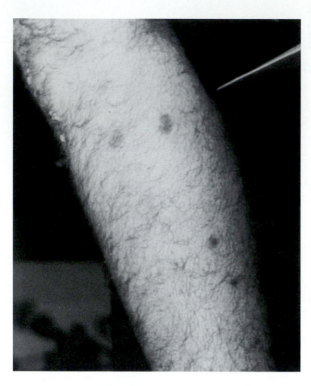

Figure 51–1. Biopsy proven erythema nodosum, unknown etiology. *(Courtesy of Scott I.M. Lim, DO.)*

TABLE 51–1. ETIOLOGIC ASSOCIATIONS WITH ERYTHEMA NODOSUM

Systemic diseases
    Sarcoidosis
    Behçet disease
    Inflammatory bowel disease
        Ulcerative colitis
        Crohn disease
Infectious diseases
    Streptococcal
    Yersina
    Tuberculosis
    Leprosy
    Psittacosis
    Histoplasmosis
    Coccidiodomycosis
    Leptospirosis
    Chlamydia
Drug Induced
    Sulfonamides
    Oral contraceptives
    Bromides
Idiopathic

erythema nodosum, streptococcus is the most common etiology; in adults, sarcoidosis and drug therapy predominate.

■ Ocular

Several of the etiologic conditions in erythema nodosum have potentially serious ocular manifestations, including sarcoidosis, Behçet disease, histoplasmosis, tuberculosis, and Crohn disease (Table 51–2). In these diseases the predominant ocular finding is an acute or chronic anterior uveitis.

DIAGNOSIS

■ Systemic

The diagnosis of erythema nodosum is made based on clinical examination and histologic features. The etiology is determined by ruling out any underlying disease. Characteristic cutaneous inflammation must be present in the commonly afflicted areas in order to diagnose erythema nodosum. Excisional biopsy of the deep skin and subcutaneous fat will identify inflammation in the septal area and in deep dermis. This will establish a definitive diagnosis of erythema nodosum and rule out other similar dermatologic inflammations, such as cutaneous polyarteritis nodosa, pancreatic panniculitis, and lupus panniculitis. Other conditions often confused with erythema nodosum include bacterial

cellulitis, primary skin infections, lymphocytic lymphoma, and giant-cell arteritis.

Laboratory evaluation shows no specific abnormalities, except those that would reflect the underlying systemic disease (eg, an elevated angiotensin-converting enzyme in active sarcoidosis). An elevated erythrocyte sedimentation

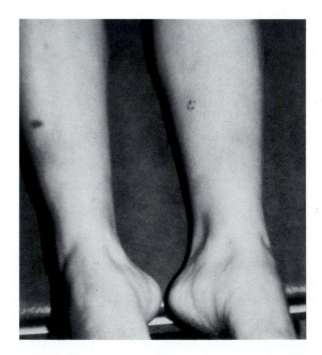

Figure 51–2. Biopsy proven erythema nodosum secondary to oral contraceptive use. *(Courtesy of Scott I.M. Lim, DO.)*

TABLE 51–2. SYSTEMIC AND OCULAR MANIFESTATIONS OF ERYTHEMA NODOSUM

- ■ **SYSTEMIC**
  - Painful, tender nodules on lower legs
  - Mild fever
  - Malaise
  - Arthralgia

- ■ **OCULAR**
  - Possible uveitic symptoms if associated with systemic inflammatory diseases (eg, sarcoidosis, Behçet disease, ulcerative colitis)

TABLE 51–3. TREATMENT AND MANAGEMENT OF ERYTHEMA NODOSUM

- ■ **SYSTEMIC**
  - Bed rest and cool compresses for lesions
  - Aspirin and nonsteroidal antiinflammatory agents
  - Proper identification and treatment of any underlying disease or infection

- ■ **OCULAR**
  - Management of the ocular manifestations of the underlying systemic disease or infection (eg, anterior uveitis with topical steroids and cycloplegics)

rate is common but not specific for any particular etiology. Mild to moderate leukocytosis with a left shift (immature cells) and a mild anemia have also been reported (O'Neill, 1991). A chest x-ray and complete blood count should always be obtained in any patient with erythema nodosum to rule out any underlying systemic disease.

Numerous other tests are indicated to help identify any underlying disease. These include antistreptolysin O titer (identifies recent staphylococcal infection), anti-DNAse B titer (helps rule out systemic lupus erythematosus), rapid plasma reagin, liver function tests, hepatitis serologies, throat culture, PPD, anergy panel, and stool culture. Depending on geographical location and the age of the patient, further serologic studies should be undertaken to rule out histoplasmosis, blastomycosis, coccidioidomycosis, or psittacosis (O'Neill, 1991).

■ Ocular

A patient presenting with uveitis and a past history of skin lesions consistent with erythema nodosum should be thoroughly evaluated for diseases such as sarcoidosis, Behçet disease, histoplasmosis, tuberculosis, and Crohn disease. Other particular ocular complications that each of these diseases may exhibit should also be carefully ruled out.

TREATMENT AND MANAGEMENT

■ Systemic

No specific treatment is indicated for erythema nodosum, because it will spontaneously resolve within 3 to 6 weeks. Depending on the level of cutaneous involvement, a combination of bed rest, aspirin, and nonsteroidal antiinflammatory therapy will help relieve patient symptoms (Sauer, 1991). Systemic steroids should be avoided because of the strong possibility of an infectious etiology. Cool compresses and wet dressings offer effective relief for large areas of tender, inflamed skin. Potassium iodide may also be beneficial

(Schulz & Whiting, 1976). Of primary importance, however, is the proper treatment and management of any underlying systemic disease.

■ Ocular

Treatment of any ocular manifestations in patients with erythema nodosum will generally involve both local and systemic management. Anterior uveitis, when present, is most often caused by systemic diseases such as sarcoidosis, tuberculosis, and Behçet manifestations. Management with topical steroids and cycloplegia will be satisfactory in most cases. Posterior segment involvement (retinal, choroidal, and vitreal) may develop secondary to histoplasmosis, sarcoidosis and Behçet disease. Therefore, treatment of the underlying disease is vital to prevent or halt further ocular complications (Table 51–3).

CONCLUSION

Erythema nodosum is a cutaneous inflammation of the lower extremities occurring in young patients. No single cause has been identified; however, there is a strong association with numerous systemic conditions. It is a self-limiting condition that resolves without any lasting tissue damage. There are no characteristic ocular findings attributable to this disease. However, many of the associated systemic diseases have important ocular manifestations that are sight threatening. A thorough ocular examination of all patients with erythema nodosum is recommended.

REFERENCES

Bondi EE, Lazarus GS. Disorders of subcutaneous tissue. In: Fitzpatrick TB, Eisen AZ, Wolff K, et al, eds. *Dermatology in General Medicine.* New York: McGraw-Hill; 1986:1141–1145.

MacPherson P. A survey of erythema nodosum in a rural community between 1954 and 1968. *Tubercule.* 1970;51:324.

Morgan GJ. Panniculitis and erythema nodosum. In: Kelly WN, Harris ED, Ruddy S, Sledge CB, eds. *Textbook of Rheumatology.* 2nd ed. Philadelphia: Saunders; 1985:1178–1179.

O'Neill JM Jr. The differential diagnosis of erythema nodosum. *Del Med J.* 1991;63:683–689.

Sauer GC. *Manual of Skin Diseases.* 6th ed. Philadelphia: Lippincott; 1991:115–116.

Schulz EJ, Whiting DA. Treatment of erythema nodosum and nodular vasculitis with potassium iodide. *Br J Ophthalmol.* 1976;94:75.

Schumacher HR. *Primer on the Rheumatic Diseases.* 9th ed. Atlanta: Arthritis Foundation; 1988:236.

52
Chapter

Cicatricial Pemphigoid

Debra Bezan

Cicatricial pemphigoid is a progressive bullous (blister-forming) disease affecting the skin and mucous membranes. Cutaneous involvement occurs in only about 25% of cases, while ocular tissue involvement occurs in approximately 75 to 85% of cases and may be the initial sign of the disease.

EPIDEMIOLOGY

Cicatricial pemphigoid is a relatively rare disorder, with an estimated prevalence in the general population ranging from 1 in 10,000 to 1 in 60,000. It may occur in young adults, but is more common in older adults, with an average age of onset between 55 and 70 years. Cicatricial pemphigoid affects women about 1.7 times more often than men. Interestingly, 14 to 32% of cicatricial pemphigoid patients also have a history of ocular hypertension or glaucoma.

NATURAL HISTORY

■ Systemic

The etiology of cicatricial pemphigoid is unknown, although it is generally thought to be an autoimmune disorder with the development of antibodies to components of the epithelia that are involved in the epithelial–connective tissue interface. These antibodies then fix complement and ultimately lead to blister formation. Some cases appear to be related to use of topical drugs, including idoxuridine, timolol, epinephrine, dipivefrin, pilocarpine, demecarium, and echothiophate iodide. There have also been a few cases reported of cicatricial pemphigold following an episode of erythema multiforme major (Stevens–Johnson syndrome).

There appears to be a genetic predisposition for developing cicatricial pemphigold because there are some HLA sub-

types that are associated with cicatricial pemphigold, including B12, DR4, DR5, DQw3, A2, B8, B35, and B49. It has been hypothesized that the drugs mentioned above may trigger cicatricial pemphigold in genetically susceptible patients.

Subepidermal blister formation is the characteristic histologic finding in cicatricial pemphigold. The histopathologic changes that occur are thought to be due to the binding of immunoglobulins (especially IgG) and complement to the basement membranes of skin and mucosa. The early or acute phases are characterized by subepithelial infiltration of T lymphocytes, macrophages, B cells, and plasma cells. Chronic phases produce some of the same inflammatory cells but also more neutrophils.

Bullous lesions of the oral mucosa are the most common systemic manifestation (Table 52–1). Other mucous membranes affected include those of the conjunctiva, nose, pharynx, larynx, esophagus, urethra, anus, and vagina. Complications associated with scarring of the respiratory or gastrointestinal structures may result in death.

Skin lesions are less common than mucosal lesions. These fall into two categories: (1) nonscarring, recurrent vesiculobullous lesions, and (2) scarring localized plaques with overlying bullae.

■ Ocular

The ocular manifestations (Table 52–2) of cicatricial pemphigoid are bilateral though not necessarily symmetric. The conjunctiva is the most commonly affected ocular tissue and is involved in approximately two thirds of cases. Two

TABLE 52–1. SYSTEMIC MANIFESTATIONS OF CICATRICIAL PEMPHIGOID

- Triggered by certain drugs
- Bullous lesions of oral and other mucous membranes are common
- Occasional bullous skin lesions
- Progressive course

systems have been developed to classify conjunctival changes that occur with cicatricial pemphigoid. The system developed by Foster and associates (1986) has the following four stages: (1) chronic conjunctivitis, rose bengal staining of the conjunctival epithelium, mucoid discharge, and subepithelial fibrosis; (2) conjunctival shrinkage and shortening of the inferior fornix; (3) development of symblepharon (Figure 52–1) along with other changes such as entropion, trichiasis, tear insufficiency, keratopathy, and corneal vascularization; and (4) severe dry eye, ocular surface keratinization, and ankyloblepharon (end stage). The system developed by Mondino and Brown (1981) grades cicatricial pemphigoid on a scale of 0 to 4 based on the percentage of visible conjunctival shrinkage: (0) no conjunctival shrinkage, (1) less than 25% shrinkage, (2) 25 to 50% shrinkage, (3) approximately 75% shrinkage, and (4) end stage with fornix obliteration.

The immunopathologic processes occurring in cicatricial pemphigoid result in hyperproliferation and poor differentiation of the conjunctival epithelial cells. There are also decreased numbers of mucin-producing goblet cells. These cellular changes cause squamous metaplasia of the epithelial cells resulting in abnormal keratinization.

These pathological changes also affect the tear film. The decreased numbers of conjunctival goblet cells result in less mucin in the tears. Conjunctival scarring blocks the ducts of the main and accessory lacrimal glands, which results in a decreased aqueous component of the tear film. In addition, entropion and trichiasis secondary to scarring cause faulty tear-spreading action.

TABLE 52–2. OCULAR MANIFESTATIONS OF CICATRICIAL PEMPHIGOID

- Chronic conjunctivitis
- Symblepharon
- Conjunctival shrinkage
- Entropion and trichiasis
- Corneal vascularization
- Severe dry eye
- Ocular surface keratinization
- Ankyloblepharon
- Restricted motility

Poor tear film quality, quantity, and spreading action result in corneal desiccation. Occasionally corneal bullae will form and erupt. These factors combined with mechanical trauma from cicatricial lid anomalies can cause significant epithelial defects and recurrent erosions. Changes in the tear film and mechanical trauma make the cornea more susceptible to secondary infection and ulceration. All of these factors may lead to corneal neovascularization, scarring, and loss of vision that can lead to legal blindness.

DIAGNOSIS

The diagnosis of cicatricial pemphigoid is based on history, clinical signs, and the progressive course of the disease. Currently there are no laboratory tests available that are specific for cicatricial pemphigoid, although tissue biopsy and impression cytology may be used to confirm the diagnosis in many cases.

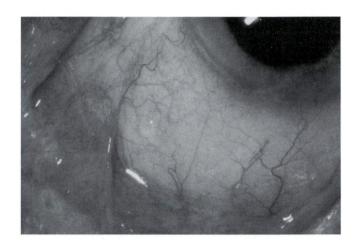

A

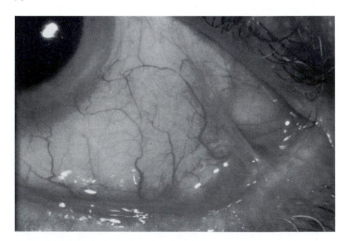

B

Figure 52–1. Symblepharon.

TABLE 52–3. TREATMENT AND MANAGEMENT OF CICATRICIAL PEMPHIGOID

- Systemic corticosteroids, immunosuppressives, and dapsone to manage inflammation
- Lubricants, topical tretinoin, bandage lenses, and punctal occlusion to manage dry eye
- Surgical management of scarred tissues

■ Systemic

The cutaneous manifestations of cicatricial pemphigoid must be differentiated from other bullous skin diseases such as bullous pemphigoid or pemphigus vulgaris.

■ Ocular

Ocular manifestations must be differentially diagnosed from other conditions that can demonstrate similar signs and symptoms. For example, symblepharon may be associated with Sjögren syndrome, sarcoidosis, keratoconjunctivitis, or erythema multiforme as well as cicatricial pemphigoid. Conjunctival scarring can be a result of chemical (especially alkali) burns, trauma, or infection by *Chlamydia trachomatis*, adenovirus 8 and 19, herpes simplex, *Corynebacterium diphtheriae*, or β-hemolytic streptococcus. In addition to cicatricial pemphigoid, conjunctival shrinkage can be associated with erythema multiforme, scleroderma (progressive systemic sclerosis), or topical drug use.

TREATMENT AND MANAGEMENT

■ Systemic

The cutaneous lesions of cicatricial pemphigoid rarely need to be treated, as they tend to resolve spontaneously, often leaving atrophic scars (Table 52–3). Medical therapy for cicatricial pemphigoid centers around controlling the chronic inflammatory process involving the mucous membranes, and in particular trying to prevent sight-threatening changes in the ocular tissues. Cytotoxic immunosuppressive drugs such as methotrexate, azathioprine, and cyclophosphamide have been used to control the inflammatory reaction in cicatricial pemphigoid with moderate success. More recently, dapsone, an antibacterial drug used to treat leprosy and dermatitis herpetiformis, has shown promise in the treatment of cicatricial pemphigoid.

■ Ocular

The signs and symptoms of dry eye are managed with ocular lubricants, moisture chambers, bandage contact lenses, and punctal occlusion. Topical tretinoin (vitamin A) therapy has been shown to be useful in reversing certain cases of squamous metaplasia. Tarsorrhaphy may be indicated for chronic corneal ulceration secondary to dry eye. Secondary infections may be managed with lid scrubs and topical and/or oral antibiotics. Topical and/or oral corticosteroids have been shown to be helpful in controlling the progression of cicatricial pemphigoid, but the ocular and systemic side effects from the dosages needed often render corticosteroids undesirable for long-term use.

When advanced cicatricial ocular changes have already occurred, surgical procedures may be performed to treat entropion, symblepharon, and ankyloblepharon. Electrocautery or cryotherapy is useful in managing trichiasis. If the cornea is severely scarred, a keratoprosthesis may be used to help the patient retain some usable vision.

CONCLUSION

Cicatricial pemphigoid is a progressive disease, presumably of autoimmune origin, that affects the skin and mucous membranes. The precise mechanism is not understood, but it is known that the use of certain topical glaucoma and antiviral medications is associated with the development of cicatricial pemphigoid in some cases.

Ocular manifestations include conjunctival inflammation, shrinkage, and scarring, entropion, trichiasis, dry eye, and corneal erosion, neovascularization, opacification, and restricted motilities. Management of this chronic, progressive disorder is often difficult. Strategies include using ocular lubricants, moisture chambers, and punctal occlusion for relief of dry eye symptoms, and using corticosteroids, cytotoxic immunosuppressive agents, or dapsone to control inflammation. In eyes with advanced scarring from cicatricial pemphigoid, surgical procedures may be needed to help the patient retain useful vision.

REFERENCES

Chan LS, Soong HK, Foster CS, et al. Ocular cicatricial pemphigoid occurring as a sequela of Stevens–Johnson syndrome. *JAMA*. 1991;266:1543–1546.

Foster CS. Cicatricial pemphigoid. *Trans Am Ophthalmol Soc*. 1986;84:527–663.

Foster CS, Shaw CD, Wells PA. Scanning electron microscopy of conjunctival surfaces in patients with ocular cicatricial pemphigoid. *Am J Ophthalmol*. 1986;102:584–591.

Kristensen EB, Norn MS. Benign mucous membrane pemphigoid: Secretion of mucous and tears. *Acta Ophthalmol*. 1974;52:266–281.

Mondino BJ, Brown SI, Lempert S, Jenkins MS. The acute manifestations of ocular pemphigoid: Diagnosis and treatment. *Ophthalmology*. 1979;86:543–552.

Mondino BJ, Brown SI. Ocular cicatricial pemphigoid. *Ophthalmology*. 1981;88:95–100.

Mondino BJ, Brown SI. Immunosuppressive therapy in ocular cicatricial pemphigoid. *Am J Ophthalmol*. 1983;96:453–459.

Mondino BJ. Cicatricial pemphigoid and erythema multiforme. *Ophthalmology.* 1990;97:939–952.

Norn MS, Kristensen EB. Benign mucous membrane pemphigoid: Cytology. *Acta Ophthalmol.* 1974;52:282–290.

Ormerod LD, Fong LP, Foster CS. Corneal infection in mucosal scarring disorders and Sjögren's syndrome. *Am J Ophthalmol.* 1988;105:512–518.

Pouliquen Y, Patey A, Foster CS, et al. Drug induced cicatricial pemphigoid affecting the conjunctiva: Light and electron microscopic features. *Ophthalmology.* 1986;93:775–783.

Sacks EH, Jakobiec FA, Wieczorek R, et al. Immunophenotypic analysis of the inflammatory infiltrate in ocular cicatricial pemphigoid: Further evidence for a T-cell-mediated disease. *Ophthalmology.* 1989;96:236–243.

Tauber J, Melamed S, Foster CS. Glaucoma in patients with ocular cicatricial pemphigoid. *Ophthalmology.* 1989;96:33–37.

Thoft RA, Friend J, Kinoshita S, et al. Ocular cicatricial pemphigoid associated with hyperproliferation of the conjunctival epithelium. *Am J Ophthalmol.* 1984;98:37–42.

Erythema Multiforme

Debra Bezan

Erythema multiforme (EM) is an acute, inflammatory condition of the skin and mucous membranes that is usually self-limiting. As the name multiforme implies, this condition takes on a number of forms. EM can be divided into two classifications: erythema multiforme minor (erythema multiforme of Hebra) and erythema multiforme major (Stevens–Johnson syndrome, ectodermosis erosiva pluriorificialis, dermatostomatitis, mucosal respiratory syndrome, or eruptive fever associated with stomatitis and ophthalmia).

EPIDEMIOLOGY

EM can occur at any age, but is most common in children and young adults. The peak occurrence is between the ages of 20 and 40. EM minor affects both sexes equally, while EM major affects males more often than females.

NATURAL HISTORY

■ Systemic

The actual mechanism is unclear but there are a number of factors that can precipitate EM, including drugs, microbial infections, and other conditions including collagen vascular diseases, vaccinations, pregnancy, neoplasms, and radiation therapy. An estimated 58% of cases of EM appear to have a drug as the precipitating factor. There are over 40 different systemic drugs that have been implicated in triggering EM. These include sulfonamides, penicillins, salicylates, barbiturates, phenylbutazone, phenytoin, arsenicals, and mercurials. Certain topical drugs of particular interest to eyecare practitioners have also been implicated, including sulfonamides, tropicamide, and proparacaine.

Microbial infections have been determined to be the precipitating factor in approximately 15% of cases, with herpes simplex and *Mycoplasma pneumoniae* infections being the best documented. Some of the other triggering microbial infections and agents mentioned in the literature include infectious mononucleosis, psittacosis, influenza, adenovirus, coxsackie virus, *Yersinia*, tuberculosis, and histoplasmosis.

What causes such a diversity of agents to trigger EM is unknown; however, there appears to be a genetic predisposition for EM based on the association of certain HLA types such as HLA-B12 and its subgroup, HLA-Bw44.

The pathophysiologic manifestations of EM are thought to be due to the deposition of immunoglobulins and complement at the dermal–epidermal junction and in the blood vessel walls of the dermis. EM is characterized by an infiltration of monocytes in the dermal layer. There is often a perivascular infiltration of lymphocytes and histiocytes around the dermal blood vessels. Subepithelial bullae form and the epidermal cells may become edematous or degenerate and become necrotic.

The systemic manifestations (Table 53–1) of EM may begin with prodromal flu-like symptoms including fever, headache, upper respiratory congestion, malaise, and prostration. These are more common with EM major than EM minor. The prodromal symptoms, if present, are followed by the characteristic dermal eruptions, which may be itchy or painful. The skin lesions are most commonly found on

TABLE 53–1. SYSTEMIC MANIFESTATIONS OF EM

- Triggered by certain drugs and microbial infections
- Prodromal flu-like symptoms
- Bull's-eye skin lesions and mucous membrane involvement are common especially in EM major (Stevens–Johnson syndrome)
- Self-limiting course

the extremities. Lesions occur more often on the trunk in EM major than EM minor. They begin as small red macules that usually develop into vesicles or bullae and may become necrotic (Figure 53–1). The lesions are termed "iris" or "target" lesions because they often have a characteristic "bull's-eye" appearance of a red center surrounded by a white zone surrounded by another red ring. Crops of skin lesions may continue to break out during the acute course of the disease.

EM minor primarily involves the skin with occasional limited involvement of the mucosa, while EM major (Stevens–Johnson syndrome) typically has both skin and mucous membrane involvement. It is more likely to affect the mouth, nose, conjunctiva, pharynx, larynx, trachea,

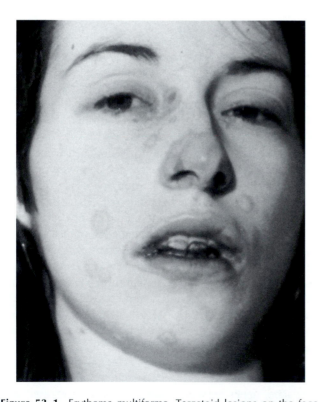

Figure 53–1. Erythema multiforme. Targetoid lesions on the face, with involvement of the oral mucous membranes and the eye (scleritis, periorbital edema, and bullae on the inner canthus). *(Reprinted with permission from Fitzpatrick TB, et al. Color Atlas and Synopsis of Clinical Dermatology: Common and Serious Diseases. 2nd ed. New York: McGraw-Hill, 1992, p 475.)*

esophagus, vagina, or urethra. Toxic epidermal necrolysis is a severe variation of EM major and characterized by widespread denuding of the epidermis.

The signs and symptoms of EM minor tend to last from 1 to 4 weeks, while EM major may last as long as 6 weeks. Both conditions usually resolve without extensive scarring of the skin, although focal areas of hyperpigmentation may remain. EM minor is more likely to recur than EM major.

Mortality is approximately 1% for EM minor but may range from 3 to 25% for EM major due to such complications as septicemia, pneumonitis, glomerulonephritis, myositis, and myocarditis.

■ Ocular

Ocular involvement is relatively common (Table 53–2) in EM major with a number of anterior segment tissues being affected (see Figure 53–1). The lids are typically affected in the acute stage, which lasts 2 to 3 weeks. They may become edematous and hyperemic and show focal ulcerating or crusting lesions. In severe cases conjunctival scarring may result in late cicatricial entropion and trichiasis.

The conjunctiva is one of the most common mucous membrane tissues to be affected by EM. Conjunctival involvement ranges from a mild transient injection to severe membrane formation and scarring. Pseudomembranes or true membranes are formed from an exudate composed of fibrin, neutrophils, other inflammatory cells, and necrotic epithelial cells. The development of later cicatricial complications of symblepharon and occasional ankyloblepharon depend on the severity of the inflammation. Episodes of conjunctival inflammation have been known to occur after EM major; however, recurrent bouts of EM major are less likely to involve the conjunctiva than the initial episode.

EM can cause a dry eye condition due to squamous metaplasia of the conjunctival epithelium and a decrease in the number of conjunctival goblet cells, resulting in poor mucin quantity and/or quality in the tear film. Scarring may also block the ducts of lacrimal glands, reducing tear production. If cicatricial entropion and trichiasis are present, the tears may not be spread properly across the ocular surface and further exacerbate a dry eye situation.

Poor tear-film quality, quantity, and spreading action can cause corneal and conjunctival desiccation. Mechanical trauma from lid abnormalities can also cause epithelial

TABLE 53–2. OCULAR MANIFESTATIONS OF EM

- Lid edema and focal ulcerations
- Conjunctival pseudomembranes or true membranes
- Occasional conjunctival scarring
- Occasional dry eye
- Occasional iritis or iridocyclitis

damage and make the cornea and conjunctiva more susceptible to secondary infection. Among the more serious infectious complications is corneal ulceration.

Although uncommon, iritis or iridocyclitis is another anterior segment manifestation of EM.

DIAGNOSIS

The diagnosis of EM is based on clinical signs and the natural history of the disease. The presence of significant mucous membrane involvement is often used to differentiate EM major from EM minor. At present there are no specific laboratory tests that are useful in the diagnosis of EM. However, a biopsy of the skin lesions has characteristic findings and helps confirm the diagnosis, although it will not identify the etiology.

■ Systemic
EM must be differentiated from other skin diseases with a similar appearance including urticarias, toxic erythemas, systemic lupus erythematosus, polyarteritis nodosa, bullous impetigo, pemphigus vulgaris, bullous pemphigoid, herpetic dermatitis, Behçet syndrome, and Reiter syndrome. A biopsy can help differentiate EM from these processes.

■ Ocular
EM must be differentially diagnosed from other conditions with similar ocular signs. Symblepharon, for example, may be associated with Sjögren syndrome, keratoconjunctivitis, sarcoidosis, or cicatricial pemphigoid in addition to EM. Conjunctival scarring similar to that seen in EM may be a result of chemical burns, trauma, trachoma, herpes simplex, diphtheria, or β-hemolytic streptococcus, and conjunctival shrinkage may be due to cicatricial pemphigoid, scleroderma, or topical drug use.

TREATMENT AND MANAGEMENT

■ Systemic
The treatment (Table 53–3) of EM involves identification and treatment of underlying factors such as *Mycoplasma pneumoniae* or *Mycobacterium tuberculosis*, if possible. If EM appears to be caused by drug use, the drug should be immediately discontinued.

Other therapies are primarily palliative or supportive. Skin lesions may be debrided, and topical and systemic antibiotics may be used to treat secondary infections. Topical and/or systemic corticosteroids may be used to control inflammation; however, there is evidence that they may prolong the course of the disease and increase the complication rate in some instances. In some severe cases (toxic epidermal necrolysis), fluid therapy may be needed to prevent systemic dehydration.

TABLE 53–3. TREATMENT AND MANAGEMENT OF EM

- ■ **SYSTEMIC**
  - Treatment of underlying microbial infection if indicated
  - Discontinue triggering drug if indicated
  - Skin lesion debridement
  - Topical and/or systemic antibiotics for secondary infection
  - Topical and/or systemic corticosteroids to manage inflammation
- ■ **OCULAR**
  - Ocular lubrication, punctal occlusion
  - Stripping of conjunctival membranes, lysis of conjunctival adhesions
  - Topical tretinoin
  - Surgical lid management

■ Ocular
Treatment of the ocular manifestations of EM includes the management of secondary dry eye with ocular lubricants, moisture chambers, bandage contact lenses, and punctal occlusion. Topical tretinoin may be helpful in reversing conjunctival squamous metaplasia by restoring normal cellular differentiation, and may also enhance goblet cell regeneration and mucin production. Stripping conjunctival membranes and frequent lysis of conjunctival adhesions with a glass rod may be of some benefit in preventing permanent scar formation. However, if cicatricial changes such as symblepharon and entropion do occur, surgical management may be indicated. Electrocautery or cryotherapy may be used to treat secondary trichiasis, and tarsorrhaphy may be indicated for cases of chronic corneal ulceration due to dry eye.

CONCLUSION

EM is a variable, self-limiting disorder that affects the skin and may also involve the mucous membranes. It can be divided into two subclassifications: EM minor and EM major (Stevens–Johnson syndrome). EM major is more likely to have ocular involvement than EM minor. Although the precise etiology is unclear, several factors are known to trigger EM, including certain systemic and topical pharmaceuticals and microbial infections. Management involves treatment of precipitating conditions, if possible, and palliative therapy for symptomatic relief. Treatment of ocular manifestations includes managing secondary dry eye and surgical repair of cicatricial conjunctival and lid anomalies.

REFERENCES

Anhalt GJ, Bahn CF, Diaz LA. Bullous diseases. *Int Ophthalmol Clin.* 1985;25:37–59.

Fitzpatrick TB, Johnson RA, Polano MK, et al. *Color Atlas and Synopsis of Clinical Dermatology: Common and Serious Diseases.* 2nd ed. New York: McGraw-Hill; 1992:474–477.

Foster CS, Fong LP, Azar D, Kenyon KR. Episodic conjunctival inflammation after Stevens–Johnson syndrome. *Ophthalmology.* 1988;95:453–462.

Genvert GI, Cohen EJ, Donnenfield ED, Blecher MH. Erythema multiforme after use of topical sulfacetamide. *Am J Ophthalmol.* 1985;99:465–468.

Huff JC, Weston WL, Tonnesen MG. Erythema multiforme: A critical review of characteristics, diagnostic criteria and causes. *J Am Acad Dermatol.* 1983;8:763–775.

Mondino BJ. Cicatricial pemphigoid and erythema multiforme. *Ophthalmology.* 1990;97:939–952.

Nelson JD, Wright JC. Conjunctival goblet cell densities in ocular surface disease. *Arch Ophthalmol.* 1984;102:1049–1051.

Ormerod LD, Fong LP, Foster CS. Corneal infection in mucosal scarring disorders and Sjögren's syndrome. *Am J Ophthalmol.* 1988;105:512–518.

Patz A. Ocular involvement in erythema multiforme. *Arch Ophthalmol.* 1950;43:244–256.

Rasmussen JE. Erythema multiforme in children: Response to treatment with systemic corticosteroids. *Br J Dermatol.* 1976;95:181–186.

Shelley WB. Herpes simplex virus as a cause of erythema multiforme. *JAMA.* 1967;201:153–156.

Soong HK, Martin NF, Wagoner MD, et al. Topical retinoid therapy for squamous metaplasia of various ocular surface disorders: A multicenter, placebo-controlled, double-masked study. *Ophthalmology.* 1988;95:1442–1446.

Tonnesen MG, Soter NA. Erythema multiforme. *J Am Acad Dermatol.* 1979;1:357–364.

Ward B, McCulley JP, Segal RJ. Dermatologic reaction in Stevens–Johnson syndrome after ophthalmic anesthesia with proparacaine hydrochloride. *Am J Ophthalmol.* 1978;86:133–135.

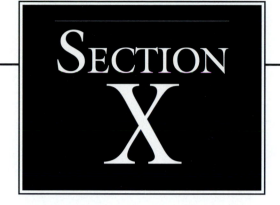

SECTION X

INFECTIOUS DISORDERS

54
Chapter

Tuberculosis

Esther S. Marks

Tuberculosis (TB) is an ancient granulomatous infection caused by *Mycobacterium tuberculosis*. Although it primarily affects the lungs, TB can attack many other tissues and organs, including most ocular structures, in particular the uvea. It has long been and continues to be a tremendous source of worldwide morbidity and mortality. In the past, a patient with consumption (TB) was relegated to a sanitorium until recovery or death occurred. Advances in medicine, both preventive and therapeutic, appeared to have set the stage for eradication of this disease. However, significant setbacks have occurred with the recent emergence of a new epidemic, AIDS, as well as a new multidrug-resistant strain of TB.

EPIDEMIOLOGY

■ Systemic

TB continues to be a serious multinational health problem with a staggering 1.7 billion persons infected worldwide, approximately one third of the world's population (Sudre et al, 1992). Twenty million persons suffer from active disease. Approximately 8 million new cases and an estimated 3 million TB-related deaths occur each year (Kochi, 1991).

From 1953 (when national reporting of TB first began) to 1984, the United States experienced a steady annual decrease in the number of cases reported to the Centers for Disease Control (CDC). However, in 1985 this downward trend halted, and beginning in 1986 actually started to reverse, with the number of cases continuing to rise ever since. The increasing numbers of persons concurrently infected with human immunodeficiency virus (HIV) or acquired immunodeficiency syndrome (AIDS) and TB has been largely blamed for this trend.

In the United States almost 70% of all TB cases involve racial minorities, and approximately 86% of infected children (14 years and younger) are from ethnic minorities. The risk of TB is greatest amongst Asians and Pacific Islanders,

followed by African-Americans, Hispanics, American Indians and Alaskan Natives, and lastly Caucasians (CDC, 1992b). The presence of HIV or AIDS appears to confer a 100 times greater risk of contracting TB, and homelessness a 150 to 300 times greater risk (Hamrick & Yeager, 1988). Although the incidence rate for the entire United States in 1992 was 10.5 per 100,000, certain geographic areas have much higher rates, such as Central Harlem in New York City, which reported 300 cases per 100,000 population in 1990 (CDC, 1992b).

Many factors are known to carry an increased risk for TB. Certain genetic factors increase patient susceptibility. Diabetes mellitus, silicosis, gastrectomy, malnutrition, alcoholism, some hematologic disorders, and certain malignancies, as well as disorders or medications resulting in immunosuppression (eg, HIV or AIDS or long-term corticosteroid use), confer poor resistance to TB infection or reactivation. Socioeconomic factors, such as low income and lack of medical attention (as with the homeless and racial minorities), and geographic factors such as poor housing or residence in shelters, correctional institutions, or healthcare facilities such as mental institutions and nursing homes also contribute to an increased risk. Persons new to the United States, born in countries where TB is more common (the countries of Asia, Africa, and South America) have a higher risk of TB.

Although TB has continued to be a disease of the elderly (primarily due to reactivation of latent infection), younger age groups have experienced enormous rises in TB. This is particularly true among those 20 to 50 years old. Men are twice as likely as women to have active TB.

Only 5% of patients infected with TB will develop active disease within 1 year. Approximately 5% more will develop clinical disease later in life. Reactivation of latent TB accounts for about 90% of active TB cases in the United States. The remaining 10% is due to primary infection.

Active TB manifests overwhelmingly as pulmonary cases in males. Extrapulmonary TB accounts for less than 20% of all cases (Rieder & Snider, 1990). Lymphatic TB and pleural TB each account for approximately 25% of cases, miliary TB (with or without meningeal TB) about 14%, genitourinary TB about 12.5%, bone and joint TB about 9%, and peritoneal, pericardial, renal, hepatic, and dermatologic TB account for the rest (Comstock & O'Brien, 1990). Overall, these extrapulmonary cases are more common in minorities, females, children (14 years and younger), and foreign-born persons.

Most alarming is the recent increase in drug-resistant TB cases, particularly multidrug resistant (MDR) TB. Most cases appear to occur in AIDS clinics or wards involving HIV or AIDS patients or healthcare workers (Beck-Sagué et al, 1992). From 1982 to 1986, MDR occurred in only 0.5% of new cases, and only 3% of recurrent cases. In 1991, MDR occurred in 3.1% of new cases and 6.9% of recurrent cases (CDC, 1992a). In a study by Frieden and associates (1993), all New York City patients with available *Mycobacterium tuberculosis* positive cultures in April 1991 were examined for TB drug susceptibility. A startling 33% were found to be resistant to one or more anti-TB medications. The main culprit appears to be prior inadequate treatment of TB, allowing reactivation and transmission of a now drug-resistant organism.

■ Ocular

The incidence of ocular manifestations of TB is extremely low at less than 1 to 2% (Gross et al, 1992).

NATURAL HISTORY

■ Systemic

The Organism

Thirty species are recognized in the genus *Mycobacterium*. Some, such as *M. avium* and *M. intracellulare*, are ubiquitous to the environment, posing a serious threat

mainly in the immunocompromised, as with the mycobacterium avium intracellulare (MAI) complex in AIDS patients. *Mycobacterium bovis* was a greater threat to humans prior to widespread dairy cattle tuberculin testing and the pasteurization of milk.

However, *M. tuberculosis* has remained a threat to humankind. An aerobic, acid-fast-staining bacillus (AFB), *M. tuberculosis* does not contain or secrete toxins. It is slow growing, requiring generation times of approximately 14 to 24 hours, and several weeks for isolation by culture.

Transmission

Mycobacterium tuberculosis most often is transmitted human to human via inhalation of aerosolized bacilli from sputum droplets. If an actively infectious patient talks, coughs, sneezes, or sings, a spray of sputum, infected with tubercle bacilli, is secreted. The larger particles expelled simply drop out of the air onto available surfaces. These particles rarely reaerosolize; therefore, it is difficult to become infected by handling an infectious patient's belongings. Smaller particles evaporate. The now desiccated and quite light bacilli may float on air currents for some time before settling very slowly. The bacilli are rapidly killed by ultraviolet radiation, including daylight. Therefore, poorly ventilated, dark rooms may aid in the transmission of this infection.

Course of the Disease

Once inhaled, the bacilli travel via the bronchi to the alveoli of the lungs. The invading bacilli are engulfed by alveolar phagocytes. These phagocytes, usually unable to destroy the microorganisms, transport the bacilli to regional lymph nodes. Along the way, the pleural space may become infected. Dissemination from the lymph nodes may occur hematogenously. Approximately 3 to 8 weeks later, a hypersensitivity reaction to TB antigens occurs. At this point the host will respond positively to a tuberculin skin test. Granuloma formation occurs as host phagocytes are activated to better entrap and kill the bacilli. The result is foci of epithelioid cells, lymphocytes, and fibroblasts surrounding a central area of caseous necrosis. Some bacilli are capable of surviving within the phagocytes and foci for years.

Primary infection rarely leads to clinical disease. Only 10% of infected patients will develop active disease. Dissemination of TB may occur during the primary infection or may occur during a reactivation of a latent infection. Most infected sites heal, leaving scar tissue and calcification.

Pulmonary TB

Active TB may present as either pulmonary or extrapulmonary TB (Table 54–1). Pulmonary TB is much more common, accounting for over 80% of all cases, and is almost always symptomatic. Patients present with a chronic productive (mucoid or mucopurulent) cough, often of

TABLE 54–1. SYSTEMIC MANIFESTATIONS OF TB

GENERAL CONSTITUTIONAL SYMPTOMS
- Low-grade fever
- Anorexia
- Weight loss
- Fatigue

PULMONARY TB
- Chronic productive (purulent or mucopurulent) cough
- Hemoptysis
- Dull aching chest pain
- Possible pleural effusion
- Rales on auscultation
- Classic x-ray: infiltrates, granulomas, with cavitation in apices of lungs
- Hilar and/or mediastinal lymphadenopathy
- (+) PPD and (+) AFB on sputum culture

EXTRAPULMONARY TB
- **Miliary TB**
  Multiple lesions on various organs
  Mild anemia and increased alkaline phosphatase
  Chest x-ray and PPD often (–)
- **TB Meningitis**
  Headache, abnormal behavior
  Altered consciousness, convulsions, coma
  (+) PPD
  CSF demonstrates increased protein, decreased glucose and chloride, pleocytosis, and (+) AFB culture
- **Pleural TB**
  Pleural effusion
  Pleuritic pain
  (+) PPD and (+) AFB cultured from pleuritic fluid
- **Lymphatic TB**
  Multiple granulomatous lymphadenitis
  Involves hilar, mediastinal, cervical, and supraclavicular nodes
  (+) PPD, and (+) AFB culture of pus or lymph biopsy
- **Genitourinary TB**
  Chronic recurrent urinary tract infections
  Nodular induration of prostate or vas deferens
  Pelvic inflammatory disease
  Amenorrhea
  Infertility
  (+) PPD, possible (+) AFB cultured from urine or biopsied from endometrium
- **Bone and Joint TB**
  Localized pain and swelling
  Possible abscesses
  Decreased joint spaces and joint damage
  (+) PPD
- **Other Organ Involvement**
  Pericardium
  Liver
  Spleen
  Brain
  Skin

several weeks duration. Hemoptysis (coughing up blood), although very common, is usually indicative of advanced disease. A low-grade fever, weight loss, anorexia, and fatigue may be present. A dull and aching chest pain may occur. Liquefaction of the caseous foci and microbial proliferation result in the formation of pulmonary cavities. Infrequently, pulmonary TB may present as an acute respiratory illness mimicking pneumonia or influenza. Pleurisy (inflammation of the pleura) with effusion (the leakage of fluid from lymphatics or blood vessels) may result (Figure 54–1).

Untreated pulmonary TB is a chronic, slowly progressive and relapsing disease, although one third of cases may develop a stable nonprogressive course (Daniel & Tripathy, 1989). An untreated patient remains infectious for about 2 years, allowing the contagious patient to infect approximately 10 other persons per year depending on the housing conditions (Chaulet & Mulder, 1987).

Extrapulmonary TB
Accounting for fewer than 20% of TB cases, extrapulmonary TB may take different forms. Hematogenous dissemination may result in miliary (millet-seed size) TB. Multiple small lesions develop in the lungs, spleen, liver, and elsewhere. More common in the young and the elderly, the diagnosis may be missed due to the nonspecific symptoms, and often negative chest x-ray and skin test. One exception is when TB meningitis occurs concurrently (usually in children). In this case (or when TB meningitis occurs in isolation), the symptoms are remarkable for headache, abnormal behavior, altered consciousness, and convulsions. Coma and death may occur without treatment.

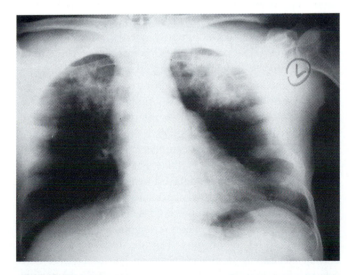

Figure 54–1. Chest x-ray of a patient with pulmonary TB revealing bilateral upper lung infiltrate, with lucencies in the infiltrate suggesting cavitation.

Lymphatic TB is characterized by multiple granulomatous lymphadenitis. The hilar and mediastinal nodes are commonly involved, followed by the cervical and supraclavicular nodes. Pleural TB (in the absence of pulmonary TB) is characterized by a pleural effusion that has progressed for 1 to 2 weeks and pleuritic chest pain.

Genitourinary TB may present in a variety of ways, because any portion of the genitourinary tract may become involved. It may manifest as chronic recurrent urinary tract infections, nodular induration of the prostate or vas deferens, pelvic inflammatory disease, or amenorrhea. Infertility may result.

Bone and joint TB is believed to occur due to reactivation of dormant foci. It most commonly involves the vertebrae of the spine (Pott disease), the large joints, and occasionally the long bones. Localized pain, swelling, and even abscess formation may occur, resulting in functional disability.

Peritoneal TB is thought to result from hematogenous dissemination, or extension from mesenteric lymph nodes or genitourinary involvement. Classically, it presents with painless ascites. However, it may also present as a fibroadhesive peritonitis, producing a tender abdomen and abdominal masses.

Other organs may become involved in TB including the pericardium, liver, spleen, brain, and skin.

■ Ocular

Ocular disease secondary to systemic TB may manifest in a wide variety of ways (Table 54–2). Virtually all ocular structures (except the crystalline lens) may be affected. Most commonly, it affects the choroid, presenting as an anterior uveitis or disseminated choroiditis. Ocular manifestations may be due to hematogenous or contiguous spread of the organism (resulting in tubercle or granuloma formation in almost any ocular tissue), or due to a hypersensitivity reaction to TB proteins (resulting in phlyctenulosis, scleritis, retinal vasculitis, or most commonly uveitis). It may present during primary, latent, or reactivation infections. There have also been reports of ocular TB with no evidence of extraocular TB (Mansour & Haymond, 1990).

Conjunctivitis may present as a unilateral red eye with a small nodule or painless ulcer on the palpebral conjunctiva. It may be surrounded by nodules or hypertrophic lesions. Regional lymphadenopathy can occur. Phlyctenular keratoconjunctivitis (Figure 54–2), once synonymous with TB, is now known to be due to a delayed hypersensitivity reaction to many different infectious organisms. The patient usually presents with a nodule on the bulbar conjunctiva, or at the limbus. The small white lesion is surrounded by an area of hyperemia. The lesion may migrate toward the central cornea, producing neovascularization and ulceration. The presentation may be unilateral or bilateral. Conjunctival injection is present, and a secondary bacterial infection may occur.

Unilateral interstitial keratitis may present acutely or as a sign of old disease. In the acute stage, the cornea will demonstrate patent stromal blood vessels, corneal edema, conjunctival injection, and possible anterior chamber reaction. In the inactive stage, the cornea will reveal stromal scarring with ghost vessels. In both stages, visual acuity may be decreased depending on the area of corneal involvement.

Scleritis may occur with usually moderate to severe pain. The conjunctival, episcleral, and scleral vessels will be inflamed diffusely or sectorally. Scleral nodules may be present, along with corneal involvement and anterior chamber reaction.

Uveitis may present acutely, chronically, or recurrently. Acute episodes are marked by typical signs: circumlimbal injection, anterior chamber reaction with possible vitreal spillover, posterior synechiae, granulomatous keratic precipitates, and iris nodules may occur. Signs and symptoms are greater in acute episodes. Choroiditis may present with mild to severe vision loss, vitritis, disc swelling, choroidal or retinal yellow-white infiltrates, and anterior chamber reaction (usually granulomatous, although nongranulomatous reaction may also occur). Periphlebitis with a macular exudative star and hemorrhages as well as neovascularization may occur.

Toxic optic neuropathy (due to the anti-TB medication ethambutol) may present with blurry vision. This may present as decreased acuity, central visual field defects, or both. Patients may also complain of altered color vision.

DIAGNOSIS

The presumptive diagnosis of TB is obtained by symptomatology, physical examination, radiographic findings, and skin testing. Definitive diagnosis requires laboratory identification and isolation of M. *tuberculosis*. Unfortunately, this organism is very slow growing, and weeks may elapse prior to definitive diagnosis.

The tuberculin skin test checks for a delayed hypersensitivity reaction of the skin to 0.1 mL (containing 5 test units) of intradermally injected purified protein derivative (PPD) of the organism. The Mantoux technique of a single puncture is preferred over the Tine method of multiple punctures in which the amount of antigen delivered is difficult to control. The injection site should raise a wheal 6 to 10 mm in diameter. It must be evaluated 48 to 72 hours later to determine the presence and amount (in mm) of induration. Erythema need not be noted. Generally, a reaction of 10 mm or greater is considered positive; however, this varies with the health of the patient, as other conditions that alter cell-mediated immunity or delayed hypersensitivity reactions can alter reaction to the PPD. Patients with HIV or AIDS are usually considered positive with an induration of

TABLE 54–2. OCULAR MANIFESTATIONS OF TB

Almost all ocular structures (except the crystalline lens) may be affected by TB

TUBERCLES (GRANULOMAS)
- May occur in lids, conjunctiva, sclera, cornea, uvea (especially the choroid), optic nerve, and orbit

CONJUNCTIVITIS
- Usually a small unilateral nodule or ulcer on the palpebral conjunctiva
- May be surrounded by nodules or hypertrophic lesions
- Local lymphadenopathy may occur
- Usually painless or foreign body sensation
- (+) AFB in conjunctival scrapings

PHLYCTENULAR KERATOCONJUNCTIVITIS
- Unilateral or bilateral white nodule on bulbar conjunctiva or at limbus (may migrate toward corneal axis)
- Discomfort, photophobia
- Tearing, blepharospasm
- Secondary bacterial infection
- Corneal ulcer and scarring may occur
- Acuity may be affected if visual axis involved

INTERSTITIAL KERATITIS
- Acute:
    Tearing, photophobic painful red eye
    Acuity variably affected depending on location of lesion
    Unilateral corneal stromal patent blood vessels
    Corneal edema and possible anterior chamber reaction
- Inactive:
    Unilateral corneal stromal scarring with ghost vessels
    Acuity variably affected depending on location of lesion

SCLERITIS
- Variably decreased acuity
- Varying pain, tearing, photophobia
- Conjunctival, episcleral, and scleral injection (diffuse or sectoral)
- Scleral nodules may be present
- Anterior chamber reaction may occur

UVEITIS WITH OR WITHOUT RETINAL VASCULITIS
- May be acute, chronic, or recurrent
- Usually granulomatous
- Variable decrease in visual acuity
- Anterior: cells, flare, keratic precipitates, iris nodules
- Disseminated: vitritis, vitreal hemorrhage, periphlebitis, macular exudative star, retinal hemorrhages, capillary closure, and neovascularization

OPTIC NEUROPATHY SECONDARY TO EMB
- Decreased visual acuity
- Visual field defects (central or peripheral)
- Abnormal color perception (especially green)

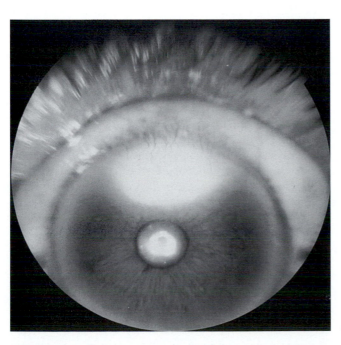

Figure 54–2. Corneal scarring secondary to old phlyctenular keratoconjunctivitis.

5 mm or greater, as are patients who have had recent and close contact with TB, or those whose chest x-ray demonstrates presumptive TB. Approximately 15% of patients acutely ill with TB will have a negative PPD. These false-negative reactions may occur due to concurrent viral, bacterial, or fungal infections, lymphatic diseases, immunosuppressive medications or illnesses, age (in very young infants and in the elderly), surgery, stress, or live virus vaccinations.

Radiographic examination is required in a suspected case of TB regardless of the results of skin testing. Chest x-ray patterns may be quite varied. The appearance of infiltrates and cavitation, especially in the apices of the lungs, is characteristic of pulmonary TB (see Figure 54–1). Hilar lymphadenopathy may or may not be present. Patients with concurrent HIV or AIDS may not demonstrate cavities, fibrosis, or granuloma formation due to their poor immune response. TB may also present in the middle or lower lobes, along with mediastinal lymphadenopathy and pleural effusion. Unfortunately, because characteristic patterns are not always seen, a misdiagnosis such as pneumonia, malignancy, or histoplasmosis may be made. Any presumptive radiologic diagnosis of TB must be confirmed by the isolation of *M. tuberculosis* in the sputum or lung tissue.

Microscopic examination of sputum, blood, pleural fluid, cerebrospinal (CSF) fluid, pus, or body tissues by biopsy may reveal the tubercle bacilli. Culturing the sample has traditionally taken several weeks (usually 6) due to the organism's slow growth. However, a new system called BACTEC (Becton Dickinson Diagnostic Instrument Systems, Towson, MD) employs special culture medium and radiometric methods to determine the presence of mycobacterial growth in 1 week, and species identification of *M. tuberculosis* within 2 weeks (Hamrick & Yeager, 1988). Drug susceptibility testing requires approximately 1 additional week.

Investigation in developing genetic and immunologic probes for the rapid but reliable identification of TB continues. Enzyme-linked immunosorbent assay (ELISA) for the measurement of IgG antibodies to antigens of *M. tuberculosis* in body fluids is being studied. Due to the variable reported sensitivity and specificity of this procedure, widespread clinical application of ELISA testing has not occurred. Polymerase chain reaction (PCR) assays are also under investigation. These DNA probes, although highly sensitive and specific, require large numbers of cells for successful identification of the organism. This requires about 2 to 3 weeks of growth (Good & Mastro, 1989).

Mycolic acids are part of all mycobacterium cells. Each species contains different amounts and types. High-performance liquid chromatography (HPLC) and gas-liquid chromatography (GLC) are two methods used to identify *M. tuberculosis* by its mycolic acid pattern. The technique requires only a couple of hours, but still must have sufficient cells (2 to 3 weeks' growth) to identify the organism (Good & Mastro, 1989).

■ Systemic

Pulmonary TB
Pulmonary TB is suspected in a patient with chronic productive cough, hemoptysis, and chest pain. Auscultation of the chest may reveal rales over the affected area. Tuberculin skin testing should be positive. Chest radiography should be abnormal. Definitive diagnosis may be obtained via smear and culture of sputum. If necessary, lung biopsy may be performed.

Extrapulmonary TB
Pleural TB may occur with or without pulmonary TB. It may be diagnosed by pleuritic chest pain and evidence of pleuritic effusion on chest x-ray. A positive PPD, and identification of the mycobacterium via culture of the pleuritic fluid, will aid in the diagnosis.

Miliary TB is characterized by persistent fever and may involve many organs. Chest x-rays are often normal, and skin testing often negative. There may be a mild anemia and mild elevation of alkaline phosphatase, but physical examination is often unrevealing. Diagnosis is difficult, and may require blood cultures, and liver or bone marrow needle biopsy.

If TB meningitis is present, the characteristic symptoms of headache and altered consciousness are present. Skin testing is usually positive. Laboratory analysis of the CSF will reveal increased protein, decreased glucose, decreased chloride, and pleocytosis. Culture of the CSF will reveal *M. tuberculosis*.

Lymphatic TB is characterized by multiple granulomatous lymphadenitis on physical examination. The tuberculin skin test is usually strongly positive. Culture of the pus from a node or biopsy of the node will reveal *M. tuberculosis*. Bone and joint TB may be diagnosed by positive skin testing, and confirmed by culture of pus from abscesses. Radiographic examination of the vertebrae and other joints will reveal decreased joint spaces and bone damage.

Genitourinary TB may present in a multitude of ways. Diagnosis relies on physical examination (pelvic, prostate) as well as potential laproscopy, endometrium biopsy, and examination and culture of the urine. Peritoneal TB may be diagnosed by the presence of a positive PPD, ascites (serous fluid-filled peritoneal cavity), and in the fibroadhesive form, may require stool cultures, digestive tract x-rays, laproscopy or laparotomy, abdominal sonograms, or computed tomography (CT).

Other forms of extrapulmonary TB require additional testing. Pericardial TB calls for an electrocardiogram, and possible pericardial puncture. Suspected tuberculomas (TB granulomas) of the brain may necessitate a variety of brain scans (CT and magnetic resonance imaging). Suspected dermatologic involvement may require skin biopsy.

■ Ocular
A good history, both medical and ocular, as well as thorough ocular examination will reveal any suspected manifestations of TB. Conjunctivitis may present as a unilateral red eye, possible foreign body sensation, a palpebral nodule, with ipsilateral lymphadenopathy. Phlyctenular disease, unilateral or bilateral, presents with tearing, discomfort or pain, and photophobia. Corneal phlyctenulosis will cause more severe symptoms than conjunctival involvement alone. Unilateral interstitial keratitis acutely presents as a tearing, photophobic, red eye. In inactive cases, the patient may be unaware of past red eyes or current corneal scarring.

Scleritis will produce a painful, diffusely or sectorally red eye. Tearing, photophobia, and decreased vision may occur. Uveitis (unilateral or bilateral) may present with a red, painful, photophobic, tearing eye, if acute. Acuity is variably affected. Chronic cases have fewer symptoms. Choroiditis may present as a blurry, painful, photophobic eye with the complaint of floaters. Sheathing of retinal vessels may be seen. In the case of choroidal or retinal manifestations, fluorescein angiography may be necessary to determine the extent of chorioretinal involvement, capillary closure, and the existence of neovascularization. Toxic optic neuropathy may be diagnosed by decreased visual acuity, visual field defects (central or peripheral), and abnormal green color vision.

Suspected ocular manifestations of TB require a systemic TB workup. At minimum, a tuberculin skin test should be performed. If positive, or if the clinician has a high index of suspicion, further testing should be done. A chest x-ray is mandated, with smears and cultures of bodily fluids or tissues performed as needed.

Ocular TB testing may include histopathologic examination of ocular tissues (eg, conjunctival scraping or chori-

oretinal biopsy). Purulent discharge from a conjunctivitis or scleritis may be cultured. If necessary, both the aqueous and vitreous may be cultured.

TREATMENT AND MANAGEMENT

Combination therapy of TB is required to avoid drug resistance problems (Table 54–3). Chemotherapy may last longer than 1 year, although multiple drug regimens have shortened treatment times. Compliance problems in some patients have led to dose adjustments from daily to twice weekly delivery under the direct supervision of a healthcare provider. Anti-TB drugs must be used with caution in patients with other

TABLE 54–3. TREATMENT AND MANAGEMENT OF TB

SYSTEMIC: PULMONARY AND EXTRAPULMONARY TB
- First-line Medications
  Therapy regimen for minimum 6 months (standard), minimum 9 months (HIV/AIDS and extrapulmonary TB), up to 18–24 months (MDR TB)
  Doses listed below are for adults; pediatric doses are similar or lower
  Isoniazid (INH) 5–10 mg/kg/d (max 300 mg/d) or 15 mg/kg (max 900 mg) twice weekly (consider adding pyridoxine 10–50 mg/d) *plus*
  Rifampin (RIF) 10 mg/kg/d (max 600 mg/d) or 10 mg/kg/d (max 600 mg) twice weekly *plus*
  Pyrazinamide (PZA) 15–30 mg/kg/d (max 2 g/d) or 50–70 mg/kg (max 4 g) twice weekly *plus*
  Ethambutol (EMB) 15–25 mg/kg/d (max 2.5 g/d) or 50 mg/kg (max 2.5 g) twice weekly *or*
  Streptomycin (SM) 15 mg/kg/d (max 1 g/d) or 25–30 mg/kg (max 1.5 g) twice weekly

- Second-line Medications
  Used in case of hypersensitivity reaction or multi-drug resistance
  Ethionamide 500–1000 mg
  Cycloserine 250–1000 mg (pyridoxine 150 mg/d recommended adjunct therapy)
  Para-aminosalicylate 10–12 g
  Capreomycin 15 mg/kg
  Kanamycin 15 mg/kg
  Amikacin 15 mg/kg

- Experimental Medications
  Spiropiperidyl rifamycin
  Fluoroquinolones
  ß-lactam agents and ß-lactamase inhibitors

- Other
  Occasional oral corticosteroid use
  Rare surgical intervention

OCULAR
- Always start with systemic treatment
- **Tubercles—Granulomas**
  Systemic treatment only
- **Conjunctivitis**
  Warm compresses
  Artificial tears
- **Phlyctenular Keratoconjunctivitis**
  Topical steroids (eg, 1.0% prednisolone acetate q2h to qid depending on severity) with rapid taper
  Broad-spectrum antibiotic if secondary bacterial infection exists
- **Interstitial Keratitis**
  Acute:
    Topical steroids (eg, 1.0% prednisolone acetate q1h to qid with slow taper)
    Topical cycloplegics (eg, 5% homatropine bid to tid)
  Inactive:
    Consider corneal transplant surgery if central cornea involved
- **Scleritis**
  NSAIDs (eg, ibuprofen 400–600 mg po qid or indomethacin 25 mg po tid × 1 week)
  Oral prednisone 60–80 mg qd with slow taper
  Note: Oral steroid treatment requires concurrent systemic anti-TB treatment
- **Anterior Uveitis**
  Topical steroids (eg, 1.0% prednisolone acetate q1h to qid)
  Cycloplegics (eg, 1.0% cyclopentolate, 2 or 5% homatropine, or 0.25% scopolamine bid to tid)
- **Disseminated Choroiditis**
  Photocoagulation may be necessary if widespread capillary dropout or neovascularization occurs
- **Retinal Vasculitis**
  Panretinal photocoagulation if widespread capillary dropout or neovascularization is present
- **Optic Neuropathy Secondary to EMB**
  Reversible with early prompt discontinuation of EMB

conditions (eg, liver or kidney dysfunction, gout, diabetes, pregnancy) due to their potentially serious side effects. The most serious and disturbing new challenge in TB today is MDR TB. This entity has created much alarm in the healthcare community, and has prompted the CDC to change drug regimen recommendations.

■ Systemic

Pulmonary TB

The first-line medications commonly used are isoniazid (INH), rifampin (RIF), pyrazinamide (PZA), ethambutol (EMB), and streptomycin (SM). Due to potential toxic side effects, baseline tests may be recommended prior to starting therapy. These may include liver and kidney function tests, complete blood count, audiometry, and visual acuity testing. INH, RIF, and PZA may each induce hepatitis. INH increases urinary excretion of pyroxidine. This may lead to pellagra (a disorder due to a deficiency of niacin), particularly in malnourished, pregnant, uremic, or diabetic patients. Therefore, these patients are often given supplemental daily pyroxidine. Gastrointestinal upset can occur with RIF and PZA. PZA may also cause hyperuricemia. EMB may cause optic neuropathy; it should therefore be avoided in very young children, because visual acuity and color testing is difficult. SM may alter hearing and vestibular function, as well as be toxic to the kidney. Hypersensitivity reactions may occur with any of the drugs. Monthly monitoring for toxic side effects is extremely important.

In the face of acquired drug resistance, second-line medications may be necessary. These include ethionamide, cyclosporine, para-aminosalicylate, capreomycin, kanamycin, and amikacin. These may also cause serious toxic side effects, requiring routine monitoring and possibly precluding their use.

The CDC-recommended drug regimens for TB in HIV negative or positive adults or children are usually the same with two exceptions. Drug doses in children are lower, and therapy lasts longer in HIV-positive patients (usually a minimum of 9 months versus the standard minimum of 6 months). There are several different options in terms of drug combinations and length of therapy. Traditionally, INH and RIF are used, along with a third medication (PZA, EMB, or SM) in order to shorten the duration of the therapeutic regimen. In response to the rise of MDR TB, the latest CDC recommendation (1993) is to initiate four-drug therapy routinely with INH, RIF, PZA, and EMB or SM. This initial four-drug regimen may be altered after drug susceptibility testing has been done.

When MDR TB is suspected in a patient, the four-drug regimen should be instituted along with one or two additional anti-TB drugs. Testing must be done to ensure that the resistant strain is susceptible to at least three of the

medications. The drug regimen must be lengthened to as long as 18 to 24 months. Cure rates, usually close to 100%, drop to 60% or less in the face of both INH and RIF resistance (CDC, 1992a). New experimental anti-TB medications are under investigation to simplify drug regimens and to aid in the treatment of drug-resistant TB. These include spiropiperidyl rifamycin, fluoroquinolones, and combinations of β-lactam agents and β-lactamase inhibitors.

Treatment during pregnancy is essential with a few provisos. SM may cause congenital deafness and therefore should be avoided, as should PZA, because its effects on the developing fetus are uncertain. With the recommended four-drug regimen now unavailable (two of the available five anti-TB drugs have been eliminated due to teratogenicity), treatment must be extended for 9 months. Despite the presence of these drugs in breast milk, the concentrations are so low that they will cause neither adverse nor therapeutic effects on a nursing infant.

Extrapulmonary TB

Extrapulmonary TB follows the same treatment regimens as pulmonary TB, although the duration of therapy may be extended to 9 months, with occasional corticosteroid use and rare surgical intervention.

■ Ocular

Ocular manifestations of TB are treated with standard systemic anti-TB regimens, along with ocular medications when indicated (Table 54–3). Conjunctivitis is treated with warm compresses and artificial tears. Phlyctenular keratoconjunctivitis is typically treated with topical steroids (with taper), and topical antibiotics for secondary infections. Acute interstitial keratitis may be managed with topical steroids (with slow taper) and cycloplegics. Corneal transplant surgery should be considered in inactive disease with central corneal scarring.

Scleritis calls for systemic medications—nonsteroidal antiinflammatory drugs (NSAIDs) or oral steroids. Oral corticosteroids, given in isolation to control severe ocular inflammation, may cause a reactivation of latent infection, and therefore should only be given after anti-TB therapy has been instituted. Chorioretinal involvement may require pan or sector retinal photocoagulation to treat or prevent neovascularization. Toxic optic neuropathy due to EMB is treated by immediate replacement of the medication. Normal visual functioning returns if the drug is discontinued early enough.

■ Prevention

Table 54–4 gives an overview of TB preventative measures.

Vaccination

Preventing the transmission or reactivation of TB involves many factors. Vaccination has long been employed

TABLE 54–4. PREVENTION OF TB

Ventilation and Housing

Good ventilation, with increased daylight, and no recirculation of air
Negative pressure hospital rooms with 6 air changes per hour
Ultraviolet irradiation
Surgical masks have questionable efficacy

Screening

PPD testing and chest x-rays of certain populations:
   HIV/AIDS patients
   Persons in close contact with suspected or known TB patients
   Persons with medical conditions known to increase risk of
     contracting TB after exposure
   Alcohol or IV drug abusers
   Foreign-born persons from countries with high TB prevalence
   Medically underserved persons
   Residents of long-term facilities (correctional facilities, mental
     institutions, nursing homes)
   Healthcare workers in repeated contact with high-risk or infected
     patients

Prophylactic Therapy

Usually INH for 6–12 months
Recommended for certain populations:
  (+) PPD ≥5 mm *plus* close recent TB contact, suspected or
    definitive HIV infection, or radiographic evidence of old
    pulmonary TB
  (+) PPD ≥10 mm *plus* other high risk factors: recent PPD
    conversion, HIV (–) IV drug abusers, or concurrent medical
    conditions increasing TB risk
  (+) PPD ≥10 mm *plus* ≤35 years and part of high incidence group:
    foreign born in high TB prevalence countries, low-income
    medically underserved or resident of long-term-care facility
  (+) PPD ≥15 mm *plus* ≤35 years with no risk factors, and of a low-
    incidence group

throughout the world to combat TB. Unfortunately, the current available vaccine, BCG (bacille Calmette-Guérin), has variable reported efficacy. Despite this, there is widespread use of BCG, particularly in countries where TB is highly prevalent. In the United States, TB is not considered a large enough health hazard to warrant implementation of a nationwide vaccination program. Derived from in vitro attenuation of *M. bovis*, BCG is a live vaccine, and therefore should be avoided in immuno-suppressed patients due to the risk of adverse reactions. Newer vaccines produced by monoclonal antibodies or recombinant DNA are under investigation (Wiegeshaus & Smith, 1989).

Ventilation and Housing

Improved ventilation with increased available daylight in public housing and institutions (correctional facilities, mental health facilities, and so on) are important in decreasing the risk of TB transmission. Hospitals should

isolate actively infectious TB patients in negative pressure rooms with six air changes per hour. Air should not be recirculated in any facility treating TB patients. Although these ventilation issues are crucial, they are also costly to institutions that may require significant remodeling in order to meet these standards. Instituting ultraviolet irradiation may be less costly and still quite effective (Iseman, 1992).

Teaching infected patients to cover their mouths when coughing or sneezing is important. Due to the minute size of the aerosolized TB-infected droplets, common surgical masking devices are not particularly effective in preventing transmission.

However, masking devices with HEPA (high efficiency particulate air) filters called particulate respirators are more effective and have been recommended for use. These devices are available as disposable respirators (with one HEPA filter) and as reusable purifying respirators (with 2 HEPA filters). Implementation has been met with some resistance due to the significantly higher cost of these devices as compared to standard surgical masks, as well as the discomfort these respirators cause the wearer.

Screening

Screening for TB through tuberculin skin testing and chest x-rays for positive reactors are key weapons in the fight against TB. The following populations should be screened: HIV-positive patients, those in close contact with suspected or known TB patients, persons with medical conditions known to increase the risk of contracting TB after exposure, alcohol and/or intravenous drug abusers, persons from countries where TB is common, medically underserved persons, residents of long-term care facilities, and healthcare workers in repeated contact with high-risk or infected populations.

Prophylactic Therapy

The goal of prophylactic therapy is to prevent reactivation of a latent infection. INH has been found to decrease the incidence of reactivation by 54 to 88% (Levin et al, 1993). The criteria for preventive TB therapy are determined by age, risk factors, and incidence group.

Therapy is recommended for persons of all ages with a positive PPD (5 mm or more) plus close recent TB contact, concurrent suspected or definitive HIV infection, or evidence of old TB on chest x-ray. Treatment is also recommended for patients of all ages with a positive PPD (10 mm or more) plus a high-risk factor. High-risk factors include recent PPD conversion, HIV-negative intravenous substance abuse, or concurrent medical conditions known to increase the risk of TB. Patients with a positive PPD (10 mm or more), no known high-risk factors, but part of a high-incidence group (foreign-born from high-prevalence country, low-income medically underserved, or resident of long-term-care institution) are candidates for therapy.

Patients with a positive PPD (15 mm or more), no risk factors, belonging to a low-incidence group, should be treated if 35 years of age or younger.

Standard prophylaxis is INH therapy for 6 to 12 months. Monthly monitoring is key to diagnosing adverse drug effects. Hepatotoxicity is more common in those 35 years and older. If the TB is INH resistant, rifampin may be used instead.

Public Health Orders

Most states have various public health orders concerning the prevention, containment, and treatment of TB. These controls may include emergency detention, medical examination, isolation, quarantine, and directly observed therapy. Many states also have the power to enforce criminal penalties (from misdemeanors to felonies) for violating a TB public health order (Gostin, 1993).

CONCLUSION

TB is no longer a vanishing disease. Its resurgence, particularly in the form of multidrug-resistant TB, is extremely troubling. Public education, widespread screening (especially of high-risk groups), and treatment are crucial to the eradication of this ancient disease. Eyecare practitioners should be alert and suspicious when confronted with an apparently idiopathic uveitis, particularly if in a patient at high risk for TB. The vigilance of all healthcare providers is necessary to successfully combat this disease.

REFERENCES

Aclimandos WA, Kerr-Muir M. Tuberculous keratoconjunctivitis. *Br J Ophthalmol.* 1992;76:175–176.

Barondes MJ, Sponsel WE, Stevens TS, Plotnick RD. Tuberculous choroiditis diagnosed by chorioretinal endobiopsy. *Am J Ophthalmol.* 1991;112:460–461.

Beck-Sagué C, Dooley SW, Hutton MD, et al. Hospital outbreak of multidrug-resistant *Mycobacterium tuberculosis* infections: Factors in transmission to staff and HIV-infected patients. *JAMA.* 1992;268:1280–1286.

Bloch AB, Reider HL, Kelly GD, et al. The epidemiology of tuberculosis in the United States: Implications for diagnosis and treatment. *Clin Chest Med.* 1989;10:297–313.

Blodi BA, Johnson MW, McLeish WM, Gass JDM. Presumed choroidal tuberculosis in a human immunodeficiency virus infected host. *Am J Ophthalmol.* 1989;108:605–607.

Braun MM, Coté TR, Rabkin CS. Trends in death with tuberculosis during the AIDS era. *JAMA.* 1993;269:2865–2868.

Brisson-Noel A, Aznar C, Chureau C, et al. Diagnosis of tuberculosis by DNA amplification in clinical practice evaluation. *Lancet.* 1991;338:364–366.

Burgoyne CF, Verstraeten TC, Friberg TR. Tuberculin skin-test-induced uveitis in the absence of tuberculosis. *Graefe's Arch Clin Exp Ophthalmol.* 1991;229:232–236.

Centers for Disease Control. Initial therapy for tuberculosis in the era of multidrug resistance. Recommendations of the Advisory Council for the Elimination of Tuberculosis. *MMWR.* 1993;42:1–8.

Centers for Disease Control. National action plan to combat multidrug resistant tuberculosis. Meeting the challenge of multidrug resistant tuberculosis: Summary of a conference; management of persons exposed to multidrug resistant tuberculosis. *MMWR.* 1992a;41:5–8, 49–57, 59–71.

Centers for Disease Control. Prevention and control of tuberculosis in U.S. communities with at-risk minority populations. Recommendations of the Advisory Council for the Elimination of Tuberculosis. Prevention and control of tuberculosis among homeless persons: Recommendations of the Advisory Council for the Elimination of Tuberculosis. *MMWR.* 1992b;41:1–15.

Centers for Disease Control. Purified protein derivative (PPD), tuberculin anergy and HIV infection: Guidelines for anergy testing and management of anergic persons at risk of tuberculosis. *MMWR.* 1991;40:27–33.

Centers for Disease Control. Screening for tuberculosis and tuberculosis infection in high risk populations. *MMWR.* 1990;39:1–7.

Centers for Disease Control. The use of preventive therapy for tuberculosis infection in the United States: Recommendations of the Advisory Committee for the Elimination of Tuberculosis. *MMWR.* 1990;39:9–12.

Chaulet P, Mulder D. Tuberculosis. In: Manson-Bahr PEC, Bell DR, eds. *Manson's Tropical Diseases.* London: Baillière-Tindall; 1987:987–997.

Comstock GW, O'Brien RJ. Tuberculosis. In: Evans AS, Brachman PS, eds. *Bacterial Infections of Humans: Epidemiology and Control.* New York: Plenum; 1990:745–771.

Cook CD, Hainsworth, M. Tuberculosis of the conjunctive occurring in association with a neighboring lupus vulgaris. *Br J Ophthalmol.* 1990;74:315–318.

Daniel TM. Rapid diagnosis of tuberculosis: laboratory techniques applicable in developing countries. *Rev Infect Dis.* 1989;11(suppl 2):S471–S478.

Daniel TM, Tripathy SP. Tuberculosis. In: Warren KS, Mahmoud AAF, eds. *Tropical and Geographical Medicine.* New York: McGraw-Hill; 1990:839–851.

Dannenberg AM. Immune mechanisms in the pathogenesis of pulmonary tuberculosis. *Rev Infect Dis.* 1989;11(suppl 2):S369–S378.

Dickensheets DL. Tuberculosis makes a comeback: Giving and interpreting the Mantoux test. *Postgrad Med.* 1989;86:97–108.

Dooley SW, Jarvis WR, Martone WJ, Snider DE. Multidrug-resistant tuberculosis. *Ann Intern Med.* 1992;117:257–259.

Edlin BR, Tokars JI, Grieco MH, et al. An outbreak of multidrug-resistant tuberculosis among hospitalized patients with the acquired immunodeficiency syndrome. *N Engl J Med.* 1992;326:1514–1521.

Fine PEM. The BCG story: Lessons from the past and implications for the future. *Rev Infect Dis.* 1989;11(suppl 2):S353–S359.

Frieden TR, Sterling T, Pablos-Mendez A, et al. The emergence of drug-resistant tuberculosis in New York City. *N Engl J Med.* 1993;328:521–526.

Gostin LO. Controlling the resurgent tuberculosis epidemic. A 50 state survey of the TB statutes and proposals for reform. *JAMA.* 1993;269:255–261.

Good RC. Serologic methods for diagnosing tuberculosis. *Ann Intern Med.* 1989;110:97–98.

Good RC, Mastro TD. The modern mycobacteriology laboratory: How it can help the clinician. *Clin Chest Med.* 1989;10:315–322.

Gross J, Gross FJ, Friedman AH. Tuberculosis. In: Tasman W, Jaeger EA, eds. *Duane's Clinical Ophthalmology.* Hagerstown, MD: Harper & Row; 1992;5:21–23.

Hamrick RM, Yeager H, Tuberculosis update. *Am Fam Physician.* 1988;38:205–213.

Hopewell PC. Impact of human immunodeficiency virus infection on the epidemiology, clinical features, management, and control of tuberculosis. *Clin Infect Dis.* 1992;15:540–547.

Iseman MD. A leap of faith: What can we do to curtail intrainstitutional transmission of tuberculosis. *Ann Intern Med.* 1992;117:251–253.

Iseman MD. Drug-resistant tuberculosis: New threats from an old disease. *Postgrad Med.* 1989;86:109–114.

Iseman MD. Treatment of multidrug-resistant tuberculosis. *N Engl J Med.* 1993;329:784–791.

Iseman MD, Goble M. Treatment of tuberculosis. *Adv Intern Med.* 1988;33:253–266.

Iseman MD, Madsen LA. Drug-resistant tuberculosis. *Clin Chest Med.* 1989;10:341–353.

Jereb JA, Kelly GD, Dooley SW, et al. Tuberculosis morbidity in the United States: Final data, 1990. CDC surveillance summaries, December 1991. *MMWR.* 1991;40:23–27.

Johnson MP, Coberly JS, Clermont HC, et al. Tuberculin skin test reactivity among adults infected with human immunodeficiency virus. *J Infect Dis.* 1992;166:194–198.

Kim JY, Carroll CP, Opremcak EM. Antibiotic-resistant tuberculosis choroiditis. *Am J Ophthalmol.* 1993;115:259–261.

Kochi A. The global tuberculosis situation and the new control strategy of the World Health Organization. *Tubercle.* 1991;72:1–6.

Levin AC, Gums JG, Grauer K. Tuberculosis: The primary care physician's role in eradication. *Postgrad Med.* 1993;93:46–60.

Lordi GM, Reichman LB. Treatment of tuberculosis. *Am Fam Physician.* 1991;44:219–224.

Mansour AM, Haymond R. Choroidal tuberculomas without evidence of extraocular tuberculosis. *Graefe's Arch Clin Exp Ophthalmol.* 1990;228:382–385.

Nanda M, Pflugfelder SC, Holand S. Mycobacterium tuberculosis scleritis. *Am J Ophthalmol.* 1989;108:736–737.

Near KA, Lefford MJ. Use of serum antibody and lysozyme levels for diagnosis of leprosy and tuberculosis. *J Clin Microbiol.* 1992;30:1105–1110.

Palittapongarnpim P, Chomy S. Fanning A, Kunimoto D. DNA fragment length polymorphism analysis of *Mycobacterium tuberculosis* isolates by arbitrarily primed polymerase chain reaction. *J Infect Dis.* 1993;167:975–978.

Parenti F. New experimental drugs for the treatment of tuberculosis. *Rev Infect Dis.* 1989;11(suppl 2):S479–S483.

Pearson ML, Jereb JA, Frieden TR, et al. Nosocomial transmission of multidrug-resistant *Mycobacterium tuberculosis. Ann Intern Med.* 1992;117:191–196.

Pérez-Stable EJ, Hopewell PC. Current tuberculosis regimens: Choosing the right one for your patient. *Clin Chest Med.* 1989;10:323–339.

Pitchenik AE, Fertel D, Bloch AB. Mycobacterial disease: Epidemiology, diagnosis, treatment, and prevention. *Clin Chest Med.* 1988;9:425–441.

Psilas K, Aspiotis M, Petroutsos G, et al. Antituberculosis therapy in the treatment of peripheral uveitis. *Ann Ophthalmol.* 1991;23:254–258.

Pust RE. Tuberculosis in the 1990s: Resurgence, regimens, and resources. *South Med J.* 1992;85:584–593.

Quinn TC. Interactions of the human immunodeficiency virus and tuberculosis and the implications for BCG vaccination. *Rev Infect Dis.* 1989;11(suppl 2):S379–S384.

Regillo CD, Shields CL, Shields JA, et al. Ocular tuberculosis. *JAMA.* 1991;266:1490.

Rieder HL, Cauthen GM, Kelly GD, et al. Tuberculosis in the United States. *JAMA.* 1989;262:385–389.

Rieder HL, Snider DE, Cauthen GM. Extrapulmonary tuberculosis in the United States. *Am Rev Respir Dis.* 1990;141:347–351.

Rosen PH, Spalton DJ, Graham EM. Intraocular tuberculosis. *Eye.* 1990;4:486–492.

Small PM, Schecter GF, Goodman PC, et al. Treatment of tuberculosis in patients with advanced human immunodeficiency virus infection. *N Engl J Med.* 1991;324:289–294.

Smith MHD. Tuberculosis in children and adolescents. *Clin Chest Med.* 1989;10:381–395.

Stead WW. Pathogenesis of tuberculosis: Clinical and epidemiologic perspective. *Rev Infect Dis.* 1989;11(suppl 2):S366–S368.

Stead WW. Special problems in tuberculosis: Tuberculosis in the elderly, and in residents of nursing homes, correctional facilities, long-term care hospitals, mental hospitals, shelters for the homeless, and jails. *Clin Chest Med.* 1989;10:397–405.

Stead WW, Dutt AK. Tuberculosis in elderly persons. *Ann Rev Med.* 1991;42:267–276.

Stead WW, Senner JW, Reddick WT, Lofgren JP. Racial differences in susceptibility to infection by *Mycobacterium tuberculosis. N Engl J Med.* 1990;322:422–427.

Sudre P, ten Dam G, Kochi A. Tuberculosis: A global overview of the situation today. *Bull WHO.* 1992;70:149–159.

Van Scoy RE, Wilkowske CJ. Antituberculous agents. *Mayo Clin Proc.* 1992;67:179–187.

Wiegeshaus EH, Smith DW. Evaluation of the protective potency of new tuberculosis vaccines. *Rev Infect Dis.* 1989;11(suppl 2):S484–S490.

55
Chapter

Leprosy (Hansen Disease)

Esther S. Marks

Leprosy is an ancient disease, first noted over 2000 years ago. It is a chronic granulomatous infection caused by the organism *Mycobacterium leprae*. It principally affects the skin and peripheral nerves of the cooler regions of the body: face, anterior portion of the eyes, upper respiratory tract, extremities, and testes. The incredible stigma once associated with leprosy and its dreaded deformities persists even today in some parts of the world. Infected persons continue to be shunned by their families and communities. Once confined to leper colonies to live out the remainder of their lives in isolation, the care of leprosy victims today is changing.

First mentioned in the United States in 1758, leprosy is believed to have made its way to the Americas through Spanish explorations and the slave trade. In 1873, Gerhard Henrik Armauer Hansen identified the organism *M. leprae* from a patient with advanced leprosy. To this day, many prefer to refer to the infection as Hansen disease, both in homage to the scientist and in recognition of the stigma attached to the word leprosy.

The disease may take several forms. The two major types are called lepromatous leprosy and tuberculoid leprosy. Lepromatous leprosy is chiefly responsible for the disfiguring deformities associated with the disease, and is considerably more infectious, with millions of organisms (multibacillary) found in the host's tissues and bodily fluids. Tuberculoid leprosy is much less infectious, with few organisms (paucibacillary) demonstrated in histopathologic examinations.

EPIDEMIOLOGY

■ Systemic

The number of registered cases of leprosy worldwide is approximately 5.5 million. This may not be a reliable indication of the true number of cases, as estimates from many countries are questionable due to poor reporting. It is estimated that 10 to 15 million cases actually exist. Most occur in endemic areas of Africa, Asia, the Pacific region, and Latin America.

In the United States, the annual incidence is about 0.07 per 100,000 (Ross & Barr, 1991). The overwhelming majority (90%) are imported cases (brought into the United States by already infected individuals from endemic countries). This was responsible for the increase of cases seen in the United States from 1975 to 1988, following waves of Southeast Asian refugees (Mastro et al, 1992) as well as increases in the number of Mexican and Caribbean immigrants (Jacobson, 1990). Most imported and indigenous cases occur in Texas, Hawaii, Louisiana, and California, although New York and Florida also report more cases than other states. There is no evidence of an imported case of leprosy resulting in transmission in the United States (Mastro et al, 1992).

The median age of onset is 20 to 30 years of age. Racial and sexual predilections vary with the type of leprosy. In lepromatous leprosy, males are affected more than females at a ratio of almost 2 to 1, whereas in tuberculoid leprosy the ratio is almost 1 to 1. Africans and Indians are more susceptible to tuberculoid leprosy, whereas Caucasians and Orientals are more susceptible to lepromatous leprosy (Ostler, 1990). In the United States, approximately 50% of all leprosy cases are the lepromatous variety. Possible genetic susceptibility has also been theorized. Household contacts of lepromatous leprosy patients run four times the risk of contracting leprosy than the household contacts of tuberculoid leprosy patients, and eight times the risk of noncontacts.

■ Ocular

Leprosy is the third leading cause of blindness worldwide (Johnstone et al, 1991). Ocular manifestations have been reported to occur in up to 90% of all leprosy patients. Although ocular manifestations occur in most forms of leprosy, they occur more frequently in lepromatous leprosy.

NATURAL HISTORY

■ Systemic

The Organism

Mycobacterium leprae is an intracellular obligate gram-positive rod 0.3 to 0.5 μm by 2 to 8 μm. An acid-fast bacillus, it cannot be cultured in vitro (only in vivo, usually using mouse footpads). It grows mainly in macrophages and Schwann cells of peripheral nerves. It prefers cooler temperatures, and therefore tends to limit itself to the skin and peripheral nerves of the extremities, ears, anterior segment of the eyes, and testes.

It is a hardy organism, surviving freezing temperatures and drying out for extended periods of time. Although it does not survive heating, its antigenic properties can continue for some time beyond death of the bacilli. The ability to oxidize dihyrophenylalanine (dopa) is one of its identifying characteristics. Probably one of the most important features of this organism, determining its natural history, is its generation times. Most bacteria have generation times counted in minutes. Some mycobacteria are slower (eg, *M. tuberculosis* can take 14 to 24 hours), *M. leprae* takes 11 to 13 days (Bullock, 1990).

Transmission

Prolonged contact with a leprosy patient has always been considered necessary to become infected. However, more recent evidence suggests that leprosy is considerably more contagious than previously believed, but that its progression to clinically evident disease is quite uncommon. Overwhelmingly, the most common vector for transmission is through the upper respiratory tract via nasal secretions. Transmission through the skin may occur via skin lesions, particularly of lepromatous (multibacillary) leprosy patients. Other vectors are possible, but much less likely (eg, via insects, or in the United States via the armadillo). Once transmitted, a patient may incubate *M. leprae* on average 1 to 7 years prior to clinical expression, although there are reports of incubation periods as short as a few months, and as long as several decades.

Course of the Disease

Although many factors are involved in disease expression (genetics, socioeconomics, environmental factors, exposure to other mycobacteria, and leprosy exposure duration), the patient's immune status is the final determinant as to what the host response will be, and therefore what form of leprosy will manifest (Table 55–1). Cell-mediated immunity (CMI) plays the key role in this determination. Once infected, the vast majority of patients (85 to 95%) will demonstrate intact CMI to leprosy, resulting in bacilli being ingested, destroyed, and disposed of by host macrophages. This occurs without any clinical signs. However, in 5 to 15% of patients, a deficient CMI exists, resulting in the ingestion of bacilli by macrophages without complete recognition of the parasite as foreign. This allows the microorganism to multiply and spread, directly and hematogenously. In this case clinical signs will develop, and the condition is called indeterminate leprosy.

Most commonly, one or more hypopigmented (or occasionally erythematous) macules will appear on the skin of the face, neck, extremities, or buttocks. The center of the lesions may be slightly hypesthetic. If biopsied, the lesions would reveal granulomatous formations but no bacilli. Approximately 75% of patients with indeterminate leprosy will heal spontaneously. The remaining 25% will progress on to another form of leprosy.

Patients with partially functioning CMI develop tuberculoid leprosy (TT). At the other end of the spectrum are patients with little or no functioning CMI to leprosy. These patients develop lepromatous leprosy (LL). The rest of the patients fall in between these two spectrums, developing borderline tuberculoid (BT), borderline (BB), or borderline lepromatous (BL) leprosy. These borderline forms are not static, but may shift toward one or the other end of the spectrum in what is called a reactional state.

Tuberculoid leprosy (TT) is characterized by one or two large skin lesions in cooler regions of the body. They are flat, hairless, hypopigmented, and hypesthetic with or without raised borders. Biopsy of the lesion will reveal epithelioid granulomas with giant cells surrounded by lymphocytes. One or two peripheral nerves may be swollen or thickened due to invasion or damage, and abscesses can occur. Sensory and motor dysfunction may result. Few bacilli are seen; therefore TT is also referred to as

TABLE 55–1. SYSTEMIC MANIFESTATIONS OF LEPROSY

INDETERMINATE LEPROSY
- Skin
    Hypopigmented skin macule on face, neck, extremities or buttocks
- Nerve
    Skin lesion may have hypesthetic center

TUBERCULOID (TT) AND BORDERLINE TUBERCULOID (BT) LEPROSY
- Skin
    Large, flat, hairless, hypopigmented lesions on cooler body regions
- Nerve
    Peripheral nerve swelling and thickening
    Sensory and motor dysfunction (eg, facial palsy and hypesthesia)
    Abscesses
    Secondary muscle atrophy

BORDERLINE (BB), BORDERLINE LEPROMATOUS (BL), AND LEPROMATOUS (LL) LEPROSY
- Skin
    Multiple, erythematous, elevated lesions (nodular, papular, or macular)
    Shiny, smooth taut appearance (resembles scleroderma)
    Thickened ears
    Leonine facies
- Mucous membranes
    Nasal stuffiness, epistaxis, mucous discharge
    Hoarseness
    Saddle nose deformity
- Extremities
    Brawny edema of lower legs, feet, hands (sausage-like fingers)
    Bone erosion and resorption in fingers and toes
- Nerve
    Swelling and thickening of peripheral nerves
    Bilateral polyneuropathy
    Hypesthesia
    Motor dysfunction with muscle atrophy
- Testes
    Atrophy and infertility
- Other
    Risk of deformity from repeated trauma due to hypesthesia
    Risk of secondary infections

REACTIONAL STATES
- **Upgrading and Downgrading Reactions**
    Fever
    Inflammation of skin lesions
    Neuritis
        Permanent sensory & motor dysfunction may occur
        Secondary muscle atrophy and hypesthesia
- **Erythema Nodosum Leprosum**
    General malaise, fever, arthralgia
    Erythematous, painful nodular rash
    Lymphadenitis, nephritis
    Orchitis, pretibial periosteitis
    Iridocyclitis
    Neuritis
        Permanent sensory and motor dysfunction may occur (eg, clawlike hand deformities or foot drop)

paucibacillary. Borderline tuberculoid leprosy (BT) involves more extensive lesions, with nerves commonly involved. Once again, few bacilli are found on biopsy; BT is also referred to as paucibacillary.

Borderline leprosy (BB) is characterized by many lesions. Usually the lesions are irregularly shaped, erythematous, and raised with punched-out centers. Numerous superficial nerves may be thickened. On biopsy, epithelioid granulomas are seen without giant cells, but with multiple bacilli. Therefore, BB is termed multibacillary.

Borderline lepromatous leprosy (BL) demonstrates multiple lesions of various forms (Figure 55–1). Nerve damage frequently occurs, resulting in both painful and hypesthetic nerves. The hands and feet become insensitive, leaving them prone to secondary infection due to trauma. Neurotrophic changes such as plantar ulcers may occur. Biopsy will demonstrate macrophage granulomas with multiple bacilli, termed multibacillary.

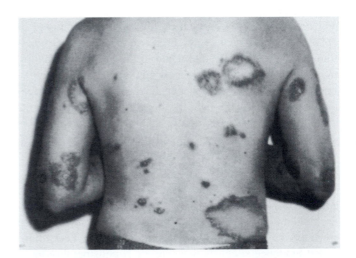

Figure 55–1. Multiple borderline lepromatous leprosy skin lesions. *(Courtesy of W. Meyers, Armed Forces Institute of Pathology.)*

Lepromatous leprosy (LL), also known as multibacillary, is characterized by disseminated and extensive progressive skin involvement (Figure 55–2). The diffuse, erythematous lesions may be macular, papular, or nodular, occurring in the cooler regions of the body. Biopsies of lesions will demonstrate macrophage granulomas and multiple bacilli. Heavy skin infiltration occurs producing a shiny, smooth appearance to the skin. The facial skin becomes thickened, deepening the natural lines of the forehead, which with thickened ears and nose produces a leonine facies. Loss of eyebrows and eyelashes may occur.

Infiltration also occurs in the mucous membranes of the upper respiratory tract, including the larynx, palate, root of the tongue, peritonsillar tissue, and nose. Patients often complain of nasal stuffiness, mucous discharge (filled with multiple bacilli), epistaxis, and hoarseness. Nasomaxillary damage occurs. The nasal cartilage and septum may be destroyed by progressive infection with edematous thickening and ulceration. The bridge of the nose may collapse, leading to a saddle nose deformity.

Edema of the lower legs, feet, and hands may occur. The fingers of the hands may become quite swollen and sausage-like, with a shiny taut appearance (resembling scleroderma) due to skin infiltration. Nerve damage occurs late in LL. Although nerve abscesses may occur, nerve damage is usually diffuse, presenting as an asymmetric polyneuropathy, with motor dysfunction and muscle atrophy. Facial palsies may occur. Insensitive hands and feet are prone to damage from repeated trauma or secondary infection, leading to bone resorption in the fingers and toes. Bone erosion in the fingers and toes may also occur due to granulomas.

Granulomatous infiltration of the testicles may occur, leading to atrophy and infertility. Secondary gynecomastia may result. Ovaries are rarely affected, being in a warmer region of the body. However, granulomatous changes have been seen in the lymph nodes, spleen, and liver (Bullock, 1990), particularly during reactional states.

Reactional states are the result of changes in the host's immune status. They may occur in treated or untreated leprosy. Upgrading reactions (type 1 or reversal reactions) and downgrading reactions occur in BT, BB, and BL leprosy. Upgrading reactions are believed to be due to an increase in CMI or a delayed hypersensitivity reaction to leprosy antigens, because on histologic examination a decrease in bacilli is noted along with increased lymphocytes. These reactions are therefore termed upgrading reactions to designate an improvement in the host's immune reaction. Downgrading reactions denote a shift towards LL due to a decrease in CMI, with resultant increase in *M. leprae* bacillary load and dissemination of the disease. Both reactions are characterized by fever, inflammation of skin lesions, and neuritis. They can lead to permanent dysfunction of motor and sensory nerves with resulting muscle atrophy, and skin hypesthesia.

Erythema nodosum leprosum (ENL, type 2 reactions) occurs in the BL and LL forms of leprosy. It may also occur in untreated or treated cases. The syndrome manifests as a general malaise, fever, and the appearance of an erythematous painful nodular rash. A proliferative vasculitis occurs. In severe cases the lesions may be large, necrotic, and ulcerative. Arthralgia, lymphadenitis, nephritis, leukocytosis, orchitis (inflammation of the testicles), pretibial periosteitis, iridocyclitis, and neuritis may occur. The neuritis may be severe leading to the same type of permanent nerve and muscle dysfunction as in reversal reactions, with claw-like hand deformities and complete foot drop (due to paralysis of the dorsiflexor muscles in the foot and ankle). Although ENL may resolve without treatment, in the more severe forms it may lead to death.

■ Ocular

Ocular involvement of any type occurs in most forms of leprosy (Table 55–2), and may be due to immune-mediated reactions or infiltration of ocular tissues by *M. leprae*. Paucibacillary forms (TT, BT) are usually characterized by eyelash and eyebrow loss, and complications secondary to fifth and seventh cranial nerve dysfunction. Multibacillary forms (BB, BL, LL) are generally characterized complications due to hematogenous and direct infiltration of anterior ocular structures. Reactional states often develop inflammatory ocular reactions.

Brow loss often begins temporally and proceeds nasally to total loss. Eyelash loss may occur on both upper and lower lids. Lids may become thickened and ptotic from

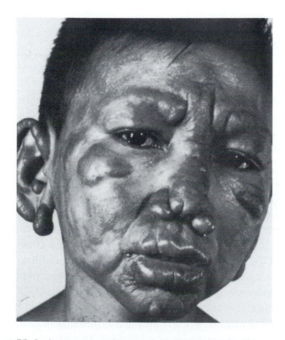

Figure 55–2. Lepromatous leprosy patient with involvement of facial features due to heavy infiltration of skin. *(Courtesy of W. Meyers, Armed Forces Institute of Pathology.)*

TABLE 55–2. OCULAR MANIFESTATIONS OF LEPROSY[a]

LID/ADNEXA
- Brow and lash loss
- Thickened lids
- Ptosis, ectropion
- Lagophthalmos secondary to seventh cranial nerve dysfunction (unilateral or bilateral)

LACRIMAL SYSTEM
- Dacryoadenitis
- Dacryocystitis

CONJUNCTIVA
- Palpebral and limbal lepromas

CORNEA
- Hypesthesia secondary to fifth cranial nerve dysfunction
- Beaded, thickened corneal nerves
- Neurotrophic keratitis with ulceration possible
- Secondary infection
- Pannus and avascular interstitial keratitis

EPISCLERA/SCLERA
- Episcleritis and scleritis due to diffuse inflammation or localized leproma
- Staphyloma or scleromalacia may develop

UVEA
- Iris pearls
- Iris atrophy with miotic pupil
- Anterior uveitis, acute or chronic
- Secondary glaucoma due to anterior or posterior synechiae formation

LENS
- Secondary cataract

[a] May occur in any form of leprosy.

skin infiltration. Infiltration of the seventh cranial nerve may lead to a facial palsy with lagophthalmos and may occur as a presenting sign of TT (Figure 55–3). This then results in a lower lid paralytic ectropion and exposure keratopathy. The cornea becomes desiccated, the conjunctiva hyperemic, and the eye is now subject to secondary infection. Infiltration of the fifth cranial nerve results in loss of corneal sensation. Direct infiltration of the corneal nerves gives rise to a beaded look due to granulomas filled with *M. leprae*. Corneal hypesthesia is quite dangerous, as it may lead to a neurotrophic keratitis, secondary trauma and infection, and even ulceration. Pannus and an avascular stromal interstitial keratitis have also been observed without loss of vision.

Infiltration and involvement of the lacrimal gland, lacrimal ducts, and meibomian glands further contribute to the dry eye. This may be due to direct involvement or secondary to lepromatous destruction of the nasomaxillary structures. Collapse of these structures may aggravate an existing dry eye with epiphora and secondary infections such as dacryoadenitis or dacryocystitis.

Conjunctival involvement is usually related to dry eye secondary to exposure. However, conjunctival and limbal nodules have been noted. These nodules are granulomas, or more specifically lepromas. Episcleritis and scleritis may occur due to a leproma or as a diffuse inflammatory reaction in ENL. Chronic or recurrent bouts may progress to more serious complications including scleromalacia and staphyloma formation.

Uveal tract involvement and its complications, usually occurring in LL or during ENL, is responsible for most of the vision loss in ocular leprosy. The presence of iris pearls is pathognomonic for ocular leprosy. These small lepromas are white particles usually located on the iris surface at the pupillary margin, which look like white grains of sand. Occasionally, they may detach from the iris surface and float in the anterior chamber. Anterior uveitis in leprosy may be chronic or acute, and may be a presenting sign of LL. The uveitis is characterized by cells and flare, and if acute in presentation a conjunctival ciliary flush, photophobia, and discomfort may be present. Chronic uveitis is usually painless unless secondary glaucoma develops due to anterior and posterior synechiae formation. Iris atrophy with miotic pupils due to the preferential destruction of dilator fibers occurs. Secondary cataracts often develop due to longstanding or recurrent inflammation.

DIAGNOSIS

■ Systemic

Inability to culture *M. leprae* in vitro, its long generation time, and its particularly long incubation time can make diagnosis difficult. A thorough physical examination and history are crucial. Key to the diagnosis are the detection of the acid-fast bacilli of *M. leprae* in skin and mucous membrane lesions as well as the demonstration of abnormal nerve function with skin hypesthesia, muscle atrophy, pareses, or paralyses. The clinician must look for characteristic skin lesions and thickened nerve trunks. The patient should be questioned concerning any history of numbness, tingling, or hot and cold sensations of the skin, particularly on the face and extremities.

Histologic examination of lesions via skin and peripheral nerve biopsies, and skin and nasal mucosal smears, should determine the bacterial index (amount of bacilli found using a logarithmic scale) and the morphologic index (indicating organism state, dead or viable). In vitro culturing is impossible, but the bacilli may be cultivated in mouse footpads for drug susceptibility studies.

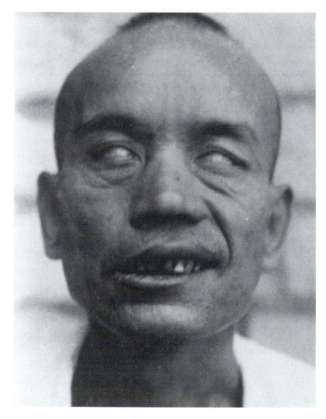 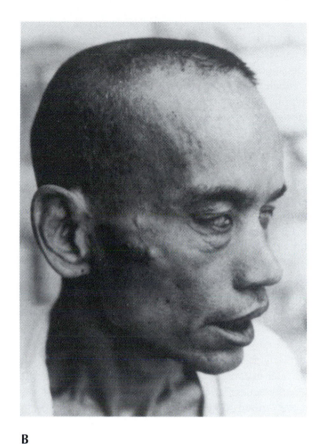

A   B

Figure 55–3. Patient with full facial palsy and resultant lagophthalmos secondary to leprosy. *(Reprinted with permission from Warren G. Facial palsy—A leprosy surgeon's viewpoint. Aus NZ J Ophthalmol. 1990;18:263.)*

The lepromin skin test reaction may be done to determine the type of leprosy. An intradermal injection of *M. leprae* is performed. An early (Fernandez) reaction occurs 48 to 72 hours later, but is of little value due to its variability. A late (Mitsuda) reaction occurs approximately 1 month later. This too is of little diagnostic value, as the majority of healthy uninfected patients will respond positively (3 mm or more induration) to this test. The issue in leprosy patients is what type of leprosy exists. A positive reaction in an infected individual indicates at least partial CMI to leprosy, and therefore it is TT or BT leprosy. A negative reaction in an infected patient indicates a lack of CMI, therefore probably indicative of LL.

Recently standardized serologic tests for leprosy include fluorescent leprosy antibody absorption (FLA-ABS) test, radioimmunoassay (RIA) for *M. leprae* antigens, enzyme-linked immunosorbent assay (ELISA) for antibodies to *M. leprae* specific phenolic glycolipid-I (PGL-I), serum antibody competition test (SACT), and passive hemagglutination (PHA) based on synthetic antigens. Tests employing recombinant DNA technology, specifically polymerase chain reaction (PCR), for the detection of *M. leprae* are under study, as are other DNA probes, such as restriction fragment length polymorphism (RFLP) (Katoch, 1991). General findings often encountered may include positive reaction to C-reactive protein, positive antinuclear antibodies, and elevated erythrocyte sedimentation rate, increased prothrombin time, proteinuria, and leukocytosis, particularly during a reactional state.

■ **Ocular**

Diagnosis of ocular manifestations usually occurs after the systemic diagnosis of leprosy, although anterior uveitis may be a presenting manifestation of previously undiagnosed LL, and lagophthalmos may be a presenting sign of TT. A thorough ocular examination will reveal the characteristic lid, corneal, and uveal involvement as well as any secondary complications. Ocular leprosy is potentially blinding; therefore all leprosy patients should have routine eye examinations.

TREATMENT AND MANAGEMENT

■ **Systemic**

It is estimated that 50% or fewer of registered leprosy cases and 20% or fewer of all leprosy cases are treated. These tremendously low figures are believed to be due to difficulty in establishing the diagnosis; lack of widespread medical care, particularly in endemic parts of the world; lack of public education; and the enormous stigma still attached to leprosy. Much work needs to be done, particularly in educating the public, because the treatment of leprosy, especially if diagnosed early, may be quite successful.

Dapsone (DDS) is a very slow-acting, antileprotic agent that has been used for years as the drug of choice. It requires prolonged treatment time to work. Unfortunately, this monotherapy has resulted in the development of DDS-resistant *M. leprae* organisms. As a result, the World Health Organization (WHO) developed a new multidrug therapy regimen for leprosy victims that requires direct supervision of monthly medications (Table 55–3). The recommendations are that paucibacillary leprosy be treated with daily self-administered doses of dapsone and monthly supervised doses of rifampin for a minimum of 6 months, and that multibacillary leprosy be treated with daily self-administered doses of dapsone, and monthly supervised doses of rifampin and clofazimine for a minimum of 2 years. The more infectious patients (particularly those with LL) are usually noncontagious 1 to 2 weeks after institution of treatment. Supervision is crucial, as the lengthy treatment regimen creates compliance problems.

In the United States, where dapsone resistance is low, standard therapy is dapsone plus rifampin for all leprosy patients. In paucibacillary patients, rifampin is discontinued after 6 months, but dapsone may be continued for several years. Treatment duration for multibacillary patients is highly individualized.

Reactional states require additional treatment, usually steroids, to decrease inflammation and avoid permanent damage. Mild ENL may respond quite well to nonsteroidal antiinflammatory drugs (NSAIDs), but severe ENL requires high-dose steroids. Thalidomide has been found to be quite effective as well. Recurrent or chronic cases should be treated with clofazimine.

Anti-leprotic drugs have different actions and may have some serious side effects. Dapsone is bacteriostatic, and may cause hemolytic anemias (particularly in patients with glucose-6-phosphate dehydrogenase deficiencies). Rifampin is bacteriocidal, and may produce a reddish-brown discoloration of urine, sputum, and sweat. It may also cause gastrointestinal upset, and rarely is hepatotoxic. Clofazimine is an antibacterial drug with antiinflammatory effects. Its main side effect is skin hyperpigmentation. GI upset may also occur. Both are dose related. Ethionamide and prothionamide are bacteriocidal. They are often used in place of clofazimine if the skin hyperpigmentation is unacceptable to the patient. They are both potentially toxic to the liver, and responsible for GI upset. Thalidomide, once used as a sedative, is now known for its teratogenic effects, and is therefore contraindicated in women of childbearing ages. It does not have antibacterial effects, but is active against ENL reactions.

A new shorter anti-leprosy regimen is under investigation by the WHO using ofloxacin and rifampin. If successful, this would be considered a major advance in the battle against leprosy. Immunotherapy is also under investigation for improving CMI.

Other medical, surgical, and rehabilitative treatments are sometimes required in leprosy. Secondary infections must be treated. Nerve abscesses may require drainage. Palsies secondary to nerve involvement may be corrected, and tendon transplantation attempted. Physical and occupational therapy for patients with deformities is important. Special care of insensitive feet is crucial in preventing trauma and secondary infection. Shoes should be fitted carefully with cushioning on the inside. Routine x-rays of the hands and feet should be performed to monitor for bone resorption.

The prognosis for leprosy patients depends on the type of leprosy and how far advanced it is. Tuberculoid leprosy generally has an excellent prognosis. Pigmentation, sensitivity, and enlarged nerves may not entirely return to normal. Patients must continue to practice care of their hands and feet even when the therapeutic drug regimen is discontinued. The relapse rate for TT patients is less than 5%, 3 to 5 years posttherapy. Lepromatous and BL leprosy patients have a more guarded prognosis. The earlier treatment is begun, the better the outcome. These patients tend to have serious deformities and are prone to relapses. However, if the patient suffers from chronic ENL, the outcomeis grave.

Prophylactic therapy is considered to confer a high degree of protection to the household contacts of leprosy patients, particularly those with borderline and lepromatous forms of leprosy. Prophylactic dapsone appears to decrease the risk of contracting leprosy by 40 to 80%. The Centers for Disease Control recommend dapsone therapy for children and young adult household contacts for 3 years, along with annual examinations for 5 years. The examiner should pay close attention to any skin, motor, or sensory changes, and biopsy any suspicious lesions.

The current vaccine available for leprosy is the baccille Calmette-Guérin (BCG). It has been reported to be quite effective (up to 80% protective), especially with several doses, in some areas of the world; however, other areas report little or no protection from leprosy with BCG. The reason for this variation is unknown. Vaccinations using BCG combined with killed *M. leprae* have been studied, with reports of 18% fewer leprosy cases with this combination vaccine. Further research is needed to develop vaccines with consistently high efficacy.

■ Ocular

Ocular treatment first relies on systemic treatment regimens for leprosy as well as for any reactional states (Table 55–3). Brow and lash loss may be cosmetically corrected with makeup, tatooing, or hair grafts. Facial palsies resulting in

TABLE 55–3. TREATMENT AND MANAGEMENT OF LEPROSY

■ **SYSTEMIC**

PAUCIBACILLARY LEPROSY (INDETERMINATE, TT,BT)
- Dapsone 100 mg po daily self-administered
- Rifampin 600 mg po monthly under supervision
    WHO standard: treatment duration 6 months minimum
    U.S. standard: treatment duration 6 months, then discontinue rifampin, but continue dapsone for up to several years

MULTIBACILLARY LEPROSY (BB, BL, LL)
- Dapsone 100 mg po daily self-administered
- Rifampin 600 mg po monthly under supervision
- Clofazimine 300 mg po monthly under supervision *plus* 50 mg po daily self-administered
- If clofazimine is not tolerated then use ethionamide/prothionamide 250–375 mg po daily self-administered
    WHO standard: treatment duration 2 years minimum
    U.S. standard: dapsone plus rifampin (duration individualized)

REACTIONAL STATES
- **Up- or Downgrading Reactions**
    NSAIDs
    Steroids
    Clofazimine 300 mg po daily
- **Erythema Nodosum Leprosum (ENL)**
    Mild: NSAIDs
    Severe: prednisone 60–80 mg po daily with slow taper
        thalidomide 300 mg po daily with slow taper

OTHER TREATMENT MODALITIES
- Medical
    Treatment of secondary infections
    Repeat x-rays to monitor bone damage
- Surgical
    Drainage of nerve abscesses
    Tendon transplantation
- Rehabilitative
    Physical and occupational therapy
    Special care of insensitive feet

PROPHYLAXIS AND PREVENTION
- Prophylaxis
    Recommended for household contacts ≤25 years old of multibacillary leprosy patients
    Treatment duration 3 years, with annual examination for 5 years
    Dose is age dependent (6 mg 3×/wk, 50 mg daily)
- Prevention
    BCG vaccination, several doses

■ **OCULAR**
- Always start with systemic therapy

LIDS/ADNEXA
- Make-up, tattoo, hair grafts
- Tarsorrhaphy

CONJUNCTIVA/CORNEA
- Lubrication: artificial tears solution and ointment prn
- Corneal transplantation

LACRIMAL SYSTEM
- Antibacterial treatment of dacryoadenitis/dacryocystitis

EPISCLERA/SCLERA
- Oral steroids (eg, prednisone 60–80 mg po daily with slow taper—usually patient already being treated with prednisone for ENL)
- Artificial tears prn
- Topical steroids (eg, prednisolone acetate 0.125% qid)

UVEA
- Topical steroids (eg, prednisolone acetate 1% q1–6 h)
- Cycloplegic (eg, homatropine 5% tid)

SECONDARY GLAUCOMA
- Laser iridotomy
- Antiglaucoma medications if necessary

SECONDARY CATARACT
- Extraction

lagophthalmos, ectropion, and exposure keratopathy require lubricating therapy with artificial tear solutions and ointments. If the palsy is permanent, surgical repair (eg, lateral tarsorrhaphy) will provide good functional and cosmetic results.

Corneal involvement requires lubricating therapy, or antibacterial therapy if a secondary infection occurs. If corneal involvement progresses to serious scarring and vision loss, corneal transplantation may be indicated. Episcleritis and scleritis respond best to systemic leprosy

and ENL therapy to decrease inflammation and eliminate lepromas. Topical steroids are of limited use.

Uveal inflammation need not lead to vision loss if appropriately treated. Anterior uveitis (especially if ENL exists concurrently) responds best to systemic leprosy/ENL therapy. Topical steroids and cycloplegics are still required to attempt to avoid anterior and posterior synechiae. Peripheral iridotomy may be required to prevent secondary glaucoma. Should cataracts result from chronic inflammation, surgery is recommended.

Conclusion

Leprosy is a worldwide health problem and has been for centuries. Prevention and control are the keys to eliminating this serious disfiguring and potentially blinding disease. Public education, widespread available medical care, prophylactic treatment, and vaccination programs are necessary to combat this infection. Research into in vitro cultivation in order to better study the organism, laboratory tests for early detection, shorter drug regimens for better compliance, and more effective leprosy vaccines hold great promise for the eradication of this ancient scourge.

References

Becx-Bleumink M. Experience with WHO-recommended multidrug therapy (MDT) for multibacillary (MB) leprosy patients in the Leprosy Control Program of the All Africa Leprosy and Rehabilitation Training Center in Ethiopia: Appraisal of the recommended duration of MDT for MB patients. *Int J Leprosy.* 1991;59:558–568.

Bullock WE. Mycobacterium leprae (leprosy). In: Mandell GL, Douglas RG, Bennett JE, eds. *Principles and Practice of Infectious Diseases.* New York: Churchill Livingstone; 1990:1906–1914.

Cohn ZA, Kaplan G. Hansen's disease, cell-mediated immunity, and recombinant lymphokines. *J Infect Dis.* 1991;163:1195–1200.

Convit J, Sampson C, Zúñiga M, et al. Immunoprophylactic trial with combined *Mycobacterium leprae*/BCG vaccine against leprosy: Preliminary results. *Lancet.* 1992;339:446–450.

Courtright P, Lewallen S, Lee HS. Comparison of the old and new W.H.O. leprosy disability grading scheme for ocular disabilities. *Int Ophthalmol.* 1991;15:295–298.

Dockrell HM, Eastcott H, Young S, et al. Possible transmission of *Mycobacterium leprae* in a group of UK leprosy contacts. *Lancet.* 1991;338:739–743.

ffytche TJ. Ocular leprosy: The continuing challenge. *Int Ophthalmol.* 1991;15:289–293.

ffytche TJ. The continuing challenge of ocular leprosy. *Br J Ophthalmol.* 1991;75:123–124.

Filice GA, Fraser DW. Management of household contacts of leprosy patients. *Ann Int Med.* 1978;88:538–542.

Gunby P. Can leprosy be neutralized by the year 2000? *JAMA.* 1992;276:2289.

Hastings RC, Franzblau SG. Chemotherapy of leprosy. *Ann Rev Pharmacol Toxicol.* 1988;28:231–245.

Hogeweg M, Faber WR. Progression of eye lesions in leprosy: Ten year follow-up study in The Netherlands. *Int J Leprosy.* 1991;59:392–397.

Jacobson RR. Leprosy. In: Evans AS, Brachman PS, eds. *Bacterial Infections of Humans: Epidemiology and Control.* New York: Plenum; 1990:349–366.

Johnstone PAS, George AD, Meyers WM. Ocular lesions in leprosy. *Ann Ophthalmol.* 1991;23:297–303.

Katoch VM. Recent advances in the development of techniques for diagnosis and epidemiology of leprosy. *Indian J Leprosy.* 1991;63:362–370.

Lewallen S, Courtright P, Lee HS. Ocular autonomic dysfunction and intraocular pressure in leprosy. *Br J Ophthalmol.* 1989;73:946–949.

Manson-Bahr PEC, Bell DR. Leprosy. In: *Manson's Tropical Diseases.* London: Baillière-Tindall; 1987:757–785.

Mastro TD, Redd SC, Breiman RF. Imported leprosy in the United States, 1978 through 1988: An epidemic without secondary transmission. *Am J Public Health.* 1992;82:1127–1130.

Meyers WM. Leprosy. *Dermatol Clin.* 1992;10:73–96.

Miller RA, Buchanan TM. Leprosy. In: Warren KS, Mahmoud AAF, eds. *Tropical and Geographical Medicine.* New York: McGraw-Hill; 1990:851–859.

Near KA, Lefford MJ. Use of serum antibody and lysozyme levels for diagnosis of leprosy and tuberculosis. *J Clin Microbiol.* 1992;30:1105–1110.

Neill MA, Hightower AW, Broome CV. Leprosy in the United States, 1971–1981. *J Infect Dis.* 1985;152:1064–1069.

Noordeen SK, Bravo LL, Sundaresan TK. Estimated number of leprosy cases in the world. *Bulletin WHO.* 1992;70:7–10.

Okoro AN. Pre-emptive diagnosis of leprosy. *Int J Dermatol.* 1991;30:767–771.

Ostler HB. Hansen's disease. *Int Ophthalmol Clin.* 1990;30:42–45.

Ross M, Barr RJ. Leprosy in the United States: Just a curiosity? *Int J Dermatol.* 1991;30:772–773.

Schwab IR, Ostler HB, Dawson CR. Hansen's disease of the eye (ocular leprosy). In: Tasman W, Jaeger EA, eds. *Duane's Clinical Ophthalmology.* Hagerstown, MD: Harper & Row; 1992;5:1–9.

Sehgal VN, Joginder, Sharma VK. Immunology of leprosy: A comprehensive survey. *Int J Dermatol.* 1989;28:574–584.

Smolin G. Hansen's disease: Have we advanced in the last 20 years? *Int Ophthalmol Clin.* 1990;30:46–48.

Spaide R, Nattis R, Lipka A, D'Amico R. Ocular findings in leprosy in the United States. *Am J Ophthalmol.* 1985;100:411–416.

Warren G. Facial palsy—a leprosy surgeon's viewpoint. *Austral NZ J Ophthalmol.* 1990;18:257–266.

Williams DL, Gillis TP, Booth RJ, et al. The use of a specific DNA probe and polymerase chain reaction for the detection of *Mycobacterium leprae. J Infect Dis.* 1990;162:193–200.

Lyme Disease

Kelly H. Thomann

Lyme disease, a multisystemic spirochetal infection, was virtually unheard of in the United States prior to 1975. Since then it has become the most common tick-borne illness in this country and now receives worldwide recognition. The disease is characterized by early and late manifestations that involve the skin, nervous system, joints, and heart. Its variability of expression, vague symptoms, and lack of a completely accurate diagnostic serologic test often delay diagnosis or lead to misdiagnosis. Recently, however, media attention and increased public awareness regarding this multifaceted disease has led to overdiagnosis, especially in endemic areas. In 1982, Lyme disease was made a reportable disease to the Centers for Disease Control (CDC), and it is now mandatory for nearly all states to report cases.

In 1975, this disease was first named Lyme arthritis when two mothers in Old Lyme, Connecticut, informed state health authorities about the large number of children in their small community who had been diagnosed with juvenile rheumatoid arthritis. This disease cluster was investigated by a group of researchers from Yale University. They soon discovered that the skin lesion, erythema migrans (originally referred to as erythema chronicum migrans), served as a clinical marker for the disease and that it was transmitted by the bite of the Ixodes tick. They described the systemic illness as well as the efficacy of antibiotics in its treatment and linked it with European literature describing a similar disease. As a result of these findings, Lyme arthritis was soon renamed Lyme disease.

EPIDEMIOLOGY

Lyme disease has now been reported in 46 states, and its distribution worldwide includes every continent except Antarctica. Three endemic areas have been identified in the United States. They are the rural areas of New York, Massachusetts, Connecticut, and Rhode Island along with coastal northeastern and middle Atlantic states; the coastal wooded areas of California and southwestern Oregon; and Wisconsin and Minnesota.

In 1982, eleven states reported 497 cases of Lyme disease to the CDC, and in 1993, approximately 8600 cases were reported, with 80 to 90% of these cases from endemic states. In the United States, the overall incidence of Lyme disease was approximately 3.5 per 100,000 in 1993. Some counties located in endemic areas have exceeded 200 cases per 100,000.

■ Systemic

The erythema migrans lesion is found in 60 to 80% of patients with Lyme disease. In more than one half of patients it is associated with flu-like illness. Secondary annular skin lesions occur in 6 to 48% of patients.

The classic neurological triad of meningitis, cranial neuritis, and motor or sensory radiculoneuritis (inflammation of the nerve root) is found in 15 to 20% of patients. Twelve to 20% of patients develop aseptic meningitis in the early stage of the disease and about 50% of these patients go on to develop facial nerve palsy. Encephalitis occurs in about two thirds of patients.

Cardiac involvement is found in 4 to 8% of patients within several weeks of disease onset. The most common abnormality is fluctuating degrees of atrioventricular block.

The number of patients with recurrence of arthritis symptoms decreases by 10 to 20% per year. Chronic arthritis (1 year or more of joint inflammation) is found in about 60% of untreated cases of Lyme disease.

■ Ocular

Current literature does not include any studies indicating overall ocular involvement, although there is a plethora of single-case reports in the ophthalmic literature. The most commonly quoted study is one by Steere and co-workers in 1983, which found conjunctivitis in 11% of patients during the early infective stage of Lyme disease. Ocular complications are most frequently encountered during the disseminated stage of infection.

NATURAL HISTORY

■ Systemic

The Organism

The pathogenic organism responsible for Lyme disease remained unknown until 1982, when a spirochete belonging to the *Borrelia* family was isolated by Willy Burgdorfer, and thus named *Borrelia burgdorferi*. Helically shaped, motile spirochetes often cause diseases with similar features. This explains why Lyme disease shares many characteristics with syphilis, which is caused by the spirochete *Treponema pallidum*.

Transmission

Ixodes ticks are the major vectors for *B. burgdorferi,* with different species found in various locations. *I. dammini* is most common in the eastern part of the United States, *I. pacificus* in the western United States, *I. scapularis* in the southeastern United States, and *I. ricinus* in Europe. There are also other, less efficient tick vectors.

The *Ixodes* tick has a 2-year life cycle (Figure 56–1) that includes three blood feedings. Adults deposit tick eggs in the spring. The larvae hatch and feed once on a small animal (most commonly the white-footed mouse) in the late summer, and then they molt into nymphs. Nymphs feed once in the following spring or early summer, usually on a small animal (again most commonly the white-footed mouse) and molt into adults late in the summer. Adult ticks

feed once on larger animals (most commonly the white-tailed deer) during the autumn. This cycle of spirochete transmission is perpetuated when an uninfected larval tick feeds on an infected mouse; the spirochetes are then stored in the midgut of the tick until the next spring, when it attaches to an uninfected mouse, feeds off it and infects it also. The cycle begins again the next year.

The white-tailed deer are not involved in the spirochete life cycle but are the preferred host for adult ticks. The prevalence of Lyme disease is most closely associated with the deer population, but many other animals also serve as hosts, the white-footed mouse in particular, but also birds and domestic animals, including dogs, cats, horses, and cattle. Reduction of the deer population in an endemic area would most likely only cause the ticks to find another preferred host. During any stage the tick can feed on humans (Figure 56–2) and transmit the disease. Because the feedings occur from spring to autumn, this disease is typically noted during these seasons. Studies have shown that the tick must feed on the host for at least 6 hours and probably longer than 24 hours before transmitting the disease. Therefore, there is a grace period during which, if a tick is found and removed promptly, the likelihood of getting the disease is small. However, only about 30% of individuals recall being bitten by a tick.

Course of the Disease

The complete natural history of Lyme disease continues to be investigated and documented. Current literature includes many single reports of varying presentations; however, these often are not clearly proven to be due to Lyme because other disease etiologies were not completely ruled out. The pathological mechanism for the multisystemic involvement of Lyme disease includes direct spirochetal invasion of tissue, vessel inflammation and perivascular infiltration, and host immunologic reaction.

Most literature divides the disease into three stages. However, the clinical manifestations of these stages tend to overlap. More recently it has been described as having early and late manifestations. Early disease, which can be broken into early infection and early disseminated infection, correlates with stages one and two; late persistent infection correlates with stage three (Table 56–1).

Early infection is characterized by a flu-like illness that occurs 3 to 30 days after the tick bite. Symptoms include fever, chills, headache, stiff neck, nausea, arthralgia, and lymphadenopathy. During this period the characteristic erythema migrans lesion (Figure 56–3) may or may not be found. The classic appearance is a flat, red spot of skin at the site of the bite, which expands and forms an erythematous, annular lesion with partial clearing in the center, giving it a "bull's-eye" appearance. The size and rate of expansion is variable. It ranges from 2 by 3 to 20 by 40 cm from 1 to 4 weeks after its appearance. It usually will fade within 3 to 4 weeks, even if

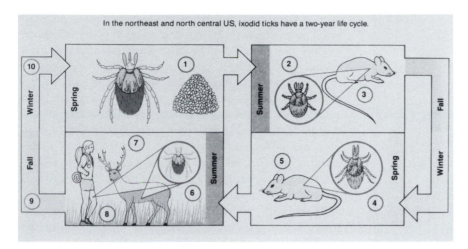

In the northeast and north central US, ixodid ticks have a two-year life cycle.

Figure 56–1. Tick life cycle. *(Reprinted with permission from Schlesinger PA. Lyme disease: Prevention and intervention. Hospital Med. 1989;25:93.)*

untreated. The lesion may feel warmer than surrounding skin but is usually asymptomatic. Burning, itching, pain, tenderness, hyperesthesia, and dysesthesia (painful impairment of the sense of touch) have all been reported. The lesion will often be found where the tick commonly feeds: the axilla, thigh, groin, buttocks, and where tight-fitting clothing begins.

The disseminated early stage of the disease (stage 2) includes more prominent symptoms involving the skin and nervous and musculoskeletal systems, and may occur several weeks to months after initial infection. Patients will often have secondary, smaller annular skin lesions, which are usually asymptomatic and tend to occur at a site other than where the initial erythema migrans lesion was found. Mild headaches and stiff neck may occur in short attacks as

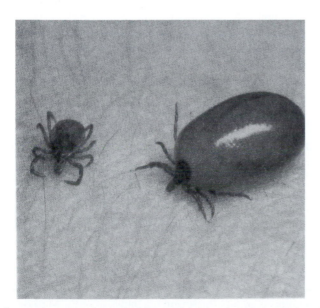

Figure 56–2. Female *Ixodes dammini* tick in the unengorged and engorged states. *(Reprinted with permission from Park M. Ocular manifestations of Lyme disease.* J Am Optom Assoc. *1989;60:286.)*

TABLE 56–1. SYSTEMIC MANIFESTATIONS OF LYME DISEASE

EARLY (ACUTE LOCALIZED) INFECTION
- Dermatologic
  - Erythema migrans
- Neurological
  - Headache, stiff neck, nausea
- General
  - Flu-like symptoms, lymphadenopathy, pharyngitis

EARLY (ACUTE DISSEMINATED) INFECTION
- Dermatologic
  - Erythema migrans, secondary annular lesions, lymphocytoma skin lesion, malar rash, diffuse skin erythema
- Neurological
  - Meningitis, cranial neuritis, motor or sensory peripheral neuritis, radiculopathy, encephalitis, mononeuritis multiplex
- Cardiac
  - Palpitations, myocarditis, A–V block, arrhythmia, pancarditis
- Rheumatologic
  - Arthralgia/musculoskeletal pain
- General
  - Malaise, fatigue, regional or generalized lymphadenopathy
- Other systems
  - Mild or recurrent hepatitis, splenomegaly, nonexudative sore throat, nonproductive cough, microscopic hematuria or proteinuria

LATE (DISSEMINATED) DISEASE
- Dermatologic
  - Acrodermatitis chronicum atrophicans
- Neurological
  - Fatigue, chronic encephalitis, chronic axonal polyneuropathy, leukoencephalopathy, subtle neuropsychologic deficits, spastic paraparesis, ataxic gait
- Rheumatologic
  - Arthritis (prolonged attacks, chronic pain)
- General
  - Fatigue

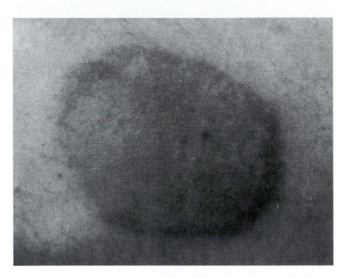

Figure 56–3. Erythema migrans lesion, which typically starts at the center of the bite and grows slowly in a circular pattern within days to weeks. *(Reprinted with permission from Park M. Ocular manifestations of Lyme disease.* J Am Optom Assoc. *1989;60:285.)*

well as transitory pain, lasting hours or days in joints, bursae, tendons, muscle, and bones. It is usually during this time that patients experience the unrelenting and debilitating malaise and fatigue commonly found with this disease.

Neurological involvement may also occur weeks to months after infection. The most common findings are meningitis and cranial or peripheral neuropathy. Unilateral or bilateral seventh (facial) nerve palsy is the most common cranial neuropathy. The peripheral neuritis is usually asymmetric and affects the motor, sensory, or both motor and sensory peripheral nerves of the limb or trunk. This usually last weeks to months, but may recur or become chronic.

Cardiac involvement may be found 4 to 8 weeks after the initial illness, and typically lasts from 3 days to 6 weeks. The most common findings are palpitations, arrythmias, myocarditis, or varying degrees of atrioventricular block. This may be mild; however, about one third of patients require a temporary pacemaker.

Musculoskeletal pain may be found from 2 weeks to 2 years after the onset of the disease. Brief attacks of asymmetric oligoarthritis after the early intermittent episodes of arthralgia and migratory musculoskeletal pain are found in 60% of patients. The large joints, especially the knee, are most commonly affected.

The liver, kidney, and respiratory and genitourinary systems may also be affected during the early disseminated stage. Signs and symptoms may include mild or recurrent hepatitis, pharyngitis, pneumonitis with dry cough, nonexudative sore throat and mild pleuritic pain, hepatosplenic tenderness, hematuria, proteinuria, and orchitis (inflammation of the testis).

Arthritis is the most prominent finding during the late persistent (stage 3) infection. During the second and third year of the illness, the arthritis found during the disseminated stage becomes chronic, lasting up to a year at a time. Usually, only one or more large joints are affected, most commonly the knee.

Chronic neurological manifestations have also been recognized in late disseminated Lyme disease, and are often associated with a mild, low-grade reversible inflammatory process in the central nervous system. Subacute encephalitis is the most common chronic symptom. It often affects memory, mood, and sleep, and may cause subtle disturbances in language. Diagnosis of this type of encephalitis is difficult due to the nonspecific symptoms.

Polyneuropathy may cause peripheral sensory symptoms such as distal paresthesias, spinal pain, or radicular (following the nerve root or pathway) pain. The shoulder girdle area is the most common radiculopathy. Halperin and associates in 1990 studied peripheral nervous system manifestations in late Lyme disease and concluded that reversible peripheral nervous system abnormalities occurred in one third of patients, and that the electrophysiologic pattern was the same for all abnormalities. This is indicative of widespread axonal damage and suggests that the varying presentations of late peripheral nervous system involvement reflects the same pathological process. Less commonly, leukoencephalopathy (inflammation of the white matter of the brain) has been reported, supported by findings of lesions and antibody to *B. burgdorferi* found within the periventricular white matter.

Six months to eight years after initial infection the skin disease, acrodermatitis chronica atrophicans may be found. This has been reported in up to 10% of patients in Europe who have Lyme disease, but much less frequently in the United States. It is most commonly found in elderly patients and is a biphasic disorder with an early inflammatory stage followed by an atrophic stage. The early stage consists of areas of swollen skin with erythematous plaques or nodules, usually found on the extremities. These lesions wax and wane over time and lead to the atrophic stage. During this stage they may be associated with pain, pruritus, hyperesthesias, or paresthesias. Other skin lesions, including those resembling scleroderma, have also been reported during this stage, although these cases are more commonly found in European literature.

Several reports have suggested that Lyme disease may cause or induce syndromes similar to multiple sclerosis, Guillain–Barré syndrome, and Alzheimer disease. These theories have recently been disputed and are now thought to be true cases of these diseases in patients who may by chance also have Lyme disease.

Transplacental transmission of *B. burgdorferi* from mother to fetus has been reported during the first trimester, with reports of fatal or severe outcomes at birth. Markowitz in 1986 reviewed 19 pregnancies complicated by Lyme disease, finding adverse outcomes in 5 of these cases.

However, each case differed and none had serologic evidence of Lyme disease. Further study is needed in this area. Prompt treatment is suggested in pregnant women when Lyme disease is suspected.

■ Ocular

A myriad of ocular complications from Lyme disease have been documented, involving virtually all parts of the eye. A nonspecific conjunctivitis, which has never been well described in the literature, is the most common ocular complication reported. It is usually short-lived and encountered during the early stage of the disease.

Other eye complications are most commonly found during the disseminated and late disease stages (Table 56–2; Figure 56–4). Intraocular inflammation in the form of granulomatous iridocyclitis, pars planitis, or vitritis have all been reported secondary to Lyme disease. The most common findings are pars planitis with posterior synechiae and granulomatous anterior chamber inflammation. *Borrelia burgdorferi* has recently been isolated from the eye (Preac-Mursic et al, 1993), thus giving concrete evidence regarding the etiology of many causes of intraocular inflammation that previously had only been supported by a causal relationship to Lyme disease. In late Lyme disease, a stromal keratitis, similar to that found in late syphilis, has also been frequently reported. This may be due to a delayed immune response.

DIAGNOSIS

Diagnosis of Lyme disease is often problematic because of its varying presentation and the present lack of a definitive laboratory test. It is typically defined by clinical presentation and supported by serologic testing. In 1991 a case definition was developed by the CDC for reporting and tracking purposes. This definition, however, is biased heavily toward diagnostic certainty, and if strictly adhered to, many cases would go undiagnosed. Clinical judgment continues to be most important in cases in which serological tests are not conclusive, yet signs and symptoms indicate Lyme disease.

Lyme disease has often been compared to syphilis as another "great imitator." Both are spirochetal in origin, multisystemic, occur in stages, and mimic other diseases. Both are acute infections initially with skin lesions, which later disseminate to involve other organ systems, especially the nervous system. Although both share many similarities, careful observation and diagnostic techniques should delineate the differences and distinguish the two diseases.

■ Systemic

The diagnosis of Lyme disease is apparent in a symptomatic patient who has the erythema migrans lesion or recalls a tick bite and has positive serology. However, these cases are rare, and diagnosis more often is dependent on clinical symptoms and serology. The patient history is particularly important and should include questions regarding any time spent in endemic areas, any exposure to animals, and recollection of a tick bite or of any lesions similar to the erythema migrans. In addition, any relationship found between symptomatology and the various stages of the disease may assist in the diagnosis. However, a tick bite alone and vague symptoms, such as headache, malaise and fatigue, although clinical manifestations of Lyme disease, are not definite indicators for the disease. The diagnosis should follow the diagnostic criteria listed in Table 56–3.

Laboratory testing for Lyme disease has improved over the past years, but still lacks a "gold standard." Current methods only indicate exposure, not active infection. In

TABLE 56–2. OCULAR MANIFESTATIONS OF LYME DISEASE

EARLY (ACUTE LOCALIZED) INFECTION
- Conjunctivitis (C)
- Photophobia (C)
- Periorbital edema (M)

EARLY (ACUTE DISSEMINATED) INFECTION
- Granulomatous iritis (C)
- Pars-planitis-like vitritis (C)
- Retinitis (included in spectrum of pars planitis like vitritis) (C)
- Oculomotor palsies (C)
- Facial palsy (C)
- Optic neuropathy (M)
- Optic neuritis (M)
- Papilledema (M)
- Pseudo tumor cerebri (M)
- Giant-cell arteritis (R)
- Macula edema (R)
- Pupil abnormalities (Horner syndrome and Argyll-Robertson-like pupils) (R)
- Blepharospasm (R)
- Anterior ischemic opthic neuropathy (R)
- Choroiditis (R)
- Retinal vasculitis (R)
- Neuro retinitis (R)
- Endophthalmitis (R)
- Orbital myositis (R)

LATE INFECTION
- Keratitis (C)
- Episcleritis (M)
- Orbital myositis (R)
- Cortical blindness (R)

C, common; M, more than one case reported; R, rare or single case report in literature.

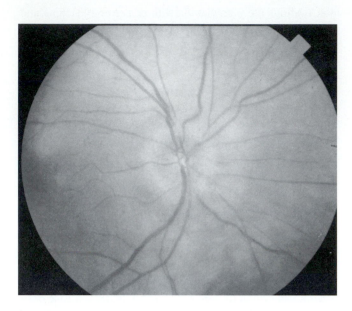

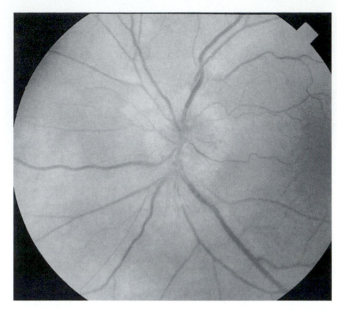

A

B

Figure 56–4. Bilateral disc edema in a patient with disseminated Lyme disease. *(Courtesy of Optometry Section, Brooklyn VAMC, NY.)*

endemic areas, asymptomatic individuals may have serological evidence of exposure without evidence of the disease. This may be as high as 10% in certain endemic regions.

The enzyme-linked immunosorbant assay (ELISA) and indirect immunofluorescence antibody (IFA) test are the most commonly used methods to detect specific antibodies against *B. burgdorferi* in the blood. ELISA is more sensitive than IFA, because it is automated and gives more objective results. Diagnosis may also be made by culture of a skin lesion or culture of serum, but this is very difficult and expensive to do. Western blot testing (protein electrophoresis) is said to be the most specific test for Lyme

antibody; however, its cost and availability make it more useful as a confirmatory test to eliminate false positive ELISA tests (Table 56–4).

Serology is less useful during early Lyme disease because it takes 2 to 4 weeks after the infection for an individual to produce detectable IgM antibody. This response peaks 6 to 8 weeks after onset of the illness, and declines to the normal range within 4 to 6 months in most patients. IgG antibody increases 6 to 8 weeks after onset of illness, peaks after 4 to 6 months, and remains elevated indefinitely in patients with continued infection. Therefore, untreated patients in later stages of the disease should show increased IgG levels.

TABLE 56–3. CDC DIAGNOSTIC CRITERIA FOR LYME DISEASE

Area	Criteria
Endemic	EM with exposure no more than 30 days prior to onset
	or
	Involvement of one or more organ system (musculoskeletal, neurologic, cardiac) and a positive antibody test
	or
Non-endemic	EM with positive antibody test
	or
	EM with involvement of two organ systems

EM, erythema migrans skin lesion.

TABLE 56–4. LYME DISEASE SEROLOGY

ELISA[a]

<1.0 = Negative
0.85–1.25 = Equivocal
>1.0 = Positive

IFA IgG/IgM[a]

IgG
<1:16 = Negative
1:16–1:32 = Equivocal
>1:32 = Evidence of past or current infection

IgM

If any present, it is considered positive

Western Blot

≤5 Bands = normal

[a] Values may differ with varying laboratories.

ELISA and IFA serology are 86 to 100% sensitive for late Lyme disease, and therefore remain the tests of choice for this stage of the disease process. Tests currently under development include the detection of *B. burgdorferi* DNA in the cerebrospinal fluid through polymerase chain reaction (PCR) amplification, T-lymphocyte cell assay, and detection of *B. burgdorferi* antigen in urine. These tests may prove to be more useful for the early detection of Lyme disease, but as of yet insufficient data exist to determine their efficacy. PCR currently holds the most promise for future use.

Problems with current serology (ELISA, IFA) include serovariability and false-negative and false-positive results. Serovariability occurs when a sample of serum tests negative at one lab and positive at another. This occurs because standardization between laboratories, although recently improved, has not been perfected. False-negative serology may be found in early Lyme disease before a full antibody response has occurred, if antibiotics were used that curtailed the immune response or if the patient is immunosuppressed (has HIV infection). False positives may occur with other treponemal infections, especially syphilis, or with conditions such as infectious mononucleosis, rheumatoid arthritis, systemic lupus erythematosus, and other spirochetal diseases such as those causing periodontal infection. Tests to rule out inflammatory conditions or syphilis are recommended if the diagnosis is questionable. The rapid plasma reagin (RPR) test is superior to the FTA-ABS test for differentiation from syphilis. Cross-reactivity of Lyme IFA and syphilis FTA-ABS has been reported to occur in 22.5 to 54% of patients. Cross-reactivity between Lyme ELISA and FTA-ABS is 32%. RPR and VDRL testing should not give false-positive results (although one case has been reported). If these are positive, then the diagnosis of syphilis rather than (or concurrent with) Lyme disease should be made.

Follow-up tests that may be helpful in seronegative cases of Lyme disease include the Western blot, PCR, and lymphocyte antigen stimulation tests. The initial use of the ELISA test, and subsequent use of the Western blot test to confirm questionable results, is presently the testing procedure of choice, because it employs the most sensitive and specific laboratory tests currently available.

■ Ocular

A patient with or without diagnosed Lyme disease may present to an eyecare practitioner with ocular manifestations of the disease. For the patient with known Lyme disease, the practitioner should be aware of the possible ocular manifestations (see Table 56–2). If a patient presents with ocular manifestations that may be due to Lyme disease, a thorough history, laboratory testing, and consideration of the differential diagnosis should be made. Referral to the appropriate physician (internist, rheumatologist, neurologist) is also indicated.

TREATMENT AND MANAGEMENT

■ Systemic

The management of tick bites and questionable Lyme disease has been problematic for many practitioners. Little research has been done regarding the effectiveness of treating tick bites prior to Lyme manifestations and positive serology. However, Magid and co-workers (1992) recently studied the efficacy of prophylactically treating patients bitten by ticks. Treatment is recommended for all tick bites in endemic areas, where the probability of becoming infected with Lyme disease is greater. This approach is more cost effective, with less potential complications than deferring treatment until absolutely indicated. In areas not endemic for Lyme disease, where the probability of getting the disease from a tick bite is less, the management of choice is to monitor the patient. In these cases, complications that result from treatment are greater than those of the disease itself. In areas where the probability of acquiring the disease through a tick bite fall between those in a non-endemic area and endemic area, the decision to treat must be weighed by both the physician and patient.

The specific antibiotic regimen, particularly its duration, has not yet been established due to varying patient responses to treatment. Early disease is usually treated with the oral antibiotics tetracycline and doxycycline (Table 56–5). In later disease, treatment protocols are less defined. Best results have been found with intravenous ceftriaxone. It has been suggested that prior treatment with steroids may predispose the patient to antibiotic failure.

Polymerase chain reaction testing, which can detect the *B. burgdorferi* antigen in the cerebrospinal fluid, may be helpful in the future to identify the persistence of spirochetal DNA after treatment and assist in determining duration and success of treatment.

The Herxheimer reaction, an increase in symptoms after administration of medication (usually encountered when treating syphilis), has been found in 15% of patients treated during early Lyme disease. The symptoms include abrupt onset of fever and chills followed by a drop in temperature and sweating within 6 hours after the first dose of antibiotics.

■ Ocular

Patients with positive Lyme serology who have otherwise unexplained ocular inflammation in which syphilis has been excluded, warrant an antibiotic trial. A seronegative patient with a high suspicion for Lyme disease should also undergo an antibiotic trial. Patients with severe ocular disease should be treated with intravenous ceftriaxone. Those with less severe ocular disease should be treated with oral tetracycline or doxycycline. If Lyme disease is

TABLE 56–5. TREATMENT AND MANAGEMENT OF LYME DISEASE: RECOMMENDATIONS FOR ANTIBIOTIC TREATMENT[a]

EARLY LYME DISEASE
- Doxycycline,[b] 100 mg twice daily for 10–21 days
- Amoxicillin, 500 mg three times daily for 10–21 days
- Erythromycin, 250 mg four times daily for 10–21 days (less effective than doxycycline or amoxicillin)

LYME CARDITIS
- Ceftriaxone, 2 g daily intravenously for 14 days
- Penicillin G, 20 million units intravenously for 14 days
- Doxycycline, 100 mg orally twice daily for 14–21 days, may suffice[c]
- Amoxicillin, 500 mg orally three times daily for 14–21 days, may suffice[c]

NEUROLOGICAL MANIFESTATIONS
- Facial nerve paralysis
  For an isolated finding, oral regimens for early disease, used for at least 21 days, may suffice
  For a finding associated with other neurologic manifestations, intravenous therapy (see below)
- Lyme meningitis[d]
  Ceftriaxone, 2 g daily by single dose for 14–21 days

Penicillin G, 20 million units daily in divided doses for 10–21 days
Possible alternatives: doxycycline, 100 mg orally or intravenously for 10–21 days; chloramphenicol, 1 g intravenously every 6 hours for 10–21 days

LYME ARTHRITIS
- Doxycycline, 100 mg orally twice daily for 30 days
- Amoxicillin and probenecid, 500 mg each orally four times daily for 30 days
- Penicillin G, 20 million units intravenously in divided doses daily for 14–21 days
- Ceftriaxone, 2 g intravenously daily for 14–21 days

IN PREGNANT WOMEN
- For localized early Lyme disease, amoxicillin, 500 mg three times daily for 21 days
- For disseminated early Lyme disease or any manifestation of late disease, penicillin G, 20 million units daily for 14–21 days
- For asymptomatic seropositivity, no treatment necessary

[a] These guidelines are to be modified by new findings and should always be applied with close attention to the clinical course of individual patients.
[b] Shorter courses are reserved for disease that is limited to a single skin lesion only.
[c] Oral regimens are reserved for mild cardiac involvement.
[d] Regimens for radiculoneuropathy, peripheral neuropathy, and encephalitis are the same as those for meningitis.
Reprinted with permission from Rahn DW, Malawista SE, Lyme disease: Recommendations for diagnosis and treatment. Ann Intern Med. 1991;114:475.

unrecognized and the eye complication is treated with steroids, it may delay the antibiotic efficacy.

■ Prevention

Advice for personal protection includes wearing lightly colored protective clothing tucked in at the ankles, wrists, and waist. Body checks for ticks should be done daily when outdoors and should become routine. The use of a repellent containing permethrin is very effective for repelling and killing ticks in states where its use is allowed.

Patient education regarding tick removal is also important. Removal should be done with tweezers, pulling slowly from the base of the tick. Antiseptic should be applied to the bite, and it should then be monitored for the appearance of an EM lesion.

An effective vaccine for humans against Lyme disease is currently being researched and tested in humans. The possibility of a vaccine in the near future looks very promising. Recent studies have successfully immunized mice and prevented infection with the *B. burgdorferi* spirochete from infected ticks. It was also discovered that this same process destroyed the infecting agent within the tick vector prior to transmission. This could be especially promising in the eradication of the disease.

Conclusion

Lyme disease, virtually unheard of in the 1970s, became a household word in the 1980s with increasing numbers of cases each year. The 1990s hold much promise for prevention, early diagnosis, treatment, and possible eradication of this troublesome multisystemic spirochetal disease. Despite its varying manifestations and the lack of a diagnostic laboratory test, an educated healthcare practitioner, using sound clinical diagnostic methodology, should be able to accurately diagnose and treat this disease.

References

Abele DC, Anders KH. The many faces and phases of borreliosis I. Lyme disease. *J Am Acad Dermatol.* 1990;23:167–185.

Banyas GT. Difficulties with Lyme serology. *J Am Optom Assoc.* 1992;63:135–140.

Centers for Disease Control. Lyme disease—United States, 1987 and 1988. *MMWR.* 1992;42:345–348.

Copelane RA. Lyme uveitis. *Int Ophthalmol Clin.* 1990; 30:291–293.

Cox J, Krajden M. Cardiovascular manifestations of Lyme disease. *Am Heart J.* 1991;122:1449–1455.

Dennis DT. Lyme disease: Tracking an endemic. *JAMA.* 1991;226:1269–1270.

Dressler F, Yoshinari N, Steere AC. The t-cell proliferative assay in the diagnosis of Lyme disease. *Ann Intern Med.* 1991;115:533–539.

Drodzicki RL, Steere AC. Comparison of immunoblotting and indirect enzyme-linked immunosorbant assay using different antigen preparations for diagnosing early Lyme disease. *J Infect Dis.* 1988;157:790–797.

Duffy J, Mertz LE, Wobig GH, Katzmann JA. Diagnosing Lyme disease: The contribution of serologic testing. *Mayo Clin Proc.* 1988;63:1116–1121.

Fikrig E, Telford SR, Barthold SW, et al. Elimination of *Borrelia burgdorferi* from vector ticks feeding on OspA-immunized mice. *Proc Natl Acad Sci USA.* 1992;89:5419–5421.

Finkel MF. Lyme disease and its neurological complications. *Arch Neurol.* 1988;45:99–104.

Finkel MF, Halperin JJ. Nervous system Lyme borreliosis—revisited. *Arch Neurol.* 1992;49:102–107.

Haberg TM. The expanding ophthalmologic spectrum of Lyme disease. *Am J Ophthalmol.* 1989;107:77–80.

Halperin J, Luft BJ, Anand AK, et al. Lyme neuroborreliosis: Central nervous system manifestations. *Neurology.* 1989;39:753–759.

Halperin J, Luft BJ, Volkman DJ, Dattwyler RJ. Lyme neuroborreliosis: Peripheral nervous system manifestations. *Brain.* 1990;113:1207–1221.

Hudacek SS. Lyme disease: Facts and essential assessments. *Adv. Clin. Care.* July/August 1990;6–9.

Keller TL, Halperin JJ, Whitman M. PCR detection of *Borrelia burgdorferi* DNA in cerebrospinal fluid of Lyme neuroborreliosis patients. *Neurology.* 1992;42:32–42.

Krupp LB, Masur D, Schwartz J, et al. Cognitive functioning in late Lyme borreliosis. *Arch Neurol.* 1991;48:1125–1129.

Lesser RL, Kornmehl MD, Pachner AR, et al. Neuro-ophthalmologic manifestations of Lyme disease. *Ophthalmology.* 1990;97:699–706.

Logican EL, Kaplan RF, Steere AC. Chronic neurologic manifestations of Lyme disease. *N Engl J Med.* 1990;323:1438–1444.

Luger SE, Krauss E. Serologic tests for Lyme disease: Interlaboratory variability. *Arch Intern Med.* 1990;150:761–763.

MacDonald AB. Lyme disease: A neuro-ophthalmologic view. *J Clin Neuro-ophthalmol.* 1987;7:185–190.

Magid D, Schwartz B, Craft J, Schwartz JS. Prevention of Lyme disease after tick bites: A cost-effectiveness analysis. *N Engl J Med.* 1992;327:534–541.

Malone MS, Grant-Kels JM, Feder HM, Luger SW. Diagnosis of Lyme disease based on dermatologic manifestations. *Ann Intern Med.* 1991;114:490–498.

Markowitz LE. Lyme disease during pregnancy. *JAMA.* 1986;255:3394–3396.

Pachner AR, Duray P, Steere AC. Central nervous system manifestations of Lyme disease. *Arch Neurol.* 1989;46:790–795.

Pachner AR, Steere AC. The triad of neurologic manifestations of Lyme disease: Meningitis, cranial neuritis, and radiculoneuritis. *Neurology.* 1985;35:47-53.

Preac-Mursic V, et al. First isolation of *Borrelia burgdorferi* from an iris biopsy. *J Clin Neuro-ophthalmol.* 1993;13:155–161.

Rahn DW, Malawista SE. Lyme disease: Recommendations for diagnosis and treatment. *Ann Intern Med.* 1991;114:472–481.

Schlesinger PA. Lyme disease: Prevention and intervention. *Hospital Med.* 1989;25:92–119.

Schned ES, Williams DW. Special concerns in Lyme disease. *Postgrad Med.* 1992;91:65–70.

Smith JL, Crumpton BC, Hummer J. The Bascom Palmer Eye Institute Lyme/syphilis survey. *J Clin Neuro-ophthalmol.* 1990;10:255–260.

Steere AC. Medical progress—Lyme disease. *N Engl J Med.* 1989;321:586–596.

Steere AC, Bartenhagen NH, Craft JE, et al. The early clinical manifestations of Lyme disease. *Ann Intern Med.* 1983;99:76–82.

Szer IS, Taylor E, Steere AC. The long term course of Lyme arthritis in children. *N Engl J Med.* 1991;325:159–163.

Williams DW, Schned ES. Lyme disease: Recognizing its many manifestations. *Postgrad Med.* 1990;87:139–146.

Winterkorn J. Lyme disease: Neurologic and ophthalmic manifestations. *Surv Ophthalmol.* 1990;35:191–204.

Winward KE, Smith JL, Culbertson WW, Paris-Hamelin A. Ocular Lyme borreliosis. *Am J Ophthalmol.* 1989;108:651–657.

Zuschke DC. Is it Lyme disease? How to interpret results of laboratory testing. *Postgrad Med.* 1992;91:48–55.

57
Chapter

Syphilis

Kelly H. Thomann

Syphilis is a slowly evolving chronic infection caused by the spirochete *Treponema pallidum*, which can affect any system in the body. At one time it was dubbed the "great pox," because it occurred in epidemic proportions in 15th-century Europe. Many people once attributed the spread of syphilis to the return of Christopher Columbus' expedition to Europe from the New World, where it was acquired in the West Indies. However, current evidence now suggests that the disease was actually present in Europe prior to this time but increased to epidemic proportions as a result of the movement of troops during the French and Spanish wars. Henry the VIII, Napoleon Bonaparte, Ludwig von Beethoven, and Florence Nightingale are just a few individuals who, throughout the past centuries, were believed to have had syphilis influence their lives. In the 1950s, penicillin treatment and preventative health programs helped lead to a significant decrease in its prevalence. However, in recent years a dramatic upswing in the number of cases has occurred. Ocular manifestations of syphilis are vast, and affect every part of the eye. The diversity of its effects explains why this disease has often been called "the great imitator."

EPIDEMIOLOGY

■ Systemic

In the early 1900s, syphilis was a major public health problem, and a significant cause of morbidity and mortality. Its incidence peaked around the time of World War II, reaching 75 cases per 100,000 persons in 1946. However, largely due to penicillin treatment, the number of cases dropped dramatically, to 4 per 100,000 persons in 1956. Beginning in the late 1970s to mid-1980s the incidence rose steadily, probably reflecting changes in sexual behavior, with a disproportionate increase in homosexual men. In 1986 the number of cases declined again, most likely because newfound public awareness of HIV led to changes in sexual behavior. However, between 1985 and 1990 there was a 75% increase in syphilis cases, rising to 20 per 100,000 persons in 1990. This increase has been particularly evident in African-American males and females, rising 126 and 231%,

respectively, from 1985 to 1990. The rates of infection in non-Hispanic Caucasian males decreased 50% during this period. A shift in occurrence to less densely populated cities, where it was previously uncommon, was also noted.

Syphilis most commonly affects the 15- to 30-year age group. Approximately one third of individuals exposed to infectious syphilis will acquire the disease. Virtually all patients with untreated primary syphilis will go on to the secondary stage, and 30% of patients with untreated secondary syphilis will go on to the tertiary stage. The disease will remain latent in the remainder of those with untreated secondary syphilis. Of those with tertiary syphilis, 10% will have cardiovascular complications, 15% will go on to have dermatologic involvement, and 10% will have neurosyphilis.

In the 1990s a tremendous increase in congenital syphilis was documented. Although the number of cases actually did rise, the data show a disproportionate increase because a new, broader case definition for congenital syphilis was adopted in 1990. In 1980, congenital syphilis was found in 0.2 per 1000 live births. In 1990, using the new definition, this rose to 6.1 per 1000 live births; however, when the former definition is applied, the frequency only rose to 1.7 per 1000 live births.

■ Ocular

Ocular involvement occurs in about 5% of untreated cases of secondary syphilis. Uveitis is the most common ocular manifestation of syphilis, and Moore (1931) reported that 4.6% of patients with secondary syphilis and 9% of patients with recurrent secondary syphilis get uveitis (Figure 57–1). Schlaegel and Kao (1982) reviewed the cases of presumptive syphilitic uveitis from 1970 to 1980 seen in their clinic and found that syphilis accounted for 1.1% of all uveitis cases. If the disease progresses to neurosyphilis, ocular involvement will occur in 10%. Hooshmand (1972) investigated ocular complications of neurosyphilis and found that of 241 cases, 44.8% had pupil abnormalities (Argyll Robertson pupil the most common), 12% had chorioretinitis, 4.6% had blepharoptosis, and 4.6% had optic atrophy.

NATURAL HISTORY

■ Systemic

The Organism

Treponema pallidum is a delicate, spiral-shaped, motile spirochete that requires a warm, moist environment to survive and whose only host is humans. Its shape enables it to move by rotating, allowing rapid penetration into mucous membranes. It is too narrow to be seen with light microscopy, but its unique shape and movement allow it to be identified by dark-field microscopy.

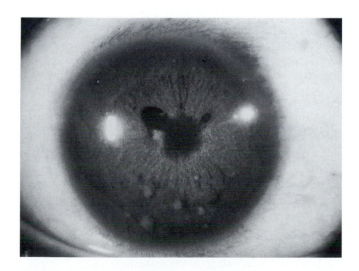

Figure 57–1. Bilateral uveitis with extensive posterior synechiae and inflammatory nodules of the iris in a patient with a positive VDRL and FTA-ABS. *(Reprinted with permission from Margo CE, Hamed LM. Ocular syphilis. Surv Ophthalmol. 1992;37:211.)*

Transmission

Transmission of *T. pallidum* primarily occurs through sexual contact, although it may also be transmitted, less frequently, via transfusion of infected blood (rare today), perinatally, and through needle sharing. The organism enters the blood through breaks in abraded areas of skin. Once it is within the tissue, it replicates locally and disseminates via the lymphatic system and bloodstream to produce systemic infection. The initial incubation period is from 9 to 90 days, with an average time of 3 weeks.

Course of the Disease

The natural history of syphilis reflects the interaction between the spirochete and the immune response of the infected individual. The first response to infection is the local infiltration of polymorphonuclear leukocytes at the site of inoculation. This leads to a cutaneous ulceration and infiltration of the lesion by lymphocytes and plasma cells. Local factors heal the lesion, but there are treponemas still present that are able to disseminate through the bloodstream, leading to the next stage of syphilis, secondary disease. The host response in this stage leads to cutaneous lesions consisting of lymphocytes and perivascular plasma cell infiltrates. Chronic inflammatory response is responsible for the tertiary stage of the disease, characterized by perivascular infiltration, which leads to obliterative endarteritis.

The course of syphilis has classically been broken into primary, secondary, latent, and tertiary stages. These most often overlap; therefore it is often easier to describe the stages of syphilis as early or late. Early disease includes primary, secondary, and early latency; late disease includes late latency and tertiary syphilis. Syphilis can also be acquired congenitally.

Primary Syphilis

Primary syphilis (Table 57–1) is characterized by the presence of a chancre at the site of treponema penetration and inoculation. The primary chancre, which may consist of one or multiple lesions, is described as a painless red papule varying in size from 0.5 to 1 cm. Within a few days of appearance its margins indurate and may become covered with a yellow or gray exudate. Because the lesion appears at the site of inoculation, it is most frequently found in genital, perineal, anal, or oral areas, although it may occur anywhere and go unnoticed if not on an exposed part of the body. The chancre will heal spontaneously in 3 to 8 weeks if untreated. It is an erosion, not an ulcer, and it therefore heals without leaving a scar. A bilateral regional lymphadenopathy may accompany the chancre.

Secondary Syphilis

Disseminated syphilis more accurately describes the secondary stage, because it is characterized by widespread dermatologic and systemic findings (see Table 57–1) due to the

TABLE 57–1. SYSTEMIC MANIFESTATIONS OF PRIMARY AND SECONDARY SYPHILIS

PRIMARY SYPHILIS
- Chancre
- Generalized lymphadenopathy

SECONDARY SYPHILIS
- **Skin**
  Early rash: macular syphilis (roseola syphilitica)
  Later rash: papular, maculopapular, or papulosquamous lesions
  Condylomata lata
  Mucous membrane lesions, especially mucous patches
  Alopecia of eyebrows, scalp, beard
- **General**
  Headache
  Lymphadenopathy
  Pruritus
  Fever
  Malaise
  Weight loss
  Arthralgia
- **Mouth/Throat**
  Tonsilitis
  Pharyngitis
  Mucous membrane lesions/mucous patches
  Ulcers/erosions
- **Genital**
  Chancre
  Condylomata lata
  Mucous patches
- **Central Nervous System**
  CSF abnormalities
  Meningismus (pain in the meningeocortical region of the brain)
  Meningitis
  Cranial nerve II–IV and VI–VIII abnormalities
- **Skeletal/Joint**
  Periostitis of the skull, tibia, sternum, ribs
- **Renal (rare)**
  Glomerulonephritis
  Nephrotic syndrome
- **Gastrointestinal (rare)**
  Invasion of intestinal wall
- **Liver (rare)**
  Hepatitis

hematogenous spread of *T. pallidum* from the primary chancre. It occurs 4 to 10 weeks after primary manifestations.

The skin manifestations of secondary syphilis are numerous and occur in almost all patients. A symmetrical, papular rash involving the entire trunk and extremities is a common finding in early secondary syphilis. It is most prominent on the palms of the hands and soles of the feet. When it first appears, the lesions usually consist of rounded, indistinct macules less than 1 cm in size, with a light pink to rose color. The rash may resolve or the lesions may go on to become scaly, reddish brown papules or maculopapules (described as a "raw ham" appearance) varying in size from 0.5 to 2 cm.

Condylomata lata skin lesions will be found in 20% of patients with secondary syphilis. These are large, relatively broad and flat, pale to grayish papules found in the folds of moist, warm locations, such as the vulva, anal area, scrotum, or perineum. They may become hypertrophic and protrude above the skin surface in some cases.

Mucous membrane lesions, which are small, superficial ulcerated areas with gray borders, frequently accompany cutaneous manifestations. They commonly occur in the tonsils and adjacent oropharynx, causing symptoms of sore throat, diffuse pharyngitis, tonsillitis, or laryngitis. Mucous patches are found in one third of patients with mucous lesions, usually in the late secondary stage. These are flat, grayish, rounded erosions covered by a membrane in the mouth or genital areas.

Alopecia of the scalp, eyebrows, eyelashes, and beard may occur, possibly as the only manifestation of this stage. This loss of hair may be diffuse or occur in a patchy distribution, causing a "moth-eaten" appearance at the involved area.

General systemic manifestations of disseminated syphilis occur in about one half of the patients as flu-like symptoms with malaise, low-grade fever, and diffuse painless lymphadenopathy. Less common symptoms include headache and arthralgia.

Bone involvement or periostitis (an inflammation of the periosteum of the bone) frequently involves the skull, tibia, sternum and ribs, rarely becoming symptomatic. Other system involvement includes the liver, kidney, intestines, and joints (see Table 57–1).

Neurological manifestations may appear late in this stage. Asymptomatic abnormalities in cerebral spinal fluid will be found in 32% of patients. A small percent will go on to have symptoms including meningitis with headache and mental changes. Cranial nerves II through IV and VI through VIII may be affected. Spinal cord or nerve root involvement may lead to tingling, weakness, and hyporeflexia.

Latent Syphilis

Untreated secondary syphilis persists 4 to 8 weeks before the patient becomes symptom and lesion free, entering the latent period. The CDC defines early latency as the first year of the latent period. During this time the patient is still considered infectious and may have a relapse back to secondary manifestations at any time. Late latency is defined as greater than 1 year after secondary syphilis. Relapse rarely occurs during this time, and the patient is considered to be noninfectious. However, pregnant women may infect the fetus during any stage of the disease.

Tertiary Syphilis

Tertiary syphilis is divided into benign late syphilis, cardiovascular syphilis, and late neurosyphilis. Cardiovascular and late neurosyphilis are the most damaging stages. Manifestations of tertiary syphilis are less frequently encountered today, probably due to antibiotic therapy for other illnesses that inadvertently treat syphilis.

Benign late syphilis involves nonvital structures. Although it is classified as "benign," the chronic destruction of this stage can lead to devastating consequences. This stage is characterized by the presence of gummas, which are localized, soft granulomas, best described as having a "gummy" consistency. Gummas represent a chronic maximum inflammatory response to a few spirochetes causing the slow destruction of tissue, eventually leading to fibrosis of the affected area. These present most commonly as isolated lesions of the skin and subcutaneous tissue, usually located on the face, neck, and extremities. They may persist several years if untreated. They may also occur in bones, commonly the tibia, fibula, clavicles, and skull, causing pain and swelling, and ultimately leading to the destruction of cartilage. Gummas may also be found in other organs (Table 57–2).

Cardiovascular tertiary syphilis results from perivascular infiltration that leads to obliterative endarteritis and ischemia. The destruction of elastic blood vessel walls can lead to medial necrosis with aneurysm formation. These effects are primarily found at the vaso vasorum of the ascending aorta, with aortic aneurysm, aortic regurgitation, and coronary artery stenosis the most common manifestations. Most of these patients are asymptomatic; however, clinical signs of cardiovascular disease may occur 10 to 40 years after primary infection.

Neurosyphilis is not actually a separate stage of the disease but a collection of syndromes spanning all stages of syphilis. However, its most devastating effects are found in tertiary syphilis; therefore it is usually classified as occurring in this stage. *Treponema pallidum* can invade the nervous system early in the disease course and cause changes in cerebrospinal fluid. These may be detected by laboratory tests, but the patient will usually be asymptomatic. However, acute syphilitic meningitis with fever, headache, stiff neck, and vomiting may occur less than 1 year after primary infection, and can be associated with acute hydrocephalus and cranial-nerve palsies. The patient with asymptomatic neurosyphilis may progress to late neurosyphilis (Table 57–3 compares early and late neurosyphilis). Symptomatic late neurosyphilis occurs after widespread damage to neuronal tissue in the brain and spinal cord, and is further broken down into meningovascular disease and parenchymal disease. These are not distinct categories, because vascular and parenchymous manifestations may occur at any time, and overlap.

Meningovascular syphilis is the result of chronic meningitis. Cerebrovascular involvement primarily manifests as strokes or seizures secondary to cerebrovascular occlusion with signs and symptoms as they relate to the particular vessel affected. Most of these patients are between the ages of 30 and 50; therefore syphilis should be considered when

TABLE 57–2. SYSTEMIC MANIFESTATIONS OF TERTIARY SYPHILIS

BENIGN LATE SYPHILIS
- Gummas of skin (common); skeletal system (common); upper respiratory tract, mouth, and tongue; lower respiratory tract; digestive system; genitourinary system; breasts

CARDIOVASCULAR SYPHILIS
- Aortic aneurysm
- Aortic regurgitation
- Coronary artery disease
- Aortic valve insufficiency
- Any of above may lead to myocardial infarction, congestive heart failure, strokes, or seizures

LATE NEUROSYPHILIS
- **Meningovascular**
  Cerebrovascular
    Strokes with signs and symptoms pertaining to the vessel distribution affected
    Seizures
  Syphilis of the spinal cord
    Syphilitic meningomyelitis: weakness and paresthesia of the legs progressing to paraparesis or paraplegia; urinary and fecal incontinence; sensory disturbance of the legs
    Spinal vascular syphilis (rare): transection of the spinal cord at the thoracic level with accompanying signs and symptoms
- **Parenchymal**
  General paresis
    Personality changes
    Speech disturbances
    Tremor of tongue, face, hands
    Hyper- or hypoactive reflexes
    Expressionless face
    Impaired handwriting
  Tabes dorsalis
    Lightning pains
    Wasting
    General paresis
    Sensory disturbances
    Loss of reflexes
    Ataxia/broad-based gait
    Bladder/bowel incontinence
    Cranial nerve II–VIII palsy
    Peripheral neuropathy
    Visceral crises (gastric crises with intense epigastric pain, nausea, and vomiting)

cerebrovascular accidents occur in a young adult. Meningovascular neurosyphilis of the spinal cord is considered separately because it presents with a different clinical picture. It occurs more than 20 years after primary infection and can be broken into syphilitic meningomyelitis, which is most

TABLE 57–3. COMPARISON OF EARLY AND LATE NEUROSYPHILIS

Early	Late
Seen in younger subjects, 1 year after infection	Seen in older subjects, 4–40 years after infection
Rare except with incomplete treatment, hence called neurorecurrence	Common (7–10%) in untreated; with treatment still seen in 1–3% from prepenicillin era; rare in penicillin era
Affects mesodermal structures: meninges, vessels	
Causes asymptomatic meningitis, cranial nerve abnormalities, strokes	Causes tabes dorsalis, paresis, dementia, stroke, death

Reprinted with permission from Musher DM, Syphilis, neurosyphilis, penicillin, and AIDS. J Infect Dis. 1991;163:1202.

commonly found, and spinal vascular syphilis (also called acute syphilitic transverse myelitis), which is rarely encountered. Syphilitic meningomyelitis has a gradual onset, beginning as weakness and paresthesia of the legs that may progress to paraphareses or paraplegia. Urinary and fecal incontinence may occur, along with variable sensory disorders of the legs. Spinal vascular syphilis has an abrupt onset with signs and symptoms associated with transection of the spinal cord, usually at the thoracic level.

General paresis and tabes dorsalis are the most common manifestations of parenchymal disease, although rarely encountered today because of the use of antibiotics. General paresis is secondary to the meningoencephalitis with direct invasion of the cerebrum by *T. pallidum*. It usually develops 15 to 20 years after primary infection and can lead to death if untreated. It is a chronic, dementing illness with psychiatric and neurologic manifestations. Tabes dorsales occurs about 20 years after the latent period and is caused by degeneration of the dorsal columns of the spinal cord and sensory nerve trunks. The classic clinical presentation includes lightning pains, paresthesia, decreased deep tendon reflexes, and abnormal pupils.

Congenital Syphilis

Maternal syphilis can adversely affect the birth of the child in many ways. Premature birth, spontaneous abortion, stillbirth, and nonimmune hydrops (abnormal serous fluid accumulation in tissues of body cavities) may occur, or the infant can be born with congenital syphilis. This is broken into early and late disease. The disease can be transmitted to an infant in two ways, most frequently through transplacental passage of *T. pallidum*, or rarely, through contact with genital lesions during the birth process. The risk of fetal infection is related directly to the stage of maternal syphilis at the time of pregnancy and the stage of pregnancy when the fetus is infected. Fetal transmission may be as high as 100% if the mother has primary or secondary syphilis. The risk of transmission is 40% when the mother is in the early latent stage, and this decreases to 10% when in the late latent stage. Fetal damage can be prevented with maternal treatment prior to the 16th week of gestation, and fetal infection usually does not occur before the 10th week of gestation. The most severely affected at birth were usually infected after the 23rd week of gestation.

Early Congenital Syphilis. Clinical manifestations appear within 3 months to the first 2 years of life in early congenital syphilis, because many treponemas are present and undergoing extensive multiplication. The typical clinical presentation is a healthy infant at birth who becomes ill several months later. The baby may also be small for gestational age. Clinical signs may include mucous patches and mucocutaneous lesions, similar to those found in secondary syphilis. A bilateral maculopapular rash, at first appearing red with oval lesions, later turning coppery brown with superficial desquamation or scaling, may be present. Vesicles and bullae are most commonly found on the palms of the hands and soles of the feet, but also may be found on the palate, perineum, and intertriginous (oppositional) body surfaces. These destructive eruptions are also called pemphigus syphiliticus, and are characterized by erythema and blister formation with eventual crusting. The blister fluid is highly contagious. These may heal and result in rhagades (scars or fissures in areas lesions were previously present). Also evident may be "snuffles" (a profuse whitish mucous nasal discharge, which is highly infectious, caused by the invasion of the nasal mucosa by *T. pallidum*); enlarged liver and spleen; and generalized lymphadenopathy.

Skeletal system involvement can be prominent and cause osteochondritis (inflammation of the cartilage and bone), periostitis, or osteitis (inflammation of the bones), especially the metaphyses of the long bones. Lesions will be painful, multiple, and symmetric, occurring in the lower limbs more often than upper extremities. The pain may be so severe that it inhibits movement and produces Parrott syphilitic pseudoparalysis, in which the child appears to be paralyzed. Other organ system involvement is listed in Table 57–4.

Late Congenital Syphilis. Fewer organisms are present at birth in late congenital syphilis; therefore obvious clinical manifestations are not yet apparent. If the ongoing inflammation continues for 6 to 12 months, the disease enters the latency stage. Beyond the age of 2 years, late congenital syphilis can manifest as clinically evident malformations affecting numerous body systems as a result of the scarring from chronic inflammation.

The teeth are prominently affected in late congenital syphilis. Hutchinson teeth are small, widely spaced permanent upper incisors with notching, thinning, and

TABLE 57–4. SYSTEMIC MANIFESTATIONS OF CONGENITAL SYPHILIS

EARLY CONGENITAL SYPHILIS
- **General**
  Small for gestational age
  Snuffles
  Enlarged liver and spleen
  Generalized lymphadenopathy
- **Cutaneous Lesions**
  Mucous patches
  Mucocutaneous lesions
  Pemphigus syphiliticus (vesicles and bullae)
  Maculopapular rash
  Rhagades (linear scars radiating from body orifices such as mouth, nostril, and anus) resulting from mucous patches and condylomata lata
- **Skeletal**
  Osteochondritis
  Periostitis
  Osteitis
  Parrott syphilitic pseudoparalysis
- **Hematologic**
  Anemia
  Leukocytosis
  Leukopenia
  Thrombocytopenia
- **Throat/Esophagus**
  Laryngitis
  Hoarse aphonia
- **Neurosyphilis**
  CSF abnormalities: pleocytosis, increased protein
  Acute syphilitic leptomeningitis: meningismus, vomiting bulging fontanelle
  Untreated neurosyphilis can lead to chronic meningovascular syphilis with progressive hydrocephalus, cranial nerve palsies, cerebral infarction, secondary endarteritis

- **Renal**
  Nephrotic syndrome
  Subacute glomerulonephritis
- **Other (uncommon)**
  Pneumonia alba (syphilitic pneumonia)
  Myocarditis
  Pancreatitis
  Fibrosis of GI tract

LATE CONGENITAL SYPHILIS
- **Dental**
  Hutchinson teeth
  Small, poorly enameled teeth
  Mulberry molars
  Prone to tooth decay
- **Hutchinson triad**
  Defective teeth, interstitial keratitis, 8th-nerve deafness
- **Skeletal system**
  Periostitis leading frontal bossing, squaring of cranium, saber shins, Higouménakis sign
  Clutton joints: caused by inflammatory lesions; painless symmetrical synovitis and hydroarthritis of the knees and sometimes elbow without involvement of adjacent bones
  Saddle nose
  Short maxilla with high palatal arch due to nasal chondritis
- **Central nervous system**
  Meningitis
  Meningovascular syphilis causing arteritis and occlusion of cerebral arteries with accompanying signs and symptoms
  Paresis (similar to that seen in adults with tertiary syphilis)
  Tabes dorsalis (rare, similar to that seen in adults with tertiary syphilis)

discoloration of the enamel caused by the vasculitis and subsequent inflammatory response to the infection in the developing permanent tooth bud prior to birth. Similar findings may also occur in the upper, lower, and lateral incisors. The canine teeth may be hypoplastic and poorly enameled. The surface of the 6-year molars may be underdeveloped with many small cusps arranged in a circle; these are known as "mulberry molars." The teeth of these children are also prone to decay due to defective enamelization.

The Hutchinson triad, another well-known manifestation of congenital syphilis, includes defective teeth, interstitial keratitis, and eighth-nerve deafness. Nerve deafness and vertigo are caused by osteochondritis of the otic capsule, leading to cochlear degeneration and fibrous adhesions. Nerve deafness is a very specific finding of congenital syphilis.

The skeletal system may be adversely affected in late congenital syphilis. Periostitis of the frontal bone may lead to rounding of the bone ("frontal bossing"), and involvement of the parietal bone may cause squaring of the cranium. Periostitis of the tibia may lead to a marked convex-

ity or bowing and is known as "saber shins." Periostitis of the clavicle can cause sternoclavicular thickening (Higouménakis sign). Chronic syphilitic rhinitis may lead to a short maxilla with a high palatal arch. Inflammation of the nasal cartilage can lead to destruction of the underlying bone and result in a saddle nose.

Congenital neurosyphilis is rare today because most children are treated prior to the serious consequences of nervous system involvement. Congenital neurosyphilis presumably follows the same course as neurosyphilis in adults. Meningitis can occur from 3 to 12 months of age and may or may not cause symptoms. Meningovascular neurosyphilis can occur in the first 2 years of life, and paresis or tabes dorsalis can manifest from about 6 to 21 years of age (see Table 57–4).

HIV and Syphilis
When *T. pallidum* infects the body, the healthy host mounts both a humoral and cell-mediated immune response, and recovery without medications can occur in many patients.

However, with HIV infection, the host response is not competent to combat the infection, creating the scene for greater severity and more frequent late complications. Neurosyphilis is the most serious consequence of syphilis, with or without concurrent HIV infection. However, due to the dysfunctional immune response in the HIV patient, rapid progression from the primary stage through neurosyphilis seems to occur more frequently both with and without adequate treatment. It has also been shown that patients who have syphilis have an increased risk of transmission and acquisition of HIV infection. A genital ulcer probably acts as an entry point for HIV transmission.

■ Ocular

There is no pathognomonic scenario for the ocular manifestations of syphilis. Ocular involvement is rarely encountered earlier than 6 months following the primary chancre, and is frequently found in secondary and tertiary syphilis. Anterior uveitis is the most common ocular complication in secondary syphilis (Table 57–5). Chorioretinitis, with varying presentations, and retinal vasculitis are also common. The chorioretinitis may be diffuse or focal (posterior pole more often than periphery), with acute vitreal inflammation usually accompanying it. One or both optic nerves may become swollen from various mechanisms with syphilis as the underlying cause. Retinal vascular lesions include angiospasm, artery or vein occlusion, and aneurysm formation. Retinal vasculitis affects the arterial supply more often, but periphlebitis and inflammation of both vessels have also been reported.

Ocular complications of late syphilis are typically found in older populations, often those who do not receive regular medical attention. In these cases, diagnosis is usually made by exclusion in a patient with positive treponemal serology. According to Schlaegel (1969), tertiary syphilis should be suspected in any patient with an unexplained pupillary abnormality, optic atrophy or neuritis, dislocated lens not related to other etiologies, apparent retinitis pigmentosa, or uveitis that is unresponsive to conventional therapy. Argyll Robertson pupils (unequal, irregular, and profoundly miotic pupils with a light-near dissociation) are most common; however, tonic pupils may also be found. The tonic pupils found in syphilis could be confused with Adie tonic pupils, but patient characteristics will help differentiate the two. Adie tonic pupils are found more commonly in females than males, and unilateral more often than bilateral, with a mean age of onset of 32 years; they are usually associated with decreased deep tendon reflexes. Syphilitic tonic pupils occur more frequently in males, are always bilateral, have a mean age of detection of 57, and usually do not have decreased deep tendon reflexes. Other common findings include retinal vascular lesions and keratitis (see Table 57–5).

Ocular disorders such as uveitis, papillitis, vitritis, optic neuritis, and retinitis are among the more prominent manifestations of syphilis in the HIV-infected individual. These are more often bilateral and follow a more aggressive course.

Ocular manifestations of congenital syphilis are similar to those in adults with secondary syphilis (see Table 57–5). Acute anterior uveitis with a secondary cataract is most common. Also, syphilis should be included in the differential diagnosis of any childhood case of chorioretinitis. The "salt-and-pepper" appearance of the retina is a classic finding. Secondary glaucoma is also commonly associated with early congenital syphilis. Interstitial keratitis is the most common late manifestation of syphilis, and can occur between the ages of 5 and 20 (Figure 57–2). After resolution, corneal opacification and ghost vessels (Figure 57–3) remain as permanent complications. Optic neuritis may also be found in late congenital syphilis.

DIAGNOSIS

■ Systemic

Primary Syphilis

Diagnosis of primary syphilis is based upon the presence of a syphilitic chancre and positive laboratory tests. The surest way to diagnose primary syphilis is through dark-field microscopy. This uses a sample from either a chancre or lymph node to identify *T. pallidum*. Identification is based on the movement and shape of the spirochete. If positive, it is the only test needed to diagnose the disease. If negative, syphilis is not ruled out, and further testing is required.

Serological testing for syphilis is divided into nontreponemal and treponemal tests. Nontreponemal (also called reaginic) tests measure antibody against a cardiolipin–lecithin cholesterol antigen known as reagin, which results from interaction of *T. pallidum* with host tissue. The venereal disease research laboratory (VDRL) and rapid plasma reagin (RPR) are the most frequently used reaginic tests, and are most useful as screening tests. These tests usually become positive within 4 to 8 weeks of infection and after 4 to 7 days of chancre appearance. However, they may be negative in 13 to 41% of patients with primary syphilis. Titers fall at a rate related to the duration of infection prior to treatment. Treatment within 6 months usually causes the patient to become seronegative in 12 months. However, it may take 2 years for later infection to seroconvert after treatment and it may never occur after treatment of late syphilis. One drawback to reaginic tests is that they are nonspecific; therefore other stimulants of antigens can give false-positive test results (eg, autoimmune disease, Lyme disease, other acute or chronic infections). Therefore, positive reaginic tests must be confirmed with treponemal serology.

Treponemal tests detect specific treponemal antibodies, and once positive remain so for life. The most common treponemal tests include fluorescent treponemal antibody test

TABLE 57–5. OCULAR MANIFESTATIONS OF SYPHILIS

PRIMARY SYPHILIS
- Chancre of the eyelid or conjunctiva (rare)

SECONDARY SYPHILIS
- Conjunctivitis
- Interstitial keratitis
- Episcleritis
- Scleritis
- Iris capillary abnormalities
    Iritis roseata—a collection of small, dilated capillaries present on the surface of the iris
    Iritis papulosa—the roseata lesions increase in size and become papule-like
    Iritis nodosa—the papulosa areas become larger and form yellow-red nodules
- Anterior uveitis
    Acute or chronic
    Recurrent
    Nongranulomatous or granulomatous
- Postinflammatory iris atrophy
- Vitritis
- Posterior uveitis
    Retinitis
    Retinal pigment epitheliitis
    Retinal vasculitis
    Necrotizing retinitis
    Choroiditis
    Serous retinal detachment
    Exudative retinal detachment
    Uveal effusion
- Optic nerve involvement
    Optic neuritis
    Papillitis
    Perineuritis
    Neuroretinitis
    Optic atrophy
    Papilledema secondary to increased ICP from meningitis or meningoencephalitis
- Pupil abnormalities
    Argyll Robertson pupils
    Tonic pupils
- Vasculitis
    Arteriolitis
    Retinal periarteritis
    Subretinal neovascularization
    Retinal necrosis
    Central retinal artery and/or central retinal vein occlusion
- Retinal involvement
    Macula edema
    Stellate maculopathy
    Disciform macular detachment

TERTIARY SYPHILIS
- Pupil abnormalities
    Argyll Robertson pupils
    Tonic pupils
- Keratitis
- Cataracts
- Lens dislocation
- Retinitis
- Optic neuritis
- Descending optic atrophy
- Optic atrophy secondary to chronic disc edema
- Papilledema due to meningitis or meningoencephalitis
- Perineuritis
- Gumma of the lids, conjunctiva, cornea, sclera, iris, ciliary body, orbit, optic nerve, superior orbital fissure

NEUROSYPHILIS
- Pupil abnormalities
    Argyll Robertson pupils
    Tonic pupils
    Dilated pupils fixed to both light and near stimuli
- Chorioretinitis
- Blepharoptosis
- Optic atrophy
- Cranial nerve palsies (3,4,6)
- Arteritis with stroke-like effects to any part of the ocular pathways

CONGENITAL
- Early
    Salt-and-pepper chorioretinitis
    Uveitis
    Secondary glaucoma
    Cataracts
    Chancre of eyelid
    Any manifestation of secondary syphilis
- Late
    Interstitial keratitis/corneal opacities
    Pupil abnormalities
    Optic atrophy
    Secondary glaucoma

(FTA-ABS), microhemagglutination *T. pallidum* assay (MHA-TP), and hemagglutination treponemal test for syphilis (HATTS). Treponemal tests are not used initially to diagnose primary syphilis because they are more expensive, have a 20% false-negative rate, and will be positive even in a patient who currently does not have the disease but was previously successfully treated for it. If dark-field microscopy is not available, diagnosis of syphilis is made by screening with nontreponemal tests and confirmation with treponemal tests.

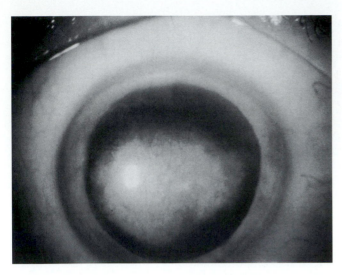

Figure 57–2. Late-onset interstitial keratitis in a patient with congenital syphilis. *(Reprinted with permission from Margo CE, Hamed LM. Ocular syphilis. Surv Ophthalmol. 1992;37:211.)*

Secondary Syphilis

The diagnosis of secondary syphilis is made based upon clinical suspicion of the disease and supporting serology. The rash found in this stage is the most prominent feature, present 75 to 100% of the time. The patient may also have flu-like symptoms or other clinical manifestations (see Table 57–1).

Sensitivity is almost 100% for nontreponemal and treponemal tests in untreated secondary syphilis. Reaginic testing can be unreliable in extremely active cases due to excessive antibody production that blocks agglutination and gives a false-negative result. This has been called the "prozone phenomenon," and may also be found in patients with concurrent HIV infection. Nontreponemal testing will usually be positive during this stage. About 30% of persons

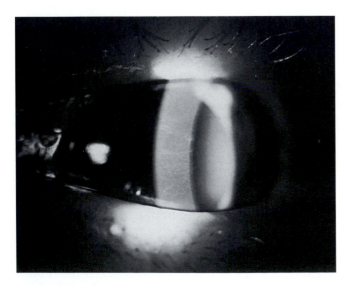

Figure 57–3. Ghost vessels secondary to interstitial keratitis in a patient with congenital syphilis.

will have cerebrospinal fluid pleocytosis with increased protein, although most of these patients will have no clinical signs of central nervous system involvement. Some controversy exists as to the usefulness of CSF evaluation in syphilis. CSF cell count and glucose level are nonspecific and cannot be used to diagnose neurosyphilis, but they may be the best indicator of disease activity. A normal cell count indicates inactive disease. Protein count greater than 45 mg/dL is consistent with active disease.

Latent Syphilis

Latent syphilis is difficult to diagnose because patients are asymptomatic and may not recall the manifestations of the primary or secondary stages that occurred previously. Often, latent syphilis is discovered inadvertently through premarital or prenatal screening. In latent syphilis, treponemal serology will be positive. Nontreponemal tests may be positive but decrease with time, and therefore can also be negative.

Controversy exists regarding the need for lumbar puncture in latent syphilis. Many currently believe the risk involved outweighs the benefits of the test. However, it is indicated when any neurological signs or symptoms are present, or in patients who have concurrent HIV infection (see "HIV and Syphilis" later in the chapter).

Tertiary Syphilis

Gummas are the presenting manifestations of benign tertiary syphilis, with the majority occurring in the skin and skeletal system. Nontreponemal and treponemal tests will usually be positive in this stage (Table 57–6). Active neurosyphilis is at best extremely difficult to diagnose. It is based on serology, after other possible disease mechanisms have been ruled out. The prozone phenomenon may also occur in tertiary syphilis; therefore a negative result with nontreponemal testing in a highly suspicious case also warrants treponemal testing or nontreponemal testing with diluted titers. The modern CSF VDRL should be the standard test for active neurosyphilis because it provides greater information than other tests. CSF pleocytosis can be indicative of neurosyphilis activity and in most cases protein will be elevated. Many recommend a CSF examination with VDRL testing in any patient with untreated syphilis whose duration is longer than 1 year and any patient with neurologic symptoms and syphilis. Positive CSF VDRL should be followed by FTA-ABS. If both are positive, they rule out a biologically false positive CSF VDRL.

Congenital Syphilis

It is vital that all pregnant women be tested for syphilis, and treated if positive to avoid the often devastating effects of congenital syphilis. Many experts feel that female patients at risk for syphilis should be tested early in the pregnancy, in the third trimester, and again at delivery. Using the 1990 CDC definition for congenital syphilis, any infant born to a

TABLE 57–6. SEROLOGY FOR SYPHILIS IN EACH STAGE OF THE DISEASE

Syphilis Stage	Nontreponemal Tests	Treponemal Tests
Primary	Positive after 4–8 weeks but up to 41% false negatives	Positive earlier than nontreponemal tests but up to 20% false negatives
Secondary	Almost always positive except with prozone phenomenon	Almost always positive; false positives possible
Latent	Usually positive	Almost always positive
Tertiary	May be positive or negative; becomes negative with time and treatment	Always positive, even if adequately treated; some false positives possible
Neurosyphilis	May be negative or weakly positive	Always positive, even if adequately treated; some false positives possible
Early congenital	Positive; role in congenital syphilis is to monitor antibody titer (can be positive due to passive transfer from mother; increasing titer implies active disease in the infant)	Always positive; may be false positive from passive transfer of antibodies from mother
Late congenital	May be negative or weakly positive	Always positive

woman with a history of untreated or inadequately treated syphilis with or without serologic confirmation is presumed to have congenital syphilis and treated as such. When this definition is not applied, diagnosis of the asymptomatic infant can be difficult because there is a passive transfer of IgG antibodies in utero and therefore false positives can occur in infants who are not infected. If not treated, the infant with positive serology must be followed over the first 3 months of life to determine if the serology titers increase or decrease. If the VDRL becomes more reactive (the titer increases), it indicates active infection, and a positive test beyond 12 to 15 months also confirms congenital syphilis. If the infant is not infected, the VDRL and FTA-ABS will eventually decrease and return to negative. Diagnosis is definitively made when the level of the nontreponemal test is fourfold or greater than the mother's serum. A probable diagnosis can be made when the infant has a reactive nontreponemal test with clinical manifestations of the disease.

Dark-field microscopy can also be used to establish the diagnosis of congenital syphilis. However, if the spirochete cannot be identified, it does not rule out infection with the disease, and serology must be used to make the diagnosis.

Polymerase chain reaction (PCR) has been shown to be highly sensitive and specific in the early detection of congenital syphilis. It holds promise for the future; however, it is not widely available at this time. Tests that specifically detect IgM antibodies (such as the FTA-ABS IgM) also are promising because IgM antibodies do not cross the placenta from the mother's blood, leading to increased accuracy in the detection of congenital infection.

HIV and Syphilis
Serologic tests for syphilis may give exaggerated results with concurrent HIV infection, and may not be as reliable as they are in other cases. Very high reaginic titers can be found when the host response is severely immunocompro-

mised. Paradoxically, the prozone phenomenon may cause serology to appear negative in secondary syphilis because of a severely immunocompromised host in late HIV disease. In these cases, the lab must be requested to do serial dilutions on the serum. Dark-field microscopy may be more valuable in these patients because it actually detects the presence of spirochetes. All patients with HIV and syphilis should have a CSF evaluation because of the increased frequency of neurosyphilis complications. Most clinicians will suspect concurrent HIV infection if syphilis is diagnosed; therefore it is recommended that all patients with syphilis should be tested for HIV, and that all patients positive for HIV should be tested for syphilis.

■ Ocular
Once a specific ocular disorder is diagnosed, the examiner must consider syphilis in the differential according to the particular manifestation, its presentation, the age of the patient, and health status along with systemic signs and symptoms. Prompt diagnosis is important because delay may lead to irreversible vision loss that was potentially treatable. The patient may need to be questioned regarding the presence of a genital chancre, a rash, or any of the other systemic manifestations. Because almost all ocular manifestations occur in secondary or tertiary syphilis, treponemal and nontreponemal tests should both be positive. However, the reactivity of nontreponemal tests decrease with time, or the prozone phenomenon may give false negatives. Tamesis and Foster (1990) found that only 68% of patients with ocular syphilis had positive VDRL versus 100% with FTA-ABS. Therefore, if the clinician is highly suspicious of syphilis, treponemal testing must be done, because ocular syphilis cannot be excluded through nontreponemal serology. Because the eye is an extension of the nervous system, the CDC recommends CSF evaluation on all patients with ocular syphilis; however, the results are often negative.

TABLE 57–7. TREATMENT AND MANAGEMENT OF SYPHILIS (CDC RECOMMENDATIONS)

PRIMARY, SECONDARY AND EARLY LATENT SYPHILIS
- Benzathine penicillin G, 2.4 million units IM, in one dose
- Contraindications: Penicillin allergies
- Follow-up: Re-examination clinically and serologically at 3 and 6 months; if nontreponemal titers have not declined fourfold by 3 months with primary or secondary syphilis, or 6 months with early latent syphilis or if signs or symptoms persist and reinfection ruled out, should have CSF examination and be retreated appropriately; all patients should be counseled and encouraged to have HIV testing

PRIMARY, SECONDARY AND EARLY LATENT WITH ALLERGY TO PENICILLIN
- Doxycyline, 100 mg orally bid for 14 days or Tetracycline, 500 mg orally qid for 14 days
- Contraindications: Pregnancy
- Follow-up: See above

LATE LATENT AND TERTIARY (GUMMATOUS AND CARDIOVASCULAR)
- Benzathine penicillin G, 7.2 million units total, administered as 3 doses of 2.4 million units IM, given 1 week apart for 3 consecutive weeks
- Contraindication: Penicillin allergy
- Follow-up: These patients all should have thorough clinical examination and CSF evaluation is strongly recommended; if CSF reveals findings consistent with neurosyphilis, treat as such

LATE LATENT AND TERTIARY WITH ALLERGY TO PENICILLIN
- Doxycycline, 100 mg orally bid for 4 weeks or Tetracycline, 500 mg orally qid for 4 weeks
- Contraindication: Pregnancy
- Follow-up: Quantitative nontreponemal tests repeated at 6 and 12 months; if titers increase fourfold or initially high titer fails to decrease or patient shows signs or symptoms attributable to syphilis, patient should be evaluated for neurosyphilis and treated appropriately; HIV testing and counseling indicated

NEUROSYPHILIS AND OCULAR SYPHILIS
- Aqueous crystalline penicillin G, 12–24 million units administered 2–4 million units every 4 hours IV, for 10–14 days
- Alternative regimen (if patient compliance ensured): Procaine penicillin, 2–4 million units IM daily and Probenecid, 500 mg orally qid; both for 10–14 days
- Adjunctive cycloplegics, oral/topical steroids are used when indicated for ocular complications
- Contraindications: Penicillin allergy: These patients should have skin tested and desensitized and managed by expert in syphilis treatment
- Follow-up: Many recommend benzathine penicillin G, 2.5 million units IM weekly for 3 doses after completion of neurosyphilis treatment regimens; follow up: CSF examination repeated every 6 months until cell count normal; if it has not decreased at 6 months, or not normal by 2 years, retreatment strongly indicated; HIV testing and counseling indicated

SYPHILIS IN PREGNANCY
- Follow the penicillin regimen appropriate for the stage of syphilis
- Contraindications: Penicillin allergy patients should be skin tested and treated or desensitized
  Women treated in the second half of pregnancy are at risk for Herxheimer reaction, which may cause premature labor and/or fetal distress
- Monthly follow-up mandatory so retreatment can be given if needed; HIV counseling and testing indicated

CONGENITAL SYPHILIS
- Aqueous crystalline penicillin G, administered as 50,000 units/kg IV every 8–12 hours or Procaine penicillin, 50,000 units/kg administered once daily for 10–14 days (if more than 1 day of therapy missed, entire treatment regimen must be reinstituted)
- Follow-up: Seropositive untreated infants must be followed closely at 1,2,3,6, and 12 months; if not infected, antibody titers must be decreasing by 3 months of age and have disappeared by 6 months; if titers stable or increasing, infant must be treated
- Treated infants: Nontreponemal titers should disappear by 6 months; infants with CSF pleocytosis should be reexamined every 6 months or until cell count normal; if cell count abnormal after 2 years or no downward trend present, treatment should be reinstituted; if CSF VDRL still reactive at 6 months, retreatment is indicated

TREATMENT AND MANAGEMENT

■ Systemic

Penicillin has long been known to be the standard treatment for all stages of syphilis. *Treponema pallidum* is most sensitive to this antibiotic, and remarkably, has not developed resistance over time. The goals of treatment are to eliminate the signs and symptoms, prevent transmission to others, and prevent the severe late sequelae of the disease. The CDC has set standards for each of the stages; however, it is almost impossible to establish a standard treatment because so many variables exist in syphilis. Most clinicians agree with the CDC protocols, but some prefer more aggressive amounts of penicillin in certain cases. Intramuscular injection is generally preferred as opposed to oral dosage primarily because it increases patient compliance. The Jarisch–Herxheimer reaction is a self-limited side effect to penicillin that occurs in some patients. When penicillin is administered, the sudden liberation of antigens or endotoxin from the spirochete causes a local anaphylactic reaction. Symptoms include fever, chills, diaphoresis, myalgia, headache, tachycardia, mild hypertension, and increased rate of respiration. It usually resolves within 24 hours and supportive care (bedrest, analgesics, antipyretics) alone is recommended. Patients should be advised of this reaction before treatment is begun. Current management of syphilis should include counseling and testing for concurrent HIV infection. The treatment of neurosyphilis is controversial because penicillin does not penetrate inflamed meninges well. Recommendations include high-dose penicillin G (Table 57–7).

It is recommended that treatment of congenital syphilis be started, even if the diagnosis is not definite. Also, any infant with the diagnosis of congenital syphilis should have radiography of the long bones, because metaphyseal changes are found in 95% of infants at the time of diagnosis. Cerebral spinal fluid examination, complete blood count including platelet count, and urinalysis should also be performed.

The CDC does not recommend any alterations from standard treatment for those concurrently infected with HIV, although some advocate more extensive dosage regimen. Serology to follow treatment of syphilis in HIV patients may be difficult because of the alterations in the test results. In order to provide long-range care, follow-up must include careful clinical evaluation and repeated CSF examinations if abnormalities were detected. Some have recommended maintenance doses of penicillin; however, it is generally accepted that rigorous follow-up is more efficacious. More studies are needed to determine optimum treatment of HIV patients with concurrent syphilis. Some vaccinations have been implicated in causing relapse to secondary syphilis in HIV patients, and it has been recommended that any unnecessary vaccination be avoided.

■ Ocular

Most experts recommend using the CDC standards for neurosyphilis to treat the ocular manifestations (see Table 57–7), even if the CSF examination is negative. Treatment of ocular syphilis may need to be prolonged in order to eradicate the disease because penicillin does not penetrate the eye very well. The Jarisch–Herxheimer reaction often occurs and may exacerbate the eye inflammation. Systemic corticosteroids can help to control this reaction. Anterior segment complications (acute interstitial keratitis, uveitis) may be treated adjunctively with cycloplegics or topical steroids, when indicated. Use of antibiotics are indicated in congenital syphilis; however, this type of keratitis does not respond to them, therefore topical steroids are needed to prevent vision loss.

CONCLUSION

Syphilis has been a known clinical entity for many centuries. It has undergone several evolutions, from occurring in epidemic proportions to becoming nearly eradicated, and is now undergoing a new resurgence along with HIV disease. Sir William Osler is often quoted as saying, "Know syphilis in all its manifestations and relations, and all other things clinical will be added unto you." This is especially true as it pertains to eyecare practitioners, because knowledge of ocular syphilis provides a wealth of information regarding ocular disease. Syphilis should be considered in almost any case of unusual ocular disease, especially in young adults with acute ocular manifestations and older adults with signs of chronic ocular disease. With the dramatic increase in the number of cases over the past years, eyecare practitioners are sure to encounter more cases of ocular syphilis in the future as the disease progresses to the secondary and tertiary stages.

REFERENCES

Alexander LL. Sexually transmitted diseases: Perspectives on this growing epidemic. *Nurse Practitioner*. 1992;17:31–42.

Ampel NM. Plagues—what's past is present: thoughts on the origin and history of new infectious diseases. *Rev Infect Dis*. 1990;13:658–665.

Arruga J, Valentines J, Mauri F, et al. Neuroretinitis in acquired syphilis. *Ophthalmology*. 1985;92:262–270.

Bos JD. Fluorescent treponemal antibody-absorption (FTA-ABS) test. *Int J Dermatol*. 1982;21:125–130.

Buckley HB. Syphilis: A review and update of this "new" infection of the '90s. *Nurse Practitioner*. 1992;17:25–32.

Centers for Disease Control. 1989 sexually transmitted diseases treatment guidelines. *MMWR*. 1989;38(S-8):5–13.

Crouch ER, Goldberg MF. Retinal periarteritis secondary to syphilis. *Arch Ophthalmol.* 1975;93:384–387.

DeLuise VP, Clark SW, Smith JL. Syphilitic retinal detachment and uveal effusion. *Am J Ophthalmol.* 1982;94:757–761.

Deschenes J, Seamone C, Baines M. Acquired ocular syphilis: Diagnosis and treatment. *Ann Ophthalmol.* 1992;24:134–138.

Deschenes J, Seamone C, Baines M. The ocular manifestations of sexually transmitted diseases. *Can J Ophthalmol.* 1990; 25:177–185.

Drusin LM. Syphilis: Clinical manifestations, diagnosis, and treatment. *Urol Clin North Am.* 1984;11:121–131.

Farnes SW, Setness PA. Serologic tests for syphilis. *Postgrad Med.* 1990;87:37–46.

Feder HM, Manthous C. The asymptomatic patient with a positive VDRL test. *Am Fam Practitioner.* 1988;37:185–190.

Fitzgerald TJ. Pathogenesis and immunology of *Treponema pallidum. Annu Rev Microbiol.* 1981;35:29–54.

Fletcher WA, Sharpe JA. Tonic pupils in neurosyphilis. *Neurology.* 1986;36:188–192.

Gregory N. Clinical problems of syphilis in the presence of HIV. *Clin Dermatol.* 1991;9:71–74.

Hart G. Syphilis tests in diagnostic and therapeutic decision making. *Ann Int Med.* 1986;104:368–376.

Hook EW, Marra CM. Acquired syphilis in adults. *N Engl J Med.* 1992;326:1060–1069.

Hooshmand H, Escobar MR, Kopf SW. Neurosyphilis: A study of 241 patients. *JAMA.* 1972;219:726–730.

Hutchinson CM, Hook EW. Syphilis in adults. *Med Clin North Am.* 1990;74:1389–1416.

Jordan KG. Modern neurosyphilis—a critical analysis. *West J Med.* 1988;149:47–57.

Kirchner JT. Syphilis—an STD on the increase. *Am Fam Practitioner.* 1991;44:843–857.

Larsen SA. Syphilis. *Clin Lab Med.* 1989;9:545–557.

Levy JH, Liss RA, Maguire AM. Neurosyphilis and ocular syphilis in patients with concurrent human immunodeficiency virus infection. *Retina.* 1989;9:175–180.

Lowhagen G. Syphilis: Test procedures and therapeutic strategies. *Semin Dermatol.* 1990;9:152–159.

Margo CE, Hamed LM. Ocular syphilis. *Surv Ophthalmol.* 1992;37:203–220.

Martin NF, Fitzgerald CR. Cystoid macular edema as the primary sign of neurosyphilis. *Am J Ophthalmol.* 1979;88:28–31.

Melvin SY. Syphilis, resurgence of an old disease. *Primary Care.* 1990;17:47–58.

Mendelsohn AD, Jampol LM. Syphilitic retinitis, a cause of necrotizing retinitis. *Retina.* 1984;4:221–224.

Moore JE. Syphilitic iritis. *Am J Ophthamol.* 1931;14:110–126.

Morgan CM, Webb RM, O'Connor GR. Atypical syphilitic chorioretinitis and vasculitis. *Retina.* 1984;4:225–231.

Musher DM. Syphilis, neurosyphilis, penicillin, and AIDS. *J Infect Dis.* 1991;163:1201–1602.

Musher DM. Syphilis. *Pediatr Infect Dis J.* 1990;9:768–769.

Musher DM. Syphilis. *Infect Dis Clin North Am.* 1987;1:83–95.

Musher DM, Hamill RJ, Baughn RE. Effect of human immunodeficiency virus (HIV) infection on the course of syphilis and on the response to treatment. *Ann Int Med.* 1990;113:872–881.

Poitevin M, Bolgert M. Syphilis in 1986. *J Clin Neuro-ophthalmol.* 1987;7:11–16.

Ross WH, Sutton HF. Acquired syphilitic uveitis. *Arch Ophthalmol.* 1980;98:496–498.

Ruder AJ, Halverson KD, Austin JK, Jones WL. Neurosyphilis with associated retinitis. *J Am Optom Assoc.* 1993;64:245–249.

Rush JA, Ryan EJ. Syphilitic optic perineuritis. *Am J Ophthalmol.* 1981;91:404–406.

Sacks JG, Osher RH, Elconin H. Progressive visual loss in syphilitic optic atrophy. *J Clin Neuro-ophthalmol.* 1983;3:5–8.

Sanchez PJ. Congenital syphilis. *Adv Pediatr Infect Dis.* 1992;7:161–180.

Schlaegel TF. *Essentials of Uveitis.* Boston: Little, Brown; 1969: 84–89.

Schlaegel TF, Kao SF. A review (1970–1980) of 28 presumptive cases of syphilitic uveitis. *Am J Ophthalmol.* 1982;93:411–414.

Spoor TC, Wynn P, Hartel WC, Bryan CS. Ocular syphilis, acute and chronic. *J Clin Neuro-ophthalmol.* 1983;3:197–203.

Tamesis RR, Foster S. Ocular syphilis. *Ophthalmology.* 1990;97:1281–1287.

Toshniwal P. Optic perineuritis with secondary syphilis. *J Clin Neuro-ophthalmol.* 1987;7:6–10.

Tramont EC. Controversies regarding the natural history and treatment of syphilis in HIV disease. *AIDS Clin Rev.* 1991:97–107.

Tramont EC. Syphilis: From Beethoven to HIV. *Mt Sinai J Med.* 1990;57:192–196.

Wellington Belin M, Baltch AL, Hay PB. Secondary syphilitic uveitis. *Am J Ophthalmol.* 1981;92:210–214.

Wooldridge WE. Syphilis, a new visit from an old enemy. *Postgrad Med.* 1991;89:193–202.

Zenker PN, Rolfs RT. Treatment of syphilis, 1989. *Rev Infect Dis.* 1990;12(suppl 6):S590–S608.

58
Chapter

HIV and AIDS

Roger Wilson

Acquired immune deficiency syndrome (AIDS) has been recognized as a new disease process since 1981. At that time, a series of rare disorders with an underlying immunodeficiency was found in previously healthy gay men. Eventually the human immunodeficiency virus (HIV) was isolated from the blood of affected patients, and was demonstrated to be responsible for the destruction of the immune system resulting in AIDS.

AIDS is not a neatly compartmentalized disease. Rather, it is the final expression of a continuum of clinical problems and conditions known as HIV disease. There are important clinical differences between a person newly infected with HIV, a person with HIV disease, and a person with AIDS. Infection with HIV may take many years to progress from wellness to the symptomatic stage. Months or years may pass before the development of life-threatening opportunistic diseases and a diagnosis of AIDS. HIV-related ocular diseases may affect any structure of the eye or visual pathways, manifesting as vascular problems, opportunistic infections, neoplasms, and neuro-ophthalmic disorders.

The clinical case definition of AIDS has undergone some revision by the Centers for Disease Control (CDC) to reflect an improved understanding of the disease process. As this scientific understanding about HIV disease has evolved, so has clinical thinking and management.

EPIDEMIOLOGY

■ Systemic

Prevalence patterns of HIV infection differ based upon country of origin, life style, sex, sexual behavior, and sexual orientation. HIV disease is most prevalent in Third World countries, particularly Africa and Asia, where 10 million people are believed to be infected. In the United States, as many as 1 million people are infected, representing a rate of about 1 in 250 in the general population. Prevalence is measured on the basis of a specific antibody response (anti-HIV Ab), as determined by an enzyme-linked immunosorbent assay test (ELISA).

The earliest cases of AIDS were diagnosed in the United States in gay men. Subsequently, cases were seen in hemophiliacs, transfusion recipients, injection drug abusers, heterosexuals, and children born to infected parent(s). As a result of ELISA testing, cases resulting from the transfusion of blood/blood products have decreased dramatically. Likewise, cases in the gay community are declining, due to the effectiveness of community-based risk reduction programs.

Globally, 60% of AIDS cases are in heterosexuals. In Africa, cases are equally distributed between men and women. African women in the childbearing years are at greatest risk, as are their unborn children.

Epidemiologic studies suggest that HIV infection patterns are changing in this country. HIV infection rates are rising in African-Americans, Latinos, injection drug abusers, women, and children. It is estimated that by the year 2005 the distribution of cases in the United States will reflect global patterns: this means that a shift is occurring toward heterosexual intercourse as the predominant mode of infection.

■ Ocular

Ocular signs and symptoms of HIV disease may manifest in up to 75% of all patients during the course of illness.

NATURAL HISTORY

The Organism—Infection and Replication

HIV is a retrovirus comprised of a core protein made up of an RNA genome. It selectively attacks a subset of lymphocytes within the cellular branch of the immune system referred to as the T4 lymphocyte. This element of infection is unusual because T cells ordinarily serve a protective function by activating and directing the immune system when a foreign microbe enters the body. The protein coat of HIV matches the receptors on the T4 cell in a lock and key fashion. This match is essential for HIV to bind to the cell.

Cellular receptors are characterized by various cluster differentiation (CD) proteins, with numeric subheadings to classify their specificity. The T4 lymphocyte is specified by the notation CD4+ to describe the type of receptor on its surface. (Thus, a T4 lymphocyte is sometimes referred to as a CD4+ lymphocyte, or simply as a T4 cell.)

Other cells besides the T4 can become infected with HIV and help transport the virus to other tissues and organs such as lymph nodes. These include monocytes and macrophages (which also exhibit the CD4+ receptor), glial cells within the central nervous system (which do not have the CD4+ receptor), and probably certain phagocytic cells (through indirect cellular mechanisms).

In order to replicate, the enzyme reverse transcriptase transforms the RNA genome core of HIV into a viral DNA copy. This viral DNA then becomes incorporated into the infected cell's nucleus, assuming part of the infected cell's genetic makeup. This stage (the latent provirus phase) is relatively quiescent, although the infection is usually advancing in other cells throughout the body. At this stage the provirus is ready for activation, but must await a replication signal. The exact trigger or mechanism involved in a change from the latent provirus stage to an active virus-replicating state is unknown. Once initiated, this process converts host cells into "virus factories." The host cells eventually die. The new virions go on to infect new cells, thereby contributing to the depletion of T4 cells. This process repeats until the immune system falters and

immune deficiency results, opening pathways for opportunistic infections (OIs) to flourish. Therefore, T4 cell counts play a vital role in the assessment and management of a patient with HIV disease.

Transmission

HIV is transmitted most commonly through sexual contact. It is readily spread through mucus membrane contact with semen and vaginal secretions. Therefore, AIDS is primarily considered to be a venereal disease.

HIV may also be transmitted via blood and blood products. Transmission via blood includes transfusion of whole blood or its components, and the practice of needle sharing by IV drug abusers.

HIV can also be transmitted during pregnancy, delivery, or rarely, after birth through breast milk. Other body fluids such as sweat, urine, saliva, feces, vomitus, nasal secretions, and tears have inconsistently contained HIV (in whole or fragments). Although the theoretical possibility exists that HIV could be transmitted via these body secretions, they are not believed to carry a sufficient innoculum to cause clinical infection.

The relative infectivity of HIV itself is an important aspect of HIV transmission that is infrequently addressed. Exposure to HIV does not always result in infection. For example, in a study by Henderson and associates (1990), the risk of HIV infection following a percutaneous needle stick injury contaminated with HIV-positive blood was calculated to be 0.3 to 0.4% per event. It also appears that HIV-infected people who engage in unprotected sexual intercourse do not always transmit the virus. In an ongoing study by Padian and co-workers (1987) of 97 unprotected female partners of 93 infected men, only 23% of the women became infected after 4 years of observation. Therefore, minimizing contact with fluids that transmit HIV should even further reduce the risk of transmission.

Course of the Disease

There are three distinct stages of HIV infection and disease manifestation; initial, chronic, and final (or crisis) stage. The early phase occurs when a person is newly infected with HIV. Upon initial infection with HIV a person may have no clinical symptoms at all. More commonly, a mild influenza-like illness develops, referred to as an acute retroviral syndrome. The person fully recovers from this illness within weeks and feels well again. However, the infection is nonetheless present and slowly taking hold within the person's immune system. Shortly after infection, the body mounts an immune response. At this point the person is HIV positive (HIV+), having produced an antibody to HIV. Although this response seems to temporarily combat the infection, it is typically not sufficient to fully clear the infection. The antibody titers are too low and lack the heterogeneity necessary to destroy genetic variations of the replicating virus. HIV begins its insidious course of destruction.

The next stage of HIV disease is the chronic phase, typically lasting years. The average time from initial infection to clinical manifestations of problems associated with HIV disease is 6.8 years. During this phase most people are reasonably healthy and feel well, but minor pathological changes are present and can be measured. These changes usually manifest as minor immune dysfunctions, abnormal blood studies, and/or mild constitutional problems. Previously it was thought that in this stage of infection, also referred to as the "latent period," HIV was dormant. However, recent studies have shown that there is progressive deterioration of the immune system during the chronic stage, with ongoing replication of the virus.

Patients in the crisis stage of HIV infection have a frank diagnosis of AIDS. The final phase may last months or years depending on the overall health of the patient and response to the various treatments. Most patients do not feel well. The T4 cell counts are far below the normal range of 800 to 1400 cells/mm^3, usually 200/mm^3 and below. Pronounced clinical manifestations develop and life-threatening OIs, diseases, and other problems emerge. Eventually, patients in the crisis stage die as a result of diseases that the body can no longer fight and therapies cannot control.

■ SYSTEMIC HIV DISEASE

Diagnosis

Primary HIV Disease

Shortly after a person becomes infected with HIV, antibodies develop against the viral core antigen and the viral envelope proteins. There is a latency period prior to the development of antibodies that ranges from 6 weeks to 6 months, and in rare cases longer than 1 year. Antibody tests that screen for antibodies to viral proteins are used to diagnose infection with HIV. The ELISA and Western blot tests are used to screen for antibodies against HIV, and thus verify that infection has occurred. Although the ELISA test is highly sensitive, the Western blot test is more specific. Two successive ELISA tests and one confirmatory Western blot test must be positive before a patient is considered HIV positive. The combined use of the ELISA and Western blot tests is the best method for establishing a definitive diagnosis of HIV infection.

Other tests are being developed to detect early signs of HIV infection during the latency period, the window of time prior to the expression of antibodies. The polymerase chain reaction (PCR), which detects HIV nucleic acids, is capable of detecting HIV infection much earlier than the ELISA and Western blot tests. However, the PCR test suffers from a high false-positive rate due to its sensitivity to cross-contamination. The antigen capture test also detects the presence

of portions of HIV earlier than antibody serologic testing, but it is not widely used because it is more valuable as a predictor of prognosis rather than early infection. Improved culture methods are now able to detect HIV in most patients who are HIV positive, but the expense and risk of culturing does not presently lend itself to clinical use.

AIDS

The CDC diagnosis of AIDS, referred to as a "case definition," has undergone revision since 1981. These changes reflect a better understanding of the natural history of HIV disease and its sequelae. AIDS is extremely complex to diagnose. The current case definition includes various categories of HIV disease that are reflective of HIV disease progression (Table 58–1). The AIDS-defining diseases and conditions vary depending on laboratory evidence of HIV infection. The list is restrictive when laboratory evidence of HIV infection is equivocal or does not exist, and broadens when a patient is confirmed as being HIV positive (Tables 58–2 to 58–4). Diseases that are strongly linked to a diagnosis of AIDS are referred to as indicator diseases. This diagnostic approach allows for a systematic classification of patients, while minimizing the likelihood of making an incorrect diagnosis.

A diagnosis of AIDS can be made on the basis of three different but highly specific sets of clinical findings (Tables 58–2 to 58–4):

- The manifestation of an indicator disease in the absence of laboratory confirmation of HIV infection (providing that the patient has no underlying problem that would otherwise contribute to the expression of the indicator disease).

TABLE 58–1. CDC DIAGNOSTIC CRITERIA FOR A CASE OF AIDS[a]

T4 Cell Categories	Clinical Categories		
≥500/mm^3	A1	B1	**C1**
200–499/mm^3	A2	B2	**C2**
<200/mm^3	**A3**	**B3**	**C3**

Bold categories A3, B3, C1, C2, and C3 represent reportable cases of AIDS.
[a]1993 CDC classification system for HIV infection and expanded AIDS surveillance case definition for adolescents and adults. Refer to clinical categories A–C (Tables 58–2 to 58–4). A case of AIDS in an adolescent or adult is diagnosed based upon the clinical category of a patient and/or the T4 lymphoctye cell count in an HIV-infected individual. A diagnosis of AIDS linked to T4 lymphocyte counts alone is not a marker for HIV infection or AIDS. HIV infection must be assured before reporting a case of AIDS to the CDC. HIV infection is defined as repeatedly reactive screening tests to HIV-1 antibody (eg, EIA) with specific HIV antibody identified by use of supplemental tests (eg, Western Blot, immunofluorescene assay). Other methods of HIV-1 diagnosis include virus isolation, antigen detection, and detection of HIV genetic material (DNA or RNA) by PCR.
Adapted from the Centers for Disease Control and Prevention. 1993 revised classification system for HIV infection and expanded surveillance case definition for AIDS among adolescents and adults. MMWR. *1992;41(No. RR-17).*

TABLE 58–2. CDC CLINICAL CATEGORY A CONDITIONS OF HIV-INFECTED ADOLESCENTS AND ADULTS[a]

Asymptomatic HIV infection

Persistent generalized lymphadenopathy (PGL)

Acute (primary) HIV infection with accompanying illness or history of acute HIV infection

[a]Category A is defined as one or more of the above conditions. However, conditions listed in categories B or C must not have occurred.
Adapted from the Centers for Disease Control and Prevention. 1993 revised classification system for HIV infection and expanded surveillance case definition for AIDS among adolescents and adults. MMWR. *1992;41(No. RR-17).*

- The manifestation of an indicator disease *with* laboratory confirmation of HIV infection regardless of the presence of other diseases or causes of immunodeficiency.
- Laboratory confirmation of HIV infection combined with a T4 lymphocyte count of <200 cell/mm³ blood (indicator disease(s) may or may not be present).

When a patient fits the case definition of AIDS, it is reported to the CDC. A diagnosis of AIDS does not mean that death is imminent. Depending on the overall health of the patient, continuation of employment and routines of daily living are generally encouraged. Close monitoring, antiretroviral medications, and prophylactic therapy are the standards of care once a diagnosis of AIDS is made.

TABLE 58–3. CDC CLINICAL CATEGORY B CONDITIONS OF HIV-INFECTED ADOLESCENTS AND ADULTS[a]

Bacillary angiomatosis

Candidiasis, oropharyngeal (thrush)

Candidiasis, vulvovaginal; persistent, frequent, or poorly responsive to therapy

Cervical dysplasia (moderate or severe)/carcinoma in situ

Constitutional symptoms, such as fever (38.5°C) or diarrhea lasting > 1 month

Hairy leukoplakia, oral

Herpes zoster (shingles), involving at least two distinct episodes or more than one dermatome

Idiopathic thrombocytopenic purpura

Listeriosis

Pelvic inflammatory disease, particularly if complicated by tubo-ovarian abscess

Peripheral neuropathy

[a] Symptomatic conditions that are not included among conditions listed in clinical category C and which meet at least one of the following criteria: the conditions are attributed to HIV infection and/or are indicative of a defect in cell-mediated immunity; or the conditions are considered by physicians to have a clinical course or management that is complicated by HIV infection. The above are examples of these conditions, but are not exhaustive.
Adapted from the Centers for Disease Control and Prevention. 1993 revised classification system for HIV infection and expanded surveillance case definition for AIDS among adolescents and adults. MMWR. *1992;41(No. RR-17).*

TABLE 58–4. CDC CLINICAL CATEGORY C CONDITIONS OF HIV-INFECTED ADOLESCENTS AND ADULTS[a]

Candidiasis of bronchi, trachea, or lungs

Candidiasis, esophageal

Cervical cancer, invasive

Coccidioidomycosis, disseminated or extrapulmonary

Cryptococcosis, extrapulmonary

Cryptosporidiosis, chronic intestinal (>1 month duration)

Cytomegalovirus disease (other than liver, spleen, or nodes)

Cytomegalovirus retinitis (with loss of vision)

HIV encephalopathy

Herpes simplex: chronic ulcer(s) (>1 month duration); or bronchitis, pneumonitis, or esophagitis

Histoplasmosis, disseminated or extrapulmonary

Isopsoriasis, chronic intestinal (>1 month duration)

Kaposi sarcoma

Lymphoma, Burkitt (or equivalent term)

Lymphoma, immunoblastic (or equivalent term)

Lymphoma, primary in brain

Mycobacterium avium complex or *M. kansasii*, disseminate or extrapulmonary

Mycobacterium tuberculosis, any site (pulmonary or extrapulmonary)

Mycobacterium, other species or unidentified species, disseminated or extrapulmonary

Pneumocystis carinii pneumonia

Pneumonia, recurrent

Progressive multifocal leukoencephalopathy

Salmonella septicemia, recurrent

Toxoplasmosis of brain

Wasting syndrome due to HIV

[a]Category C includes any conditions listed in the 1987 surveillance case definition for AIDS. The conditions in clinical category C are strongly associated with severe immunodeficiency, occur frequently in HIV-infected individuals, and cause serious morbidity and mortality.
Adapted from the Centers for Disease Control and Prevention. 1993 revised classification system for HIV infection and expanded surveillance case definition for AIDS among adolescents and adults. MMWR. *1992;41(No. RR-17).*

Treatment and Management

There is presently no cure for AIDS. The ideal therapy against HIV is a vaccine to protect a person from becoming infected. Vaccination (acquired immunity) enables the body to mount a virocidal response before an infection is established. Researchers have thus far been unable to develop an effective vaccine against HIV. One major obstacle is the multitude of genetic variations that HIV produces as it replicates. Therefore, in order to be effective an HIV vaccine must be capable of mounting a multiple immune response to protect against viral heterogeneity.

Current management protocols include treatment of primary HIV disease, prophylaxis against opportunistic diseases, and prompt, aggressive treatment of any problems when they present. Medical therapy has been particularly challenging because HIV, like other viruses, depends on the internal metabolism of an infected cell for replication. Inhibiting cellular processes with medications often causes damage to the host cell as well as others that are not infected. Present investigations include attempts to develop therapies against various aspects of HIV's life cycle (such as inhibiting binding to T4 cells, inhibiting viral enzymes, disrupting the assembly of new viruses, or killing virions as they bud from host cells). Additionally, because patients with HIV disease tend to be on multiple medications, close monitoring for drug interactive side effects is required.

Treatment of Primary HIV Disease

The mainstay of therapy against HIV are the antiretroviral medications that act by inhibiting the enzyme reverse transcriptase. Reverse transcriptase is required in the first phase of viral replication, the conversion of viral RNA to DNA for incorporation into the T4 cell's nucleus. Interfering with this process results in inhibition of viral replication. Included in this group are the FDA approved drugs zidovudine (AZT), dideoxyinosine (ddI), and dideoxycytidine (ddC), and other compounds under investigation.

Zidovudine was approved for treatment of HIV disease in 1987 and is the most widely prescribed antiretroviral. Numerous studies have demonstrated the effectiveness of AZT in slowing the progression of HIV disease, reducing the number of OIs, prolonging life, increasing the number of circulating T4 lymphocytes, decreasing the concentration of circulating viral protein in the blood, and reversing central nervous system problems in people whose T4 lymphocyte cell counts are below 200/mm^3 of blood. Patients on AZT also regain weight and some immune function. The dosage for patients who are symptomatic but not critical is one 200 mg tablet every 4 hours for the first month followed by a reduction to 100 mg every 4 hours. Up to 45% of patients taking AZT experience side effects, especially bone marrow depression manifesting as granulocytopenia and anemia. Severe headache, nausea, insomnia, myalgias, seizures, and neurotoxicity have occurred in some patients. Another drawback is the development of AZT-resistant strains of HIV. This problem occurs in some patients after more than 1 year of AZT therapy. AZT is also frequently prescribed when a patient's T4 count drops below 500/mm^3 blood in an attempt to slow HIV disease progression and/or the development of OIs. However, recent studies suggest that the clinical outcome for patients receiving this earlier intervention with AZT may be no different than those starting it when the T4 lymphocyte cell count drops below 200/mm^3 blood.

Dideoxyinosine (ddI), another reverse transcriptase inhibitor, was approved in 1991 for the treatment of advanced HIV disease. It is indicated in cases where a patient is intolerant of AZT, has had significant clinical deterioration on AZT, or demonstrates signs of drug resistance. In addition to its effects in lymphocytes, ddI also possesses anti-HIV activity in monoctyes and macrophages. Like AZT, it slows the progression of HIV disease, delays the onset of OIs, increases the number of lymphocytes, decreases the amount of circulating viral antigens, and produces weight gain in patients. The dosage is weight dependent. For adults weighing 50 to 74 kg, the dose is two 100 mg tablets twice a day. Primary side effects are peripheral neuropathy and pancreatitis. Hyperurecemia, headaches, hepatitis, diarrhea, and insomnia have also been reported.

Dideoxycytidine (ddC), a third reverse transcriptase inhibitor, gained FDA approval in 1992. It is prescribed in combination with AZT in patients who have T4 lymphocyte cell counts ≤300/mm^3 blood in the presence of advancing HIV disease or in those who are deteriorating immunologically. When compared to AZT monotherapy, ddC appears to produce a more lasting increase in T4 lymphocyte cell counts. Short-term clinical data have also revealed reduced plasma viral antigens in patients on ddC therapy. The recommended initial dosage in patients weighing more than 30 kg is 0.75 mg po every 8 hours in combination with 200 mg of AZT three times daily. The primary dose-limiting side effect is peripheral neuropathy, and infrequently pancreatitis.

Adverse ocular reactions can also occur as a result of antiretroviral therapy. One case of macular edema and one report of excessive growth of the eyelashes have been attributed to AZT. Patients taking AZT have presented with flame hemorrhages, Roth spots, and cotton-wool spots. These retinal changes were caused by drug-induced anemia rather than HIV-related pathology. Geier and associates (1993) reported two cases of temporary tritan color vision defects following AZT administration. Lafeuillade and colleagues (1991) reported one case of optic neuritis associated with ddI therapy in an adult. Some children treated with ddI demonstrate retinal toxicity manifested as degeneration of the peripheral retinal pigment epithelium. Additional ocular side effects resulting from antiretroviral therapy will likely emerge as more patients receive these medications over extended periods of time.

Due to the problems of systemic toxicity and drug resistance, combination therapies are gaining in popularity. Multidrug therapeutic approaches aim to prescribe reduced dosages of two or more antiretrovirals, affecting HIV at either various stages of replication or through interfering with one stage repeatedly (eg, reverse transcription). For example, AZT has demonstrated antiviral activity when combined with acyclovir, dideoxyadenosine (ddA), ddC, ddI, interferon alfa, granulocyte-macrophage colony-stimulating factor (GM-CSF), granulocyte colony-stimulating factor (G-CSF), erythropoietin, and other experimental compounds. Advantages of this approach include reduction of toxic reactions through reduced concentrations of doses, prevention of HIV-resistant strain formation, synergistic or additive effects of some combinations, and the ability to attack HIV in multiple stages of its life cycle. Disadvantages of combination therapies include compounding multidrug side effects and drug interactions. No combination to date has effected a cure. Nevertheless, multidrug therapy shows great promise in the future management of HIV disease.

Prophylaxis

The second level of management of HIV-related diseases is through prophylaxis. Clinical experience has proven that patients benefit from this preventive therapeutic approach. The T4 lymphocyte count serves as a valuable guide in the initiation of prophylactic therapy for many conditions. Prophylaxis against *Pneumocystis carinii* pneumonia (with medications such as trimethoprim-sulfamethoxazole, pentamidine, and dapsone) typically begins at T4 counts ≤200; for disseminated fungal diseases prophylaxis is begun at ≤150. Toxoplasmosis prophylaxis also begins at T4 counts of 200 or less. *Mycobacterium avium–intracellulare* complex (MAc) prophylaxis with rifabutin begins at T4 counts of 100 or less. Broad spectrum macrolide antibiotic prophylaxis is being studied. Tuberculosis prophylaxis (with isoniazid) is initiated in patients with positive skin tests or those at high risk for tuberculosis, or both. Prophylaxis against CMV is at the investigational stage. Prophylactic approaches will likely undergo close scrutiny and change as knowledge about HIV expands.

Psychosocial Needs

A frequently overlooked aspect of care is the psychosocial needs of the patient with HIV disease. Patients may suffer loss of independence (physical, financial); rejection (family, job, housing); depression; prejudice; and other personal and social problems. Sensitivity to these issues and knowledge of community resources may greatly enhance the quality of life for some patients.

■ SYSTEMIC HIV-RELATED DISEASES AND OPPORTUNISTIC INFECTIONS

The systemic problems associated with AIDS are virtually endless due to the patient's inability to fight disease. For adults and adolescents the CDC classifies HIV infection into three clinical categories: (1) general manifestations of HIV disease (see Table 58–2, clinical category A); (2) symptomatic conditions that contribute to or are complicated by HIV infection (see Table 58–3, clinical category B); and (3) those that are associated with severe immunodeficiency and occur frequently in persons with HIV infection (see Table 58–4, clinical category C). A review of some of the more commonly occurring systemic problems associated with a diagnosis of AIDS follows.

Kaposi Sarcoma

Kaposi sarcoma (KS) is a multicentric neoplasm characterized by a proliferation of spindle cells with neovascularization, edema, and various infiltrative cell types that fuse to form the lesions. KS is the most common neoplasm in AIDS. Before AIDS, KS was a rare, relatively benign, and slowly-growing lesion affecting only older men from Eastern Europe, Mediterranean regions, and of Jewish ancestry.

KS was initially seen in up to 40% of AIDS patients, primarily in homosexual and bisexual men. The incidence of KS in AIDS has declined over the years, and is now seen in only 15% of newly diagnosed cases. The etiology of KS is unclear, as is the reason for the decline in new cases. Recent research is challenging the notion that KS is a true malignancy. An infectious co-factor may be involved.

KS is an indicator disease for AIDS when it presents in a patient under 60 years of age, or at any age in conjunction with laboratory evidence of HIV infection. It can manifest in the visceral organs, lungs, brain, lymph nodes, skin, and eye. KS can be fatal, particularly when the lungs are involved. Treatment of KS is aimed at ameliorating symptoms and complications. Systemic therapies consist of chemotherapy, immunotherapy, immune enhancement therapy, and growth inhibition factors. Local therapies are comprised of radiation therapy, strontium-90 therapy, excision, and cryotherapy.

Pneumocystis carinii Pneumonia

Pneumocystis carinii is a ubiquitous organism. It is an opportunistic protozoan, but also shares some properties of fungi. In immunocompetent people, it is a benign organism. It causes the most common OI in AIDS, a serious and often fatal pneumonia in up to 85% of patients. *P. carinii* was originally thought to be a pulmonary OI. However, since the late 1980s, numerous cases of disseminated *P. carinii* have been reported that involve other organs, including the eye.

Diagnosis of *P. carinii* pneumonia is made via x-ray of the lungs, examination of bronchial secretions, bronchoscopy, and (rarely) lung biopsy. In extrapulmonary disease, radiography, sonography, and computed tomography are used in the diagnosis.

Treatment of primary disease is with either pentamadine or trimethoprim-sulfamethoxazole (TMP-SMX). In moderate to severe cases corticosteroids may be added, the rationale being that the antiinflammatory effect of the corticosteroids limits the amount of pulmonary compromise caused by the dying organisms.

Prophylaxis against *P. carinii* is given to patients who have had pneumonia or who demonstrate T4 cell counts below 200 to 250/mm^3 of blood. Systemic prophylactic therapy with TMP-SMX or dapsone is preferred over aerosolized pentamidine, as either one is more effective in curbing dissemination of the disease than aerosolized pentamidine, which is site specific (pulmonary) in it effects.

Tuberculosis

Mycobacterium tuberculosis (TB) is relatively common in AIDS, affecting up to 35% of patients. Pulmonary TB alone is not an indicator disease for AIDS. However, disseminated (extrapulmonary) TB (with or without concurrent pneumonia) is an AIDS-defining disease. TB is rapidly becoming an important OI in AIDS because it can be spread to the normal population. Although most cases are still readily treatable, resistant and fatal strains are developing. (See chapter 54.).

Mycobacterium avium–intracellulare Complex

Disseminated *Mycobacterium avium-intracellulare* complex (MAC), an indicator disease for AIDS, is a bacterial syndrome that affects up to 40% of AIDS patients. MAC complex tends to occur very late in the disease. Most patients have T4 cell counts below 50/mm³ blood at diagnosis. Symptoms include fever, night sweats, and generalized wasting syndrome. Single-agent therapy (rifabutin) and combination therapies are often used.

Cytomegalovirus Disease

Cytomegalovirus (CMV) is a DNA virus and a member of the herpes family. Latent CMV infection (as measured by anti-CMV antibody) is quite high in the adult population, ranging from 50 to 100% depending on country of origin, general health, immune status, and personal habits. CMV is transmitted perinatally, sexually, through tissue transplantation, exposure to blood and blood products, and through contact with a variety of body fluids including urine, saliva, and tears.

In immunocompetent people CMV infection rarely causes severe clinical disease. More often, patients will complain of a typical, self-limiting viral syndrome. Cytomegalovirus disease is a late complication of AIDS, presenting most often when the T4 cell count drops below 100/mm³ blood. In order to be classified as an indicator disease for AIDS, it must manifest in a patient over 1 month old in an organ other than the liver, spleen, or lymph nodes. In people with AIDS, CMV causes pneumonitis, colitis, esophagitis, gastritis, hepatitis, adrenalitis, nephritis, and retinitis.

Management of CMV disease requires a systemic approach. Currently there are two medications that are FDA approved: ganciclovir and foscarnet. Both are virostatic agents, administered intravenously through a permanent indwelling catheter, and require an initial induction followed by lifelong maintenance therapy. Immunoglobulin therapy is occasionally added to treat systemic disease. Oral prophylactic therapies are under investigation.

HIV Encephalopathy

The central nervous system (CNS) is yet another site of infection for HIV. Neurological abnormalities affect up to 40% of patients, manifesting as peripheral neuropathies, myelopathies, and encephalopathies. HIV-related encephalopathy is the most commonly occurring problem within the CNS. Cognitive dysfunction, seizures, headaches, confusion, affective disorders, depression, and impaired motor abilities are common symptoms. Advanced cases present with a progressive psychomotor deficit and dementia. Treatment with AZT may slow progression of the problem and in some cases restore cognitive functions.

HIV Wasting Syndrome

A complicated group of clinical findings constitute the HIV wasting syndrome. These include (1) involuntary weight loss (exceeding 10% of baseline), (2) fevers lasting longer than 1 month, (3) persistent diarrhea (>1 month) and, (4) the lack of a diagnosis linked to these symptoms. Because many other problems can account for these symptoms, HIV wasting syndrome is a diagnosis of exclusion. Management of the condition is based on treatment of any co-existing problem(s) and supportive therapy of individual symptoms.

Syphilis

Infection with *Treponema pallidum* in people with AIDS advances quickly to neurosyphilis in a majority of cases. Therefore, it is extremely important to diagnose syphilis in HIV-infected persons. Any patient with HIV disease who has syphilis should be treated as if they have neurosyphilis. (See chapter 57.)

Toxoplasmosis

Infection of the brain with *Toxoplasma gondii* is an AIDS-defining disease. It is the most common OI of the CNS in people with AIDS, producing profound morbidity and death in up to 35% of cases. (See chapter 64.)

Other Diseases and Conditions Indicative of AIDS

Depending on laboratory evidence of HIV infection and qualifying characteristics, numerous other problems present in patients that contribute to a diagnosis of AIDS (Tables 58–2 and 58–3). To simplify the case-reporting process and to be inclusive of conditions that pose significant public health concerns in the HIV epidemic, the CDC's most recent revision also added pulmonary tuberculosis, recurrent pneumonia, and cervical dysplasia and cancer.

■ OCULAR HIV-RELATED DISEASE

There is an incomplete understanding of the etiology, natural history, and prognostic value of the ocular manifestations of HIV disease. HIV has been isolated in the cornea, conjunctiva, tears, aqueous, vitreous, and retina of some patients with AIDS. Some ocular manifestations of AIDS may be due to HIV alone; others (eg, retinal OIs) result from the immunodeficiency caused by HIV; and some may be due to a combination of factors. HIV-related ocular diseases affect all aspects of the eye (including the adnexa, orbit, anterior segment, posterior segment, and visual pathways), and may manifest as vascular problems, opportunistic infections, neoplasms, or neuro-ophthalmic disorders.

Adnexal and Anterior Segment Disorders

Table 58–5 summarizes adnexal and anterior segment HIV manifestations.

Vascular

Conjunctival microvasculopathy is seen in HIV positive patients with T4 cell counts below 400/mm³ of blood. These microvascular changes are most pronounced in the perilimbal region of the bulbar conjunctiva. They manifest as irregular coma-shaped vascular fragments (commonly affecting venules), a sludging of the blood flow column, and a granular appearance to the blood. The presence of conjunctival microvasculopathy is probably linked to the blood flow disruption that is seen in the retinal circulation. These changes have also been observed in patients with other vascular diseases including diabetes mellitus and sickle-cell anemia. The cause of conjunctival vascular abnormalities is unknown, but may be due to the same pathological processes that cause posterior segment ischemia.

Opportunistic Infections

The development of ocular OIs tends to occur as a later process of immunodeficiency. Patients will usually demonstrate a T4 count below 200/mm³ of blood before the expression of ocular OIs. This process parallels the expression of OIs elsewhere in the body.

Viral

Molluscum contagiosum. Molluscum contagiosum disease of the eyelids is commonly seen in patients with AIDS. The DNA virus that causes this condition is sometimes seen on the margins of the lids in immunocompetent persons, presenting as raised white vesicular lesions. It causes a low-grade, chronic follicular conjunctivitis that is cured by either lancing and expressing the lesions or excising them. In people with AIDS, molluscum contagiosum can cause far greater clinical disease. The lesions are often 2 to 3 mm in size and greater in number than in immunocompetents. Response to conventional therapy is excellent.

Herpes zoster ophthalmicus. Reactivation of the herpes zoster virus ordinarily occurs in immunocompetent people older than 60 years of age, presenting as either shingles or herpes zoster ophthalmicus (HZO). However, in HIV dis-

ease reactivation may be seen in younger patients, affecting as many as 21% during their illness. In a 1986 study by Sandor and co-workers of patients under the age of 44 years presenting with herpes zoster ophthalmicus, 61% were found to be HIV positive. This finding has been duplicated in other studies.

HZO in HIV disease presents in the usual fashion with a hemifacial vesiculobullous rash that does not cross the midline. As in traditional HZO, if the nasociliary branch of the ophthalmic division of the trigeminal nerve is involved, the chance of ocular complications is great. Ophthalmic problems may include ptosis, proptosis, blepharitis, conjunctivitis, keratitis, uveitis, retinitis (acute retinal necrosis), optic neuropathy, oculo-motor palsies, and vasculitis (including central retinal artery occlusion).

HZO in HIV disease is treated with analgesics for pain, intravenous acyclovir (oral acyclovir is under investigation), palliative therapy for skin lesions, ocular lubricants, and occasionally prophylactic antibiotics to diminish the chance of secondary bacterial infections. Vidarabine and interferon therapy have also been used with limited success. Uveitis is treated with cycloplegics and steroids, although steroids may be of little value due to a diminished inflammatory response. Patients with HIV disease may require longer and more aggressive therapy than immunocompetent persons. Some people with AIDS who develop shingles have been successfully treated with foscarnet.

Apparently healthy patients under the age of 45 who present with herpes zoster ophthalmicus should be referred for a complete physical examination, including blood studies, to rule out HIV disease as the trigger for this bout of reactivation.

Herpes simplex virus. Herpes simplex virus (HSV) disease occurs in some patients with AIDS. HIV will cause a slow decline in the immune system's ability to control latent infections. Therefore, in people with HIV disease, HSV can cause chronic lesions on the skin of the eyelids and mucous membranes of the conjunctiva, as well as the typical HSV keratitis, stromal disease, and uveitis.

Ocular HSV disease is treated with antiviral preparations, with acyclovir being the treatment of choice. If needed, cycloplegics and steroids are added (once the keratitis resolves) to control any accompanying uveitis. As in HZO, HSV disease may linger in people with AIDS, requiring closer follow-ups and extended therapy.

Resistant strains of HSV are developing in some people with AIDS. Foscarnet has been used to treat these cases with limited success. Experimentation involving acyclovir in combination with other substances is also underway in the treatment of resistant strains.

Parasitic Disease. Microsporidial protozoal parasites have been isolated in HIV positive patients and people with

TABLE 58–5. OCULAR ADNEXAL AND ANTERIOR SEGMENT MANIFESTIONS OF HIV

LOCATION	PROBLEM	FREQUENCY[a]
● Adnexa / orbit	● Viral	
	Molluscum contagiosum	C
	Herpes zoster ophthalmicus	C
	● Neoplastic	
	Kaposi sarcoma	VC
	Primary non-Hodgkin lymphoma	R
	Burkitt lymphoma	R
	● Histiocytosis-X	
	Eosinophilic granuloma	R
	● Inflammatory	
	Ocular myositis	R
● Conjunctiva	● Vascular	
	Microvasculopathy	VC
	● Neoplastic	
	Kaposi sarcoma	VC
	● Bacterial	
	Nonspecific conjunctivitis	C
● Cornea	● Autoimmune	
	Ocular surface disease	VC
	● Viral	
	Herpes zoster keratitis	R
	Herpes simplex keratitis	R
	● Parasitic	
	Microsporidial keratitis	R
	● Fungal	
	Candida albicans ulcers	R
	● Bacterial	
	Pseudomonas aeruginosa ulcers	R
● Anterior chamber	● Inflammatory	
	Primary HIV-related uveitis	R–C
	● Angle-closure glaucoma	R

[a]VC, very common (>25%); C, common (10–25%); R, rare (<10%).

AIDS. These organisms have caused keratoconjunctivitis in some of these patients. There is currently no effective treatment. Ocular lubricants, steroids, sulfa drugs, and broad-spectrum antibiotics have been used with varying success.

Fungal Disease. Spontaneous fungal ulcers of the cornea have been infrequently reported in people with advanced HIV disease. Heinemann and associates (1987) reported a case of *Candida albicans* endophthalmitis in a patient with AIDS. Conventional therapies such as topical and intravenous amphotericin-B and pimaricin have been successful in treating these infections.

Bacterial Disease. Chronic conjunctivitis has been reported in AIDS patients. The prevalence is not known, as no study has been conducted to investigate this problem. Culture and sensitivity studies often fail to isolate a specific organism, so broad-spectrum antibiotics are used to treat these cases.

Although a few cases of *Pseudomonas aeruginosa* infections of the cornea have been reported in both HIV+ and AIDS patients, this problem is rare. The observed cases represented apparently either spontaneous or contact lens associated etiologies.

Medications used in the treatment of bacterial diseases of the anterior segment in people with HIV disease is the same as in immunocompetent people. For patients responding poorly to standard therapy, management may require hospitalization with extended therapy.

Autoimmune-like Disease
A generalized sicca complex develops in some people with HIV disease. Ocular involvement is possible. In a 1990 study of 42 HIV-positive men (with and without a diagnosis of AIDS) by Lucca and colleagues, 21% had both signs and symptoms of keratoconjunctivitis sicca (KCS), including a positive Schirmer test. Additionally, increased tear

osmolarity was seen in 89% of this group compared to 0% of the control group (who were also HIV-positive men, but had no dry eye complaints). Lucca and Farris repeated this study in 1992 with women and found 17% of HIV-positive women had signs and symptoms of clinical dry eye as opposed to 0% of the matched HIV-negative control group. These studies demonstrate that KCS occurs more frequently in HIV-infected persons than in the general population. Therefore, HIV-positive patients with complaints of dry eye should be carefully evaluated for clinical evidence of keratitis sicca.

Patients with dry eyes secondary to HIV disease are managed utilizing topical lubricants, ointments, and sometimes punctal occlusion. Bandage contact lenses should be used with caution due to an increased risk of bacterial keratitis and ulcers in immunocompromised people.

Inflammatory Disorders

Primary HIV-related uveitis is seen in some people with AIDS. Many cases of anterior, intermediate, and posterior uveitis have been linked to ocular OIs. Others have no apparent cause other than HIV itself. Because the inflammatory response is greatly diminished in AIDS, treatment of the underlying primary disease is usually sufficient to clear the uveitis. Corticosteroids are of limited therapeutic value. Some cases have responded to antiretroviral therapy (AZT) alone, supporting the notion that HIV is the primary etiology.

Neoplasms

Although Kaposi sarcoma (KS) is typically a late manifestation of AIDS, ocular KS is the initial manifestation of AIDS in 4 to 10% of cases. KS presents most frequently in the conjunctiva, with a predilection for the inferior cul-de-sac (Figure 58–1). It can easily be confused with a red eye of infectious or inflammatory origin such as chronic lid edema, blepharitis, subconjunctival hemorrhage, pyogenic or foreign body granuloma, malignant melanoma, metastatic disease, squamous cell carcinoma, lymphangioma, hordeolum, chalazion, or cavernous hemangioma.

Patients with ocular KS may report symptoms affecting comfort, function, or visual acuity. Lesions may interfere with the eyelids (entropion or ectropion), the tear film (incomplete blinks), the cornea (trichiasis, exposure keratitis and secondary infections), and motility (orbital lymphedema). Initial treatment of ocular KS is palliative unless pain, functional, cosmetic, or visual deficit is present. Palliative treatments include artificial tears, bland ointment, epilation of eyelashes if superficial keratitis secondary to trichiasis is present, and sunglasses for cosmesis. Chemotherapy and immunotherapy have been used for systemic KS. Periorbital and conjunctival lesions also diminish when systemic treatment is successful. Radiation therapy and strontium-90 therapy have been successful in treating periocular and conjunctival lesions. However, these tech-

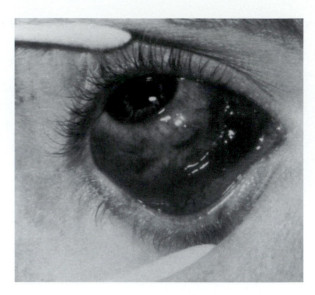

Figure 58–1. KS of the eyelid and conjunctiva. *(Courtesy of Brian DenBeste, OD.)*

niques do not offer a permanent cure. Lesions will recur and new ones continually appear. Surgical excision and cryotherapy have met with limited success.

Other types of adnexal and orbital neoplasms are rarely encountered in patients with AIDS. Goldberg and associates (1992) documented a case of primary eyelid non-Hodgkin's lymphoma (B-cell type) in a patient with AIDS. Antle and co-workers (1990) reported a case of large-cell orbital lymphoma (non-Hodgkin's lymphoma), and Brooks and colleagues (1984) reported a case of orbital Burkitt lymphoma. Both were in patients with AIDS.

Posterior Segment and Orbit

Table 58–6 summarizes posterior segment HIV manifestations.

Vascular

Cotton-wool spots (CWS) were the first lesions to be documented as an ocular change in patients with AIDS (Figure 58–2). They are the most common ocular manifestation of HIV disease, occurring in 50 to 90% of patients. Although seen in patients at all stages of the disease, CWS are rare in clinically well HIV-positive patients, and common in people with a diagnosis of AIDS. CWS usually do not manifest until T4 cell counts fall below 200 to 400/mm³ blood.

CWS in HIV disease are smaller and resolve more quickly than CWS seen in other ischemic processes (such as diabetes mellitus). They tend to present most often in the posterior pole, have a variable clinical course, and usually resolve in 4 to 6 weeks. As old lesions resolve, new lesions may appear (proximal or distal to the resolving lesion). These microinfarctions of the nerve fiber layer are a manifestation of an underlying retinal microvascular

TABLE 58–6. OCULAR POSTERIOR SEGMENT MANIFESTIONS OF HIV

LOCATION	PROBLEM	FREQUENCY[a]
● Retina / choroid	● Vascular	
	Noninfectious retinopathy	VC
	● Viral	
	Cytomegalovirus	VC
	Necrotizing retinitis	R
	● Parasitic	
	P. carinii choroidopathy	R
	Toxoplasmosis retinochoroiditis	R
	● Fungal	
	Cryptococcus sp. chorioretinitis	R
	Histoplasmosis chorioretinitis	R
	Candida sp. chorioretinitis	R
	Aspergillus funigatus	R
	● Bacterial	
	Syphilitic retinitis	R–C
	Tubercular choroiditis	R
	Endogenous bacterial retinitis	R
	M. avium–intracellulare	R
	● Neoplastic	
	Primary malignant lymphoma	R
	● Inflammatory	
	Primary HIV-related uveitis	R–C

[a]VC, very common (>25%); C, common (10–25%); R, rare (<10%).

ischemic/occlusive process. Therefore, it is common to see associated superficial and intraretinal dot and blot hemorrhages as well as microaneurysms, intraretinal microvascular abnormalities, and nonperfusion of capillary beds. On fundus fluorescein angiography, characteristic hypo- and hyperfluorescence is seen, corresponding to these various retinal lesions.

When seen together these retinal manifestations are commonly referred to as noninfectious AIDS-related retinopathy, although this terminology is often used interchangeably with the presence of CWS alone. Noninfectious AIDS-related retinopathy is not associated with the presence of a retinal opportunistic infection. There are a number of theories about the etiology of noninfectious AIDS-related retinopathy, including immune complex deposition on the walls of the retinal vessels, direct infection of the retinal vessels with HIV, hemorheolic abnormalities, or any combination of those factors. There is no treatment for noninfectious AIDS-related retinopathy. It tends to wax and wane without direct bearing on a patient's systemic condition.

An indirect prognostic relationship of noninfectious AIDS-related retinopathy to systemic health has been inferred in some studies. There may be a relationship (at least temporally) between CWS and the subsequent development of *P. carinii* pneumonia (PCP). Several clinicians have reported that some patients develop PCP within a few weeks of the appearance of the CWS. The reason(s) for this relationship are presently unknown. As yet, no research has been conducted to study this potential relationship. CWS have also been correlated with decreased cerebral blood flow. As the number of CWS increase, the cerebral blood flow decreases. This finding suggests a strong relationship between ocular microangiopathy and systemic microvascular changes, particularly in the central nervous system.

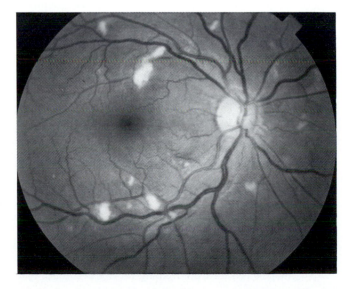

Figure 58–2. Cotton-wool spots in AIDS. *(Courtesy of David Lampariello, OD.)*

Because noninfectious AIDS-related retinopathy is a sign of damage to the blood–retina barrier and may be a sign of worsening clinical condition, coordination of care among all healthcare providers is important. Dilated fundus examinations are indicated in these patients every 3 to 6 months to rule out the development of ocular OIs, especially CMV retinitis.

Opportunistic Diseases

Viral Diseases

Cytomegalovirus retinitis. The most common ocular OI in AIDS is cytomegalovirus (CMV), which causes a relentless retinitis in 12 to 46% of cases. Patients who have immunosuppression from other causes (for example, secondary to chemotherapy or immunosuppression during organ transplantation) infrequently develop CMV retinitis. The reasons for this are currently unknown.

The pathophysiology of CMV retinitis follows a similar course to that of other blood-borne pathogens. CMV is believed to infect the retina through hematologic processes (a break in the blood–retina barrier secondary to microangiopathy), or directly through the optic nerve. Although CMV retinitis can present as the initial manifestation of AIDS, this is clinically rare, occurring in about 1% of cases. Typically CMV retinitis presents as a late manifestation of AIDS, particularly in patients with ≤50 T4 cells/mm³ of blood, or in patients with a T4 lymphocyte/T8 lymphocyte cell ratio below 0.11. CMV retinitis is considered to be a negative prognostic sign. In 1991, the survival time after a diagnosis of CMV retinitis in a person with AIDS averaged approximately 8 months.

CMV retinitis is bilateral as often as it is unilateral. Untreated unilateral disease will progress to a bilateral presentation because it is a systemic infection. Depending on the location of the lesion(s), visual complaints range from significant floaters to mild photopsia to metamorphopsia, or visual field defects. Visual acuity may be normal or reduced. Peripheral lesions may be symptom free or produce only mild complaints such as floaters. Lesions of the macula will cause diminished visual acuity secondary to tissue necrosis and macular edema. Optic nerve involvement and lesions of the papillomacular bundle and of the fovea will all cause profound loss of vision and eventually irreversible blindness.

The diagnosis of CMV retinitis is primarily based upon clinical (ophthalmoscopic) appearance. Laboratory tests that can detect CMV include biopsies, viral culture and isolation studies, serologic testing, and viral genome studies. Each has drawbacks and generally does not provide useful information for a clinical diagnosis. The differential diagnosis of CMV retinitis includes myelinated nerve fibers, cotton-wool spots, other types of infectious retinitis, vascular problems, and neoplastic diseases. Vascular diseases such as diabetic retinopathy, hypertensive retinopathy, and retinal vein occlusion must be ruled out as they can mimic the hemorrhagic variety of CMV retinitis. Infectious and neoplastic diseases should also be ruled out through diagnostic testing and clinical observation.

The most characteristic feature of CMV retinitis is the appearance of one or two granular lesions presenting along the major vascular arcades of the retina or near the optic nervehead. The lesions eventually involve all layers of the retina and become discrete, white patches with granular borders. The Bruch membrane apparently prevents penetration of the infection into the choroid. Hemorrhage and vasculitis may accompany the lesions. The lesions slowly enlarge and spread through cell-to-cell transmission. If left untreated, total retinal destruction will result within months. Occasionally the early lesions of CMV retinitis may be confused with cotton-wool spots; however, they are readily differentiated by depth and clinical course. CMV involves all layers of the retina and is progressive, whereas CWS are superficial and resolve within weeks.

As the disease progresses inflammatory cell migration and subretinal fluid will produce a slight elevation to the lesion. Eventually the lesions take on a hazy, gray-white appearance. This opacification is due to edema and tissue necrosis, which affects retinal transparency. The retinal necrosis is replaced by mottling and clumping of the retinal pigment epithelium, and scarring. Small areas of vessel occlusion and capillary nonperfusion will also develop, resulting in further destruction of the retina. CMV retinitis is rarely accompanied by vitritis or an anterior segment inflammation (due to a diminished immune response).

Although cytomegalovirus retinitis has somewhat clinically variable presentations, granular borders and minimal intraocular inflammation are the hallmarks of the diagnosis. A fulminant/edematous form has been identified consisting of intraretinal, blotchy hemorrhages and vasculitis (Figure 58–3). This presentation, having a "catsup and cottage cheese" appearance, is the most common. A granular/indolent variety has also been observed. This is less dense, not as opaque, and has little hemorrhage. The distinction between the two types should be viewed as academic because its distinction conveys little information about management.

Retinal detachment (RD) can develop as a late complication of CMV retinitis in 15 to 34% of patients. Rhegmatogenous and nonrhegmatogenous RDs have been seen in AIDS. Rhegmatogenous detachments usually occur in peripheral areas of healing, where thinning and atrophy exist; whereas nonrhegmatogenous RDs occur more posteriorly, in conjunction with exudative processes.

Treatment of CMV retinitis depends on various factors. Some clinicians refrain from treating unilateral disease that has destroyed the fovea, or small peripheral lesions because

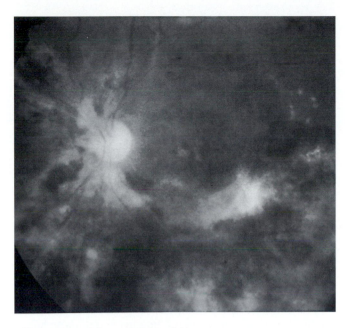

Figure 58–3. Advanced CMV retinitis. *(Courtesy of Brian DenBeste, OD.)*

of the numerous side effects associated with treatment. Sight-threatening lesions in one or both eyes, or extensive peripheral lesions, are always treated. Preterminal patients may forego treatment in favor of other quality of life issues. Treatment options are limited. Currently there are two medications approved by the Federal Drug Administration (FDA): ganciclovir and foscarnet. Both of these medications are virostatic and must be administered intravenously for life. Neither will effect a cure. Each has had relatively good success in controlling CMV retinitis, with 80 to 100% of patients showing a positive response within 3 weeks of treatment. After the initial induction dose, individual maintenance schedules are developed.

Ganciclovir (9-1[1,3-dihydroxy-2-propoxymethyl]-guanine) is a nucleoside analog, and is similar to acyclovir. The main action of ganciclovir is to inhibit viral DNA polymerase. Ganciclovir is used to treat both disseminated CMV infections and retinitis. The dosage for patients with normal renal function consists of 5 mg/kg of body weight for a 2-week induction period twice a day, infused over 1 hour. A maintenance schedule follows consisting of 5 mg/kg once daily for 7 days or 6 mg/kg for 5 days. Maintenance therapy must be continued indefinitely to decrease the chances for reactivation of the CMV retinitis. Reactivation or breakthrough retinitis can occur in any patient on full or maintenance therapy. It is seen along borders of previously inactive sites as white lesions. This is contrasted to the opaque and scarred regions of retina that were previously active. Breakthrough retinitis requires reinduction therapy.

Bone marrow suppression, which induces neutropenia, is the main side effect of ganciclovir in up to 50% of patients. Bacterial infections, phlebitis at the infusion site, and sepsis can result as a consequence of long-term maintenance therapy. Patients taking AZT generally do not tolerate ganciclovir. AZT causes neutropenia and anemia in some patients. Potentially fatal bone-marrow suppression could occur from co-administration. Granulocyte macrophage-colony stimulating factor (GM-CSF) is under investigation as an adjunct to ganciclovir. GM-CSF stimulates the growth of granulocytes and macrophages, thereby reducing the neutropenia caused by ganciclovir.

Intravitreal injections and sustained release intraocular implants of ganciclovir have been used with good results on some patients who have sight-threatening lesions and cannot tolerate this drug intravenously, or those who need to continue taking AZT. Endophthalmitis and retinal detachment have been associated with intravitreal injections. Intraocular administration has the drawback of not treating systemic CMV infection.

Foscarnet (trisodium phosphonoformate hexahydrate) is the other intravenously administered virostatic agent approved for the treatment of CMV retinitis. Foscarnet has a similar mode of action to that of ganciclovir. Like ganciclovir, it requires an initial induction, followed by indefinite maintenance therapy. The induction dosage most often used is an initial bolus of 20 mg/kg of body weight, followed by a 2- to 3-week infusion of 230 mg/kg per day.

It is likely that foscarnet will be the first choice to treat CMV retinitis. The preliminary results from the Foscarnet–Ganciclovir Cytomegalovirus Retinitis Study showed that patients treated with foscarnet survived 4 months longer than those treated with ganciclovir. Foscarnet also has a greater compatibility with AZT than ganciclovir because it does not cause bone marrow suppression. Its major toxicity is renal, although several other side effects have also been reported. Problems associated with ganciclovir, such as breakthrough retinitis and complications related to long-term intravenous infusions, also occur with foscarnet.

Laser therapy has not been successful in management of CMV retinitis. The theory was that laser burns to healthy retina would prevent further spread of the infection. However, research continues to study the role of laser treatment in the management of CMV retinitis.

In general, patients with CMV retinitis should be seen every 2 weeks to 1 month. However, patients with sight-threatening lesions must be followed more closely than those with peripheral lesions. After induction, patients on ganciclovir or foscarnet should be evaluated at 2 weeks. Thereafter, visits should be based upon response to treatment. Serial photographs are required in managing patients, particularly when assessing therapeutic response. Sequential visual field testing has also been used to confirm ophthalmoscopic success of therapy.

Necrotizing retinitis. Necrotizing retinitis with an acute onset is a newly defined clinical problem that can present in both immunocompetent and immunocompromised individuals. Although relatively rare, the prevalence of necrotizing retinitis in patients with HIV disease is increasing. It shares clinical similarities with the acute retinal necrosis (ARN), but has some important differences. In immunocompetent patients, necrotizing retinitis is linked temporally to the reactivation of herpes zoster virus. In HIV disease, it is also associated with herpes zoster virus diseases, but CMV and HSV have also been implicated.

Classic ARN is characterized by severe vaso-occlusion of the peripheral retina. White necrotic retina overlies the occluded vessels. There is a sharp line of demarcation between the normal and involved retina. Necrotizing retinitis in AIDS differs from ARN in that the necrosis begins in the posterior pole rather than the periphery, there is minimal or no intraocular inflammation, and involvement of the vasculature and peripheral retina occurs late. Progression is more rapid than ARN, acyclovir therapy yields a poor response, vitreoretinal bands and retinal detachments rarely occur, and a cherry-red spot in the macula is common. In some cases it may present as an outer retinal necrosis with later inner retinal involvement. Occasionally small white granulomatous infiltrates are noted at the level of the choroid.

It is vitally important to rule out CMV retinitis in the differential of this entity, as the two problems are sight threatening and require vastly different therapies. Necrotizing retinitis in AIDS is distinguished from CMV retinitis in that it often presents bilaterally, usually has deep and diffuse retinal opacification, does not have granular borders, has less hemorrhage, and progresses more rapidly. Also, necrotizing retinitis in AIDS can present at any time during the course of illness, unlike CMV retinitis, which typically presents as a late manifestation.

Treatment for AIDS-related necrotizing retinitis is limited. Most cases are refractory to any therapy. Some cases have been treated with intravenous acyclovir, acyclovir in combination with vidarabine, ganciclovir, and laser therapy. All techniques have met with limited success. The prognosis for patients with necrotizing retinitis is poor. Retinal obliteration with detachment and blindness almost always results.

Parasites

Pneumocystis choroidopathy. Pneumocystic choroidopathy is one of several problems resulting from dissemination of pulmonary *Pneumocystis carinii* infection. Patients who are taking aerosolized pentamadine for prophylaxis are at greatest risk for the development of Pneumocystic choroidopathy, because this medication is administered locally (to the lungs), and therefore cannot adequately provide systemic prophylaxis. Pneumocystic choroidopathy

presents without ocular symptoms. This is true even when lesions appear subfoveally. The rare exception is in cases where a secondary serous retinal detachment occurs. Due to the disseminated nature of the disease, the lesions are often bilateral and multifocal. They are round or oval, may be multilobular and confluent, yellow-white or gray in color, may be elevated, and number from 1 to greater than 20. Some lesions are well circumscribed, while others have irregular borders. They present in all quadrants of the posterior pole without vasculitis or vitreous inflammation. They range in size from one-third to 2 disk diameters. On fundus fluorescein angiography the lesions demonstrate early blockage (hypofluorescence at the choroid), and late staining. Visual field studies sometimes demonstrate depressed sensitivity corresponding to the lesions.

The differential diagnosis of Pneumocystic choroidopathy includes secondary syphilis, histoplasma chorioretinitis, *M. avium–intracellulare* infection, cryptococcus chorioretinitis, ocular toxoplasmosis, *M. tuberculosis* choroiditis, reticulum cell sarcoma, central nervous system lymphoma, septic choroiditis, metastatic carcinoma, sarcoidosis, Vogt–Koyanagi–Harada syndrome, and sympathetic ophthalmia.

Patients with *P. carinii* choroidopathy require systemic treatment. The lesions will regress over a period of weeks to months when treated systemically. Long-term systemic therapy may be required to prevent reinfection. Pneumocystic choroidopathy is an important marker for disseminated Pneumocystic infection. Its presence requires immediate referral for systemic evaluation and treatment.

Toxoplasmosis. Toxoplasma gondii, an obligate intracellular protozoan parasite, can cause fatal toxoplasmosis in AIDS patients. CNS toxoplasmosis is an indicator disease in AIDS, affecting as many as 35%. Ocular toxoplasmosis occurs in approximately 2% of patients with AIDS.

In an immunocompetent person, ocular toxoplasmosis typically presents as a result of reactivation of a congenital infection. In a person with AIDS, it is more likely an acquired problem, although it can develop from reactivation of a latent infection.

Ocular toxoplasmosis in a patient with AIDS presents differently than in an immunocompetent person. The size of the lesions are larger in a person with AIDS, most likely reflecting impaired ocular immunity. There is usually a minimal or reduced inflammatory response of the vitreous and anterior segment unlike the dense vitritis ordinarily seen. The lesions may be multiple and bilateral. The retinal necrosis can involve large areas of the periphery, posterior pole, or peripapillary area as opposed to the focal lesion(s) normally encountered. Retinal detachment can be a late complication. Ocular toxoplasmosis needs to be carefully differentiated from CMV retinitis, syphilitic retinitis, and necrotizing retinitis.

Ocular toxoplasmosis in AIDS is treated similarly to that in the immunocompetent patient with either pyrimethamine and sulfadiazine, clindamycin, or tetracycline, but may require sustained therapy. Due to a diminished inflammatory response, corticosteroid therapy is generally not necessary. It frequently recurs when treatment ceases.

Fungi

Cryptococcus chorioretinitis. Cryptococcus neoformans primarily causes disease of the central nervous system in people with AIDS. However, these organisms are capable of causing ocular disease through systemic dissemination, primarily in injection drug abusers and patients with indwelling catheters. A few cases of Cryptococcus choroiditis and chorioretinitis have been reported. Infection produces deep, multifocal, discrete yellow-white spots from one-fifth to one disk diameter in size. Perivasculitis, vitritis, anterior uveitis with mutton-fat keratic precipitates, and sometimes papilledema accompany these lesions. Treatment includes amphotericin B and 5-fluorocytosine.

Ocular histoplasmosis. A few cases of disseminated ocular histoplasmosis to the retina have been reported, producing the characteristic creamy white intraretinal and subretinal lesions.

Candida species. Rare cases of Candida retinitis and chorioretinitis with overlying inflammation of vitreous have been reported in people with AIDS.

Bacteria

Syphilis. Syphilis, a sexually transmitted disease, is caused by the spirochete *Treponema pallidum*. In the eye, syphilis causes uveitis as well as optic nerve disease, scleritis, retinitis, interstitial keratitis, and retinal vasculitis. In HIV disease, a diagnosis of syphilis can be complicated by many factors. Concomitant infection with HIV often leads to an accelerated course of illness that can be difficult to eradicate. Conventional penicillin therapy tends to be insufficient in the treatment of an HIV-infected syphilitic patient. Diagnoses have been missed due to false negatives in laboratory tests, which occur commonly in patients co-infected with HIV. Also, neurosyphilis, which is quite common in HIV disease, presents earlier than in non-HIV-infected patients. Syphilitic ocular disease in AIDS is common. As in immunocompetent people, the most common ocular manifestations of AIDS-related syphilis include uveitis, optic nerve disease, and retinitis.

Primary syphilitic disease should be treated in conjunction with the ocular disease. Prolonged and aggressive intravenous treatment may be required.

Tubercular choroiditis. Pulmonary tuberculosis (TB), caused by *Mycobacterium tuberculosis*, is an increasing problem in HIV-infected people. Extrapulmonary (disseminated) TB, such as tubercular choroiditis, is an AIDS-defining disease and thus has special significance to the eyecare provider. Although tubercular choroiditis is still rare, it is extremely important to consider it in the differential of the chorioretinal opportunistic diseases of AIDS. The multiple choroidal infiltrates cause a vitritis, are yellowish in color, and are of varying size. The prevalence of tubercular choroiditis may be increasing, mirroring the increased incidence of TB in the AIDS population. Tuberculosis in AIDS requires prolonged treatment with isozianid, rifampin, and pyrazinamide. (See chapter 54.)

Endogenous bacteria. Rare cases of bacterial infection of the retina have been reported. These cases present similarly to other infections of the retina with multifocal, yellow-white exudates. They are often misdiagnosed as viral, fungal, or parasitic disease. They do respond to antibiotic therapy.

Neoplasms

Intraocular tumors are rare in AIDS. A case of primary ocular malignant lymphoma was reported by Schanzer and associates (1991). The incidence of neoplastic eye disease in AIDS (other than Kaposi sarcoma) may rise as medical advancements enable patients to live longer. This will likely result in an increasing window of time for these diseases to manifest.

Neuro-Ophthalmic Disorders

Table 58–7 summarizes neuro-ophthalmic HIV manifestations.

A spectrum of neuro-ophthalmic problems is seen in up to 8% of people with HIV disease. All aspects of the visual system are affected, including the ocular motor system and visual pathways. Etiologies include direct infection with HIV, opportunistic infections, and malignancies. Toxoplasmosis of the central nervous system, cryptococcal meningitis, primary lymphoma of the brain, neurosyphilis, progressive multifocal leukoencephalopathy (PML), and a myriad of retinal OIs contribute to the development of the neuro-ophthalmic disorders.

Within the eye, optic nerve problems including optic neuropathies, primary atrophy of the optic nerve, optic neuritis, papillitis, and papilledema may occur as primary or secondary problems. Deficits in contrast sensitivity and color vision, and abnormalities in visual fields, electroretinograms, and electro-oculograms have been found in patients with HIV disease. In general, the more advanced the HIV disease, the more profound is the visual dysfunction.

Neuro-ophthalmic problems of the ocular motor system manifest as cranial nerve palsies, rotary nystagmus,

TABLE 58–7. NEURO-OPHTHALMIC MANIFESTATIONS OF HIV

LOCATION	PROBLEM	FREQUENCY[a]
● Cranial nerves	Palsies of CN III, IV, VI	R–C
	Optic neuritis	C
	Neuropathies	C
● Extraocular muscles	Abnormal saccades	VC
	Abnormal pursuits	R–C
	Skew deviations	R
	Rotary nystagmus	R
	Convergence insufficiency	R
● Visual pathways	Visual field defects	R
	Pupillary abnormalities	R
	Papilledema	R

[a]VC, very common (>25%); C, common (10–25%); R, rare (<10%).

problems with convergence, and abnormalities in tracking. Recent studies have shown that many HIV-positive persons demonstrate abnormal ocular motilities, primarily seen as dysfunctions in pursuits and saccades. It is noteworthy that these problems present in clinically healthy patients. When the clinical reliability of ocular motility testing is fully established, these techniques will likely have a significant role for eyecare providers in the early identification of HIV-infected patients.

Management of Ocular Manifestations

Patient management protocols for patients with ocular manifestations of HIV disease have not been finalized. At the 1991 International AIDS conference in Florence, Italy some recommendations for ophthalmic care did emerge. Annual eye exams for HIV positive patients and semiannual exams for patients with AIDS were recommended. Another general approach is to link the frequency of eye exams in patients with known retinal disease to patient symptoms and T4 cells/mm^3 of blood as follows:

Number of T4/mm^3	Frequency of Eye Exam
Unknown or at diagnosis	Baseline, follow as appropriate
200–500	6–12 months[a]
< 200	2–6 months[a]
New symptom	Stat, follow as appropriate

[a]*Frequency of examination depends on overall patient health.*

Linking the frequency of eye examinations to the number of T4 cells is reasonable, because ocular manifestations begin to present around the 400/mm^3 mark. This schedule allows eyecare providers to take a proactive role in the management of patients with HIV disease. Furthermore,

because changes in the systemic condition of some patients are mirrored through the manifestation of eye disease (eg, CMV retinitis, PC choroidopathy), routine eye exams may serve as another patient management tool.

INFECTION CONTROL

General Guidelines

HIV infection poses many concerns for healthcare workers, including the potential for inadvertent transmission during a patient care procedure. Since 1985 the CDC has issued several sets of infection control protocols governing the examination of patients before settling on a rational approach, referred to as universal precautions. The universal precautions system assumes that all patients are capable of transmitting infectious diseases, and therefore recommends that all patients be treated exactly the same way.

Infection control protocols recommended for HIV are based upon the likelihood of contact with various fluids. Procedures involving exposure to high-risk fluids such as blood, semen, and vaginal secretions may require numerous precautions. This could include specific barriers such as gloves, gowns, masks, and eye shields. Because tears pose virtually no transmission risk, nonsurgical eye care requires only simple universal precautions as follows:

- Handwashing between examinations.
- Disinfection of instruments (such as tonometer tips or fundus contact lenses); rinse with water to remove organic debris, soak 5 to 10 minutes in one of the following solutions: 70% isopropyl alcohol, 70% ethanol, 1 to 10 dilution of sodium hypochlorite (household bleach), or 3% hydrogen peroxide. (Thorough wiping with an isopropyl alcohol-soaked pad also disinfects against HIV, but this technique is not approved by the CDC.)

- Disinfection of trial contact lenses; either hydrogen peroxide or heat systems, depending on compatibility with the lens material. (Other systems that are not listed in the CDC recommended guidelines also appear adequate. See next section on contact lenses for additional information.)
- Latex gloves are worn if the doctor has any break on the skin that could make contact with the tears or mucous membranes of a patient, or if the patient has an open or weeping lesion that the doctor might touch.

Contact Lenses

Patients with known HIV infection who desire (or already wear) contact lenses should be assessed on an individual basis. Factors to consider include general health, ability to comply with follow-up schedules, and ocular and corneal health. Fitting HIV-infected patients with extended-wear lenses may be contraindicated due to the potential risk for corneal disease in an immunocompromised person.

Guidelines have not been established for monitoring patients with HIV disease who wear contact lenses. The CDC has not reported large numbers of problems associated with contact lenses in patients with HIV disease. Until studies are conducted to identify issues relating to HIV-positive contact lens patients, detailed patient education about potential risks, documentation of problems, and frequent monitoring are indicated.

There are no known cases of HIV transmission from doctor to patient or vice versa resulting from contact lens practice. Routine disinfection of contact lenses against HIV appears to be effective. Currently, only hydrogen peroxide and heat systems (whichever one is most appropriate for the material) are included in CDC guidelines for disinfection of trial contact lenses.

Conclusion

The natural history of HIV disease is still evolving. Even after an effective vaccine and/or curative medications are discovered, people who are already infected with HIV will continue to require specialized care. HIV disease will be responsible for much illness and death into the 21st century.

The natural history of the ocular problems of HIV disease is not well understood. The identification of visual problems associated with HIV infection may prove valuable in the earlier diagnosis of HIV disease. Clinical studies are needed to assess the relationship between ocular problems in HIV and advancing systemic disease. Additionally, the preliminary research on eye movements, contrast sensitivity, and visual fields in HIV positive patients require follow-up studies. Clinical studies of the anterior segment, in

particular the tear film and corneal physiology, will be needed to address the questions relating to contact lens wear and HIV. Prophylaxis and a cure for CMV retinitis are urgently needed. Infection control guidelines also need refinement and updating, although simple, universal precautions are adequate for nonsurgical eye care.

Due to the development of life-threatening problems in HIV disease, baseline evaluations for other potential problems are sometimes forgotten, resulting in fragmentation of care. To solve this problem, the multidisciplinary team approach has emerged in which a case manager coordinates all aspects of care and stays in constant communication with the various providers.

Given the clinical correlations that are emerging between systemic HIV disease and its ocular manifestations, regular eye exams are indicated in the multidisciplinary management of these patients. Perhaps the most important role that eyecare providers can play in the HIV epidemic is to educate patients as well as the healthcare community about the value of regular eye exams for people with HIV disease.

References

American Academy of Ophthalmology. Updated recommendations for ophthalmic practice in relation to the human immunodeficiency virus. Clinical alert 2/4. San Francisco: AAO; August 1988.

American Academy of Optometry, section on public health and occupational vision. AIDS task force policy statement. *Am J Optom Physiol Opt*. 1988;65:559–601.

Ammann AJ. The immunology of AIDS. *Int Ophthalmol Clin*. 1989;29:77–82.

Anand R, Nightingale SD, Fish RH et al. Control of cytomegalovirus retinitis using sustained release of intraocular ganciclovir. *Arch Ophthalmol*. 1993;111:223–227.

Antle CM, White VA, Horsman DE, et al. Large cell orbital lymphoma in a patient with acquired immune deficiency syndrome. *Ophthalmology*. 1990;97:1494–1498.

Bachman DM, Brune LM, DiGioia RA, et al. Visual field testing in the management of cytomegalovirus retinitis. *Ophthalmology*. 1992;99:1393–1399.

Baltimore D, Feinberg MB. HIV revealed. Toward a natural history of the infection. *N Engl J Med*. 1989;321:1673–1675. Editorial.

Barnes PF, Bloch AB, Davidson PT, et al. Tuberculosis in patients with human immunodeficiency virus infection. *N Engl J Med*. 1991;324:1644–1650.

Becerra LI, Ksiazek SM, Savino PJ, et al. Syphilitic uveitis in human immunodeficiency virus-infected and noninfected patients. *Ophthalmology*. 1989;96:1727–1730.

Blodi BA, Johnson MW, McLeish WM, et al. Presumed choroidal tuberculosis in a human immunodeficiency virus infected host. *Am J Ophthalmol*. 1989;108:605–607.

Bozzette SA, Sattler FR, Chiu J, et al. A controlled trial of early adjunctive treatment with corticosteroids for *Pneumocystis carinii* pneumonia in the acquired immunodeficiency syndrome. *N Engl J Med*. 1990;323:1451–1457.

Brodie SE, Friedman AH. Retinal dysfunction as an initial ophthalmic sign in AIDS. *Br J Ophthalmol*. 1990;74:49–51.

Brooks HL Jr, Downing J, McClure JA. Orbital Burkitt's Lymphoma in a homosexual man with acquired immune deficiency. *Arch Ophthalmol*. 1984;102:1533–1537.

Butler GA, Friedman AH. Screening indices for cytomegalovirus retinitis in patients with human immunodeficiency virus. *Mt Sinai J Med*. 1992;59:61–65.

Cali A, Meisler DM, Rutherford I, et al. Corneal microsporidiosis in a patient with AIDS. *Am J Trop Med Hyg*. 1991;44:463–468.

Cantrill HL, Henry K, Jackson B, et al. Recovery of human immunodeficiency virus from ocular tissues in patients with acquired immune deficiency syndrome. *Opththalmology*. 1988;95:1458–1462.

Caskey PJ, Ai E. Posterior segment manifestations of AIDS. *Ophthalmol Clin North Am*. 1990;3:393–412.

Cellini M, Baldi A. Vitreous fluorophotometric recordings in HIV infection. *Int Ophthalmol*. 1991;15:37–40.

Centers for Disease Control. 1993 revised classification system for HIV infection and expanded surveillance case definition for AIDS among adolescents and adults. *MMWR*. 1992;41:1–19.

Centers for Disease Control. The HIV/AIDS epidemic: The first 10 years. *MMWR*. 1991:40:357–363, 369.

Centers for Disease Control. Recommendations for preventing the transmission of human immunodeficiency virus and hepatitis B virus to patients during exposure-prone invasive procedures. *MMWR*. 1991;40:1–9.

Centers for Disease Control. Update: Universal precautions for prevention of transmission of human immunodeficiency virus, hepatitis B virus, and other bloodborne pathogens in health-care settings. *MMWR*. 1988;37:377–382, 387–388.

Centers for Disease Control. Recommendations for prevention of HIV transmission the health-care settings. *MMWR*. 1987;37:S2–S18.

Centers for Disease Control. Revision of the CDC surveillance case definition for acquired immunodeficiency syndrome. *MMWR*. 1987;36:1S–15S.

Chang SW, Katz MH, Hernandez SR. The new AIDS case definition. Implications for San Francisco. *JAMA*. 1992;267:973–975.

Chess J, Marcus DM. Zoster-related bilateral acute retinal necrosis syndrome as presenting sign in AIDS. *Ann Ophthalmol*. 1988;20:431–438.

Chow Y-K, Hirsch MS, Merrill DP, et al. Use of evolutionary limitations of HIV-1 multidrug resistance to optimize therapy. *Nature*. 1993;361:650–654. Letter.

Cohen JI, Saragas SJ. Endophthalmitis due to *Mycobacterium avium* in a patient with AIDS. *Ann Ophthalmol*. 1991;22:47–51.

Colin J, Malet F, Chastel C. Acyclovir in herpetic anterior uveitis. *Ann Ophthalmol*. 1991;23:28–30.

Cooley TP, Kunches LM, Saunders CA, et al. Treatment of AIDS and AIDS-related complex with 2',3'-dideoxyinosine given once daily. *Rev Infect Dis*. 1990;12(suppl 5):S552–S560.

Coombs RW, Collier AC, Allain JP, et al. Plasma viremia in human immunodeficiency virus infection. *N Engl J Med*. 1989;321:1626–1631.

Cooney TG. Clinical management of the complications of HIV infection. *J Gen Intern Med*. 1991;6(suppl):S12–S18.

Cotton P. Medicine's arsenal in battling "dominant dozen," other AIDS-associated opportunistic infections. Medical news & perspectives. *JAMA*. 1991;266:1476–1481.

Croxatto JO, Mestre C, Puente S, et al. Nonreactive tuberculosis in a patient with acquired immune deficiency syndrome. *Am J Ophthalmol*. 1986;102:660–661. Letter.

Culbertson WW. Infections of the retina in AIDS. *Int Ophthalmol Clin*. 1989;29:108–118.

Davis JL. Human immunodeficiency virus-related uveitis. *Curr Opin Ophthalmol*. 1991;2:471–479.

Davis JL, Nussenblatt RB, Bachman DM, et al. Endogenous bacterial retinitis in AIDS. *Am J Ophthalmol*. 1989;107:613–623.

De Smet MD. Differential diagnosis of retinal and choroiditis in patients with acquired immunodeficiency syndrome. *Am J Med*. 1992;92(suppl 2A):17S–21S.

Douglas RG Jr. Antimicrobial agents. In: Gilman AG, Rall TW, Nies AS. Taylor P, eds. *Goodman and Gilman's Pharmacological Basis of Therapeutics*. 8th ed. New York: Pergamon; 1991:1182–1184.

Antiviral agents. Zidovudine. In: Olin BR, ed. *Drug Facts and Comparisons*. 45th ed. Philadelphia: Lippincott; 1991:1779–1782.

Dugel PU, Rao NA, Forster DJ. *Pneumocystis carinii* choroiditis after long-term aerosolized pentamidine therapy. *Am J Ophthalmol*. 1990;110:113–117.

Duker JS, Shakin EP. Rapidly progressive outer retinal necrosis in the acquired immunodeficiency syndrome. *Am J Ophthalmol*. 1991;111:255–256. Letter.

Erlich KS, Mills J, Chatis P, et al. Acyclovir-resistant herpes simplex virus infections in patients with the acquired immunodeficiency syndrome. *N Engl J Med*. 1989;320:293–296.

Fabricius E-M, Hoegl I, Pfaeffl W. Ocular myositis as first presenting symptom of human immunodeficiency virus (HIV-1) infection and its response to high-dose cortisone treatment. *Br J Ophthalmol*. 1991;75:696–697.

Farizo KM, Buehler JW, Chamberland ME, et al. Spectrum of disease in persons with human immunodeficiency virus infection in the United States. *JAMA*. 1992;267:1798–1805.

Farrell PL, Heinemann MH, Roberts CW, et al. Response of human immunodeficiency virus-associated uveitis to zidovudine. *Am J Ophthalmol*. 1988;106:7–10.

Fauci AS. The human immunodeficiency virus: Infectivity and mechansims of pathogenesis. *Science*. 1988;239:617–622.

Fijikawa LS, Salahuddin SZ, Ablashi D, et al. HTLV-III in the tears of AIDS patients. *Ophthalmology*. 1986;93:479–481.

Fischl MA. Antiretroviral therapy in combination with interferon for AIDS-related Kaposi's sarcoma. *Am J Med*. 1991;90(suppl 4A):2S–7S.

Forster DJ, Dugel PU, Frangieh GT. Rapidly progressive outer retinal necrosis in the acquired immunodeficiency syndrome. *Am J Ophthalmol*. 1990;110:341–348.

Foster RE, Lowder CY, Meisler DM, et al. Presumed *Pneumocystis carinii* choroiditis. Unifocal presentation, regression, with intravenous pentamidine, and choroiditis recurrence. *Ophthalmology*. 1991;98:1360–1365.

Freeman WR, Gross JG, Labelle J, et al. *Pneumocystis carinii* choroidopathy. *Arch Ophthalmol*. 1989;107:863–867.

Freeman WR, Henderly DE, Lipson BK. Retinopathy before the diagnosis of AIDS. *Ann Ophthalmol*. 1989;21:468–474.

Freidberg DN, Stenson SM, Orenstein JM. Microsporidial kerato-conjunctivitis in acquired immunodeficiency syndrome. *Arch Ophthalmol*. 1990;108:504–508.

Friedman DI. Neuro-ophthalmic manifestations of human immunodeficiency virus infection. *Neurol Clin*. 1991;9:55–72.

Friedman Y, Franklin C, Freels S, et al. Long-term survival of patients with AIDS, *Pneumocystis carinii* pneumonia, and respiratory failure. *JAMA*. 1991;266:89–92.

French PD, Murphy SM, Forster SM. Retinal changes associated with severe anaemia in the acquired immunodeficiency syndrome. *Int J STD AIDS*. 1990;1:211–212.

Gabrieli CB, Angarano G, Moramarco A, et al. Ocular manifestations in HIV-seropositive patients. *Ann Ophthalmol*. 1990;22:173–176.

Gagliuso DJ, Teich SA, Friedman AH, et al. Ocular toxoplasmosis in AIDS patients. *Trans Am Ophthalmol Soc*. 1990;88:63–88.

Gerberding JL, Schecter WP. Surgery and AIDS. *JAMA*. 1991;265:1572–1573. Editorial.

Geier SA, Held M, Bogner JR, et al. Impairment of tritan colour vision after initiation of treatment with zidovudine in patients with HIV disease or AIDS. *Br J Ophthalmol*. 1993;77:315–316.

Geier SA, Schielke E, Klauss V, et al. Retinal microvasculopathy and reduced cerebral blood flow in patients with acquired immunodeficiency syndrome. *Am J Ophthalmol* 1992;113:100–101. Letter.

Goldberg SH, Fieo AG, Wolz DE. Primary eyelid non-Hodgkin's lymphoma in a patient with acquired immunodeficiency syndrome. *Am J Ophthalmol*. 1992;113:216–217. Letter.

Goldschmidt RH, Dong BJ, Johnson MAG, et al. Evaluation and treatment of AIDS-associated illnesses: An approach for the primary physician. *JABFP*. 1988;1:112–130.

Groopman JE. Treatment of AIDS with combinations of antiretroviral agents: a summary. *Am J Med*. 1991;90 (suppl 4A):27S–30S.

Gross FJ, Waxman JS, Rosenblatt MA, et al. Eosinophilic granuloma of the cavernous sinus and orbital apex in an HIV-positive patient. *Ophthalmology*. 1989;96:462–467.

Harkins T, Herriott KB. Medical management of acquired immune deficiency syndrome patients: A review. *J Am Optom Assoc*. 1992;63:35–42.

Haseltine WA. Molecular biology of the AIDS virus: Ten years of discovery: Hope for the future. Plenary lecture, international AIDS symposium, Florence, Italy 1991:1–54.

Heinemann M-H, Bloom AF, Horowitz J. *Candida albicans* endophthalmitis in a patient with AIDS. *Arch Ophthalmol*. 1987;105:1172–1173. Letter.

Henderson DK, Fahey BJ, Willy M, et al. Risk for occupational transmission of human immunodeficiency virus type-1 (HIV-1) associated with clinical exposures: A prospective evaluation. *Ann Intern Med*. 1990;113:740–746.

Hersh EM, Brewton G, Abrams D, et al. Ditiocarb sodium (diethyldithiocarbamate) therapy in patients with symptomatic HIV infection and AIDS. A randomized, double-blind, placebo-controlled, multicenter study. *JAMA*. 1991;265:1538–1544.

Ho DD, Moudgh T, Alam M. Quantitation of human immunodeficiency virus type I in the blood of infected persons. *N Engl J Med*. 1989;321:1621–1625.

Holland GN. Focal points. An update on AIDS-related cytomegalovirus retinitis. Clinical modules for ophthalmologists. *Am Acad Ophthalmol*. 1991;9:1–12.

Holland GN, Engstrom RE, Glasgow BJ, et al. Ocular toxoplasmosis in patients with the acquired immunodeficiency syndrome. *Am J Ophthalmol*. 1988;106:653–657.

Jabs DA, Green R, Fox R, et al. Ocular manifestations of acquired immune deficiency syndrome. *Ophthalmology*. 1989;96:1092–1099.

Kaslow RA, Blackwelder WC, Ostrow DG, et al. No evidence for a role of alcohol or other psychoactive drugs in accelerating immunodeficiency in HIV-1 positive individuals. A report from the multicenter AIDS cohort study. *JAMA*. 1989;261:3424–3429.

Keane JR. Neuro-ophthalmologic signs of AIDS: 50 patients. *Neurology*. 1991;41:841–845.

Kestelyn P. Ocular problems in AIDS. *Int Ophthalmol*. 1990;14:165–172.

Kestelyn P, Stevens AM, Bakkers E. Severe herpes zoster ophthalmicus in young African adults: A marker for HTLV-III seropositivity. *Br J Ophthalmol*. 1987;71:806–809.

Klutman NE, Hinthorn DR. Excessive growth of eye lashes in a patient with AIDS being treated with zidovudine. *N Engl J Med*. 1991;325:1896. Letter.

Koser MW, Jampol LM, MacDonell K. Treatment of *Pneumocystis carinii* choroidopathy. *Arch Ophthalmol*. 1990;108:1214–1215.

Kramer T, Grossniklaus HE. Ocular manifestations of fungal and parasitic diseases. *Curr Opin Ophthalmol*. 1991;2:212–219.

Kreiger AE, Holland GN. Ocular involvement in AIDS. *Eye*. 1988;2:496–505.

Kuppermann BD, Pteey JG, Richman DD, et al. Correlation between CD4+ counts and prevalence of cytomegalovirus retinitis and human immunodeficiency virus-related noninfectious retinal vasculopathy in patients with acquired immunodeficiency syndrome. *Am J Ophthalmol*. 1993;115:575–582.

Kwok S, O'Donnell JJ, Wood IS. Retinal cotton-wool spots in a patient with *Pneumocystis carinii* infection. *N Engl J Med*. 1982;307:184–185. Letter.

Lafeuillade A, Aubert L, Chaffanjon P, et al. Optic neuritis associated with dideoxyinosine. *Lancet*. 1991;337:615–616. Letter.

Lalonde RG, Deschênes JG, Seamore C. Zidovudine-induced macular edema. *Ann Int Med*. 1991;114:297–298.

Levy JA. Human immunodeficiency viruses and the pathogenesis of AIDS. *JAMA*. 1989;261:2997–3006.

Levy JH, Liss RA, Maguire AM. Neurosyphilis and ocular syphilis in patients with concurrent human immunodeficiency virus infection. *Retina*. 1989;9:175–180.

Liesegang TJ. Diagnosis and therapy of herpes zoster ophthalmicus. *Ophthalmology*. 1991;98:1216–1229.

Lifson AR. Do alternate modes for transmission of human immunodeficiency virus exist? A review. *JAMA*. 1988;259:1353–1356.

Lo B, Steinbrook R. Health care workers infected with the human immunodeficiency virus. The next steps. *JAMA*. 1992;267:1100–1105.

Lowenfels AB, Wormser G. Risk of transmission of HIV from surgeon to patient. *N Engl J Med*. 1991;325: 888–889.

Lucca JA, Farris RL. Keratoconjunctivitis sicca (KCS) in HIV-positive female individuals. *Association for Research in Vision and Ophthalmology*. 1992;2975. Abstract.

Lucca JA, Farris RL, Bielory L, et al. Keratoconjunctivitis sicca in male patients infected with human immunodeficiency virus type 1. *Ophthalmology*. 1990;97:1008–1010.

Mansour AM. Neuro-ophthalmic findings in acquired immunodeficiency syndrome. *J Clin Neuro-ophthalmol.* 1990;10:167–174.

Mansour AM. Orbital findings in acquired immunodeficiency syndrome. *Am J Ophthalmol.* 1990;110:706–707. Letter.

Margolis TP, Lowder CY, Holland GN, et al. Varicella-zoster virus retinitis in patients with acquired immunodeficiency syndrome. *Am J Ophthalmol.* 1991;112:119–131.

McLeish WM, Pulido JS, Holland S, et al. The ocular manifestations of syphilis in the human immunodeficiency virus type 1-infected host. *Ophthalmology.* 1990;97:196–203.

Merigan TC. Treatment of AIDS with combinations of antiretroviral agents. *Am J Med.* 1991;90(suppl 4A):8S–17S.

Mills J, Masur H. AIDS-related infections. *Sci Am.* August 1990;263:50–57.

Morinelli EN, Dugel RU, Riffenburgh R, et al. Infectious multifocal choroiditis in patients with acquired immune deficiency syndrome. *Ophthalmology.* 1993;100:1014–1021.

Nanda M, Pflugfelder SC, Holland S. Fulimant pseudomonal keratitis and scleritis in human immunodeficiency virus-infected patients. *Arch Ophthalmol.* 1991;109:503–505.

National Institutes of Health conference. Immunopathic mechanisms in human immunodeficiency virus (HIV) infection. *Ann Int Med.* 1991;114:678–693.

National Institutes of Health conference. Antiretroviral therapy in AIDS. *Ann Int Med.* 1990;113:604–618.

National Institutes of Health–University of California. Special report: Consensus statement on the use of corticosteroids as adjunctive therapy for pneumocystis pneumonia in the acquired immunodeficiency syndrome. *N Engl J Med.* 1990;323:1500–1504.

Nelson MR, Erskine D, Hawkins DA, et al. Treatment with corticosteroids: A risk factor for the development of clinical cytomegalovirus disease in AIDS. *AIDS.* 1993;7:375–378.

Newsome DA. Noninfectious ocular complications of AIDS. *Int Ophthalmol Clin.* 1989;29:95–97.

Nguyen N, Rimmer S, Katz B. Slowed saccades in the acquired immunodeficiency syndrome. *Am J Ophthalmol.* 1989;107:356–360.

Northfelt DW, Clement MJ, Safrin S. Extrapulmonary pneumocystosis: Clinical features in human immunodeficiency virus infection. *Medicine.* 1990;69:392–398.

Nussenblatt RB, Palestine AG. Human Immunodeficiency virus, herpes zoster, and the retina. *Am J Ophthalmol.* 1991;112:206–207. Editorial.

O'Donnell JJ, Jacobson MA. Cotton-wool spots and cytomegalovirus retinitis in AIDS. *Int Ophthalmol Clin.* 1989;29:105–107.

O'Hara MA, Raphael SA, Nelson LB. Isolated anterior uveitis in a child with acquired immunodeficiency syndrome. *Ann Ophthalmol.* 1991;23:71–73.

Padian N, Marquis L, Francis DP, et al. Male-to-female transmission of human immunodeficiency virus. *JAMA.* 1987;258:788–790.

Palestine AG, Frishberg B. Macular edema in acquired immunodeficiency syndrome-related microvasculopathy. *Am J Ophthalmol.* 1991;111:770–771. Letter.

Parrish CM, O'Day DM, Hoyle TC. Spontaneous fungal corneal ulcer as an ocular manifestation of AIDS. *Am J Ophthalmol.* 1987;104:302–303. Letter.

Pepose JS. Contact lens disinfection to prevent transmission of viral disease. *CLAO J.* 1988;14:165–168.

Pertel P, Hirshtick R, Phair J, et al. Risk of developing cytomegalovirus retinitis in persons infected with the human immunodeficiency virus. *J AIDS.* 1992;5:1069–1074.

Pezzi PP, Tamburi S, D'offizi GP, et al. Retinal cotton-wool-like spots: A marker for AIDS? *Ann Ophthalmol.* 1989;21:31–33.

Pflugfelder SC, Saulson R, Ullman S. Peripheral corneal ulceration in a patient with AIDS-related complex. *Am J Ophthalmol.* 1987;104:542–543. Letter.

Pillai S, Mahmood MA, Limaye SR. Herpes zoster ophthalmicus, contralateral hemiplegia, and recurrent ocular toxoplasmosis in a patient with acquired immune deficiency syndrome-related complex. *J Clin Neuro-ophthalmol.* 1989;9:229–233.

Pomerantz RJ, Kuritzkes DR, de la Monte SM, et al. Infection of the retina by human immunodeficiency virus type I. *N Engl J Med.* 1987;317:1643–1647.

Quiceno JI, Capparelli E, Sadun AA, et al. Visual dysfunction without retinitis in patients with acquired immunodeficiency syndrome. *Am J Ophthalmol.* 1992;113:8–13.

Redmond R, Wilson R. Neurological manifestations of AIDS: *J Am Optom Assoc.* 1990;10:760–767.

Reynolds JEF, ed. *Martindale The Extra Pharmacopoeia.* 30th ed. London: Pharmaceutical Press; 1993:560.

Rosenblatt MA, Cunningham C, Teich S, et al. Choroidal lesions in patients with AIDS. *Br J Ophthalmol.* 1990;74:610–614.

Rozencweig M, McLaren C, Beltanagady M, et al. Overview of phase I trials of 2',3'-dideoxyinosine (ddI) conducted on adult patients. *Rev Infect Dis.* 1990;12(suppl 5):S570–S575.

Salahuddin SZ, Palestine AG, Heck E, et al. Isolation of the human T-cell leukemia/lymphotroic virus type III from the cornea. *Am J Ophthalmol.* 1986;101:149–152.

Sandor EV, Millman A, Croxson TS, et al. Herpes zoster ophthalmicus in patients at risk for the acquired immune deficiency syndrome (AIDS). *Am J Ophthalmol.* 1986;101:153–155.

Santos C, Parker J, Dawson C, et al. Bilateral fungal corneal ulcers in a patient with AIDS-related complex. *Am J Ophthalmol.* 1985;102:118–119. Letter.

Schanzer MC, Font RL, O'Malley RE. Primary ocular malignant lymphoma associated with the acquired immune deficiency syndrome. *Ophthalmology.* 1991;98:88–91.

Schuman JS, Orellana J, Freidman AH, et al. Acquired immunodeficiency syndrome. *Surv Ophthalmol.* 1987;31:384–410.

Seiff SR, Margolis T, Graham SH, et al. Use of intravenous acylovir for treatment of herpes zoster ophthalmicus in patients at risk for AIDS. *Ann Ophthalmol.* 1988;20:480–482.

Shami MJ, Freeman W, Friedberg D. A multicenter study of *Pneumocystis* choroidopathy. *Am J Ophthalmol.* 1991;112:15–22.

Shelton MJ, ODonnell AM, Morse GD. Zalcitabine. *Ann Pharmacother.* 1993;27:480–489.

Shuler JD, Engstrom RE, Holland GN. External ocular disease and anterior segment disorders associated with AIDS. *Int Ophthalmol Clin.* 1989;29:98–104.

Shuler JD, Holland GN, Miles SA, et al. Kaposi's sarcoma of the conjunctiva and eyelids associated with the acquired immunodeficiency syndrome. *Arch Ophthalmol.* 1989;107:858–862.

Sidikaro Y, Silver L, Holland GN. Rhegmatogenous retinal detachment in patients with AIDS and necrotizing retinal infections. *Ophthalmology.* 1991;98:129–135.

Sloand EM, Pitt E, Chiarello RJ, et al. HIV testing. State of the art. *JAMA.* 1991;266:2861–2866.

Smith RE. Toxoplasmic retinochoroiditis as an emerging problem in AIDS patients. *Am J Ophthalmol.* 1991;106:738–739. Editorial.

Specht CS, Mitchell KT, Bauman AE, et al. Ocular histoplasmosis with retinitis in a patient with acquired immune deficiency syndrome. *Ophthalmology.* 1991;98:1356–1359.

Tamesis RR, Foster CS. Ocular syphilis. *Ophthalmology.* 1990;97:1281–1287.

Tenhula WN, Xu S, Madigan MC, et al. Morphometric comparisons of optic nerve axon loss in acquired immunodeficiency syndrome. *Am J Ophthalmol.* 1992;113:14–20.

Tunis SW, Tapert MJ. Acute retrobulbar neuritis complicating herpes zoster ophthalmicus. *Ann Ophthalmol.* 1987;19:453–460.

Ullman S, Wilson RP, Schwartz L. Bilateral angle-closure glaucoma in association with the acquired immune deficiency syndrome. *Am J Ophthalmol.* 1986;101:419–424.

Van De Perre P, Simonon A, Msellati P. Postnatal transmission of human immunodeficiency virus type I from mother to infant. A prospective cohort study in Kigali, Rwanda. *N Engl J Med.* 1991;325:593–598.

Vogt MW, Ho DD, Bakar SR. Safe disinfection of contact lenses after contamination with HTLV-III. *Ophthalmology.* 1986;93:771–774.

Wachter RM, Luce JM, Hopewell PC. Critical care of patients with AIDS. *JAMA.* 1992;267:541–547.

Whitcup SM, Butler KM, Caruso R, et al. Retinal toxicity in human immunodeficiency virus-infected children treated with 2',3'-dideoxyinosine. *Am J Ophthalmol.* 1992;113:1–7.

Wilson R. Cytomegalovirus retinitis in AIDS. *J Am Optom Assoc.* 1992;63:49–58.

Wilson R. HIV and contact lens wear. *J Am Optom Assoc.* 1992;63:13–15. Editorial.

Yarchoan R, Mitsuya H, Thomas RV, et al. In vivo activity against HIV and favorable toxicity profile of 2',3'-dideoxyinosine. *Science.* 1989;245:421–425.

Young TL, Robin JB, Holland GN. Herpes simplex keratitis in patients with acquired immune deficiency syndrome. *Ophthalmology.* 1989;96:1476–1479.

59
Chapter

Herpes Simplex

Christine M. Dumestre

Herpes simplex virus (HSV) is one of the most common infectious agents known to humans. The word herpes, meaning "to creep" in Greek, was used to describe the spreading nature of the cutaneous lesions back in the time of Hippocrates in 400 BC. It remains latent in neurons of sensory ganglia after primary infection, allowing it to reactivate at any time during the life of the host.

HSV is divided into two different serotypes, type 1 (HSV-1) and type 2 (HSV-2). It can range in manifestations from asymptomatic infections and self-limiting "cold sores" to fatal encephalitis. HSV-1 is usually responsible for infections above the waist such as labial, oral, upper respiratory tract infections, eye infections, encephalitis, and some cases of generalized herpes simplex. HSV-2 is primarily responsible for infections affecting areas below the waist such as venereally transmitted genital herpes and infections affecting newborns via transmission through the mother's infected birth canal. However, HSV-1 and HSV-2 are not limited to these sites.

Ocular HSV, although commonly misdiagnosed, is the most common cause of severe ocular infection in the United States. Ocular herpes simplex infections are usually due to HSV-1, although HSV-2 can cause some cases of neonatal infection or be secondary to autoinoculation from genital herpes. HSV can cause blepharitis, conjunctivitis, keratitis, uveitis, and retinitis, depending on whether the infection is primary or recurrent.

EPIDEMIOLOGY

■ Systemic
HSV infections are found throughout the world with humans being the only known natural host. HSV-1 is generally acquired during early childhood years, whereas HSV-2 infection occurs predominantly in sexually active adolescents and young adults. After primary infection, the virus becomes latent in sensory ganglia. Recurrent infection occurs with both HSV-1 and HSV-2. Approximately 20 to 40% of the population experience recurrent labial herpes or "cold sores" from HSV-1. After a primary genital herpes infection (HSV-2), recurrence is approximately 60 to 80%.

Up to 50 to 100% of the adult population has antibodies to HSV, indicating previous exposure to the virus.

Newborns are usually infected with HSV-2 from mothers with genital herpes. Dental and medical personnel are at increased risk of acquiring HSV from patients with oral or genital HSV infections. Also, wrestlers have acquired HSV from contact with superficial abrasions.

■ Ocular
Epidemiology of herpetic ocular disease has been less thoroughly investigated, although it is known to be the most common cause of corneal blindness. Ocular infection is primarily due to HSV-1, although HSV-2 can also be respon-

sible. There are 500,000 cases of ocular HSV reported each year in the United States. The recurrence rate following initial herpetic keratitis is about 25% in 2 years. The most common cause of visual loss from HSV keratitis is from involvement of the corneal stroma, which occurs in 10 to 48% of recurrent HSV keratitis infections. Ocular involvement occurs in 20% of neonatal HSV infections.

NATURAL HISTORY

■ Systemic

The Organism
Herpes simplex virus is a member of the herpes viridae family. It is a linear, double-stranded DNA virus with two serotypes, HSV-1 and HSV-2. Infection begins with the spread of virus from one person to another.

Transmission
Transmission occurs by direct contact with actively infected symptomatic or asymptomatic individuals, although those with active lesions are much more infectious. HSV-1 is usually transmitted through contact with oral secretions, and HSV-2 through contact with genital secretions. The virus enters the host through the mucosal surfaces or breaks in the skin. Upon entry, the virus infects localized epithelial cells and uses the cell for its own replication. Once replication is complete, the host cells are lysed, releasing replicated virions and causing a localized inflammatory response. This inflammatory response is what is seen in both the primary infection (although generally subclinical), and reactivation.

Course of the Disease
Primary HSV-1 infection is commonly acquired during childhood and is usually asymptomatic or may present as a nonspecific upper respiratory tract infection. Gingivostomatitis (inflammation of the gums and mouth) and pharyngitis (inflammation of the pharynx) are the most common clinical presentation of primary HSV-1 infection. The incubation period is 3 to 5 days, and patients may suffer from fever, malaise, myalgia, inability to eat, irritability, and cervical adenopathy. Signs include lesions or vesicles involving intraoral membranes, lips, and facial area (Figure 59–1). This acute primary infection is self-limiting and recovery is complete within 1 to 2 weeks.

Herpes simplex infection varies widely in severity and duration. Neonates as well as immunocompromised patients (eg, secondary to AIDS, chemotherapy, malnutrition) suffer more severe and prolonged HSV infections.

After primary infection, the virus is transported intraaxonally to the nerve cell bodies of regional ganglia, where it resides in a latent state. It remains controversial as to whether this latent state is one of no replication or one of very low continuous replication of the virus. The virus can remain latent for the lifetime of the host, or it can reactivate, causing recurrent infection. Reactivation occurs by virus transportation from the regional ganglia to the body surface along sensory nerves by anterograde axoplasmic transport. This leads to a recurrent infection of the same or neighboring site as that affected during primary infection. There are precipitating factors associated with HSV recurrence. These precipitating "trigger" factors include sun

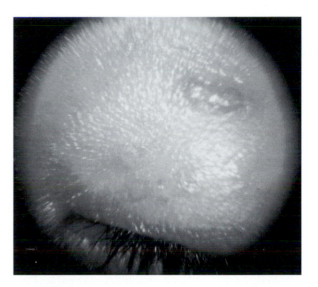

A

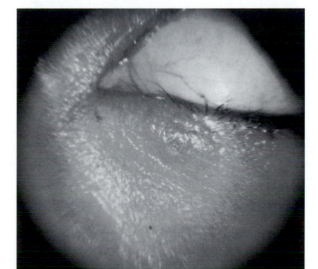

B

Figure 59–1. Recurrent ocular HSV infection with upper and lower lid vesicles. *(Courtesy of Susan P. Schuettenberg, O.D.)*

exposure, wind, fever, local trauma, menstruation, emotional stress, and decreased immunity.

Herpes labialis or "cold sores" is the most frequent clinical manifestation of recurrent HSV-1 infection. Reactivation of latent virus in the trigeminal nerve can produce intraoral mucosal ulcers, or more commonly a herpetic ulceration at the vermillion border of the lip known as the herpetic cold sore. Prodromal itching, tingling, or burning sensation is commonly described before the formation of vesicles on the lip border. Once the vesicles form, they progress to an ulcer, and then crust, and heal without scarring within a few days. Studies have shown that through asymptomatic viral shedding, persons can be infectious without the presence of the labialis lesion. However, the presence of the lesion makes the person far more infectious. Recurrent infections usually occur at the same site and are associated with precipitating factors such as stress, menstruation, fever, sun and wind exposure, direct trauma, and immunosuppression. Oral facial HSV infection is self-limiting in the immunocompetent, but may produce severe infection in the immunocompromised if left untreated.

HSV-2 infection is usually acquired by sexual contact via infected genitalia. It usually occurs in young adulthood as a primary infection, with an incubation period of 2 to 7 days. Genital herpes as a primary infection is associated with fever, malaise, headache, myalgia, and bilateral inguinal adenopathy. Pain and itching of genitalia develop into vesicular lesions and painful erythematous ulcers. Prodromal neuralgic type pain is sometimes described as radiating to the lower back and hips. Patients may also present with dysuria and vaginal or urethral discharge. Lesions of primary infection may last several weeks before completely healing. Recurrent genital herpes occurs from reactivation of HSV-2 in the sacral ganglia. HSV-2 genital infections have a recurrence rate of 80% within 12 months. Recurrent infections have a similar but milder course, and healing occurs within 5 to 10 days.

Primary oral or genital HSV can also cause a finger infection known as herpetic whitlow. This HSV infection is usually acquired by medical or dental personnel who are in contact with patients' active lesions. Signs and symptoms include abrupt onset of edema, erythema, and localized tenderness at the base of the cuticle in the infected finger. Fever and lymphadenitis are also not uncommon.

Visceral HSV infections are rare and most commonly seen in immunosuppressed patients. Immunodeficient patients are more likely to develop disseminated HSV infection involving visceral organs. Visceral HSV infections may include the esophageal mucosa, lungs, and liver (Table 59–1).

Herpes simplex meningitis is usually associated with primary genital herpes infection. The course of the disease is acute, self-limiting, and benign. Symptoms include headache, fever, and mild photophobia that lasts 2 to 7 days.

Although uncommon, HSV infections can spread from a peripheral site to the brain, causing HSV encephalitis. HSV is the most common etiology of acute sporadic viral encephalitis in the United States. It is usually associated with HSV-1. Symptoms include acute onset fever, headache, and neurological disturbances similar to those seen with temporal lobe dysfunction. There are no clinical signs indicative of herpetic etiology. Only the detection of HSV from brain biopsy is diagnostic. Untreated patients deteriorate rapidly, and mortality is as high as 60 to 80%.

Neonatal HSV infections are acquired by newborns from the infected birth canal of the mother during delivery. Most neonatal HSV infections are type 2. Infected newborns can present with self-limiting skin infections, conjunctivitis, or fatal disseminated disease with or without CNS involvement. Of those with CNS involvement, neurological sequelae include lethargy, cranial nerve palsies, and seizures. Untreated neonatal HSV disseminates and develops into CNS infection in 70% of cases, and results in death in 65% of cases.

■ Ocular

Ocular HSV infections usually present as recurrent infection and are primarily due to HSV-1. HSV-2 can sometimes cause ocular infection by secondary spread from genital herpes or as a part of widespread infection with neonatal HSV.

Ocular herpes can be acquired as a primary infection from contact with an infected individual, or it can be mechanically transferred to the eye from other HSV-infected sites on the same individual. More commonly, HSV infection is acquired affecting a nonocular site (skin or mouth), which later spreads to the eye by recurrent infection of the latent virus. Reactivation affecting the eye is usually in the form of a keratitis.

Although rare, HSV-1 can occur as a primary ocular infection. Primary ocular HSV infection is mainly associated with unilateral blepharitis and/or conjunctivitis (see Figure 59–1). Patients can experience fever, malaise, and tenderness of preauricular nodes. Vesicles form on lids and lid margins, ulcerate within days, and heal without scarring. Conjunctivitis is acute and follicular, with the presence of mucoid discharge. Approximately 20% of primary ocular infections involve the cornea. Primary HSV is self-limited and lasts 2 to 3 weeks, although in the presence of keratitis it may last longer.

Recurrent ocular HSV infections occur by reactivation of latent virus from the trigeminal, superior cervical, or ciliary ganglion. The most common target of recurrent ocular HSV disease is the cornea, although the lids may also be affected. Epithelial keratitis begins with fine superficial punctate lesions caused by actively replicating virus. These fine lesions increase in size to form the classic dendritic

TABLE 59–1. SYSTEMIC MANIFESTATIONS OF HSV

	SYMPTOMS	SIGNS
• Oral Facial HSV		
1. Primary infection: gingivostomatitis and pharyngitis	• Fever, malaise, myalgia, inability to eat, irritability	• Lesions of hard and soft palate, gingiva, tongue, lip, facial area, and cervical adenopathy
2. Recurrent herpes labialis	• Itching, burning or tingling on the mucocutaneous junction of the lip	• Vesicles that rupture to form an ulcer that will crust without scarring
• Genital HSV		
1. Primary infection	• Fever, headache, malaise, myalgia, pain, itching, dysuria, vaginal and urethral discharge	• Lesions of external genitalia, form vesicles, pustules, to painful erythematous ulcers and tender inguinal adenopathy
2. Recurrent infection	• Same as above with a milder course	
• Herpetic Whitlow	• Tenderness of infected finger, and fever	• Abrupt onset of edema, and erythema of finger and lymphadenitis
• CNS HSV		
1. Encephalitis	• Acute onset of fever and focal neurological symptoms, especially temporal lobe	• No clinical signs upon which herpetic etiology can be established
2. Meningitis	• Acute onset of fever, headache, and mild photophobia	
• Neonatal HSV	• Infection can be localized, disseminated, or involve the CNS	• Newborns often present with vesicles or conjunctivitis or neurological dysfunction such as seizures, CN palsies, and lethargy
• Visceral HSV		
1. Esophagitis	• Dysphagia, substernal pain, and weight loss	• Ulcerations of esophagus seen with endoscopy
2. Pneumonitis	• Fever, cough, dyspnea	• Mucosal lesions or tracheobronchitis
3. Hepatitis	• Fever	• Abrupt elevations of bilirubin and serum transaminase

ulcer with its characteristic branching and terminal end bulbs (Figure 59–2). Signs and symptoms include irritation, tearing, photophobia, blurred vision, and decreased corneal sensation. Dendritic ulcers usually heal spontaneously within 5 to 12 days, but can progress to larger, slower-healing geographic ulcers.

In cases of recurrent HSV infection, HSV particles may extend into the stroma, causing stromal keratitis. HSV stromal disease is thought to be due to a hypersensitivity reaction in response to viral particles that have settled into the stroma. Disciform keratitis is a round pattern of stromal edema, usually found under intact epithelium, which may heal after several months. Interstitial keratitis presents with areas of stromal infiltration from inflammatory cells and tends to be chronic and persistent. Complications from recurrent HSV stromal keratitis include vascularization, necrosis, scarring, stromal thinning, and perforation, which

may result in blindness. Symptoms of stromal keratitis include photophobia, lacrimation, blurred vision, and variable pain, depending on the severity.

Postinfectious herpetic ulcers may follow epithelial or stromal disease and are known as metaherpetic or trophic ulcers. The ulcer is sterile and occurs due to basement membrane disruption, similar to recurrent corneal erosions. The ulcer is characterized as round with rolled edges from epithelial cells that cannot adhere well to basement membrane. They can persist from weeks to months, and re-epithelialization is limited until basement membrane healing occurs. Symptoms are limited by decreased corneal sensation, but can involve tearing, foreign body sensation, and pain upon awakening.

Uveitis can occur as a sequela to stromal and endothelial inflammation or as a direct site of recurrent HSV infection. It can present as a mild to severe anterior chamber reaction. Secondary glaucoma may occur following uveitis.

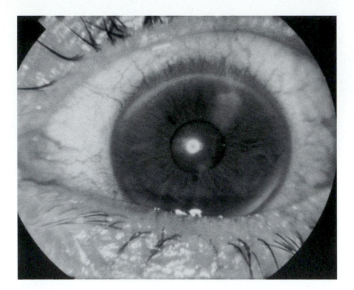

Figure 59–2. Classic appearance of HSV dendritic keratitis with characteristic branching, terminal end bulbs, and fluorescein stain pattern.

Herpes simplex retinitis is the least common ocular manifestation of HSV infection, and is limited to neonates and immunocompromised patients (Table 59–2). It manifests as an acute retinal necrosis or a chorioretinitis.

DIAGNOSIS

■ Systemic

The diagnosis of HSV infection is usually based on clinical presentation, particularly the appearance of characteristic vesicular lesions. In addition, several laboratory methods are used in the diagnosis of HSV. The "gold standard" or definitive diagnosis is made by isolating the virus itself in tissue cultures inoculated with vesicular scrapings or fluid. This method is expensive, time consuming, and not readily available. Another method is by cytological examination of lesion scrapings with Giemsa stain for multinucleated epithelial giant cells or intranuclear eosinophilic inclusion bodies. This is a good, quick, in-office procedure used to confirm diagnosis, but is not very sensitive and cannot differentiate between HSV and varicella zoster. A variety of serological tests are available to detect HSV antibodies; however, these are only useful for the diagnosis of primary infection by documenting rising antibody titers. Recently, monoclonal antibodies have been used for the detection of HSV antigen. New commercially available HSV antigen detection tests (DuPont Herpchek) have shown to be rapid (4 hours) and similar in sensitivity to tissue cultures. This test has proven reliable in diagnosis of HSV infection of the skin, genitourinary system, and eyes.

■ Ocular

Ocular HSV infection is usually diagnosed by clinical examination. The unilateral presence of lid vesicles with follicular conjunctivitis, dendritic or geographic ulcers, or disciform or interstitial keratitis can all indicate HSV ocular infection. The diagnosis of HSV keratitis can be made on the characteristic fluorescein staining appearance of the dendritic epithelial lesion with its branching nature and terminal end bulbs. Central epithelium is lost and stains with fluorescein, while the periphery of the lesion consists of infected cells and stains with rose bengal. HSV keratitis does not always present with a characteristic dendritic lesion; sometimes only a superficial punctate keratitis is noted. The history of recurrent disease, unilateral presentation, decreased corneal sensation, and the involvement of multiple corneal layers are all suggestive of HSV ocular infection. Reduced corneal sensation can be tested and serve as a diagnostic tool for HSV keratitis. A cotton wisp used to touch the cornea can grossly qualify asymmetry in corneal sensation. There are also commercially available corneal sensation devices that can quantify corneal sensation. Reduced corneal sensation is noted in the eye with HSV even after the acute condition is resolved. Diagnosis is not always readily available by clinical examination; therefore, laboratory testing may be necessary. As mentioned previously, Herpchek is a reliable diagnostic test for detecting HSV antigen. Tear film swabs used with viral transport media (Herptran media) can be sent to hospitals or reference labs where Herpchek assay is readily available to confirm the diagnosis of HSV infectious keratitis. These laboratory tests are valuable to confirm the diagnosis, but treatment should be instituted upon clinical presentation.

TREATMENT AND MANAGEMENT

There are a number of antiviral agents available for the treatment of HSV infections. These agents are nucleoside derivatives that work by interfering with the synthesis of HSV DNA. They include idoxuridine, vidarabine, trifluridine, and acyclovir.

■ Systemic

The course of labial or genital herpetic infections is usually self-limiting and benign; however, complications do exist and can be quite severe. This holds especially true for the immunocompromised and the neonate. In severe and life-threatening cases, antiviral therapy becomes essential. Vidarabine and acyclovir (ACV) are both useful in treating systemic HSV infections. Intravenously they are effective in reducing mortality associated with HSV encephalitis and disseminated neonatal infection. Oral or intravenous ACV is effective against mucocutaneous HSV infections in

TABLE 59–2. OCULAR MANIFESTATIONS OF HSV

	SYMPTOMS	SIGNS
• **Blepharitis** (Usually with primary infection)	• Itching, irritation, and swelling of lids	• Unilateral, vesicles on lid and lid margins, which ulcerate, crust, and heal without scarring
• **Conjunctivitis** (Usually with primary infection)	• Redness, lacrimation, discharge	• Acute follicular conjunctivitis with preauricular lymphadenopathy; may be associated with lid or corneal involvement
• **Keratitis**		
1. Epithelial keratitis	• Irritation, lacrimation, photophobia, blurred vision	• SPK, dendritic lesions, geographic ulcers, decreased corneal sensation
2. Stromal keratitis	• Photophobia, lacrimation, mild pain, blurred vision	• Stromal edema, stromal infiltration, vascularization, necrosis
3. Trophic ulcer	• Slight tearing, foreign body sensation, pain upon awakening, symptoms limited by decreased corneal sensation	• Loss of corneal sensation, round ulcer with rolled edges from epithelial cells that cannot adhere to damaged basement membrane
• **Uveitis**	• Photophobia, pain, blurred vision	• Mild to severe anterior chamber reaction, ciliary injection, small KPs
• **Glaucoma**		• Secondary glaucoma from uveitis
• **Retinitis**		• Choroidal hemorrhage, exudates, fine vitreal opacities, retinal edema, narrowing of arterioles

immunocompromised patients, and can also prevent the frequency of reactivation. Oral ACV is also used to shorten the duration and symptoms of genital herpes as well as prophylactically to prevent genital HSV recurrence. Topical ACV is available for use on genital herpes lesions and other localized external lesions (Table 59–3).

Along with antiviral therapy, preventative measures can also be used to reduce HSV infection. Sunblock on lips can be used to prevent recurrent labial herpes. Condoms should be used to prevent sexual transmission. Medical and dental workers should wear gloves when in contact with oral or genital secretions. Cesarean section delivery may be considered to avoid neonatal HSV in those infected with genital herpes. Antiviral treatment has no effect on viral latency.

■ Ocular

The three antiviral agents approved for the treatment of HSV ocular infection in the United States are idoxuridine (IDU) 0.5% ointment and 0.1% solution, vidarabine (Vira-A) 3% ointment, and trifluridine (Viroptic) 1% solution. ACV (Zovirax) 3% ointment has also shown to be quite effective in the treatment of ocular herpes, but is not commercially available in the United States. Idoxuridine and vidarabine are equally effective in treating epithelial kerati-

tis. They both have poor corneal penetrance and therefore are not very effective in treating HSV stromal keratitis. Trifluridine is currently the drug of choice in the United States in the treatment of HSV epithelial keratitis. It is more potent and has better ocular penetration than idoxuridine or vidarabine. All three antiviral agents present with the common side effects of ocular toxicity, especially with long-term application. Toxicities include superficial punctate keratitis, lid margin thickening, narrowing of lacrimal puncta, follicular conjunctivitis, and contact dermatitis (see Table 59–3).

Topical ACV is as effective, if not better, than other antiviral medications in the treatment of epithelial keratitis. ACV is more effective than other agents because the nature of its chemical structure makes it more specific in its action towards the virus. It is highly potent, less toxic to the ocular surface, and penetrates the cornea topically. One disadvantage of ACV is its greater potential in developing resistance. It therefore should be used with caution in those countries where it is available.

Treatment of ocular HSV depends on its presentation. It is necessary to establish which ocular structures are effected by the virus and whether the infection is primary or recurrent. The immune status of the patient is also contributory in deciding the mode of treatment.

TABLE 59–3. TREATMENT AND MANAGEMENT OF HSV

■ **SYSTEMIC**
- **Vidarabine (Vira–A)**
  15 mg/kg/d IV for 10 days
  Indication: Systemic treatment of HSV encephalitis
  Contraindication/side effect: May produce nausea, diarrhea, GI disturbance, bone marrow depression, CNS toxicity
- **Acyclovir (Zovirax)**
  Ointment: 5% cream applied 4–6 times a day for 10 days
  Oral: 200 mg tablets po 5 times a day for 2 weeks
  Intravenous: 5–10 mg/kg IV q8h for 5–7 days
  Indication: Topical ointment used for genital herpes lesions or immunosuppressed patients with localized external lesions
  Oral ACV used for treatment of genital herpes and also used prophylactically to prevent recurrence
  IV ACV is useful to treat immunocompromised patients, neonates, and patients with progressive cutaneous, CNS, or visceral dissemination of HSV infection
  Contraindication/side effect: Oral: nausea, headache, diarrhea, anorexia, leg pain, rash, renal dysfunction
  IV: local phlebitis, nausea, vomiting, hypotension, diaphoresis, renal toxicity, rash, headache, hematuria

■ **OCULAR**
  CONJUNCTIVITIS/BLEPHARITIS
- Supportive therapy
- Prophylactic antiviral or antiviral/antibiotic combination may be used

  EPITHELIAL/STROMAL KERATITIS AND UVEITIS
- **Trifluridine (Viroptic)**
  1% solution 9 times a day for 2 weeks
  Indications: Topical treatment of HSV keratitis; currently drug of choice in U.S.
  Contraindication/side effects: Most toxic of the ocular agents used, may result in SPK, follicular conjunctivitis, punctal occlusion, thickening and keratinization of lid margins, meibomian gland pouting, ptosis, contact dermatitis
- **Idoxuridine (IDU)**
  1% solution q2h or 0.5% ointment 5 times a day for 2 weeks

  Indication: Topical treatment of HSV epithelial keratitis
  Contraindication/side effect: Toxicity due to adverse effect on host cells; may result in SPK, follicular conjunctivitis, lid margin thickening and keratinization, punctal occlusion, conjunctival cicatrization, corneal scarring, ptosis, contact dermatitis
- **Vidarabine (Vira–A)**
  3% ointment 5 times daily for 2 weeks
  Indication: Topical treatment of HSV epithelial keratitis
  Contraindication/side effects: Similar side effects to IDU, although less toxic
- **Acyclovir (Zovirax)**
  3% ointment 5 times daily for 2 weeks
  Indication: Topical ophthalmic ointment; not FDA approved in U.S.
  Contraindication/side effect: Almost no adverse side effects; occasional punctate keratitis, conjunctivitis
- **Debridement**
  Indication: Was once the only effective treatment of HSV epithelial keratitis and remains a safe, effective alternative to antiviral agents

  STROMAL HERPETIC DISEASE AND METAHERPETIC ULCER
- **Referral to corneal specialist**
- **Cycloplegics**
  5% Homatropine tid
  Indication: Treatment of uveitis
- **Cortocosteroids**
  0.125–1% prednisolone acetate 2–4 times a day with tapering
  Indication: Treatment of stromal keratitis and uveitis
  Contraindication/side effect: Contraindicated for epithelial keratitis; complications include progression of epithelial infection, stromal ulceration, glaucoma, cataract, microbial superinfection, steroid dependence
- **Lubricants**
  Artificial tears igtt qid to q2h for symptomatic relief
  Indication: Used in the treatment of metaherpetic or trophic ulcers
  Contraindication/side effect: None

  PENETRATING KERATOPLASTY, IF INDICATED

Herpes simplex blepharoconjunctivitis is usually self-limiting and warrants no treatment. Some believe that antiviral therapy should be used prophylactically to prevent corneal involvement. Using an antiviral agent may shorten the course of the disease. Sometimes a combination antiviral and antibiotic ointment is used on lid vesicles to avoid secondary bacterial infection.

Herpes simplex epithelial disease (dendritic, geographic) is treated with antiviral medications to destroy the active virus that has invaded epithelial cells. Viroptic is the current treatment of choice (see Table 59–3 for specific dosages). Debridement was the sole mode of treatment prior to the availability of antiviral therapy. It is effective in removing infected epithelial cells and currently is used alone or in combination with antiviral therapy. Virus-laden cells have poor adherence to the basement membrane of the epithelium and are easily removed with a cotton-tip applicator. Regeneration of the surrounding noninfected epithelium promotes healing.

Corticosteroids should not be used in the presence of an epithelial defect where there is active viral replication such as dendritic (epithelial) keratitis. This enhances viral replication and can lead to geographic ulceration.

Stromal herpetic disease (disciform, interstitial keratitis) is more complicated to treat, and specific guidelines are difficult to give. Corticosteroids are used when there is involvement of the visual axis, but only with an intact epithelium. Their use is indicated when the keratitis is solely due to the host immunologic response, as in disciform (stromal) keratitis in which inflammation that is potentially destructive to the cornea can be suppressed. Disciform keratitis tends to be more responsive to steroids than interstitial keratitis. When corticosteroids are used to treat stromal keratitis, low dosages should be used with careful follow-up. An example would be 0.125 to 1% prednisolone acetate two to four times a day with tapering to avoid rebound inflammation, once the desired effect is achieved. The side effects of steroids include glaucoma, cataract, secondary microbial infection, and steroid dependence. One should also use an antiviral concurrently to prevent the reactivation of epithelial disease. In herpetic stromal disease, corticosteroids can potentially reduce pain, edema, scarring, and vascularization, and improve vision.

Metaherpetic or trophic ulcers are recurrent corneal erosions due to persistent epithelial defects caused by poor adherence to a damaged basement membrane from repeated HSV attacks; thus they will be easily distinguished from active herpes simplex lesions (through the history of corneal lesions). Antiviral agents do not help in these cases because there is no active viral replication. These ulcers are best managed with lubricating agents, patching, or bandage contact lenses to help promote reepithelialization. Referral to a corneal specialist may be indicated. Low-dose steroids may also be used. Close follow-up is necessary to avoid stromal thinning and to ensure that epithelial healing is taking place. Surgical treatment should be considered if medical treatment is unsuccessful. Conjunctival flaps are an alternative to provide a stable epithelial surface.

In severe cases of chronic ocular HSV infection where medical treatment has failed, penetrating keratoplasty may be necessary. Keratoplasty should be considered in patients who have corneal scarring, corneal perforation, or irreversible corneal edema. Corneal transplantation may preserve vision and/or the integrity of the eye. Corneal transplants are most successful when performed on a quiet nonactively infected eye. Recurrent ocular HSV infection can present itself even after corneal transplantation.

Whenever there is involvement of the anterior chamber (uveitis), in ocular HSV infection, cycloplegics are indicated. Corticosteroids may be used, but should be avoided if there is an epithelial defect or stromal ulceration. Antiviral treatment is also needed, preferably one that can penetrate the cornea, such as topical acyclovir or trifluridine. Oral acyclovir is also effective, although not approved for this use in the United States.

Acute retinal necrosis and chorioretinitis caused by HSV are treated with intravitreal, intravenous, and /or oral ACV.

Immunocompromised patients who have ocular HSV infections in general should be treated more aggressively. Because of their immunodeficiency, the course of disease is generally longer and recurrent infections more frequent. Educating the patient on trigger factors and how to avoid them can be helpful. Some even recommend the use of oral ACV prophylactically to prevent recurrent episodes.

CONCLUSION

HSV, one of the most common infectious agents, is diverse in its clinical presentation and severity. Its benign manifestations are universal and felt by nearly everyone. Unfortunately, the more severe clinical consequences can be life- or sight-threatening. Eyecare professionals must have knowledge of the various manifestations of HSV to be able to diagnose and treat properly to help avoid a poor outcome.

REFERENCES

Alexander LJ. Diseases of the retina. In: Bartlett JD, Jaanus DS, eds. *Clinical Ocular Pharmacology*. Boston: Butterworth; 1984.

Arffa RC, ed. *Graysons Diseases of the Cornea*. 3rd ed. St. Louis: Mosby; 1991.

Baker DA, Pavan-Langston D, Gonik B, et al. Multicenter clinical evaluation of the DuPont Herpchek HSV ELISA, a new rapid diagnostic test for the direct detection of herpes simplex virus. *Adv Exp Med Bio*. 1990;263:71–76.

Blodi MD, Frederick C, eds. *Herpes Simplex Infections of the Eye*. New York: Churchill Livingstone; 1984.

Collum L, Akhtar J, McGettrick P. Oral acyclovir in herpetic keratitis. *Trans Ophthalmol Soc UK*. 1985;104:629–632.

Corey L, Spear PG. Infections with herpes simplex virus. *N Engl J Med*. 1986;318:749–756.

Dascal A, Chan-Thim J, Morahan M, et al. Diagnosis of herpes simplex virus infection in a clinical setting by a direct antigen detection enzyme immunoassay kit. *J Clin Microbiol*. 1989;27:700–704.

Dawson CR. The herpetic eye study. *Arch Ophthamol*. 1990;8:191–192.

Eggleston M. Therapy of ocular herpes simplex infections. *Infection Control*. 1987;8:294–296.

Evans AS, ed. *Viral Infections of Humans: Epidemiology and Control*. 3rd ed. New York: Plenum; 1989.

Falcon MG. Rational acyclovir therapy in herpetic eye disease. *Br J Ophthalmol*. 1987;71:102–106.

Fingeret M, Casser L, Woodcome HT. *Atlas of Primary Eyecare Procedures*. Norwalk, CT: Appleton & Lange; 1990.

Glaser R, Gotlieb-Stematsky T. *Human Herpes Virus Infections: Clinical Aspects*. New York: Marcel Dekker; 1982.

Gordon JY. Pathogenesis and latency of herpes simplex virus type 1(HSV-1): An ophthamologist's view of the eye as a model for the study of virus–host relationship. *Adv Exp Med Biol*. 1990; 278:205–209.

Ho M. Interferon as an agent against herpes simplex virus. *J Invest Dermatol*. 1990;95:158s–160s.

Langston D, Dunkel EC. A rapid clinical diagnostic test for herpes simplex infectious keratitis. *Am J Ophthamol*. 1989;107:675–677.

Lee SF. Comparative laboratory diagnosis of experimental herpes simplex keratitis. *Am J Ophthamol*. 1990;109:8–12.

Leisegang TJ. Ocular herpes simplex infection: Pathogenesis and current therapy. *Mayo Clinic Proc*. 1988;63:1092–1105.

Mannis MJ, Plotnick RD, Schwab IR, Newton RD. Herpes simplex dendritic keratitis after keratoplasty. *Am J Ophthamol*. 1991;111:480–484.

Monnickendam MA. Herpes simplex virus ophthalmia. *Eye*. 1988; 2:s56–s69.

Pavan-Langston D. Herpes simplex virus ocular infections: Current concepts of acute, latent and reactivated disease. *Trans Am Ophthamol Soc*. 1990;88:727–793.

Pavan-Langston D, Dunkel EC. *Handbook of Ocular Drug Therapy and Ocular Side Effects of Systemic Drugs*. Boston: Little, Brown; 1991:158–181.

Pepose JS. External ocular herpes infections in immunodeficiency. *Curr Eye Res*. 1991;10:87–95.

Pepose JS. Herpes simplex keratitis: Role of viral infection versus immune response. *Surv Ophthamol*. 1991;35:345–352.

Sillis M. Clinical evaluation of enzyme immunoassay in rapid diagnosis of herpes simplex infection. *J Clin Pathol*. 1992;45: 165–167.

Wilhelmus KR. Diagnosis and management of herpes simplex stromal keratitis. *Cornea*. 1987;6:286–291.

60
Chapter

Herpes Zoster

Diane T. Adamczyk

Varicella zoster is a highly contagious virus that causes an infection, usually during childhood, known as varicella or chickenpox. It is characterized by a vesicular skin rash. Once the primary infection runs its course, the virus remains dormant in the sensory ganglia. Later in life the latent virus may reactivate as a secondary infection, herpes zoster (HZ) or shingles. The name is derived from the Greek word "herpein," which means to spread or to creep, and "zoster," which means girdle, zone, or sword belt.

Classically HZ manifests as a vesicular skin eruption along a dermatome or cranial nerve, with the potential for various complications, including painful postherpetic neuralgia (PHN). Most commonly, HZ affects the thoracic dermatome. Herpes zoster ophthalmicus (HZO) occurs when the virus affects the trigeminal nerve, specifically the ophthalmic division, with the potential for ocular complications.

EPIDEMIOLOGY

■ Systemic

Varicella/herpes zoster viral infection occurs worldwide. In the United States, almost all adults carry the HZ virus in a latent state, with serological evidence of a previous infection found in 95% (Liesegang, 1984).

In Western countries, the initial infection of varicella usually occurs in those younger than 15 years of age. In tropical or semitropical countries, varicella infection does not occur until an older age. This is particularly important in the development of congenital HZ, where the initial infection of varicella affects the pregnant woman, and subsequently the developing fetus.

In the United States, approximately 3 million cases of chickenpox occur per year, more commonly in the spring. Varicella results in approximately 100 deaths per year. Death occurs in 2 per 100,000 cases of healthy children, with more than a 15 times greater risk present in adults (Straus et al, 1988).

HZ has no sexual, racial, or seasonal predilection. It occurs more frequently in the immunocompromised and elderly populations. HZ usually affects those older than 50, with about 2.5 cases per 1000 from ages 20 to 49 years, 5 cases per 1000 for those 50 to 59, and 10 per 1000 for those 80 years and older (Hope-Simpson, 1965). There is an overall age-adjusted incidence of 130 cases per 100,000, with at least 300,000 cases per year occurring in the United States (Ragozzino et al, 1982). The chance of a patient experiencing a second attack of HZ is probably the same as a person of the same age, in the general population, experiencing a first attack. Up to 4% of patients with HZ have a second attack (Marsh, 1992).

HZ affects the thoracic region in over half of cases, followed by the cranial nerves in approximately 20% of cases, and then the cervical or lumbar region, with the sacral region least affected (Burgoon et al, 1957).

Complications of HZ, such as postherpetic neuralgia (PHN), occur in up to 14.3% of patients. PHN is found to increase with age, affecting 50% of those at 60 years and 75% of those at 70 (Watson & Evans, 1986). Cutaneous dissemination may occur in up to 26% of patients. Approximately half of these cases will have systemic involvement, that is, visceral (eg, pneumonitis) or neurologic (Straus et al, 1988).

■ Ocular

The range of involvement of the ophthalmic division of the trigeminal nerve varies from 8 to 56%, depending on the study. All or some of the branches of the ophthalmic division may be affected, with the frontal nerve (the supraorbital branch and then the supratrochlear) most commonly affected, followed by the nasociliary nerve. Occasionally the ophthalmic, along with the maxillary (second division), are involved, with all three divisions rarely affected (Edgerton, 1945).

Herpes zoster ophthalmicus (HZO) is almost always unilateral. Ocular complications may occur in 50 to 72% of the cases. In a series by Womack and Liesegang in 1983, ocular complications included lids (28% with only vesicle involvement and 13% with other lid involvement), cornea (55%), uveitis (43%), and postherpetic neuralgia (17%). Ophthalmoplegia may occur in up to one third of patients. In a study by Liesegang (1985), corneal involvement occured in 65% of HZO patients. This involvement included punctate epithelial keratitis (51%), pseudodendrites (51%), corneal scarring (51%), anterior stromal infiltrates (41%), keratouveitis/endotheliitis (34%), neurotrophic keratitis (25%), mucous plaques (13%), exposure keratitis (11%), and disciform keratitits (10%).

NATURAL HISTORY

■ Systemic

The Organism

The varicella zoster virus (human herpes virus 3) is a double-stranded DNA virus, surrounded by an envelope. Only one serotype for varicella exists, with the possibility of minor variations. In HZ, the virus can be isolated from the papules and clear vesicles up to 7 days after the rash, and longer in the immunosuppressed. The virus sheds up to 14 days. Crusted skin lesions do not contain any viable virus. The only natural host is humans.

Transmission

The primary infection of varicella occurs when the virus is spread by direct contact with a skin lesion of either varicella or herpes zoster, or is transmitted by inhaling infected airborne droplets (eg, from nasal or pharyngeal secretions). Varicella is highly contagious; however, moderately close contact must take place in order for transmission to occur. Transmission occurs in 61 to 87% of uninfected siblings, with less transmission occurring at school (Weller, 1983b). The incubation period is 14 to 17 days. The contagious period ranges from 2 days prior to the onset of the rash to the time the lesions are crusted.

Viral infection can occur only through enveloped virions, which are susceptible to physical or chemical agents. It is believed that the sensory ganglion is infected either through a hematogenous route or by the virus traveling from the skin to the nerves to the ganglion of the spinal or cranial nerves. It then remains in the ganglion in a latent state, unless reactivated.

HZ or shingles (the secondary infection) is a reactivation of the latent varicella virus. Effective regulatory mechanism and lack of susceptibility to trigger factors in HZ prevents frequent reactivation, as compared to herpes simplex (HS) (Straus, 1989). Viral reactivation is initiated when immunity is decreased. This occurs most commonly in a generally healthy elderly patient who has a normal age-related decrease in immunity. Reactivation also may occur with illnesses such as AIDS, tuberculosis, or syphilis; or chemotherapy, steroid use, irradiation, anticancer treatments, poisons, malignancy, physical or emotional trauma, stress, or surgery.

Although contact with a patient with varicella or HZ may result in HZ, it is unlikely, because lifelong immunity results from the initial infection. However, HZ may occur in a reexposed patient who, although previously infected with varicella, did not develop adequate immunity.

With reactivation, the virus replicates, follows the sensory nerve to the epidermis and dermis, accompanied by inflammation. Viral replication is greatest within the first 72 hours, and then decreases. HZ patients do not have infectious respiratory secretions and therefore are less contagious than varicella patients.

Course of the Disease

Varicella. Varicella is characterized by itching, fever, and vesicular skin lesions. The skin lesions affect the epidermis and heal within 2 weeks usually without scarring. The lesions initially present as macules with edema, followed by papules, and then vesicles with a surrounding red areolar area, and finally crusting, without sequelae. However, occasionally the lesions become pustular, punched out, painful ulcers. An uncomplicated, self-limiting course of varicella usually occurs in healthy children. Infants, adults, and immunocompromised individuals may be at increased risk for complications (eg, encephalitis, pneumonia, and death).

Herpes Zoster. With reactivation of the varicella virus, HZ manifestations may be categorized into prodromal, acute, and postherpetic phases (Table 60–1). The prodromal phase may precede the acute phase by hours to days.

The acute phase is characterized by grouped skin lesions that follow the affected dermatome (Figure 60–1) or cranial nerve, with the potential to affect adjacent areas. The lesions are usually unilateral and rarely bilateral. An occasional vesicle may affect an area other than the dermatome, possibly resulting from a hematogenous spread of the virus. Skin hypersensitivity (hyperesthesia) is usually present

TABLE 60–1. PHASES OF HZ (SHINGLES)

Prodromal Phase

Malaise	GI disturbance (eg, nausea)
Headache	Chills
Fever	Anorexia
Dysethesia/hyperestheia	Itch
Tingling	Increased skin temperature
Burning	Pain (deep, boring, sharp, lancing;
Redness	constant or intermittent)

Acute Phase

Variable patterns of pain
Hypersensitivity and decreasing dysethesia
Unilateral, grouped skin lesions, following a dermatome[a]
   Erythematous papules and edema (in 12–24 hours)
   Vesicular lesion, with erythematous base (in 72 hours), may have
     turbid yellow fluid or hemorrhagic changes
   Pustule, with less erythema (in 7–8 days)
   Crust (in 10–12 days)
   Crust falls off (in 14–21 days)

Postherpetic Neuralgia

Steady, boring, burning, lancing pain
May be accompanied by insomnia, anorexia, lassitude, or depression

[a]In part modified from Burgoon et al, 1957.

with the rash. Because both the dermis and epidermis are involved, scarring may result in HZ because of involvement of the deeper skin layers.

In mild cases, vesicles may not form, with only an erythematous maculopapule forming that resolves in 7 to 10

days. In severe cases the lesions may become gangrenous, sometimes taking weeks to heal. Generally, the cutaneous lesions are self-limiting, clearing within 1 to 3 weeks. The severity and duration is usually less in the young. Occasionally no skin lesions form, but reactivation occurs, with positive serologic evidence, which is called zoster sine herpete.

Accompanying the acute phase is an increase in the antibody titers of IgG, IgM, and IgA. These are present for 2 to 5 days after the skin rash, peaking at 2 to 3 weeks (Weller, 1983a). Also present is an acute inflammation that usually lasts 8 to 14 days, accompanied by pain. The acute pain may be the result of viral invasion to the nerve and from the associated inflammatory reaction. This inflammatory process may explain why pain is more common and severe in HZ than herpes simplex. The pain is often greater and lasts longer in the elderly. There is no apparent association with the skin lesions, and it may be brought on by simply touching the area.

A serious complication of HZ is postherpetic neuralgia, which affects the thoracic dermatome and the ophthalmic nerve most commonly. This is a persistent, boring pain that follows (usually 1 month after) the acute phase of the disease. PHN increases with age, and is rarely seen in those younger than 40 years. It may occur spontaneously or be precipitated by light touch or clothing. This unrelenting pain may result in mood changes, antisocial behavior, and severe depression or suicidal tendencies. It is not known if the depression is part of the disease process or a result of the severe pain. PHN resolves in 1 to 3 months in approximately half the patients. About 20% continue to suffer with PHN beyond a year.

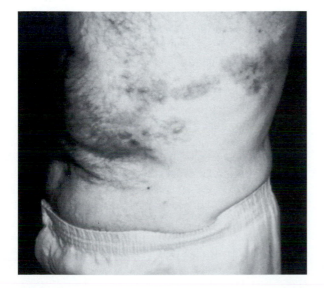

A

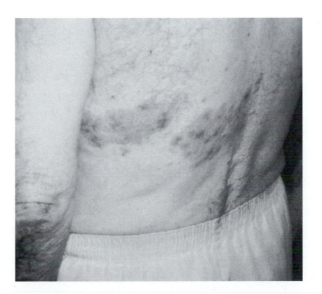

B

Figure 60–1. Acute HZ following the thoracic dermatome.

Generally HZ is a self-limited disease. In those younger than 20 years, the course is usually less severe and of a shorter duration (approximately 2 weeks), than that seen in older patients (in which the disease may persist for months). After resolution, reduced sensitivity or numbness may continue over the affected areas, along with a tingling or painful sensation brought on by wind or cold air.

HZ is usually a localized disease. However simultaneous, multiple areas (eg, ophthalmic and thoracic) may rarely be involved (HZ generalisatus). Disseminated disease, which may include multisystemic involvement, increases with age, resulting from viral spread either through direct or hematogenous routes (Table 60–2). Rarely, dissemination may result in cerebral angiitis, myelitis, or meningoencephalitis, leading to death. In the immunosuppressed, HZ may occur more commonly, with severe skin dissemination and neurological complications.

■ Ocular

Varicella. The primary infection of varicella may involve the ocular area. Ocular involvement may commonly

TABLE 60–2. SYSTEMIC MANIFESTATIONS OF VARICELLA AND HZ

VARICELLA (CHICKENPOX)
- Itch
- Fever
- Vesicular lesions
- Complications: encephalitis, pneumonia

HERPES ZOSTER (SHINGLES)
- Vesicular rash along a dermatome
- Fever
- Headache
- Depression
- Lymphadenopathy
- Mucous membrane lesions
- Complications
    Visceral organs (rare)
        Lungs—pneumonitis
        Liver—hepatitis
        Bladder—urinary retention
        Heart—myocarditis, endocarditis
    Central nervous system
        Bell palsy
        Myelitis (rare)
        Meningoencephalitis (rare)
    Vasculitis
        Cerebral angiitis: stroke or contralateral
            hemiplegia (unique to HZO)
        Segmental granulomatous arteritis (carotid or
            internal cerebral artery)
    Skeleton—arthritis
    Miscellaneous: delirium and hallucination

include conjunctivitis along with other manifestations (Table 60–3).

Herpes Zoster. Herpes zoster ophthalmicus (HZO) results from a reactivation of the virus in the trigeminal/gasserian ganglion, affecting the ophthalmic division. This division may be more commonly affected because of the increased potential for it to be exposed to trauma. However, the nasociliary nerve of the ophthalmic division is often the site for the most serious ocular complications. HZO is classically characterized by unilateral skin lesions that do not cross the midline, accompanied by hyperesthesia and preauricular lymphadenopathy.

Viral dissemination occurs more commonly in HZO than any other HZ presentation. Viral spread may affect adjacent areas to the trigeminal ganglion such as the brainstem or carotid artery. Death may rarely result.

Ocular structures are affected by HZ from direct viral invasion and replication into the eye, secondary inflammation, or autoimmune reactions. Ocular complications are not dependent on age and affect up to 70% of patients. They usually occur during or after the skin involvement, within the first 2 weeks. These complications may resolve without sequelae or may result in a poor visual outcome. Specific areas of ocular involvement or those unique to HZO will be described below (see Table 60–3).

Pain. Postherpetic neuralgia is common and especially severe in those affected by HZO. The elderly and those who have persistent, moderate to severe pain at presentation may be more inclined to PHN. However, PHN may still occur even in the absence of acute pain.

Skin/Lid. The vesicles found in HZO are usually smaller and more numerous than those found elsewhere (Figure 60–2). Although the lesions do not cross the midline, the edema may. An acute inflammation may accompany the skin lesions, along with a secondary staphylococcal aureus infection. A classic sign of nasociliary nerve involvement is Hutchinson sign (a vesicle at the tip of the nose).

Other lid involvement of HZ includes scarring, often more severe in this area, and ptosis. Lid scarring may result in a number of manifestations such as entropion, ectropion, exposure keratitis, and trichiasis, with a secondary epithelial keratopathy. Ptosis may occur secondary to the edema or from affected sympathetic innervation to the levator. Usually the ptosis is transient, but occasionally it may be permanent.

Conjunctiva. Conjunctivitis is a common ocular manifestation of HZO. It usually has a rapid resolution that does not require treatment.

Cornea. Corneal involvement is a frequent ocular manifestation of HZO. It is uncertain if the virus arrives via the

TABLE 60–3. OCULAR MANIFESTATIONS OF VARICELLA AND HZ

VARICELLA
- Conjunctivitis
- Eyelid vesicular lesions
- Limbal/conjunctival vesicles
- Superficial punctate keratopathy
- Stromal disciform keratitis
- Rare: anterior uveitis, retinitis, secondary glaucoma, optic neuritis, cataract

HERPES ZOSTER
- **Ophthalmic Division of the Trigeminal Nerve[a]**
  Frontal nerve
    Upper lid
    Superior conjunctiva
    Forehead
    Midline of scalp
  Lacrimal nerve
    Lacrimal gland
    Conjunctiva
    Skin of the upper lid (external 1/3 of eyelid)
  Nasociliary nerve
    Choroid
    Conjunctiva
    Cornea
    Lacrimal sac
    Sclera
    Iris
    Skin of the lids (inner 1/3 of the upper lid)
    Anterior and posterior ethmoid sinuses
    Vesicle tip of the nose (Hutchinson sign)
- **Ocular complications**
  Skin/lids
    Skin lesions (papule, vesicle, pustule, crust)
    Ptosis
    Secondary staphylococcal aureus infection
    Complications secondary to scarring: ectropion, entropion, punctal eversion, madarosis, poliosis, trichiasis, distichiasis, lagophthalmos, exposure keratitis, lid retraction, meibomian damage
  Conjunctiva
    Conjunctivitis (mucopurulent)
    Mucous membrane lesions: conjunctiva, nose, and mouth
    Conjunctival vesicles (associated pain, photophobia, lacrimation)
    Petechial hemorrhages
    Pseudomembrane (rare)
    Symblepharon (rare)

- **Ocular complications (con't)**
  Cornea, early
    Punctate epithelial keratitis (first week)
    Pseudodendrite (first 2 weeks)
  Cornea, late
    Anterior stromal infiltrates (1–3 weeks)
    Mucous adherent plaques (any time, usually 8–12 weeks)
    Sclerokeratitis (1–3 months) (rare)
    Keratouveitis/endotheliitis (1–21 days) (may last days to years)
    Serpiginous ulcerations (2–20 weeks) (rare)
    Disciform keratitis (1–9 months)
    Neurotrophic keratitis (3–21 days)
    Exposure keratitis (anytime, usually 2–3 months)
    Corneal scarring
  Inflammation
    Episcleritis
    Iritis
    Scleritis: (rare) diffuse or nodular
  IOP
    Hypotony
    Acute and chronic glaucoma
  Pupil
    Pupil distortion
    Horner syndrome
    Light-near dissociation
  EOM
    Ophthalmoplegia—3rd (most common), 6th, or 4th nerve palsy
  Retina/optic nerve (rare)
    Acute retinal necrosis
    Neuroretinitis
    Vascular occlusion
    Choroidal/retinal detachment
    Choroiditis
    Optic neuritis
    Thrombophlebitis
  Miscellaneous
    Iris sector atrophy
    Iris cyst formation
    Hypopyon
    Cataract
    Sympathetic ophthalmia/phthisis bulbi (rare)
    Heterochromia irides
    Proptosis
    Anterior chamber hemorrhage
    Dacryoadenitis, canaliculitis

[a] When the maxillary division is affected, the skin and conjunctiva of the lower lid may be affected, along with other structures in this region.

lid margin, conjunctiva, or from the corneal nerves. Corneal complications may result from viral replication, denervation, lid abnormalities, decreased blink, abnormal tear film, hypoesthesia, neurotrophic damage, corneal exposure, and inflammation. Localized decreased corneal sensation is a hallmark of HZO. Many corneal manifesta- tions will resolve without treatment or sequelae (Figure 60–3); others however, if left untreated, could potentially lead to vision loss.

Corneal involvement may be divided into early (2 to 4 weeks) manifestations, which are generally self-limited; and late manifestations. Early involvement may be the

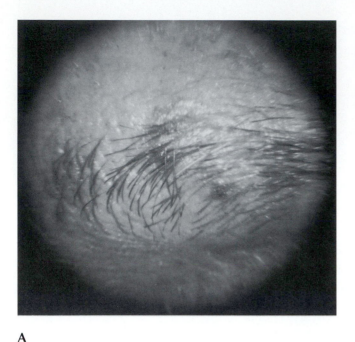

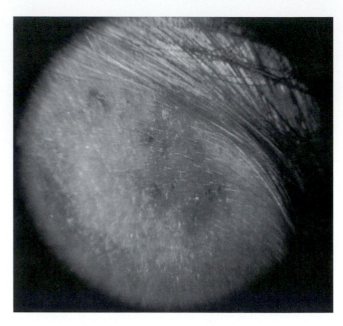

A

B

Figure 60–2. HZO affecting the frontal nerve of the ophthalmic division.

result of direct viral assault and its sequelae. Late involvement may reflect an immune reaction or an inflammatory response.

The following discussion of corneal complications is a compilation from Liesegang (1985) and Cobo (1988) (see Table 60–3). Early corneal manifestations include punctate epithelial keratitis (PEK) and zoster pseudodendrites. Both involve corneal epithelial cells, which are

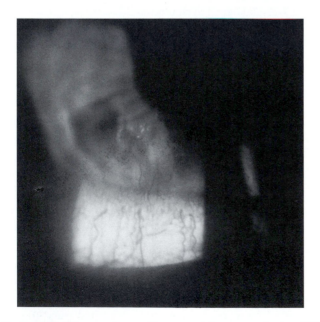

Figure 60–3. HZ corneal scar. *(Courtesy of Optometry Service, FDR VA Hospital, Montrose, NY.)*

probably where viral replication occurs. Positive viral cultures still occur at this stage.

Punctate epithelial keratitis is an area of elevated, swollen epithelial cells, with or without stromal edema, which are usually multiple and peripherally located. PEK is self-limiting and is believed to be an early form of a pseudodendrite. The pseudodendrite is composed of peripherally located swollen epithelial cells, with a gray-white, dendritic pattern. Pseudodendrites are self-limited, usually resolving within days or up to a month.

Mucous adherent plaques are sometimes confused with the early zoster pseudodendrite. They may occur anywhere on the cornea, or can be found over the areas of chronic stromal inflammation. It is believed that tear film instability and epithelial changes play a role in their formation. No viruses are found in these self-limited lesions. They are flat to slightly elevated, gray-white plaques, sharply demarcated, and variable in size and configuration (eg, linear or branched).

Anterior stromal infiltrates, which are an early form of stromal keratitis, also known as nummular keratitis, are often associated with a pseudodendrite or PEK. These lesions are located in the periphery, under the Bowman membrane, and are 1 to 2 mm in diameter. When the subepithelial infiltrates are limited to a sector of the cornea, a branch of the corneal nerve may be affected. They may follow a variable course, but usually resolve with minimal treatment. Nummular scars usually do not affect vision.

Disciform keratitis may result from stromal keratitis, weeks to months after the initial onset. It presents clinically as a focal, well-demarcated, mid to deep stromal infiltration, with localized stromal edema, located either centrally or peripherally. Disciform keratitis may lead to interstitial keratitis, with neovascularization and scarring.

Rarely will corneal involvement include serpiginous ulcers or sclerokeratitis. Serpiginous ulcers are crescent shaped, peripherally located, and can potentially lead to thinning and perforation.

Decreased corneal sensation is usually localized, may be brief or last months to years, and may lead to neurotrophic keratopathy. Neurotrophic keratopathy can lead to a pannus or scar formation, or an ulcer with the potential for decreased vision, perforation, or loss of the eye.

Inflammation and Intraocular Pressure. Inflammation, particularly of the anterior segment, is a common clinical manifestation of HZO. It may occur any time in the disease process. Iritis/iridocyclitis occurs in less than half the patients. It is associated with the classic signs and symptoms, and is usually mild and self-limited (in 6 to 12 months), with only the severe cases resulting in serious sequelae. The intraocular pressure may be either increased, from inflammation, debris, or synechiae, or decreased, from necrosis of the ciliary body. Pressure increases may manifest acutely or chronically, with glaucoma resulting from chronically increased IOP.

Pupil. Localized ischemic changes may result in pupil distortion. Sympathetic nerve and ciliary ganglion involvement may result in Horner syndrome or a light near dissociation pupil, respectively.

Extraocular Muscle. Extraocular muscle (EOM) involvement is generally seen in patients who are older than 40 years. It may occur at any time in the disease process, even weeks or months after the onset, but it usually takes place when the skin lesions scar. The patient may be asymptomatic or complain of diplopia. The third cranial nerve (total or partial involvement) is most frequently affected, followed by the sixth or the fourth nerves. It generally is self-limited, resolving in 2 months, although rarely it may be permanent.

Retina and Optic Nerve. Retinal and optic nerve manifestations of HZO are generally rare, with poor visual prognosis.

DIAGNOSIS

The diagnosis of HZ, in most instances, is made based on the characteristic skin lesions and their distribution, along with history and physical exam. Other tests, though less frequently used, may assist in the diagnosis. These include the Tzanck technique, a nonspecific test for herpetic infection, which stains material from the base of the vesicle; skin biopsy; viral culture (which is definitive, but slow); serum conversion; antibody titers; enzyme-linked immunosorbent assay (ELISA), used for serodiagnosis; fluorescein antibody membrane antigen test (FAMA), used for serodiagnosis; serological tests; and immunofluorescent and immunoenzyme stains.

■ Systemic

A general physical exam, including chest x-ray and blood workup, should be a part of the management of a HZ patient. This will assist in ruling out any underlying systemic disease with associated decreased immunity. When dissemination has occurred, referral and workup by the appropriate specialist is recommended. In addition, HZ in a patient younger than 45 may indicate underlying HIV infection (Sandor et al, 1986).

■ Ocular

Diagnosis of specific ocular manifestations of HZ is made through a complete eye health evaluation. Corneal evaluation includes biomicroscopy and use of fluorescein and rose bengal dyes, along with testing for corneal anesthesia (eg, esthesiometer). Diagnostic features of specific corneal involvement is as follows.

PEK stains poorly with fluorescein or rose bengal. Pseudodendrites differ from the true dendrite of simplex, in that they are broader, without central ulceration and rounded raised borders. Consequently pseudodendrites do not stain with fluorescein and stain more with rose bengal. Herpes simplex stains centrally with fluorescein, in an area excavated, with no epithelium, and with rose bengal at the ulcer border. Mucous adherent plaques of HZ stain uniformly with rose bengal, but poorly with fluorescein.

TREATMENT AND MANAGEMENT

Table 60–4 summarizes varicella and HZ treatment and management.

■ Systemic

Varicella
Treatment and management of the primary infection of varicella or chickenpox is nonspecific, including palliative measures, compresses, and appropriate hygiene. Because varicella is highly contagious, measures should be taken to prevent spread to noninfected or immunocompromised individuals, such as isolation of the infected patient or prophylactic use of varicella-zoster immune globulin. In addi-

TABLE 60–4. TREATMENT AND MANAGEMENT OF VARICELLA AND HZ

VARICELLA
- Supportive palliative care
- Isolation of patient
- Analgesics (avoid aspirin)

HERPES ZOSTER
- Complete physical, if <45 years, rule out concurrent HIV infection
- **General Therapies**
  Acyclovir: 800 mg, 5 times/day, for 7–10 days; (within 72 hours of skin lesions)
    Side effects: GI disturbances (nausea, vomiting, diarrhea), headache, bone marrow suppression, lethargy, seizure, transient increases serum creatinine, and nephrotoxicity. If concurrent HIV infection, hospitalize for IV acyclovir
  Steroid: Immunocompetent, <60 years: 60–80 mg/day, for 7–10 days, then taper over additional 2 weeks
    Use with caution, questionable efficacy
      >60 years: treat concurrently with ACV, to decrease the risk of dissemination
    Side effects: viral dissemination, cataracts, increased IOP, recurrences, prolonged disease, decreased immunity, risk of concurrent bacterial, fungal or herpes simplex disease, others
- **Skin Lesions**
  Cloth soaked with cool/warm water
  Burow solution (5% aluminum acetate)
  Calamine lotion
  Silver nitrate 0.25%
  Oral antihistamine
  Topical antibiotic ointment
- **Acute Pain**
  ACV
  Analgesics
  Capsaicin cream (zostrix)
  Steroid
  Nonsteroidal antiinflammatory drugs
  Narcotics
  Antidepressants
  Anticonvulsants
  Unsubstantiated use: amantadine, cimetidine
  Local anesthetics (eg, stellate ganglion block)
- **Postherpetic Neuralgia**
  Steroid
  Capsaicin cream (Zostrix)
  Tricyclic antidepressants (eg, amitriptyline HCL, 10 mg/d initial, increase to 50–75 mg/d prn)
  Combination anticonvulsant and tricyclic antidepressant (eg, amitriptyline HCl, 25 mg/d, plus carbamazepine 200 mg/d)
  Local anesthetics (eg, somatic or sympathetic block)
  Surgery
- **Miscellaneous Treatments**
  Pain
    Neuroaugmentation (eg, ultrasound, acupuncture)

Neurosurgical procedures (eg, neurectomy)
Cryoanalgesia (dry ice)
Experimental antiviral agents
  6-deoxy ACV
  BVDU [5-(2-bromovinyl)-2 deoxyuridine]
  2-fluoro-5-iodoarabinosylcytosine (FIAC)
- **Ocular Treatment**
  Note: concentration and frequency of topical agents are dependent on the severity of the disease, with topical ACV 3% prescribed 5 times per day
  Lids
    Trichiasis: cryotherapy
    En/ectropion: lid surgery
    Skin lesions/scarring: oral ACV
  Cornea
    Epithelial disease: topical and oral ACV
    Punctate epithelial keratopathy: monitor
    Pseudodendrite: monitor, oral ACV
    Mucoid adherent plaques: monitor, topical steroids, lubricants, mucolytics (acetylcysteine)
    Keratitis: oral and topical ACV; steroid
    Stromal disease: monitor (eg, anterior stromal infiltrates), steroids, oral ACV
    Ulcer: steroid, topical ACV
    Disciform keratopathy: steroid
    Neurotrophic keratopathy: lubricants, mucolytic agents, soft contact lens, tape lids or for more severe cases; tarsorrhaphy, cyanoacrylate glue patch conjunctival flap or botulinous toxin induced ptosis, (steroids should be avoided or used with caution), patient education.
    Exposure keratopathy: tarsorrhaphy, conjunctival flap
    Corneal perforation: penetrating keratoplasty
    Corneal scar: penetrating or lamellar keratoplasty
    Patient education: monitor for redness, decreased vision, lack of corneal luster
  Inflammation
    Episcleritis: monitor, topical vasoconstrictor, steroid
    Keratouveitis: topical ACV, steroid
    Iritis: steroids, mydriatics
    Secondary glaucoma: eg, beta blocker, epinephrine; topical steroid
    Scleritis: steroid, NSAIDs
    Uveitis: oral ACV, steroid, cycloplegic
    Optic neuritis: ACV, steroid
  Ophthalmoplegia
    Monitor
    Persistent diplopia: prism or occlusion
    Proptosis, contralateral hemiplegia: oral steroid
  Retina
    Acute retinal necrosis: IV ACV, steroids (oral prednisone), aspirin, laser photocoagulation

tion, aspirin should not be used because of its association with Reye syndrome. The exact pathogenesis of Reye syndrome is not known, but it has been associated with influenza or varicella and the use of salicylates, often leading to death.

Herpes Zoster

Management of HZ may include monitoring the patient or use of antiviral medications. As with varicella, appropriate hygiene and precautions should be taken. These include patient isolation from those never infected with the virus or from those immunocompromised, along with the use of gloves, until the lesions have crusted and the potential for spread has decreased.

The treatment of herpes zoster has been revolutionized with the antiviral agent acyclovir (ACV). ACV affects DNA synthesis through inhibition of DNA polymerase, resulting in decreased viral replication. ACV has replaced other antiviral medications as the drug of choice, with oral treatment generally safe for both the immunocompetent and immunosuppressed. Unlike ACV, other antiviral drugs such as idoxuridine are nonselective. Vidarabine has the same mechanism of action as ACV, but is not as specific.

ACV affects viral cells as opposed to host cells. This specificity decreases its toxic side effects (see Table 60–4), making it a well-tolerated drug. ACV is most effective when used early in the course of the disease, within 3 days of the onset of the skin lesions, when it inhibits viral replication and dissemination. Although ACV's action is on the family of herpes viruses, a much higher concentration is needed for the varicella virus than the simplex virus. Consequently, high dosage is most effective in HZ.

ACV decreases acute pain (with no evidence of an affect on PHN), skin dissemination and duration, as well as providing a more expedient resolution of the signs and symptoms. Disseminated disease (eg, central nervous system involvement) or concurrent infection with HIV is usually treated with intravenous ACV.

Steroids used during the acute phase of HZ decrease inflammation, necrosis, and scarring. However, steroids have questionable effectivity, and can possibly cause numerous side effects. Oral ACV may be used in conjunction with steroids to decrease the potential of dissemination. In the immunosuppressed, steroids are generally contraindicated. However, if their use is needed, discontinuation with tapering should begin as soon as possible.

Skin Lesions

Specific lotions, ointments, or solutions may be used to sooth and soften the crusts of skin lesions. These include Burow solution (5% aluminum acetate), which provides a mildly antiseptic, drying effect; silver nitrate 0.25%, which provides a germicidal, astringent effect, but stains the skin brown; calamine lotion; and a cloth soaked with water to

help remove exudates. In addition, oral antihistamines may be used to decrease itching, and antibiotic ointments may be used if bacterial infection is present.

Acute Pain and Postherpetic Neuralgia

Treatment for pain in HZ, both acute and postherpetic, remains a clinical challenge, often being ineffective or lacking supportive studies. Topical capsaicin (derived from the nightshade plant) cream (Zostrix) has been promising in decreasing acute and persistent pain. Its mechanism of action is related to substance P (a sensory or pain transmitter), which capsaicin depletes within several weeks of use (2 to 4 weeks), resulting in pain relief. The patient may continue to be pain free after discontinuation of capsaicin. However, some, particularly the elderly suffering from PHN, may need to continue with treatment indefinitely.

Local anesthetics, such as stellate ganglion blocks, appear to have good results in acute pain and should be reserved for use in certain cases not successfully treated by other means. The administration of local anesthetics, however, should be done by one experienced with the technique, such as an anesthesiologist. Neurosurgical techniques, as with sympathetic blocks, should only be considered as a final alternative in the most debilitating cases.

Disseminated Disease

For disseminated HZ disease, co-management with the respective specialist for the area involved is appropriate. In addition, a complete physical, with blood workup and chest x-ray should be done to rule out underlying disease, such as tuberculosis and malignancy. In patients younger than 45 years with no apparent cause for HZ, an evaluation should be done to rule out HIV infection.

■ Ocular

Varicella

The ocular treatment of varicella is as described in the systemic section. Iritis and keratitis may be treated with mydriatics. Cautious use of steroids may be efficacious for late interstitial keratitis.

Herpes Zoster

Ocular complications of HZ may be managed with systemic antivirals, steroids (topical or systemic), or specific treatment modalities dependent on the type of manifestation (see Table 60–4).

ACV has been noted to influence the incidence and severity of eye complications, including anterior uveitis, corneal disease, and lid scarring. Prompt ACV treatment is important for effectivity and is as discussed previously. Topical ACV 3% has shown inconsistent but favorable results in corneal disease. It is well tolerated, with few side effects including punctate keratopathy and burning. It is the antiviral drug of choice based on its ocular penetrance, where available.

Treatment with ACV is specific for the herpes virus; therefore, any inflammatory or immunologic process would need steroidal treatment. Steroids should be used cautiously, as noted previously, particularly in the immunosuppressed and in those with the potential for exacerbating a herpes simplex infection.

Pain

For control of pain (acute and persistent), stellate ganglion blocks have shown positive results in HZO. Ganglion blocks appear to decrease the course of the disease, relieve pain, and prevent PHN. Patients usually show relief of pain after 1 to 5 blocks (Currey & Dalsania, 1991). The mechanism of action is not known.

Lids and Skin

Lotions or ointment may be used for the periocular cutaneous lesions. If cicatricial lid retraction is present, skin graft or tarsorrhaphy may be needed.

Cornea

Punctate epithelial keratopathy and pseudodendrites are generally self-limited. However, because of viral presence, oral ACV may act prophylactically to decrease the progression of PEK to pseudodendrites.

Mucoid adherent plaques, sometimes associated with stromal inflammation and tear abnormalities, are also often self-limiting. Treatment ranges from monitoring only, to lubricants and mucolytics, or topical steroids.

Stromal involvement (anterior stromal infiltrates) may only need to be monitored. Topical steroids should only be used in cases of decreased vision, associated uveitis, secondary increased IOP from inflammation, and chronic stromal disease.

Various treatment modalities are recommended for neurotrophic keratopathy. Patients with decreased corneal sensation should be closely monitored and educated to the possible sequelae of neurotrophic complications (eg, redness, decreased VA, change in corneal luster).

Penetrating keratoplasty was once not considered a treatment option for certain corneal manifestations because HZ patients were considered poor candidates because of affected corneal sensation and associated lid and tear disturbances. However, studies (Reed et al, 1989; Soong et al, 1989) have shown promising results in select patients, who receive careful postoperative management.

CONCLUSION

Almost every person is infected with the varicella-zoster virus in childhood, which usually follows a benign course.

Reactivation of the latent virus, herpes zoster, occurs more commonly in the elderly and immunosuppressed population, and follows a more debilitating course, with the potential for long-standing sequelae. HZ has a number of clinical manifestations, including painful postherpetic neuralgia. Herpes zoster ophthalmicus occurs when reactivation affects the ophthalmic division of the trigeminal nerve, with the potential for sight-threatening complications.

Treatment of HZ, using the antiviral drug acyclovir, has significantly improved the course of the disease. Prompt treatment can help to greatly minimize serious general and ocular sequelae.

REFERENCES

Amanat LA, Cant JS, Green FD. Acute phthisis bulbi and external ophthalmoplegia in herpes zoster ophthalmicus. *Ann Ophthalmol.* 1985;17:46–51.

Archambault P, Wise JS, Rosen J, et al. Herpes zoster ophthalmoplegia. Report of six cases. *J Clin Neuro-ophthamol.* 1988;8:185–191.

Atmaca LS, Ozmert E. Optic neuropathy and central retinal artery occlusion in a patient with herpes zoster ophthalmicus. *Ann Ophthalmol.* 1992;24:50–53.

Borruat FX, Herbort CP. Herpes zoster ophthalmicus. Anterior ischemic optic neuropathy and acyclovir. *J Clin Neuro-ophthalmol.* 1992;12:37–40.

Browning DJ, Blumenkranz MS, Culbertson WW, et al. Association of varicella zoster dermatitis with acute retinal necrosis syndrome. *Ophthalmology.* 1987;94:602–606.

Bucci FA, Gabriels CF, Krohel GB. Successful treatment of postherpetic neuralgia with capsaicin. *Am J Ophthalmol.* 1988;106:758–759.

Büchi ER, Herbort CP, Ruffieux C. Oral acyclovir in the treatment of acute herpes zoster ophthalmicus. *Am J Ophthalmol.* 1986;102:531–532.

Burgoon CF, Burgoon JS, Baldridge GD. The natural history of herpes zoster. *JAMA.* 1957;164:265–269.

Chess J, Marcus DM. Zoster-related bilateral acute retinal necrosis syndrome as presenting sign in AIDS. *Ann Ophthalmol.* 1988;20:431–438.

Cobo LM. Corneal complications of herpes zoster ophthalmicus. Prevention and treatment. *Cornea.* 1988;7:50–56.

Cobo LM, Foulks GN, Liesegang T, et al. Observation on the natural history of herpes zoster ophthalmicus. *Curr Eye Res.* 1987;6:195–199.

Cobo LM, Foulks GN, Liesegang T, et al. Oral acyclovir in the therapy of acute herpes zoster ophthalmicus. *Ophthalmology.* 1986;93:763–770.

Cobo LM, Foulks GN, Liesegang T, et al. Oral acyclovir in the therapy of acute herpes zoster ophthalmicus. An interim report. *Ophthalmol.* 1985;92:1574–1583.

Cole EL, Meisler PM, Calabrese LH, et al. Herpes zoster ophthalmicus and acquired immune deficiency syndrome. *Arch Ophthalmol.* 1984;102:1027–1029.

Cooper M. The epidemiology of herpes zoster. *Eye.* 1987; 1:413–421.

Culbertson WW, Blumenkranz MS, Pepose JS. et al. Varicella zoster virus is a cause of the acute retinal necrosis syndrome. *Ophthalmology.* 1986;93:559-569.

Currey TA, Dalsania J. Treatment for herpes zoster ophthalmicus: Stellate ganglion block as a treatment for acute pain and prevention of postherpetic neuralgia. *Ann Ophthalmol.* 1991;23:188–189.

Edgerton AE. Herpes zoster ophthalmicus. *Arch Ophthalmol.* 1945;34:40–62, 114–153.

Harding SP, Lipton JR, Wells JCD. Natural history of herpes zoster ophthalmicus: Predictors of postherpetic neuralgia and ocular involvement. *Br J Ophthalmol.* 1987;71:353–358.

Harding SP, Porter SM. Oral acyclovir in herpes zoster ophthalmicus. *Curr Eye Res.* 1991;10(suppl):177–182.

Hoang-Xuan T, Büchi ER, Herbort CP, et al. Oral acyclovir for herpes zoster ophthalmicus. *Ophthalmology.* 1992;99:1062–1071.

Hope-Simpson RE. The nature of herpes zoster: A long-term study and a new hypothesis. *Proc Royal Soc Med.* 1965;58:9–20.

Jessell TM, Iverson LL; Cuello AC. Capsaicin-induced depletion of substance P from primary sensory neurones. *Brain Res.* 1978;152:183–188.

Karbassi M, Raizman MB, Schuman JS. Herpes zoster ophthalmicus. *Surv Ophthalmol.* 1992;36:395–410.

Karlin JD. Herpes zoster ophthalmicus: The virus strikes back. *Ann Ophthalmol.* 1993;25:208–215.

Karlin JD. Herpes zoster ophthalmicus and iris cysts. *Ann Ophthalmol.* 1990;22:414–415.

Kothe AC, Flanagan J, Trevino RC. True posterior ischemic optic neuropathy associated with herpes zoster ophthalmicus. *J Am Acad Optom.* 1990;67:845–849.

Liesegang TJ. Diagnosis and therapy of herpes zoster ophthalmicus. *Ophthalmology.* 1991;98:1216–1229.

Liesegang TJ. Ophthalmic herpes zoster: Diagnosis and antiviral therapy. *Geriatrics.* 1991;46:64–71.

Liesegang TJ. Corneal complications from herpes zoster ophthalmicus. *Ophthalmology.* 1985;92:316–324.

Liesegang TJ. The varicella-zoster virus: Systemic and ocular features. *J Am Acad Dermatol.* 1984;11:165–191.

Lightman S, Marsh JR, Powell D. Herpes zoster ophthalmicus: A medical review. *Br J Ophthalmol.* 1981;65:539–541.

Marsh RJ. Ophthalmic zoster. *Br J Ophthalmol.* 1992;76:244–245.

Marsh RJ, Cooper M. Double-masked trial of topical acyclovir and steroids in the treatment of herpes zoster ocular inflammation. *Br J Ophthalmol.* 1991;75:542–546.

Marsh RJ, Cooper M. Ophthalmic zoster: Mucous plaque keratitis. *Br J Ophthalmol.* 1987;71:725–728.

McGill J. The enigma of herpes stromal disease. *Br J Ophthalmol.* 1987;71:118–125.

Mondino BJ, Farley MK, Aizuss DH. Sectorial corneal infiltrates and pannus in herpes zoster ophthalmicus. *Clin Exp Ophthalmol.* 1986;224:313–316.

Ostler H, Thygeson P. The ocular manifestations of herpes zoster, varicella, infectious mononucleosis and cytomegalovirus disease. *Surv Ophthalmol.* 1976;21:148–159.

Pavan-Langston D. Varicella-zoster ophthalmicus. *Int Ophthalmol Clin.* 1975;15:171–185.

Ragozzino MW, Melton J, Kurland CT, et al. Risk of cancer after herpes zoster. A population-based study. *N Engl J Med.* 1982;307:393–397.

Reed JW, Joyner SJ, Knauer WJ. Penetrating keratoplasty for herpes zoster keratopathy. *Am J Ophthalmol.* 1989;107:257–261.

Ross JVM. Herpes zoster ophthalmicus sine eruptione. *Arch Ophthalmol.* 1949;42:808–812.

Sandor EV, Millman A, Croxson S, Mildvan D. Herpes zoster ophthalmicus in patients at risk for the acquired immune deficiency syndrome (AIDS). *Am J Ophthalmol.* 1986;101: 153–155.

Seiff SR, Margolis T, Graham SH, O'Donnell JJ. Use of intravenous acyclovir for treatment of herpes zoster ophthalmicus in patients at risk for AIDS. *Ann Ophthalmol.* 1988;20:480–482.

Soong HK, Schwartz AE, Meyer RF, Sugar A. Penetrating keratoplasty for corneal scarring due to herpes zoster ophthalmicus. *Br J Ophthalmol.* 1989;73:19–21.

Straus SE. Clinical and biological differences between recurrent herpes simplex virus and varicella-zoster virus infections. *JAMA.* 1989;262:3455–3458.

Straus SE, Ostrove JM, Inchauspe G, et al. Varicella-zoster virus infections. Biology, natural history, treatment and prevention. *Ann Int Med.* 1988;108:221–237.

Strommen GL, Pucinol F, Tight RR, Beck CL. Human infection with herpes zoster: Etiology, pathophysiology, diagnosis, clinical course and treatment. *Pharmacotherapy.* 1988;8:52–68.

Thibodeaux D. Herpes zoster ophthalmicus. In: Onofrey BE, ed. *Clinical Optometric Pharmacology and Therapeutics.* Philadelphia: Lippincott; 1991.

Tunis SW, Tapert MJ. Acute retrobulbar neuritis complicating herpes zoster ophthalmicus. *Ann Ophthalmol.* 1987; 19:453–460.

Verghese A, Sugar AM. Herpes zoster ophthalmicus and granulomatous angiitis. An ill-appreciated cause of stroke. *J Am Geriatr Soc.* 1986;34:309–312.

Watson PN, Evans RJ. Postherpetic neuralgia. *Arch Neurol.* 1986;43:836–840.

Weller TH. Varicella and herpes zoster. Changing concepts of the natural history, control, and importance of a not-so-benign virus (first of two parts). *N Engl J Med.* 1983a;309:1362–1368.

Weller TH. Varicella and herpes zoster. Changing concepts of the natural history, control, and importance of a not-so-benign virus (second of two parts). *N Engl J Med.* 1983b;309:1434–1440.

Wilson CA, Wander AH, Choromokos EA. Central retinal artery obstruction in herpes zoster ophthalmicus and cerebral vasculopathy. *Ann Ophthalmol.* 1990;22:347–351.

Womack LW, Liesegang TJ. Complications of herpes zoster ophthalmicus. *Arch Ophthalmol.* 1983;101:42–45.

61
Chapter

Rubella

Diane T. Adamczyk

Rubella, also known as German measles, was first recognized in the 1800s. It is a relatively benign viral disease when it occurs postnatally, usually affecting children and young adults. However, when a pregnant woman is infected, its most damaging effects are to the developing fetus. The classic rubella triad of cataract, heart disease, and deafness in infants born during a rubella epidemic was first described in the 1940s. Congenital rubella syndrome encompasses a variety of systemic and ocular abnormalities that occur as a result of fetal infection.

EPIDEMIOLOGY

■ Systemic

Rubella occurs worldwide, affecting all races and sexes equally. Specific patterns of infection are determined by population density, location, and climate, often taking either an endemic or epidemic form. For example, endemic infections occur in large continental populations, with occasional epidemics occurring every 6 to 9 years, whereas epidemics generally affect island populations at less frequent intervals (Boniuk, 1975). In the United States, major epidemics have occurred in 1917, 1935, 1943, and 1964, with less severe epidemics in 1952 and 1958. Many of the epidemics in the United States have coincided with war and military movement.

Rubella occurs more frequently in the winter and the spring. It generally affects children, with 15% immune to rubella when they enter school, 74% immune by adolescence, and 90% immune by adulthood (Calvert, 1969). The rate of infection is high for those who are not immune and have extended exposure to individuals who are actively infected with the virus, whereas brief exposure results in only 20% becoming infected. A typical annual incidence of 2000 was once reported in New York City, with a tenfold increase to more than 20,000 cases occurring during the 1964 to 1965 epidemic (Cooper & Krugman, 1967). With consistent vaccination programs, the epidemiologic trends have shown a decline. It was estimated 5 years after vaccination programs were instituted, 10,000 to 20,000 cases of congenital rubella were avoided (Krugman & Katz, 1974).

The incidence of rubella in pregnancy is 10 cases per 100,000 during nonepidemic years, becoming 30 times higher in epidemic years (Boniuk, 1975). Fetal exposure to rubella may result in an abnormal outcome (eg, stillbirth, spontaneous abortion) or malformation, with the exact incidence difficult to determine because years may pass before a congenital defect is discovered. The chance of the fetus being affected decreases as the pregnancy progresses. Although reports vary, infection in the first month of pregnancy may affect up to half the fetuses; in the second month up to one quarter; and in the third month approximately 10%. Infection that occurs in the second trimester may result in a fetal defect in up to 10% of cases.

Fetal survival is approximately 20% when infection occurs in the first month of pregnancy, and 50% in the second month, with most surviving in the third month (Tate, 1969). Death occurs in up to 20% in the first 18 months of life (Boniuk, 1975). Postnatal complications of rubella infection are generally rare, with encephalitis occurring in 1 of 5000 cases. The fatality rate is 1.8 per 100,000 (Boniuk, 1972b, 1975).

Systemic manifestations of congenital rubella are numerous, with the heart and hearing most commonly involved. Heart disease occurs in 52 to 61%, with patent ductus the most common heart manifestation. Hearing loss occurs in 29 to 52%, psychomotor retardation in up to 40%, low birthweight in 40%, thrombocytopenic purpura in up to 31%, and transient bone changes in 40 to 50%.

■ Ocular

Ocular manifestations may occur in 30 to 60% of infants exposed congenitally to rubella (Rudolph & Desmond, 1972). A common manifestation is cataracts, affecting 63 to 82%, with bilateral involvement in 50 to 80%. Retinopathy has been reported to occur in 13 to 88% of cases, with the actual incidence difficult to determine, particularly when the fundus is obscured by media opacities. Glaucoma has been reported to occur in 2 to 15%; strabismus in 35% in the first 6 months, and in 60% by 18 months; nystagmus in 38%; iris hypoplasia in 33%; and microphthalmia in 60%.

Associated systemic findings with ocular manifestations of congenital rubella include heart defects in 96% and hearing loss in 50%.

NATURAL HISTORY

■ Systemic

The Organism

The rubella virus, identified in 1962, belongs to the togavirus group of viruses. It consists of a RNA core, with only one antigenic type. Its infectivity is affected by higher temperatures and extremes of pH. Humans are the natural host of rubella, although animals may be artificially infected.

The virus replicates in the cell cytoplasm. Hemagglutinins and complement-fixing and immunoprecipitating antigens are produced. Infected cells have been found to have prolonged doubling time.

Transmission

Postnatally, the virus may be introduced to those who have no antibodies to rubella from clinically or subclinically infected individuals or from inoculation through vaccination. Viral spread from actively infected individuals occurs through airborne respiratory particles (eg, nasopharyngeal droplets from a cough or sneeze), with spread from those vaccinated less likely to occur.

Once infected, lifelong immunity usually results. However, reinfection may occur in those with low antibody levels, as may be found in those vaccinated. With rare exception, reinfection in a pregnant woman appears to have a significantly lower risk to the fetus than a primary infection.

Once infected, incubation time is 10 to 16 days. It is believed that the virus replicates in upper respiratory mucosa, and then spreads to the lymph nodes where it continues to replicate. The virus is found in the nasopharynx secretions for approximately 2 weeks. Prenatally, the virus is transmitted to the embryo from the infected mother through the placenta. The time during the pregnancy when the viral infection occurs is important, because those developing tissues and organs are affected and damaged. The virus may be found in many tissues, sometimes months after birth.

Course of the Disease

Postnatal rubella infection generally has a benign clinical course. Children generally present with less symptoms than adults, particularly after inoculation with a vaccination. Clinical presentation (Table 61–1) typically includes a maculopapular rash, lymphadenopathy, headache, swollen joints, and a mild fever. Adults may experience arthralgic symptoms. The infection may also manifest subclinically or present with mild symptoms, without a rash. The rash follows viral spread through the blood (viremia), usually 2 to 3 weeks after the infection. The rash presents more frequently with increasing age of infection.

Viral antibodies are found to occur at the same time as the rash. An immunologic mechanism may be related to the appearance of the rash. Antibody titers peak at 7 to 10 days, initially consisting of IgM and IgG. IgM is present for about 1 month after the rash, with IgG present for years. Once infected, the individual usually maintains lifelong immunity.

Complications of postnatal infection include a transient rheumatoid-like arthritis, thrombocytopenic purpura, and rarely encephalitis, necrotizing vasculitis, or neurologic deficit.

The course of congenital rubella is significantly different than that of postnatal infection. The fetus may potentially be affected from maternal infection that occurs during or just prior to pregnancy. Fetal infection may result in spontaneous abortion, stillbirth, malformations, or multiple organ involvement, or may have no significant effect.

The time of the maternal infection influences how the virus affects the developing fetus. A first-trimester infection has the greatest risk to fetal viability and malformation, because the virus influences multiplying and differentiating cells. Fetal malformations may result from prolonged cell doubling time, cell death, continued viral presence, or effect on chromosomes (Rawls, 1972). It is during this time that cardiac, hearing, and psychomotor defects are most likely to occur. Second- and third-trimester infections may have less apparent manifestations. If infection occurs toward the end of the pregnancy, the infant may be born with rubella resembling a postnatal infection.

Unique to congenital rubella is the persistence of the infection. This may be the result of an immune mechanism or continued production of the virus. The virus has been found in various newborn excretions and secretions. Viral

TABLE 61–1. SYSTEMIC MANIFESTATIONS OF RUBELLA

POSTNATAL INFECTION
- Upper respiratory tract inflammation
- Constitutional symptoms: fever, malaise, muscle ache, headache
- Lymphadenopathy
- Viremia
- Rash
    Initially: transient blush
    Maculopapular rash
- Antirubella virus antibodies
- Swollen joints
- Complications
    Rheumatoid-like arthritis, thrombocytopenic purpura
    Rare: encephalitis, necrotizing vasculitis, or
        neurologic deficit

CONGENITAL RUBELLA MANIFESTATIONS
- Cardiac
    Patent ductus arteriosus (with or without stenosis of
        pulmonary artery or its branches)
    Atrial and ventricular defects
    Coarctation of the aorta, aortic stenosis
    Congestive heart failure
    Murmur
    Necrotizing myocarditis
- Hearing loss
    Mild or severe
    Unilateral or bilateral
    Sensory damage
    Impaired vestibular function
- Psychomotor retardation
    Spastic quadriparesis
    Mental retardation
    Focal neurologic deficits and seizures (uncommon)
- Miscellaneous
    Thrombocytopenic purpura
    Long bone lesions—evident on x-ray (transient)
    Expanded rubella syndrome (usually transient):
        hepatosplenomegaly, hepatitis, hemolytic anemia,
        bulging anterior fontanelle, with or without
        pleocytosis
    Bleeding tendencies
    Low birthweight
    CNS: microcephaly, mental disability, impaired
        motor development, neurosensory impairment,
        meningitis, encephalitis
    Pneumonia
    Dental defects
    Cleft palate
    Encephalomyelocele, meningocele
    Esophageal atresia
    Pancreatic insufficiency

isolation occurs in 60 to 80% of infants, during the first month of life, and occasionally in some beyond 1 year.

Systemic manifestations of congenital rubella most commonly include cardiac involvement and loss of hearing. Cardiac involvement may present without symptoms, or

may develop into congestive heart failure within the first months of life, sometimes resulting in death. Hearing loss is sensorineural, probably secondary to damage to the organ of Corti. Central nervous system infection may result in psychomotor retardation (see Table 61–1).

Death in congenital rubella syndrome usually occurs within the first 6 months of life, especially in the first 3 months. Death may result from pneumonia, congestive heart failure, encephalitis, or hepatitis, and sometimes following heart surgery.

■ Ocular

Ocular complications of postnatal rubella are rare; therefore this discussion will be limited to congenital rubella, in which ocular manifestations are common (Table 61–2). These include most classically cataracts and retinopathy, along with microphthalmia, iris changes, and glaucoma. Ocular involvement results from maternal infection that occurs during the first trimester of pregnancy. Each eye may be affected differently because of a slower development or greater viral affect in one eye versus the other.

The susceptibility of the lens to viral infection during the first trimester may be related to a number of developmental factors, such as lack of protection from the virus provided by the eyelid and lens capsule. A cataract results from viral encroachment in the lens. The primary and secondary lens fibers are affected by degeneration, liquefaction, and vacuolization, especially in the equatorial area. This may result in a more oval, spherophakic lens, that is smaller than usual. Although usually a bilateral manifestation, unilateral cataracts may occur (Figure 61–1).

TABLE 61–2. OCULAR MANIFESTATIONS OF CONGENITAL RUBELLA SYNDROME

- Cataract
- Retinopathy
    Pigment changes
    Retinal folds
    Subretinal neovascularization
    Pallor of optic nerve
- Nystagmus (pendular or searching type)
    Associated with cataracts or microphthalmia
- Iris
    Pupil: miotic (thin sphincter), poor dilation (absent
        dilator), poor light reactions
    Iridocyclitis
    Transillumination defects
- Cornea
    Clouding
    Microcornea
- Microphthalmia
    Often associated with cataracts
- Glaucoma

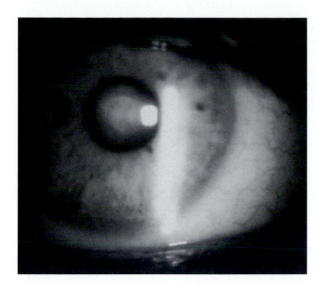

Figure 61–1. Central, white opacified area seen in rubella cataracts. *(Courtesy of Dr. Scott Richter, SUNY, College of Optometry.)*

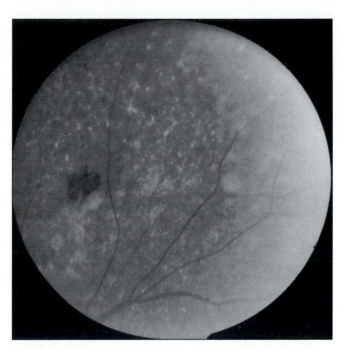

Figure 61–2. Retinal pigmentary variations. *(Courtesy of Dr. Scott Richter, SUNY, College of Optometry.)*

Clinically, the rubella cataract has a central, pearly, white area. A less dense cortical opacity surrounds the nuclear area. The cataract may also present as a more uniformly dense opacity.

The cataract is usually present at birth, and may continue to progress. Decreased vision and nystagmus may result from the cataract. Although rare, the lens may spontaneously absorb, either completely or partially (Boger et al, 1981). The cataract is frequently associated with microphthalmia.

Retinal manifestations in congenital rubella are common. These may occur unilaterally or bilaterally, as hypopigmentation or hyperpigmentation (Figure 61–2). The characteristic appearance is a fine, granular, mottled, pepper-like pigment clumping, of variable size. This can affect any or all parts of the retina, possibly involving a sector, the periphery, or more commonly involving the posterior pole and macula. Generally these retinal changes are not progressive, although rarely the virus may continue to affect the pigment epithelium after birth. In addition, retinal folds may occur, particularly in microphthalmic eyes. Subretinal neovascularization also may develop, with resultant decreased vision. Most commonly, however, visual acuity is unaffected with rubella retinal manifestations. Electrodiagnostic testing including electroretinogram and electrooculogram are unaffected. Based on this, it is suggested that the classic rubella pigment retinopathy affects pigment distribution, rather than its function (Krill, 1972).

Glaucoma can also present in congenital rubella, either at birth or during infancy. It may result from abnormal angle development, secondary to inflammation, pupillary block, or cataract surgery. Glaucoma is usually not associated with cataracts.

Strabismus appears to be the result of other ocular manifestations that occur in congenital rubella, such as cataracts or central nervous system involvement (brain damage). The strabismus is initially an eso or convergent deviation, often intermittent, later possibly becoming exo or divergent. The more severely affected eye deviates.

Microphthalmic eyes result from abnormal development in congenital rubella. Vision is always poor, with an abnormal electroretinogram.

DIAGNOSIS

■ Systemic

Diagnosis of postnatal rubella infection is based on a history of exposure, clinical presentation or methods that detect either the virus or its antibodies. Cultures from pharyngeal secretions may be taken 1 week prior to the rash, and 2 weeks after the rash. Blood cultures may be done 1 week prior to the rash, and are best done 2 days after the rash appears.

Serological testing for rubella antibodies include complement-fixing serum antibody, inhibition of hemagglutination, direct immunofluorescence technique, or immunoprecipitating reaction. Rubella antibodies may be found 2 to 4 days after the rash, and are present throughout life. However, the complement-fixing antibody decreases with time, so it is an effective test for only 1 to 2 years after the infection.

Congenital rubella may be diagnosed based on clinical presentation (eg, heart defect, low birthweight, cataract) or through viral isolation. The virus may be found beyond a year in the infant's throat, cerebrospinal fluid, stool, urine, conjunctiva, and lens. Tissue suspension, culture, and complement-fixation serum antibodies can be used in the diagnosis. A positive complement-fixing serum antibody test in an infant older than 6 months indicates congenital rubella.

Diagnosis of systemic manifestations of congenital rubella are made based on complete physical evaluation. In addition, observing the child for unusual or abnormal behavior may indirectly indicate undetected manifestations, such as hearing loss. This should then prompt further testing, such as audiometry.

■ Ocular

Diagnosis of ocular manifestations of congenital rubella is often based on the overall clinical presentation, associated systemic findings, and specific evaluation of the eye.

Cataracts often present as an obvious dense opacity in the pupil. Differential diagnosis includes retinoblastoma, as well as other causes of congenital leukocoria. History and use of ultrasonography will assist in making the appropriate diagnosis.

Diagnosis of retinal changes secondary to congenital rubella may be difficult, because these changes are often obscured by a cataract. Sometimes retinal changes may be the only manifestation of the infection, making the diagnosis even more difficult. In addition, because these pupils are often difficult to dilate, installation of mydriatics prior to the exam may be necessary in order to maximize dilation. Differential diagnosis of the retinal changes include retinitis pigmentosa, syphilis, Leber congenital amaurosis, and radiation exposure. History, visual acuity, electrodiagnostic testing, and serological testing will assist in differentiating these entities from rubella. Associated hearing loss is also indicative of rubella infection.

Diagnosis of microphthalmia may be difficult, particularly if it is bilateral and not severe. It is made by measuring the horizontal corneal diameter. Normal findings are 10.5 to 11.5 mm, but may be 8 to 10 mm in congenital rubella.

Diagnosis of glaucoma can be elusive. Intraocular pressure is difficult to measure in infants. Other signs of increased IOP (eg, buphthalmos) may not be evident in these eyes because of associated small corneas. When corneal changes are present, (eg, edema and breaks in the Descemet membrane), it may help with the diagnosis, but differentiation from other possible etiologies such as corneal haze from microphthalmos or corneal touch from the lens, must be made. When infantile glaucoma is associated with cerebral palsy and deafness, rubella is usually the underlying etiology.

Observing the child for unusual behavior may indicate an underlying ocular problem. For example, various types of autostimulation have been noted in infants with congenital cataracts, who are trying to stimulate their retinas. These may include oculodigital phenomenon (producing pressure phosphenes, by pressing on the globe) or hand wagging phenomenon (hand waving over the eyes to change light intensity, while looking at a bright light; Roy, 1967).

TREATMENT AND MANAGEMENT

Table 61–3 gives an overview of rubella treatment and management.

■ Systemic

The best management for rubella is prevention of the infection. This may be done with the use of a vaccination. All nonimmune individuals, particularly children (older than 1 year of age) should be vaccinated. However, immunization should be avoided in those with depressed immune status. Nonimmune women should be immunized at least 2 to 3 months before pregnancy. Actively infected individuals should be isolated from pregnant women, particularly during the first trimester. An injection of human gammaglobulin may be considered if exposure during pregnancy occurs,

TABLE 61–3. TREATMENT AND MANAGEMENT OF RUBELLA

■ **SYSTEMIC**
- Vaccination (prevention)
- Postnatal
  Palliative measures
- Congenital
  Gammaglobulin (injection during pregnancy)
  Multidisciplinary care
  Hearing aids
  Special education/rehabilitation
  Counseling

■ **OCULAR (CONGENITAL)**
- Cataract
  Extraction
  Appropriate refractive correction
- Strabismus
  Remove cataract
  Refractive correction
  Vision therapy (eg, occlusion)
  Strabismic surgery (if necessary)
- Glaucoma
  Medical (eg, timolol, carbonic anhydrase
    inhibitor)
  Surgical (eg, goniotomy, filtering,
    cyclocryotherapy)

in order to prevent infection. Results, however, vary as to its effectiveness. Counseling on the potential affects of rubella on the developing fetus and subsequent management options are necessary.

For postnatal infection, treatment is generally palliative, based on symptoms.

For children of congenital rubella syndrome, the potential for multisystem involvement requires multispecialist care. Occasionally cardiac involvement requires surgery. Hearing loss can be managed with hearing aids. In addition, special education or rehabilitation programs for children may need to be considered.

■ Ocular

Treatment and management of ocular manifestations of congenital rubella syndrome is primarily aimed at optimizing and preserving visual function. Cataract extraction is important to improve vision and visual development in the infant. Surgery may be complicated by other ocular manifestations of rubella such as microphthalmia, along with viral persistence. Surgery may be recommended as early as 3 months. Following surgery, appropriate refractive correction is essential. Associated nystagmus may subsequently show improvement.

Strabismus, which is often secondary to the poor image in a cataractous eye, is often corrected after the lens is removed. Appropriate vision therapy including occlusion may subsequently be necessary.

Glaucoma is initially treated with medical therapy. If uncontrolled, consideration for surgery may be necessary.

CONCLUSION

Rubella is a viral infection that can follow a benign course in individuals affected postnatally, or follow a more devastating course in the developing fetus affected by maternal infection. Congenital rubella syndrome classically includes hearing loss and cardiac and ocular involvement. Optimal care includes comanagement of these patients with the appropriate specialists. Ultimately the best treatment for the disease is its prevention. Since the discovery and use of a vaccination in the late 1960s, the potential for rubella epidemics has decreased; however, the threat of the disease to unborns will continue until everyone is immunized.

REFERENCES

Boger WP. Late ocular complications in congenital rubella syndrome. *Ophthalmology*. 1980;87:1244–1252.

Boger WP, Peterson RA, Robb RM. Spontaneous absorption of the lens in the congenital rubella syndrome. *Arch Ophthalmol*. 1981;99:433–434.

Boniuk M. Glaucoma in the congenital rubella syndrome. *Int Ophthalmol Clin*. 1972a;12:121–136.

Boniuk M, Zimmerman LE. Ocular pathology in the rubella syndrome. *Arch Ophthalmol*. 1967;77:455–473.

Boniuk V. Rubella. *Int Ophthalmol Clin*. 1975;15:229–241.

Boniuk V. Systemic and ocular manifestations of the rubella syndrome. *Int Ophthalmol Clin*. 1972b;12:67–76.

Bonomo PP. Involution without disciform scarring of subretinal neovascularization in presumed rubella retinopathy. *Acta Ophthalmol*. 1982;60:141–146.

Calvert DR. The rubella epidemic of 1964. *J Am Optom Assoc*. 1969;40:794–798.

Collis WJ, Cohen DN. Rubella retinopathy. A progressive disorder. *Arch Ophthalmol*. 1970;84:33–35.

Cooper LZ, Krugman S. Clinical manifestations of postnatal and congenital rubella. *Arch Ophthalmol*. 1967;77:434–439.

Fleet WF, Benz EW, Karzon DT, et al. Fetal consequences of maternal rubella immunization. *JAMA*. 1974;227:621–627.

Geltzer AI, Guber D, Sears ML. Ocular manifestations of the 1964-65 rubella epidemic. *Am J Ophthalmol*. 1967;63:221–229.

Gregg NM. Further observations on congenital defects in infants following maternal rubella. *Trans Ophthalmol Soc Aust*. 1944;4:119–130.

Gregg NM. Congenital cataract following german measles in the mother. *Trans Ophthalmol Soc Aust*. 1941;3:35–46.

Hertzberg R. Congenital cataract following german measles in the mother. *Aust NZ J Ophthalmol*. 1985;13:303–309.

Hertzberg R. Twenty-five year follow-up of ocular defects in congenital rubella. *Am J Ophthalmol*. 1968;66:269–271.

Krill AE. Retinopathy secondary to rubella. *Int Ophthalmol Clin*. 1972;12:89–103.

Krugman S, Katz SL. Rubella immunization: A five year progress report. *N Engl J Med*. 1974;290:1375–1376.

Murphy AM, Reid RR, Pollard I, et al. Rubella cataracts. Further clinical and virologic observations. *Am J Ophthalmol*. 1967;64:1109–1119.

O'Neill JF. Strabismus in rubella syndrome. *Int Ophthalmol Clin*. 1972;12:111–120.

O'Neill JF. Strabismus in congenital rubella. *Arch Ophthalmol*. 1967;77:450–454.

Orth DH, Fishman GA, Segall M, et al. Rubella maculopathy. *Br J Ophthalmol*. 1980;64:201–205.

Rawls WE. Virology and epidemiology of rubella virus. *Int Ophthalmol Clin*. 1972;12:21–66.

Romano A, Weinberg M, Bar-Izhak R, et al. Rate and various aspects of eye infection resulting from congenital rubella. *J Pediatric Ophthalmol Strabismus*. 1979;16:26–30.

Roy FH. Microsurgery of congenital rubella cataract. *Am J Ophthalmol*. 1968;65:81–90.

Roy FH. Ocular autostimulation. *Am J Ophthalmol*. 1967;63:1776–1777.

Roy FH, Fuste F, Hiatt RL, et al. The congenital rubella syndrome with virus recovery. *Am J Ophthalmol*. 1966;62:222–232.

Roy FH, Hiatt RL, Korones SB, Roane J. Ocular manifestations of congenital rubella syndrome. *Arch Ophthalmol*. 1966;75:601–607.

Roy FH, Deutsch AR. The congenital rubella syndrome. *Am J Ophthalmol*. 1966;62:236–238.

Rudolph AJ, Desmond MM. Clinical manifestations of the congenital rubella syndrome. *Int Ophthalmol Clin*. 1972;12:3–19.

Scheie HG, Schaeffer DB, Plotkin SA, Kertesz ED. Congenital rubella cataracts. Surgical results and virus recovery from intraocular tissue. *Arch Ophthalmol*. 1967;77:440–444.

Sears ML. Congenital glaucoma in neonatal rubella. *Br J Ophthalmol*. 1967;51:744–748.

Slusher MM, Tyler ME. Rubella retinopathy and subretinal neovascularization. *Ann Ophthalmol*. 1982;14:292-294.

Tate HR. Congenital rubella syndrome. *Eye, Ear, Nose Throat Month*. 1969;48:33–41

Weiss DI, Ziring PR, Cooper LZ. Surgery of the rubella cataract. *Am J Ophthalmol*. 1972;73:326–332.

62
Chapter

Histoplasmosis

Taryn Mathews

Histoplasmosis is a systemic disease caused by the fungus *Histoplasma capsulatum*. Although infection occurs throughout the world, it is endemic to the United States, particularly in the Ohio and Mississippi River valley regions. It is acquired by inhalation of fungal spores. The primary focus of infection is the lungs, but the fungus can also disseminate to other organs throughout the body, particularly the liver, spleen, and lymph nodes. Depending on the immune status of the patient, the disease manifests in a variety of ways, ranging from a benign, asymptomatic infection to a fatal disseminated disease.

The presumed ocular histoplasmosis syndrome (POHS) is a granulomatous choroiditis believed to result from dissemination of the fungus via the bloodstream during the primary systemic infection. It is characterized and diagnosed by the clinical presentation of peripapillary choroiditis, peripheral atrophic lesions, and exudative maculopathy. Although clinical and epidemiologic studies support *H. capsulatum* as the cause of the ocular syndrome, diagnosis remains presumptive until the organism is definitively isolated.

EPIDEMIOLOGY

■ Systemic

Systemic histoplasmosis occurs throughout the world, particularly in temperate and tropical areas. It is most frequently found in the river valleys of the central eastern United States. It is estimated that 50 million people in the United States have been infected. In highly endemic regions, over 80% of the population reacts positively to the histoplasmin skin test. However, the actual prevalence of infection is not known, because the skin test can become negative as a person ages.

Systemic histoplasmosis affects all age groups, but it is most prevalent at the extremes of life. Incidences of positive skin tests are the same for males and females, but the clinical disease is more common in adult men. Caucasians and African-Americans have equal rates of positive skin tests; however, the clinical disease is more common in Caucasians.

■ Ocular

The geographic distribution of POHS is consistent with the distribution of the systemic disease. This prevalence of POHS in endemic areas helps to substantiate the possible role of *H. capsulatum* in the syndrome.

POHS has been seen in patients ranging in age from 7 to 77 years, with most cases occurring from 20 to 50 years of age. Initial infection resulting in peripheral atrophic scars is believed to occur in childhood or early adulthood. About 70% of POHS patients have peripapillary changes. Macular manifestations normally occur 10 to 30 years after infection, with maculopathy most commonly seen in the fourth decade.

Macular involvement in POHS is more common in Caucasians than African-Americans by a ratio of 6 to 1. However, the frequency of peripheral histo spots is equal for the two races. Maculopathy, particularly bilateral, along with a greater sensitivity to histoplasmin are more often found in men than women.

In endemic regions, up to 12% of adults have peripheral histo scars and 1 per 1000 adults is afflicted with maculopathy. Bilateral peripheral scars are present in 52% of patients with macular involvement. It is estimated that both maculas are involved in 10% of the patients. The average amount of time before the second macula becomes affected is 4.8 years. The incidence of pulmonary calcification on x-ray increases from 12.5 to 80% when patients have maculopathy as opposed to peripheral scars without macular involvement.

NATURAL HISTORY

■ Systemic

The Organism

Histoplasma capsulatum is a dimorphic fungus, meaning that it exists as both a mold and yeast. At room temperature (23°C) and in its natural habitat, it exists as a mold. However, at 35 to 37°C and in vivo, it exists as the unicellular yeast. Its natural habitat is rich, moist, surface soil. Growth requirements, such as organic nitrogen, explain the high concentration of histoplasmosis in areas infested with the fecal material of birds and bats. Epidemics of histoplasmosis occur following the disturbance of areas where birds have roosted and in caves inhabited by bats.

Transmission

When contaminated soil is disturbed, the spores are released into the environment. Human infection only occurs when the tiny aerosolized spores are inhaled into the distal air spaces of the lung. In the alveoli, spores convert to the yeast form, the pathogenic form of *H. capsulatum*. Histoplasmosis is not contagious; transmission only occurs through inhalation of *H. capsulatum* spores.

Course of the Disease

The yeast cells proliferate in the lung parenchyma by budding or fission. The initial response by the lung tissue is the infiltration of polymorphonuclear leukocytes (PMNs). The PMNs are rapidly followed by the accumulation of macrophages, which phagocytize the yeasts. The yeasts then undergo an intense multiplication inside the macrophages, which results in the production of a pneumonitis. The yeast-laden macrophages are spread, via the lymphatics, to the regional hilar lymph nodes. From the lymph nodes, the fungus enters the circulation and is spread throughout the body, particularly to the liver and spleen.

Two to three weeks after the initial infection, a lymphocyte cellular immune response develops at the primary and metastatic infection sites. An intense inflammatory reaction occurs, followed by granuloma formation, caseation necrosis, and fibrotic encapsulation. Months to years later, the necrotic foci may undergo calcification. The healed encapsulated foci of infection are called histoplasmomas. Often, it is difficult to distinguish them from carcinoma, and in the past they were believed to be secondary to tuberculosis.

Prior to the histoplasmin skin test, histoplasmosis was considered to be a rare, fatal disease, and its detection occurred primarily at autopsies. The combination of positive histoplasmin skin test reactions, pulmonary calcifications, and negative tuberculin skin tests revealed histoplasmosis to be a common disease, particularly in an asymptomatic, benign form.

Benign Histoplasmosis

More than 90% of the infections in normal hosts caused by *H. capsulatum* are benign, asymptomatic, and resolve without treatment. Because these patients do not seek medical care, they are discovered inadvertently by a positive reaction to the histoplasmin skin test or by the presence of calcified lesions on a routine chest x-ray. However, when the lesions heal without the formation of fibrosis or calcification, the chest radiograph is normal. Asymptomatic reinfection may occur. It is believed that the POHS develops in people that have the benign form of the systemic disease. The remaining 5 to 10% of patients with symptomatic infection fall into three categories: primary acute histoplasmosis, disseminated histoplasmosis, and chronic pulmonary histoplasmosis (Table 62–1).

Primary Acute Histoplasmosis

Primary acute symptomatic histoplasmosis is uncommon and usually occurs in infants and children, possibly secondary to their immature immune systems. Three to 14 days after their initial exposure, these individuals present with a respiratory illness similar to the presentation of influenza, with varying severity. When the chest x-ray is abnormal, it shows one or more soft pulmonary infiltrates and enlargement of the hilar and mediastinal lymph nodes. In the acute form of histoplasmosis, it is common for the infection to spread without complication to extrapulmonary sites such as the liver, spleen, and lymph nodes.

A primary acute histoplasmosis infection usually resolves with no residual effects in 2 weeks to 3 months. Complete recovery without therapeutic intervention usually occurs, even when the patient appears to be very ill. During the illness, the histoplasmin skin test becomes positive. The lesions in the lungs, lymph nodes, and extrapulmonary organs can resolve completely, but they often calcify 6 months to several years after the symptomatic infection.

Although the acute form is usually benign, a severe pulmonary illness can occur in individuals who have inhaled a massive number of spores. These patients present with diffuse infiltrates, dyspnea, hypoxia, and acute respiratory distress. Early diagnosis and treatment are necessary to prevent death from respiratory insufficiency.

TABLE 62–1. SYSTEMIC MANIFESTATIONS OF HISTOPLASMOSIS

SIGNS
- Benign systemic histoplasmosis
  Chest x-ray may be (+) or (–) for pulmonary calcification
- Primary acute histoplasmosis
  Pulmonary infiltration, calcification, cavitation
  Enlargement and calcification of lymph nodes, liver, spleen
- Disseminated histoplasmosis
  Pulmonary infiltration, calcification, cavitation
  Enlargement and calcification of lymph nodes, liver, spleen
  Adrenal gland insufficiency
  Anemia, leukopenia, thrombocytopenia,
  Ulcerations of the mouth, tongue, nose, larynx, intestines
- Chronic pulmonary histoplasmosis
  Cavitation, histoplasmomas, bronchiectasis

SYMPTOMS
- Benign systemic histoplasmosis
  None
- Primary acute histoplasmosis
  Fever, chills, dry cough, malaise, myalgia, arthralgia, headache
- Disseminated histoplasmosis
  Fever, cough, chills, malaise, headache, diarrhea, weight loss, dyspnea
- Chronic pulmonary histoplasmosis
  Weight loss, fever, chronic cough, chest pain

Disseminated Histoplasmosis

In disseminated histoplasmosis the T-cell immune response is weak or absent, and so the parasitic intracellular yeasts cannot be killed. The fungus undergoes extensive and uncontrolled multiplication inside the macrophages of the reticuloendothelial system. As the yeast continues to grow in multiple organs, additional macrophages are necessary to contain the organisms. The failure of the cell-mediated immune response results in a severe disseminated systemic illness.

Disseminated histoplasmosis can occur at any age, but usually affects young infants and the aged. In adults, disseminated histoplasmosis is a complication of immunosuppressive conditions such as underlying diseases, chemotherapy for hematologic malignancies, glucocorticoid therapy, therapy for organ transplant recipients, and acquired immunodeficiency syndrome. Some patients become ill when immunosuppressive therapy is initiated. This suggests that dormant *H. capsulatum* organisms within the body become active when the immune system falters.

Patients with disseminated histoplasmosis experience fever, cough, chills, malaise, headache, diarrhea, weight loss, and dyspnea. The widespread dissemination throughout the body has an effect on many organs. The uncontrolled growth of the fungus places extraordinary demands on the phagocyte system. The resulting suppression of the bone marrow causes anemia, leukopenia, and thrombocytopenia. Pulmonary involvement is variable, but the most common presentation on the x-ray is diffuse interstitial infiltrates. Many of these patients have adrenal gland involvement; approximately 20% go on to develop Addison disease. Other findings include hepatosplenomegaly, lymphadenopathy, and ulcerations of the mouth, tongue, nose, larynx, and intestines. On rare occasions there is the presentation of chronic meningitis and endocarditis.

In addition to the disseminated form of histoplasmosis seen in infants and immunosuppressed patients, there is a chronic disseminated form that is found in healthy adults. These patients appear to have normal T-cell function. One explanation speculates that the development of this chronic form results from a temporary suppression of immunity secondary to an underlying viral infection. The clinical presentation of the two disseminated forms is similar. Both presentations of the disseminated disease can be devastating, but the chronic form tends to run a slower course.

If antifungal therapy is not instituted, up to 80% of patients suffering from disseminated histoplasmosis die. About 50% of the patients have negative skin tests. If left untreated, patients die within 4 to 10 months. Adrenal insufficiency is believed to be the most common cause of death in the disseminated form of the disease.

Chronic Pulmonary Histoplasmosis

Chronic pulmonary histoplasmosis results from the infection of lung tissue that has already been compromised by another disease process such as chronic obstructive pulmonary disease in older Caucasian males. Radiography shows the formation of histoplasmomas, cavitation (the formation of cavities), and bronchiectasis (dilation of the bronchial tubes). Symptoms associated with this form are weight loss, fever, chronic cough, and chest pain. The infection may resolve over a period of 1 to 3 months. Some patients suffer with progression of the disease, but it is difficult to separate the effects of histoplasmosis from the coexisting pulmonary disease.

◼ Ocular

In 1959, Woods and Wahlen described presumed ocular histoplasmosis syndrome (POHS) as the clinical triad of circumpapillary choroiditis, peripheral atrophic chorioretinal scars (histo spots), and exudative maculopathy. The syndrome is also characterized by clear media and linear streak lesions (Table 62–2). The typical patient is healthy, resides in an area endemic for histoplasmosis, and ranges in age from 20 to 50 years.

When *H. capsulatum* is disseminated throughout the body via the bloodstream, it is believed that the fungus

TABLE 62–2. OCULAR MANIFESTATIONS OF HISTOPLASMOSIS

SIGNS
- Circumpapillary choroiditis
- Peripheral atrophic choroidal scars (histo spots)
- Exudative maculopathy
- No inflammatory reaction (no cells or flare)
- Linear streak lesions

SYMPTOMS
- Decreased VA
- Metamorphopsia
- Photopsia

STAGES OF MACULOPATHY
- Stage 1: Macular yellow-white lesion of active choroiditis
- Stage 2: Neovascularization, macular pigment ring with overlying sensory retinal detachment
- Stage 3: Subretinal or subretinal pigment epithelial hemorrhage from the neovascular net
- Stage 4: White, edematous lipid exudates around area of serous detachment
- Stage 5: White elevated scar

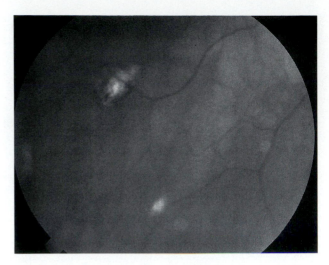

Figure 62–1. Peripheral atrophic histo spots. *(Courtesy of the Optometry Service, FDR VA Hospital, Montrose, NY.)*

enters the choroid through the choroidal vessels. The resulting POHS usually occurs after the benign form of the systemic disease. After becoming entrapped in the choroid, it is hypothesized that the fungus replicates during a period of transient immunosuppression. The clinical picture of this process is focal areas of chorioretinitis resulting in the formation of a granulomatous mass. The presence or absence of symptoms will depend on whether these areas are located in the macula or the peripheral retina, respectively.

With the emergence of the lymphocytic immune response, the focal chorioretinitis begins to resolve as the fungal organisms are killed and healing takes place over a few weeks. During the inflammatory and healing processes, breaks may occur in the Bruch membrane, and there is atrophy and metaplasia of the surrounding retinal pigment epithelium (RPE), giving rise to the classic "histo spots." The disruption of the Bruch membrane and RPE is a precursor for the development of a subretinal neovascular membrane, particularly in the macula.

Peripheral Atrophic Chorioretinal Scars

The peripheral atrophic histo spots are healed lesions most often found posterior to the equator, away from the macula (Figure 62–1). The number of scars per eye varies from 0 to 70. The spots are typically 0.2 to 0.7 DD in size, yellow-orange in color, bilateral, and depigmented. When pigment is present, it occurs in clumps at the borders of the histo spots. When the histo spots are outside of the disc and macular regions, visual loss does not occur. These lesions usually heal

without neovascularization. The presence of inflammatory cells in the choroid and evidence of spots changing or disappearing suggest that these histo spots may be active. The random distribution of the histo spots in both eyes in areas of the fundus with greater blood supply supports the hypothesis of the fungus reaching the choroid through the bloodstream.

Peripapillary Choroiditis

The choroiditis surrounding the disc is important for making the diagnosis of POHS. These scars are in the choroid and RPE, and the degree of involvement of these two areas is variable. The area involved can have a diffuse and/or nodular appearance extending from 0.125 to 0.5 DD from the disc. At the level of the RPE there is a pigment line located at the inside border of the area of peripapillary depigmentation. The outer margin has an irregular and indistinct appearance (Figure 62–2).

In most cases, the peripapillary changes are inactive and the patient is usually asymptomatic. However, these changes will always cause an increase in the blind spot on visual field testing. Ten percent of POHS patients become symptomatic when the scars around the disc become activated. Activation involves disruption of the RPE and Bruch membrane with subsequent neovascularization and possible hemorrhage. Hemorrhage leads to detachment of the sensory retina and/or the RPE, which can extend from the disc out to the macula. Visual prognosis is poor in patients that develop a hemorrhage. If left untreated, about half of these patients will become legally blind.

Maculopathy

The development of maculopathy (see Figure 62–2) occurs 10 to 30 years after the peripheral histo spots have formed

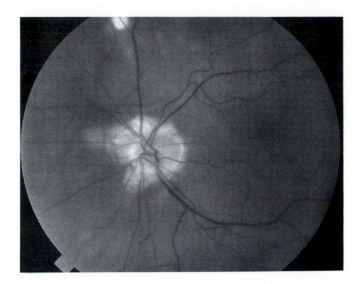

Figure 62–2. Peripapillary RPE changes secondary to histoplasmosis. *(Courtesy of the Optometry Service, FDR VA Hospital, Montrose, NY.)*

and healed. There have been a number of speculations to explain this reactivation process. Because macular lesions usually originate from areas of previous scarring, vascular decompensation may be the mechanism of reactivation. Another possibility is that the unique structure of the macular region predisposes the area to neovascularization. An immunologic mechanism is a more likely etiology, because lymphocytes have been found to persist in the choroid many years after the primary active disease. It is hypothesized that these T lymphocytes remain sensitized from the primary infection. When the antigen or part of the antigen is reintroduced to the choroid, either from active foci in the body or from an outside source, the sensitized T cells react and an inflammatory reaction results.

The problem with the immunologic explanation is that no organism has ever been found in the choroid or retina of patients with the POHS. Yet patients with the benign form of systemic histoplasmosis are found to have old dead organisms in the granulomatous lesions in their lungs. The reason for the difference is not known. One hypothesis is the pathogenesis of the ocular lesions is different from that of the lung lesions. When granulomas form in the lung, the fibrotic scar tissue encapsulates the dead fungal organisms. In the eye, the scarring process in POHS does not result in the Histoplasma organisms being walled off in the lesions. Researchers continue to search for the fungus in the ocular lesions.

It is involvement of the macula, particularly the fovea, that causes ocular symptoms. The patient is usually not aware of the histo spots in the periphery. It is believed that the maculopathy does not occur until after the peripheral histo lesions have become atrophic. The patient presents

with symptoms of decreased visual acuity, metamorphopsia, and photopsia. Often, the symptoms of a developing lesion precede the ophthalmoscopic signs.

The maculopathy of POHS passes through a number of stages. In the first stage, there is a yellow-white spot, which represents an area of active choroiditis. The lesion may stabilize, but usually progresses to the later stages, eventually resulting in exudative macular disease.

In this early, mild stage, the choroiditis is most often due to the activation of an old histo scar. A granulomatous mass forms in the choroid with overlying disruption of the Bruch membrane and depigmentation of the RPE. These early lesions often have the following characteristics: locations near the macular periphery; completely flat, fuzzy white borders, less than 1 DD in size; and a window defect without leakage or late staining on fluorescein angiography. On rare occasions, these histo spots may become elevated with an underlying neovascular net and/or enlarge laterally.

The main feature in the second stage of maculopathy is a pigment ring in the macula with an overlying sensory retina detachment. The inflammatory process in the choroid causes a hole in the Bruch membrane and the pigment epithelium. This hole allows the ingrowth of neovascularization from the choroid. The pigment ring represents hyperpigmentation of the RPE in its attempt to stop the growth of the neovascular net. When the choroiditis does not produce a hole, a gray nodule may form. This nodule is believed to be a localized area of RPE detachment that later converts to a pigment ring.

Blood vessel growth starts inside the pigment ring and then radiates outward in a sea fan fashion under the sensory retina or in the subpigment epithelial space. It is difficult to determine if the vessels lie under the sensory retina or RPE, because the RPE is usually depigmented from the choroiditis.

The combination of blood vessel growth and leakage causes the sensory retina to elevate and detach. Because the bond between the sensory retina and RPE is weak, the area of sensory retina detachment is usually much greater than the original area of choroiditis and RPE detachment. The size of the detachment corresponds to the size of the scotoma. This stage is similar to stage one in that it can stop or undergo regression.

Stage three of POHS maculopathy consists of subretinal or subretinal pigment epithelial hemorrhage from the neovascular net. When the sensory retinal detachment is extensive, the underlying hemorrhage is difficult to view even on fluorescein angiography.

Stage three progresses to stage four maculopathy with the addition of white edematous residues such as lipid exudates around the area of serous detachment. The hemorrhaging and accumulation of exudates recur and persist for 2 years or longer. Finally, in stage five, there is a white elevated scar. The size of the scar ranges from 0.33 to 1 DD. The scar can be atrophic, fibrous, or microcystic (Figure 62–3). Microcystic degeneration occurs when there is chronic sensory retina detachment with minimal hemorrhage. Fibrosis of the scar develops when there has been a great deal of blood under the retina.

Other Manifestations

An important part of the clinical presentation of POHS is lack of an inflammatory reaction in the aqueous or vitreous. If cells are seen in the anterior chamber or the vitreous, then the diagnosis is not POHS and another cause should be considered, such as inflammatory pseudohistoplasmosis syndrome. Here, patients present with the triad of signs classic for POHS along with inflammatory cells in the ocular media. Although the cause of this syndrome is not known, it is believed to be the manifestation of inflammatory ocular diseases caused by sarcoidosis, tuberculosis, or syphilis.

Another sign that occurs in approximately 5% of POHS patients is linear streak lesions. They usually run parallel to the ora serrata at the equator in both eyes. All four quadrants can be affected. Their length varies from half a clock hour to 11 clock hours. The degree of pigmentation is variable, but most are completely depigmented. Often, large choroidal vessels can be seen running perpendicular to these streaks. These streaks seem to be the result of loss of choriocapillaris and RPE. Many believe that they are simply a linear aggregation of peripheral histo spots. The differential diagnosis includes lattice degeneration.

Prognosis

Visual prognosis depends on the degree of macular involvement, frequency of recurrent macular detachment, and duration of detachment. The most important factor is the distance of the neovascular membrane from the fovea. The prognosis is good when the choroidal neovascular membrane is located greater than 1 DD from the foveal center, even with a macular detachment. On rare occasions, a patient with foveal involvement will spontaneously recover with good acuity. Patients with sensory retina detachments and choroidal neovascular membranes outside the foveal avascular zone have a 60 to 70% chance of retaining 20/40 vision or better. If the neovascularization is inside the foveal avascular zone, the chance of good vision is 15% or less. Without treatment, approximately 59% of patients become legally blind.

Studies have shown that histo spots are not static; they change in size, shape, and density. A patient with scars in the macula has a one in four chance of developing problems over the next 3 years. If the macula is unaffected, the chance of developing visual symptoms is reduced to one in fifty.

If a patient has symptomatic macular involvement in one eye, the fellow eye has a 20 to 30% chance of developing symptoms. The risk of developing symptoms in the second

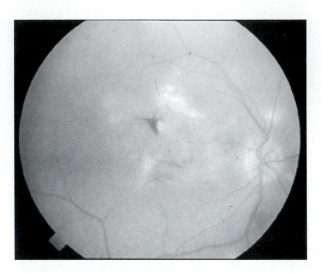

Figure 62–3. Macular scarring in histoplasmosis. (*Courtesy of the Optometry Service, FDR VA Hospital, Montrose, NY.*)

eye increases if the patient has circumpapillary and macular scars. Some patients report an improvement in acuity in the first eye when the second eye becomes symptomatic.

The relationship between the systemic and ocular forms of histoplasmosis is uncertain. Exposure to the fungus rarely results in visual loss. The classic ocular syndrome only seems to occur in the benign form of the disease. It is hypothesized that certain individuals are predisposed or genetically susceptible to the visual syndrome. Support can be found in studies that have shown that patients with the POHS are more likely to have the HLA-B7 and HLA-DRw2 antigens.

DIAGNOSIS

■ Systemic

Making the diagnosis of systemic histoplasmosis begins with a careful and thorough history. If the patient presents with a respiratory infection, histoplasmosis should be considered as a cause, particularly in patients who live or have lived in an endemic region. If histoplasmosis is suspected, questions should be directed at determining if the patient has been exposed to the fungus, particularly at potential exposure sites such as chicken coops, caves inhabited by bats, storm cellars, gardens, and construction sites. Often diagnosis is difficult because histoplasmosis can mimic tuberculosis, influenza, sarcoidosis, and other fungal infections. In addition, it is important to consider that histoplasmosis can coexist with other infections.

A definitive diagnosis of histoplasmosis is made when the fungus is isolated by culture or histology. Culturing is the preferred method, because direct examination of the fungus is difficult due to its small size and intracellular location. Smears of bone marrow and blood may also be useful for diagnosing patients with disseminated disease. If body secretions do not reveal the fungus, then the visceral organs involved should be biopsied.

Obtaining the results of a culture can take from 5 days to 6 weeks because *H. capsulatum* is a slow-growing organism. The culture time lessens as the number of organisms in the specimen increases.

The histoplasmin skin test cannot be used to diagnose histoplasmosis, with two exceptions. The first is in a young infant with active infection, and the second is in a previously known negative skin reactor who tests positive after a recent exposure to the fungus. In all other cases, a positive skin test simply indicates that at some time in the patient's life, infection with the fungus occurred. It provides no information concerning age or activity of the disease. In endemic areas, up to 90% of the population tests positive to histoplasmin. In addition, a negative skin test occurs in many patients with disseminated histoplasmosis due to their weakened immune systems. Despite its limitations in diagnosing histoplasmosis, the histoplasmin skin test has been and continues to be invaluable in epidemiologic studies of the disease.

Because isolation of the fungus by culture is slow and a positive skin test is not diagnostic, serologic tests are helpful in making a presumptive diagnosis. The serologic tests most commonly used for histoplasmosis are the complement-fixation test, immunodiffusion, and radioimmunoassay. The complement-fixation test is considered to be more specific than the others, and some consider it to be the best serologic test. However, it is negative in 30% of patients with acute histoplasmosis and in approximately 50% of patients with disseminated disease. In addition, a previously performed histoplasmin skin test can induce antibody production, resulting in a false-positive result on the complement-fixation test. The immunodiffusion test is not as sensitive as the complement-fixation test and is negative in up to 50% of patients with acute histoplasmosis. Radioimmunoassay is the most sensitive test, which makes it very useful in screening for histoplasmosis.

Unfortunately, all of the serologic tests have limited usefulness in diagnosing histoplasmosis because of the large number of false negatives and false positives. Another disadvantage is the 2- to 3-week wait for test results. Patients with the acute form of the disease often show signs of recovery before the test results are known, and severely ill patients require immediate therapy.

Another important diagnostic tool is an x-ray examination. The classic x-ray picture of healed histoplasmosis is multiple calcified foci in both lungs. These lesions can be distinguished from those caused by tuberculosis because they are larger in size. These pulmonary foci are often found during routine examination in patients who are totally asymptomatic.

Patients who are under 30 years of age and nonsmokers should be monitored with repeat chest films every 3 to 6 months. Histoplasmomas and cavitations may require more invasive procedures to confirm the diagnosis and to rule out carcinoma and tuberculosis.

■ Ocular

The diagnosis of ocular histoplasmosis is presumptive, because *H. capsulatum* has never been definitively identified in the eye of a patient with the POHS. There have been a handful of cases in which the investigators claim to have isolated the organism, but none of these cases have been substantiated. The diagnosis is made mainly by finding the classic clinical presentation of the syndrome.

When Woods and Wahlen (1959) described the clinical syndrome, they established criteria for a diagnosis of POHS. Their findings were categorized based on those patients who were most likely to have a choroiditis due to histoplasmosis, to those least likely to be associated with the disease. In addition to the classic fundoscopic findings, the diagnostic criteria include clear media, a positive histoplasmin skin test, pulmonary calcifications on the x-ray, and a negative tuberculin reaction.

Because the clinical picture of POHS is so typical, the other tests are more useful in establishing past exposure to the fungus rather than in making a diagnosis. As with systemic histoplasmosis, the histoplasmin skin test is not very useful because the majority of the endemic population tests positive. Negative reactions do occur in patients with the syndrome, and no relationship between skin sensitivity and chorioretinitis has actually been established. Also, the test causes 7% of the patients to suffer a recurrence of their maculopathy.

The differential diagnosis includes other causes of inflammatory disease of the fundus such as toxoplasmosis, syphilis, sarcoidosis, toxocariasis, multifocal choroiditis, and vitiliginous chorioretinitis. Noninflammatory conditions such as myopic degeneration, drusen of the optic disc, and angioid streaks can also mimic ocular histoplasmosis. When the syndrome is found in patients who reside in nonendemic regions and have negative skin tests, other causative organisms should be considered.

TREATMENT AND MANAGEMENT

■ Systemic

The treatment regimen for systemic histoplasmosis (Table 62–3) depends on the form of the disease and the status of the patient's immune system. When antifungal therapy is required, amphotericin B is the primary antifungal drug. Amphotericin B is a polyene antibiotic that binds to the cell membrane and disrupts the cell's metabolic activity. It is administered intravenously and is very toxic. Because

TABLE 62–3. TREATMENT AND MANAGEMENT OF HISTOPLASMOSIS

■ **SYSTEMIC**
- Antifungal drugs: amphotericin B, ketoconazole, itraconazole
- Corticosteroids
- Pulmonary surgery (rare)

■ **OCULAR**
- Patient monitoring: home Amsler grid
- Avoidance of stress, aspirin, and the Valsalva maneuver
- Corticosteroids when indicated
   200 mg/d for 2–3 weeks in divided dosages, then in single dose every other day at breakfast; taper gradually
- Fluorescein angiogram
   Performed (when neovascular net is suspected) less than 72 hours prior to laser treatment and within 2 weeks after treatment
- Laser photocoagulation
   Of neovascular membranes 200 μm or more from foveal center
- Surgical removal of subfoveal neovascular nets
   Experimental

human and fungal cytoplasmic membranes are similar, antifungal drugs that act on these membranes can cause toxicity in humans. Side effects include hypotension, thrombophlebitis, chills, fever, nausea, anemia, and nephrotoxicity. Because amphotericin B has severe adverse effects, ketoconazole is considered by some to be the preferred drug because of its effectiveness with less toxicity. Ketoconazole is an oral imidazole that can cause nausea, vomiting, liver dysfunction, and abnormal synthesis of steroids. A promising third drug, itraconazole, is currently under investigation. To reduce inflammation, corticosteroids may be administered in conjunction with the antifungal drugs.

Because the vast majority of acute pulmonary histoplasmosis infections are benign and resolve without complications, treatment is usually not indicated. Patients with the severe life-threatening form of acute histoplasmosis require antifungal therapy with amphotericin B. Disseminated histoplasmosis also requires aggressive antifungal therapy, because without medication, this form of the disease is fatal. With treatment, mortality is reduced from 85% to 15%. Chronic pulmonary histoplasmosis responds well to both amphotericin B and ketoconazole. On rare occasions, surgery is required for cavitations and lesions indistinguishable from pulmonary carcinoma. About half of the patients with AIDS relapse after treatment. Investigators have found that immunosuppressed patients respond well to a maintenance dose of amphotericin B.

■ **Ocular**
It is essential that ocular management (see Table 62–3) includes daily monitoring with an Amsler grid, because the patient often notices changes in vision prior to the appearance of ophthalmoscopic signs. Emotional or physical stress, aspirin, and the Valsalva maneuver should be avoided because they may reactivate or aggravate maculopathy.

Medical therapy, particularly the antifungal agents discussed in the treatment of symptomatic systemic histoplasmosis, has been found to be ineffective in the treatment of POHS. The use of oral and periocular corticosteroids is controversial, but patients often report improved vision after being treated with them. The main concern is determining if the benefits from steroid treatment outweigh the potential risks and side effects.

The infiltration of T lymphocytes to combat the choroiditis of POHS has been hypothesized. Steroids indirectly interfere with the T lymphocyte immune reaction by adversely affecting the ability of macrophages to phagocytize and process antigens. In addition, by reducing the permeability of capillaries, steroids decrease leakage from the choroidal neovascular net. In suppressing the inflammatory reaction, corticosteroids possibly prevent the progression to the destructive later stages of maculopathy.

Because steroid therapy suppresses the inflammatory reaction before the macula is severely damaged, patients are instructed to take prednisone immediately after noticing a change in vision. Once patients learn to properly assess their symptoms, they are quite reliable in determining a recurrence of macular involvement and usually can be trusted to initiate their own therapy.

Oral and periocular steroids can be given separately or simultaneously. Because patient reaction to steroids varies, it is advantageous to administer tablets and injections at the same time. This allows the determination of the best route according to the patient's experience. If the patient is compliant, tablets are the preferred route, because they are easy to take and are less costly. Advantages of steroid injection include placing the drug directly at the site of inflammation, uniocular treatment, and avoidance of most systemic effects.

The clinical presentation of each individual patient will determine the recommended dosage, tapering regimen, and duration of treatment. An initial choroiditis is believed to be active for 8 weeks. If choroidal neovascularization has developed, treatment may be required for 2 years. The patient will require close monitoring for the potential development of increased intraocular pressure and posterior subcapsular cataracts from long-term corticosteroid use.

If the patient does not improve or worsens on corticosteroid therapy after 2 to 3 weeks of treatment, then photocoagulation should be considered. Laser treatment is used to prevent further visual loss and to maintain and prolong the vision that remains. Vision may be worse after treatment, and even when treatment is successful, the visual field defect will be larger. Because the underlying disease process still exists, recurrences of choroidal neovascularization can occur after laser therapy.

A thorough examination should be performed to aid in the preparation and planning of the laser treatment. Tests of particular importance are the Amsler grid, a visual field, and fluorescein angiography. Because a neovascular net can change and grow rapidly, the fluorescein must be performed less than 72 hours before treatment. In fact, it is best to do the fluorescein angiogram on the day of treatment, using it as a guide to make certain that the entire choroidal neovascular net is localized and destroyed.

The goal of photocoagulation is to aggressively and completely ablate the entire neovascular net without damaging the fovea. The use of partial photocoagulation is controversial. However, the overriding consensus is that it is contraindicated, because it may stimulate the remaining net to grow. To ensure that the entire area is obliterated, the laser burns are applied 100 to 150 μm beyond the border of the choroidal neovascularization.

Inactive histo lesions are not prophylactically treated, because treatment can result in activation and histo spots can disappear on their own. In some cases, laser is used in conjunction with corticosteroids. Studies have shown that when active maculopathy is left untreated, 59% of the eyes have 20/200 vision or worse results. The effectiveness of argon laser photocoagulation of choroidal neovascular membranes 200 μm or more from the foveal center has been proven by the Macular Photocoagulation Study. Lasering of neovascularization inside the foveal avascular zone is not recommended, because the resulting visual acuity is poor with or without therapy.

Both the blue-green argon laser and the red krypton laser have been shown to be effective in destroying the choroidal neovascular net in the POHS. It has been determined that the argon laser should be used on neovascularization that is greater than 0.25 DD away from the fovea. The blue-green laser is more damaging as it is absorbed by macular pigment and blood; the krypton laser is therefore preferred for treating areas less than 0.25 DD from the fovea. The red wavelength penetrates deeper to destroy the underlying neovascular membrane, causing less damage to the inner macular layers.

After treatment, careful follow-up examinations are performed. The patient uses the Amsler grid daily to detect visual change due to a persistent or recurrent net. Within 2 weeks after the treatment, a fluorescein angiogram is performed. If leakage is detected, the patient is retreated. These patients must be monitored carefully for the rest of their lives, because recurrent neovascular nets can occur years after laser treatment.

Visual prognosis following corticosteroid and/or laser therapy depends on both the condition of the patient before treatment and the possible side effects of the treatment. If the patient has symptoms of maculopathy for more than 6 months, a large neovascular membrane, or a neovascular membrane close to the fovea, then the visual prognosis after treatment is poor. Adverse effects of laser treatment include choroidal bleeding, thermal vasculitis, retinal edema, and internal limiting membrane wrinkling.

Another form of treatment, presently in the experimental stage, involves the surgical removal of the subfoveal nets. Thomas and Kaplan (1991) successfully performed this surgery on two patients with improved visual acuity and no recurrence. Despite the unknown long-term effects, intraocular surgery holds great promise as a choice of therapy in the near future.

CONCLUSION

The presumed ocular histoplasmosis syndrome is a common cause of visual loss in endemic areas. Despite the understanding of the systemic disease from its benign to fatal presentations, the relationship between the ocular and nonocular forms remains uncertain. Epidemiologic and experimental studies have provided some answers, but they have not substantiated *Histoplasma capsulatum* as the cause of the ocular syndrome. However, both forms of the disease can be devastating. As researchers continue to look for a correlation, the focus should be on proper diagnosis, management, and treatment.

REFERENCES

Beck RW, Sergott RC, Barr CC, Annesley WH. Optic disc edema in the presumed ocular histoplasmosis syndrome. *Ophthalmology* 1984;91:183–185.

Bindschadler D. Fungal diseases. In: Mitchell R, Petty T, Schwarz M, eds. *Synopsis of Clinical Pulmonary Disease*, 4th ed. St. Louis: Mosby; 1989:106–117.

Bottoni FG, Deutman AF, Aandekerk AL. Presumed ocular histoplasmosis syndrome and linear streak lesions. *Br J Ophthalmol.* 1989;73:528–535.

Braley RE, Meredith TA, Aaberg TM, et al. The prevalence of HLA-B7 in presumed ocular histoplasmosis. *Am J Ophthalmol* 1978;85:859–861.

Campochiaro PA, Morgan KM, Conway BP, Stathos J. Spontaneous involution of subfoveal neovascularization. *Am J Ophthalmol.* 1990;109:668–675.

Chandler FW, Watts JC. Fungal infections. In: Dail DH, Hammar SP, eds. *Pulmonary Pathology.* New York: Springer-Verlag; 1988;189–201.

Check IJ, Diddie KR, Jay WM, et al. Lymphocyte stimulation by yeast phase histoplasma capsulatum in presumed ocular histoplasmosis syndrome. *Am J Ophthalmol.* 1979;87:311–316.

Deutsch TA, Tessler HH. Inflammatory pseudohistoplasmosis. *Ann Ophthalmol.* 1985;17:461–465.

Dreyer RF, Gass DM. Multifocal choroiditis and panuveitis. *Arch Ophthalmol.* 1984;102:1776–1784.

Feman SS, Tilford RH. Ocular findings in patients with histoplasmosis. *JAMA.* 1985;253:2534–2537.

Fountain JA, Schlaegel TF. Linear streaks of the equator in the presumed ocular histoplasmosis syndrome. *Arch Ophthalmol.* 1981;99:246–248.

Gass JD. *Stereoscopic Atlas of Macular Diseases.* 3rd ed. St. Louis: Mosby; 1987:112–128.

Graybill JR. Infections caused by fungi and the higher bacteria (actinomycoses and norcardia). In: Stein JH, ed. *Internal Medicine.* Boston: Little, Brown; 1990:1556–1562.

Han DP, Folk JC. Internal limiting membrane wrinkling after argon and krypton laser photocoagulation of choroidal neovascularization. *Retina.* 1986;6:215–219.

Han DP, Folk JC, Bratton AR. Visual loss after successful photocoagulation of choroidal neovascularization. *Ophthalmology.* 1988;95:1380–1384.

Holland GN. Endogenous fungal infections of the retina and choroid. In: Ryan SJ, ed. *Retina.* vol. 2. St. Louis: Mosby; 1989;2:625–635.

Johnston RL, Mitchell PC, Berman AM. Presumed ocular histoplasmosis syndrome. *J Am Optom Assoc.* 1988;59:401–405.

Joondeph BC, Tessler HH. Clinical course of multifocal choroiditis: Photographic and angiographic evidence of disease recurrence. *Ann Ophthalmol.* 1991;23:424–429.

Kleiner RC, Ratner CM, Enger C, Fine SL. Subfoveal neovascularization in the ocular histoplasmosis syndrome. *Retina.* 1988;8:225–229.

Klintworth GK, Hollingsworth AS, Lusman PA, Bradford WD. Granulomatous choroiditis in a case of disseminated histoplasmosis. *Arch Ophthalmol.* 1973;90:45–48.

Lewis ML, Van Newkirk MR, Gass JD. Follow-up study of presumed ocular histoplasmosis syndrome. *Ophthalmology.* 1980;87:390–399.

Louria DB. Fungus, actinomyces, and nocardia infections of the lungs. In: Baun GL, Wolinsky E, eds. *Textbook of Pulmonary Diseases.* Boston: Little, Brown; 1983;459–467.

Macular Photocoagulation Study Group. Argon laser photocoagulation for ocular histoplasmosis. *Arch Ophthalmol.* 1983; 101:1347–1357.

Meredith TA, Smith RE, Duquesnoy RJ. Association of HLA-DRw2 antigen with presumed ocular histoplasmosis. *Am J Ophthalmol.* 1980;89:70–76.

Negroni P. *Histoplasmosis.* Springfield, IL: Thomas; 1965.

Olk RJ, Burgess DB. Treatment of recurrent juxtafoveal subretinal neovascular membranes with krypton red laser photocoagulation. *Ophthalmology.* 1985;92:1035–1046.

Olk RJ, Burgess DB, McCormick PA. Subfoveal and juxtafoveal subretinal neovascularization in the presumed ocular histoplasmosis syndrome. *Ophthalmology.* 1984;91:1592–1602.

Roth AM. Histoplasma capsulatum in the presumed ocular histoplasmosis syndrome. *Am J Ophthalmol.* 1977;84:293–298.

Sabates FN, Lee KY, Ziemianski MC. A comparative study of argon and krypton laser photocoagulation in the treatment of presumed ocular histoplasmosis syndrome. *Ophthalmology.* 1982;89:729–734.

Sarosi GA, Davies SF. Histoplasmosis. In: Fishman A, ed. *Pulmonary Diseases and Disorders.* 2nd ed. New York: McGraw-Hill; 1988;1775–1781.

Sarosi GA, Davies SF, eds. *Fungal Diseases of the Lung.* Orlando: Grune & Stratton; 1986.

Sawelson H, Goldberg RE, Annesley WH, Tomer TL. Presumed ocular histoplasmosis syndrome: The fellow eye. *Arch Ophthalmol.* 1976;94:221–224.

Schlaegel TF. Presumed ocular histoplasmosis. In: Tasman W, Jaeger EA, eds. *Duane's Clinical Ophthalmology.* Philadelphia: Lippincott; 4:1991.

Schlaegel TF. *Update on Ocular Histoplasmosis.* Boston: Little, Brown; 1983.

Schlaegel TF. *Ocular Histoplasmosis.* New York: Grune & Stratton; 1977.

Scholz R, Green WR, Kutys R, et al. Histoplasma capsulatum in the eye. *Ophthalmology.* 1984;91:1100–1104.

Schwarz J. *Histoplasmosis.* New York: Praeger; 1981.

Sheffer A, Green R, Fine SL, Kincaid M. Presumed ocular histoplasmosis syndrome–A clinicopathologic correlation of a treated case. *Arch Ophthalmol.* 1980;98:335–340.

Singerman LJ. Important points in management of patients with choroidal neovascularization. *Ophthalmology.* 1985;92:610–614.

Singerman LJ, Wong B, Ai E, Smith S. Spontaneous visual improvement in the first affected eye of patients with bilateral disciform scars. *Retina.* 1985;5:135–143.

Thomas MA, Kaplan HJ. Surgical removal of subfoveal neovascularization in the presumed ocular histoplasmosis syndrome. *Am J Ophthalmol.* 1991;111:1–7.

Watzke RC. Histoplasmosis. In: Gold DH, Weingeist TA, eds. *The Eye in Systemic Disease.* Philadelphia: Lippincott; 1990:200–202.

Wilkinson CP. Presumed ocular histoplasmosis. *Am J Ophthalmol.* 1976;82:140–142.

Woods AC, Wahlen HE. The probable role of benign histoplasmosis in the etiology of granulomatosis uveitis. *Trans Am Ophthamol Soc.* 1959;57:318.

Yassur Y, Gilad E, Ben-Sira I. Treatment of macular subretinal neovascularization with the red-light krypton laser in presumed ocular histoplasmosis syndrome. *Am J Ophthalmol.* 1981;91:172–176.

63
Chapter

Chlamydia

Taryn Mathews

For thousands of years, humans have suffered from systemic and ocular infections caused by the intracellular parasite chlamydia. The genus *Chlamydia* has two species, *C. trachomatis* and *C. psittaci*, and each species has a number of serotypes responsible for various chlamydial diseases. This chapter will be restricted to diseases caused by *C. trachomatis*.

In the developing world, the severest form of chlamydia, called trachoma, is the greatest cause of preventable vision loss despite improvements in living conditions. In the industrialized world, chlamydia causes the most common sexually transmitted disease. Genital chlamydial infections are transmitted to the eye, causing adult inclusion conjunctivitis and neonatal conjunctivitis. Oculogenital chlamydial infections can be difficult to diagnose, because many of those afflicted are asymptomatic and clinical features are shared with other common infections.

The term TRIC, which stands for trachoma-inclusion conjunctivitis, is a name given to all the serotypes that cause trachoma, inclusion conjunctivitis, and the associated systemic complications. Recognizing the clinical presentation in combination with appropriate testing allows for the correct diagnosis and choice of treatment. Reinfection and further spread of the disease can be prevented by examining the patient and the sexual partners.

EPIDEMIOLOGY

■ Systemic

Each year, there are three to four million new cases of genital infection caused by *C. trachomatis*. In fact, it is the most common sexually transmitted disease in the United States. A significant number of patients infected with *Neisseria gonorrhoeae* have a concurrent chlamydial infection. Approximately 25% of heterosexual men suffer with concurrent infection. In women, 30 to 50% with gonorrhea also have a chlamydial infection. Combined infections are more prevalent in single, noncaucasian or Asian females in their late teens and early 20s. In industrialized countries, chlamydial infections are more prevalent than gonorrhea because routine diagnostic testing and treat-

ment of gonorrhea (in both sexual partners) has been more effectively instituted.

Chlamydial cervicitis develops in 60% of women who engage in sexual activity with infected men. In sexually transmitted disease (STD) clinics, over 20% of women have cervical infection from chlamydia. In the United States, chlamydial cervicitis in pregnant women is 5 to 10 times greater than gonorrhea. Infants exposed during birth have a 60% chance of developing a chlamydial infection. Approximately 10 to 20% of these newborns develop pneumonia.

Thirty-five to fifty percent of patients with nongonococcal urethritis (NGU) test positive for *C. trachomatis*, making it the leading cause of NGU and of postgonococcal urethritis (PGU). In the United States, the number of new NGU cases increases by half a million each year.

Chlamydia causes two thirds of epididymitis cases. Homosexual males have rectal infections more often than urethral infections due to anorectal intercourse. Although chlamydia has not been established as the cause of Reiter syndrome, 40 to 70% of male patients with this syndrome have *C. trachomatis* in their urethras.

■ Ocular

Trachoma

Trachoma is one of the major causes of blindness throughout the world. Although blindness is preventable, approximately 200 million of the estimated 700 million cases of trachoma involve blindness or severe visual loss. The blinding form, known as endemic trachoma, is most prevalent in countries of low socioeconomic status with a dry, sandy climate. Trachoma is associated with impoverished rural communities of underdeveloped countries plagued with poor sanitation, overcrowding, and unhealthy living conditions. Today, the regions most affected by trachoma include North Africa, sub-Saharan Africa, the Middle East, and parts of the Indian subcontinent, Asia, Latin America, Australia, and the Pacific Islands. In the United States, trachoma is prevalent in southwestern American Indians, Mexicans, and the states of Arkansas, Missouri, Oklahoma, West Virginia, and Kentucky.

Adult Inclusion Conjunctivitis

The typical patient with inclusion conjunctivitis is a young, sexually active adult ranging in age from 18 to 35 years. In many cases, the patient reports having a new sexual partner. It is more frequently seen in industrialized countries, and all social classes are known to be affected by the disease. But like trachoma, it is more prevalent in people with poor hygiene. In about 70% the condition affects only one eye. Recurrences occur when both sexual partners are not treated. The incidence of inclusion conjunctivitis has increased dramatically with the rise in chlamydial genital infections and other venereal diseases. Each year, over 4 million Americans contract genital chlamydial disease. Approximately 1 in 300 of these patients develop inclusion conjunctivitis.

Neonatal Inclusion Conjunctivitis

Neonatal inclusion conjunctivitis or blennorrhea is the most common form of eye disease caused by chlamydia. The number of cases in industrialized countries is on the rise. Two to six percent of all newborns in the United States contract chlamydia as a result of exposure to infected birth canals. Children born to infected mothers have a 50% chance of developing inclusion conjunctivitis.

NATURAL HISTORY

■ Systemic

The Organism

Chlamydia is an obligate, intracellular parasite that possesses characteristics of bacteria and viruses. For many years, this parasite was considered to be a virus, but is now classified as a bacterium with a separate order, genus, and species. Similar to a bacterium, chlamydia possesses DNA and RNA, divides by binary fission, and is sensitive to antibiotics. However, like a virus, chlamydia is unable to produce ATP, and is therefore dependent on the host epithelial cell for energy. *C. trachomatis* is subdivided into several serotypes. Sexually transmitted diseases and neonatal infections are caused by serotypes D through K, whereas trachoma is caused by serotypes A through C.

Transmission

Chlamydia has a unique life cycle that involves two forms, the elementary body (EB) and the reticulate or initial body (RB). A brief description of the life cycle provides an explanation for the basis of diagnostic testing. The EB is the infectious form, which is phagocytized by its target, the epithelial cell (genital or ocular). After it enters the cell, it changes into the larger RB. The RB then multiplies into aggregates of EBs near or attached to the nucleus. An aggregate of EBs is called an inclusion body. When the cell ruptures, the EBs are released to infect other epithelial cells. The life cycle requires about 48 hours.

Chlamydia, transmitted via sexual contact, results in genital infection. Newborns of infected mothers acquire the parasite through exposure to the infected birth canal. Transmission of the oculogenital disease is primarily through sexual contact, either from the genital tract to the fingers and then to the eye, or directly from the genitals to the eye. It is very rare for transmission of inclusion conjunctivitis to occur through eye to eye contact. Before chlorination, adult inclusion conjunctivitis was transmitted from genital secretions in swimming pools. Today, swimming pool conjunctivitis is rare and is caused by adenovirus.

The transmission of trachoma occurs by eye-to-eye or hand-to-eye contact via flies, fomites, contaminated towels, and water. It is believed that trachoma develops after repeated, prolonged exposure to the organism over months or years.

Course of the Disease

C. trachomatis is a major cause of a number of genital infections in men and women (Table 63–1). In men, it has been associated with a large percentage of the NGU and PGU cases. Nongonococcal urethritis, as the name implies,

TABLE 63–1. SYSTEMIC MANIFESTATIONS OF CHLAMYDIA

NONGONOCOCCAL URETHRITIS (NGU)
- May or may not be asymptomatic
- Mucopurulent discharge
- Dysuria
- Pruritus
- Meatal erythema and tenderness
- Possible association with Reiter syndrome: urethritis, uveitis, conjunctivitis, arthritis

POSTGONOCOCCAL URETHRITIS (PGU)
- Persistent urethral discharge despite PCN treatment for gonorrhea
- Epididymitis
- Proctitis
  Rectal mucopurulent discharge
  Rectal mucosa erythema
  Constipation
  Tenesmus
  Pruritus

COMPLICATIONS IN WOMEN
- Cervicitis
  Often concurrently infected with *N. gonorrhea*
  Yellow, mucopurulent discharge
  Erythematous, edematous cervix
  Bleeds easily with minor trauma
- Salpingitis
  Subsequent fallopian tube scarring and sterility may result

- Pelvic inflammatory disease
  Multiple infecting organisms
  Cervicitis
  Endometritis (vaginal bleeding, abdominal pain, uterine tenderness)
  Endosalpingitis (subsequent scarring and sterility may result)
  Pelvic peritonitis
  Perihepatitis (also known as Fitz–Hugh–Curtis syndrome, characterized by inflammation of the liver capsule with fibrinous adhesions and pleuritic upper abdominal pain and tenderness)

COMPLICATIONS IN PREGNANT WOMEN
- Increased risk of ectopic pregnancy
- Premature delivery
- Postpartum endometritis

COMPLICATIONS IN NEWBORNS
- Pneumonia: afebrile, coughing, tachypneic
- Otitis with potential hearing loss
- Vaginitis

LYMPHOGRANULOMA VENEREUM (LGV)
- Painless genital ulcer or vesicle which heals without scarring
- Regional (groin) lymphadenopathy called bubos
- Skin over involved lymph nodes thins, becomes inflamed, with fistula formation and scarring
- Symptoms: fever, myalgia, malaise
- Complications: hemorrhagic proctitis, genital elephantiasis, strictures, fistulas (penis, urethra, rectum)

is urethritis not caused by gonorrhea but with the clinical presentation of gonorrhea. PGU is a type of NGU that develops 2 to 3 weeks after successful gonorrhea treatment.

One to three weeks after exposure, NGU patients present with a mucopurulent discharge. The presentation is similar to gonorrhea, but chlamydial urethritis is not as severe. Other symptoms include dysuria and urethral pruritus. Meatal erythema and tenderness are found upon examination. However, in about one third of men diagnosed with chlamydial urethritis, there are no signs or symptoms. PGU patients complain of a persistent urethral discharge after being treated with penicillin for gonorrhea. These patients had concurrent infection that was unknown until the gonorrhea was treated. Epididymitis is a complication that often occurs secondary to chlamydial urethritis. Patients with Reiter syndrome have urethritis, arthritis, conjunctivitis, and a rash. The relationship of chlamydia to Reiter syndrome is unknown, but a genital infection caused by *C. trachomatis* often precedes the syndrome.

Proctitis caused by chlamydia occurs in men or women who have anorectal intercourse. It is an inflammatory condition that is often asymptomatic or mild. Examination reveals rectal mucosa erythema and a mucopurulent discharge. Patients complain of anorectal discharge, constipation, tenesmus (the unsuccessful urge to void), and pruritus.

In women, the most common complication of chlamydial infection is a mucopurulent cervicitis. Some patients have mild symptoms, many others have no symptoms. The cervix becomes red and edematous, bleeds easily from minor trauma, and produces a yellow mucopurulent discharge. As with urethritis in men, many patients have simultaneous infections from *C. trachomatis* and *N. gonorrhoeae*.

Further complications of chlamydial infection in women include urethritis, salpingitis (inflammation of the fallopian tubes), pelvic inflammatory disease, secondary peritonitis, and fallopian tube scarring with subsequent sterility. Tubal scarring from chlamydia may be a contributing factor in the increase of ectopic pregnancies. Chlamydial infection during pregnancy may also lead to premature delivery and postpartum endometritis.

Pelvic inflammatory disease is caused by multiple organisms, particularly *N. gonorrhoeae* and *C. trachomatis*. Microorganisms travel from the lower genital tract to the fallopian tubes and endometrium. The disease is characterized by cervicitis, endometritis, endosalpingitis, and pelvic peritonitis. In endometritis, patients suffer with vaginal bleeding, abdominal pain, and uterine tenderness. Perihepatitis (inflammation of the liver capsule) may also occur.

Systemic complications in newborns infected during delivery include pneumonia, otitis, vaginitis, and hearing loss. The development of pneumonia occurs from 2 to 12 weeks of age. Clinical examination reveals afebrile, coughing, and tachypneic (breathing very rapidly) newborns.

Lymphogranuloma venereum (LGV) is a systemic sexually transmitted disease caused by *C. trachomatis* serotypes L1, L2, and L3. Although still endemic in tropical countries, LGV is rare in the United States, and rarely causes ocular manifestations. Therefore, this chlamydial disease will not be discussed.

■ Ocular
Table 63–2 summarizes the ocular manifestations of chlamydia.

Trachoma
The clinical presentation of trachoma is variable due to differences in the various strains, the occurrence of concurrent bacterial infections, and the climate. In endemic regions, trachoma primarily affects young children. In fact, almost all the children acquire the infection by the age of 1 or 2 years, and then the disease slowly runs its course through the adult years. It is uncommon for the infection to start during adulthood. Relapses or recurrences of disease may occur due to latency or the failure to develop immunity. It is common to see recurrent disease in children, even after they have been treated. The severe blinding complications of trachoma are more common in adults.

Endemic trachoma is a chronic, bilateral follicular keratoconjunctivitis. The layer most involved in trachoma infections is the epithelium of the conjunctiva and cornea. The pathologic changes of the conjunctival epithelium include weakened cell to cell adhesions, hyperplasia, irregularity of cell size, and the infiltration of lymphocytes and polymorphonuclear leukocytes. The area of the conjunctiva most affected is the upper tarsal plate.

Following the epithelial changes is a chronic inflammatory reaction in the subepithelial tissues. The infiltration of inflammatory cells results in edema, hyperemia, papillary hypertrophy, and the formation of follicles. Follicles do not form during the first year of life. A unique feature

of trachomatous follicles is their softness, allowing their contents of lymphocytic cells to be easily expressed onto the conjunctiva, resulting in necrosis and scarring. Scarred follicles at the limbus form depressions called Herbert pits. These pits have a serrated appearance and are pathognomonic of trachoma. The follicular response is sometimes masked by the papillary hypertrophy and inflammation.

MacCallan, in 1931, was the first to classify the clinical features of the conjunctiva in trachoma into four stages (see Table 63–2). The first three stages, lasting months to years, are characterized by follicles in the superior palpebral conjunctiva, superior limbus, and caruncle. Serous exudation is usually present. Papillary hypertrophy eventually obscures the follicles. Cicatricial or conjunctival scarring eventually occurs. The inflammatory reaction, follicles, and papillae subside and are replaced by scar tissue in the final stage. The amount of scarring varies depending on the severity of the inflammatory reaction in the earlier stages. The MacCallan system is limited as it only addresses the conjunctival involvement. The World Health Organization (WHO) developed a grading system to enable personnel (other than eyecare providers) to assess the degree of severity of trachoma within a community. The system is based on the number of upper tarsal follicles and the degree of upper tarsal papillary hypertrophy (see Table 63–2).

Endemic trachoma has a gradual onset. The typical patient is less than 2 years of age. The presenting symptoms are redness, tearing, photophobia, pain, mucopurulent discharge, swollen lids and conjunctiva, and a tender preauricular lymph node. The degree of pain and photophobia depends on the extent of corneal involvement. The amount of discharge will vary depending on the development of secondary bacterial infection.

Visual impairment in trachoma results from complications of the active disease. As the inflammation subsides, the conjunctiva becomes severely scarred and fibrotic. Damage to the goblet cells and the ductules of the lacrimal gland lead to dry eye syndromes. Dacryocystitis often occurs from scarring of the lacrimal sac. The scarred conjunctiva shrinks and contracts, forming a white horizontal scar across the upper tarsal plate approximately one third of the distance from the lid margin. These linear scars, called Arlt lines, contract to produce entropion. Scarring at the lid margin results in further distortion and deformity of the lids and trichiasis.

Blindness in trachoma ultimately is due to the effects of the secondary complications on the cornea (Figure 63–1). In fact, entropion and trichiasis are the most common causes of severe visual loss. Recurrent abrasion of the cornea by the lashes combined with keratitis sicca and abnormal lid closure result in corneal ulceration and scarring. In addition, the compromised cornea is more susceptible to secondary bacterial infections. A concurrent bacterial

TABLE 63–2. OCULAR MANIFESTATIONS OF CHLAMYDIA

TRACHOMA
- MacCallan trachoma grading
  - Stage I: Soft, immature follicles in the upper palpebral conjunctiva without scarring
    Serous exudation of variable degree is usually present
    Follicles may be present at limbus (especially superior) and caruncle
  - Stage IIA: Mature upper tarsal plate follicles and moderate papillary hypertrophy
  - Stage IIB: Papillary hypertrophy predominates resulting in obscuration of follicles
  - Stage III: Cicatricial or conjunctival scarring
  - Stage IV: Healed trachoma (the inflammatory reaction, follicles, and papillae have subsided and are replaced by scar tissue)
- The WHO trachoma grading
  Based on number of follicles and the degree of papillary hypertrophy
- Symptoms
  Erythema, tearing, mucopurulent discharge
  Photophobia, pain
  Edematous lids and conjunctiva
  Tender preauricular lymph node
- Complications
  Vision loss secondary to conjunctival (Arlt lines) and corneal scarring
  Dry eye syndrome secondary to lacrimal gland and goblet cell damage
  Dacryocystitis secondary to lacrimal sac damage
  Lid deformities (entropion, ectropion, trichiasis)
  Corneal ulceration and scarring secondary to trichiasis
  Secondary bacterial infections

ADULT INCLUSION CONJUNCTIVITIS
- Symptoms
  Mild irritation, foreign body sensation, tearing, photophobia
  Conjunctival erythema, mild mucopurulent discharge
  Lid edema, lids sealed shut in AM
  (+) or (–) genital symptoms

- Signs
  Ipsilateral tender palpable preauricular node
  (–) fever, (–) upper respiratory infection
  Hyperemic, edematous conjunctiva
  Follicular/papillary palpebral conjunctiva hypertrophy (especially lower tarsal conjunctiva and fornix)
  Superiorly located keratitis with yellow subepithelial infiltrates (peripheral > central cornea)
  Corneal vascularization, limbal swelling, and micropannus formation (resolves with treatment)
- Less common findings
  Pseudoptosis
  Mild anterior uveitis
  Association with Reiter syndrome
  Ipsilateral otitis media

NEONATAL INCLUSION CONJUNCTIVITIS
- Usually presents bilaterally 5 days after birth
- Signs
  Profuse mucopurulent discharge
  Edematous lids
  Hyperemic conjunctiva
  Papillary hypertrophy
  Inflammatory pseudomembrane
  Corneal infiltration and pannus formation

LYMPHOGRANULOMA VENEREUM (LGV)—OCULAR FINDINGS RARE
- Follicular conjunctivitis or granulomatous reaction
- Preauricular lymphadenopathy
- If lymphatic drainage obstructed, elephantiasis of lids occurs
- Rare corneal involvement with superior peripheral infiltrates spreading to central cornea
- Rare episcleritis, sclerokeratitis, interstitial keratitis, anterior uveitis, optic neuritis

infection increases the severity of the disease. The presentation of disease can range from very mild with few or no complications to complete degeneration of the cornea and conjunctiva.

Adult Inclusion Conjunctivitis
Adult inclusion conjunctivitis is an oculogenital disease, affecting the conjunctiva and the genital or urinary tract. It is caused by *C. trachomatis* serotypes D through K. The ocular clinical presentation has a similar appearance to the early stages of trachoma, but the condition is benign and

self-limiting without the scarring and other severe complications. To differentiate the condition from endemic trachoma, it is sometimes referred to as paratrachoma.

One to two weeks after exposure, adults present with an acute follicular conjunctivitis. Symptoms include mild irritation, foreign body sensation, tearing, photophobia, redness, lid swelling, and mild mucopurulent discharge. Patients report sticky eyelids sealed shut upon awakening. Upper respiratory symptoms and fever are absent, helping to differentiate inclusion conjunctivitis from conjunctivitis caused by viruses, especially adenovirus. However, a

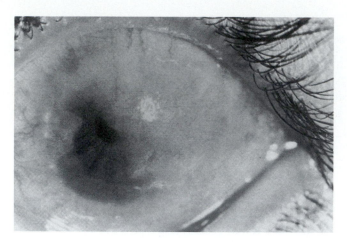

Figure 63–1. Severe corneal pannus and scarring in endstage trachoma. *(Reprinted with permission from Mandel ER, Wagoner MD.* Atlas of Corneal Disease. *Philadelphia: WB Saunders Co, 1989.)*

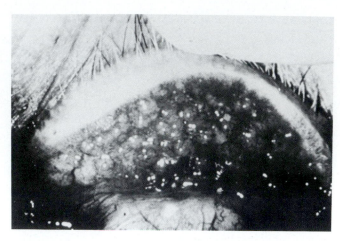

Figure 63–2. Mixed follicular and papillary hypertrophy in adult inclusion conjunctivitis. *(Reprinted with permission from Wallace W.* Diseases of the conjunctiva. In: Bartlett JD, Jaanus SD, eds. Clinical Ocular Pharmacology. *Boston: Butterworths 1989:546.)*

small, mildly tender preauricular node does occur on the affected side. Symptoms of systemic or genital manifestations consistent with chlamydia may or may not be present.

The conjunctiva is injected, hyperemic, and edematous with a combination of follicular and papillary hypertrophy in the upper and lower conjunctiva (Figure 63–2). In contrast to endemic trachoma, the conjunctival response is greatest in the lower tarsal conjunctiva and fornix, and the follicles may take up to 3 weeks to appear.

Corneal involvement usually occurs during the second week of the disease. The keratitis occurs in the superficial epithelium and is usually localized to the superior cornea. Subepithelial infiltration and opacification occur in the peripheral and central cornea, although the marginal infiltrates are more common. The infiltrates have a yellow appearance and stain with fluorescein. Superior superficial corneal vascularization and limbal swelling occur, followed by the formation of a micropannus of 1 to 3 mm. Most of the corneal changes resolve with treatment.

Additional less common clinical findings include a pseudoptosis, persistent superficial punctate keratitis, mild anterior uveitis, Reiter syndrome, and (in 14% of cases) otitis media on the involved side. There have been reports of patients with genital chlamydia having inclusion conjunctivitis without symptoms. On occasion, inclusion conjunctivitis can become a chronic condition.

Untreated, inclusion conjunctivitis has a natural course of 6 to 18 months. The disease resolves without complications, although a few cases of conjunctival scarring have been reported. With topical and systemic treatment, the disease resolves over a 3-week period. Patients report feeling better after 1 week of treatment.

Neonatal Inclusion Conjunctivitis
Neonatal inclusion conjunctivitis usually presents bilaterally on the fifth day after birth. However, the duration of incubation is variable, with a range of 3 to 21 days. The clinical presentation is indistinguishable from other forms of acute neonatal conjunctivitis without diagnostic testing. The signs include edematous lids, conjunctival hyperemia, papillary hypertrophy, and a profuse mucopurulent discharge. Corneal pannus and infiltration are also seen.

The clinical presentation of the neonatal form is similar to the adult form of inclusion conjunctivitis. However, there are a number of distinguishable differences. Because newborns lack mature conjunctival lymphoid tissue, follicles cannot develop until 4 or 5 months of age. Therefore, the conjunctival reaction is primarily one of papillary hypertrophy rather than follicular. Newborns have more mucopurulent discharge than adults. In severe cases, infants can develop an inflammatory pseudomembrane in the palpebral conjunctiva. Membranes are not seen in the adult form. Newborns have more intracytoplasmic inclusion bodies. Lastly, the infant form responds better to topical medication than the adult variety.

When infected infants are not treated both orally and topically, they are more likely to develop conjunctival scarring and pannus. Untreated neonates are also more likely to develop chlamydial pneumonia.

Diagnosis

■ Systemic
Despite the availability of many diagnostic techniques, chlamydial infections are often difficult to diagnose. Many cases go unnoticed because of their mild or asymptomatic

nature. Furthermore, chlamydial infections are often masked by a concurrent infection, especially gonorrhea. The variability and limitations of the various tests also hinder the diagnostic process. Therefore, the clinical presentation plays a crucial part in chlamydial diagnosis. Patient history, genital examination, cultures, smears, routine blood work, urinalysis, serologic tests, and in the case of suspected pneumonia, chest x-ray are all employed in the diagnosis.

Before present-day diagnostic tests were available, chlamydia was cultured by inoculating the yolk sac of embryonated chicken eggs. Today, the standard diagnostic test is the McCoy cell tissue culture. In this test, irradiated tissue culture cells, called McCoy cells, are inoculated with the presumed infected specimens. After a 3-day incubation, iodine or Giemsa stain is applied to identify inclusion bodies. Although the McCoy cell tissue culture is the definitive test for the diagnosis of chlamydia, there are a number of disadvantages associated with it. It is expensive, not readily available, and can be negative in half the cases.

Due to the problems associated with culturing, antigen detection tests for diagnosing chlamydial infections were developed. The most sensitive test for diagnosis is the fluorescein-conjugated monoclonal antibody test. The technique entails fixing the genital or ocular specimens on a slide and then incubating it with the fluorescein-conjugated monoclonal antibody. When the antibodies bind to the chlamydial inclusions, they become bright fluorescent green in the cytoplasm. This test is highly sensitive and specific for diagnosing urethral, cervical, and ocular infections. A main advantage of this technique, in addition to reliability, is that results are obtained in as little as 30 minutes.

In urethritis, the specimen should be obtained by inserting the swab at least 2 cm into the urethra. To diagnose cervicitis, a Pap smear should be performed. The cervix should be cleaned first and the swab should be rotated inside the cervix. An increase in neutrophils and inflammatory cells will also be found on Pap smears.

The other antigen test is the serologic technique called enzyme-linked immunosorbent assay (ELISA). It is rapid, inexpensive, relatively sensitive and specific, and especially useful in screening large numbers of specimens. Other serologic tests can also be used to diagnose chlamydia, but are only useful for certain conditions. The micro-immunofluorescence test, which allows the differentiation of the various serotypes of chlamydia, is useful for infant pneumonia and salpingitis.

Newborns suspected to have systemic complications from chlamydia should be examined for pneumonia, genital infection, and ear involvement. Chest x-ray will demonstrate mild interstitial infiltrates and hyperexpansion of the lungs. Also, there is an increase in immunoglobulins and eosinophilia.

■ Ocular

The diagnosis of ocular chlamydial infections (trachoma or inclusion conjunctivitis) relies on patient history and ocular examination with thorough slit-lamp evaluation of the anterior segment. If a chlamydial infection is suspected, a conjunctival scraping should be obtained. The purpose of scraping is to collect epithelial cells, not the mucopurulent discharge. If this is not possible, diagnosis may be made by clinical presentation. For example, endemic trachoma has a number of distinguishing signs that are useful for clinical diagnosis. The signs are lymphoid follicles on the superior tarsal conjunctiva, conjunctival scarring, vascular pannus, and limbal follicles or Herbert pits. The presence of two of the four signs is sufficient for diagnosis of trachoma. The patient should be questioned concerning the presence of eye disease in family members or friends. In suspected inclusion conjunctivitis the patient, or in the case of a newborn, the mother, should be questioned concerning the presence of genital infection.

The main method for diagnosing chlamydial ocular infections is by Giemsa staining of the typical inclusion bodies. When Giemsa stain is applied to a smear of conjunctival scrapings, the cytoplasmic inclusions of the epithelial cells appear reddish blue. The singular or multiple inclusions are seen next to the nucleus. Occasionally, elementary bodies can be seen from ruptured epithelial cells. The cytology of the smear becomes important in old cases of trachoma or inclusion conjunctivitis that lack the classic inclusion bodies. Diagnosis in these cases depends on the presence of PMNs, plasma cells, Leber cells (giant macrophages with phagocytized debris), and lymphocytes.

Giemsa staining is especially useful for the diagnosis of ocular conjunctivitis in newborns because they have large numbers of inclusions. Giemsa staining is not as useful a diagnostic test in adult inclusion conjunctivitis and systemic chlamydial disease because the sensitivity is low and false positives are high. Furthermore, in trachoma and inclusion conjunctivitis, the inclusions appear the same on Giemsa staining. Therefore, the test cannot be used to differentiate the two conditions.

The fluorescein-conjugated monoclonal antibody test (MicroTrak, Syva) is the preferred test over the Giemsa stain for evaluating adult inclusion conjunctivitis and trachoma. The test results are reliable and are obtained quickly, especially important in cases such as newborn conjunctivitis where treatment should be administered rapidly.

If diagnostic testing is not readily available or affordable, the Centers for Disease Control (CDC) recommend instituting treatment without confirmation through diagnostic techniques. This approach (for both systemic and ocular infections) involves oral treatment for 6 days. If there is significant improvement within 3 to 4 days, then the clinician may assume that the suspicion of chlamydial infection was correct and therapy should be continued. However, it is better to confirm the diagnosis with testing rather than relying on the clinical presentation.

TREATMENT AND MANAGEMENT

■ Systemic

The treatment of choice for adult chlamydial genital infections, as well as all other chlamydial infections, is oral tetracyclines (Table 63–3). Chlamydial infections require a minimum of 7 days of treatment and often need 2 to 3 weeks of therapy. *C. trachomatis* infections may also be treated with oral doxycycline, or erythromycin. The treatment for infected pregnant women is erythromycin, or amoxicillin.

A crucial part of the treatment of genital chlamydial infections is the education and treatment of the patient's sexual partners. When treatment is unsuccessful, it is often due to reinfection by the untreated partner. Even if the sexual partner of an infected patient is asymptomatic, treatment should still be instituted.

Because tetracyclines cause skeletal and dental defects in the fetus and in children less than 8 years old, neonates with chlamydial infections (ocular and/or systemic) should be treated with erythromycin ethylsuccinate or estolate. Absorption of this antibiotic is enhanced by milk. Both parents of the infected infant should also be tested and treated if necessary.

■ Ocular

Trachoma

Mass treatment programs with topical tetracycline or erythromycin have been instituted for endemic trachoma. The ointment is applied to the eyes of all the infected children. Topical therapy alone does not eradicate trachoma, but does prevent the blinding complications. Ideally, topical

TABLE 63–3. TREATMENT AND MANAGEMENT OF CHLAMYDIA

GENITAL CHLAMYDIAL INFECTIONS
- Adults
  - Tetracycline hydrochloride 500-mg tabs po qid × minimum 1 wk (max 3 wks), OR
  - Doxycycline 100-mg tabs po bid × minimum 1 wk OR
  - Erythromycin 500-mg tabs po qid × minimum 1 wk
  - Surgical aspiration of bubos in LGV may be indicated to prevent rupture
  - *Sexual partners must be tested and treated if indicated*
- Pregnant women
  - Erythromycin 500-mg tabs po qid × 10–14 days OR
  - Amoxicillin 500-mg tabs po tid × 10 days
  - *Sexual partners must be tested and treated if indicated*
- Neonates (all chlamydial infections)
  - Erythromycin ethylsuccinate or estolate 50 mg/kg body weight/day × 14 days
  - *Parents and their sexual partners must be tested and treated if indicated*

OCULAR CHLAMYDIAL INFECTIONS
- **Trachoma**
  - Medical Therapy
    - Adults
      - Tetracycline 250-mg tabs po qid × 3 wks
    - Pregnant women
      - Erythromycin 500-mg tabs po qid × 3 wks
    - Children
      - Tetracycline or erythromycin ung bid to tid × 21–60 days PLUS
      - Tetracycline 250-mg tabs po qid × 3 wks (if child > 8 years old) OR
      - Erythromycin 500-mg tabs po qid × 3 wks (if child < 8 years old)

Surgical Therapy
  - Corrective lid surgery may be indicated
- **Adult Inclusion Conjunctivitis**
  - Adults
    - Tetracycline 250-mg tabs po qid × 3 wks or 500mg qid × 2 wks OR
    - Doxycycline 100-mg tabs po qd × 2 wks PLUS
    - Tetracycline, erythromycin, or sulfacetamide ung bid to tid × 2–3 wks
    - *Patients and their sexual partners must be tested for genital infection and treated if indicated*
  - Pregnant women
    - Erythromycin 500 mg tabs po qid × 2 wks PLUS
    - Erythromycin or sulfacetamide ung bid to tid × 2–3 wks
    - *Patients and their sexual partners must be tested for genital infection and treated if indicated*
- **Neonatal Inclusion Conjunctivitis**
  - Erythromycin ethylsuccinate 50 mg/kg body weight/day × 2 wks PLUS
  - Erythromycin or sulfacetamide ung qid × 2 wks
  - *Parents and their sexual partners must be tested for genital infection and treated if indicated*
- **Lymphogranuloma Venereum (LGV)**
  - Tetracycline 250-mg tabs po qid × 3 wks or 500-mg qid × 2 wks OR
  - Doxycycline 100-mg tabs po qd × 2 wks PLUS
  - Tetracycline, erythromycin, or sulfacetamide ung bid to tid × 2–3 wks
  - *Patients and their sexual partners must be tested for genital infection and treated if indicated*

treatment should be combined with systemic antibiotics. Unfortunately, it is difficult and potentially dangerous to administer mass treatment with systemic antibiotics.

The treatment for adult trachoma is oral tetracycline. For pregnant women and children under 8 years old, the treatment of choice is oral erythromycin. Sulfonamides may also be used, but the toxic and allergic side effects make them a secondary choice. In addition to medical therapy for trachoma, surgery may be necessary to correct entropion and trichiasis.

The rise of industrialization with improved living conditions has also contributed to the decline of the incidence and severity of trachoma in many parts of the world. Basic improvements in living standards, and personal hygiene (particularly face washing), are helping to decrease the prevalence of trachoma. Research is ongoing to develop a vaccine for trachoma.

Adult Inclusion Conjunctivitis

The treatment of choice for adult inclusion conjunctivitis is oral tetracycline. In patients that are not compliant, it may be better to prescribe doxycycline, as it only requires single daily doses. Pregnant women should be given erythromycin. Topical medications (erythromycin, tetracycline, or sulfacetamide ointment) do not cure inclusion conjunctivitis, but their use may reduce the duration of the infection. It is important to emphasize to the patient that sexual partners must be evaluated and treated if necessary.

Neonatal Inclusion Conjunctivitis

Neonatal inclusion conjunctivitis is treated with topical erythromycin or sulfacetamide ointment as well as oral erythromycin ethylsuccinate. Inadequate treatment of neonatal conjunctivitis can lead to the development of pneumonia. The infant's parents (and their sexual partners) must be evaluated for infection and treated if necessary.

CONCLUSION

Chlamydial infections in humans are common throughout the world. The clinical presentation is quite variable, ranging from trachoma, which causes severe visual loss in millions of people, to oculogenital infections, which usually resolve with treatment, leaving few or no complications. The clinical presentation, diagnostic testing, and evaluation of both the patient and the source of infection are important in the treatment and management of chlamydial disease.

REFERENCES

Arffa RC. Chlamydial infections. In: Kist K, ed. *Grayson's Diseases of the Cornea*. St. Louis: Mosby-Year Book; 1991:151–162.

Bialasiewicz AA, Jahn GJ. Evaluation of diagnostic tools for adult chlamydial keratoconjunctivitis. *Ophthalmology*. 1987;94:532–537.

Cotran RS, Kumar V, Robbins SL. Chlamydial diseases. In: Cotran RS, Kumar V, Robbins SL, eds: *Robbins Pathologic Basis of Disease*. 4th ed. Philadelphia: Saunders; 1989:326–328.

Dawson CR. Pathogenesis and control of blinding trachoma. In: Tasman W, Jaeger EA, eds. *Duane's Clinical Ophthalmology*. Philadelphia: Lippincott; 1991;5.

Dawson CR, Sheppard JD. Follicular conjunctivitis. In: Tasman W, Jaeger EA, eds. *Duane's Clinical Ophthalmology*. Philadelphia: Lippincott; 1991;4.

Forster RK, Dawson CR, Schachter J. Late follow-up of patients with neonatal inclusion conjunctivitis. *Am J Ophthalmol*. 1970;69:467–472.

Harrison HR, Phil D, English MG, et al. Chlamydia trachomatis infant pneumonitis. *N Engl J Med*. 1978;298:702–708.

Hawkins DA, Wilson RS, Thomas BJ, Evans RT. Rapid, reliable diagnosis of chlamydial ophthalmis by means of monoclonal antibodies. *Br J Ophthalmol*. 1985;69:640–644.

Holmes KK. Pelvic inflammatory disease. In: Jeffers JD, Boynton SD, eds. *Harrison's Principles of Internal Medicine*. New York: McGraw-Hill; 1991:533–537.

Holmes KK. The chlamydia epidemic. *JAMA*. 1981;245:1718–1723.

Milano M, Gorini G, Olliaro P, et al. Evaluation of diagnostic procedures in chlamydial eye infection. *Ophthalmologica*. 1991;203:114–117.

Quinn TC, Bender B. Sexually transmitted diseases. In: Harvey AM, Johns RJ, McKusick VA, et al, eds. *The Principles and Practice of Medicine*. Norwalk, CT: Appleton & Lange; 1988:657–659.

Peterson HB, Walker CK, Kahn JG, et al. Pelvic inflammatory disease. *JAMA*. 1991;266:2605–2611.

Polack FM. *External Diseases of the Eye*. Barcelona: Ediciones Scriba; 1991:49–56.

Sanders LL, Harrison HR, Washington AE. Treatment of sexually transmitted chlamydial infections. *JAMA*. 1986;255:1750–1756.

Schachter J. Chlamydial infection (first of three parts). *N Engl J Med*. 1978;298:428–435.

Sheppard JD, Dawson CR. Chlamydial infections. In: Gold DH, Weingeist TA, eds. *The Eye in Systemic Disease*. Philadelphia: Lippincott; 1990:169–174.

Stamm WE, Holmes KK. Chlamydial infections. In: Jeffers JD, Boynton SD, eds. *Harrison's Principles of Internal Medicine*. New York: McGraw-Hill; 1991:764–772.

Stenberg K, Mardh PA. Chlamydial conjunctivitis in neonates and adults. *Acta Ophthalmologica*. 1990;68:651–657.

Terry JE. Diseases of the cornea. In: Bartlett JD, Jaanus SD, eds. *Clinical Ocular Pharmacology*. Boston: Butterworths; 1989:570–572.

Wallace W. Diseases of the conjunctiva. In: Bartlett JD, Jaanus SD, eds. *Clinical Ocular Pharmacology*. Boston: Butterworths; 1989:544–547.

Whitcher JP. Chlamydial diseases. In: Smolin G, Thoft RA, eds. *The Cornea*. Boston: Little, Brown; 1983:210–220.

Yanoff M, Fine BS. Specific inflammations. In: Cooke DB, Patterson D, Anderson W, eds. *Ocular Pathology*. Philadelphia: Lippincott; 1989:221–224.

64
Chapter

Toxoplasmosis

Sherry J. Bass ▪ Jerome Sherman

Toxoplasmosis is a disease that is caused by infection with the protozoal organism, *Toxoplasma gondii*. This organism is ubiquitous in the environment, and is the most common cause of infection in the human retina (Tabbara, 1983). In addition to the retina, it can also affect the brain. Without treatment, it can lead to blindness and even death. Toxoplasmosis can be transmitted to a fetus or it can be acquired during life, manifesting most often in the immunosuppressed.

EPIDEMIOLOGY

▪ Systemic

Toxoplasmosis is most prevalent in warm, humid climates. However, evidence of infection with toxoplasma is common and widespread. Seropositivity by the fourth decade of life is approximately 50% in the United States, and reaches greater than 90% in France, El Salvador, and Tahiti (McCabe & Remington, 1990).

The reported rates of congenital infection in the United States vary according to the study, from as low as 1 in 10,000 (Alexander, 1994) to as high as 13 in 10,000 (McCabe & Remington, 1990). Only a toxoplasma infection acquired during gestation will result in fetal infection. Future offspring from a previously infected mother will not be affected due to maternal immunity that develops subsequent to the initial infection.

▪ Ocular

Retinochoroiditis will develop in fewer than 1% of patients with acquired toxoplasma infection as compared to greater than 80% of patients with congenital toxoplasmosis (Alexander, 1994). The estimates of the percentage of all cases of uveitis that are due to toxoplasmosis infection range from a low of 16% (Schlaegel, 1978) to a high of 70% (Cassady, 1960). A conclusive diagnosis of ocular toxoplasmosis in the adult is difficult, because it requires isolation of toxoplasma organisms from ocular tissue in the patient suffering from the active form of the disease.

NATURAL HISTORY

The Organism

Toxoplasma gondii is an obligate intracellular parasite and as such requires a host to sustain its existence. The organism exists in three different life forms: tachyzoite, bradyzoite, and sporozoite. The tachyzoite is the most mobile and reproductive form. When conditions become unfavorable, the organism becomes encysted to form the bradyzoite. Many bradyzoites are contained within a single cyst. These cysts enlarge over time as the bradyzoites slowly reproduce and increase in number. They can ultimately burst, releasing bradyzoites, which then transform into the active tachyzoite. Sporozoites (another reproductive form) exist within the oocyst, which is produced within the intestines of the definitive host, the cat.

Entry into the host is extremely important to the survival of the organism. The tachyzoite is the mobile form, which gains entry into the host cell by releasing enzymes that disrupt the host cell membrane. Once entry is achieved, it begins to multiply within the host cell, eventually destroying it and leading to the release of more *Toxoplasma* protozoans.

Domestic and some wild cats are the definitive hosts of *T. gondii*. The organism can also survive in intermediate hosts, which include many animals as well as humans. The life cycle begins when cats either ingest meat from animals chronically infected with tissue cysts or pick it up from soil contaminated with oocysts. Once ingested, gastric enzymes digest the oocyst or cyst wall, releasing sporozoites from the oocyst and bradyzoites from the tissue cyst. The bradyzoites then turn into the mobile form, the tachyzoite, and invade the mucosal cells of the small intestine. They then reproduce asexually and sexually, forming zygotes, which develop into oocysts. The oocysts are then passed out with the feces (Figure 64–1). An infected cat can shed as many as 10 million oocysts in a single day (Schlaegel, 1978). Once excreted, the oocysts mature and can remain viable and infectious in the soil for years. The warmer and wetter climates are more favorable environments for survival. Colder and dryer regions have less cases of human infection. Only freezing to below 20° C or heating above 66° C will destroy the oocyst.

Other animals, including humans, can acquire the parasite from the soil. In addition to reproducing within the feline intestines, in other species the organism is disseminated to other parts of the body via the bloodstream and invades other tissues as well, including muscle, heart, lung, liver, retina, and brain. As the definitive host, the cat is the only animal in which *T. gondii* reproduces within the intestine (enteroepithelial). In the intermediate hosts, including humans, the organism reproduces outside the intestine, in other tissues of the body (extraintestinal).

The immune system, if normal, battles against the invasion of *T. gondii*. As a result, the tachyzoites transform into the bradyzoite form, which will then become encysted to form dormant, inactive tissue cysts. These cysts remain in the host tissue for the life of the host and only reactivate when the immunity of the host is suppressed (Schlagel, 1978).

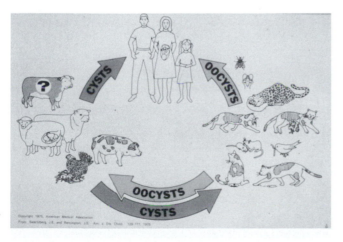

Figure 64–1. Life cycle of *Toxoplasma gondii*. (*Reprinted with permission from Am J Dis Child. 1975;129:777–779. Copyright 1975 American Medical Association.*)

Transmission

There are many different ways humans can acquire *T. gondii*; ingestion of the oocyte is the most common. This occurs when undercooked infected meat, and contaminated vegetables and food are eaten (Frenckel, 1985), and ingestion of raw milk (Sacks et al, 1982). Handling infected cats, infected litter boxes, sandboxes, or soil may also result in the transmission of *T. gondii*. Accidental needle pricks have been reported to result in infection (Shoukrey & Tabbara, 1986), as have blood transfusions and organ transplants (McCabe & Remington, 1984; Ryning et al, 1979). *T. gondii* can cross the placenta in a pregnant woman (usually unaware of the infection) to infect the developing fetus (Desmonts & Couvreur, 1974; Desmonts et al, 1985; Perkins, 1973).

Course of the Disease

Clinically, toxoplasmosis infection in humans may be divided into the following types: acquired toxoplasmosis, congenital toxoplasmosis, and toxoplasmosis in the immunosuppressed individual (Table 64–1).

■ Systemic

Acquired Toxoplasmosis

Once infected, the majority of human hosts is rarely symptomatic, with only 10 to 20% reporting symptoms (Remington & Desmonts, 1983). Some of the symptoms, such as fever, malaise, sore throat, and myalgia can mimic influenza or infectious mononucleosis. The most common systemic manifestation of acquired toxoplasma infection is cervical lymphadenopathy. This can be associated with fever, malaise, myalgia, fatigue, headache, sore throat, and a maculopapillar rash. Some of the symptoms can last for several months. Fatigue is the earliest symptom and often the last to subside. The liver and spleen may also be affected. Central nervous system infection may lead to encephalitis, particularly in immunosuppressed individuals, and is often fatal (Parke & Font, 1986).

■ Ocular

Acquired Toxoplasmosis

The organism in its mobile tachyzoite form reaches the ocular structures via the bloodstream, and enters the retinal cells, causing a retinitis, which can then affect the choroid, leading to a retinochoroiditis. The organism primarily affects the retina, resulting in consequent inflammation of the choroid and sclera. Therefore, this process is termed "retinochoroiditis" as opposed to "chorioretinitis" seen in other inflammatory conditions.

The retinochoroiditis creates a vitreous reaction or vitritis, due to the release of inflammatory cells and *Toxoplasma* antigens into the vitreous. This can spill over into the anterior chamber, resulting in an anterior uveitis.

TABLE 64–1. SYSTEMIC MANIFESTATIONS OF TOXOPLASMOSIS

TYPE OF TOXOPLASMOSIS	SYMPTOMS	SIGNS
• Acquired systemic toxoplasmosis	• Fever • Malaise • Sore throat • Myalgia	• Cervical lymphadenopathy • Maculopapillar rash • Liver and spleen enlargement • Rising toxoplasma antibody titers
• Congenital toxoplasmosis	• Rash • Fever • Psychomotor retardation • Jaundice	• Hydro- or microcephaly • CSF abnormalities • Cerebral calcifications • Lymphadenopathy • Enlarged spleen
• Toxoplasmosis in the immunocompromised	• Same as in acquired toxoplasmosis PLUS • Confusion • Headache	• Same as in acquired toxoplasmosis EXCEPT serologic tests may show elevated rather than changing antibody titers PLUS • Encephalitis • Coma • Myositis • Myocarditis • Pneumonitis (rarely)

The mobile tachyzoite eventually reverts into the less active bradyzoite, which becomes encysted. These cysts remain within the ocular tissue and can lie dormant for years. Eventually they burst, releasing multiple bradyzoites. If an individual has normal immunity, the protozoans can be controlled. If immunity is compromised, because of immunosuppressive drugs, stress, or HIV infection, recurrences of previous infections may occur.

Patients with acquired toxoplasmosis may develop a retinochoroiditis (usually unilateral) months to years after the initial onset of the disease. Reduced visual acuity is usually the presenting symptom. This may be the only manifestation of infection and has also been reported as an initial manifestation of AIDS (Weiss et al, 1986).

The retinochoroiditis consists of focal white fluffy lesions affecting the inner retinal layers. These lesions are often surrounded by edema resulting in hazy borders (Figure 64–2). They may be single or multiple and can vary in size as well as location. Some can be so large as to form granulomas, associated with marked vitritis, which can make visualization of the fundus difficult. Visual acuity will be affected depending on the degree of vitritis and location of the lesions. If the lesions affect the macula, papillomacular bundle, and/or optic nerve, there will be a subsequent loss of visual acuity even without much vitritis. Some lesions affect the outer retinal layers and are more gray-white in appearance. These lesions are not, as a rule, associated with much overlying vitritis.

Healing of the retinochoroiditis lesions results in a punched-out scar with sclera visible in the center and pigment heaped up on the sides (Figure 64–3). Once the inflammatory reaction has subsided, including any vitritis, visual acuity will improve, unless the macula or optic nerve has been adversely affected from the infection. The scars harbor *Toxoplasma* cysts. Therefore, over time, recurrences of the retinochoroiditis will occur at the edge of previous scars to form satellite lesions. The exception to this is in

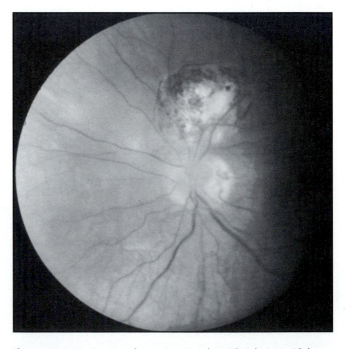

Figure 64–2. Active toxoplasmosis retinochoroiditis lesion with hazy borders.

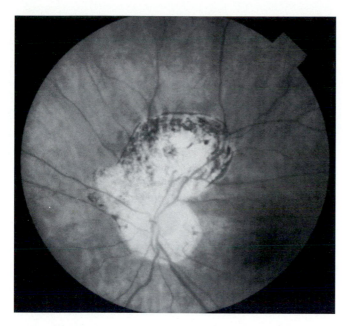

Figure 64–3. Healed toxoplasmosis retinochoroiditis lesion with pigmented borders and sclera and large choroidal vessels visible in the center.

acquired toxoplasmosis in the immunosuppressed patient. In these patients, toxoplasmosis is a more diffuse disease. Therefore, lesions can appear anywhere in the retina and are not necessarily associated with old lesions. All inactive toxoplasmosis scars need to be examined annually for signs of recurring retinochoroiditis.

The optic nerve can develop an optic neuritis or papillitis with no other evidence of retinal involvement. A rare case of neuroretinitis has been reported as a manifestation of ocular toxoplasmosis in which a patient presented with a swollen disk and a macular star (Moreno, 1992).

Patients with active ocular toxoplasmosis must also be closely monitored for the development of retinal tears and subsequent retinal detachment. The etiology of these tears is believed to be due to the increased vitreal traction on the retina from the vitritis.

There appears to be an association between Fuchs heterochromic cyclitis and ocular toxoplasmosis, but the reason is not well known (De Abreu et al, 1982; Schwab, 1991). It has been suggested (Schwab, 1991) that the toxoplasmosis causes an anterior segment inflammation that can lead to heterochromia, posterior cataract, and iridocyclitis that looks like Fuchs heterochromic disease but that may actually have a different pathogenesis.

■ Systemic

Congenital Toxoplasmosis
The highest incidence of transmission of *T. gondii* from mother to developing fetus is in the third trimester, and the

lowest is in the first trimester of pregnancy (Desmonts & Couvreur, 1974). Approximately 60% of fetuses will be affected when *T. gondii* is acquired during pregnancy, especially during the third trimester (Remington et al, 1983). However, the earlier in pregnancy the disease is acquired, the more severe the manifestations of the disease.

Clinical systemic signs of congenital toxoplasmosis in the newborn can vary and may include hydrocephaly or microcephaly, cerebral calcifications, rash, fever, psychomotor retardation, jaundice, lymphadenopathy, enlarged spleen, and cerebrospinal fluid abnormalities.

■ Ocular

Congenital Toxoplasmosis
Ocular signs include microphthalmia, enophthalmos, ptosis, nystagmus, strabismus, and iris and lens abnormalities. The most common finding, however, is the ocular manifestation of retinochoroiditis, especially affecting the maculas in both eyes (Figure 64–4), which can develop weeks after the onset of systemic symptoms.

Retinochoroiditis lesions often occur in the maculas in congenital toxoplasmosis probably because the *Toxoplasma* tachyzoite becomes trapped in the small terminal perifoveal capillaries (Tabbara, 1987). Some macular toxoplasmosis lesions have been erroneously diagnosed as macular colobomas. The condition can reactivate years later, resulting in the formation of new lesions adjacent to previously healed scars.

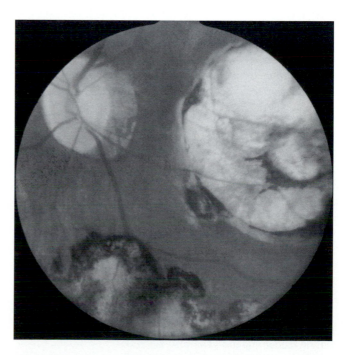

Figure 64–4. Macular toxoplasmosis retinochoroidal lesions usually signify congenital infection.

■ Systemic

Toxoplasmosis in the Immunosuppressed Patient

In a healthy individual, it is rare for acquired toxoplasmosis to manifest any clinical signs, and infected people are often never aware they have acquired the disease. However, the immunocompromised patient presents another picture. In contrast to a healthy individual, the immunocompromised patient will manifest systemic signs and symptoms of this disease. This has become more of a clinical dilemma in the last several years with the development and progression of AIDS in the population.

Those with compromised immune systems chiefly suffer from *T. gondii* infection (acquired or reactivation) of the central nervous system and the eyes (Gaglioso & Teich, 1990). *T. gondii* also affects the liver, spleen, lung, heart, and lymph nodes.

■ Ocular

Toxoplasmosis in the Immunosuppressed Patient

The ocular involvement is similar to previously described ocular manifestations of acquired toxoplasmosis, and will consist of one or more retinochoroidal lesions or massive areas of retinal necrosis (Holland, 1989), which may affect one or both eyes. Unlike toxoplasmosis in immunocompetent patients, these lesions arise in areas unassociated with previously healed toxoplasmosis scars, suggesting acquired infection or dissemination of the organism. The lesions also do not pigment as well as they do in the congenital and acquired immunocompetent forms. The explanation for this is as yet unclear. Due to their immunocompromised state, there is a minimal amount of vitritis and uveitis in these patients.

In addition, *T. gondii* may infect the iris, choroid, and vitreous. These areas are not usually affected in persons with normal immunity. The ocular lesions respond to standard treatment; however, the very immunocompromised host must be kept on a maintenance dose to prevent reactivation.

DIAGNOSIS

■ Systemic

The most common clinical sign of systemic toxoplasmosis is cervical lymphadenopathy. This may be associated with flu-like symptoms such as fever, headache, sore throat, and fatigue. Sometimes mistaken for infectious mononucleosis, systemic toxoplasmosis can also simulate lymphomas and Hodgkin disease. The palpable lymph nodes may or may not be tender and are generally discrete.

Serologic tests are used in the differential diagnosis of acquired systemic toxoplasmosis, because it can simulate other diseases. These tests have their limitations, mainly because some give false-positive results and because antibodies to *Toxoplasma* organisms are highly prevalent in certain areas. However, in some situations, the clinical picture may not easily define the diagnosis therefore requiring the use of serologic tests.

Following acute infection, antibody titers go from negative or a low of 1 in 16 to a high of 1 in 1024 in 6 to 8 weeks. These levels then gradually decrease over months to years. A rising antibody titer indicates acute infection.

The main serologic tests used in the diagnosis of active *Toxoplasma* infection, whether systemic or ocular, are the Sabin–Feldman or methylene blue dye test, indirect fluorescent antibody (IFA) test, indirect hemagglutination test, and enzyme-linked immunosorbent assay (ELISA). Other serologic tests may be used, but only the most widely used will be discussed here.

The Sabin–Feldman or methylene blue dye test is a sensitive and specific test and is the reference against which all other serologic tests are evaluated. Methylene blue dye will not stain *Toxoplasma* organisms following lysis of their cell membranes with sera containing *Toxoplasma* antibodies. This test is not carried out in many hospitals because it is necessary to maintain a live supply of *Toxoplasma* organisms.

The indirect fluorescent antibody (IFA) test is a widely used serologic test and has good sensitivity, specificity, and reproducibility. It is more widely used than the dye test because it does not require living parasites. It detects the presence of IgG and IgM antibodies. This test is useful in diagnosing congenital toxoplasmosis infection because of its ability to detect IgM antibodies not normally found in the newborn. It is positive in the majority of infants born with congenital toxoplasmosis. It will be negative in immunosuppressed patients, and false-positive results can be caused by the presence of antinuclear antibodies or rheumatoid factors.

The indirect hemagglutination test is popular because of its ease of use. Its only drawback appears to be an inability to detect antibodies early in the active stage of infection (Schlaegel, 1978).

The ELISA test is both sensitive and specific for the serodiagnosis of toxoplasmosis (Milatovic & Bravery, 1980). It can detect the presence of IgG and IgM antibodies as well as antigens produced by the organism. It can also test the presence of antibodies in serum and in ocular fluids and is helpful in making the differential diagnosis in some cases (Rollins et al, 1983). The ELISA test can detect 70 to 80% of congenitally infected infants.

There are different techniques for performing an ELISA test depending upon whether testing for the presence of antibodies or antigens. The ELISA test can detect antigens and is therefore useful in determining if the organism is still present. This may be advantageous in cases of panuveitis where the fundus may not be well visualized. Furthermore, the

TABLE 64–2. OCULAR MANIFESTATIONS OF TOXOPLASMOSIS

TYPE OF TOXOPLASMOSIS	SYMPTOMS	SIGNS
• Acquired systemic toxoplasmosis	• Reduced visual acuity • Photophobia • Subsequent to infection	• Retinochoroiditis • Vitritis • Anterior uveitis • Optic neuritis or papillitis • Retinal tears • Retinal detachments • Well-pigmented chorioretinal scars • New lesions originating near old scars
• Congenital toxoplasmosis	• Reduced vision from birth or shortly after birth	• Retinochoroiditis (often bilateral macular lesions) • Microphthalmia • Enophthalmos • Ptosis • Nystagmus • Strabismus
• Toxoplasmosis in the immunocompromised	• Reduced vision if lesions affect macula, optic nerve or papillomacular bundle	• Retinochoroiditis • Poorly pigmented scars • Minimal vitritis • New lesions unassociated with previous scars

ELISA test will not test false-positive with antinuclear antibodies or rheumatoid factor. As a result, in most clinical settings, ELISA is the first test of choice to use when determining acute infection.

Neuroradiologic techniques are not usually ordered except when a child is born with manifestations suggesting congenital infection or in the immunocompromised patient. In such cases, a CT scan would reveal areas of calcification within the brain. CNS involvement can be detected using CT scan and MRI with contrast in which multiple, diffuse ring-shaped lesions become evident (Gaglioso et al, 1990). CT and MRI testing in the AIDS patient with toxoplasmosis encephalitis may reveal a multitude of these lesions.

■ Ocular

The presenting symptom of active ocular toxoplasmosis is reduced visual acuity caused by vitritis and/or inflammatory retinochoroidal lesions affecting the macula and/or optic nerve. The diagnosis of ocular infection is based on the clinical presentation and supporting lab work (Table 64–2).

TREATMENT AND MANAGEMENT

The drug regimen to treat toxoplasmosis can be complicated and is not without side effects. Therefore, prevention is the rule. The consumption of raw or undercooked meat should be avoided. Hands should be washed after handling cats, litter boxes and sandboxes, uncooked meat, and soil. Pregnant women who do not have antibodies against the disease should try to avoid contact with cats.

If and when to treat an infected patient depends upon the activity of the disease. Newborns with congenital toxoplasmosis are treated. Adults with ocular toxoplasmosis are treated during recurrence of retinochoroiditis when lesions threaten the macula, papillomacular bundle, or optic nerve. Individuals with AIDS suffering from CNS and/or ocular toxoplasmosis receive similar treatment as well, which has been shown to be effective in over 75% of patients (Gaglioso et al, 1990).

■ Systemic

The standard agents currently used in the treatment of toxoplasmosis include pyrimethamine (Daraprim), sulfadiazine or trisulfapyrimidine, clindamycin, folinic acid, and corticosteroids (Table 64–3). These medications act to kill the active tachyzoite and suppress inflammation, but there is no effective agent to wipe out the inactive bradyzoite. Pyrimethamine and sulfadiazine are used in conjunction and operate at different steps in the synthesis of nucleic acid.

Pyrimethamine may induce leukopenia and thrombocytopenia; therefore, patients on this regimen must have their blood counts monitored. Folinic acid should be added to counteract the effects of pyrimethamine-induced folate deficiency. Clindamycin, unlike pyrimethamine, does not cross the blood–brain barrier. Hence, it should not be used in the treatment of congenital toxoplasmosis or in toxoplasmosis encephalitis. Its systemic side effects include pseudomembranous colitis.

TABLE 64–3. TREATMENT AND MANAGEMENT OF TOXOPLASMOSIS (SYSTEMIC AND OCULAR)

ADULT PATIENT
1. Pyrimethamine
   Loading dose 75 mg po × 2 days
   Then 25 mg/d × 3–6 wks
   Monitor blood counts for leukopenia and
      thrombocytopenia
   combined with sulfadiazine *or* trisulfapyrimidine
   Loading dose 2g po followed by 1g qid × 3–6 wks
   adjunct: folinic acid
   3–5 mg IM or po 2 x/wk
                       or
   Clindamycin:
   300 mg po qid × 3–6 wks
   Does not cross blood–brain barrier, do not use in toxo
      encephalitis
   May cause colitis
   combined with sulfadiazine *or* trisulfapyrimidine
   Loading dose 2g po followed by 1g qid × 3–6 wks
                       plus
   Prednisone
   20–80 mg po daily with 3–6 wks taper
   May cause increased IOP, and/or cataracts
                       OR
2. Trimethoprim–sulfamethoxazole
   160 mg (trimeth) plus 800 mg (sulfameth) po bid 4–6
      wks
   May cause skin rash and/or mild diarrhea
   alone or combined with clindamycin
   300 mg qid × 2 wks

                       plus
Prednisone:
   80 mg qd × 2 days, tapered 20 mg qid to 20 mg qd ×
      4 wks
   May cause increased IOP and/or cataracts
3. Ocular topical agents used in cases of anterior uveitis
   Prednisolone acetate
   0.5–1.0% frequency variable
   Homatropine
   2–5% bid—qid

IMMUNOCOMPROMISED PATIENT
1. Same regimen as adult patient (doses may be increased)
2. *Exception:* Prednisone is contraindicated

INFANT PATIENT
1. Pyrimethamine
   1mg/kg/d po once every 3 days
   Monitor blood counts for leukopenia and
      thrombocytopenia
   Combined with sulfadiazine
   50–100 mg/kg/d po in 2 divided doses × 3 wks

PREGNANT PATIENT
1. Pyrimethamine
   Not advised because it is teratogenic during the first
      trimester
2. Sulfadiazine
   Loading dose 2 g po followed by 1g qid × 4 wks
3. Abortion (if indicated)

The immunosuppressed patient with toxoplasmosis encephalitis may be treated with the same drugs (although possibly in higher doses) as other individuals with the exception of corticosteroid use, which in general is contraindicated in immunosuppression. In addition, persons with AIDS must be on a maintenance dose once the condition resolves or else a relapse will occur. Treatment with pyrimethamine alone as maintenance therapy for CNS toxoplasmosis in persons with AIDS has been shown to be effective (DeGans et al, 1992).

Infants with congenital toxoplasmosis are treated with a lighter drug regimen (see Table 64–3). Women who contract toxoplasmosis during the early stages of pregnancy may be advised to consider abortion because of the severity of the disease on the developing fetus, even though the risk of infection is lower in the earlier stages of pregnancy. Treatment during pregnancy is limited to sulfadiazine, because pyrimethamine is teratogenic during the first two trimesters.

■ Ocular

The treatment for systemic toxoplasmosis and ocular toxoplasmosis are the same. Systemic medication is essential due to the poor penetration of topically applied agents into the vitreous. If, in rare cases, there is a spillover of any vitreal reaction into the anterior chamber, then topically

applied antiinflammatory and cycloplegic agents may be added to the systemic regimen.

Corticosteroids are also used only when the retinochoroiditis lesions affect the optic nerve, papillomacular bundle, or macula, thus threatening vision (see Table 64–3). In a recent study of common treatment modalities for ocular toxoplasmosis, nearly 95% of respondants used corticosteroids as part of their initial treatment regimen (Engstrom et al, 1991). Other antiparasitic agents sometimes used in the treatment of toxoplasmosis include tetracycline, spiramycin (available in Europe only), and minocycline.

Recently, the increasing difficulty in obtaining the standard medications for the treatment of ocular toxoplasmosis led to a study by Opremcak and associates (1992) investigating the efficacy of a fixed-combination antibiotic called trimethoprim–sulfamethoxazole (Bactrim DS). Sixteen patients with active toxoplasmosis were treated with either trimethoprim–sulfamethoxazole alone, or in combination with clindamycin and prednisone. All 16 patients demonstrated improved acuity and resolution of the retinochoroiditis. However, the investigators cautioned that further research is needed to firmly establish trimethoprim–sulfamethoxazole as an effective substitute for conventional therapy.

Treatment of ocular toxoplasmosis may not be necessary when retinochoroiditis foci lie outside the vascular arcades and do not threaten the optic nerve, macula, or papillomacular bundle and when the vitreal reaction does not obscure vision to worse than about 20/70. These lesions, however, must be monitored frequently to assess progression.

Other treatment modalities may include vitrectomy in cases where vitreous exudation and vitreous membranes result in decreased vision and retinal traction. Photocoagulation and cryotherapy have also been used in the treatment of toxoplasmosis, but there are complications such as hemorrhage and retinal detachment associated with both procedures. In addition, although these two procedures can focally obliterate the live tachyzoite as well as the cysts, the organism may occur elsewhere in the retina; hence total eradication is not possible.

The follow-up of the patient with active toxoplasmosis includes frequent (weekly) measures of visual acuity, anterior chamber evaluation for possible spillover of the vitritis, measurement of intraocular pressure, and dilated fundus examinations. Once lesions have healed (or in the case of a new patient having healed retinochoroiditis lesions), visual fields should be performed to assess any defects resulting from the lesions. Lesions affecting the papillomacular bundle may result in field defects disproportionate with the size of the lesion. Patients with inactive toxoplasmosis should be monitored annually.

CONCLUSION

Despite all that is known about the transmission of *Toxoplasma gondii*, toxoplasmosis is still prevalent. With the development and progression of AIDS, it is no longer a rarity to see patients with the acquired form of this disease. Future research must concentrate on the development of a vaccine against the disease as well as less teratogenic therapeutic agents that can also be effective against the inactive cysts. More sensitive and specific serologic tests need to be developed to detect the antibodies and *Toxoplasma* antigens in blood serum as well as in ocular fluids. In addition, the causative mechanisms of recurrences need to be investigated. Research also needs to address toxoplasmosis in the immunosuppressed patient in terms of the role of the immune system and how infection can best be prevented and controlled.

REFERENCES

Alexander L. *Primary Care of the Posterior Segment*. 2nd ed. Norwalk, CT: Appleton & Lange; 1994:315–319, 324.

Anderson S. *Toxoplasma gondii*. In: Mandell GL, Douglas RG Jr, Bennett JE, eds. *Principles and Practice of Infectious Diseases*. New York: Wiley; 1979:2127.

Cassady JV. Toxoplasmic retinochoroiditis. *Trans Am Ophthalmol Soc*. 1960;58:392.

De Abreu MT, Belfort R, Hirata PS. Fuchs' heterochromic cyclitis and ocular toxoplasmosis. *Am J Ophthalmol*. 1982;93:739–44.

DeGans J, Portegres P, Reiss P, et al. Pyrimethamine alone as main therapy for central nervous system toxoplasmosis in 38 patients with AIDS. *J AIDS*. 1992;5:137–142.

Desmonts G, Couvreur J. Congenital toxoplasmosis: A prospective study of 378 pregnancies. *N Engl J Med*. 1974;290:1110.

Desmonts G, Forestier F, Thulliez P, et al. Prenatal diagnosis of congenital toxoplasmosis. *Lancet*. 1985;1:500.

Engstrom RE Jr, Holland GN, Nussenblatt RB, Jabs DA. Current practices in the management of ocular toxoplasmosis. *Am J Ophthalmol*. 1991;111:601–610.

Feldman HA, Miller LT. Serological study of toxoplasmosis prevalence. *Am J Hyg*. 1956;64:320.

Frenkel JK. Toxoplasmosis. *Pediatr Clin North Am*. 1985;32:917.

Gaglioso DJ, Teich SA, Friedman AH, Orellana J. Ocular toxoplasmosis in AIDS patients. *Trans Am Ophthalmol Soc*. 1990;88:63–86.

Holland GN. Ocular toxoplasmosis in the immunocompromised host. *Int Ophthalmol*. 1989;13:399–402.

McCabe RE, Remington JS. Toxoplasmosis. In: Warren KS, Mahmoud AAF, eds. *Tropical and Geographical Medicine*. New York: McGraw-Hill; 1984:281.

McCabe RE, Remington JS. Toxoplasma gondii. In: Mandell GL, Douglas RG, Bennett JE, eds. *Principles and Practice of Infectious Diseases*. 3rd ed. New York: Churchill Livingstone; 1990:2090–2103.

Milatovic D, Bravery I. Enzyme-linked immunosorbent assay for the serological diagnosis of toxoplasmosis. *J Clin Pathol*. 1980;33:841–844.

Moreno RJ. Neuroretinitis: An unusual presentation of ocular toxoplasmosis. *Ann Ophthalmol*. 1992;24:68–70.

Nicolle C, Manceaux L. Sur une infection a corps de Leishman (ou organismes voisins du gondi). *Compt Rend Acad Sci*. 1908;147:763.

Opremcak EM, Scales DK, Sharpe MR. Trimethoprim–sulfamethoxazole therapy for ocular toxoplasmosis. *Ophthalmology*. 1992;99:920–925.

Parke DW II, Font RL. Diffuse toxoplasma retinochoroiditis in a patient with AIDS. *Arch Ophthalmol*. 1986;104:571.

Perkins ES. Ocular toxoplasmosis. *Br J Ophthalmol*. 1973;57:1.

Remington JS. Toxoplasmosis in the adult. *Bull NY Acad Med*. 1974;50:211–227.

Remington JS, Desmonts G. Toxoplasmosis. In: Remington JS, Klein JO, eds. *Infectious Diseases of the Fetus and Newborn Infant*. 2nd ed. Philadelphia: Saunders; 1983:143.

Rollins DF, Tabbara KF, O'Connor GR, et al. Detection of toxoplasmal antigen and antibody in ocular fluids in experimental ocular toxoplasmosis. *Arch Ophthalmol*. 1983;101:455.

Ryning FW, McLeod R, Maddox, JC, et al. Probable transmission of *Toxoplasma gondii* by organ transplantation. *Ann Intern Med*. 1979;90:47.

Sacks JJ, Roberto RR, Brooks NF. Toxoplasmosis infection associated with raw goats milk. *JAMA*. 1982;248:1728.

Schlaegel TF. *Ocular Toxoplasmosis and Pars Planitis*. New York: Grune & Stratton; 1978:8.

Schwab IR. The epidemiological association of Fuchs' heterochromic iridocyclitis and ocular toxoplasmosis. *Am J Ophthalmol*. 1991;111:356–362.

Shoukrey N, Tabbara KF. Eye related parasitic diseases. In: Tabbara KF, Hyndiuk RA, eds. *Infections of the Eye*. Boston: Little, Brown; 1986:167.

Tabbara KF. Toxoplasmosis. In: Tasman W, Jaeger EA, eds. *Clinical Ophthalmology*. Philadelphia: Harper & Row; 1987; 4.

Tabbara KF. Management of ocular toxoplasmosis. *Trans Pacific Coast Ophthalmol Soc*. 1983;63:23.

Weiss A, Margo CE, Ledford, DK, et al. Toxoplasmic retinochoroiditis as an initial manifestation of AIDS. *Am J Ophthalmol*. 1986;101:248.

65

Chapter

Toxocariasis

Diane T. Adamczyk

Toxocariasis is caused by the parasite *Toxocara canis*, a roundworm commonly found in dogs. Human infection occurs most frequently in children, who often have a history of eating dirt that is contaminated with parasite eggs, from dog excrement. Once infected, *Toxocara* in humans manifests as either the systemic disease, visceral larva migrans (VLM), or the ocular disease, ocular larva migrans. VLM may involve multiple organs (eg, the liver, lungs, and heart) along with the central nervous system. Ocular manifestations vary from minimal or no symptoms to marked symptomatology. Correct diagnosis is important, particularly with ocular involvement, because appropriate management can preserve both vision and the eye.

EPIDEMIOLOGY

■ Systemic

Toxocara is a common, global parasitic infection that occurs in domestic animals, particularly dogs. Reports worldwide indicate that 13.5 to 93% of dogs may be infected. Puppies in particular are at greatest risk of infection, with more than 80% found to be infected between 2 and 6 months of age, decreasing to less than 20% in those older than 1 year. Transmission of *Toxocara* eggs may occur through dog excretion, with the eggs often found in dirt. Soil contaminated with *Toxocara* may be found in 10 to 30% of public areas (parks and playgrounds), while 11% of private areas (backyards and gardens) are contaminated (Childs, 1985). VLM is found more commonly in the south central and southeastern part of the United States, possibly because soil and climatic conditions harbor *Toxocara* eggs better.

The risks of infection, particularly for children, are high, especially in those with a history of pica or geophagia (eating dirt) or owning a puppy. Although any age may be affected, VLM occurs most commonly in children between 1 and 4 years, with an average age of 2 years. Although both sexes and all races are affected, boys,

African-American children, and children of parents with an education below high school level are more commonly infected. Although studies are inconsistent, those individuals having greater contact with dogs through occupations such as dog breeding may have increased exposure to *Toxocara*.

The exact incidence of *Toxocara* infection in humans is not known, because many cases go undiagnosed or unrecognized. Serologic evidence of infection may be found in up to 6.5% of the general population, with up to 30% in children. Systemic involvement commonly includes hepatomegaly in 87% and pulmonary manifestations in approximately 50%, with *Toxocara* reported in 13.6% of patients with poliomyelitis and 7.5% of patients with epilepsy (Mok, 1968).

■ Ocular

As with VLM, ocular involvement from *Toxocara* occurs most commonly in children, but at a slightly older age. Although any age may be affected, ocular manifestations are seen in 4 to 8 year olds, with an average age of 7.5 years. Central lesions occur more commonly in children 6 to 14 years of age, with peripheral lesions more common in adolescents and adults (Wan et al, 1991).

493

Usually one eye is affected, with 2.4% having bilateral involvement (Brown, 1970). Ten percent of uveitis in children may be secondary to *Toxocara* (Perkins, 1966). Ocular and systemic disease rarely occur together.

NATURAL HISTORY

The Organism

Toxocara is a roundworm that infects domestic animals, with *T. canis* commonly infecting the dog. The complete life cycle of *T. canis* occurs in the dog, its natural host. Infection in the dog may occur through reactivation of larvae from hormonal changes in a pregnant bitch, with transplacental transfer to the puppy; from a nursing bitch's milk; from a nursing bitch licking her young; from ingesting feces; or from eating an infected mouse or rabbit. In the prenatally infected puppy, at birth, a third-stage larva is formed in the lungs, which the puppy coughs up and swallows. This then goes to the small intestine, maturing to adult worms in approximately 3 weeks. The adult worm sheds 200,000 eggs per day through the puppy's feces, until 4 to 6 months of age, when the infection decreases. Eggs are also shed through a lactating bitch's feces. These eggs become infectious in 2 to 7 weeks, and may remain viable, dependent on soil type and climate, for months to years. The adult dog may ingest the eggs, which hatch in the small intestine, with second-stage larvae passing through the intestinal wall. These travel to various organs and tissues (liver, lungs, brain, eye), usually remaining in these tissues, instead of completing the cycle as in a puppy.

Transmission

Humans are infected through pica or geophagia, poor hygiene (particularly after playing or working in dirt or around infected puppies), or sometimes by ingesting food contaminated with eggs from infected soil, such as lettuce. In the small intestine the ova hatch, with the larvae going through the intestinal wall, traveling to various tissues and organs, via the blood or lymphatic system. When the larvae cannot pass through the blood vessel because of its size, they travel through the blood vessel wall into the surrounding tissue. Larvae may remain viable in these tissues for weeks, months, or even years, eventually dying. The larvae may become dormant, later to reactivate. In humans, a complete life cycle to mature adult worms does not occur, which explains why human feces lack ova. Inflammation, hemorrhage, necrosis, or an eosinophilic granulomatous response may occur with infection in either systemic or ocular disease.

Course of the Disease

■ Systemic

As the life cycle of *Toxocara* evolves in humans, various organs and tissues may be affected, with numerous systemic manifestations resulting (Table 65–1) in visceral larva migrans (VLM). These manifestations are related to larval migration and its sequelae, along with larval death, which may produce more severe reactions than the live larva. Eosinophils surround the larva, with the development of an inflammatory, granulomatous reaction along with fibrous tissue. Clinical manifestations most commonly include fever, fatigue, lymphadenopathy, and eosinophilia. Toxocariasis generally follows an unremarkable course, resolving in weeks, with an incubation time of days to months. Eosinophilia may last for years, with the antibody titer often decreasing over time. Rarely, the course of the disease results in death, which is usually from complications of myocarditis or encephalitis.

■ Ocular

The effect of *Toxocara* in the eye (Table 65–2) differs in a number of respects from systemic involvement. Ocular symptoms may result from just one or two larvae, whereas many larvae are needed to elicit symptoms from larger organs, such as the liver. Ocular manifestations occur at a later age than VLM. This may be due to a latent period that follows the initial infection. Reactivation occurs years later, resulting in ocular manifestations.

The larva enters the eye through the choroidal (posterior ciliary) and retinal circulation, migrating to the subretinal area or vitreous. The incubation period may take

TABLE 65–1. SYSTEMIC MANIFESTATIONS OF TOXOCARIASIS (VISCERAL LARVAL MIGRANS)

SIGNS/SYMPTOMS
- Fever, abdominal pain, fatigue/malaise, headache, pallor, anemia, anorexia/weight loss, irritability, sleep/behavioral disturbances, nausea, vomiting, pharyngitis, limb pains, dizziness, constipation, poliomyelitis
- Eosinophilia, leucocytosis, elevated isohemagglutinations, increased serum gammaglobulin (IgG, IgM)
- Lymphadenopathy

VISCERAL INVOLVEMENT
- Splenomegaly
- Hepatomegaly
- Pulmonary involvement
    Pneumonia, cough, wheeze, bronchitis, asthma, transient pulmonary infiltrates on chest films
- Neurologic involvement
    Seizures or epilepsy, behavior disorders, increased eosinophils in cerebrospinal fluid
- Dermatologic involvement
    Urticarial, pruritic, or nodular skin rash
- Cardiac involvement
    Myocarditis

TABLE 65–2. OCULAR MANIFESTATIONS OF *TOXOCARA*

VITREORETINAL INVOLVEMENT
- Retinochoroiditis
- Vitritis
- White mass/granuloma (1/2 to 4 disk diameters)
- Retinal traction
- Vitreous bands
- Traction bands (extend from lesion to disk or macula)
- Retinal folds
- Heterotropic macula
- Tortuous/deviated vessels
- Distorted optic nervehead
- Macular granuloma, associated with hemorrhages or serous detachment
- Peripheral–falciform fold, unilateral pars planitis, retinal fold from peripheral mass to optic nervehead
- Other: retinal hemorrhage, retinal edema, papillitis (rare), secondary retinal artery occlusion

ENDOPHTHALMITIS
- Minimal pain or photophobia
- Leukocoria
- Cyclitic membrane
- Eosinophils in vitreous
- Vitritis
- Keratic precipitates
- Hypopyon (rare)
- Anterior chamber reaction (less common)
- Secondary cataract and glaucoma, synechiae, iris bombe, phthisis bulbi

MISCELLANEOUS
- Strabismus, keratitis (rare), conjunctivitis, larva in lens (rare), iris nodules (rare), diffuse unilateral subacute neuroretinitis

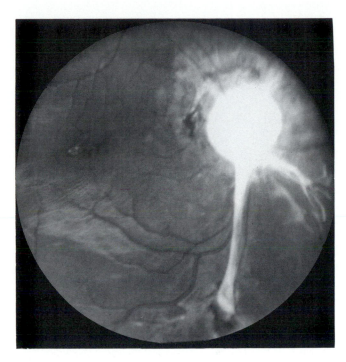

Figure 65–1. *T. canis* vitreoretinal band to the optic nervehead. *(Photo courtesy of Dr. Jerome Sherman, SUNY, College of Optometry.)*

Endophthalmitis is usually associated with minimal pain and photophobia, possibly resulting in leukocoria, retinal detachment, retrolental mass, or cyclitic membrane. Visual prognosis with cyclitic membranes is generally poor, requiring prompt surgical intervention.

DIAGNOSIS

■ Systemic

Many cases of VLM may be misdiagnosed or go undetected. The definitive diagnosis of *Toxocara* is made based on tissue biopsy; however, this is often not possible. A history of geophagia, exposure to dogs, suggestive clinical manifestations, and other testing procedures will support the diagnosis. *Toxocara* infection should be ruled out in children with seizures or epilepsy.

Enzyme-linked immunosorbent assay (ELISA) has proven to be one of the most reliable and sensitive tests for *Toxocara*. ELISA may indicate past or present infection. The recommended titer for diagnosis of VLM is 1 in 32, which has a sensitivity of 78% and specificity of 92%.

Eosinophilia is frequently present in *Toxocara*. However, its absence does not preclude the diagnosis. When eosinophilia is present, it may remain for months, possibly years after the initial infection. Leukocytosis, elevated serum gamma globulin (IgG and IgM), and isohemaglutinin titers against A and B blood may be found.

months to years, with death of the larva eventually occurring. *Toxocara* causes damage to the eye by direct affect of the larva to the eye and/or from the inflammatory response. Larval death results in a more marked inflammatory response than that of the live larva.

Toxocara usually affects only one eye, manifesting as a focal retinal granuloma, peripheral inflammatory mass, and/or endophthalmitis. As the larva migrates through the choroid and retina, a retinochoroiditis with an overlying vitreous reaction may occur, either centrally or peripherally. A granulomatous reaction and a white fibrous mass may result. The granuloma most commonly is found in the macular or peripapillary area, but may also occur in the periphery. Eventually this lesion takes on a more glistening white or gray appearance, with the inflammation subsiding. Vitreous bands, retinal dragging, strabismus, heterotropia of the macula, and vision loss may subsequently occur (Figures 65–1 and 65–2). Vision may be preserved in cases of peripheral lesions.

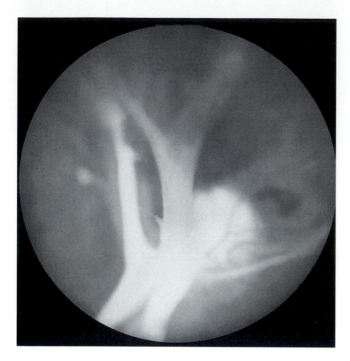

Figure 65–2. Marked vitreous band in suspected *T. canis. (Photo courtesy of Dr. Scott Richter, SUNY, College of Optometry.)*

Other tests must be interpreted with caution because of cross-reactions with other parasites, and lack of sensitivity and specificity (eg, fluorescent antibody and hemagglutinin tests). Stool and urine testing does not assist in the diagnosis, since *Toxocara* is not excreted in humans.

■ Ocular

Ocular diagnosis of *Toxocara* is based on clinical presentation, history, and a complete eye evaluation. A unilateral inflammation, pars planitis, or leukocoria in a child should make the practitioner suspicious of *Toxocara*. Definitive diagnosis, although not always determined, is made through histologic evidence of the organism in an enucleated eye.

Diagnosis may be relatively easy, based on the classic clinical presentation of a granuloma, with associated retinal manifestations. However, the use of specific tests (eg, for eosinophilia or ELISA), which are often helpful in VLM, may be equivocal in ocular disease. Antibody levels in ocular *Toxocara* are weaker than in VLM. An ELISA of 1 in 8 is the criterion for ocular diagnosis. With this criteria, ELISA has a 90% sensitivity and 91% specificity for ocular *Toxocara* (Pollard, 1979). However, the presence of an elevated titer does not provide a definitive diagnosis, but in the presence of clinical signs may be supportive of one. When the diagnosis is questionable, aqueous or vitreous samples should be taken, which may demonstrate eosinophils and positive ELISA findings, along with absence of tumor cells that may be present in retinoblastoma.

History, associated findings, computed tomography (CT), and ultrasound may assist in the differential diagnosis of *Toxocara* from other ocular diseases. For example, the CT and ultrasound may show calcification in retinoblastoma, but this is rarely found in *Toxocara*. Microphthalmia is an associated finding in persistent primary hyperplastic vitreous, but not in *Toxocara*. Correct diagnosis is essential, because many cases of *Toxocara* are misdiagnosed, resulting in inappropriate management, as evidenced by cases of enucleation when a misdiagnosis of retinoblastoma is made.

TREATMENT AND MANAGEMENT

■ Systemic

The optimal management of *Toxocara* is prevention. This may include deworming puppies and appropriate hygiene when dealing with soil and dogs (Table 65–3).

When VLM does occur, mild disease may simply be monitored, with referral to a pediatrician who is trained to deal with any potential complications, such as pulmonary, hepatic, neurologic, or cardiac involvement.

TABLE 65–3. TREATMENT AND MANAGEMENT OF *TOXOCARA*

■ **SYSTEMIC**
PREVENTION
- Deworm dogs
- Hygiene (when dealing with soil, dogs)
- Educate dog owners
- Enforce pooper scooper/leash laws
- Keep children from contaminated areas

VISCERAL LARVA MIGRANS
- Monitor
- Referral to physician or pediatrician with appropriate training to deal with potential complications (pulmonary, hepatic, neurologic, or cardiac)
- Severe respiratory and myocardial involvement: steroids
- Anthelminthic drugs (eg, diethylcarbamazine, thiabendazole)

■ **OCULAR**
- Inflammation
    Steroids (topical, subconjunctival, subtenon, oral), cycloplegic agents
- Anthelminthics
    (variable success), used with steroids
- Surgical
    Vitrectomy, laser photocoagulation/cryotherapy, pars plana vitrectomy, secondary cataract removal
- Secondary glaucoma
    Medication, surgery (eg, trabeculectomy)

Specific treatment is determined by patient symptomatology, disease severity and organ involvement. Steroids may be used for severe respiratory and myocardial involvement. Anthelminthic drugs, such as diethylcarbamazine and thiabendazole, may relieve symptoms and duration by killing the larvae. However, these drugs should be used sparingly and in those who are very sick, because severe side effects may result. Often the organism is best left untreated.

■ Ocular

Treatment of ocular involvement of *Toxocara* is dependent on the severity and potential threat to the eye and vision. For example, monitoring the patient with a nonthreatening peripheral granuloma may be the best treatment option. Steroid treatment may be necessary for some cases of inflammation. Although the use of anthelminthics in ocular disease is of questionable value, they may be used in conjunction with steroids. Surgical intervention may ultimately be necessary. Pars plana vitrectomy may be needed in cases of chronic endophthalmitis, to remove vitreous bands and to prevent the possible sequelae of retinal detachment, phthisis bulbi, or amblyopia. Photocoagulation or cryotherapy may be used to kill the larvae; however, this treatment is reserved for those cases where the resultant inflammatory response to the dead larvae outweighs the risk of no treatment.

CONCLUSION

Toxocara is a parasitic infection that occurs commonly in its natural host, the domestic dog, with infection and an incomplete life cycle occurring in humans. The disease in humans affects children most commonly, resulting in systemic (visceral larva migrans) or ocular manifestations (ocular larva migrans), with each rarely occurring concurrently. *Toxocara* usually follows a benign course, or may manifest in ways such that the underlying cause may go undiagnosed. Correct diagnosis may therefore prevent inappropriate treatment and allow prompt management when indicated.

REFERENCES

Arpino C, Curatolo P. Toxocariasis in children. *Lancet.* 1988;1:1172.

Arpino C, Gattinara GC, Piergili D, Curatolo P. *Toxocara* infection and epilepsy in children: A case-control study. *Epilepsia.* 1990;31:33–36.

Belmont JB, Irvine A, Benson W, O'Connor R. Vitrectomy in ocular toxocariasis. *Arch Ophthalmol.* 1982;100:1912–1915.

Berrocal J. Prevalence of *Toxocara canis* in babies and in adults as determined by the ELISA test. *Trans Am Ophthalmol Soc.* 1980;78:376–413.

Biglan AW, Glickman LT, Lobes LA. Serum and vitreous toxocara antibody in nematode endophthalmitis. *Am J Ophthalmol.* 1979;88:898–901.

Brown DH. Ocular *Toxocara canis. J Pediatr Ophthalmol.* 1970;7:182–191.

Brown GC, Tasman WS. Retinal arterial obstruction in association with presumed *Toxocara canis* neuroretinitis. *Ann Ophthalmol.* 1981;13:1385–1387.

Byers B, Kimura SJ. Uveitis after death of a larva in the vitreous cavity. *Am J Ophthalmol.* 1974;77:63–66.

Caucanas JP, Magnaval JF, Pascal JP. Prevalence of toxocaral disease. *Lancet.* 1988;1:1049.

Childs JE. The prevalence of *Toxocara* species ova in backyards and gardens of Baltimore, Maryland. *AJPH.* 1985;75:1092–1094.

Clemett RS, Allardyce RA, Williamson HJE, et al. Ocular *Toxocara canis* infections: Diagnosis by enzyme immunoassay. *Aust NZ J Ophthalmol.* 1987;15:145–150.

Cox TA, Haskins GE, Gangitano JL, Antonson DL. Bilateral *Toxocara* optic neuropathy. *J Clin Neuro-ophthalmol.* 1983;3:267–274.

Dernouchamps JP, Verougstraete C, Demolder E. Ocular toxocariasis: A presumed case of peripheral granuloma. *Int Ophthalmol.* 1990;14:383–388.

Dinning WJ, Gillespie GH, Cooling RJ, Maizels RM. Toxocariasis: A practical approach to management of ocular disease. *Eye.* 1988;2:580–582.

Duguid IM. Features of ocular infestation by *Toxocara. Br J Ophthalmol.* 1961;45:789–796.

Ellis GS, Pakalnis VA, Worley G. *Toxocara canis* infection. Clinical and epidemiological associations with seropositivity in kindergarten children. *Ophthalmology.* 1986;93:1032–1037.

Ferguson EC, Olson LJ. *Toxocara* ocular nematodiasis. *Int Ophthalmol Clin.* 1967;7:583–603.

Gill D, Dunne K, Kenny V. Toxocariasis in children. *Lancet.* 1988;1:1172.

Jones WL. *Toxocara canis. J Am Optom Assoc.* 1979;4:450–454.

Kennedy JJ, Defeo E. Ocular toxocariasis demonstrated by ultrasound. *Ann Ophthalmol.* 1981;13:1357–1358.

Kielar RA. *Toxocara canis* endophthalmitis with low ELISA titer. *Ann Ophthalmol.* 1983;15:447–449.

Kirber WM, Nichols CW, Braunstein SN. Unusual presentation of ocular toxocariasis in friends. *Ann Ophthalmol.* 1979;11:573–576.

Liesegang TJ. Atypical ocular toxocariasis. *J Pediatr Ophthalmol.* 1977:14:349–353.

Maguire AM, Zarbin MA, Connor TB, Justin J. Ocular penetration of thiabendazole. *Arch Ophthalmol.* 1990;108:1675.

Maguire AM, Green WR, Michels RG, Erozan YS. Recovery of intraocular *Toxocara canis* by pars plana vitrectomy. *Ophthalmology.* 1990;97:675–680.

Marmor M, Glickman L, Shofer F, et al. *Toxocara canis* infection of children: Epidemiologic and neuropsychologic findings. *Am J Public Health.* 1987;77:554–559.

Mok CH. Visceral larva migrans. A discussion based on review of the literature. *Clin Pediatr.* 1968;7:565–573.

Molk R. Ocular toxocariasis: A review of the literature. *Ann Ophthalmol.* 1983;15:216–231.

Molk R. Treatment of toxocaral optic neuritis. *J Clin Neuro-ophthalmol.* 1982;2:109–112.

O'Connor PR. Visceral larva migrans of the eye. *Arch Ophthalmol.* 1972;88:526–529.

Perkins ES. Pattern of uveitis in children. *Br J Ophthalmol.* 1966;50:169–185.

Pollard ZF. Long-term follow-up in patients with ocular toxocariasis as measured by ELISA titers. *Ann Ophthalmol.* 1987;19:167–169.

Pollard ZF. Ocular *Toxocara* in siblings of two families. *Arch Ophthalmol.* 1979;97:2319–2320.

Pollard ZF, Jarrett WH, Hagler WS, et al. ELISA for diagnosis of ocular toxocariasis. *Ophthalmology.* 1979;86:743–752.

Richer SP, Stiles WR. Presumed *Toxocara canis* with peripheral retinal granuloma and secondary macular hole. *J Am Optom Assoc.* 1987;58:404–407.

Rodriguez A. Early pars plana vitrectomy in chronic endophthalmitis of toxocariasis. *Graefe's Arch Clin Exp Ophthalmol.* 1986;224:218–220.

Schantz PM, Glickman LT. Toxocaral visceral larva migrans. *N Engl J Med.* 1978;298:436–439.

Schantz PM, Weis PE, Pollard ZF, White MC. Risk factors for toxocaral ocular larva migrans: A case control study. *Am J Public Health.* 1980;70:1269–1272.

Schimek RA, Perez WA, Carrera GM. Ophthalmic manifestations of visceral larva migrans. *Ann Ophthalmol.* 1979;11:1387–1390.

Searl SS, Moazed K, Albert DM, Marcus LC. Ocular toxocariasis presenting as leukocoria in a patient with low ELISA titer to *Toxocara canis. Ophthalmology.* 1981;88:1302–1306.

Sharkey JA, McKay PS. Ocular toxocariasis in a patient with repeatedly negative ELISA titre to *Toxocara canis. Br J Ophthalmol.* 1993;77:253–254.

Shields JA. Ocular toxocariasis. A review. *Surv Ophthalmol.* 1984;28:361–381.

Shields JA, Felberg NT, Federman JL. Discussion of presentation by Dr Zane F. Pollard, et al. *Ophthalmology.* 1979;86:750–752.

Taylor MRH, Keane CT, O'Connor P, et al. The expanded spectrum of toxocaral disease. *Lancet.* 1988:692–694.

Wan WL, Cano MR, Pince KJ, Green RL. Echographic characteristics of ocular toxocariasis. *Ophthalmology.* 1991;98:28–32.

Zinkham WH. Visceral larva migrans. A review and reassessment indicating two forms of clinical expression: Visceral and ocular. *Am J Dis Child.* 1978;132:627–633.

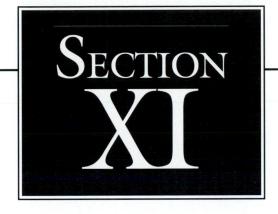

SECTION XI

HEMATOLOGIC DISORDERS

66
Chapter

Anemias

Holly Myers

Anemia is a deficiency in quantity or quality of erythrocytes, and may be classified based on morphologic or etiologic differences (Table 66–1). Morphologic classification may be divided into microcytic, normocytic, or macrocytic. Etiologic classification may be based on rapid loss of red blood cells (RBCs), the slow production of RBCs, or abnormal RBCs. In general, anemias will result in pallor, fatigue, irritability, bruising, and dyspnea. In addition, systemic findings may include lymphadenopathy, bone tenderness, enlargement of the spleen and liver, and abnormalities of the epithelium and mucosa, such as brittle nails, pallor of mucous membranes, and sore tongue.

Ocular findings associated with anemia involve many tissues. Retinal and optic nerve changes are probably the most significant, with superficial and deep retinal hemorrhages, cotton-wool spots, exudates, and dilated tortuous retinal veins all common findings. Central retinal vein occlusion, vitreous hemorrhages, and optic neuropathy with resultant pallor and atrophy may develop. Conjunctival pallor may occur, as well as subconjunctival hemorrhages.

This chapter will be limited to a discussion of iron-deficient anemia, aplastic anemia and pernicious anemia.

■ IRON-DEFICIENT ANEMIA

Iron-deficient anemia is the most common anemia in the United States (Linker, 1993). An inadequate iron level is most frequently caused by a chronic recurrent hemorrhage, usually from the gastrointestinal tract in males and from the genitourinary tract in females. Decreased levels of iron may also occur secondary to dietary deprivation, malabsorption from small intestine disease, and physiologic loss. Anemia results from a disruption in the balance between iron absorption and loss. Pregnancy, for example, often interrupts the balance as iron requirements increase to 2 to 5 mg per day during pregnancy and lactation (Bridges & Bunn, 1991). Iron-deficient anemia is usually mild; however it may become severe enough to be life threatening.

The author would like to acknowledge Patricia Leggin for assisting in the preparation of this chapter.

EPIDEMIOLOGY

Iron-deficient anemia is generally more common in women than men because of the greater physiological demand. As many as 40% of all women of childbearing years are iron depleted, and almost 20% actually develop anemia (Bridges & Bunn, 1991). No information is available on specific incidence of systemic or ocular manifestations of iron deficiency.

NATURAL HISTORY

Iron is required for the synthesis of hemoglobin, myoglobin, and enzymes needed for oxygen transport. Iron is stored in the body but must be replaced because of loss due to growth, small blood loss, and loss of desquamated cells.

501

TABLE 66–1. CLASSIFICATION OF ANEMIAS

Etiologic

Inadequate Erythropoiesis
Aplastic anemia
Myelophthisic anemia
Bone marrow carcinoma
Iron-deficiency anemia
Thalassemia
Anemia of chronic disease

Excessive Blood Loss
Hemorrhagic anemia

Excessive Blood Destruction
Congenital hemolytic and acquired anemias
Sickle cell anemia

Morphological

Microcytic
Iron-deficient anemia
Thalassemia
Anemia of chronic disease

Normocytic
Aplastic anemia
Infectious anemia
Pure red cell aplasia
Inflammation
Renal disease
Neoplasms
Pituitary/thyroid failure
Starvation

Macrocytic
Megaloblastic
  Vitamin B_{12} deficiency
  Folate deficiency
Nonmegaloblastic
  Myelodysplasia
  Chemotherapy
  Myxedema

The average American diet provides 10 to 30 mg of iron per day, of which 10% is absorbed (Cook, 1992). The intake of iron through the diet occurs in two forms, heme iron and nonheme iron. Heme compounds are absorbed relatively efficiently (15 to 35%) through the upper small intestine. Nonheme iron is absorbed much less efficiently (2 to 20%) (Cook, 1992). It is generally in the oxidized ferric form and is therefore insoluble in the upper intestine, where iron absorption primarily occurs. The acid in the stomach will aid absorption of ferric iron by maintaining it in a soluble form. Different foods may chelate insoluble iron and reduce its absorption. The daily requirement of iron varies with gender, age, and in females, menses (Table 66–2).

■ Systemic

Iron-deficient anemia may be considered in three clinical stages. The first stage is storage iron depletion, with storage iron depleted but hemoglobin normal. The next stage is early iron-deficient erythropoiesis. In this stage the erythroid iron supply is reduced, but anemia is not yet present. The final stage is the presence of iron-deficiency anemia. Here the red cells become severely hypochromic and microcytic.

Systemic symptoms (Table 66–3) may result from mild cases of iron deficiency and may include palpitations, increased fatigability, headache, irritability, and light-headedness. An uncommon but very specific symptom of iron-deficiency anemia is pica. Pica is the bizarre ingestion of large quantities of ice, clay, or laundry starch. In profound iron depletion, epithelial and mucosal changes occur including inflammation of the tongue, brittle nails, and koilonychia (spoon-shaped nails). In severe cases dysphagia may occur secondary to the formation of mucosal adhesions in the esophagus called esophageal webs.

■ Ocular

Ocular manifestations are not usually present unless anemia is severe (Table 66–4). In severe cases, conjunctival pallor may be present, but this sign is neither sensitive nor specific. With a sudden massive hemorrhage in the body, significant fundus findings may occur within weeks with bilateral vision loss. Retinal hemorrhages (superficial and deep), cotton-wool spots (Figure 66–1), exudates, dilated and tortuous retinal veins, and retinal edema are often present with pallor of the optic disc. These changes usually resolve over the course of days or weeks; however, restoration of vision may not occur.

Altitudinal hemianopsia, peripheral field constriction, isolated scotomas, or complete blindness may result. Similar visual field loss may be seen in patients who have recently undergone vigorous pressure-reduction therapy for severe arterial hypertension (Cove et al, 1979). The field defects may resemble those found in chronic open-angle glaucoma and normotensive glaucoma, with the patient also presenting with a concurrent history of hemodynamic crisis.

DIAGNOSIS

■ Systemic

Bone marrow iron stain, plasma ferritin studies, and iron-binding capacity tests are performed to diagnose iron deficiency (Table 66–5). Iron-deficient anemia is characterized by the lack of stainable iron in the bone marrow, and impaired hemoglobin synthesis that results in microcytic, hypochromic red cells. The clinical signs will vary, depending on the severity of the anemia, from virtually no symptoms to pallor of mucous membranes, abnormalities of the nails, and the formation of esophageal webs. Laboratory

TABLE 66–2. NORMAL RED CELL BLOOD AND IRON VALUES FOR ADULTS

	Males	Females
Normal Red Blood Cell Values		
Hematocrit (Hct)	47% ±7	42% ±5
Hemoglobin (Hgb)	16 g/dL ±2	14 g/dL ±2
Red blood cell count (RBC)	$5.4 \times 10^6/\mu L$ ±0.8	$4.8 \times 10^6/\mu L$ ±0.6
Mean cell volume (MCV)	90 fL ±8	90 fL ±8
Mean cell hemoglobin (MCH)	29 pg/cell ±2	29 pg/cell ±2
MCH concentration (MCHC)	33.5 g/dl ±2	33.5 g/dl ±2
Normal Iron Balance		
Normal Hgb	16 g/dL	14 g/dL
Hgb iron	2500 mg	1900 mg
Iron intake per day	10–15 mg	10–15 mg
Storage iron	1000 mg	500 mg
Iron absorbed per day	1.0 mg	1.0–2.5 mg
Iron loss per day	1.0 mg	1.0–2.5 mg

Adapted from Spivak JL, The anemic patient. In: Harvey AM, et al, eds. The Principles and Practice of Medicine. 2nd ed. Norwalk, CT: Appleton & Lange; 1988:310–322.

testing will solidify the diagnosis as well as quantify the relative degree of iron depletion in the body.

The most reliable test in detecting iron deficiency is a bone marrow iron stain. A number of other tests are useful, including plasma iron, total iron-binding capacity (TIBC), transferring saturation, plasma ferritin, erythrocyte-free protoporphyrin, and mean corpuscular volume (MCV) tests. Many of these tests are neither sensitive nor specific and may be subject to alteration by inflammation and infection. The most conclusive evidence for iron deficiency is a therapeutic trial of iron. The success of a therapeutic trial must not stop the clinician from determining the exact cause of the iron deficiency whether nutritional, physiological, hemorrhagic, or secondary to another disease process.

■ Ocular

Diagnosis of iron-deficient anemia usually relates to systemic manifestations. However, ocular findings, such as a pale conjunctiva or retinal hemorrhage, may indicate potential iron-deficient anemia.

TREATMENT AND MANAGEMENT

Iron-deficient anemia is treated with iron replacement therapy (Table 66–6). The ferrous form is given as a daily supplement on an empty stomach to enhance absorption. Patients who cannot tolerate iron on an empty stomach should take it with food. Hematologic values should return to normal after 2 months of treatment. Because of possible severe hypersensitivity reactions, parenteral iron therapy

should only be given when every attempt at oral therapy has been made.

■ APLASTIC ANEMIA

Aplastic anemia is the result of bone marrow dysfunction, whose etiology may be idiopathic or secondary to external chemical or physical agents. Approximately one half of patients with aplastic anemia will have hemorrhage in the retina, skin, or mucous membranes at the time of diagnosis. Cotton-wool spots and dilated retinal veins are also frequently seen.

Many systemic drugs have been noted to cause aplastic anemia. Several ocular medications have been implicated as well, including topical ocular chloramphenicol, carbonic anhydrase inhibitors such as acetazolamide (Diamox) and methazolamide (Neptazane).

EPIDEMIOLOGY

Aplastic anemia can occur at any age and in both sexes. In over half the cases it is idiopathic, with the remaining cases secondary to irradiation, chemical agents, and other disease processes. Mortality associated with aplastic anemia is greater than 80%, with a 50% mortality rate within 3 months of diagnosis. Aplasia secondary to drugs or hepatitis has an even poorer prognosis (Bridges & Bunn, 1991). Specific incidence of ocular and systemic findings are unknown.

TABLE 66–3. SYSTEMIC MANIFESTATIONS OF ANEMIAS

GENERAL SYSTEMIC SIGNS AND SYMPTOMS OF ANEMIA
- Pallor
- Weakness
- Lethargy
- Dyspnea
- Tachycardia
- Palpitations
- Tachypnea (very rapid breathing) on exertion
- Cutaneous hemorrhage (bruise)
- Lymphadenopathy
- Bone tenderness
- Hepatosplenomegaly
- Epithelial abnormalities

SYSTEMIC SIGNS AND SYMPTOMS OF SPECIFIC ANEMIAS
- **Iron-Deficient Anemia**
  Headache
  Light-headedness
  Pica
  Glossitis
  Koilonychia
  Dysphagia
- **Aplastic Anemia**
  Easy bruisability
  Epistaxis
  Increased menstrual flow
  Bacterial infections of mouth and perirectal area
- **Pernicious Anemia**
  Glossitis
  GI disturbances
    Atrophic gastritis
    Anorexia
    Diarrhea
  Neurogenic disturbances
    Subacute combined degeneration
  Autoimmune diseases

TABLE 66–4. OCULAR MANIFESTATIONS OF ANEMIAS

IRON-DEFICIENT ANEMIA
- Conjunctival findings
  Pallor
  Hemorrhage
- Retinal findings
  Hemorrhages
  Cotton-wool spots and exudates
  Blood accumulation under the internal limiting
    membrane
  Vitreous hemorrhage from internal limiting
    membrane breaks
  Dilated tortuous veins
  Central retinal vein occlusion with or without
    macular edema
- Cranial nerve palsies

APLASTIC ANEMIA
- Conjunctival pallor
- Subconjunctival hemorrhage
- Hyphema
- Retinal findings
  Retinal and preretinal hemorrhages
  Cotton-wool spots
  Optic disc swelling
  Pallor of the optic discs

PERNICIOUS ANEMIA
- Conjunctival pallor
- Retinal findings
  Dilated veins
  Hemorrhages
  Pallor of the fundus
  Retinal edema
- Optic nerve findings
  Pallor
  Optic neuropathy

NATURAL HISTORY

■ Systemic

Aplastic anemia may present insidiously or acutely, and because of its high mortality must be addressed promptly. Patients typically experience bone pain and enlargement of the spleen. In addition, bacterial infections of the mouth and perirectal area, bruising, nosebleeds, and increased menstrual flow in women are commonly seen. Mucous membranes and nailbeds are often pale (see Table 66–3).

■ Ocular

Typical ocular findings (see Table 66–4) associated with aplastic anemia include conjunctival pallor, subconjunctival hemorrhage, retinal and preretinal hemorrhage, cotton-wool spots, optic disc swelling (Figure 66–2), and pallor. Hyphema rarely occurs (Lilley et al, 1990).

DIAGNOSIS

■ Systemic

Diagnosis of aplastic anemia is made based on clinical presentation, blood workup, and aspiration and biopsy of the bone marrow (see Table 66–5). Bone marrow biopsy will show a severely hypocellular or aplastic marrow, with an increase in the number of fat cells.

■ Ocular

Although a number of ocular manifestations may be associated with aplastic anemia, they are not common occurrences.

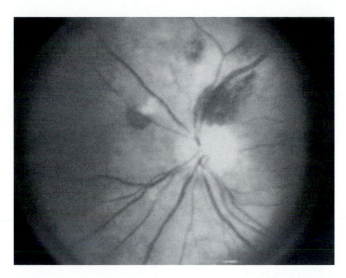

Figure 66–1. Fundus of a patient with severe anemia. Note intraretinal hemorrhages and cotton-wool spots. *(Reprinted with permission from Lowenstein JI. Retinopathy associated with blood anomalies. In: Albert DM, Jacobiec FA, eds.* Principles and Practices of Ophthamology. *Vol 2, Clinical Practice. Philadelphia: Saunders; 1994:399–408.)*

Conjunctival pallor, retinal hemorrhage, and optic disc abnormalities may occur. These findings are common in all forms of anemia, and a definitive diagnosis of aplastic anemia cannot be made based on their presence or character alone. Because the patients are usually profoundly ill, diagnosis is based on systemic manifestations along with bone marrow biopsy.

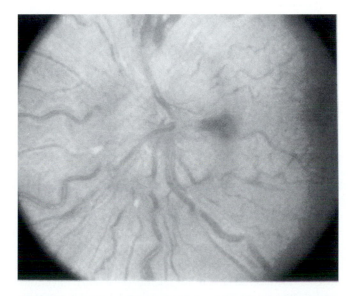

Figure 66–2. Disc swelling and flame-shaped hemorrhages in a patient with aplastic anemia. *(Reprinted with permission from Lilley ER, Bruggers CS, Pollock SC. Papilledema in a patient with aplastic anemia. Case report.* Arch Ophthalmol. *1990;108:1674.)*

TABLE 66–5. LABORATORY FINDINGS IN ANEMIAS

Iron-Deficient Anemia

	Normal	Iron Deficient
MCV(fL)	80–99	< 80
Plasma iron(μg/dL)	65–175	< 30
Iron-binding capacity(μg/dL)	300–360	400
Transferrin saturation(%)	25–50	< 16
Plasma ferritin(μg/L)	20–250	< 12
Erythrocyte-free protoporphyrin(μg/dL)	27–61	180
Basophilic stippling	Absent	Absent
Marrow iron stores	Present	Absent

Aplastic Anemia

Severe
Platelet count <20,000/μL
Reticulocyte count <60,000/μL
Granuloctye count <500/μL
Bone marrow biopsy: hypocellular or aplastic
Mild
Platelet count <1800/μL
Hematocrit <38%
Granuloctye count <1800/μL
Bone marrow biopsy: at least one hypocellular biopsy

Pernicious Anemia

Peripheral blood	Bone marrow
Oval macrocytes	Hypercellularity
Anisocytosis	Erythroid hyperplasia
Poikilocytosis	Giant metamyelocytes
Howell–Jolly bodies	Neutrophil hypersegmentation
Neutrophil hypersegmentation	

TREATMENT AND MANAGEMENT

■ Systemic

The treatment of aplastic anemia is bone marrow transplantation. Should a specific etiologic agent be identified, it should be removed immediately (see Table 66–6). Patients must also receive supportive care, which in very early aplastic anemia may be all that is required. Patients should be protected from infection and any bleeding whether from disease or physiological (eg, menstruation should be suppressed). Fifty percent of patients receiving transplantation treatment survive, remaining disease free for 2 years.

■ Ocular

There is no specific ocular treatment for aplastic anemia. However, when the systemic manifestations are treated, ocular findings tend to resolve, with the exception of nerve damage severe enough to be permanent.

■ PERNICIOUS ANEMIA

Pernicious anemia is a hereditary autoimmune disorder of the gastric mucosa. The gastric mucosa is unable to secrete the glycoprotein "intrinsic" factor that is necessary for the absorption of vitamin B_{12} (cyanocabalmin). Cyanocabalmin plays a critical role in the synthesis of nucleic acids, which is involved in the formation of blood precursors.

EPIDEMIOLOGY

■ Systemic

Pernicious anemia is typically present in elderly patients with northern European ancestry, and is almost as common in African-Americans and Latin Americans. It is the most common cause of vitamin B_{12} deficiency in the Western world. It is a disease of the elderly, with the average patient presenting around age 60. Pernicious anemia can occur in young people and is especially common in African-American women between 30 and 40 years of age. It is slightly more common in women.

■ Ocular

Specific incidence of ocular manifestations are unknown.

NATURAL HISTORY

■ Systemic

Patients with pernicious anemia exhibit symptoms of palpitations, increased fatiguability, headache, irritability, and light-headedness. Changes in mucosal cells lead to glossitis as well as other gastrointestinal disturbances such as diarrhea. The deficiency in vitamin B_{12} causes a complex neurologic syndrome. The peripheral nerves are affected first, followed by the posterior spinal column and finally involvement of the cerebral function. Initially patients will have paresthesias in the feet and hands and a loss of fine touch and vibratory sense. As it progresses, weakness and advancement of paresthesis occur with difficulty in balance, and dementia and other neuropsychiatric abnormalities may occur in more advanced cases (see Table 66–3).

Other abnormalities associated with pernicious anemia include Hashimoto thyroiditis, hyperthyroidism, vitiligo, Addison disease, and hypoparathyroidism. Gastric polyps and carcinoma occur with increased incidence. Life expectancy is slightly shorter than normal, which may be secondary to the predisposition to gastric cancer, an increased risk associated with the severe, irreversible neurologic damage, and coexisting diseases.

■ Ocular

The ocular findings in pernicious anemia are consistent with those associated with anemia (see Table 66–4). Retinopathy with dilated veins and hemorrhage may be seen. Less commonly present are extraretinal hemorrhages, pallor of the fundus and optic nerveheads, and retinal edema. Although not common, the major impact on the visual system is optic neuropathy. Vision loss is usually bilateral, slightly asymetric, and gradual, resulting in 20/40 to 20/200 VA. The typical visual field defect is either a central or centrocecal scotoma. Dyschromatopsia is often present and is believed to be due to optic nerve dysfunction or to retinal abnormalities.

DIAGNOSIS

■ Systemic

Diagnosis of pernicious anemia is primarily based on laboratory findings (see Table 66–5). Careful observation of a peripheral blood smear will show macrocytes with a characteristic oval shape and lack of central pallor and hypersegmented neutrophils. The blood smear will also show an excessive variation in erythrocyte size (anisocytosis) and an abnormal variation in shape (poikilocytosis), although the oval shape predominates. Serum vitamin B_{12} levels are usually less than 100 pg/mL, but a variety of factors may give falsely high or low levels. Orally administered radioactive vitamin B_{12} (Schilling test) is used to document the impaired absorption of B_{12}. The bone marrow is abnormal with marked erythroid hyperplasia.

■ Ocular

Ocular manifestations may be suggestive of pernicious anemia, but diagnosis is based on the associated laboratory and systemic findings. These include retinal hemorrhages, pallor of the fundus or disc, and the presence of optic neuropathy.

TREATMENT AND MANAGEMENT

■ Systemic

Because patients with pernicious anemia cannot absorb oral vitamin, the treatment (see Table 66–6) is with intramuscular injections of vitamin B_{12}, preferably hydroxocobalamin. A recommended treatment regimen is once daily injections for 2 weeks, twice daily for an additional 4 weeks, and then monthly for the lifetime of the patient. With therapy, the neurological abnormalities are reversible provided no permanent axonal damage has occurred.

TABLE 66–6. TREATMENT AND MANAGEMENT OF ANEMIAS (SYSTEMIC AND OCULAR)

IRON-DEFICIENT ANEMA
- 200 mg elemental iron (3 tab ferrous sulfate daily on an empty stomach)

APLASTIC ANEMIA
- Remove causative agent
- Bone marrow transplant

PERNICIOUS ANEMIA
- 1000-mg IM injections of vitamin B_{12}
  Daily for 2 weeks
  Then twice daily for 4 weeks
  Then continued monthly for life

■ Ocular

The retinopathy is reversible once the hemoglobin is restored to normal levels. The optic neuropathy is also reversible, but permanent damage to axons can result, with associated visual loss.

CONCLUSION

The anemias encompass a wide variety of specific disorders that result from a decrease in the number and/or functioning of red blood cells. Systemic manifestations associated with anemia depend on the severity, cause, and rapidity of onset. Other associated disorders occurring with anemia may also vary the presentation of the disease. The disease may follow an insidious course, with symptoms so nonspecific that the presence of the anemia may go unrecognized. Fatigue, headache, and dyspnea are common symptoms. Systemic features may include jaundice, petechiae, bruising, and lymphadenopathy. Laboratory studies are necessary to identify the specific type and etiology of the anemia.

Ocular abnormalities of the fundus are common manifestations of anemia. These may include dilatation of the venous system, retinal hemorrhages, cotton-wool spots, and exudates. Patients presenting with these ocular findings, along with vague systemic complaints, should alert the eyecare practitioner to consider anemia in the differential diagnosis.

REFERENCES

Adams P, Chalmers TM, Foulds WS, et al. Megaloblastic anemia and vision. *Lancet.* 1967;2:229–231.

Aisen ML, Bacon BR, Goodman AM, Chester EM. Retinal abnormalities associated with anemia. *Arch Ophthalmol.* 1983;101:1049–1052.

Bridges KR, Bunn HF. Anemias with disturbed iron metabolism. In: Wilson JD, Braunwald E, Isselbacher KJ, et al, eds. *Harrison's Principles of Internal Medicine.* New York: McGraw-Hill; 1991:1518–1522.

Carmeil R. Megaloblastic anemias. In: Kelley WN, ed. *Textbook of Internal Medicine.* Philadelphia: Lippincott; 1992:1303–1307.

Cook JD. Iron deficiency and iron leading anemias. In: Kelley WN, ed. *Textbook of Internal Medicine.* Philadelphia: Lippincott; 1992:1300–1303.

Cove D, Seddon M, Fletcher R, et al. Blindness after treatment for malignant hypertension. *Br Med J.* 1979;2:245.

Drance S. The visual field of low-tension glaucoma and shock-induced optic neuropathy. *Arch Ophthalmol.* 1977;95:1359.

Foulds WS, Chisolm IA, Stewart JB, Wilson TM. The optic neuropathy of pernicious anemia. *Arch Ophthalmol.* 1969;82:427–432.

Furuse N, Hayasaka S, Yamamoto Y, Setogawa T. Retinal microaneurysms in a patient with drug-induced aplastic anemia. *Ophthalmologica.* 1987;195:188–191.

Kirkham TH, Wrigley PFM, Holt JM. Central retinal vein occlusion complicating iron deficiency anemia. *Br J Ophthalmol.* 1971;55:777–780.

Klewin K, Appen R, Kaufman P. Amaurosis and blood loss. *Am J Ophthalmol.* 1978;86:669.

Lerman S, Feldmann AL. Centrocecal scotoma as the presenting sign in pernicious anemia. *Arch Ophthalmol.* 1961;65:381–385.

Lilley ER, Bruggers CS, Pollock SC. Papilledema in a patient with aplastic anemia. Case report. *Arch Ophthalmol.* 1990;108:1674–1675.

Linker CA. Blood. In: Tierney LM, McPhee SJ, Papadkis MA, et al, eds. *Current Medical Diagnosis and Treatment.* 32nd ed. Norwalk, CT; Appleton & Lange: 1993:399–408.

Loewenstein JI. Retinopathy associated with blood anomalies. In: Albert DM, Jacobiec FA, eds. *Principles and Practices of Ophthalmology.* Vol 2, *Clinical Practice.* Philadelphia: Saunders; 1994:995–1000.

Mansour AM. Aplastic anemia simulating central retinal vein occlusion. *Am J Ophthalmol.* 1985;100:478–479.

Merin S, Freund M. Retinopathy in severe anemia. *Am J Ophthalmol.* 1968;66:1102–1106.

Motolko M, Drance S, Douglas G. Visual field defects in low-tension glaucoma. *Arch Ophthalmol.* 1982;100:1074.

Rubenstein RA, Yanoff M, Albert DM. Thrombocytopenia, anemia, and retinal hemorrhage. *Am J Ophthalmol.* 1968;65:435–439.

Shorb SR. Anemia and diabetic retinopathy. *Am J Ophthalmol.* 1985;100:434–436.

Spivak JL. The anemic patient. In: Harvey AM, Johns RJ, McKusick WA, et al, eds. *The Principles and Practice of Medicine.* 2nd ed. Norwalk, CT: Appleton & Lange; 1988:310–322.

Williamson J, Cant JS, Mason DK, et al. Sjögren's syndrome in relation to pernicious anemia and idiopathic Addison's disease. *Br J Ophthalmol.* 1970;54:31–36.

67
Chapter

Polycythemia

Holly Myers

Polycythemia ("many cells") is an increase in red blood cells (RBCs), and is characterized by an increase in blood volume and viscosity and a decrease in blood flow, resulting in systemic and ocular findings.

There are two classifications of polycythemia: polycythemia vera (erythema vera, primary polycythemia, Vasquez disease) and secondary polycythemia (erythrocytosis, physiologic polycythemia). Polycythemia vera refers to an increase in the absolute number of RBCs and in the total blood volume without a known physiological cause. Secondary polycythemia refers to an increase in the number of RBCs as a response to increased erythropoietin level, from an underlying disorder. A third term, relative polycythemia (spurious polycythemia), refers to conditions in which a reduction in plasma volume, rather than an increase in RBC mass, results in an elevated hematocrit. Polycythemia can affect the tissues of the conjunctiva, retina, and optic nerve due to increased RBC mass with resultant tissue hypoxia. This chapter will be limited to a discussion of polycythemia vera and secondary polycythemia.

EPIDEMIOLOGY

■ Systemic
Polycythemia vera most commonly affects the middle-aged and the elderly, although it may occur at any age. It is slightly more common in males than females. The incidence is reported at 5 per million (Frenkel and Fleischman, 1992). Caucasians are most commonly affected, particularly Jews of European extraction. Polycythemia vera is uncommon in African-Americans.

■ Ocular
There are no contemporary studies that include the incidence or prevalence of ocular findings within the polycythemia vera or secondary polycythemia groups.

The author would like to acknowledge Christopher Adsit for assisting in the preparation of this chapter.

NATURAL HISTORY

■ Systemic
Polycythemia vera has an insidious onset, running a chronic course, with arterial thrombosis its major cause of morbidity and mortality. Its specific etiology is unknown, but evidence suggests that its underlying cause is a neoblastic disorder of stem cells.

The disease is characterized by an increase in RBCs. Bone marrow hyperplasia and an increase in white blood cells and platelets may also be present. These blood cell changes lead to a total blood volume increase and an intense engorgement of the entire vascular system. The viscosity of blood sometimes increases from a normal value of 3 times the viscosity of water to 15 times the viscosity of water. Capillaries become plugged by the very viscous blood.

Symptoms of polycythemia are caused by diminished cerebral blood flow and the tendency to hemorrhage and form a thrombus (Table 67–1). Limb pain is common. The skin and mucous membranes are affected, and the liver and spleen are enlarged.

In the initial stages of the disease, before the red cell mass has increased, symptoms may be few. These initial symptoms may include redness after bathing, along with occasional burning of the palms and soles. As the red cell mass increases, the classic presentation of polycythemia emerges. This includes hemorrhage, in the mucosa or skin; occlusive vascular lesions such as cerebral or myocardial infarction; peripheral venous thrombosis; enlargement of the spleen (in 70 to 90% of cases); and enlargement of the liver (in 40%) (Berlin, 1975; Frenkel & Fleischman, 1992).

As the disease progresses, significant thrombocytosis occurs and asymptomatic leukocytosis is usually present. In about 20% of patients, weakness, fatigue, weight loss, progressive enlargement of the spleen, and increasing anemia and hemorrhage occur. These patients usually die of clinical complications within 3 years (Frenkel & Fleischman, 1992).

In the final stages of the disease, some may convert to myelofibrosis or acute myelogenous leukemia. Although the frequency of the disorder progressing to acute myelogenous leukemia varies, it has been reported from 10 to 36% (Frenkel & Fleischman, 1992; Lawerence & Goetsch, 1950).

TABLE 67–1. SYSTEMIC MANIFESTATIONS OF POLYCYTHEMIA

SYMPTOMS
- Secondary to decreased cerebral blood flow
  Headache, paralysis, vertigo, various psychological disturbances, weight loss, dizziness, tinnitus, weakness/fatigue, myoclonus, grand mal seizures
- Limb pain (common)
- Miscellaneous
  Dyspnea
  Hoarseness
  GI problems

SIGNS
- Skin
  Intense red color of the lips, cheeks, and tip of nose
  Bluish cyanotic color on skin of distal extremities
  Ecchymosis
  Intense itching (especially after a hot bath)
  Dry skin, eczema, acne, urticaria
- Mucous membranes
  Deep red color
  Bleeding of the nose and gums
  GI or genitourinary bleeding
- Hemorrhagic phenomenon
  Hemothorax
  Hemoptysis
- Enlargement of the spleen
- Enlargement of the liver

Secondary polycythemia results in an increase in RBCs from tissue hypoxia or disorders that cause an increase in erythropoietin production. Erythropoietin is a hormone secreted primarily by the kidney in the adult, which acts on stem cells of the bone marrow to stimulate RBC production. Many factors may indirectly cause an RBC elevation, including an inappropriate quantity of erythropoietin, an abnormal affinity for oxygen, erythrocytosis caused by carboxyhemoglobin or methemoglobin, or secondary hypoxia caused by an underlying condition such as congenital heart disease (Table 67–2). Carboxyhemoglobin or methemoglobin is a compound formed from hemoglobin by oxidation. It does not function as an oxygen carrier and is normally present in the blood in small amounts; however, toxic agents increase its amount.

Systemic characteristics of secondary polycythemia are varied but are similar to those in polycythemia vera. Hyperplasia of the bone marrow is not seen in secondary polycythemia. Transition to leukemia does not occur in secondary polycythemia as it may in polycythemia vera.

The median survival of untreated patients with polycythemia vera is about 18 months. Appropriate therapy results in survival approaching that of those expected for age-matched normals (Frenkel & Fleischman, 1992).

■ Ocular

Polycythemia slows blood flow and causes subsequent tissue hypoxia. Ocular tissues affected include the conjunctiva (Figure 67–1), optic nerve, and retina. Retinal manifestations may occur early in the disease possibly as a result of the retina's high oxygen demand.

Symptoms include blurred vision, along with problems secondary to cerebrovascular insufficiency, such as visual field defects, amaurosis fugax, and visual hallucinations (Table 67–3).

Although polycythemia vera tends to have higher blood cell counts compared to secondary polycythemia, the retinal changes are identical and only vary in degree.

TABLE 67–2. ETIOLOGIES OF SECONDARY POLYCYTHEMIA

Hypoxia caused by
  decrease in the atmospheric oxygen (high altitudes), pulmonary disease, congenital heart disease, hypoventilation syndromes (eg, Pickwickian syndrome)

Inherited or acquired abnormalities of the hemoglobin

Erythrocytosis induced by carboxyhemoglobin or methemoglobin
  Carboxyhemoglobin and hematocrit increased in smokers, return to normal 3–6 months after smoking cessation

Abnormal affinity for oxygen
  Increased red cell mass from hypoxia, secondary to hemoglobinopathies

Inappropriate erythropoietin production
  Secondary to tumors, cysts, vascular anomalies

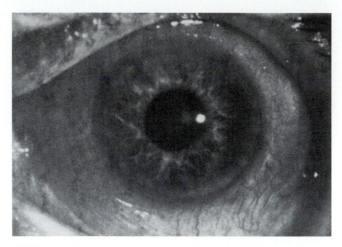

Figure 67–1. Conjunctival vascular engorgement in a patient with primary polycythemia. *(Reprinted with permission from Lindsey J, Insler S, Polycythemia rubra vera and conjunctival vascular congestion.* Ann Ophthalmol. *1985;17:62.)*

The initial retinal changes noted include dilated, darkened and tortuous retinal veins. These findings resemble those found in frank vascular occlusion, with early disease resembling a partial central retinal vein occlusion (CRVO). Following this, the optic nerve becomes hyperemic, with the entire fundus becoming a deeper darker color. In very severe polycythemia, the retinal veins will appear dilated and tortuous, and become darker; hemorrhages will appear, edema may be seen, and finally thrombus of the central retinal vein

may occur. The optic nerve will be florid in color and exhibit moderate to severe edema. In 10% of cases, the optic disc swelling may be 3 diopters or more. Disc swelling may be the presenting sign in this disorder (Wagener & Rucker, 1948).

The most serious ocular sequelae of polycythemia is CRVO. It may occur in one or both eyes, but it is rare. The prognosis for a CRVO is better when secondary to polycythemia than when secondary to the typical etiology of arteriosclerosis and hypertension (Ballantyne & Michaelson, 1980).

Ocular manifestations also include the conjunctival vessels. Vascular congestion of the conjunctiva is usually equal to that of congestion in the skin. This conjunctival presentation may be mistaken for a conjunctivitis.

DIAGNOSIS

■ Systemic

Polycythemia may be diagnosed by complete physical examination, history, and laboratory workup (Table 67–4). A physical examination may reveal involvement of the skin, mucous membranes, neuromuscular system, and enlargement of the spleen and liver. Diagnosis may also be assisted by a history of associated systemic symptoms such as vertigo, weight loss, dyspnea, and gastrointestinal difficulties. The bone marrow shows nearly 100% hyperplasia of cellular elements.

TABLE 67–3. OCULAR MANIFESTATIONS OF POLYCYTHEMIA

SYMPTOMS
- Decreased vision
- Cerebrovascular insufficiency
   Amaurosis fugax
   Visual field loss (hemianopic and scotomas)
   Visual hallucinations

SIGNS
- Retina
   Darkening, dilation, and tortuosity of retinal veins
   Deeper, darker purple hue
   Small scattered superficial and deep retinal
      hemorrhages
   Retinal edema
   Bilateral thrombus of the central retinal vein
   CRVO
- Optic nerve
   Florid color
   Moderate to severe edema
- Conjunctival vessels
   Dilation and tortuousity of the vessels

TABLE 67–4. DIAGNOSIS OF POLYCYTHEMIA

Polycythemia Vera Diagnosis Criteria

Category A
   Measured increase in red cell mass: men >36 mL/kg,
      women >30 mL/kg
   Normal arterial oxygen saturation >92%
   Splenomegaly
Category B
   Thrombocytosis: platelet count >400,000/µL
   Leukocytosis: white blood cell >12,000/mL (in absence of
      fever or infection)
   Elevated serum vitamin B_{12} content
   >900 pg/mL and unbound vitamin B_{12}-binding
      capacity: >2200 pg/mL
Diagnosis of polycythemia vera if all three in category A are present, or only one or two in category A are present with at least two criteria from category B

Tests

	Normal	Polycythemia
RBC count	4.5 million/mm³ PV	6–8 million/mm³
Red cell volume		3 × normal
Blood viscosity		Up to 8 × normal
Hematocrit		70 to 80%
Red cell structure		Normal

Adapted from Wasserman LR, The management of polycythemia vera. Br J Hematol. *1971;21:371.*

Laboratory workup may identify abnormal RBC count, hemoglobin, and hematocrit. Platelet abnormalities may be present and correlate with an increased risk of thrombohemorrhagic phenomena. An increased platelet count (>400,000/µL) is often present at the initial diagnosis. Because leukocytosis occurs in almost 50% of patients, serum B_{12} levels are elevated, which is secondary to an associated increase in leukocyte alkine phosphatase activity and production of vitamin B_{12}-binding proteins.

■ Ocular

Although not usually found in isolation of the systemic manifestations, ocular findings may present initially. Conjunctival vascular congestion, hyperemia, and edema of the optic disc and retinal venous abnormalities may be seen early in the disease and assist the diagnosis.

TREATMENT AND MANAGEMENT

Table 67–5 summarizes the treatment and management of polycythemia.

■ Systemic

Treatment is based on the severity and nature of the symptoms and physical findings, particularly on the potential of cardiovascular burden from increased blood viscosity. Phlebotomy and myelosuppressive agents (eg, chlorambucil or radioactive phosphorus) may be needed to manage polycythemia. In secondary polycythemia, the underlying disease is treated first, when possible.

■ Ocular

The treatment of ocular manifestations is directed at the underlying systemic disease.

TABLE 67–5. TREATMENT AND MANAGEMENT OF POLYCYTHEMIA

■ SYSTEMIC
- General
  Phlebotomy alone
  Phlebotomy with myelosuppressive agents
  (radioactive phosphorus, chlorambucil)
- Secondary polycythemia
  Underlying disease is always treated first when possible

■ OCULAR
- Treatment of underlying systemic condition

CONCLUSION

Patients with polycythemia are generally diagnosed by the systemic manifestations of the disease, specifically postbathing redness, splenomegaly, and thrombohemorrhagic symptoms. The patient may, however, be identified by early ocular signs and symptoms. Conjunctival vascular congestion, blurred vision, and dilation of the retinal venous system may all present early in the disease. Because intervention may significantly increase the patient's survival time, appropriate diagnosis is critical for these patients.

REFERENCES

Ascher K. Eye manifestations in polycythemia. *JAMA*. 1971;215:295. Letter.

Ballantyne AJ, Michaelson IC. *The Fundus of the Eye*. Baltimore: Williams & Wilkins; 1980:342–343.

Berk PD, Goldberg JD, Donovan PB, et al. Therapeutic recommendations in polycythemia vera based on Polycythemia Vera Study Group protocols. *Semin Hematol*. 1986;23:132.

Berlin NI. Diagnosis and classification of the polycythemias. *Semin Hematol*. 1975;12:339.

Christian A. The nervous system of polycythemia vera. *Am J Med Sci*. 1917;154:547.

Cohen M. Fundus changes in polycythemia. *Arch Ophth*. 1937;17:817.

Freedman B. Papilledema, optic atrophy and blindness due to emphysema. *Br J Ophthalmol*. 1963;47:290.

Frenkel EP, Fleischman RA. Polycythemia vera. In: Kelley WN, ed. *Textbook of Internal Medicine*. Philadelphia: Lippincott; 1992;1084–1087.

Hocking WG, Golde DW. Polycythemia: Evaluation and management. *Blood*. 1989;3:59.

Hoffman R, Wasserman LR. Natural history and management of polycythemia vera. *Adv Intern Med*. 1979;24:255.

Lawrence JH, Goetsch AT. Familial occurrence of polycythemia and leukemia. *Calif Med*. 1950;73:361.

Lindsey J, Insler M. Polycythemia rubra vera and conjunctival vascular congestion. *Ann Ophthalmol*. 1985;17:62.

Modan B. An epidemiological study of polycythemia vera. *Blood*. 1965;26:657.

Modan B, Kallner H, Zemer D, Yornan C. A note on the increased risk of polycythemia vera in Jews. *Blood*. 1971;37:172.

Rothstein T. Bilateral central retinal vein closure as the initial manifestation of polycythemia. *Am J Ophthalmol*. 1972;74:256–260.

Silverstein MN, Lanier AP. Polycythemia vera, 1935–1969: An epidemiologic survey in Rochester, Minnesota. *Mayo Clin Proc*. 1971;4B:751.

Thomas DJ, Marshall J, duBoulay GH, et al. Cerebral blood-flow in polycythemia. *Lancet*. 1977;23:161–163.

Wagener HP, Rucker CW. Lesions of the retina and optic nerve in association with blood dyscrasias. In: Sorsby A, ed. *Modern Trends in Ophthalmology*. London: Butterworth; 1948:300.

Wasserman LR. The management of polycythemia vera. *Br J Hematol*. 1971;21:371.

68
Chapter

Sickle Hemoglobinopathies

Holly Myers

The hemoglobinopathies are a group of disorders, usually inherited, that have abnormal erythrocyte function under certain conditions. This is caused by abnormalities in hemoglobin structure, function, or production. Abnormal hemoglobin usually occurs because of a substitution of a single amino acid in one of its polypeptide chains. There are over 300 types of hemoglobinopathies. This chapter will be limited to a discussion of sickle-cell syndromes.

Normal adult hemoglobin is pliable and flexible and flows easily through capillaries. It delivers oxygen to tissues. In sickle-cell syndromes, the hemoglobin becomes elongated and more rigid. This is referred to as "sickled" or a "sickle cell." In this state its movement through small blood vessels is slowed and an increase in viscosity results. The most significant ocular manifestation is sickle retinopathy. This retinopathy is characterized in part by venous tortuosity and occlusions, retinal pigment epithelial hyperplasia and hypertrophy, arteriolar occlusion, vitreous hemorrhage, and neovascularization.

EPIDEMIOLOGY

■ Systemic

Hemoglobinopathies are common where malaria is endemic because they provide protection against the lethal effects of malaria. Sickle-cell syndromes are present in 10% of African-Americans. Of this group, 80% have sickle-cell trait (SA), 10% sickle-cell thalassemia (SThal), 4% sickle-cell anemia (SS), and 2% sickle-cell hemoglobin C disease (SC) (Goldberg, 1992).

■ Ocular

Proliferative sickle-cell retinopathy (PSR) is primarily seen in those between 40 and 50 years of age and is rare in patients under 20 years of age. Vision loss occurs in 34% of patients with PSR and only 2% in patients without PSR (Moriarty et al, 1988).

In SS, the ocular complications are less severe, with proliferative sickle-cell retinopathy present in only about 10% of the population (Siegel, 1988). Persons carrying the genotype SA normally do not express significant variation in function and ocular findings are uncommon. SC has a significantly higher incidence of proliferative retinopathy at 32% (Moriarty et al, 1988). SThal has a higher incidence of retinopathy than sickle-cell anemia. Ocular findings are rare in hemoglobin C trait (AC) (Goldberg, 1992).

Vitreous hemorrhage has been reported in 23% of SC patients and is infrequent in SS or SA. Retinal detachment is most common in SC, and again, is rare in SS or SA.

NATURAL HISTORY

■ Systemic

Specific inheritance patterns are associated with the different sickle-cell syndromes (Table 68–1). These inheritance

The author would like to acknowledge Christopher Adsit for assisting in the preparation of this chapter.

TABLE 68–1. SICKLE-CELL HEMOGLOBINOPATHIES

Normal Hemoglobin

Hemoglobin F (HbF): fetal hemoglobin
Hemoglobin A (HbA): normal adult hemoglobin

Abnormal Hemoglobin

Hemoglobin S (HbS): valine is substituted for glutamic acid
Hemoglobin C (HbC): lysine is substituted for glutamic acid
Thalassemia (Thal): disorder of the rate of globin chain synthesis

Inheritance

HbS + HbS = SS	Sickle-cell anemia
HbS + HbA = SA	Sickle-cell trait
HbS + HbC = SC	Sickle-cell C disease
HbS + Thal = SThal	Sickle-cell thalassemia
HbA + HbC = AC	Hemoglobin C trait

TABLE 68–2. SYSTEMIC MANIFESTATIONS OF SICKLE-CELL SYNDROMES

ACUTE SICKLE-CELL CRISIS
- Extreme pain
  Back
  Chest
  Extremities
- Complications
  CVA
  Acute chest syndrome from involvement of the pulmonary vessels
  Hepatic crisis
  Acute renal failure

CHRONIC ORGAN DAMAGE
- Chronic skin ulcers
  Particularly the legs
- Bone infarcts
  Associated with bone pain
- Microinfarct of the renal medulla
  Inability to concentrate urine
- Papillary infarcts
  Prolonged painless hematuria
- Autosplenectomy
  Common in patients with SS

ADDITIONAL MANIFESTATIONS (NOT RELATED TO VASOOCCLUSION)
- Increased susceptibility to infections
- Gallstone formation
- Abnormal growth and development

patterns form five major hemoglobinopathies that have a wide range of systemic and ocular complications (Table 68–2). They are sickle-cell anemia (SS), sickle-cell trait (SA), sickle-cell C disease (SC), thalassemia (SThal), and hemoglobin C trait (AC).

Of the sickle-cell syndromes, SS has the most acute life-threatening systemic manifestations. Persons carrying the genotype SA normally do not express significant variation in function and systemic findings are uncommon. SC and SThal have relatively fewer systemic complications compared to SS. Systemic findings are rare in AC.

Sickle-cell anemia is homozygous for hemoglobin S and causes an unrelenting hemolytic anemia. The clinical manifestations appear after the newborn period when HbF is replaced by HbS. Most manifestations of the disease are related to the vasoocclusive phenomena that result because of the elongated or sickling characteristics of the abnormal hemoglobin in the presence of decreased oxygen. As the oxygenation of tissue decreases from a vascular occlusive phenomenon, acidosis develops, with further sickling occurring and increased occlusion. This cycle of erythrostasis is characteristic throughout the body. Cardinal manifestations of SS are chronic infection and vasoocclusive episodes with end-organ damage.

High mortality rate in early childhood is associated with "acute sickle-cell crisis." These crises are periodic occurrences of acute pain and fever, and are caused by recurrent vasoocclusive events that affect various parts of the body (back, chest, extremities). The episode may last from hours to days. Various conditions may precipitate the crisis, such as influenza, trauma, surgery, dehydration, extreme psychological or physical stress, and exposure to heat or cold. This crisis may cause complications including cerebrovascular accident (CVA), hepatic crisis, acute renal infarction, and acute chest syndrome from involvement of pulmonary vessels.

Recently, survival rates have improved, with increasing numbers of patients reaching 50 years of age and beyond. This is thought to be due to improvements in nutrition and more adequate prevention, such as partial exchange transfusions (Benz, 1992).

Due to the ongoing nature of the disease, chronic damage may occur. Skin ulcers, bone infarcts, microinfarcts of the renal medulla, papillary infarcts, and autosplenectomy may be found. Individuals may have increased susceptibility to infection and gallstone formation and have abnormal growth and development.

Patients with sickle-cell trait are typically asymptomatic. Clinical manifestations may appear when unusual circumstances foster sickling. Congenital heart disease, travel in an unpressurized air craft, and pregnancy may cause clinical manifestations.

Sickle-cell C disease and sickle-cell thalassemia are associated with mild anemia and patients may be asymptomatic. Splenomegaly is common and infarction may occur in some cases. Infarcts of the bone and bone pain may occur. Anemia may complicate pregnancy. The vasoocclusive manifestations from sickling are in general less frequent and less severe than those seen in SS. Patients with

SC and SThal may also present with systemic complications, as previously described for the SS patient.

■ Ocular

In contrast to the systemic manifestations, the ocular findings are more common and more severe in SC and in SThal, less severe in SS, and rare in SA (Table 68–3). The expected degree of ocular involvement cannot be based upon the severity of the systemic disease. Patients who have SS with the most acute life-threatening systemic manifestations have fewer ocular complications than patients with SC and SThal disease. Although SC and SThal patients have fewer systemic complications, they demonstrate a much higher incidence of proliferative retinopathy.

The ocular manifestations of sickle-cell syndromes are secondary to the effect of arteriolar, capillary, and venule occlusions. Ocular manifestations are many and affect virtually every tissue. The conjunctiva, iris, uvea, optic nerve, and retina are all possible sites of disease expression. Retinal changes are of primary concern because it is the proliferative retinopathy that causes the most profound and permanent visual impairment. The anterior segment may, however, be the initial site of the sickling process.

The capillaries in the conjunctiva, particularly in the inferior quadrant, appear comma shaped. These may appear isolated because the efferent and afferent vessels lack red blood cells. This may even be observed with the naked eye. Heat from slit-lamp examination may warm the conjunctiva, dilate the vessels, and subsequently hide the sign, whereas a topical vasoconstrictor such as phenylephrine will enhance the sign. This finding is a very reliable indicator of sickle-cell disease. It is observed in 97% of SS patients, 80% of SC patients, and 64% of SThal patients. The severity of the conjunctival sign has been shown to correlate with the severity of the disease (Comer & Fred, 1964; Nagpol et al, 1977b; Paton, 1961).

Microhyphemas from trauma are normally benign, but in patients with sickle-cell syndromes a small hyphema may cause a severe secondary glaucoma. The sickling seems to be increased as a result of stagnation, hypoxia, and acidosis in the anterior chamber. These sickled cells obstruct the aqueous outflow and result in an increased IOP.

The uveal tract is well vascularized and can be affected by the blood sludging from the sickled cells. Focal iris atrophy, rubeosis iridis with secondary glaucoma, and choroidal vessel occlusion have all been observed.

Transient plugs of deoxygenated erythrocytes are seen in small vessels on the surface of the optic nerve. No functional visual impairment occurs. They are most common in SS (29%) and SThal (10%) and do occur in SC (2%) (Goldbaum et al, 1978).

A variety of retinal findings may occur in many different combinations. Retinal changes not associated with proliferative retinopathy include venous tortuosity, black sun-

TABLE 68–3. OCULAR MANIFESTATIONS IN SICKLE-CELL SYNDROMES

GENERAL
- Conjunctival sickling sign
- Focal iris atrophy
- Refractory increase in IOP with microhyphemias
- Rubeosis irides
- Optic disc sign
- Choroidal vascular occlusion

RETINOPATHY
- **Nonproliferative**
  Venous tortuosity
  Black sunbursts
  Refractile deposits
  Silver-wire arterioles
  Salmon-patch hemorrhages
  Retinal holes/tears
  CRAO
  Macular arteriole occlusions
  Retinal venous occlusions
  Angioid streaks
  Macular holes
  Dark without pressure
- **Proliferative**
  Stage I: Peripheral Arteriolar Occlusions
    Capillary bed and venule fail to fill
    Grayish-brown coloration of retina
    Silver-wire or chalky white arterioles
    Interface of perfused to nonperfused retina visible with FA
  Stage II: Peripheral Arteriolar–Venule Anastomoses
    Anastomoses at interface of nonperfused retina, blood shunted from occluded arterioles to nearest venule
    Enlargement of preexisting capillaries
    Resemble telangiectases and microaneurysms
  Stage III: Neovascular Proliferation
    Neovascular capillary buds from perfused to nonperfused retina
    Attempt to revascularize ischemic retina
    Fan-shaped neovascularization
    FA: vitreous leakage
  Stage IV: Vitreous Hemorrhage
    Due to minor ocular trauma, vitreous collapse, or traction on adherent neovascular tissue
    Small and localized or massive
    Clotted hemorrhage becomes organized to form white fibrous tissue
    Intermittent bleed in fibrovascular area
  Stage V: Retinal Detachment
    Rhegmatogenous and/or nonrhegmatogenous
    Associated retinal holes
    Vitreous hemorrhage

bursts, dark without pressure, refractile deposits, salmon patch hemorrhages, and retinal holes and tears.

Tortuosity of the venous system is a common characteristic of sickle-cell syndromes, present in 47% of patients with SS and 32% of patients with SC. It is uncommon in SA or SThal. It may not be considered diagnostic because it is associated with so many other diseases (Goldberg, 1992).

"Sunbursts" are black fundus lesions with stellate borders (Figure 68–1). Usually 0.5 to 2.0 disc diameters in size, they are focal areas of RPE migration, hyperplasia, and hypertrophy. These are thought to be the result of acute vascular occlusion of the retina that lead to deep retinal hemorrhage near the RPE.

Granular, refractile substance is often seen in the retinal periphery and is associated with arteriolar occlusions. In addition, when hemoglobin degrades, small schisis cavities are formed intraretinally and hemosiderin is trapped within these spaces. This rarely involves the macular area. These are a prognostic sign for the subsequent development of neovascularization.

Dark-without-pressure appears as geographic brown mottled areas in the retina. It is found in SC, SS, and SThal. The etiology is unclear, but it is believed to be the sequel to vascular occlusive events in the area.

Salmon-patch hemorrhages are located in the midperipheral retina usually within the sensory retina but may break through the internal limiting membrane into the subretinal space. The appearance is oval or round with defined borders, and is bright red when recent, changing to an orange and then to a yellow or white nodule. The hemorrhage normally measures between 0.25 and 2.0 disc diameters. Usually, a sudden occlusion of an adjacent arteriole is the cause. The hemor-

rhage may last days to weeks, and will result in a retinoschisis cavity or a focal thinned patch. Refractile bodies are often found within this cavity.

Retinal holes or tears may be found in the equatorial region or slightly posterior to the equator. Small to moderate in size, these are usually oval or horseshoe shaped. There may be adjacent or overlying vitreous traction bands. The patient is normally without symptoms until vitreous hemorrhage or retinal detachment occurs.

Various vascular occlusions occur in sickle hemoglobinopathies. Central retinal artery occlusion (CRAO) has been reported in SA, SS, and SC, but is infrequent. Macular arteriole occlusions have been reported with SS and SThal. Discrete occlusions of the capillary network causes pathological avascular zones and an enlargement of the foveal avascular zone, which may result in significant visual defects. Venous occlusions have only rarely been reported. Extensive vaso-occlusion of the choroid or posterior ciliary vessel may occur. This has been reported in SA, SC, and SThal.

Angioid streaks are not frequently seen, and when present rarely cause visual disability. These are most frequently seen in SS disease, but have been reported in each major sickle-cell hemoglobinopathy. It is unclear as to whether the brittleness of the Bruch membrane is caused by the deposition of iron or calcium in the membrane (Jampol et al, 1987).

Proliferative sickle-cell retinopathy occurs primarily between 40 and 50 years of age and is rare in patients under 20 years. Vision loss occurs in 34% of patients with PSR and only 2% of patients without PSR. Proliferative disease is classically characterized by seafan neovascularization (Figure 68–2). Seafans may spontaneously regress, with resulting fibrous tissue or progress to ultimately result in a retinal

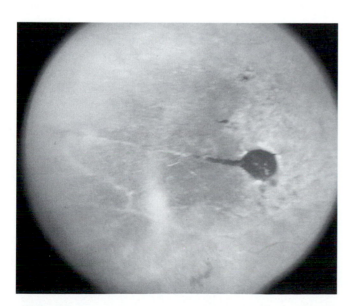

Figure 68–1. Patient with SS disease. Note vascular nonperfusion, pigment clumping, and large "black sunburst." *(Courtesy of Jane Stein, The Eye Institute, Pennsylvania College of Optometry.)*

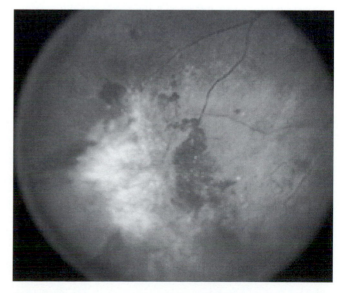

Figure 68–2. Patient with SC disease. Note seafan-like neovascularization, hemorrhage, and fibrosis. *(Courtesy of Jane Stein, The Eye Institute, Pennsylvania College of Optometry.)*

detachment. Vitreous hemorrhage and retinal detachment are common is SC and occur rarely in SS or SA.

Proliferative sickle-cell retinopathy may be divided into five stages that mark its progression. Peripheral arteriolar occlusion marks stage I, peripheral arteriolar-venule anastomoses stage II, neovascular proliferation stage III, vitreous hemorrhage stage IV, and retinal detachment stage V. Table 68–3 details these stages (Goldberg, 1971a).

DIAGNOSIS

■ Systemic
A sickle-cell syndrome should be suspected in African-American patients with repeated episodes of bone, joint, abdominal, or thoracic pain, accompanied by hemolytic anemia.

A blood cell count will typically show moderately severe anemia. A "sickle-cell preparation" consists of blood mixed with a solution of sodium metabisulfate. This will deoxygenate the blood and induce sickling, if abnormal hemoglobin is present. It is important to determine the phenotype and then identify the type of hemoglobin. Hemoglobin electrophoresis is done for the diagnosis of the different sickle-cell syndromes (Table 68–4).

■ Ocular
Diagnosis of a sickle-cell syndrome may begin with observations during ocular examination. Anterior segment evaluation may show iris atrophy that occurs from the pupillary border to the collarette. When comma-shaped vessels on the conjunctiva are observed, the diagnosis of a sickle-cell syndrome should be considered, because these are a reliable indicator of the disease. However, differential diagnosis should consider other etiologies associated with conjunctival vascular changes and sludging of blood (eg, polycythemia).

Retinal findings are often characteristic such that diagnosis of sickling can be made based on clinical grounds. The presence of black sunbursts, salmon-patch hemorrhages, vascular occlusions, or seafan neovascularization are suggestive

of sickle-cell syndromes. Other retinopathies that are characterized by closure of retinal vessels may have a similar appearance. These retinopathies include sarcoidosis, chronic myelogenous leukemia, Takayasu pulseless disease, retinopathy of prematurity, branch retinal vein occlusion, Eales disease, and diabetes mellitus. Fluorescein angiography may assist in the diagnosis and treatment of proliferative disease.

TREATMENT AND MANAGEMENT

■ Systemic
When patients experience acute sickle cell pain crisis, treatment is necessary and is dependent on the severity of the event (Table 68–5). Therapy may include analgesics, bed rest, and vigorous hydration. When hypoxia occurs, oxygen should be administered. Transfusions have a limited role in the management of sickle-cell syndromes, but may be particularly helpful during periods of increased risk, such as surgery.

Treatment includes supportive management and routine physicals, along with good nutrition that includes folic acid supplements. Patient education includes genetic counseling and advising the patient of the importance of prompt medical attention for symptoms of pain, fever, or infection.

■ Ocular
Indications for treatment include retinal neovascularization, vitreal hemorrhage that does not resolve, retinal detachment, and secondary glaucoma (Table 68–6).

Treatment is indicated when the proliferative neovascular stages III and IV are reached. This includes direct focal ablation and panretinal photocoagulation. When a feeder vessel is treated, there is a higher risk of choroidal neovascularization and retinal detachment. The effectiveness of the therapy is determined with the use of fluorescein angiography.

Persistent hemorrhage may necessitate a vitrectomy. When retinal detachment occurs, standard corrective techniques may be used, along with appropriate management to prevent anterior segment ischemia.

TABLE 68–4. DIFFERENTIAL DIAGNOSIS OF SICKLE-CELL SYNDROMES

Genotype	Clinical Condition	Hemoglobin Electrophoresis Findings (%)					Other Assoc. Findings
		HbA	HbS	HbA2	HbF	HbC	
SA	Sickle-cell trait		55–60	40–45	2–3	1	Asymptomatic, no anemia
SS	Sickle-cell anemia	0	85–95	2–3	5–15	—	Usually clinically severe
S/B⁰-thal	Sickle-cell/B-thalassemia	0	70–80	3–5	10–20	—	Moderate severity, >50% splenomegaly, hypochromia and microcytosis
S/B⁺-thal	Sickle-cell/B-thalassemia	10–20	60–75	3–5	10–20	—	As above
SC	HbSC disease	0	45–50	2–3	1	45–50	Moderate severity, splenomegaly

TABLE 68–5. SYSTEMIC TREATMENT AND MANAGEMENT OF SICKLE-CELL SYNDROMES

- Acute pain crisis
    - Treatment varies depending on the severity: vigorous hydration, analgesics, bed rest
- Hypoxia
    - Oxygen
- Supportive management
    - Good nutritional state
    - Folic acid supplements
    - Education: genetic counseling, importance of prompt medical care

Treatment of glaucoma in those with sickle-cell disease may warrant special considerations. Topical agents are generally good treatment options for sickle-cell patients, but carbonic anhydrase inhibitors and oral osmotic agents are contraindicated. Carbonic anhydrase inhibitors increase hemoconcentration and blood viscosity, resulting in systemic acidosis, which potentiates sickling. Oral osmotic agents should be avoided because these also may result in increased blood viscosity. In sickle-cell patients with hyphema and acute increased intraocular pressure uncontrolled by topical agents, paracentesis may be the most effective treatment (Wax et al, 1982). Extra consideration should be given to the sickle-cell patient with hyphema, because the hypoxia in the anterior chamber increases cell sickling, with a greater risk for severe secondary glaucoma. Because of this risk, all African-American patients who present with hyphema should be screened for sickle-cell disease.

TABLE 68–6. OCULAR TREATMENT AND MANAGEMENT OF SICKLE-CELL SYNDROMES

- Retinal pre-neovascularization (stages I and II)
    - No preventative treatment has been shown to prevent retinal neovascularization in sickle-cell patients
- Retinal neovascularization (stages III–V)
    - Treatment forms: direct focal ablation, feeder vessel treatment, panretinal scatter
- Vitreal hemorrhage (nonresolving)
    - Vitrectomy
- Retinal detachment
    - Standard techniques with special consideration to prevent anterior ischemia
- Hyphema/secondary glaucoma
    - Topical agents
    - Carbonic anhydrase inhibitors and oral osmotic agents are contraindicated
    - Paracentesis (effective for secondary glaucoma with hyphema)

CONCLUSION

Sickle-cell syndromes are relatively common in African-Americans. Dependent on the type, sickle-cell syndromes have the potential for severe systemic or ocular manifestations. Patients with sickle-cell anemia are at greatest risk to develop life-threatening systemic manifestations. Patients with sickle-cell hemoglobin C disease and sickle-cell thalassemia should be monitored closely for evidence of proliferative retinopathy and treated when appropriate, in an attempt to prevent a catastrophic event such as a retinal detachment. The role of the eyecare practitioner in both diagnosis and treatment is paramount to the care of these patients.

REFERENCES

Benz EJ. Hemoglobinopathy: Genetics, pathophysiology and clinical features. In: Kelley WN, ed. *Textbook of Internal Medicine.* Philadelphia: Lippincott; 1992:1293–1299.

Bonanomi MT, Cunha SL, de Aravjo JT. Funduscopic alterations in SS and SC hemoglobinopathies. *Ophthalmology.* 1988;197: 26–33.

Carney MD, Jampol LM. Epiretinal membranes in sickle cell retinopathy. *Arch Ophthalmol.* 1987;105:214–217.

Comer PB, Fred HL. Diagnosis of sickle cell disease by ophthalmoscopic inspection of conjunctiva. *N Engl J Med.* 1964;271: 544–545.

Condon PI, Jampol LM, Farber MD, et al. A randomized clinical trial of feeder vessel photocoagulation of sickle cell retinopathy 2. Update and analysis of risk factors. *Ophthalmology.* 1984; 91:1496–1498.

Condon PI, Serjeant GR. Ocular findings in sickle cell thalassemia in Jamaica. *Am J Ophthalmol.* 1972;74:1105.

Gartaganis S, Ismiridis K, Papageorgiou O, et al. Ocular abnormalities in patients with B-thalassemia. *Am J Ophthalmol.* 1989;108:699–703.

Goldbaum MH, Jampol LM, Goldberg MF. The disc signs in sickling hemoglobinopathies. *Arch Ophthalmol.* 1978;96:1597–1600.

Goldberg MF. Sickle cell retinopathy. In: Tasman W, Jaeger EA, eds. *Duane's Clinical Ophthalmology.* Philadelphia: Lippincott; 1992;3.

Goldberg MF. Classification and pathogenesis of sickle retinopathy. *Am J Ophthalmol.* 1971a;71:649.

Goldberg MF. Natural history of untreated proliferative sickle retinopathy. *Arch Ophthalmol.* 1971b;85:428.

Goldberg MF, Acacio I. Argon laser photocoagulation of proliferative sickle retinopathy. *Arch Ophthalmol.* 1973;90:35

Isenberg SJ, McRee WE, Jedrzynski MS, et al. Effects of sickle cell anemia on conjunctival oxygen tension and temperature. *Arch Intern Med.* 1987;147:67–69.

Jampol LM, Acheson R, Eagle RC, et al. Calcification of Bruch's membrane in angioid streaks with homozygous sickle cell disease. *Arch Ophthalmol.* 1987;105:93–98.

Jampol LM, Condon P, Farber M, et al. A randomized clinical trial of feeder vessel photocoagulation of sickle cell retinopathy, 1. Preliminary results. *Ophthalmology*. 1983;90:540–545.

Jampol LM, Goldbaum MH. Peripheral proliferative retinopathies. *Surv Ophthalmol*. 1980;25:1–14.

Jampol LM, Green JL, Goldberg MF, et al. An update: Vitrectomy surgery and retinal detachment repair in sickle cell disease. *Arch Ophthalmol*. 1982;100:541–593.

Moriarty BJ, Acheson RW, Condon PI, Serjeant GR. Patterns of visual loss in untreated sickle cell retinopathy. *Eye*. 1988; 2:330–335.

Nagpol KC, Goldberg MF, Rabb MF. Ocular manifestations of sickle hemoglobinopathies. *Surv Ophthalmol*. 1977a;21:391.

Nagpol KC, Asdourian GK, Goldbaum MH, et al. The conjunctival sickling sign, hemoglobin S, and irreversibily sickled erythrocytes. *Arch Ophthalmol*. 1977b;95:808–811.

Paton D. The conjunctival sign of sickle cell disease. *Arch Ophthalmol*. 1961;66:90–94.

Paylor RR, Carney MD, Ogura K, et al. Alteration of the blood–retinal barrier and vitreous in sickle cell retinopathy. *Int Ophthalmol*. 1986;9:103–108.

Peachey NS, Gagliano DA, Jacobson MS, et al. Correlation of electroretinographic findings and peripheral retinal nonperfusion in patients with sickle cell retinopathy. *Arch Ophthalmol*. 1990;108:1106–1109.

Roth SE, Magargal LE, Kimmel AS, et al. Central retinal-artery occlusion in proliferative sickle-cell retinopathy after retrobulbar injection. *Ann Ophthalmol*. 1988;20:221–224.

Serjeant BE, Mason KP, Acheson RW, et al. Blood rheology and proliferative retinopathy in homozygous sickle cell disease. *Br J Ophthalmol*. 1986;70:522–525.

Siegel D. Diagnosis and treatment of sickle cell retinopathy. *J Am Optom Assoc*. 1988;59:885–888.

Rednam KRV, Jampol LM, Goldberg MF. Scatter retinal photocoagulation for proliferative sickle cell retinopathy. *Am J Ophthalmol*. 1982;93:594.

Wax MB, Ridley ME, Magargal LE. Reversal of retinal and optic disc ischemia in a patient with sickle cell trait and glaucoma secondary to traumatic hyphema. *Am Acad Ophthalmol*. 1982;89:845–851.

Welch RB, Goldberg MF. Sickle-cell hemoglobin and its relation to fundus abnormality. *Arch Ophthalmol*. 1966;75:353.

69
Chapter

Leukemias

Connie L. Chronister

Leukemia is a neoplastic disease of the bone marrow, with the neoplasm consisting of abnormal proliferation of lymphocytes and their precursors. This proliferation occurs throughout the body, especially in the bone marrow, spleen, and lymph nodes.

Leukemia can be classified as chronic or acute. Further classification of the common acute forms include acute lymphocytic leukemia (ALL) and acute myelocytic leukemia (AML). The common chronic forms include chronic lymphocytic leukemia (CLL) and chronic myelocytic leukemia (CML).

All ocular tissues, especially those that are vascularized, may be affected by leukemia. The presence of systemic leukemia can often be detected by ocular examination. The ocular sequelae of leukemia emphasize the important role that the eyecare practitioner plays in its detection, diagnosis, and management.

EPIDEMIOLOGY

■ Systemic

The incidence of all leukemias is 13 per 100,000 persons per year, and is slightly higher in men than women (Champlin & Golde, 1991). The acute leukemias affect women and men equally. ALL primarily affects children and young adults, while AML can occur in all ages, particularly adults. Although AML is often idiopathic, it may occur in patients with increased exposure to high doses of radiation or to alkylating agents (Fishman et al, 1991). The elderly are more likely to exhibit chronic lymphocytic and chronic myelogenous leukemia, with men affected more often than women.

■ Ocular

The prevalence of ocular involvement in patients with leukemia ranges from 9 to 90 percent (Guyer et al, 1989). This variation is due to the many different types of leukemia, in addition to when the study was performed,

(pre- or postmortem). Allen and Straatsma (1961) found that of all leukemic eyes, 80% with ocular findings were those with acute leukemia. Kincaid and Green (1983) found that 75% of chronic leukemic autopsied eyes exhibited ocular involvement. A postmortem study by Leonardy and colleagues (1990) showed infiltrates in the eyes of 31% of leukemic patients, with the choroid being the most frequently involved ocular tissue.

NATURAL HISTORY

■ Systemic

The etiologies of the leukemias remain unknown. Sandler (1990) reviewed the possibilities, which include exposure, either occupational or environmental, to ionizing radiation or toxins. The human T-cell leukemia is associated with exposure to a retrovirus (HTLV-I). Other associations with leukemia include chromosomal or genetic abnormalities, along with implications of smoking as a possible cause.

Leukemic cells overgrow normal cells in the bone marrow. These neoplastic cells have a slower cycle, remain immature, and never stop dividing. As a result, leukemic cells take over the bone marrow and invade other tissues. Death may commonly result from infection due to malfunctioning leukocytes that leave the patient immunocompromised from hemorrhaging and anemia secondary to lack of platelets and red blood cells (Kincaid, 1990).

Prior to chemotherapy, many patients died before central nervous system (CNS) involvement. Because the CNS is less accessible to chemotherapy, leukemia can thrive there (Champlin; 1991). Symptoms of CNS leukemia include nausea, vomiting, lethargy, and seizures.

Acute Leukemias

Acute leukemias have a rapid, progressive, declining course that often causes death within months if left untreated. Blood analysis reveals immature leukocytes. These immature leukocytes are from proliferation of myeloid or lymphoid cells. These cells accumulate in the bone marrow, circulate in the blood, and may infiltrate into lymph nodes, spleen, skin, viscera, and the CNS. These blood-borne cells can circulate, accumulate in, and affect any organ site, including ocular tissues. The organs affected may be characteristic of the type of leukemia. Leukemic infiltration rarely affects organ function except for the bone marrow and CNS. The end result can be meningeal infiltration with increasing intracranial pressure. Disruption of normal hematopoiesis causes anemia, thrombocytopenia, and granulocytopenia. Without treatment, the average survival rate of patients with acute leukemia is 4 months (Berkow & Fletcher,1992).

The signs and symptoms (Table 69–1) of systemic acute leukemias include bleeding, pallor, fever, petechiae, mucous membrane hemorrhage, and easy bruisability. All of these signs and symptoms are due to the failure of normal hematopoiesis seen in leukemic patients. If the CNS becomes involved, the patient may experience headaches, vomiting, and irritability. Some patients complain of joint and bone pain.

Chronic Leukemia

Chronic leukemia can have an insidious onset with nonspecific symptoms (see Table 69–1) of fatigue, weakness, anorexia, weight loss, fever, night sweats, and a sense of abdominal fullness. Patients may remain asymptomatic for some time. Unlike acute leukemia, chronic leukemia rarely causes pallor, bleeding, and easy bruisability at the onset of the disease, but these do manifest with disease progression, along with fever and marked lymphadenopathy. Some patients, especially with CML, experience weight loss and hepatosplenomegaly.

Chronic leukemias show a more prolonged clinical course. The disease is characterized by excessive produc-

TABLE 69–1. SYSTEMIC MANIFESTATIONS OF LEUKEMIA

ACUTE LEUKEMIA
- Failure of normal hematopoiesis
  - Bleeding
  - Petechiae
  - Pallor
  - Fever
  - Easy bruisability
  - Mucous membrane hemorrhage
- Infection
- CNS involvement
  - Headaches
  - Vomiting
  - Irritability
- Joint and bone pain

CHRONIC LEUKEMIA
- Possibly asymptomatic in early stages
- Insidious onset of nonspecific symptoms
  - Fatigue
  - Weakness
  - Fever
  - Night sweats
  - Anorexia
  - Weight loss
  - Sense of abdominal fullness
- With disease progression
  - Pallor
  - Fever
  - Marked splenomegaly
  - Marked lymphadenopathy
  - Bleeding
  - Easy bruisability

tion of granulocytes in the bone marrow, spleen, and liver. This excessive production progresses to an accelerated phase, and patients can develop myeloblast tumors in the bone, CNS, lymph nodes, and skin. The course is indolent and chemotherapy rarely prolongs life. The median survival time in CML is 3 to 4 years after clinical onset (Berkow & Fletcher, 1992). However, in CLL a much more benign course may occur, with survival possibly as long as 10 to 15 years. These patients are usually elderly and often die of other disease processes.

■ Ocular

Ocular manifestations of leukemia (Table 69–2) are numerous, with all the ocular tissues, particularly those vascularized, affected. Generally, ocular involvement is more common in the acute than chronic forms of leukemia. In chronic leukemia, ocular findings can regress and then reappear, possibly missed by the eyecare practitioner. Ocular symptoms of CNS leukemia include blurring of vision, diplopia, extraocular muscle palsies from cranial nerve involvement, and papilledema. Leukemic infiltrates

TABLE 69–2. OCULAR MANIFESTATIONS OF LEUKEMIA

- **Ocular Adnexa**
  Lacrimal gland infiltration (dry eye)
  Dacryocystitis secondary to infiltration (epiphora)
  Extraocular muscle infiltration (paresis)
  Infiltration of skin of lid (lid swelling)
- **Orbit**
  Infiltration with associated exophthalmos, lid edema, chemosis, pain
- **Conjunctiva**
  Infiltrates in perivascular regions
  Conjunctival swellings
  Subconjunctival hemorrhage
  Necrosis secondary to ischemia
- **Cornea**
  Sterile peripheral corneal ulcers with pannus
- **Episcleral/Sclera**
  Episcleritis
  Infiltrates in perivascular regions (rare)
- **Iris and Ciliary Body**
  Infiltration
  Iris color change
  Associated pseudohypopyon (gray-yellow in color)
- **Retina**
  Dilated and tortuous venules
  Yellowing of vascular reflex

Hemorrhages (flame, dot, blot, white-centered)
Retinal leukemia infiltrates (perivascular gray-white sheathing)
Retinal infiltration tumors
Vitreal infiltrates
Cotton-wool spots
Microaneurysm
Peripheral retinal neovascularization
- **Choroid**
  Serous sensory retinal detachment
  RPE hypertrophy, hyperplasia, atrophy
  Photoreceptor disruption
  Cystoid retinal edema
  Drusen
- **Optic Nerve**
  Direct infiltration of optic nerve (vision loss, field loss)
  Papilledema secondary to CNS infiltration
- **Opportunistic Infections**
  Cytomegalovirus
  Herpes simplex
  Herpes zoster ophthalmicus
  Mumps
  Toxoplasmosis
  Bacterial infection
  Fungal infection (eg, *Candida, Aspergillus*)

have been found in the optic nerve, choroid, retina, ciliary body, anterior chamber, conjunctiva, limbus, sclera, and lacrimal apparatus.

Eye and adnexal involvement in leukemia is due most commonly to direct infiltration of neoblastic cells, along with secondary hematologic changes and infection. The orbit and ocular adnexa can be infiltrated with leukemic cells that lead to exophthalmos, lid edema, chemosis, EOM restrictions, dry eye, dacryoadenitis, dacryocystitis, and pain. Granulocytic sarcomas in AML often seen in children are a poor prognostic sign. Orbital tumors or masses can erode into the cranial cavity. Lacrimal gland infiltration can cause an associated dry eye. Rarely, EOM infiltration can lead to paresis. Dacryocystitis due to infiltration of the lacrimal sac and duct along with infiltration of the skin of the lid are rare occurrences in leukemia patients.

Conjunctival involvement is most often seen in lymphocytic leukemia. Infiltration occurs at all levels of this highly vascularized tissue. Infiltrates tend to aggregate in perivascular regions. The clinical picture of infiltration includes episcleritis, conjunctival swellings, and subconjunctival hemorrhages (Figure 69–1).

The cornea is normally an avascular tissue, with direct infiltration of leukemic cells not found beyond the limbus. Corneal involvement includes direct infiltration of the limbus and sterile peripheral corneal ulcers, with pannus.

Anterior segment involvement includes infiltration of the iris, ciliary body, and anterior chamber structures. Iris infiltration is characterized by a change in iris color that is not always clinically evident, and is often associated with a hypopyon that is gray-yellow in color.

Iritis can rarely occur due to compromised vascular perfusion of the limbal vessels. With anterior chamber

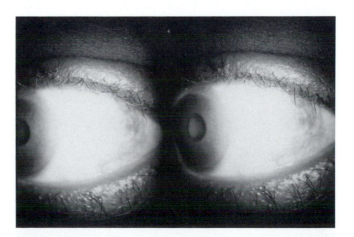

Figure 69–1. Stereophotograph of subconjunctival hemorrhage that can occur in patients with leukemia. *(Courtesy of Jane Stein, The Eye Institute, Pennsylvania College of Optometry.)*

involvement increased intraocular pressure often occurs. Trabecular meshwork infiltration may cause moderate elevation of IOP and secondary glaucoma. Rarely, anterior segment necrosis occurs secondary to ischemia.

Ocular involvement of the retina is more common in the acute leukemias. Retinal hemorrhage, cotton-wool spots (Figure 69–2), microaneurysms, peripheral neovascularization, and infiltrates are all associated with leukemic retinopathy. The choroid, due to its vast vascularity, commonly contains leukemic infiltration, but this is often difficult to detect clinically. Leukemia affects the CNS and consequently the optic nerve. Papilledema due to increased intracranial pressure can also be seen secondary to leukemic CNS involvement.

Early retinal findings include dilated and tortuous veins. The color of the venule and arteriolar reflex changes to a more yellow color, reflecting the decreased red cell count and increased white cell count. Hemorrhage is usually found in the posterior pole and in all of the retinal layers. Flame-shaped dot and blot hemorrhages frequently with a white center (Roth spot) are often seen in leukemic patients (Figure 69–3). The white center of the hemorrhage usually consists of leukemic cells, infiltrate, debris, platelet–fibrin aggregates, or septic emboli. Occasionally a vitreal hemorrhage can be found. During a relapse, leukemic hemorrhaging is usually not directly related to prognosis but is related to coexisting anemia.

Smaller infiltrates can be found perivascularly (sheathing), and may appear as gray-white streaks along the vessels. Massive infiltrates or tumors may destroy normal retinal architecture, with some infiltrates occasionally reaching the vitreous through breaks in the internal limit-

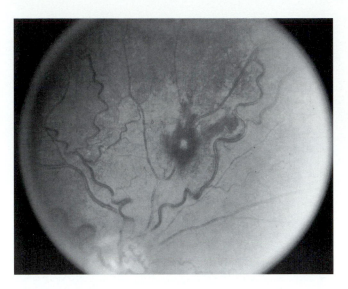

Figure 69–3. Fundus photography of a white-centered hemorrhage. The white center usually consists of leukemic cells. *(Courtesy of Jane Stein, The Eye Institute, Pennsylvania College of Optometry.)*

ing membrane. Leukemic retinal infiltration with a high leukocyte count is a poor prognostic sign (Rosenthal, 1983).

Cotton-wool spots are often found in leukemic patients and are due to ischemia caused by the anemia. Microaneurysms, a less common finding in leukemic retinopathy, are more often found in the peripheral retina and are most likely related to increased viscosity from elevated white cell count. Microaneurysms may be mistaken for dot hemorrhages and are underdiagnosed in leukemic patients that do not undergo fluorescein angiography (Kincaid & Green, 1983).

Peripheral retinal neovascularization, although a rare finding, is more commonly seen in chronic leukemic patients. The appearance is similar to the sea fans in sickle-cell disease. This is also related to increased white cell count. Leukemic therapy reduces the risk of neovascularization.

The choroid most consistently shows leukemic infiltration, but this is difficult to detect clinically. The leukemic infiltration tends to be perivascular and the choroidal infiltration may disrupt overlying retinal pigment epithelium (RPE), causing RPE atrophy, hypertrophy, hyperplasia, and migration into sensory retina, secondary photoreceptor disruption, drusen, serous detachments, and cystoid retinal edema. Serous sensory retinal detachment is the most common clinical presentation of choroidal infiltration. The detachment most commonly occurs in the posterior pole and is generally shallow. Occasionally a serous detachment is the first observed manifestation of the leukemic process (Kincaid & Green, 1983).

Optic nerve involvement includes direct infiltration of the optic nerve and papilledema due to increased intracranial

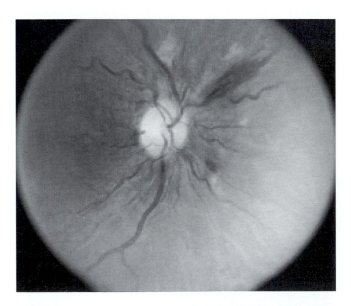

Figure 69–2. Fundus photograph of retinal hemorrhages and cotton-wool spots commonly seen in leukemic retinopathy. *(Courtesy of Jane Stein, The Eye Institute, Pennsylvania College of Optometry.)*

pressure from CNS leukemic infiltration. Direct invasion may be difficult to differentiate from papilledema; in addition, there is the possibility of both increased intracranial pressure and direct invasion of the nerve occurring concurrently. Acuity may remain fairly good even with direct infiltration of the optic nerve. Optic nervehead infiltration appears as a fluffy infiltrate superficial to lamina cribrosa. Nervehead swelling from retrolaminar leukemic invasion can cause profound vision loss and may require prompt irradiation to save vision.

Opportunistic ocular infections occur due to immunosuppression in patients with leukemia. The most common viral infection seen in leukemia patients is cytomegalovirus (Kincaid & Green, 1983). Other ocular viral infections occurring in these patients include herpes simplex (corneal ulcer), herpes zoster ophthalmicus, and mumps (granulomatous uveitis). Fungal infections seen in leukemic patients include *Candida* and cryptococcal retinitis, uveitis, and vitritis, as well as *Aspergillus* choroiditis and vitritis. Toxoplasmosis is a protozoal ocular infection which may occur in these immunocompromised patients. These patients are also vulnerable to a variety of bacterial ocular infections.

DIAGNOSIS

Table 69–3 gives an overview of leukemia diagnosis.

■ Systemic

Acute Leukemias
Diagnosis of acute leukemia is based on patient history, clinical presentation, and laboratory testing for anemia, thrombocytopenia, and leukemic blast cells in a bone mar-

TABLE 69–3. DIAGNOSIS OF LEUKEMIA

Acute Leukemia

Anemia

Thrombocytopenia

Leukemic blast cells usually found in blood smear

Bone marrow biopsy differentiates types of acute leukemias

Chronic Leukemia

White blood cell count
    Asymptomatic patient: <50,000/μL
    Symptomatic patient: 200,000–1,000,000/μL

Platelet count normal to slightly elevated

Hemoglobin greater than 10 gm/dL

Blood smears
    Increase in absolute eosinophil and basophils

Bone marrow biopsy and aspirate hypercellular

row smear. A bone marrow biopsy confirms the diagnosis and differentiates ALL from AML. CNS involvement may be diagnosed by examination of the CSF for leukemic cells.

Chronic Leukemia
The diagnosis of chronic leukemia is based on patient history; clinical presentation, particularly the delay of pallor, bleeding, and bruisability at the early stages of the disease; along with blood workup. Laboratory testing includes complete blood count, and blood smears. Bone marrow is hypercellular on both aspirate and biopsy.

■ Ocular
Diagnosis of ocular involvement is often made by the ophthalmoscopic appearance of the retina. In addition, fluorescein angiography can assist in the diagnosis of retinal manifestations, including microaneurysms and serous detachment. Aspiration of the anterior chamber may reveal leukemic cells.

TREATMENT AND MANAGEMENT

Table 69–4 describes leukemia treatment and management.

■ Systemic
Chemotherapy is the primary treatment modality for leukemia patients. Adjunct radiation to treat accumulations of leukemic cells is also used. Bone marrow transplantation may be done after the bone marrow has been destroyed by irradiation and chemotherapy. The optimal bone marrow donor includes an HLA-compatible sibling.

The acute leukemias are treated in three phases. This includes induction, which is the first phase of chemotherapy. When the patient goes into remission, a continued intensive period of chemotherapy follows during the consolidation phase. This is followed by the maintenance phase, which consists of a lower chemotherapy dose that may continue for several years. Treatment of the acute leukemias results in remission in approximately 75% of cases, with an even better prognosis in children suffering from ALL. In AML, remission usually lasts 2 years, and in ALL, relapse may occur years after remission (Fishman et al, 1991).

Because CLL usually follows a benign course, treatment is withheld until the patient experiences severe symptomatology, bone marrow or autoimmune involvement. Then an alkylating agent or chemotherapy may be instituted. CML may be treated with busulfan and bone marrow transplantation.

■ Ocular
Irradiation with systemic chemotherapy is utilized for leukemic infiltration of the eye (infiltration of iris, pseudo-

TABLE 69–4.   TREATMENT AND MANAGEMENT OF LEUKEMIA

■ **SYSTEMIC**
- Chemotherapy
- Radiation
- Bone marrow transplantation

AML
- Three phases of chemotherapy: induction consolidation, and maintenance
- Chemotherapy (cytarabine with doxorubicin or daunorubicin)
- Bone marrow transplant
- Chemotherapy and/or radiation followed by bone marrow transplantation
- Monitor for infection and potential antibiotic treatment
- Monitor for potential of increased bleeding (eg, care with brushing teeth, stool softener, hormonally suppressed menstruation)

ALL
- Three phases of chemotherapy: induction, consolidation, and maintenance
- Prednisone; vincristine; doxorubicin; L-asparaginase
- Prophylaxis for potential meningeal involvement (radiation, intrathecal methotrexate, or cytarabine)
- Monitor for infection and bleeding as above

CLL
- Monitor
- Alkylating agent
- Chemotherapy
- Steroid

CML
- Cytotoxic agent (Busulfan)
- Bone marrow transplantation

■ **OCULAR**
- Systemic chemotherapy (for ocular leukemic infiltration)
- Irradiation and intrathecal chemotherapy (for retrolaminar infiltration)
- Bone marrow transplantation

OCULAR SIDE EFFECTS OF TREATMENT
- **Cytotoxic Drugs**
  Cataracts, cranial nerve palsy, optic atrophy, intraocular inflammation
- **Bone Marrow Transplantation, With Chemotherapy**
  Graft-versus-host disease (Sjögren- or scleroderma-like illness: dry eye, conjunctival keratinization, ectropion, uveitis

hypopyon with increased IOP). Irradiation and intrathecal injection of chemotherapy is critical in the treatment of retrolaminar infiltration (Nikaido et al, 1988). Bone marrow transplantation can improve ocular and systemic sequelae.

There can be some ocular side effects from the treatments for leukemia. Cytotoxic drugs have caused cataracts (usually posterior subcapsular cataracts), cranial nerve palsies (nerves III to VII), optic atrophy, and intraocular inflammation (Kincaid & Green, 1983). The side effects of bone marrow transplantation with associated chemotherapy can cause acute graft-versus-host disease (GVHD) (Jabs et al, 1983). GVHD occurs with graft rejection and causes a Sjögren-syndrome-like or scleroderma-like illness that includes severe dry eye, conjunctival keratinization, ectropion of the eyelid, and uveitis (Jabs et al, 1983).

CONCLUSION

Leukemia is a serious disease that is very difficult to treat and can cause significant ocular side effects. All of the ocular tissues can be affected, most commonly the well-vascularized tissues of the retina and uveal tract. The prompt

diagnosis and treatment of leukemia patients is critical. Therefore, eyecare practitioners need to be aware of the systemic as well as the ocular manifestations of leukemia, so that they are able to properly diagnose, treat, and manage these severely ill patients.

REFERENCES

Allen RA, Straatsma BR. Ocular involvement in leukemia and allied disorders. *Arch Ophthalmol.* 1961;66:490–508.

Berkow R, Fletcher AJ. *The Merck Manual.* 16th ed. Rahway, NJ: Merck Research Laboratories; 1992:1233–1245.

Champlin R, Golde D. The leukemias. In: Wilson JD, Braunwald E, Isselbacher KJ, et al, eds. *Harrison's Principles of Internal Medicine.* New York: McGraw-Hill; 1991:1552–1561.

Currie JN, Lessell S, Lessell IM, et al. Optic neuropathy in chronic lymphocytic leukemia. *Arch Ophthalmol.* 1988;106:654–60.

Fishman MC, Hoffman AR, Klausner RD, Thaler MS. Leukemia and lymphoma. In: Fishman MC, Hoffman AR, Klausman RD, Thaler MS, eds. *Medicine.* Philadelphia: Lippincott; 1991:398–405.

Fonken HA, Ellis PP. Leukemic infiltrates in the iris. *Arch Ophthalmol.* 1966;76:32–6.

Guyer DR, Schachat AP, Vitale S, et al. Leukemic retinopathy: Relationship between fundus lesions and hematologic parameters at diagnosis. *Ophthalmology.* 1989;96:860–864.

Jabs DA, Hirst W, Green WR, et al. The eye in bone marrow transplantation. *Arch Ophthalmol.* 1983;101:585–90.

Johnston SS, Ware CF. Iris involvement in leukemia. *Br J Ophthal.* 1973;57:320–324.

Kincaid MC. Leukemia. In: Gold DH, Weingeist TA, eds. *The Eye in Systemic Disease.* Philadelphia: Lippincott; 1990:138–140.

Kincaid MC, Green WR. Ocular and orbital involvement in leukemia. *Surv Ophthalmol.* 1983;27:211–232.

Leonardy NJ, Rupani M, Dent G, Klintworth GK. Analysis of 135 autopsy eyes for ocular involvement in leukemia. *Am J Ophthalmol.* 1990;109:436–444.

Nikaido H, Mishima H, Ono H, et al. Leukemic involvement of the optic nerve. *Am J Ophthalmol.* 1988;105:294–298.

Rosenthal AR. Ocular manifestations of leukemia. *Ophthalmology.* 1983;90:899–905.

Sandler DP. Epidemiology and etiology of leukemia. *Curr Opin Oncol.* 1990;2:3–9.

Schachat AP, Markowitz JA, Guyer DR, et al. Ophthalmic manifestations of leukemia. *Arch Ophthalmol.* 1989;107:697–700.

70
Chapter

Dysproteinemias

Holly Myers

Dysproteinemia (paraproteinemia) is the disease process that results from an abnormal amount or nature of protein. Primary dysproteinemias are due to neoplastic proliferation of reticuloendothelial cells, which have protein-producing abilities. Common secondary etiologies of dysproteinemia include cirrhosis, nephrosis, and collagen disease. Systemic manifestations of dysproteinemia vary depending on the specific etiology. Hyperviscosity syndrome, hepatosplenomegaly, pallor, peripheral lymphadenopathy, and abnormal bone marrow morphology are all typically seen. In Waldenström macroglobulinemia and multiple myeloma, monoclonal paraprotein is seen in serum or urine protein electrophoresis. This chapter will discuss two primary dysproteinemias: Waldenström macroglobulinemia and multiple myeloma. These conditions more commonly cause ocular manifestations such as bilateral hyperviscosity retinopathy, or present clinically as a complete central retinal vein occlusion.

■ WALDENSTRÖM MACROGLOBULINEMIA

Waldenström macroglobulinemia is a malignant proliferation of lymphocytes of unknown etiology that secrete the macroglobulin immunoglobulin M (IgM). A macroglobulin is a protein with high molecular weight. The increased secretion of this high-molecular-weight protein causes an increase in serum viscosity. Waldenström first described the disease and its ocular findings in 1944. In one patient, the initial complaint was a decrease in vision secondary to a central retinal vein occlusion, and in a second patient, prominent dilated veins with hemorrhages around the optic nerves were described. Systemically, the disease is associated with lymphadenopathy and enlargement of the spleen and liver, but the major clinical manifestation is hyperviscosity syndrome.

EPIDEMIOLOGY

■ Systemic
Waldenström macroglobulinemia is slightly more common in men and its incidence increases with age. The median age of onset is 64 years (Longo, 1991). Approximately 33% of patients have renal disturbances and 25% have neurological disturbances (Longo, 1991).

■ Ocular
The incidence of hyperviscosity retinopathy in Waldenström macroglobulinemia ranges from 30 to 67% (Ackerman, 1962; Holt & Gordon-Smith, 1969). Common retinal findings include venous dilation and tortuosity, hemorrhages, retinal edema, exudates, branch or central retinal vein occlusion, and disc edema. Central retinal artery occlusions, arterial changes, capillary microaneurysms, and vitreous hemorrhages are less commonly seen. Specific incidence for these ocular findings are not available.

Preparation of the chapter was assisted by Patricia Leggin.

NATURAL HISTORY

■ Systemic

Waldenström macroglobulinemia presents insidiously with symptoms of weakness, fatigue, and epistaxis (Table 70–1). Patients tend to have weight loss, dyspnea, recurrent infections, neurologic and renal disturbances, and recurrent episodes of congestive heart failure. Neurological disturbances may include dizziness, vertigo, headache, nystagmus, ataxia, and seizures. Upon physical examination, it is common to find pallor, hepatosplenomegaly, purpura, and peripheral lymphadenopathy. In patients with increasing serum viscosity it is also common to observe bleeding gums and epistaxis. The median survival time is over 3 years (Longo, 1991; Michaeli & Durie, 1992).

■ Ocular

Many ocular tissues are affected in Waldenström macroglobulinemia due to the involvement of the vascular system (Table 70–2). The conjunctiva, cornea, and retina are among the tissues typically showing changes secondary to the disease.

In the conjunctiva, the blood within the vessels will appear segmented and sluggish. Fine, iridescent, crystalline bodies may be seen deposited diffusely in the conjunctiva and cornea. Nonspecific keratoconjunctivitis has been reported (Boniuk & Friedman, 1981).

The retinal changes are consistent with those seen in hyperviscosity retinopathy (Figure 70–1). The earliest signs include mild venous dilation and small hemorrhages in the peripheral retina without a reduction in visual acuity. As the viscosity increases, the hemorrhages increase in number, appearing in the posterior pole, along with exudates. The venous system becomes more engorged with compressions at arteriovenous crossings.

With these changes, associated retinal thickening and lack of retinal perfusion, a decrease in visual acuity may result. These findings will be progressive if effective therapy is not initiated. Cotton-wool spots are seen as the number of hemorrhages and microvascular abnormalities increase. The veins continue to dilate, developing a "sausage-string appearance." Ultimately, the retinal vein will occlude, and retinal edema, subretinal fluid, and exudates become marked. Disc congestion is common. An exudative detachment may occur with vitreal hemorrhage.

With progressive ischemia, rubeosis irides and secondary glaucoma may result. Because of the very high level of macroglobulin production, a subsequent decrease in antibody synthesis occurs, which reduces the patient's ability to fight infection; patients can then develop orbital cellulitis from a simple sinus infection.

TABLE 70–1. SYSTEMIC MANIFESTATIONS OF DYSPROTEINEMIAS

WALDENSTRÖM MACROGLOBULINEMIA
- General findings
  - Weakness / fatigue
  - Epistaxis / bleeding gums
  - Weight loss
  - Pallor
  - Peripheral lymphadenopathy
  - Purpura
  - Recurrent infections
  - Dyspnea
  - Congestive heart failure
- Neurological findings
  - Headache
  - Dizziness / vertigo
  - Seizures
- Visceral findings
  - Renal abnormalities
  - Hepatosplenomegaly

MULTIPLE MYELOMA
- Bone findings
  - Pain/tenderness
  - Pathological fractures
  - Punched-out lesions of the skull, vertebrae, and ribs
- Laboratory findings
  - Proteinuria
  - Normocytic normochromic anemia
  - Hypercalcemia
- Neurological findings
  - Encephalopathy
  - Carpal tunnel syndrome
- Cardiovascular findings
  - Congestive heart failure
  - Orthostatic hypotension
- Visceral findings
  - GI obstruction
  - Hepatosplenomegaly
  - Renal failure
- General findings
  - Purpura
  - Increased susceptibility to infections

DIAGNOSIS

■ Systemic

The diagnosis of Waldenström macroglobulinemia is based upon physical findings and laboratory diagnostic testing. The typical clinical presentation is pallor, hepatosplenomegaly, purpura, peripheral lymphadenopathy, bleeding gums, and epistaxis. Plasma electrophoresis and bone marrow morphology are also diagnostic. A serum M component is present in excess of 30 g/L. Pleomorphic "lymphoid" cells predominate, and are found to infiltrate the marrow, lymph nodes, liver, and

TABLE 70–2. OCULAR MANIFESTATIONS OF DYSPROTEINEMIAS

WALDENSTRÖM MACROGLOBULINEMIA
- Conjunctiva
  Sludging of the blood
- Retina
  CRVO: visual acuity loss, dilation and tortuosity of retinal veins, diffuse hemorrhages, posterior pole exudates
- Neurological
  EOM palsies from compression of cranial nerves
  Loss of vision from compression of optic nerve

MULTIPLE MYELOMA
- Orbit/neurological
  Orbital bone involvement (proptosis may be the initial presentation)
  Optic nerve compression with vision loss
  Cranial nerve III, IV, VI compression causing EOM palsies

- Conjunctiva
  Sludging of blood
  Iridescent crystalline deposits
- Cornea
  Iridescent crystalline deposits: may be presenting sign; light scattering may cause significant impairment of vision
- Retina
  Less severe retinopathy than in Waldenström macroglobulinemia
- Uvea
  Ciliary body cysts
- Other tissues that may be infiltrated by myeloma cells
  Optic nerve
  Lacrimal gland
  Sclera
  Iris

spleen. These cells have been shown to synthesize the macroglobulins.

■ Ocular

The sign of sludging blood within the conjunctiva may be exaggerated by applying ice on the closed eyelid. Upon fundus evaluation, the signs of vascular changes, particular in the venous system, will be present. The retinopathy will correlate with the high blood viscosities and diminish markedly or disappear when the viscosity is reduced.

TREATMENT AND MANAGEMENT

Table 70–3 summarizes dysproteinemia treatment and management.

■ Systemic

Plasmapheresis or medical therapy with chlorambucil will decrease IgM levels and in turn decrease serum viscosity. About 80% of patients respond to chemotherapy, with the median survival greater than 3 years.

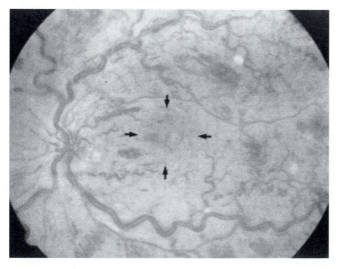

A

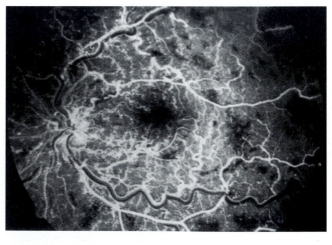

B

Figure 70–1. A. The fundus of a patient with Waldenström macroglobulinemia. Note the severe venous engorgement, flame-shaped, dot-and-blot hemorrhages, and the serous detachment of the macula. **B**. Fluorescein angiogram of fundus in **A**. *(Published courtesy of* Brit J Ophthalmol *[1983; 67: 103].)*

TABLE 70–3. TREATMENT AND MANAGEMENT OF DYSPROTEINEMIAS

WALDENSTRÖM MACROGLOBULINEMIA
- **Systemic**
  Plasmapheresis OR medical therapy with chlorambucil
- **Ocular**
  Treatment of underlying systemic condition
  Secondary glaucoma: topical or oral antiglaucoma medication
  Rubeosis iridis, retinal ischemia, retinal breaks: photocoagulation

MULTIPLE MYELOMA
- **Systemic**
  Radiotherapy
  Chemotherapy: melpalan, other alkylating agents, and prednisone
- **Supportive Therapy for Complications of Myeloma**
  Hypercalcemia: corticosteroid, hydration
  Bone resorption: calcitonin, dichloromethane diphosphonate
  Bone weakness: fluorides, calcium, vitamin D
  Iatrogenic impairment of renal function: allopurinol during chemotherapy, high fluid intake
  Acute renal failure: plasmapheresis
  Infection: antibiotics prn
  Hyperviscosity syndromes: plasmapheresis
  Pain: analgesics
  Anemia: identification of pathogenesis and subsequent therapy
- **Ocular**
  Treatment of underlying systemic condition
  Band keratopathy: penetrating or lamellar keratoplasty
  Orbital infiltration: local irradiation

■ Ocular

Most ocular findings will resolve with systemic treatment. Secondary glaucoma should be addressed as necessary, and may require topical and systemic agents. Photocoagulation may be indicated should neovascularization of the iris, retinal ischemia, or retinal breaks occur. Vigorous treatment for orbital cellulitis may be necessary and should be directed at the causative agent.

■ MULTIPLE MYELOMA

Multiple myeloma is a dysproteinemia that results from neoplastic formation of the myeloma cell. The specific etiology is not known. The abnormally elevated protein in this disease is usually in the immunoglobulin G (IgG) fraction of plasmaglobulins. IgG is the elevated protein 70% of the time, IgA 29% of the time, and IgD in 1% of cases, with IgE rarely elevated (Boniuk & Friedman, 1981).

The malignant proliferation of cells, along with tumor formations and tumor products, result in a number of organ and organ system dysfunctions. Common are bone pain and fracture, renal failure, susceptibility to infection, hypercalcemia, anemia, neurologic symptoms, and manifestations secondary to hyperviscosity syndrome. Myeloma may involve many ocular tissues including the conjunctiva, cornea, uvea, retina, and sclera. Infiltration around the globe along with orbital involvement can occur.

EPIDEMIOLOGY

■ Systemic

Multiple myeloma is the most common dysproteinemia (Longo, 1991). It typically affects persons between 40 and 70 years of age, with 64 years the median age at diagnosis. It is rare before age 30. The yearly incidence is around 3 per 100,000 (Longo, 1991; Michaeli & Durie, 1992). Males are affected slightly more than females, and African-Americans are twice as likely to be affected as Caucasians (Longo, 1991). Neurologic signs and symptoms occur in about 33% of patients (Michaeli, 1992).

■ Ocular

The most common ocular tissues involved in multiple myeloma are the retina, ciliary epithelium, iris, choroid, and conjunctiva. The cornea and orbit are thought to be rarely involved. Baker and Spencer (1974) found cysts of the ciliary epithelium in 33 to 50% of patients with multiple myeloma. Holt and Gordon-Smith (1969) noted retinopathy in 8 of 22 patients with myeloma.

NATURAL HISTORY

■ Systemic

The systemic manifestations of multiple myeloma (see Table 70–1) are similar to macroglobulinemia; however, in multiple myeloma extensive bone involvement occurs. Pain, tenderness, and pathological fractures can be present. In 70 to 90% of cases, punched-out lesions of the skull, vertebrae, and ribs occur (Knapp, 1987; Longo, 1991). In addition, proteinuria is present in 50% of cases at the time of diagnosis, with 90% of cases developing proteinuria sometime during the course of the disease. Neurological manifestations are a result of nerve compression from vertebral collapse, encephalopathy in the hyperviscosity syndrome, or amyloid infiltration of peripheral nerves (Michaeli & Durie, 1992).

Deposits of amyloid and infiltration of myeloma cells affect other organs and tissues, causing congestive heart failure, orthostatic hypotension, carpal tunnel syndrome, gastrointestinal obstruction, and hepatosplenomegaly. Purpura, mainly in the folds of the skin, may also be seen from this infiltration. Affected persons may have normocytic normochromic anemia, hypercalcemia, and increased susceptibility to infections.

The prognosis is affected by the number of diagnostic features. Patients with high paraprotein spikes, hypercalcemia, renal failure, or extensive bone disease have shorter survival time. Approximately 10% of patients will progress slowly over many years. About 15% of patients die within the first 3 months after diagnosis, with rate of death about 15% per year thereafter (Longo, 1991; Michaeli & Durie, 1992). The disease usually follows a chronic course for 2 to 5 years before developing into an acute terminal phase. The median survival is 3 years (Longo, 1991).

■ Ocular

Ocular findings (see Table 70–2) in multiple myeloma are the result of associated serum or hematologic disorders or of myeloma infiltrates. Many tissues are involved, including the conjunctiva, cornea, orbital structures, and retina. Compression of the cranial nerves may cause loss of vision and extraocular muscle (EOM) palsies.

Sludging of the blood within the vessels of the conjunctiva is present because of increased blood viscosity. Iridescent crystalline deposits may be seen, representing immunoglobulin deposition. These crystals may also be present within the corneal epithelium or stroma (Figure 70–2). The resultant light scattering may cause a significant but reversible impairment of vision. Band keratopathy may also be present, and is associated with hypercalcemia.

The secondary retinopathy is less severe than that of macroglobulinopathy because the IgG molecules are of a much lower molecular weight and thus do not induce as marked an increase in blood viscosity (Figure 70–3). In the uvea, multiple, visible cavities are filled with a proteinaceous material. This protein is the same myeloma protein (IgG) as that found in the serum, and is deposited between the pigmented and nonpigmented epithelial layers of the pars plana. Choroidal tumors, infiltrates, and destruction have also been reported. Other tissues may be infiltrated by myeloma cells, such as the optic nerve, lacrimal gland, sclera, and iris.

DIAGNOSIS

■ Systemic

Bone pain, fatigue, anemia, and increased erythrocyte sedimentation rate may suggest the diagnosis of multiple

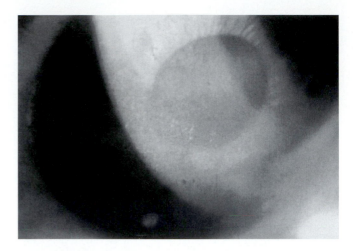

Figure 70–2. Paraproteinemic crystalline keratopathy. *(Reprinted with permission from Omerod LD, et al. Paraproteinemic crystalline keratopathy. Opthalmol. 1988;95:202–212.)*

myeloma. Other findings contributing to the diagnosis include multiple osteolytic lesions, pathological fractures, bone tumors, osteoporosis, hypercalcemia, cryoglobulinemia, pyroglobulinemia, hyperglobulinemia, and Bence–Jones proteinuria. In most cases, myeloma is widely disseminated at the time of diagnosis (Knapp, 1987). The presence of a paraprotein on serum electrophoresis is the hallmark of the disease.

When a paraprotein is present, myeloma must be differentiated from benign monoclonal gammopathy, which is an adenoma of plasma cells and is present in 1% of adults (Longo, 1991). Myeloma differs from benign monoclonal

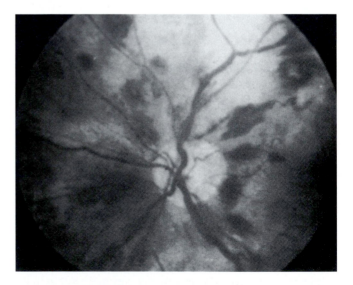

Figure 70–3. Fundus of a patient with multiple myeloma. Note the dilation of veins and flame-shaped hemorrhages. *(Reprinted with permission from Orallana J, Friedman AH. Ocular manifestations of multiple myeloma, Waldenström's macroglobulinemia. Surv Ophthalmol. 1981;26:161.)*

gammopathy by the presence of Bence–Jones protein, anemia, renal failure, bone lesions, and hypercalcemia.

■ Ocular

Ocular findings consistent with multiple myeloma aid in the diagnosis. These include crystalline deposits in the conjunctiva and cornea, sludging of the conjunctival blood, and mild hyperviscosity retinopathy. Corneal and conjunctival crystals may also be present in benign monoclonal gammopathy, but the retinal findings are typically absent.

TREATMENT AND MANAGEMENT

Table 70–3 summarizes treatment and management recommendations for the dysproteinemias.

■ Systemic

Tumor mass may be reduced with chemotherapy and radiotherapy. Melpalan and other alkylating agents, along with prednisone, are recommended (Knapp 1987; Longo, 1992). Supportive care is necessary to prevent serious morbidity from the complications of the disease.

■ Ocular

Most ocular manifestations improve with systemic treatment. Band keratopathy may be treated by penetrating or lamellar keratoplasty if visual function is greatly impaired. Infiltration of myeloma cells to the orbit may respond to local irradiation.

CONCLUSION

Waldenström macroglobulinemia and multiple myeloma are examples of plasma disorders or types of dysproteinemia. Waldenström macroglobulinemia is a disease recognized by the presence of monoclonal IgM paraprotein, infiltration of bone marrow by plasmacytic lymphocytes, and enlargement of the spleen. The macroglobulin IgM is responsible for many of the systemic and ocular findings, including the hyperviscosity retinopathy. Multiple myeloma is characterized by bone pain, replacement of bone marrow by malignant plasma cells, and the presence of monoclonal paraprotein. As in Waldenström macroglobulinemia, the primary ocular manifestation of the disease is hyperviscosity retinopathy, with myeloma protein also infiltrating various ocular tissues such as the choroid, orbit, and optic nerve. Patients with dysproteinemia who have ocular manifestations require careful co-management to ensure optimal care.

REFERENCES

Ackerman AL. The ocular manifestations of Waldenström's macroglobulinemia and its treatment. *Arch Ophthalmol.* 1962;67:39–45.

Aronson SB, Shaw R. Corneal crystals in multiple myeloma. *Arch Ophthalmol.* 1959;61:541–546.

Ashton N. Ocular changes in multiple myelomatosis. *Arch Ophthalmol.* 1965;73:487–494.

Auran J, Dann A, Hyman GA. Multiple myeloma presenting as vortex crystalline keratopathy and complicated by endocapsular hematoma. *Cornea.* 1992;11:584–585.

Avashia JH, Fath DF. Bilateral central retinal vein occlusion in Waldenström's macroglobulinemia. *J Am Optom Assoc.* 1989;60:657–658.

Baker TR, Spencer WH. Ocular findings in multiple myeloma. *Arch Ophthalmol.* 1974;91:110–113.

Beebe WE, Webster RG. Atypical corneal manifestations of multiple myeloma. A clinical, histopathologic and immunohistochemical report. *Cornea.* 1989;8:274–280.

Boniuk MM, Friedman AH. Ocular manifestations of multiple myeloma, Waldenström's macroglobulinemia and benign monoclonal gammopathy. Clinical pathological review. *Surv Ophthalmol.* 1981;26:157–169.

Carr RE, Henkind P. Retinal findings associated with serum hyperviscosity. *Am J Ophthalmol.* 1963;56:23–31.

Delaney WV. Chorioretinal destruction in multiple myeloma. *Am J Ophthalmol.* 1968;66:52–55.

Eiferman RA, Rodrigus MM. Unusual superficial stromal corneal deposits in IgG K monoclonal gammopathy. *Arch Ophthalmol.* 1980;98:78–81.

Friedman AH, Marcheusky A, Odel JG, et al. Immunofluorescent studies of the eye in Waldenström's macroglobulinemia. *Arch Ophthalmol.* 1980;98:743–746.

Green ED, Morrison LK, Love PE, et al. A structurally aberrant immunoglobulin paraprotein in a patient with multiple myeloma and corneal crystal deposits. *Am J Med.* 1990;88:304–311.

Hill JC. Subepithelial corneal deposits in IgG myeloma. *Br J Ophthalmol.* 1989;73:552–554.

Holt JM, Gordon-Smith EC. Retinal abnormalities in diseases of the blood. *Br J Ophthalmol.* 1969;53:145–160.

Johnson BL, Storey JO. Proteinaceous cysts of the ciliary epithelium. *Arch Ophthalmol.* 1970;84:166–170.

Knapp AJ, Gartner S, Henkind P. Multiple myeloma and its ocular manifestations. A clinical review. *Surv Ophthalmol.* 1987;31:343–351.

Kremer I, Wright P, Merin S, et al. Corneal subepithelial monoclonal kappa IgG deposits in essential cryoglobulinemia. *Br J Ophthalmol.* 1989;73:669–673.

Longo DL. Plasma cell disorders. In: Wilson JD, Braunwald E, Isselbacher KJ, et al, eds. *Harrison's Principles of Internal Medicine.* New York: McGraw-Hill; 1991:1410–1417.

Luxenberg MN, Mausolf FA. Retinal circulation in the hyperviscosity syndrome. *Am J Ophthalmol.* 1970;70:588–598.

Michaeli J, Durie BGM. Plasma cell disorders. In: Kelley WN, ed. *Textbook of Internal Medicine.* 2nd ed. Philadelphia: Lippincott; 1992:1087–1092.

Ormerod LD, Collin HB, Dohlman CH, et al. Paraproteinemic crystalline keratopathy. *Ophthalmology.* 1988;9:202–212.

Piette WW, Blodi CS. Multiple myeloma and other plasma cell dyscrasias. In: Gold DH, Weingeist TA, eds. *The Eye in Systemic Disease.* Philadelphia: Lippincott; 1990;134–138.

Pinkerton RMH, Robertson DM. Corneal and conjunctival changes in dysproteinemia. *Invest Ophthalmol.* 1969; 8:357–364.

Sanders TE, Podos SM, Rosenbaum LJ. Intraocular manifestations of multiple myeloma. *Arch Ophthalmol.* 1967;77:789–794.

Sanders TE, Podos S. Pars plana cysts in multiple myeloma. *Trans Am Acad Ophthalmol Otol.* 1966;70:954–957.

Schwab PJ, Okun E, Fahey JL. Reversal of retinopathy in Waldenström's macroglobulinemia by plasmapheresis. *Arch Ophthalmol.* 1960;64:515–522.

Thomas E, Olk J, Markman M. Irreversible visual loss in Waldenström's macroglobulinemia. *Br J Ophthalmol.* 1983;67:102–106.

Yassa NH, Font RL, Fine BS, et al. Corneal immunoglobulin deposition in the posterior stroma. A case report including immunohistochemical and ultrasound observations. *Arch Ophthalmol.* 1987;105:99–103.

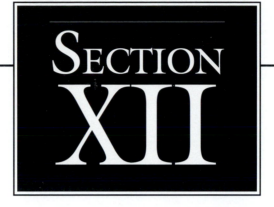

SECTION XII

ONCOLOGIC DISORDERS

Metastases of Systemic Malignancies

Leonard J. Oshinskie

Metastasis occurs when malignant cells separate from a primary site and establish a new colony of cells through adherence and invasion at a secondary site. This dissemination occurs through interstitial spread of tumor cells at the primary site followed by circulation of these cells via the blood stream or lymphatic system. Two general forms of malignant neoplasms—carcinomas or sarcomas—have the ability to metastasize to the eye and orbit although sarcomas rarely do so. Carcinomas are neoplasms that originate from epithelial tissue. Examples include lung carcinoma or basal cell epithelioma. Sarcomas generally arise from bone or soft tissue. Examples are osteogenic sarcoma or rhabdomyosarcoma.

Recognition of ocular metastasis is important since it is sometimes the first sign of an otherwise occult systemic neoplasm that requires additional evaluation and treatment by an oncologist or internist. Ocular metastasis may indicate relapse in a patient who has otherwise received fully effective treatment for a systemic malignancy. Diagnosis of ocular metastasis is also important in patient care because additional therapy may be helpful in preventing vision loss or alleviating pain.

Metastasis to neurological structures involving the visual system, such as cranial nerves or visual pathways, frequently occurs and should be suspected in patients with a history of cancer who present with diplopia or homonymous visual field defects.

Although metastasis can involve many body systems, this chapter will discuss systemic carcinomas (neoplasms of epithelial origin) that are metastatic to intraocular and orbital structures.

Rare dissemination of systemic carcinoma to the eyelids or conjunctiva is not discussed, nor does this chapter discuss primary ocular cancer, such as choroidal melanoma, that is metastatic to other body systems.

EPIDEMIOLOGY

■ Systemic

Nearly one million Americans are afflicted each year with cancer, the second leading cause of death in the United States. Although almost any body tissue can harbor neoplasms, the most common primary sites for neoplasms in adults are the lung, breast, colon and rectum, prostate, urinary tract, and uterus. About 60% of patients with cancer have systemic metastatic disease at the time of diagnosis of their primary disease. Certain organs are prone to harboring metastasis, such as the lungs, liver, and bone.

■ Ocular

Fortunately only a small percentage (0.5 to 12%) of cancer patients present with ocular metastasis. However, ocular metastasis is considered the most common form of intraocular cancer, occurring more commonly than choroidal melanoma. Ocular metastasis usually occurs in the first 2 to 3 years following diagnosis of the systemic malignancy. The most commonly involved site of ocular metastasis is the choroid. The orbit may also be involved. The retina, optic nerve, extraocular muscles, iris and ciliary body, and sclera are much less likely to be involved (Figure 71–1). Metastasis is bilateral in about 10% of patients and seems to affect either eye with equal frequency. Affected patients are most often 40 to 60 years of age. Ocular metastasis is unusual in children and almost entirely limited to the orbit.

The overall incidence for ocular metastasis shows no sex predilection, but lung cancer is the most common primary tumor metastatic to the eye in males. In females breast cancer is, by far, the most common form of ocular metastatic disease. Other primary sites less commonly metastatic to the eye include the gastrointestinal and genitourinary systems. The thyroid gland, cutaneous melanoma, and uterus are rarely metastatic to the eye. For orbital metastasis, Goldberg and associates (1990) report the most common primary tumors to the orbit are breast (42%), lung (11%), unknown (11%), prostate (8.3%), cutaneous melanoma (5.2%), and gastrointestinal (4.4%). Although the majority of patients with ocular metastasis already carry a diagnosis of cancer, 10 to 42% of patients present with ocular metastasis before the primary cancer is discovered. Certain primary sites such as the lung have an affinity for intraocular metastasis compared to the orbit; others, such as the prostate, occur more often in the orbit than intraocularly. Metastasis from the breast seems to occur with equal frequency to the eye or orbit.

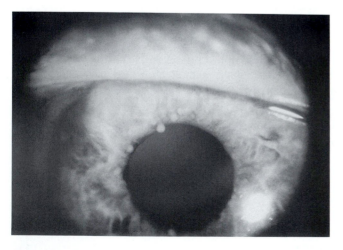

Figure 71–1. Metastatic iris nodules in patient with lung carcinoma. (*Reprinted with permission from Teague BL, Oshinskie LJ, Stoj MJ. Ocular metastasis of pulmonary oat cell carcinoma. J Am Optom Assoc. 1991;61:124–130.*)

NATURAL HISTORY

■ Systemic

Unfortunately, once ocular metastasis has occurred the prognosis for survival is usually poor. This is because the primary disease or other metastatic disease has advanced to cause complications such as pneumonia and hemorrhage or compression of structures vital to life such as the central nervous system, heart, or lungs. In general, lung cancer metastasizes to ocular structures earlier than breast cancer following primary diagnosis. Patients with ocular metastasis from the lung have a mean survival time of about 6 months, while those with spread from the breast survive about 9 months on average. A few patients, however, have survived for years following ocular metastasis. The prognosis for younger patients found to have new intraocular metastasis is poorer than for older patients with ocular involvement.

■ Ocular

Ocular signs that should raise suspicion of systemic malignancy or metastasis include Horner syndrome, cranial nerve palsies, and homonymous hemianopsia. Intraocular involvement often leads to a nonrhegmatogenous retinal detachment and decreased vision. Orbital metastasis often results in strabismus, ptosis, and proptosis.

The most common form of intraocular metastasis, choroidal involvement, often presents in the posterior pole due probably in part to the rich blood supply in this tissue. These lesions can appear yellow or yellow-gray with variable coloration and pigment. They are relatively flat compared to primary tumors of the eye. Multiple sites within one eye are possible. An associated, overlying, nonrhegmatogenous retinal detachment is typical and may appear gray or pigmented rather than yellow. Any patient, especially one with a history of cancer, who presents with nonrhegmatogenous detachment or choroid mass should be suspected to have metastasis (Figure 71–2).

Other signs more frequently found in patients with intraocular metastasis are uveitis, conjunctival erythema, and disc edema. Less common signs include increased intraocular pressure, vitreous hemorrhage, and retinal hemorrhage.

DIAGNOSIS

■ Systemic

The general signs or symptoms of systemic cancer are listed in Table 71–1. Patients with suspected ocular metastasis should be questioned appropriately and referred to an internist for a general physical as well as diagnostic testing.

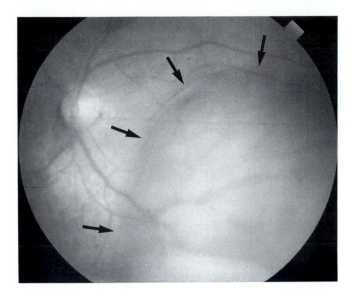

Figure 71–2. Nonrhegmatogenous retinal detachment overlying choroidal metastasis from lung carcinoma. Patient had no previous history of cancer at time of presentation. (*Reprinted with permission from Teague BL, Oshinskie LJ, Stoj MJ. Ocular metastasis of pulmonary oat cell carcinoma. J Am Optom Assoc. 1991; 61:124–130.*)

TABLE 71–2. MANIFESTATIONS OF METASTATIC DISEASE TO INTRAOCULAR AND ORBITAL STRUCTURES

INTRAOCULAR
- Decreased vision
- Visual field defect
- Floaters
- Headache/pain
- Conjunctival erythema
- Uveitis
- Disc edema
- Nonrhegmatogenous RD

ORBITAL
- Ptosis
- Proptosis
- Headache/pain
- Diplopia
- Decreased vision
- Conjunctival erythema

Adapted from: Freedman MI, Folk JC. Metastatic tumors to the eye and orbit. Arch Ophthamol. 1987;105:1215–1219.

Depending on the malignancy suspected these tests might include CT of the abdomen, CT or MRI of the brain, bone scan, chest x-ray, or lumbar puncture. Laboratory tests, referred to as tumor markers, may be helpful as adjunctive diagnostic tests in identifying the primary tumor site. These include plasma carcinoembryonic antigen (CEA), prostate-specific antigen (PSA), mucin-type glycoproteins such as CA 15-3 or CA-125, and others.

Ocular

Any patient presenting with a history of cancer, particularly types that are more commonly metastatic to the visual system, should be carefully examined to exclude the signs and symptoms of ocular involvement. If the patient does not have a history of cancer and presents with ocular signs that suggest ocular metastasis, the patient should be questioned about the general systemic signs and symptoms of cancer (see Table 71–1).

TABLE 71–1. MANIFESTATIONS SUGGESTIVE OF VARIOUS TYPES OF SYSTEMIC CANCER

- Unexplained weight loss
- Persistent cough
- Dysphagia
- Irregular bowel or bladder habits
- Loss of appetite
- Lump in the breast
- Blood in the feces or urine

Decreased vision is most often the initial symptom that causes the patient to seek eyecare in cases of intraocular metastasis (Table 71–2). At a minimum, comprehensive ocular examination with quantitative visual fields should be performed.

Diagnosis can be assisted with additional testing such as fluorescein angiography, ultrasonography, and CT or MRI imaging; however, these tests are not always conclusive (Figure 71–3). Fine needle biopsy can help identify the primary site. A retinal specialist or retinal oncologist is often consulted.

Differential diagnosis includes amelanotic melanoma, exudative age-related macular degeneration, choroidal osteoma, localized choroidal hemangioma, choroiditis, nonrhegmatogenous retinal detachment, and posterior scleritis.

Orbital involvement should be suspected if a patient with cancer presents with proptosis, diplopia, or new-onset strabismus, ptosis, pain or headache, decreased vision, or conjunctival erythema or cellulitis. Interestingly, enophthalmus has also been reported to occur in some patients, particularly patients with breast cancer, due to loss of bony orbit or fibrous tissue pulling the globe posteriorly. CT scanning and needle biopsy are often used in diagnosis of orbital metastasis.

TREATMENT AND MANAGEMENT

■ Systemic

Therapy of systemic cancer is through the use of a variety of chemotherapeutic or hormonal agents, irradiation, and surgery (Table 71–3).

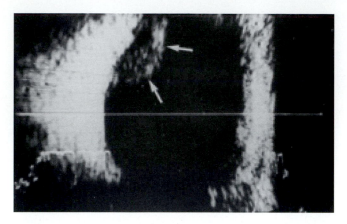

Figure 71–3. B-scan ultrasonography of retinal detachment and thickened choroid of patient in Figure 71–2. (*Reprinted with permission from Teague BL, Oshinskie LJ, Stoj MJ. Ocular metastasis of pulmonary oat cell carcinoma. J Am Optom Assoc. 1991; 61:124–130.*)

■ Ocular

The most commonly involved sites of ocular metastasis are the choroid and the orbit. The retina, optic nerve, extraocular muscles, iris and ciliary body, and sclera are much less likely to be involved (see Figure 71–1). Metastasis is bilateral in about 10% of patients and seems to affect either eye with equal frequency.

Patients with a known history of cancer and ocular metastasis should return to their oncologist for palliative care. If the systemic malignancy is expected to be responsive to chemotherapy, then this therapy is generally used for choroidal disease that is small and relatively non-progressive. Radiation is commonly used in patients with larger tumors that have caused vision loss, if the malignancy is known to be resistant to chemotherapy or if other intraocular complica-

TABLE 71–3. TREATMENT AND MANAGEMENT OF OCULAR METASTASIS

- Referral to oncologist or internist for diagnosis of primary site if unknown
- Chemotherapy (agent varies by cancer type)
- Radiation in divided doses if unresponsive to chemotherapy
- Hormonal therapy in cases of prostate or breast cancer
- Debulking of tumor in orbital cases causing proptosis and exposure
- Enucleation for patient in intractable pain
- Fundus/biomicroscopic photography
- Visual fields
- Ultrasonography
- Fluorescein angiography
- Lubrication for exposure secondary to proptosis
- Fresnal prism or patching for diplopia

tions such as glaucoma are present. Radiation is particularly therapeutic in cases of orbital involvement. Hormonal therapy is employed to control tumor growth in cases of prostate or breast cancer. Enucleation is sometimes done if the patient has intractable pain. Lubrication or orbital surgery may be helpful to alleviate exposure due to proptosis. Fresnel prisms or patching can be prescribed for diplopia associated with extraocular muscle involvement.

Virtually any portion of the visual system can be affected by chemotherapy, so the clinician should consult a reference such as Imperia and co-workers (1989) to specifically identify which side effects are known to be associated with each type of chemotherapeutic agent. Radiation therapy of the head, eye, or orbit is reported to cause a retinopathy that often appears similar to diabetic retinopathy with cotton-wool spots, exudates, and hemorrhages. Optic atrophy, dry eyes, and cataracts are also side effects of radiotherapy.

CONCLUSION

Any patient with a history of systemic cancer, particularly breast or lung cancer, should be evaluated for ocular signs of metastasis including nonrhegmatogenous detachment, choroidal masses, uveitis, conjunctival erythema, and disc edema. Metastatic disease to the eye is seldom the initial sign of systemic cancer, but may indicate relapse of an already known cancer. If metastasis is suspected, a retinal consultation is appropriate. The patient's internist or oncologist should be consulted for appropriate therapy.

REFERENCES

Ferry AP, Font RL. Carcinoma metastatic to the eye and orbit: A clinicopathologic study of 227 cases. *Arch Opthalmol.* 1974;92:276–286.

Freedman MI, Folk JC. Metastatic tumors to the eye and orbit. *Arch Ophthalmol.* 1987;105:1215–1219.

Gartner S. Metastatic Carcinoma to the eye and adnexa. In: Duane TD, ed. *Clinical Ophthalmology.* Philadelphia: Harper & Row; 1979;5.

Goldberg RA, Rootman J, Cline RA. Tumors metastatic to the orbit: A changing picture. *Surv Ophthalmol.* 1990,35:1–24.

Imperia PS, Lazarus HM, Lass JH. Ocular complications of systemic cancer chemotherapy. *Surv Ophthalmol.* 1989;34:209–230.

Jakobiec FA, Rootman J, Jones IS. Secondary and metastatic tumors of the orbit. In: Duane TD, ed. *Clinical Ophthalmology.* Hagerstown, MD: Harper & Row, 1979;2.

Merrill CF, Kaufman DI, Dimitrov NV. Breast cancer metastatic to the eye is a common entity. *Cancer.* 1991;68:623–627.

Purtilo DT, Purtilo RB. *A Survey of Human Diseases.* Little, Brown: Boston; 1989.

Ratanatharathorn V, Powers WE, Grimm J, et al. Eye metastasis from carcinoma of the breast: Diagnosis, radiation treatment and results. *Cancer Treatment Reviews.* 1991;18:261–276.

Ruddon RW, Norton SE. Use of biological markers in diagnosis of cancers of unknown primary tumor. *Semin Oncol.* 1993;20:251–260.

Shields JA. Metastatic tumors of the uvea. *Int Ophthalmol Clin.* 1993;33:155–161.

Shields JA, Shakin EP, Shields CL. Metastatic malignant tumors. In: Gold DH, Weingeist TA, eds. *The Eye in Systemic Disease.* Philadelphia: Lippincott; 1990.

Swanson MW. Metastatic tumor formation: Processes within the visual system. *J Am Optom Assoc.* 1990;61:296–308.

72
Chapter

Non-Hodgkin Lymphoma and Intraocular Lymphoma

Leonard J. Oshinskie

Lymphomas represent a group of diseases that are the result of abnormal arrest and clonal proliferation of T or B lymphocytes. These malignant cells infiltrate tissues throughout the body with morbid consequences such as lymphadenopathy, splenomegaly, and hematologic or immunologic abnormalities.

Lymphomas are generally classified as either Hodgkin or non-Hodgkin (NHL). Although the systemic clinical findings of these two subgroups may be similar, Hodgkin lymphoma is differentiated from NHL histologically by the presence of multinucleated, giant cells called Reed–Sternberg cells. These two general subgroups of lymphoma will be briefly discussed prior to the detailed discussion of the specific topic of this chapter, intraocular lymphoma.

The nomenclature of ocular lymphomatous disease has recently been re-examined in the literature. Until recently, the term ocular reticulum cell sarcoma (RCS) has been used to describe malignant neoplasms of the NHL type found in the eye. However, this term is a misnomer because the cells found on vitreous biopsy do not arise from reticulum cells and are not sarcomas. They are instead usually large cell lymphocytes of the B-cell type. Therefore, the terms of large cell lymphoma or intraocular lymphoma have been used in recent reports to categorize patients with lymphomatous disease of the eye. Non-Hodgkin lymphoma or a subgroup of NHL, large-cell lymphoma or diffuse large-cell lymphoma, are the terms now used in the literature when discussing the systemic disorder associated with intraocular lymphoma.

HODGKIN DISEASE

Hodgkin disease presents with progressive enlargement of the cervical nodes as well as other lymph nodes and can eventually cause enlargement of the internal organs. The etiology of Hodgkin disease is unknown. Males are affected more commonly, and patients tend to be ages 15 to 35 or older than 50. Systemic diagnosis is often by biopsy of involved sites. Ocular complications, which are rare, include decreased visual acuity, visual field defects, swelling of the optic nerve head, central retinal artery occlusion, uveitis, retinal vasculitis, and orbital infiltrates.

Treatment of Hodgkin disease is by radiation and combination chemotherapeutic regimens. One group of these agents, known as MOPP, includes mechlorethamine, Oncovin (vincristine), procarbazine, and prednisone. The 10-year survival rate of patients with stage I or II Hodgkin disease who are treated with radiation is approximately 85 to 90%. For patients with more advanced stages who are treated with chemotherapy and radiation, the long-term survival rate varies depending on the chemotherapeutic agent or agents used, the particular histopathologic type of Hodgkin disease, and organs involved. In many cases, however, a cure is obtained.

■ NON-HODGKIN LYMPHOMA

Non-Hodgkin lymphoma (NHL) represents a group of diseases diverse in their histopathology and natural course. Various classification systems have existed for NHL, but the preferred system for classifying NHL has been established by the Non-Hodgkin's Lymphoma Pathologic Classification Project (1982). The characteristics of cell size, nuclear configuration, cell type (T- or B-cell origin), and growth pattern are used to separate NHL types. Whereas only 5% of all newly diagnosed cancer is the NHL variety, lymphomas are among the leading causes of cancer death in males under 55. The annual incidence of this group of diseases is approximately 7 in 100,000 in the United States. The etiology of the group of diseases may be multifactorial and includes viruses, immunodeficiency, geographic location, and environmental and genetic factors. Patients may present with weight loss, malaise, fever, or night sweats. Systemic findings in NHL are quite varied. General findings include enlargement of lymph nodes and other organs as the result of infiltration, as well as abnormalities of blood elements.

Patients with low-grade types of NHL may survive for years. Those with aggressive forms may succumb very quickly although advances in chemotherapy have made some forms curable. Diagnosis is assisted by biopsy of involved lymph nodes and imaging studies. Treatment is by chemotherapy, radiation, and surgery.

EPIDEMIOLOGY

■ Systemic
The subgroup of NHL, diffuse large-cell lymphoma (DLCL), is among the most common forms of NHL lymphoma in adults; however, it is still a rare disease in the general population. The systemic form can occur at any age, but affects patients ages 50 to 60 most often with a slight predilection for males. Immunocompromised patients are at higher risk for primary CNS lymphoma.

■ Ocular
When intraocular lymphoma is found in isolation, it is referred to as the primary ocular form. It is also found commonly in association with the CNS lymphoma and, less commonly, with the systemic forms. Intraocular lymphoma is often a harbinger of undetected CNS or systemic lymphoma. In a group of patients reported to have intraocular

lymphoma (referred to as "ocular RCS" by Freeman and associates [1987]) 22% had the ocular form alone, 56% had the CNS and ocular forms together, 16% had both the systemic and ocular forms, and 6% had all three forms simultaneously. Bilateral ocular involvement was found in 44% of patients, but has been found by others in up to 80% of cases and is often asymmetric. Most studies have found females were much more commonly affected than males, while others show a similar distribution. The average age of patients with a diagnosis of intraocular lymphoma is 60, although it has been reported in much younger patients.

NATURAL HISTORY

■ Systemic
Clinical findings of DLCL are lymphadenopathy, splenomegaly, and bone marrow failure. CNS involvement includes cranial nerve palsies, usually nerves III and VI, and compression of the spinal cord by infiltrative masses with accompanying findings of back pain, paralysis or weakness of limbs, and bowel or bladder dysfunction (Table 72–1). Survival rates range widely depending on the stage of DLCL, organ systems involved, and chemotherapeutic regimen.

■ Ocular
Ocular manifestations of intraocular lymphoma are often the first sign of generalized lymphoma, often preceding CNS or systemic involvement by months or years. Posterior uveitis and vitritis are common ocular findings. Initial symptoms include decreased vision and floaters. Other eye signs are keratic precipitates, anterior chamber reaction, hypopyon, subretinal infiltrates, exudative retinal detachment, vitreous hemorrhage, neovascular glaucoma, and optic nerve swelling. Orbital infiltration in NHL results in proptosis, palpable orbital masses, eyelid swelling, and pain (Table 72–2). Patients with intraocular lymphoma and CNS involvement generally have an average life expectancy

TABLE 72–1. MANIFESTATIONS OF SYSTEMIC DIFFUSE LARGE CELL LYMPHOMA

- Local lymphadenopathy in early stages
- Paralysis or weakness of limbs
- Bowel or bladder dysfunction
- Lymphadenopathy
- Splenomegaly
- Gastrointestinal masses
- Cranial nerve palsies
- Spinal cord compression

TABLE 72–2. MANIFESTATIONS OF INTRAOCULAR AND ORBITAL LYMPHOMA

INTRAOCULAR
- Blurred vision/floaters
- Posterior uveitis
- Vitritis
- Keratic precipitates
- Anterior uveitis
- Hypopyon
- Exudative retinal detachment
- Neovascular glaucoma
- Optic nerve head swelling
- Subretinal infiltrates
- Cranial nerve palsies (with CNS involvement)

ORBITAL
- Proptosis
- Orbital mass
- Eyelid edema
- Pain

of about 3 years, although a few patients have enjoyed long-term survival with intrathecal chemotherapy and irradiation.

DIAGNOSIS

■ Systemic
Because the signs of intraocular lymphoma often precede systemic involvement, if the diagnosis is suspected following eye examination the patient should be referred to an internist or oncologist for further evaluation. Workup should include CT or MRI imaging to rule out infiltrates of the CNS or internal organs, lumbar puncture, or biopsy of the lymph nodes.

■ Ocular
Intraocular lymphoma can present initially as a uveitis. Therefore it is important to consider this disease in the differential diagnosis of any older patient with an apparently

TABLE 72–3. TREATMENT AND MANAGEMENT OF INTRAOCULAR AND ORBITAL LYMPHOMA

- Local radiation treatment to eye
- Radiation treatment to local CNS sites
- Chemotherapy of systemic cases with CHOP therapy (cyclophosamide, hydroxyldaunomycin, Oncovin, prednisone) and bleomycin
- Refer for vitreous biopsy for definitive diagnosis
- Fundus photography
- Referral to oncologist for radiation and/or chemotherapy

idiopathic uveitis, particularly if it is unresponsive to steroids. Definite diagnosis is assisted by vitreous biopsy, which will demonstrate large pleomorphic cells with irregular nuclear contours and coarse chromatin. Several reports suggest that repeat biopsies, biopsies of chorioretinal lesions, and special handling of biopsies assist accurate diagnosis.

Because the fundus findings in intraocular lymphoma often appear as multifocal yellow or creamy lesions, this condition has also been confused with several of the multifocal chorioretinopathies such as acute posterior multifocal placoid pigment epitheliopathy, or birdshot chorioretinopathy. It is also important to consider intraocular lymphoma in the differential diagnosis of AIDS patients thought to have CMV retinitis.

TREATMENT AND MANAGEMENT

■ Systemic
Several factors are considered before treatment begins, including cell type, tumor staging, tumor site, age, and general systemic condition (Table 72–3). Treatment for systemic DLCL often includes irradiation and combination chemotherapy. One such regimen is referred to as CHOP (cyclophosphamide, hydroxyldaunomycin, Oncovin, and prednisone). Other chemotherapeutic agents used in various combinations for treatment of NHL include bleomycin, methotrexate, procarbazine, and etoposide. If the CNS involvement is minimal, combination irradiation and chemotherapy may extend life substantially. Patients with significant CNS lymphoma and concurrent intraocular lymphoma have a poor prognosis.

■ Ocular
Ocular therapy includes local irradiation in fractionated doses of approximately 35 to 40 Gy. If concurrent CNS involvement is found, chemotherapy and irradiation of the CNS are also used. Fundus photography is used to monitor the effect of treatment.

CONCLUSION

Intraocular lymphoma is a rare condition that typically presents in older adults as posterior uveitis and vitritis, unresponsive to treatment with steroids. Diagnosis is assisted by vitreous biopsy. Systemic or CNS disease is often found in association with intraocular lymphoma, and any patient with the ocular form needs a systemic evaluation to rule out these conditions. Treatment is by irradiation often in combination with chemotherapy.

REFERENCES

Armitage JO. Treatment of non-Hodgkin's lymphoma. *N Engl J Med.* 1993;328:1023–1030.

Buettner H, Bolling JP. Intravitreal large-cell lymphoma. *Mayo Clin Proc.* 1993;68:1011–1015.

Char DH, Ljung BM, Miller T, Phillips T. Primary intraocular lymphoma (ocular reticulum cell sarcoma) diagnosis and management. *Ophthalmology.* 1988;95:625–630.

Char DH. *Clinical Ocular Oncology.* New York: Churchill Livingstone; 1989.

Farah R, Weichselbaum RR. Management of stage I and II Hodgkin's disease. In: *Hematology/Oncology Clinics of North America.* 1989;3:253–264.

Freeman LN, Schachat AP, Knox DL, Michels DG. Clinical features, laboratory investigations and survival in ocular reticulum cell sarcoma. *Ophthalmology.* 1987;94:1631–1639.

Margolis L, Fraser R, Litcher A, Char DH. The role of radiation therapy in the management of ocular reticulum cell sarcoma. *Cancer.* 1980;45:688–692.

Magrath I, Wilson W, Horvath K, et al. Clinical features and staging. In: Magrath I, ed. *The Non-Hodgkin's Lymphomas.* Baltimore; Williams & Wilkins; 1989.

Miller NR. *Clinical Neuro-ophthalmology.* 4th ed. Baltimore; Williams & Wilkins: 1988.

Non-Hodgkin's Lymphoma Pathologic Classification Project. National Cancer Institute sponsored study of classifications of non-Hodgkin's lymphomas: Summary and description of a working formulation for clinical usage. *Cancer.* 1982;49:2112–35.

Velasquez WS, Fuller LM, Kong JS, Jagannath. Diffuse large cell lymphoma: Stages I and II in adults. In: Fuller LM, Hagemeister FB, Sullivan MP, Velasquez WS, eds. *Hodgkin's and Non-Hodgkin's Lymphomas in Adults and Children.* New York; Raven: 1988.

Vose JM, Bierman PJ, Weisenburger DD, Armitage JO. The therapy of non-Hodgkin's lymphoma: Introduction and Overview. In: Armitage JO, ed. *Hematology/Oncology Clinics of North America.* 1991;5:845–852.

Whitcup SM, de Smet MD, Rubin BI, et al. Intraocular lymphoma: Clinical and histopathologic diagnosis. *Ophthalmology.* 1993;100:1399–1406.

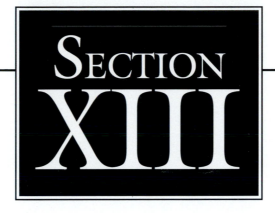

SECTION XIII

METABOLIC DISORDERS

73
Chapter

Hyperlipidemia

Esther S. Marks

Hyperlipidemia refers to an elevation in one or both of the major classes of circulating lipids: cholesterol and triglycerides. Primary (genetic) lipid disorders are due to inherited or sporadic inborn errors of lipid metabolism. Secondary (acquired) lipid disorders are due to an underlying disease such as diabetes mellitus, dietary excess, or medications such as diuretics, β-blockers, and steroids.

The potential consequences of hyperlipidemia, whether primary or secondary, are similar: most importantly, an increased risk for atherosclerosis and its vascular complications (mainly coronary artery disease), as well as the cutaneous manifestation of xanthomas, and pancreatitis. The number one cause of death in the United States for both men and women is coronary heart disease; therefore much research has been devoted to the association between lipid disorders and atherosclerotic cardiovascular disease. Coronary heart disease morbidity and mortality is a heavy economic burden, costing billions of dollars each year in hospitalizations, medical procedures, and lost productivity.

Lipid disorders have well-documented ocular manifestations. Corneal arcus has been studied extensively as a potential identifiable risk factor in coronary heart disease and cardiovascular disease mortality. Other ocular manifestations include xanthelasmas and lipemia retinalis.

EPIDEMIOLOGY

■ Systemic

The incidence and prevalence of hyperlipidemia are difficult to extract from the literature. This is due to the enormous variety of hyperlipidemias, the varying laboratory and clinical guidelines for the definition of hyperlipidemia, and the tendency to discuss these conditions in terms of their relationship (especially hypercholesterolemia) to coronary artery disease.

However, using the criteria established by the National Cholesterol Education Program, it is believed that 36% of the United States population (between the ages of 20 and 74 years) suffers from hypercholesterolemia. In terms of gender, 41% of men and 32% of women are hypercholesterolemic. The incidence increases with age from 20% in ages 20 to 39 years, to 47% in ages 40 to 59 years, to 58% in ages 60 to 74 years (Sempos et al, 1989). African-Americans and Caucasians appear to have similar cholesterol levels. Increased cholesterol levels (both primary and secondary forms) are strongly associated with an increased risk for atherosclerotic vascular disease and its complications. Xanthomas are usually associated with only the primary forms of elevated cholesterol.

The heterozygous form of familial hypercholesterolemia affects 1 in 500 persons, with anywhere from 40 to 90% developing xanthomas. Premature coronary artery disease often occurs by the fourth decade. The homozygous form affects only 1 per million persons, with profound premature coronary artery disease and aortic stenosis by age 20 years. Nonfamilial hypercholesterolemia is a common form of primary hyperlipidemia with both genetic and environmental components. Although not associated with xanthoma formation, it is associated with an increased risk for premature coronary artery disease.

Hypertriglyceridemia is usually more common in men than women, and generally more common in Caucasians than African-Americans. Acute pancreatitis and eruptive xanthomas along with lipemia retinalis (known as the chylomicronemia syndrome) most commonly result from the coexistence of a primary and secondary form of hypertriglyceridemia. Familial hypertriglyceridemia affects approximately 1 in 200 persons.

Combined hyperlipidemia, in which both cholesterol and triglyceride levels are elevated, may be familial or acquired. The familial form affects about 1 in 100 persons. Greater than 15% of patients with premature coronary artery disease have familial combined hyperlipidemia. Dysbetalipoproteinemia (type III hyperlipidemia), although phenotypically distinct from familial combined hyperlipidemia, is also characterized by elevated cholesterol and triglyceride levels, and affects 1 in 10,000 persons. Approximately 25% of these patients develop tendon xanthomas, 64% have palmar xanthomas, and 80% develop tuberous xanthomas.

■ Ocular

Corneal arcus exists in 20 to 30% of the population. Its incidence increases with age. It is more common in men than women, and appears at a younger age in African-Americans than Caucasians. Although over 50% of patients with corneal arcus are normolipidemic, the presence of arcus in patients under 50 years may suggest hyperlipidemia and a risk for coronary artery disease. Fifty percent of patients with heterozygous familial hypercholesterolemia will demonstrate arcus after 30 years of age.

Xanthelasmas are associated with elevated blood lipid levels in only 30 to 50% of patients. They are increasingly more common with age, and are highly associated with corneal arcus. The younger the patient with xanthelasmas, the more likely a lipid disorder exists. Xanthelasmas occur in 23% of patients with familial hypercholesterolemia.

The incidence of lipemia retinalis, a rare phenomenon, is not available in the literature. However, it only occurs in patients with extremely high triglyceride levels.

NATURAL HISTORY

Lipoproteins are complex macromolecules composed of a core of cholesterol and triglycerides, surrounded by phospholipids and apolipoproteins. Lipoproteins may be catego-

rized by several different methods: ultracentrifugation, electrophoresis, or immunologic techniques. Ultracentrifugation divides the lipoproteins by density into their familiar classes of chylomicrons, very-low-density lipoproteins (VLDL), intermediate-density lipoproteins (IDL), low-density lipoproteins (LDL), and high-density lipoproteins (HDL). Electrophoresis separates the lipoproteins by electrical charge and size into beta, prebeta, and alpha lipoproteins. Immunologic techniques separate the lipoproteins by their apolipoprotein categories. The eleven major apolipoproteins are apo A-I, apo A-II, apo A-IV, apo (a), apo B-48, apo B-100, apo C-I, apo C-II, apo C-III, apo D, and apo E.

Triglycerides are the major lipid in chylomicrons and VLDLs. Synthesized from carbohydrates, triglycerides are stored in adipose and muscle tissue to serve as an energy source. Cholesterol, the major lipid in LDL and HDL, is a structural component of all cell membranes, and is a precursor for liver bile acids as well as steroid hormones. Cholesterol and triglycerides are obtained by diet and by synthesis in the liver.

Chylomicrons transport the exogenous lipids from the small intestine into the circulation. Triglycerides are released into the peripheral tissues when the chylomicrons are exposed to the enzyme lipoprotein lipase. Special receptors on the liver take up the chylomicron remnants. These remnants may then be excreted into the bile, or used to form VLDL. VLDL may then be degraded into IDL for hepatic removal, or converted into LDL. LDL, a cholesterol-rich lipoprotein, is then delivered to receptors in peripheral tissues and organs. HDL, synthesized both by the liver and intestine, facilitates the removal of peripheral cholesterol to the liver, and has therefore always been viewed as cardioprotective. This occurs via the enzyme lethicin-cholesterol acyltransferase (LCAT), which allows the transfer of cholesterol to IDL. IDL is then converted to LDL, which is excreted by the liver via bile into the intestine. The apolipoproteins are largely responsible for the rate of lipoprotein biosynthesis and breakdown.

■ Systemic

Hyperlipidemia, an elevation in cholesterol and/or triglycerides, may be primary or secondary (see Table 73–1 for an abbreviated list). The primary forms are due to an inborn error of lipid metabolism as a result of structural defects or deficiencies in apolipoproteins, enzymes, lipid transfer proteins, or receptors. The secondary forms are due to underlying conditions or diseases that alter lipid metabolism, such as diabetes mellitus, obesity, hypothyroidism, renal failure, nephrotic syndrome, and obstructive liver disease. Drugs such as alcohol, β-blockers, diuretics, glucocorticoids, estrogen, and progestogens may also alter lipid profiles resulting in secondary hyperlipidemias.

The manifestations of hyperlipidemia (Table 73–2) may be due directly to the elevated lipid levels themselves.

TABLE 73–1. TYPES OF HYPERLIPIDEMIAS (ABBREVIATED LIST)

Primary[a]

Familial hypercholesterolemia, heterozygous and homozygous
Nonfamilial hypercholesterolemia
Familial hypertriglyceridemia
Familial combined hyperlipidemia
Familial dysbetalipoproteinemia

Secondary[b]

Diet
    Excessive intake of saturated fats
    Excessive intake of cholesterol
    Excessive caloric intake
Diseases
    Diabetes mellitus
    Obesity
    Hypothyroidism
    Systemic lupus erythematosus
    Renal failure
    Nephrotic syndrome
    Obstructive liver disease
    Cushing syndrome
    Acromegaly
    Anorexia nervosa
    Porphyria
Drugs
    Alcohol
    Estrogen
    β-blockers
    Diuretics
    Glucocorticoids
    Progestogens
    Anabolic steroids
    Retinoids
    Phenytoin

[a]Due to inherited or sporadic inborn error of lipid metabolism.
[b]Due to underlying conditions or drugs.

TABLE 73–2. SYSTEMIC AND OCULAR MANIFESTATIONS OF HYPERLIPIDEMIAS IN GENERAL

- ■ **SYSTEMIC**
  - Elevated lipid levels
  - Atherosclerosis and its thromboembolic vascular complications
    Cardiovascular: angina, myocardial infarction
    Peripheral vascular: Intermittent claudication
    Cerebrovascular: Transient ischemic attacks, cerebrovascular accidents
  - Xanthomas
    Planar, palmar, tendon, subperiosteal, eruptive, tuberous, mediastinum, retroperitoneum
  - Abdominal pain
  - Chylomicronemia syndrome
    Pancreatitis, hepatomegaly, eruptive xanthomas, lipemia retinalis, neurologic involvement

- ■ **OCULAR**
  - Corneal arcus
  - Xanthelasma
  - Lipemia retinalis

Systemically, this may present as xanthomas and pancreatitis; and ocularly, as corneal arcus, xanthalasmas, and lipemia retinalis. Often, the manifestations are due to a condition to which hyperlipidemia contributes—atherosclerosis and its complications. The manifestations may vary with each type of lipid disorder (Table 73–3). Finally, the hyperlipidemia may manifest secondary to or as a sign of an underlying condition such as diabetes mellitus.

Xanthomas are deposits of lipids that occur most commonly in the skin and tendons, although they may also develop in the mediastinum, retroperitoneum, and bone. Although the presence of such lesions suggests a lipid disorder (primary or secondary), patients with normal lipid profiles may also demonstrate these findings. More importantly, the absence of xanthomas does not eliminate the presence of a lipid disorder.

Planar xanthomas are flat or slightly raised cutaneous yellowish to yellowish-orange lesions associated with the homozygous form of familial hypercholesterolemia. They may occur throughout the body, especially on the knees, ankles, upper trunk, neck, face, and dorsal aspects of the hands. Palmar xanthomas are flat yellowish-orange cutaneous lesions occurring in the creases of the palms and on the palmar surface of the fingers, and are usually associated with familial dysbetalipoproteinemia.

Tendon xanthomas are nontender, firm, smooth, elevated nodular lesions within the tendon. They may occur in any tendon, although the Achilles and the extensor tendons of the fingers appear to be the most common. If particularly large, the overlying skin may break down due to mechanical irritation. Tendon xanthomas are of particular importance, as their size often parallels that of underlying coexistent atherosclerotic plaques.

Eruptive xanthomas (Figure 73–1) are multiple, small, yellowish-orange lesions usually associated with profound hypertriglyceridemia (a condition that may occur in uncontrolled diabetes mellitus). They usually develop on extensor surfaces, the buttocks, and the trunk. Tuberous xanthomas are believed to arise when eruptive xanthomas coalesce into soft, elevated papules. They are found on extensor surfaces, knees, elbows, buttocks, and palmar surfaces of the hands. These usually occur in primary hypertriglyceridemias.

The chylomicronemia syndrome, most commonly caused by the simultaneous presence of both a primary and secondary form of hypertriglyceridemia, results in a constellation of clinical signs and symptoms. These include acute pancreatitis, abdominal pain, hepatomegaly, eruptive xanthomas, lipemia retinalis, memory loss,

TABLE 73–3. SYSTEMIC AND OCULAR MANIFESTATIONS SPECIFIC TO TYPE OF HYPERLIPIDEMIA

PRIMARY HYPERLIPIDEMIAS
- **Familial Hypercholesterolemia**
  - Systemic
    - Elevated plasma LDL cholesterol
    - Premature coronary artery disease
    - Myocardial infarction, especially in males in early 40s
    - Tendon xanthomas usually on extensor surfaces
  - Ocular
    - Premature corneal arcus
    - Xanthelasma common in heterozygotes only
- **Nonfamilial Hypercholesterolemia**
  - Systemic
    - Plasma LDL cholesterol 160–220 mg/dL
    - Increased risk of premature coronary artery disease
  - Ocular
    - Corneal arcus
    - Xanthelasma possible
- **Familial Hypertriglyceridemia**
  - Systemic
    - Elevated triglyceride levels
    - Usually asymptomatic
    - May develop chylomicronemia syndrome, especially if diabetes is present
  - Ocular
    - Lipemia retinalis possible
- **Familial Combined Hyperlipidemia**
  - Systemic
    - Elevated triglyceride and cholesterol levels
    - Premature coronary artery disease
    - Myocardial infarction at around age 40 years
    - May develop chylomicronemia syndrome, especially if diabetes is present
  - Ocular
    - Corneal arcus and xanthelasma possible
    - Lipemia retinalis possible

- **Familial Dysbetalipoproteinemia**
  - Systemic
    - Elevated triglyceride and cholesterol levels
    - Atherosclerosis: in men prematurely, in women after menopause
    - Xanthomas: tendon, tuberous, or palmar
    - Peripheral vascular disease predominates
    - Coronary artery disease may also occur
  - Ocular
    - Premature corneal arcus
    - Xanthelasma and lipemia retinalis possible

SECONDARY HYPERLIPIDEMIAS
- **Acquired Hypercholesterolemia**
  - Systemic
    - Elevated plasma cholesterol levels
    - May be due to dietary excess, anorexia nervosa, porphyria, or diuretic drugs
  - Ocular
    - Corneal arcus and xanthelasma possible
- **Acquired Hypertriglyceridemia**
  - Systemic
    - Elevated plasma triglyceride levels
    - May be due to uncontrolled diabetes mellitus, obesity, estrogen use, alcohol, retinoids, or β-blockers
    - In severe cases may develop chylomicronemia syndrome, especially if diabetes and a primary form of hypertriglyceridemia are present
  - Ocular
    - Lipemia retinalis possible
- **Acquired Combined Hyperlipidemia**
  - Systemic
    - Elevated plasma cholesterol and triglyceride levels
    - May be due to hypothyroidism, nephrotic syndrome, and excess glucocorticoid
  - Ocular
    - Corneal arcus and xanthelasma possible

dementia, peripheral neuropathy, and paresthesias. Either the inflamed pancreas (irritated by chemicals released by chylomicrons) and/or the enlarged liver (due to fatty infiltration) causes the abdominal pain. It may be mild to severe, and may extend into the chest area. Xanthomas erupt over the extensor surfaces and the buttocks. Lipemia retinalis may be observed. Dementia in the form of memory loss occurs. The peripheral neuropathy and paresthesias may present like a carpal tunnel syndrome. All of these manifestations are reversible with treatment.

It is not hyperlipidemia itself that leads to increased morbidity and mortality, but rather the interaction of hyperlipidemia with multiple other factors such as genetics, atherosclerosis, hypertension, cigarette smoking, obesity, lack of physical exercise, alcohol abuse, certain med-ications, and other diseases. Hyperlipidemic states will aggravate and accelerate the atherosclerotic process, thereby increasing the risk for vascular disease and its complications. There is clear evidence that elevated total cholesterol levels as well as elevated LDL cholesterol levels play significant roles in the development of coronary heart disease. Low HDL cholesterol levels have also been shown to increase the risk for cardiac complications due to atherosclerosis. Although elevated triglyceride levels have been increasingly recognized as playing a role in the atherogenic process, controversy still exists concerning their importance.

It is well known that the process of atherosclerosis is lifelong, commencing in childhood and progressing into adulthood until it becomes clinically apparent. Fatty

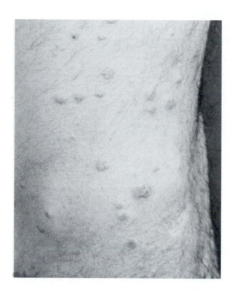

Figure 73–1. Eruptive xanthomas on the leg of a diabetic patient with uncontrolled diabetes and hypertriglyceridemia. (*Reprinted with permission from Steiner G, Shafrir E. Primary Hyperlipoproteinemias. New York: McGraw-Hill, 1991.*)

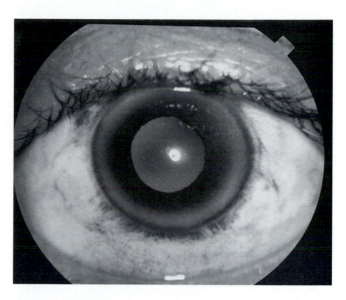

Figure 73–2. Prominent corneal arcus in a patient with elevated cholesterol levels.

streaks appear initially in the aorta of children, and then spread to the coronary arteries, with eventual potential involvement of the peripheral and cerebrovascular systems. The progression of these streaks to fibrous plaques usually occurs in adulthood (20 years or older).

If the atherosclerotic lesions develop sufficiently, the clinical signs and symptoms of a thromboembolic occlusive state become evident. The type of signs and symptoms depend on the vascular system involved; for example, for the cardiovascular system, angina, or myocardial infarction; for the peripheral vascular system, intermittent claudication; for the cerebrovascular system, transient ischemic attacks and cerebrovascular accidents.

The lipid profile in women deserves special consideration given the changes that occur during menstrual cycles, pregnancy, and menopause. Estrogen increases both VLDL and HDL levels, whereas progestogens decrease the cardioprotective HDL levels. Women have significant increases in cholesterol and triglyceride levels during pregnancy, yet there is considerable disagreement concerning whether or not this increases their risk for coronary artery disease. Oral contraceptives as well as menopause appear to alter the lipid profile to a more atherogenic state. However, postmenopausal estrogen replacement dramatically reduces mortality (30 to 60%) from coronary artery disease.

■ Ocular

The ocular manifestations of hyperlipidemia include corneal arcus, xanthelasmas, and lipemia retinalis. Corneal arcus is a grayish-white ring of lipid deposition in the corneal stroma (Figure 73–2). It occurs at the limbus with a clear interval (0.3 to 1.0 mm) between the limbus and the

lesion, never involves the central cornea, and therefore never affects visual acuity. Arcus usually starts superiorly, and then continues inferiorly, slowly progressing completely around the corneal circumference. It is almost always a bilateral phenomenon. Although more common with increasing age in all populations, arcus may occur prematurely in lipid disorders, particularly the genetic forms. It is felt to be primarily due to elevated cholesterol levels. A study by Varnek and associates (1979) suggested that marked nasal arcus in particular is linked to high cholesterol levels. Below the age of 50 years (in men) the presence of corneal arcus has been shown to be a risk factor for coronary heart disease mortality, especially in the presence of a hyperlipidemic state (Chambless et al, 1990).

Xanthelasmas are a form of xanthoma (Figure 73–3). Located on the eyelids, they are yellowish, slightly elevated soft lesions of lipid deposition. As with corneal arcus, they are seen more commonly with age, and the majority occur in the normolipidemic population. However, the younger the patient with xanthelasma, the more likely it is due to a lipid disorder, particularly elevated cholesterol levels.

Lipemia retinalis occurs in the presence of extremely elevated triglyceride levels (usually exceeding 1000 mg/dL). It tends to occur in the retinal periphery first, and then as triglyceride levels continue to rise, it extends back to involve the posterior pole and the optic disc. The retinal vessels become salmon or creamy, milky white in color. As the triglyceride levels are brought under control, the color recedes first from the disc and posterior pole, and then from the peripheral fundus. Visual impairment or complications, either transient or permanent, have rarely been noted.

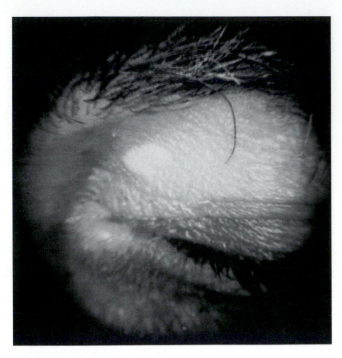

Figure 73–3. Xanthelasma of the upper lid in a 44-year-old patient with hypercholesterolemia.

DIAGNOSIS

■ Systemic

The diagnosis of hyperlipidemia (primary or secondary) should include a full history (including family), a physical examination, and laboratory evaluation. The history should inquire about diet, underlying diseases (eg, diabetes or hypothyroidism), drugs, hyperlipidemia in the family, as well as any premature heart disease or deaths. A routine physical examination should be performed noting body weight and the presence of any xanthomas. Laboratory lipid diagnosis may be obtained by ultracentrifugation, electrophoresis, or immunologic techniques. Other laboratory tests, such as blood glucose, thyroid profile, and liver function tests, may be warranted in patients suspected of having an underlying disease giving rise to a secondary hyperlipidemia.

A fasting lipid profile (including no alcohol intake 24 to 48 hours prior to testing) should include total cholesterol, triglycerides, HDL cholesterol, and LDL cholesterol. Although there is variation in suggested laboratory values and clinical application, the National Cholesterol Education Program (NCEP), under the auspices of the National Heart, Lung and Blood Institute (NHLBI), developed guidelines in 1988 for the classification of cholesterol levels in adults age 20 years and older (Table 73–4). As a general rule, total cholesterol levels of 240 mg/dL or above and LDL cholesterol levels of 160 mg/dL or above are considered

TABLE 73–4. NHLBI GUIDELINES FOR THE LABORATORY DIAGNOSIS OF HYPERLIPIDEMIA AND THE RISK FOR CORONARY HEART DISEASE

Total Cholesterol

Desirable	<200 mg/dL
Borderline high	200–239 mg/dL
High	>239 mg/dL

LDL Cholesterol

Desirable	<130 mg/dL
Borderline high	130–159 mg/dL
High	>159 mg/dL

HDL Cholesterol

Recommended	>35 mg/dL

Atherosclerosis Risk Ratios (average risk = 20–25% chance of developing coronary heart disease by age 60 years)

Risk	LDL/HDL (female, male)	Total Cholesterol/HDL (female, male)
1/2 average	1.47, 1.00	3.27, 3.43
average	3.22, 3.55	4.44, 4.97
2 × average	5.03, 6.25	7.05, 9.55
3 × average	6.14, 7.99	11.04, 13.39

Triglycerides

Common laboratory values 30–150 mg/dL
NHLBI guidelines:

Normal	<250 mg/dL
Borderline high	250–500 mg/dL
High	>500 mg/dL

high and place the patient at increased risk for coronary artery disease. These values will be lower with children, and higher with older adults. HDL cholesterol levels below 35 mg/dL are considered risky for coronary heart disease, but research into further categorization has been limited. Atherosclerosis risk ratios were also developed using LDL, HDL, and total cholesterol. The higher the LDL/HDL and total cholesterol/HDL ratios, the higher the risk for developing coronary heart disease.

The role triglyceride levels play in atherosclerotic disease is still controversial; therefore, fewer guidelines exist for identifying different levels of risk. Many laboratories consider approximately 30 to 150 mg/dL desirable. Levels are slightly lower for women and children. However, the National Institutes for Health (NIH) Consensus Development Conference on Treatment of Hypertriglyceridemia, sponsored by the NHLBI in 1984, concluded that in the presence of normal cholesterol levels, triglyceride levels below 250 mg/dL may be considered normal because little evidence exists predicting an increased risk for coronary heart disease. Triglyceride levels are considered borderline high at 250 to 500 mg/dL, and high at above 500 mg/dL. Levels above 500 mg/dL run increasingly higher risks for pancreatitis.

■ Ocular

External and biomicroscopic examination will easily reveal palpebral xanthelasmas and corneal arcus. Lipemia retinalis may be observed as salmon- to milky-colored retinal blood vessels on dilated fundus examination.

TREATMENT AND MANAGEMENT

■ Systemic

The treatment of hyperlipidemia is essentially similar whether primary or secondary in nature (Table 73–5). Any underlying systemic condition that contributes to the lipid disorder must be controlled. Any medications that adversely affect lipid levels should be changed if possible. Diet and body weight management are crucial to lipid level control. Physical activity, the cessation of smoking, and limited alcohol intake should be encouraged. When these measures fail to lower lipid levels sufficiently, pharmacologic intervention may be required.

Caloric intake should be adjusted to achieve appropriate body weight. Daily cholesterol intake should be restricted to less than 200 to 300 mg. Total fat intake should be limited to less than 30% of total calories, with polyunsaturated fat 10% or less, monounsaturated fat 10 to 15%, and saturated fat less than 7 to 10% of total fat. Carbohydrates should make up 50 to 60%, and protein should make up 10 to 20% of total calories (National Cholesterol Education Program Expert Panel, 1988). Studies have found that the daily addition of 25 to 35 g of fiber (psyllium, Metamucil) to a low-fat, low-cholesterol diet, is efficacious in further lowering cholesterol levels (Lipsky et al, 1990). Compliance is the most difficult aspect of the dietary regimen, requiring the combined efforts of the patient, physician, and often a nutritionist or dietician.

If a patient has desirable cholesterol levels (below 200 mg/dL), general dietary and risk reduction information should be provided. Remeasurement is advised in 5 years. Borderline high cholesterol levels (200 to 239 mg/dL) in the absence of coronary heart disease and risk factors requires slightly stricter dietary and risk reduction information, along with remeasurement in one year. Risk factors include male sex, family history of premature coronary heart disease, cigarette smoking, hypertension, low HDL cholesterol (below 35 mg/dL), diabetes mellitus, history of cerebrovascular or peripheral vascular disease, and severe obesity (defined as 30% or more overweight). Borderline high cholesterol levels in the presence of coronary heart disease or two risk factors requires lipoprotein analysis. High cholesterol levels (240 mg/dL and above) also require lipoprotein analysis.

Upon analysis, if LDL cholesterol levels are desirable (below 130 mg/dL), once again simple dietary and risk reduction information should be provided, with remeasure-

TABLE 73–5. TREATMENT AND MANAGEMENT OF HYPERLIPIDEMIAS

■ **SYSTEMIC**
- **Nonpharmacologic Modalities—All of the Following**
  Physical activity recommended
  Cessation of cigarette smoking
  Dietary regimen
      Limitation or elimination of alcohol
      Adjust caloric intake to achieve appropriate body weight
      Daily cholesterol intake <200–300 mg
      Total fat intake <30% of total caloric intake
        Polyunsaturated fat ≤10%
        Monounsaturated fat 10–15%
        Saturated fat <7–10%
      Carbohydrates 50–60% of total caloric intake
      Protein 10–20% of total caloric intake
      25–35 g/d fiber (psyllium)

IF INSUFFICIENT, ADD:
- **Pharmacologic Modalities**
  Control any underlying disease
  Change any medication that adversely affects lipid levels if possible
  Plus one or two of the following
  Bile-acid resins
      Cholestyramine or colestipol: 4–5 g up to 24–30 g/d bid
  Nicotinic acid
      100–250 mg up to 3g/d tid
  HMG-CoA reductase inhibitors
      Lovastatin (Mevacor): 20 mg up to 80 mg/d qd
      Others: pravastatin, simvastatin
  Fibric acids
      Gemfibrozil (Lopid): 600 mg bid
  Probucol
      500 mg bid

■ **OCULAR**
- Treatment of underlying lipid disorder, if present
  Corneal arcus
      No direct treatment
  Xanthelasma
      No direct treatment necessary
      May be surgically removed for cosmesis
  Lipemia retinalis
      No direct treatment

ment within five years. Borderline high LDL cholesterol levels (130 to 159 mg/dL) in the absence of coronary heart disease and risk factors requires slightly stricter dietary and risk-reduction information, along with remeasurement in 1 year. Borderline high LDL cholesterol levels in the presence of coronary heart disease or two risk factors, and high LDL cholesterol levels (160 mg/dL or above) both require a full clinical evaluation. Special care should be taken to rule out the presence of underlying diseases, or primary lipid disorders.

In the absence of coronary heart disease and risk factors, the goal is LDL cholesterol below 160 mg/dL and total cholesterol below 240 mg/dL. In the presence of coronary heart disease or two risk factors, the goal is LDL cholesterol below 130 mg/dL and total cholesterol below 200 mg/dL. The first step is strict dietary management. If the cholesterol goals are met within 3 months, long-term monitoring is suggested by remeasurement of lipid levels four times the first year and two times per year thereafter. If the cholesterol goals are not met within the first 3 months, then even stricter dietary management is required under supervision. If the cholesterol goals are met within 6 months, long-term monitoring again is suggested. If the goal is not met, medication must be considered.

Treatment modalities for hypertriglyceridemia are less clear due to controversy concerning the role triglycerides play in cardiovascular disease. If nonpharmacological modalities fail (eg, diet, exercise, weight reduction), drug therapy should be considered. Patients with severe hypertriglyceridemia must follow an extremely restrictive diet, limiting fat intake to less than 20% of total calories. Should chylomicronemia syndrome occur, strict elimination of all oral intake and alcohol will quickly decrease triglyceride levels. Refeeding may be initiated with severe fat intake reduction. Drug therapy may be required.

The type of lipid disorder determines the appropriate medication(s), as some of the drugs affect cholesterol only, triglycerides only, or both. Hypercholesterolemia is treated with bile-acid resins, nicotinic acid, HMG-CoA (3-hydroxy-3-methylglutaryl coenzyme A) reductase inhibitors, or probucol. Combined hyperlipidemia is treated with nicotinic acid, HMG-CoA reductase inhibitors, or fibric-acid derivatives. Hypertriglyceridemia is treated with nicotinic acid or fibric-acid derivatives.

Bile-acid resins (eg, cholestyramine and colestipol) reduce total and LDL cholesterol levels by removing bile acids from the intestine. This prevents reabsorption by the liver, dropping cholesterol levels and increasing LDL receptor synthesis. Circulating LDL cholesterol levels drop. Its major side effect is constipation. These drugs may also interfere with the absorption of other drugs (eg, warfarin, thyroxine, thiazide diuretics, β-blockers).

Nicotinic acid inhibits the production of VLDL and triglycerides, which also lowers the level of LDL. Frequent side effects occur, including skin rashes, flushing, gastrointestinal symptoms, hyperglycemia, hyperuricemia, fatigue, and liver toxicity. Therefore, nicotinic acid is contraindicated in peptic ulcer disease, gouty arthritis, hyperuricemia, and liver disease. Patients on nicotinic acid should have uric acid, liver function, and glucose levels monitored.

HMG-CoA reductase inhibitors (eg, lovastatin, pravastatin, or simvastatin) inhibit the synthesis of cholesterol in the liver, stimulating the synthesis of LDL receptors. Circulating LDL and VLDL levels drop, as do triglyceride levels. Diarrhea, insomnia, liver toxicity, and muscle pain may occur. Liver function and creatinine kinase levels should be monitored. Lovastatin has produced cataracts in studies using dogs (Fraunfelder, 1988). The evidence in humans is inconclusive; therefore, prior to initiating lovastatin therapy, an examination of the crystalline lens is recommended, with routine annual examinations thereafter.

Fibric acids (eg, gemfibrozil, known as Lopid) lower triglyceride levels by increasing the activity of lipoprotein lipase. Cholesterol gallstones, gastrointestinal symptoms, skin rashes, leukopenia, and muscle pain may occur. Care should be taken with patients on oral anticoagulants because gemfibrozil potentiates their effects.

Probucol lowers cholesterol levels by promoting LDL clearance through the liver. It may also cause gastrointestinal symptoms as well as disturb the cardiac rhythm. Therefore, probucol is contraindicated in patients with ventricular irritability.

■ Ocular

There is no treatment for corneal arcus. Although it has no adverse effect on ocular structures, arcus noted in patients under age 50 is a strong risk factor for coronary heart disease mortality. Therefore, arcus noted in any patient younger than 50, particularly if unaware of their lipid levels, warrants a blood cholesterol test.

Xanthelasmas, although cosmetically unappealing, also have no adverse effect on the ocular adnexa. However, these patients also warrant blood cholesterol testing, particularly if arcus and xanthelasma coexist. With antilipidemic medications, the xanthelasmas may slowly regress. Surgical removal of these lid lesions is feasible; however, approximately 40% recur.

Lipemia retinalis itself requires no treatment as it rarely adversely affects the eye. However, its presence occurs only with triglyceride levels well over 1000 mg/dL. Lipemia retinalis in patients with a known lipid disorder warrants referral back to their physician for immediate control. Clearly, if a patient presents with lipemia retinalis, and is unaware of an existing lipid disorder, urgent referral to a lipid metabolism specialist is warranted, considering the risk of developing pancreatitis.

CONCLUSION

Hyperlipidemia is often labelled a disease of modern civilization with its high-cholesterol, high-fat diet. Both primary and secondary forms of hyperlipidemia demonstrate clear associations with atherosclerotic cardiovascular disease, particularly coronary heart disease. Due to the significant morbidity and mortality associated with such thromboembolic heart disease, patients suspected of hyperlipidemia warrant, at minimum, a test of cholesterol levels, if not an entire lipid profile. The ocular manifestations of hyperlipidemia, in particular corneal arcus, are potential prognostic factors for coronary heart disease. Thus, the eye-care practitioner plays an integral role in the potential diagnosis, treatment, and management of lipid disorders.

REFERENCES

Alexander LJ. The prevalence of corneal arcus senilis in known insulin-dependent diabetic patients. *J Am Optom Assoc.* 1985;56:556–559.

Alexander LJ. Ocular signs and symptoms of altered blood lipids. *J Am Optom Assoc.* 1983;54:123–126.

Assman G, Betteridge DJ, Gotto AM, Steiner G. Management of hypertriglyceridemic patients: A. Treatment classifications and goals. *Am J Cardiol.* 1991;68:30A–34A.

Assman G, Brewer HB. Genetic (primary) forms of hypertriglyceridemia. *Am J Cardiol.* 1991;68:13A–16A.

Barchiesi BJ, Eckel RH, Ellis PP. The cornea and disorders of lipid metabolism. *Surv Ophthalmol.* 1991;36:1–22.

Breslow JL. Genetics of lipoprotein disorders. *Circulation.* 1993;87(suppl 3):III-16–III-21.

Brunzell JD. The hyperlipoproteinemias. In: Wyngaarden JB, Smith LH, eds. *Cecil Textbook of Medicine.* Philadelphia: Saunders; 1988:1137–1144.

Carmena R, Grundy SM. Management of hypertriglyceridemic patients: B. Dietary management of hypertriglyceridemic patients. *Am J Cardiol.* 1991;68:35A–42A.

Castelli WP, Garrison RJ, Wilson PWF, et al. Incidence of coronary heart disease and lipoprotein cholesterol levels: The Framingham study. *JAMA.* 1986;256:2835–2838.

Chait A, Brunzell JD. Acquired hyperlipidemia (secondary hyperlipoproteinemias). *Endocrinol Metabol Clin North Am.* 1990;19:259–278.

Chambless LE, Fuchs FD, Linn S, et al. The association of corneal arcus with coronary heart disease and cardiovascular disease mortality in the Lipid Research Clinics mortality follow-up study. *Am J Public Health.* 1990;80:1200–1204.

Davidson MH. Implications for the present and direction for the future. *Am J Cardiol.* 1993;71:32B–36B.

Drood JM, Zimetbaum PJ, Frishman WH, et al. Nicotinic acid for the treatment of hyperlipoproteinemia. *J Clin Pharmacol.* 1991;31:641–650.

Dunn FL. Management of hyperlipidemia in diabetes mellitus. *Endocrinol Metabol Clin North Am.* 1992;21:395–414.

Franklin FA, Brown RF, Franklin CC. Screening, diagnosis, and management of dyslipoproteinemia in children. *Endocrinol Metabol Clin North Am.* 1990;19:399–449.

Fraunfelder FT. Ocular examination before initiation of lovastatin (Mevacor) therapy. *Am J Ophthalmol.* 1988;105(1):91–92.

Ginsberg HN. Lipoprotein physiology in nondiabetic and diabetic states: Relationship to atherogenesis. *Diabetes Care.* 1991;14:839–855.

Ginsberg HN. Lipoprotein physiology and its relationship to atherogenesis. *Endocrinol Metabol Clin North Am.* 1990;19:211–228.

Goodman DS. New guidelines for lowering blood cholesterol. *Clin Lab Med.* 1989;9:17–27.

Gordon DJ. Role of circulating high-density lipoprotein and triglycerides in coronary artery disease: risk and prevention. *Endocrinol Metabol Clin North Am.* 1990;19:299–309.

Gotto AM. Dyslipidemia and atherosclerosis: A forecast of pharmaceutical approaches. *Circulation.* 1993;87(suppl 3):III-56–III-59.

Gotto AM. Overview of current issues in management of dyslipidemia. *Am J Cardiol.* 1993;71:3B–8B.

Gotto AM. Hypertriglyceridemia: Risks and perspectives. *Am J Cardiol.* 1992;70:19H–25H.

Gotto AM. Rationale for treatment. *Am J Med.* 1991;91(suppl 1B):31S–36S.

Gotto AM, LaRosa JC, Hunninghake D, et al. The cholesterol facts. A summary of evidence relating dietary fats, serum cholesterol, and coronary heart disease. A joint statement by the American Heart Association and the National Heart, Lung, and Blood Institute. *Circulation.* 1990;81:1721–1733.

Grundy SM. Cholesterol lowering drugs as cardioprotective agents. *Am J Cardiol.* 1992;70:27I–32I.

Grundy SM. Cholesterol and coronary heart disease: A new era. *JAMA.* 1986;256:2849–2858.

Hunningshake DB. Drug treatment of dyslipoproteinemia. *Endocrinol Metabol Clin North Am.* 1990;19:345–360.

Jones PH. A clinical overview of dyslipidemias: Treatment strategies. *Am J Med.* 1992;93:187–198.

Lavie CJ, O'Keefe JH, Blonde L, Gau GT. High density lipoprotein cholesterol: Recommendations for routine testing and treatment. *Postgrad Med.* 1990;87:36–51.

Levy RI, Troendle AJ, Fattu JM. A quarter century of drug treatment of dyslipoproteinemia, with a focus on the new HMG–CoA reductase inhibitor fluvastatin. *Circulation.* 1993;87(suppl 3):III-45–III-53.

Lipid Research Clinics Program. The lipid research clinics coronary primary prevention trial results, 1. Reduction in incidence of coronary heart disease. *JAMA.* 1984;251:351–364.

Lipid Research Clinics Program. The lipid research clinics coronary primary prevention trial results, 2. The relationship of reduction in incidence of coronary heart disease to cholesterol lowering. *JAMA.* 1984;251:365–374.

Lipsky H, Gloger M, Frishman WH. Dietary fiber for reducing blood cholesterol. *J Clin Pharmacol.* 1990;30:699–703.

Malenka DJ, Baron JA. Cholesterol and coronary heart disease: The attributable risk reduction of diet and drugs. *Arch Intern Med.* 1989;149:1981–1985.

Mancini M, Betteridge DJ, Pometta D. Acquired (secondary) forms of hypertriglyceridemia. *Am J Cardiol.* 1991;68:17A–21A.

McNamara DJ, Howell WH. Epidemiologic data linking diet to hyperlipidemia and arteriosclerosis. *Semin Liver Dis.* 1992;12:347–355.

Miller VT. Dyslipoproteinemia in women: special considerations. *Endocrinol Metabol Clin North Am.* 1990;19:381–398.

Montalto SJ. Lovastatin and cataracts: An update. *Clin Eye Vision Care.* 1989;1:212–217.

National Center for Health Statistics, National Heart, Lung, and Blood Institute Collaborative Lipid Group. Trends in serum cholesterol levels among U.S. adults aged 20 to 74 years. *JAMA.* 1987;257:937–942.

National Cholesterol Education Program Expert Panel. Report on detection, evaluation, and treatment of high blood cholesterol in adults. *Arch Intern Med.* 1988;148:36–69.

National Heart, Lung, and Blood Institute Consensus Development Panel. Treatment of hypertriglyceridemia. *JAMA.* 1984;281:1196–1200.

Nishimoto JH, Townsend JC, Selvin GJ, DeLand PN. Corneal arcus as an indicator of hypercholesterolemia. *J Am Optom Assoc.* 1990;61:44–49.

Pearson TA. Therapeutic management of triglycerides: An international perspective. *Am J Cardiol.* 1992;70:26H–31H.

Phillips CI, Tsukahara S, Gore SM. Corneal arcus: Some morphology and applied pathophysiology. *Jpn J Ophthalmol.* 1990;34:442–449.

Schonfeld G. Inherited disorders of lipid transport. *Endocrinol Metabol Clin North Am.* 1990;19:229–257.

Scott D, Kurenitz M. Using lipid lowering agents effectively: When diet is not enough. *Postgrad Med.* 1990;87:171–186.

Segal P, Insull W, Chambless LE, et al. The Lipid Research Clinics Program Prevalence study: The association of dys-lipoproteinemia with corneal arcus and xanthelasma. *Circulation.* 1986;73(suppl I):108–118.

Sempos C, Fulwood R, Haines C, et al. The prevalence of high blood cholesterol levels among adults in the United States. *JAMA.* 1989;262:45–52.

Stamler J, Wentworth D, Neaton JD. Is the relationship between serum cholesterol and risk of premature death from coronary heart disease continuous and graded? *JAMA.* 1986;256:2823–2838.

Stein EA. Management of hypercholesterolemia: Approach to diet and drug therapy. *Am J Med.* 1989;87(suppl 4A):20S–27S.

Stein EA, Steiner PM. Triglyceride measurement and its relationship to heart disease. *Clin Lab Med.* 1989;9:169–185.

Steiner G, Shafrir E. *Primary Hyperlipoproteinemias.* New York: McGraw–Hill; 1991.

Varnek L, Schnohr P, Jensen G. Presenile corneal arcus in healthy persons. A possible cardiovascular risk indicator in younger adults. *Acta Ophthalmol.* 1979;57:755–765.

Wilson PWF. The epidemiology of hypercholesterolemia: A global perspective. *Am J Med.* 1989;87(suppl 4A):5S–13S.

Working Group on Management of Patients with Hypertension and High Blood Cholesterol. National Education Programs Working Group report on the management of patients with hypertension and high blood cholesterol: *Ann Int Med.* 1991;114:224–237.

74

Chapter

Sphingolipidoses

Kelly H. Thomann

The sphingolipidoses are a group of inherited disorders also known as lysosomal storage diseases. Each disease has a specific dysfunctional lysosomal hydrolase along the intricate pathway of sphingolipid metabolism. Sphingolipids are essential components of membranes in tissues, especially the nervous system. Due to a defect, a sphingolipid particular to each disease accumulates pathologically in organs and tissues, leading to the clinical manifestations of the disease (Table 74–1).

Ocular manifestations in this group of diseases may involve the cornea, conjunctiva, lens, retina, and eye movements (Table 74–2). However, often the noteworthy ocular involvement occurs in the most devastating subgroups of these diseases in which the lifespan of the patient is very limited.

This chapter will be limited to discussions of Gaucher disease, Tay–Sachs disease, Niemann–Pick disease, and Fabry disease.

■ GAUCHER DISEASE

Gaucher disease is characterized by accumulation of the extremely insoluble glycolipid, glucocerebroside, in the lysosomes of macrophages in the body. Enlarged liver and spleen (hepatosplenomegaly) are the most prominent clinical manifestations. Gaucher disease exists in three forms (types I, II, and III). Affected patients may be relatively asymptomatic with a normal lifespan, or the disease may follow a rapidly progressive course leading to death in the first few years of life.

Ocular involvement in type I is minimal and rarely found, but may include ocular motor apraxia and yellow-brown conjunctival pingueculae. Type II always manifests with severe neurological abnormalities, including abnormalities to the cranial nerve innervation of the extraocular muscles. Type III may also show the same motility dysfunction as type II. White retinal lesions have also been reported in types II and III.

EPIDEMIOLOGY

■ Systemic

Type I Gaucher disease makes up greater than 99% of all cases and is found in approximately 1 in 2000 Jewish persons in the United States and 1 in 40,000 in the general population. It has a carrier frequency of 1 in 13 to 1 in 20 in those of Ashkenazi Jewish heritage. Types II and III each occur in less than 1 in 100,000 people and show no ethnic predilection, except for a subgroup of type III found in a northern district of Sweden where all persons with the disease can be traced to the same family tree.

■ Ocular

There is no epidemiological information available regarding ocular manifestations in Gaucher disease.

TABLE 74–1. SYSTEMIC MANIFESTATIONS OF THE SPHINGOLIPIDOSES

GAUCHER DISEASE
- **Type I**
  Liver: hepatomegaly, abnormal liver function, hepatic failure
  Spleen: splenomegaly, anemia, thrombocytopenia, hypersplenism
  Skeletal system: Erlenmeyer flask deformity, aseptic necrosis of the femoral heads, bone infarcts, fractures of long bones, recurrent pain and swelling
  Pulmonary dysfunction
- **Type II**
  Liver dysfunction (see type I)
  Spleen dysfunction (see type I)
  Strabismus
  Retroflexion of the head
  Dysfunction of all cranial nerves
  Extrapyramidal dysfunction
- **Type III**
  Manifestations variable and similar to types I and II

TAY–SACHS DISEASE
- **Early Signs**
  Increased startle reflex
  Hypotonia
- **Progression To**
  Myoclonus
  Pyramidal dysfunction
  Spasticity of the limbs
  Seizures
  Psychomotor arrest
  Progressive mental deterioration

- **Terminal Stage**
  Megalencephaly
  Amaurosis
  Deafness
  Spastic and vegetative state

NIEMANN–PICK DISEASE
- **Type A**
  Hepatomegaly
  Splenomegaly
  Severe CNS involvement
  Pulmonary infiltration
- **Type B**
  Hepatomegaly
  Splenomegaly
- **Type C**
  Mild to moderate hepatosplenomegaly
  Progressive ataxia and mental retardation
  Seizures
  Other neurological involvement: abnormal muscle tone, dysarthria, movement disorders
- **Type D**
  Similar manifestations to type C but in individuals with Nova Scotian lineage; laboratory testing does not show evidence of sphingomyelinase deficiency

FABRY DISEASE
- Pain in extremities and abdomen
- Angiokeratomas
- Hypohydrosis leading to anhydrosis
- Renal dysfunction

NATURAL HISTORY

■ Systemic

Gaucher disease has an autosomal recessive inheritance pattern. Glucocerebrosidase, the deficient enzyme, is necessary to catalyze the hydrolysis of glucocerebroside to glucose and ceramide. The macrophages that become engorged with glycolipid are responsible for the pathology in various tissues and organs of the body. Involvement of the spleen macrophages causes anemia, thrombocytopenia, and other signs of hypersplenism. Involvement of the liver Kupffer cells causes hepatomegaly, abnormal liver function, and rarely, hepatic failure. Deficient bone marrow cells may commonly lead to bone manifestations. Erlenmeyer-flask deformity, a flaring of the distal femur, is a classic sign of bone involvement. Other frequent complications of the bones include aseptic necrosis of the femoral heads, bone infarcts, pathologic fractures of long bones, and recurrent episodes of pain and swelling. The pul-

monary parenchyma may be involved and cause lung dysfunction or predispose individuals to pneumonia.

The most common form of Gaucher disease is known as type I, adult or non-neuropathic. It presents as a disease of the visceral organs with a wide array of clinical severity and rarely involves the nervous system. Genetic and environmental factors that are not fully understood influence the degree of involvement. Severely affected patients may die in their third decade, often due to pneumonia. Less severe, asymptomatic patients may be diagnosed in middle or old age when the bone marrow is examined for an unrelated disorder or during the workup of a blood disorder such as thrombocytopenia. These patients may show minimal skeletal changes or spleen enlargement, usually do not require treatment, and may have a normal lifespan with death from unrelated factors.

Type II (infantile or neuropathic) Gaucher disease has a more stereotypical presentation than type I. It is characterized by extensive nervous system involvement presenting very early in life, with death most commonly occurring

TABLE 74–2. OCULAR MANIFESTATIONS OF THE SPHINGOLIPIDOSES

GAUCHER DISEASE
- **Type I**
  Ocular motor apraxia
  Pigmented pingueculae
- **Types II & III**
  Eye movement paralysis
  White retinal spots

TAY–SACHS DISEASE
- Macular cherry red spot

NIEMANN–PICK DISEASE
- **Types A & B**
  Macular cherry red spot
  Corneal opacification
  Lenticular opacities
- **Types C & D**
  Ocular motility dysfunction; especially supranuclear gaze paresis

FABRY DISEASE
- Corneal verticellata
- Posterior cataracts
- Retinal and conjunctival angiokeratomas

before age 2. It presents with a painless enlargement of the liver and spleen followed by neurologic involvement. Trismus, a prolonged jaw muscle spasm due to dysfunction of the motor division of the trigeminal nerve; strabismus due to disturbance of the oculomotor, trochlear, and/or abducens nerves; and retroflexion of the head comprise the classic triad found in this form. Extensive cranial nerve and extrapyramidal dysfunction follows, leading to progressive spasticity and hyperreflexia. Death most commonly occurs from anoxia or infection due to pulmonary involvement.

A third form, type III (juvenile or subacute neuropathic), also exists, but is the least frequently encountered and is actually a continuum between types I and II, not a distinct disorder. It appears as a chronic disorder with progressive neurologic dysfunction and death usually occurring in early adulthood.

■ Ocular

The ocular findings in type I include ocular motor apraxia and yellowish brown conjunctival pingueculae. Each is a consequential finding and does not affect ocular function. The more obvious ocular manifestations are found in types II and III when the cranial nerves become affected, manifesting as a supranuclear palsy. Cortical blindness has also been documented in type II. Discrete white spots in or on the superficial retina have been reported in types II and III. These spots are composed of swollen histiocytes (known as

Gaucher cells), and seem to appear more frequently temporal to the macula in an arcuate pattern. Some references have classified Gaucher disease as one of the sphingolipidoses that causes a macular cherry red spot; however, this is incorrect.

DIAGNOSIS

■ Systemic

Type I Gaucher disease is usually diagnosed following unexplained splenomegaly. These patients generally will have a mild to moderate anemia and thrombocytopenia. Bone fractures and thinning of the cortices of long bones may also lead to suspicion of the disease. The most reliable and easiest way to diagnose Gaucher disease is to measure leukocyte β-glucosidase activity in blood. It can also be confirmed by examination of bone marrow aspirate; however, it is not necessary if other tests have already been done. Diagnosis can also be made through cultured skin fibroblasts and cultured amniotic fluid cells prenatally.

■ Ocular

If present, the ocular motor apraxia in type I Gaucher disease will be evident on extraocular motility testing during routine examination. Pigmented pingueculae may be seen on slit-lamp examination. Supranuclear palsies, found in Gaucher types II and III, may be evident on external and motility examination, if possible. White retinal lesions will be seen on fundus examination.

TREATMENT AND MANAGEMENT

■ Systemic

Up until recently, the only therapy for Gaucher disease has been supportive, in an effort to lessen the impact of the disease manifestations. This includes repair of fractured bones, removal of an enlarged spleen to control anemia and thrombocytopenia, and treatment of intercurrent infections with antibiotics. There are a number of definitive approaches to the management of this disease, some of which are being applied today. Replacement of the deficient enzyme has been very encouraging but extremely expensive. Currently, approaches to administer the enzyme in a more cost-efficient manner are under investigation. Marrow transplantation, gene transfer, and organ allografts are other ways that could theoretically cure the disease. However, it is not entirely clear on whom these should be performed, because mild cases do not warrant aggressive treatment and more severe cases have greater risks involved.

Genetic and prenatal testing is possible to detect couples who are each heterozygous for Gaucher types I, II, and III disease.

■ Ocular

There is no treatment indicated for any of the ocular manifestations of Gaucher disease. Types II and III will seldom be followed in a primary care practice due to their rarity, severity of manifestations, and the short lifespan of the patients affected.

■ TAY–SACHS DISEASE

Tay–Sachs disease, which is also classified as one of the gangliosidoses, is considered the prototypical sphingolipid disorder. This disease appears early, with affected persons having a very short lifespan and displaying progressive mental deterioration, loss of motor skills, and seizures. The classic ocular manifestation, seen in almost all cases of this disease, is the macular cherry red spot.

EPIDEMIOLOGY

■ Systemic

Ninety percent of patients afflicted with Tay–Sachs disease are of Jewish descent. It is estimated that 1 out of 27 individuals of Ashkenazi Jewish heritage and 1 out of 30 French-Canadian Jewish persons are carriers for the disease. In New York City, the frequency of the Tay–Sachs gene in the Jewish population has been estimated to be 1 in 30 compared to 1 in 300 Jewish persons in the entire United States.

■ Ocular

It is estimated that 90% of children with Tay–Sachs disease have the characteristic cherry red macula.

NATURAL HISTORY

■ Systemic

Tay–Sachs disease is transmitted with an autosomal recessive inheritance pattern and caused by the absence of hexosaminidase A, which causes abnormal concentrations of G_{M2} ganglioside, and ceramide trihexoside (a derivative of G_{M2} ganglioside) in the central nervous system and viscera. There are several subclasses of G_{M2} gangliosidoses. Tay–Sachs disease is infantile neuronal G_{M2} gangliosidoses type 1. Other subclasses of Tay–Sachs exist, with variant B the most common.

Abnormal sphingolipid accumulation in Tay–Sachs disease causes all cells of the nervous system to take on a characteristic appearance. The cytoplasm swells and the cells become extremely enlarged. Morphologically, this causes a marked increase in brain weight and volume, which in turn causes prominent megalencephaly and results in overall nervous system dysfunction. As opposed to the other sphingolipid diseases, organomegaly is uncommon.

Tay–Sachs disease usually manifests between 3 and 7 months of age. At 2 to 3 months, an increased startle reaction and hypotonia may be the first signs in those affected. By 12 to 18 months these signs progress to segmental and diffuse myoclonus, pyramidal dysfunction, spasticity of the limbs, and prolonged seizures. Also very prominent is an early psychomotor arrest along with progressive mental deterioration, usually evident at 4 to 6 months. Previous milestones that the child had attained quickly are lost. By about 18 months, the child reaches a terminal state in which he or she is megalencephalic, amaurotic, deaf, spastic, and in a vegetative state, out of contact with the environment. Death usually occurs between 3 and 5 years of age, most commonly due to overall poor health, organ dysfunction, or aspiration pneumonia.

■ Ocular

The most obvious ocular finding is the macular cherry red spot and it is often a major component in the diagnosis of Tay–Sachs disease. It is caused by the retinal ganglion cells accumulating G_{M2} ganglioside. The cherry red spot is described as a white halo that is opaque, slightly elevated, and about 1½ disc diameters in size. The outer border is less sharply demarcated than the inner border. The red spot is actually the normal choroidal color, which is seen more prominently centrally where no ganglion cells are located. The surrounding ganglion cells are swollen from the accumulation of lipid products causing a loss of retinal transparency. In the periphery, where there is only one layer of ganglion cells, the swollen area is less obvious. With time, blindness occurs secondary to ganglion cell and nerve fiber layer death, with subsequent optic atrophy. These patients are usually blind by 18 months of age.

DIAGNOSIS

■ Systemic

Diagnosis of Tay–Sachs disease is made through the obvious clinical manifestations. Enzymatic diagnosis most commonly utilizes serum cultured fibroblasts. It may also be diagnosed through analysis of other enzyme sources such as serum, urine, and tears. Mass screening of high-risk populations is possible using automated procedures. Amniotic fluid may be analyzed to make a diagnosis prenatally.

■ Ocular

Macular cherry red spot will be evident on fundus examination and in some cases may contribute to the conclusive diagnosis of Tay–Sachs disease.

TREATMENT AND MANAGEMENT

■ Systemic

Currently there is no treatment for this disease. Genetic counseling is now available to detect homozygous carriers as well as to make the diagnosis prenatally.

■ Ocular

There is no treatment for the macular cherry red spot.

■ NIEMANN–PICK DISEASE

Niemann–Pick disease is generally characterized by a deficiency of sphingomyelinase, the enzyme that catalyzes the first step in the degradation of sphingomyelin. Sphingomyelin, a phospholipid, is an important component of the plasma membrane of cells and organelles such as the endoplasmic reticulum, mitochondria, and erythrocyte stroma. A deficiency of its catalytic enzyme will result in an accumulation of sphingomyelin in body tissues. Cholesterol is also prominently accumulated cellularly, especially in particular subtypes of Niemann–Pick disease. Each subtype varies in severity of manifestations according to the amount of sphingomyelin accumulation. Ocular involvement includes motility dysfunction, macular cherry red spots, and less rarely, corneal and lenticular opacities.

EPIDEMIOLOGY

■ Systemic

Niemann–Pick disease has been reported in all races, but more than 50% of cases are of Ashkenazi Jewish heritage. Its incidence in the United States is said to be 1 out of 100,000 persons of Ashkenazi heritage.

■ Ocular

Macular cherry red spot is found in approximately 50% of Type A Niemann–Pick patients.

NATURAL HISTORY

■ Systemic

Niemann–Pick disease includes a wide array of clinical and biochemical heterogeneity. This disease is broken into two main categories: one with total or nearly total deficiency of sphingomyelinase and the other in which the activity of sphingomyelinase is slightly reduced or normal, despite prominent signs of the disease and consistent increases in tissue cholesterol. The first group is further broken down into the acute neuropathic form (also known as type A), which is the most common variant; and the chronic, visceral form (also known as type B). Both show an autosomal recessive pattern of inheritance. Type A has an early onset and rapid course, with death occurring between 1 to 4 years of age. These patients show prominent hepatosplenomegaly by 6 months of age, severe central nervous system involvement and frequent complications due to heavy pulmonary infiltration. Type A also has other variants with minimal neurological sequelae and mostly visceral symptomatology. The prognosis depends on the progression of lipid storage. Type B (the visceral form) displays a slower clinical course in which patients often reach adulthood, and mental retardation, which is common in type A, is not a characteristic. A variable degree of sphingomyelinase deficiency exists. These patients have extensive visceral involvement with manifestations apparent by infancy or childhood. The first sign is usually an enlarged spleen with the liver becoming involved later in the disease. The lungs are often diffusely infiltrated, with patients complaining of dyspnea on exertion, along with having an increased susceptibility to respiratory infections and pneumonia. The liver is usually not impaired functionally, but abdominal distention due to enlargement may be distressing to the patient. Except for visceral organ enlargement, these patients usually reach adulthood with reasonably good health.

The second subgroup of Niemann–Pick disease, which is also inherited in an autosomal recessive fashion, is comprised of those who show moderate deficiency of sphingomyelinase and are currently believed to have an altered ability to process cholesterol. This group is broken into the chronic neuropathic form (type C) and the Nova Scotia variant (type D). In these types, there is both visceral and nervous system involvement that may be subacute or chronic. Type D shows almost identical manifestations to type C, but is found in a particular group of Nova Scotia persons and lacks evidence of sphingomyelinase deficiency. There is also a type E in which patients exhibit an elevated level of sphingomyelin in one or more organs but no family history of the disease. This subtype will not be discussed in this chapter.

Types C and D Niemann–Pick disease show variable age of onset from late infancy to early adulthood. They are characterized by mild to moderate hepatosplenomegaly, sea-blue histiocytes in the bone marrow, supranuclear vertical gaze paresis, slowly progressive ataxia and mental retardation. These signs are all caused by abnormal intracellular cholesterol homeostasis. Ataxia is the most notable neurologic feature. Clumsiness of gait may be a first sign of the disease, and these patients may also show decreased ability to tandem walk. As the disease progresses, the ataxia becomes profound and includes all extremities. Learning impairment and progressive dementia are inevitable. They are the most distressing part of the disease. The dementia may eventually include psychosis, behavioral disturbances, hallucinations, and delusions. Other neurological signs include dystonia (abnormal muscle tone), movement disorders, dysarthria (abnormal speech or articulation), and seizures. The peripheral nervous system is spared. Death usually occurs by age 20, and may be due to aspiration pneumonia.

■ Ocular

A cherry red spot in the macula is found in the first group of Niemann–Pick disease, especially the acute neuropathic form (type A). Abnormal lipid accumulation occurs in retinal ganglion, amacrine, receptor, and retinal pigment epithelial cells. However, ganglion cell function is preserved, which accounts for the delayed visual loss as opposed to Tay–Sachs disease, which displays amaurosis as an early sign. The cherry red macula resembles that seen in Tay–Sachs disease except the white ring that surrounds the spot is less sharply demarcated and extends peripherally as a generalized, mild retinal opacification. Another differing factor is that the ring in Niemann–Pick disease remains until death, while in Tay–Sachs disease it usually becomes smaller.

A mild opacification of the corneal stroma may be found. Brown, granular discoloration of the anterior lens and round, flat, white spots on the posterior lens capsule have also been documented.

Several cases of what has been called "macular halo" have been documented in Niemann–Pick disease type B. The halo consists of symmetrical punctate crystal-like opacities in a ring around the fovea. Vision is not impaired.

The second group of Niemann–Pick disease (including types C and D) does not have any retinal or macular manifestations, but shows characteristic ocular motility dysfunction. Most characteristic is a supranuclear vertical gaze paresis. It is usually absent in the early course of the disease. It may first manifest as a loss of downward volitional saccades and progress to total loss, followed by a complete loss of vertical volitional movements. Eventually the horizontal saccades will be affected. Slow vertical pursuits and reflex eye movements are usually preserved, even late in the disease.

Diagnosis

■ Systemic

The constant features of all variants of Niemann–Pick disease are hepatosplenomegaly and foam cells in the bone marrow. Diagnosis can be made by measuring sphingomyelinase

activity in tissue samples or homogenates of cultured skin fibroblasts. Currently, the easiest method to decisively diagnose this disease is by assessing the level of sphingomyelinase in white blood cell preparations. These patients will show a level markedly lower than normal. This technique, however, will not show heterozygous carriers.

■ Ocular

The macular cherry red spot will be seen on fundus evaluation. It may go unnoticed if vision is normal. Corneal and lenticular opacities will be seen with biomicroscopy. Eye movement abnormalities, present in types C and D, are apparent on ocular motility and electrodiagnostic testing. Early impairment may be apparent with optokinetic nystagmus testing.

Treatment and Management

■ Systemic

No specific therapy exists for Niemann–Pick disease. Various measures to modify cholesterol intake and processing hold promise for the management of types C and D. Enzyme replacement trials as well as organ allografts are being investigated.

■ Ocular

There is no treatment for the ocular manifestations of Niemann–Pick disease.

■ Fabry Disease

Fabry disease is the only sphingolipid disease with an x-linked recessive mode of inheritance. This disease is caused by defective activity of the enzyme α-galactosidase A and is characterized by lesions of the skin and dysfunction of the kidneys, heart, and central nervous system. Ocular manifestations are a prominent component of this disease. They include whorled corneal opacities (verticellata) and posterior cataracts.

Epidemiology

■ Systemic

The incidence of Fabry disease is 1 in 40,000 persons.

■ Ocular

Corneal verticillata are found in over 90% of patients and often appear prior to the dermatologic and visceral signs of the disease. It has also been found that 80% of females heterozygous for this disease have corneal verticillata. Posterior lenticular opacities may develop in half of the patients and up to 60% demonstrate dilation and tortuosity of the conjunctival and retinal vessels. Periorbital edema has been described in 25% of patients with this disease.

NATURAL HISTORY

■ Systemic

The deficiency of α-galactosidase A results in accumulation of ceramide trihexoside in the lysosomes of endothelial cells, especially those found in the tissues of the kidneys, skin, blood vessels, and corneal epithelium. Fabry disease often affects males early in childhood. Heterozygous female carriers may be affected by the disease to a lesser extent, they may be asymptomatic, or rarely, severely affected. Pain in the extremities and abdomen is usually the initial as well as most prominent and debilitating manifestation. The pain may be associated with chronic paresthesias of the limbs, myalgia, and polyarthralgia. It is often initially misdiagnosed as juvenile rheumatoid arthritis. The attacks are often triggered by exercise, temperature changes, fatigue, and emotional stress. They persist throughout life.

Cutaneous telangiectasias (a dilation of capillaries and small arteries), called angiokeratomas, usually appear at about 7 to 10 years as dark red to black, nonblanching macules and papules ranging in size up to 4 mm in diameter. They are typically located on the lower abdomen, genitals and upper thighs, and also found in the gastrointestinal, genitourinary, and respiratory tracts. They increase in number with time and persist throughout life. They are due to the cellular accumulation of glycosphingolipid.

Hypohydrosis (decrease in sweating) usually begins at puberty and progresses to complete lack of sweating (anhydrosis) by the third decade. This, and other impaired autonomic functions and paresthesias, are presumably due to the glycolipid deposits in the sensory and autonomic ganglia.

By adolescence, renal function deteriorates, leading to hypertensive renal insufficiency and uremia by the third and fourth decades. Ceramide trihexoside accumulates in the blood vessel walls and can cause premature myocardial infarction or cerebrovascular disease. Most will die by their fourth to fifth decade from chronic renal failure or cardiovascular disease.

■ Ocular

The most noteworthy ocular feature in Fabry disease is corneal verticelatta (Figure 74–1). It consists of prominent cream-colored intraepithelial lines in a whorled configuration radiating from a central nodal point. The extent is variable and not related to the severity of the disease. It does not impair vision. Another ocular sign is a star-shaped posterior

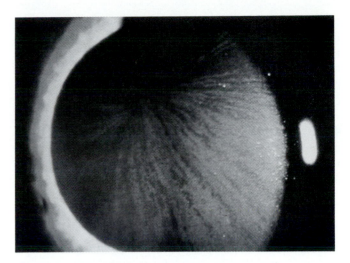

Figure 74–1. *The whorled configuration of corneal verticellata. (Reprinted with permission from Mandel ER, Wagoner MD.* Atlas of Corneal Disease. *Philadelphia: Saunders; 1987, p 47.)*

cataract, found in both men with the disease and female carriers. Retinal and conjunctival tortuosity (which are actually cutaneous angiokeratomas) have also been noted.

DIAGNOSIS

■ Systemic

Patients will show elevated levels of ceramide trihexoside concentrations in plasma. Diagnosis can also be made by demonstration of a deficiency of the enzyme α-galactosidase-A. The most common enzyme sources are the leukocytes and skin fibroblasts of these patients, but organ tissue and urine may also be used. Urinalysis may be used to detect heterozygous carriers and prenatal diagnosis can be made with cultured amniotic cells.

■ Ocular

Diagnosis of corneal verticellata and conjunctival angiokeratomas may be made with biomicroscope examination and may be the first sign of this disease. Fleischer vortex dystrophy, and corneal pigmentation secondary to usage of amiodarone or indomethacin, may resemble the corneal opacities, and are included in the differential diagnosis. The retinal angiokeratomas will be seen on fundus evaluation.

TREATMENT AND MANAGEMENT

■ Systemic

Medication to decrease the frequency and severity of pain may be utilized. Hemodialysis for the chronic renal disease or renal transplant may be considered, but are often contraindicated or complicated by cardiovascular disease. Enzyme replacement and organ allografts as a prospective mode of treatment are currently being investigated and may be promising in the future. Genetic counseling and prenatal diagnosis are available.

■ Ocular

No treatment is necessary for the ocular manifestations of Fabry disease, because ocular function is not impaired. Routine ocular examinations are recommended.

CONCLUSION

The sphingolipidoses are a group of diseases that when taken individually, are relatively rare. However, their sometimes devastating effects have made it important for the medical community to understand these complex disorders. Over the last two decades, the enzyme defect for each disease has been located and characterized. This has lead to genetic testing to detect carriers of these traits as well as prenatal testing to detect the diseases. New management strategies, which may eventually involve cures, are being investigated at this time. Ocular involvement ranges from subtle to those manifestations that are a vital part of the diagnosis of the particular disorder; hence the eyecare practitioner may play an important role in the management of these diseases.

REFERENCES

Adachi M, Schneck L, Volk BW. Progress in investigations of sphingolipidoses. *Acta Neuropathol.* 1978;43:1–18.

Brady RO. Sphingolipidoses. *Ann Rev Biochem.* 1978;47:687–713.

Brady RO. Genetics and the sphingolipidoses. *Med Clin North Am.* 1969;53:827–838.

Brady RO, James SP, Barranger JA. The liver in lipid storage disease: Biochemical basis of pathogenesis and clinical features. *Prog Liver Dis.* 1982;7:331–346.

Cogan DC, Chu FC, Reingold D, Barranger J. Ocular motor signs in some metabolic diseases. *Arch Ophthalmol.* 1981;99:1802–1808.

Glew RH, Basu A, Prence EM, Remalay AT. Biology of disease, lysosomal storage diseases. *Lab Invest.* 1985;53:250–269.

Larsen H, Ehlers N. Ocular manifestations in Tay–Sachs' and Niemann–Pick's diseases. *Acta Ophthalmologica.* 1966;43:285–293.

Pilz H, Heipertz R, Seidel D. Basic findings and current developments in sphingolipidoses. *Hum Genetics.* 1979;47:113–134.

Sandhoff K. The biochemistry of sphingolipid storage diseases. *Angewandse Chemie.* 1977;16(5):273–285.

Suzuki K: Enzymatic diagnosis of sphingolipidoses. *Meth Enzymol.* 1978;50:456–488.

Gaucher Disease

Beutler E. Gaucher disease: New molecular approaches to diagnosis and treatment. *Science.* 1992;256:794–799.

Beutler E. Gaucher's disease. *N Engl J Med.* 1991;325:1354–1360.

Beutler E. Gaucher disease. *Blood Rev.* 1988;2:50–70.

Cogan DG, Chu FC, Gittanger J, Tychsen L. Fundal abnormalities of Gaucher's disease. *Arch Ophthalmol.* 1980;98:2202–2203.

Goldblatt J. Type I Gaucher disease. *J Med Genet.* 1988;25:415–418.

Martin BM, Sidransky E, Ginns EI. Gaucher's disease: Advances and challenges. *Adv Pediatr.* 1989;36:277–306.

Peters SP, Lee RE, Glew RH. Gaucher's disease: A review. *Medicine.* 1977;56:425–442.

Niemann–Pick Disease

Brady RO, Filling-Katz MR, Barton NW, Pentchev PG. Niemann–Pick disease types C and D. *Neurogenet Dis.* 1989;7:75–88.

Elleder M. Niemann–Pick disease. *Path Res Pract.* 1989;185:293–328.

Francois J. Metabolic tapeto retinal degenerations. *Surv Ophthalmol.* 1982;26:293–333.

Grover WD, Naimann JL. Progressive paresis of vertical gaze in lipid storage disease. *Neurology.* 1971;21:896–899.

Vanier MT, Pentchev P, Rodriguez-Lafrasse C, Rousson R. Niemann–Pick disease type C: An update. *J Inher Metab Dis.* 1991;14:580–595.

Walton DS, Robb RM, Crocker AC. Ocular manifestations of group A Niemann–Pick disease. *Am J Ophthalmol.* 1978;85:174–180.

Fabry Disease

Dufier J. Ophthalmologic involvement in inherited renal disease. *Adv Nephrol.* 1992;21:143–156.

Goldberg MF. A review of selected inherited corneal dystrophies associated with systemic diseases. *Birth Defects.* 1971;7:13–25.

Kato H, Sato K, Hattori S. Fabry's disease. *Int Med.* 1992;31:682–685.

Paller AS. Metabolic disorders characterized by angiokeratomas and neurologic dysfunction. *Neurol Clin.* 1987;5:441–446.

Stanbury JB, Wyngaarden JB, Frederickson DS, et al. *The Metabolic Basis of Inherited Disease.* New York: McGraw-Hill; 1982:803–969.

75
Chapter

Albinism

Jerome Sherman ▪ Sherry J. Bass

Albinism is a congenital deficiency in pigment that has been recognized since ancient times. Early writings suggest that Noah of the Biblical period was an albino. In contrast to the generalized or universal form of albinism, albinism affecting only the eye was not recognized until the beginning of the 20th century.

When the enzyme tyrosinase is present and functioning properly, tyrosine is converted into melanin, resulting in normal skin and eye color. In all forms of albinism, melanocytes are present but are amelanotic due to absent, relatively deficient, or poorly functional tyrosinase (Carr & Siegel, 1981). When tyrosinase is absent, the term used is tyrosinase-negative. In this case, hair, skin, and ocular findings are more prominent than in the tyrosinase-positive form, in which at least some tyrosinase can be demonstrated. Other forms of albinism exist, such as cutaneous albinism, ocular albinism, and the rarer Hermansky–Pudlak (HP) and Prader–Willi (PW) syndromes.

EPIDEMIOLOGY

Cutaneous Albinism
No epidemiological data are available in the literature concerning cutaneous albinism.

Oculocutaneous Albinism
There are four subtypes of oculocutaneous albinism. All are inherited as autosomal recessive traits. Each subtype is relatively rare, and the incidence in the United States and Europe ranges from 1 in 10,000 to 1 in 40,000.

Ocular Albinism
Ocular albinism had been thought to be inherited as an X-linked trait. In the late 1970s, a new form of ocular albinism, inherited as an autosomal recessive trait, was reported (O'Donnell et al, 1976). The incidence of X-linked ocular albinism is 1 in 50,000, and although the incidence of autosomal recessive ocular albinism is not known

with certainty, it is probably the more common form of ocular albinism (O'Donnell & Green, 1987).

Hermansky–Pudlak and Prader–Willi Syndromes
In Puerto Rico the prevalence of HP syndrome is 1 in 1800 people with albinism. The incidence of PW syndrome is estimated to be 1 in 25,000 people with albinism.

NATURAL HISTORY

Cutaneous Albinism
Although not frequently encountered by the eyecare practitioner, these individuals typically have hypopigmentation of the skin but normally pigmented and functioning eyes. The most obvious finding is a white frontal hair lock with occasional hypopigmentation on the forehead. Visual function is normal.

Oculocutaneous Albinism

The hereditary pattern is mostly autosomal recessive, although the tyrosinase-negative and tyrosinase-positive forms represent different genotypes. Thus, it is possible for a tyrosinase-negative albino married to a tyrosinase-positive albino to have all "normal" children, although they will all be carriers of two different recessive genes. In Caucasians the skin is quite light and sometimes described as milk white (Figure 75–1). In African-American albinos, the skin color is lighter than unaffected family members but slightly darker than most Caucasians.

Most individuals with oculocutaneous albinism (especially the complete or tyrosinase-negative type) burn in the sun and never tan. Slow tanning does occur, however, in the mild forms of the tyrosinase-positive or incomplete albinism. Although the underlying condition changes little over time, continued exposure to ultraviolet rays may lead to precancerous keratosis, and squamous and basal cell carcinoma. Amelanotic malignant melanomas also have been reported. Those with the mild form of tyrosinase-positive albinism who tan slowly, appear to be at a lower risk of serious dermatologic consequences.

The hair of the tyrosinase-negative albino is usually described as straw or platinum in color. The hair of the tyrosinase-positive albino may be nearly as light in the early years of life, but generally darkens with age.

Ocular findings include reduced central vision, nystagmus, iris transillumination (Figure 75–2), decreased pigmentation of the fundus, poor foveal development, and ill-defined macular landmarks (Figure 75–3).

Ocular Albinism

Although the skin and hair appear normal in ocular albinism, the same ocular manifestations seen in oculocutaneous albinism are clearly present. Some patients with ocular albinism have jet-black hair, dark skin, brown eyes that

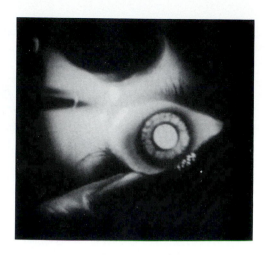

Figure 75–2. Iris transillumination.

demonstrate iris transillumination, and macular hypoplasia with resultant nystagmus and reduced visual acuity.

Clinically, ocular albinism appears limited to the eyes, but skin biopsies reveal unusual macromelanosomes (abnormally formed melanin granules) in the dermis and epidermis. These diagnostic macromelanosomes appear only in X-linked ocular albinism and have not been found in autosomal recessive ocular albinism (Creel et al, 1974).

The impaired ocular function in autosomal recessive ocular albinism may be due to altered neuroectoderm (the retinal and iris pigment epithelium), whereas the skin, hair,

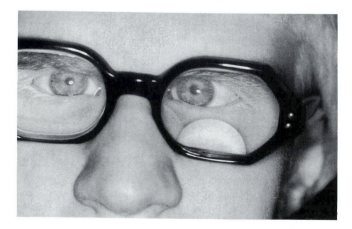

Figure 75–1. Classic tyrosinase-negative oculocutaneous albinism showing hair, skin, eyes. *(Courtesy of Bruce Rosenthal, OD.)*

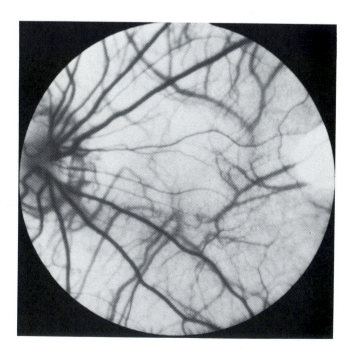

Figure 75–3. Macular hypoplasia in an albinotic fundus.

and iris stroma are normal due to intact neural-crest derived melanocytes.

On rare occasion, nystagmus may decrease slowly in time, with subtle improvement in visual acuity. Clinically, overall visual function generally remains unchanged, in spite of electroretinogram (ERG) amplitudes that begin supernormal in the early years and slowly decrease to an abnormal range. This suggests slow destruction of the photoreceptors, most likely due to excessive light exposure.

HP and PW Syndromes

Several rare syndromes with life-threatening manifestations exist. HP syndrome is the association of oculocutaneous albinism with defective platelet function leading to an increased bleeding tendency. Easy bruisability and gum bleeding are common in HP syndrome.

HP in Puerto Rican albinos should be suspected because they appear to be at a higher risk. Aspirin use can be life threatening in HP patients, and death can be caused by fibrotic restrictive pulmonary disease. Ceroid (yellowish-brown lipid end-products of unsaturated fatty acid metabolism) may accumulate in tissues in HP, and an enteropathic disorder resembling Crohn disease has also been reported (Simon et al, 1982). It is unclear whether this disorder is actually caused by the ceroid.

PW syndrome is characterized by muscular hypotonia, hypogenitalism, obesity, mental retardation, short stature, and diminished sensitivity to pain. A single chromosomal abnormality has been demonstrated as a frequent cause of PW (Ledbetter et al, 1981). This subtle abnormality, an interstitial deletion on the proximal long arm of one of the number 15 chromosomes, can be easily missed unless specifically considered during chromosomal analysis. In 1982, a previously missed component of the PW syndrome was recognized, that of oculocutaneous albinoidism (Hittner et al, 1982). Nine patients were found with PW who also had decreased tyrosinase activity in isolated hair bulbs, light hair and skin, decreased pigmentation of the iris stroma, and variable amounts of iris translucency. However, none had reduced vision, nystagmus, photophobia, or foveal hypoplasia; hence the term "albinoidism."

DIAGNOSIS

When a patient presents with congenital nystagmus and reduced best corrected visual acuity, albinism is one of several conditions to consider in the differential diagnosis. The tyrosinase-negative oculocutaneous albino, with platinum hair and diaphanous blue eyes, is easily diagnosed. However, albinism is best considered a syndrome with a variety of clinical expressions (Table 75–1). Some patients with albinism present with findings so subtle that the correct

TABLE 75–1. SYSTEMIC MANIFESTATIONS OF ALBINISM

CUTANEOUS ALBINISM
- White frontal hair lock
- Hypopigmentation of skin—occasionally of forehead

OCULOCUTANEOUS ALBINISM
- **Tyrosinase Negative**
  Light skin (burns easily)
  White hair
  (–) tyrosinase activity in hair bulbs
  No melanin
- **Tyrosinase Positive**
  Light skin (burns easily)
  White to yellow hair
  Normal to increased tyrosinase activity in hair bulbs
  Trace melanin

OCULAR ALBINISM
- **X-linked**
  Light skin (may or may not tan)
  Normal hair
  Normal tyrosinase activity in hair bulbs
  Abnormally formed melanin
- **Autosomal Recessive**
  Light skin (may or may not tan)
  Normal hair
  Normal tyrosinase activity in hair bulbs
  Normal melanosomes in skin

HP SYNDROME
- Light skin (freckles, burns easily)
- White to brown hair
- Normal tyrosinase activity in hair bulbs
- Incompletely melanized melanosomes in skin
- Other: easy bruisability, gum bleeding, platelet function defect (prolonged bleeding time), enteropathic disorder

PW SYNDROME
- Light skin
- Light hair
- Decreased tyrosinase activity in hair bulbs
- Other: interstitial deletion on long arm of chromosome #15, muscular hypotonia, hypogenitalism, obesity, mental retardation, short stature, diminished sensitivity to pain

diagnosis is often overlooked. Occasionally the examination of family members becomes essential if the actual diagnosis is ever to be appreciated. If viewed as a syndrome, as few as two but often all of the components listed in Table 75–2 under "oculocutaneous albinism" will be identifiable.

The typical patient with albinism presents at a young age with photophobia and reduced vision. Nystagmus is usually of the horizontal pendular variety, but a rotary component may be observed. The nystagmus may lessen at near, and with a very reduced reading distance the child may be able

TABLE 75–2. OCULAR MANIFESTATIONS OF ALBINISM

CUTANEOUS ALBINISM
- Normal ocular structures and normal visual functioning

OCULOCUTANEOUS ALBINISM
- Light blue irides
- Nystagmus—congenital, bilateral and usually pendular
- Reduced visual acuity (20/20– to 20/800–) almost always bilateral
- Photophobia
- Iris transillumination, occasionally very subtle
- Foveal hypoplasia
- Macular hypoplasia
- Small capillary free zone in posterior pole
- Hypopigmentation of choroid and retinal pigment epithelium
- Prominent observable choroidal vessels
- Bihemispheric VEP asymmetries

OCULAR ALBINISM
- Normal irides *plus* any of the other manifestations listed under OCA

HP SYNDROME
- Blue to brown irides *plus* any of the other manifestations listed under OCA

PW SYNDROME
- Blue to brown irides
- Variable iris transillumination

to distinguish reading material. This may be due to the accommodative and vergence system coming into play as well as the change in head position. Color vision testing and visual fields are generally normal and are most useful in ruling out some other conditions causing nystagmus and reduced visual acuity, such as achromatopsia, optic nerve hypoplasia, retinal degeneration (Leber congenital amaurosis), and macular scar.

Iris transillumination is a translucency of the iris due to defects in the iris pigment epithelium (Figure 75–2). Variable amounts of iris transillumination should be present in every albino. Testing should occur in a completely black room after 30 seconds of dark adaptation, and a well-charged halogen transilluminator should be ideally placed directly on the globe near the equator. Grading the transillumination is useful, because the greater the transillumination, the more likely the diagnosis of albinism. None, trace, and 1+ through 4+ are the grades suggested.

Although a positive iris transillumination is most helpful in diagnosing the subtle forms of albinism, it is not pathognomonic. It may occur in pigmentary glaucoma, pigmentary dispersion syndrome, pseudo-exfoliation, chronic open-angle glaucoma, and chronic recurrent uveitis (Krill,

1972). Lightly pigmented, nonalbinotic patients may exhibit trace to 1+ iris transillumination as well.

Visual acuity is quite variable in albinism and ranges from 20/20 to 20/800. Most albinos have visual acuity in the 20/100 to 20/400 range. The patient with only trace nystagmus, and visual acuity of 20/20, 3 to 4+ transillumination, poor foveal and macular landmarks, and siblings with albinism might be considered a forme fruste albino by some. Others may use the term "albinoidism" to describe this clinical presentation. Of particular interest are a few asymptomatic individuals with normal visual acuity but no identifiable fovea amongst family members with albinism.

Most patients with albinism have no clinically demonstrable fovea, poorly defined macular landmarks and capillaries that appear to traverse the macula, sometimes encroaching on the spot where the foveal reflex should be present. Minimal retinal and choroidal pigment allows the large choroidal vessels to be easily observed.

Refractive error measurements in albinism are widely scattered and thus are not diagnostic. Fonda (1962) reported that well over one third of nearly 300 albino eyes had astigmatism greater than three diopters. In addition, over one third had moderate to high myopia and over one third had mild to moderate hyperopia. Strabismus was also present in over one third of the sample as well, with exotropia diagnosed in 83 patients and esotropia in 28.

In questionable cases, the diagnosis can be supported by a specific electrophysiological profile. The electroretinogram (ERG) shows large supernormal responses in essentially all young albinos. This is probably due to the light energy of the flash bouncing around the eye until much of it is eventually absorbed by the photoreceptors. In a normally pigmented eye, light absorbed by the retinal and choroidal pigment have no influence on the size of the ERG. As the albino ages, the ERG amplitude gradually drops to the normal range and then often to the subnormal range, possibly due to chronic overexposure to light and eventual retinal degeneration.

Clinically, ERGs are not particularly useful in the diagnosis of albinism, and reductions in amplitude over time do not appear to have a clinical correlate with age. Most albinos report that their vision either has remained the same or has actually gotten somewhat better as they get older. Visual acuity measurements generally appear unchanged with time. Occasionally, an albino may form pigment at the macula as he or she grows older, and demonstrate an improvement in visual acuity.

The electrooculogram (EOG) is the best clinical test of retinal pigment epithelial function. Available data suggest large amplitudes during light adaptation and larger than normal Arden ratios. Like the ERG, the EOG is not used for the clinical diagnosis of albinism.

The visual evoked potential (VEP), in contrast to ERGs and EOGs and when performed under appropriate conditions, is quite useful in the diagnosis of albinism. Standard pattern VEPs using only one occipital electrode will reveal the typical VEP profile found in any macular abnormality. VEPs to fine checks or gratings will be flat because VEPs under these conditions reflect the foveal and macular pathways. As the pattern size increases, generally the VEP amplitude increases. But albinos have a unique feature that can be elegantly demonstrated with VEPs using bihemispheric recordings. During the past three decades a wealth of scientific reports have shown that the human albino, like the albino rat, pig, and Siamese cat, have disorganized uncrossed retinogeniculate striate projections. In normal humans, about half of the optic nerve crosses at the chiasm, allowing all nasal fibers to decussate. However, in albinos not only do the nasal fibers cross, but many temporal fibers do as well. VEPs recorded from both occipital hemispheres in normal patients are quite symmetric, because half of the optic nerve fibers project to the right hemisphere while the other half project to the left hemisphere. Asymmetry of the VEPs using bihemispheric recordings appears to be a universal finding in all forms of albinism. Some clinical researchers claim they can diagnose all cases of albinism solely on the basis of bihemispheric VEP recordings (P. Apkarian, personal communication). Although brain tumors, cerebrovascular accidents, and aneurysms can also cause asymmetric VEPs, the diagnosis of albinism is generally made in the very young, who are not likely to be suffering from such neurological problems. In addition, these conditions can be diagnosed based on other signs and symptoms.

The importance of viewing albinism as a continuum has been well demonstrated by a study of albinotic characteristics of 13 family members who were graded clinically, electrophysiologically, and biochemically. The authors (Simon et al, 1982) point out that the correlation between visual acuity and nystagmus was "particularly strong," and suggest that nystagmus imposes a visual deficit beyond that related to foveal hypoplasia alone. Thus the "variable expression of albinism," an expression used by Simon and associates (1982), should be recognized by clinicians, and in difficult cases examination of family members is clearly indicated. Even monocular albinism appears possible (Sherman, 1991).

HP and PW

HP syndrome should be considered in Puerto Rican albinos and in those albinos who bruise easily and report excessive bleeding. A hematologist should be consulted. The diagnosis is based upon prolonged bleeding time with a normal platelet count, normal prothrombin time (PT), normal partial thromboplastin time (PTT), and normal factor VIII determinations accompanied by a platelet function defect characterized by diminished platelet aggregation and serotonin uptake (Simon et al, 1982). The diagnosis of PW can be supported by chromosome analysis (Hittner et al, 1982).

TREATMENT AND MANAGEMENT

Table 75–3 summarizes the treatment and management of albinism.

■ Systemic
Due to unpredictable breaks in the ozone layer, essentially everyone should limit exposure to sunlight and artificial

TABLE 75–3. TREATMENT AND MANAGEMENT OF ALBINISM

CUTANEOUS ALBINISM
- Systemic
  Protective sunwear
  Sunblock lotion
- Ocular
  None

OCULOCUTANEOUS ALBINISM
- Systemic
  Protective sunwear
  Sunblock lotion
- Ocular
  Protective sunshades with side shields
  Correction of refractive error
  Low-vision devices
  Auditory feedback to reduce nystagmus

OCULAR ALBINISM
- Systemic
  Protective sunwear
  Sunblock lotion
- Ocular
  Protective sunshades with side shields
  Correction of refractive error
  Low-vision devices
  Auditory feedback to reduce nystagmus

HP SYNDROME
- Systemic
  Protective sunwear
  Sunblock lotion
  Hematology consult
  Avoidance of antiplatelet drugs (eg, aspirin)
  Avoidance of surgery unless essential
- Ocular
  Protective sunshades with side shields
  Correction of refractive error
  Low-vision devices
  Auditory feedback to reduce nystagmus

PW SYNDROME
- Systemic
  Protective sunwear
  Sunblock lotion
- Ocular
  Protective sunshades with side shields

sources of ultraviolet rays. However, the albino is at an even greater risk of precancerous keratosis, squamous cell and basal cell carcinoma, and amelanotic malignant melanomas. The use of sunscreen products, umbrellas, hats, and other protective clothing should be emphasized.

If the diagnosis of HP syndrome is established, antiplatelet drugs such as aspirin must be avoided. Surgery should be avoided unless essential. There are no known treatment recommendations for PW syndrome. However, because of the chromosomal abnormality found in this disease, genetic counseling should be offered to affected patients.

■ Ocular

Various absorptive lenses in addition to frames with side shields should be considered or advised. Light tints are sometimes adequate to lessen photophobia and occasional glare. Many albinos have large refractive errors requiring correction with spectacles or contact lenses. The young albino generally needs only to move closer to printed material. Based upon the patient's age and visual acuity, adds from +2.00 to +10.00 should be attempted. Telescopes and microscopes are often helpful. Low-vision specialists (B. Rosenthal, personal communication) report that virtually all albinos can be helped visually with various tints and low-vision devices.

Auditory biofeedback for the amelioration of nystagmus has met with some success (S. Goldrich, personal communication).

Conclusion

Albinism is actually a spectrum of diseases with many different presentations. Although all forms of albinism have in common some problem with pigmentation in the skin and eye, these structures may be variably affected. Even within families, members may be affected differently.

The eyecare practitioner must consider albinism when presented with any patient with either reduced vision from birth and/or nystagmus. Albinos, especially the ocular types, are easy to miss. Because some forms of albinism are associated with other systemic problems, the proper diagnosis becomes extremely important.

References

Butler MG. Prader–Willi syndrome. Current understanding of cause and diagnosis. *Am J Med Genet.* 1990;35:319–332.

Carr RE, Siegel IM. The retinal pigment epithelium in ocular albinism. In: Duane TD, ed. *Clinical Ophthalmology.* Philadelphia: Harper & Row; 1981;4:413–423.

Creel D, O'Donnell E Jr, Witkop C Jr. Visual system anomalies in human ocular albinos. *Science.* 1978;201:931–933.

Creel D, Witkop C Jr, King RA. Asymmetric visually evoked potentials in human albinos: Evidence for visual system anomalies. *Invest Ophthalmol.* 1974;13:430–440.

Donaldson DD. Transillumination of the iris. *Trans Am Ophthalmol Soc.* 1974;72:89–105.

Fonda G. Characteristics and low vision corrections in albinism. *Arch Ophthalmol.* 1962;68:754.

Hittner HM, King RA, Riccardi VM, et al. Oculocutaneous albinoidism as a manifestation of reduced neural crest derivatives in the Prader–Willi syndrome. *Am J Ophthalmol.* 1982;94:328–337.

Krill AE. Albinism. In: Krill AE, ed. *Krill's Hereditary Retinal and Choroidal Diseases.* Philadelphia: Harper & Row; 1972:645–663.

Ledbetter DH, Riccardi VM, Airhardt SD, et al. Deletions of chromosome 15 as a cause of the Praeder–Willi syndrome. *N Engl J Med.* 1981;304:325.

O'Donnell FE, Green WR. The eye in albinism. In: Duane TD, ed. *Clinical Ophthalmology.* Philadelphia: Harper & Row; 1987;4:6.

O'Donnell FE, Hambrick GW Jr, Green WR, et al. X-linked ocular albinism. An oculotaneous macromelanosomal disorder. *Arch Ophthalmol.* 1976;94:1883–1892.

Sherman J. Patient management: The case of the colorful patient. *Optom Management.* 1991;26:56–57.

Simon JW, Adams RJ, Calhoun JH, et al. Ophthalmic manifestations of the Hermansky–Pudlak syndrome (oculocutaneous albinism and hemorrhage diathesis). *Am J Ophthalmol.* 1982;93:71–77.

Witkop CJ, Pineiro B, Almadovar C, Nunez-Babcock M. Hermansky–Pudlak syndrome. An epidemiologic study. *Ophthal Pediatr Genet.* 1990;11:250–295.

76
Chapter

Homocystinuria

Esther S. Marks

Homocystinuria is one of the most common treatable inborn errors of amino acid metabolism. Discovered in 1962, both in Northern Ireland and in the United States, homocystinuria is characterized by skeletal, vascular, and ocular abnormalities, as well as mental retardation. Although there is an extremely wide range of clinical expression, the typical presentation is of a young, tall individual with very long limbs, generalized osteoporosis, and bilateral ectopia lentis, who has suffered one or more thromboembolic episodes. The striking similarity to Marfan syndrome, a connective tissue disorder, is probably one reason for the relatively recent recognition of homocystinuria as a completely unrelated and distinct disorder.

EPIDEMIOLOGY

■ Systemic
There are various reports concerning the incidence and prevalence of homocystinuria. It is believed to affect from 1 in 40,000 to 1 in 200,000 newborns. Approximately 1 in 100 persons carry the gene for this disease (Capoferri et al, 1990). About 50% of patients suffer some degree of mental retardation. Conversely, only 0.021% of the mentally retarded population suffers from homocystinuria (Nelson & Maumenee, 1982). By age 15 years, 50% will demonstrate spinal osteoporosis. There is a 40% probability of a thromboembolic event by age 20 years (van den Berg et al, 1990). Death from thromboses occurs in approximately 70% (Mudd et al, 1985).

■ Ocular
Ectopia lentis, the ocular hallmark of homocystinuria, occurs in approximately 90% of patients, with close to 70% occurring by age 10 years (Mudd et al, 1985). Conversely, of all nontraumatic cases of ectopia lentis, 5% are due to homocystinuria (Nelson & Maumenee, 1982). Although several other ocular manifestations are associated with this disease, the incidences and prevalences are not available in the literature.

NATURAL HISTORY

■ Systemic
Homocystinuria is an error of metabolism of sulfur-containing amino acids. It is an autosomal recessive disorder that has been mapped to the long arm of chromosome 21. There is considerable variety of clinical expression, ranging from very mild to quite severe.

There are several known enzymatic defects that result in homocystinuria. The most common is a deficiency of cystathionine beta-synthetase. This enzyme normally catalyzes homocysteine to cystathionine on the pathway to cysteine. Its deficiency results in elevated plasma levels of homocystine and methionine, as well as urinary excretion of homocystine. Homocystine is a disulfide oxidation product composed of two molecules of homocysteine. Methionine is an amino acid present in almost all foods ingested by humans. Although used in the production of body proteins, the vast majority is degraded to cystine via transsulfuration in the liver.

There are a variety of systemic manifestations in homocystinuria (Table 76–1). The skeletal abnormalities are due to homocystine preventing normal connective tissue formation by interfering with the cross-linking of collagen. Generalized osteoporosis, especially of the spine, followed by the long bones, is very common. This results in vertebral collapse and frequent fractures. The limbs and fingers are excessively long and narrow, and the patient is often described as having a Marfanoid body habitus (see Chapter 40). Scoliosis is common but kyphosis (hunchback) is infrequent. The anterior chest is prone to deformity, either pectus excavatum (a depression of the sternum) or pectus carinatum (an outpouching of the sternum). Genu valgum (knocked knees) may occur. Joints are usually quite lax although upon passive flexion they may feel tight. Reports of pancreatitis and gastrointestinal involvement (diarrhea) are rare (Ilan et al, 1993).

The vascular damage in homocystinuria is the most serious and life threatening of all the systemic manifestations. It has been suggested that these abnormalities may be related to the elevated levels of plasma homocysteine causing arteriosclerotic lesions (McCully, 1992). Also, there have been contradictory reports concerning the effect of plasma homocystine on platelet adhesiveness. Intimal and endothelial vascular changes occur, along with disruption of the elastic lamellae. This leads to thrombotic lesions and embolic episodes. These thromboembolic events (Figure 76–1) may occur in any vessel in the body—cerebral, cardiac, peripheral, and so forth. The natural progression of the disease results in early death, often by age 30 years, usually due to a thrombotic vascular occlusion.

The cutaneous manifestations of homocystinuria include fair hair and fair skin. Many patients demonstrate a pinkish to purplish discoloration of the skin of the cheeks (malar flush), trunk, and limbs (livedo reticularis). This is due to dilated capillaries and venules.

Mental retardation occurs often insidiously in homocystinuria. Its slow progression means that it often goes unnoticed for the first year or two of life. Other central nervous system features include seizures and psychiatric disturbances.

TABLE 76–1. SYSTEMIC MANIFESTATIONS OF HOMOCYSTINURIA

LABORATORY TESTS
- Elevated levels of plasma homocystine and methionine
- Urinary excretion of homocystine

SKELETAL ABNORMALITIES
- Generalized osteoporosis especially of the spine
- Vertebral collapse and frequent fractures
- Excessively long and narrow limbs and fingers (Marfanoid body habitus)
- Genu valgum
- Scoliosis with infrequent kyphosis
- Deformities of anterior chest: pectus excavatum or pectus carinatum
- Increased joint mobility, although tight on passive flexion

VASCULAR ABNORMALITIES
- Thromboembolic lesions may occur in any artery or vein in any part of the body, with resulting bruits, loss of pulses, and ischemic symptoms such as intermittent claudication
- Cardiac murmurs, cardiomegaly, myocardial infarctions, hypertension

CUTANEOUS ABNORMALITIES
- Fair skin and hair
- Malar flush
- Livedo reticularis of trunk and limbs

CENTRAL NERVOUS SYSTEM ABNORMALITIES
- Mental retardation
- Seizures
- Psychiatric disorders

VISCERAL ABNORMALITIES
- Gastrointestinal involvement (eg, diarrhea)
- Pancreatitis

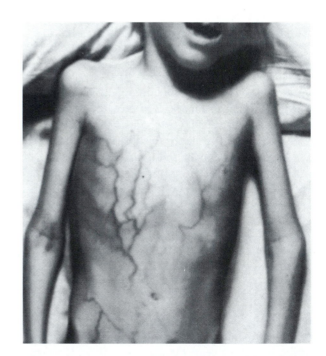

Figure 76–1. Dilated veins in homocystinuric patient with thrombosis of the inferior vena cava. *(Reprinted with permission from Schimke RN, McKusick VA, Huang T, Pollack AD. Homocystinuria: Studies of 20 families with 38 affected members. JAMA. 1965;193:713.)*

■ Ocular

Although there are several ocular features of homocystinuria (Table 76–2), the classic ocular manifestation is bilaterally subluxated lenses (ectopia lentis; Figure 76–2). Although usually described as dislocating inferiorly or inferonasally, this is not diagnostic. The lens zonules are believed to be adversely affected by the defective cross-linkage of collagen, leading to progressive spherophakia with increased myopia and eventual dislocation of the lenses.

The subluxated lens is quite mobile, with visible phakodonesis and iridodonesis on ocular examination. There have also been reports of congenital cataracts and rare reports of aniridia. The typical presentation is of a myopic patient with blue irides and bilateral ectopia lentis.

Secondary glaucoma is not uncommon. Although the anterior chamber angles are normal, the subluxated lens may induce a pupillary block. An acute glaucomatous attack also may occur due to dislocation of the lens into the anterior chamber.

Retinal involvement in homocystinuria includes retinal detachments and increased peripheral retinal degenerations. Retinal vascular complications have been

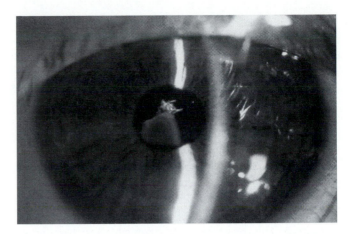

Figure 76–2. Ectopia lentis in a 15-year-old female patient with homocystinuria. *(Reprinted with permission from Hagee MJ. Homocystinuria and ectopia lentis.* J Am Optom·Assoc. *1984;55:270.)*

reported such as central retinal artery occlusions, presumably by the same thromboembolic process that affects the rest of the body. Other less commonly mentioned ocular manifestations include staphylomas, strabismus, and buphthalmos from pupillary-block glaucoma at an extremely young age.

TABLE 76–2. OCULAR MANIFESTATIONS OF HOMOCYSTINURIA

LENTICULAR FEATURES
- Progressive myopia probably secondary to spherophakia
- Bilateral ectopia lentis (usually down and in)
- Phakodonesis
- Congenital cataracts

IRIS AND ANGLE FEATURES
- Blue irides
- Iridodonesis
- Rare aniridia
- No angle abnormalities

SECONDARY GLAUCOMA
- Pupillary-block glaucoma (with buphthalmos if occurs in the very young)
- Glaucoma secondary to anterior subluxation of the lens

RETINAL AND OPTIC NERVE FEATURES
- Retinal detachment
- Peripheral retinal degenerations
- Central retinal artery occlusion
- Optic nerve atrophy
- Staphyloma

OTHER FEATURES
- Strabismus

DIAGNOSIS

■ Systemic

Diagnosis of a patient suspected of homocystinuria requires a thorough medical and ocular examination for demonstration of the systemic and ocular homocystinuria features. Special attention should be given to the patient and family history: in particular any mental retardation, skeletal, vascular, or ocular abnormalities. The healthcare provider should also inquire as to any early family deaths.

Diagnosis may be established at birth when routine screening of newborns is performed to rule out metabolic and endocrine disorders. The infants are screened for hypermethioninemia. However, false negatives do occur (Cacciari & Salardi, 1989).

Plasma levels of methionine and homocystine may be determined. The normal person has less than 0.45 mg/100 mL plasma methionine, with homocystine undetectable. A person with homocystinuria has up to 30 mg/100 mL plasma methionine and up to 5.4 mg/100 mL plasma homocystine. Urinary excretion of homocystine is undetectable in the normal person, whereas in a person with homocystinuria, it may exceed 270 mg/d (Abel et al, 1978).

The cyanide–nitroprusside reaction tests for the presence of homocystine in the urine. Sodium cyanide is mixed with a sample of urine and allowed to react for 10 minutes at room temperature. A small quantity of sodium nitroprusside solution is added. If the sample turns a pink to purple color, the test is considered positive for an excess disulfide compound. In order to confirm and identify the specific amino acid, the sample may then be submitted to chromatography (paper, thin-layer, or ion-exchange) or electrophoresis (Cacciari & Salardi, 1989; Presley & Sidbury, 1967).

A new fluorescent thiol reagent, dansylaminophenylmercuric acetate (DAPMA), has recently been designed and clinically tested for the detection and diagnosis of homocystinuria using the urine of patients (Maddocks & MacLachlan, 1991). The reagent was tested on urine samples from 102 patients and successfully detected the only 4 with homocystinuria. No false positives or negatives occurred. This test appears to be much more specific and sensitive, not to mention safer to perform, than the standard cyanide–nitroprusside urine test.

The diagnosis of homocystinuria may also be confirmed with cultured skin fibroblasts revealing greatly reduced cystathionine beta-synthetase enzyme activity. This may also be shown with hepatocytes or phytohemagglutinin (a plant protein that causes agglutination) stimulated lymphocytes.

The differential diagnosis for homocystinuria is chiefly Marfan syndrome. It is an important distinction, because homocystinuria is treatable. Although these two diseases are similar superficially, there are some distinct differences, both in etiologies and in manifestations (Table 76–3).

■ Ocular

The ocular features of homocystinuria will be revealed in a thorough ocular examination, including keratometry (to distinguish corneal from lenticular astigmatism), refraction, gonioscopy, and indirect ophthalmoscopy. Care should be taken when dilating the pupils of any patient with ectopia lentis, to avoid inducing pupillary block. Some clinicians advocate reclining the patient while dilating using milder mydriatics (eg, 0.5% tropicamide; Hagee, 1984).

Ultrasound may be considered when faced with a young patient with progressive myopia. This allows for the determination of lenticular versus axial myopia. Any patient with nontraumatic ectopia lentis should be considered suspect for homocystinuria, particularly if any other manifestations, systemic or ocular, are present.

TREATMENT AND MANAGEMENT

Table 76–4 gives an overview of homocystinuria treatment and management.

■ Systemic

Newborns identified with homocystinuria should be immediately put on a low-methionine diet with cystine supplements under the supervision of a physician and nutritionist or dietician. The objective is to prevent or minimize mental retardation, lens dislocations, osteoporosis, and thromboembolic episodes. Although it does appear to reduce mental retardation and thromboembolic events, it is questionable how helpful it is in reducing ectopia lentis (van den Berg et al, 1990).

In infants a failure to gain weight is a serious complication. A sufficient intake of amino acids despite a low-methionine diet is essential for growth. The infants must also obtain sufficient calories from fat and carbohydrates to meet their energy requirements. If not, their bodies will break down their own proteins, resulting in increased levels of methionine.

Follow-up of plasma methionine and homocystine levels should occur weekly until the infant is 6 weeks old. Then

TABLE 76–3. A COMPARISON OF HOMOCYSTINURIA AND MARFAN SYNDROME

Major Features	Homocystinuria	Marfan Syndrome
Inheritance	Autosomal recessive	Autosomal dominant
Etiology	Inborn error of amino acid metabolism	Inborn error of connective tissue proteins
Skeletal	Tall stature	Tall stature
	Generalized osteoporosis	Hyperextensible joints
	Prone to vertebral collapse and repeated fractures	Prone to repeated dislocations
	Scoliosis	Scoliosis
	Pectus excavatum or pectus carinatum	Pectus excavatum or pectus carinatum
Vascular	Thromboembolic events	Dissecting aortic aneurysms
Cutaneous	Fair skin and hair	Skin folds and stretch marks
Mental retardation	May be present	Absent
Ectopia lentis	Usually down and in	Usually up and out
Other ocular	Lenticular myopia	Axial myopia
	Normal angle	Angle anomalies
	Secondary glaucoma	Secondary glaucoma

TABLE 76–4. TREATMENT AND MANAGEMENT OF HOMOCYSTINURIA

■ **SYSTEMIC**

DIET RESTRICTIONS AND SUPPLEMENTS
- Low-methionine intake
- Cystine supplement
- Multivitamin supplements

PHARMACOLOGIC AGENTS
- Pyridoxine 500 to 1000 mg/d
- Betaine 8 g/d
- Acetylsalicylic acid and dipyridamole

SURGERY OR INVASIVE DIAGNOSTIC PROCEDURES
- Avoided unless absolutely necessary due to high risk of thromboembolism

GENETIC COUNSELING

■ **OCULAR**

EYEWEAR
- Spectacle or contact lens correction of refractive error
- Protective eyewear
- Avoid contact sports

SURGERY
- Avoided unless acuity decreased or ocular emergency (eg, retinal detachment or anterior subluxation of lens)

the checkups should occur biweekly until the child is 1 year old. If well controlled, monthly checkups should follow. To ensure against overtreatment, height, weight, and head circumference should be measured at each visit until the child is 3 years old. Skeletal and bone age should be measured yearly (Abel et al, 1978).

A low-methionine diet is difficult to follow. As mentioned previously, almost all foods ingested by humans contain some level of methionine. Eggs, meats, chicken and turkey, milk and milk products, peanut butter, fish, noodles, rice, and cereals are all high in methionine. In contrast, fruits and vegetables have a relatively low content.

Diet alone is usually insufficient treatment. Multivitamin supplements are recommended. Pharmacological amounts of pyridoxine (vitamin B$_6$) provide partial biochemical and clinical improvement in approximately 50% of patients. Pyridoxine, a coenzyme necessary to activate cystathionine beta-synthetase, appears to help reduce thromboembolic episodes. Betaine, which helps reduce levels of homocysteine by accelerating its methylation, also appears to be useful (Rubba, 1989). To help provide protection against thrombus formation, the use of acetylsalicylic acid (aspirin) and dipyridamole also have been advocated.

Arteriography, cardiac catheterization, and general anesthesia should be avoided due to the significant risk of thromboembolic crises. Genetic counseling is recommended.

■ **Ocular**

Patients should be given full spectacle or contact lens corrections. Protective eyewear and counseling against participation in contact sports (to avoid ocular trauma resulting in further subluxation, anterior subluxation, or retinal detachment) should be considered. Usually, surgery to remove a subluxated lens is avoided due to the ocular and systemic risks involved, unless visual acuity is seriously affected, or in an ocular emergency such as an anteriorly subluxated lens or retinal detachment.

CONCLUSION

Homocystinuria is an inherited metabolic disorder of sulfur-containing amino acids. In many respects it is similar to Marfan syndrome, with skeletal, vascular, and ocular abnormalities. However, the distinction is important because homocystinuria, unlike Marfan syndrome, is treatable. Due to the wide variety of clinical expression, an astute eyecare practitioner may provide the initial diagnosis in a child or young adult presenting with bilateral ectopia lentis.

REFERENCES

Abel E, Michell M, Ekvall S. Homocystinuria. In: Palmer S, Ekvall S, eds. *Pediatric Nutrition in Developmental Disorders.* Springfield, IL: Thomas; 1978.

Burke JP, O'Keefe M, Bowell R, Naughten ER. Ocular complications in homocystinuria—early and late treated. *Br J Ophthalmol.* 1989;73:427–431.

Cacciari E, Salardi S. Clinical and laboratory features of homocystinuria. *Haemostasis.* 1989;19(suppl 1):10–13.

Capoferri C, Pierro L, Brancato R. Echobiometry in homocystinuria. *Optom Vision Sci.* 1990;67:566.

Cross HE, Jensen AD. Ocular manifestations in the Marfan syndrome and homocystinuria. *Am J Ophthalmol.* 1973;75:405–420.

Hagee MJ. Homocystinuria and ectopia lentis. *J Am Optom Assoc.* 1984;55:269–276.

Ilan Y, Eid A, Rivkind AI, et al. Gastrointestinal involvement in homocystinuria. *J Gastroenterol Hepatol.* 1993;8:60–62.

Maddocks JL, MacLachlan J. Application of new fluorescent thiol reagent to diagnosis of homocystinuria. *Lancet.* 1991;338:1043–1044.

McCully KS. Homocystinuria, arteriosclerosis, methylmalonic aciduria, and methyltransferase deficiency: A key case revisited. *Nutrition Rev.* 1992;50:7–12.

Mudd SH. Homocystinuria. In: Wyngaarden JB, Smith LH, eds. *Cecil Textbook of Medicine.* Philadelphia: Saunders; 1988;1160–1161.

Mudd SH, Levy HL, Skovby F. Disorders of transsulfuration. In: Scriver CR, et al, eds. *The Metabolic Basis of Inherited Disease.* 6th ed. New York: McGraw-Hill; 1989;693–734.

Mudd SH, Skovby F, Levy HL. et al. The natural history of homocystinuria due to cystathionine β-synthetase deficiency. *Am J Hum Genet.* 1985;37:1–31.

Nelson LB, Maumenee IH. Ectopia Lentis. *Surv Ophthalmol.* 1982;27:143–160.

Presley GD, Sidbury JB. Homocystinuria and ocular defects. *Am J Ophthalmol.* 1967;63:1723–1727.

Rubba P. Ultrasonographic detection of arterial disease in treated homocystinuria. (Letter) *N Engl J Med.* 1989;321: 1759–1760.

Schimke RN, McKusick VA, Huang T, Pollock AD. Homocystinuria: Studies of 20 families with 38 affected members. *JAMA.* 1965;193:711–719.

van den Berg W, Verbraak FD, Bos PJM. Homocystinuria presenting as central retinal artery occlusion and long-standing thromboembolic disease. *Br J Ophthalmol.* 1990;74:696–697.

Warburg M. *Diagnosis of Metabolic Eye Disease.* Munksgaard, Denmark: Scandinavian University Books; 1972:56–58.

77
Chapter

Wilson Disease

Kelly H. Thomann

Wilson disease, also called hepatolenticular degeneration, is an inherited autosomal recessive disorder of copper metabolism and excretion. The liver's ability to transport and store copper in the bile is impaired, resulting in toxic accumulations in the liver, central nervous system, cornea, kidney, and other organs.

The systemic manifestations and severity of Wilson disease are variable. These include liver, neurologic, psychiatric, blood, kidney, bone, and joint disturbances. Females present more often with liver disease and males with neurological features.

The Kayser–Fleischer ring, a deposition of copper in the cornea, is the classic feature of Wilson disease. Copper deposition is also seen in the lens and is known as a "sunflower cataract."

EPIDEMIOLOGY

■ Systemic

Wilson disease occurs equally in males and females, in every ethnic group, and in all geographic locations. Incidence is not accurately known; however, various sources list the range from 1 in 30,000 to 1 in 200,000 live births. Prevalence is thought to be 3 in 100,000 people. It is estimated that from 1 in 100 to 1 in 200 persons is a heterozygous carrier for the disease.

■ Ocular

The Kayser–Fleischer ring is present in all cases with neurological involvement and in 70 to 90% of cases with diagnosed liver disease. It is absent in over 30% of children who present with acute liver disease. The sunflower cataract is present in 15 to 20% of patients.

NATURAL HISTORY

■ Systemic

Copper balance in the body is regulated by the liver. It is excreted in the stool primarily via the bile. The site of the primary defect in Wilson disease is the liver lysosome. Its malfunction causes the liver to decrease the incorporation of copper into ceruloplasmin, the major copper transport protein. The excess copper binds either to albumin or other cellular groups in the liver. This results in toxicity, which is manifested as either acute liver disease or chronic liver disease from years of excess storage. When the capacity to store copper in the liver becomes exceeded, it is released into the blood and excreted through the kidneys. The excess copper also becomes deposited in other sites, most notably the brain, kidney, and eyes.

Wilson disease may manifest between the ages of 5 and 50. However, most patients become symptomatic during adolescence, or in their 20s or 30s. It can be progressive and fatal if treatment is delayed. Its clinical manifestations may be reversible even after severe functional impairment but not after permanent damage has occurred to the brain or liver. The first expression of this disease is always a deposition of copper in the liver. In half of the patients, this may cause asymptomatic liver damage. In the other half, it may be symptomatic and manifest as a form of liver disease. This may be encountered as acute hepatitis (often mistaken for viral hepatitis or infectious mononucleosis), which is self-limited; fulminant hepatitis (which is generally lethal);

chronic active hepatitis (parenchymal liver disease); or cirrhosis (chronic, progressive liver disease).

Neurologic disease, in the form of extrapyramidal or cerebellar dysfunction, may also be encountered as the first clinical sign of this disease. Primary neurologic manifestations include resting and intention tremors of the head and limbs, spasticity, rigidity, choreic movements, slowness of movement, excess salivation, dysphagia, dysarthria, and hoarseness. As the disease progresses, the "classic" neurologic syndrome seen includes dysphagia and drooling, rigidity and slowness of movement of limbs, fixed posture and facial muscles with the mouth agape, and dysarthria and a coarse wing-beating tremor.

Psychiatric disturbances may be found and are sometimes indistinguishable from schizophrenia, mania, depression, psychoses, classic neurosis, and bizarre behavioral disturbances.

Occasionally blood, joint, bone, and kidney disease are encountered as the initial manifestations, but they are more frequently encountered later in the course of the disease (Table 77–1). Primary or secondary amenorrhea in young females, as well as repeated spontaneous abortions secondary to excess free copper in intrauterine secretions, have also been documented as an initial sign of this disease.

If untreated, Wilson disease ultimately will lead to death due to irreversible liver failure.

■ Ocular

The Kayser–Fleischer ring (Figure 77–1) is seen as a golden brown, ruby-red or green-brown band that is often visible grossly (without the biomicroscope). Its size ranges from 1.0 to 3.0 mm, starting at the limbus at the level of the Descemet

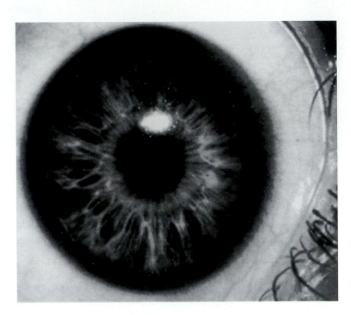

Figure 77–1. Kayser–Fleischer ring located in the Descemet membrane can be identified by external inspection. *(Reprinted with permission from Finley TF. Wilson's disease.* J Am Optom Assoc. *1988;59:1119.)*

membrane. It is most pronounced peripherally and tends to fade toward the center of the cornea. The ring consists of nonuniform layers of unequal-size granules rich in copper and sulfur and separated by clear intervals of variable width. Its color is probably due to the scattering and reflection of light created by the layer of copper granules. The varying appearances may be due to the differences in size, shape, and density of the copper granules. The copper in the Descemet membrane that produces the Kayser Fleisher ring is actually only a small percentage of the total corneal copper present. However, color change is produced only by deposits at this layer. The earliest site of pigment deposition is an arc in the superior periphery of the cornea from the 10 o'clock to the 2 o'clock meridian; the arc spreads slowly toward the horizontal plane and gradually broadens. Later, a band appears inferiorly as a crescent from the 5 o'clock to the 7 o'clock position and in time the arcs meet.

The "sunflower" cataract is a much less common ocular sign in Wilson disease. It appears as a centrally pigmented opacity of the lens with tapering extensions that resemble the petals of a sunflower. It has been shown to consist of copper granules located in the anterior subcapsular lens and occasionally the posterior lens capsule. It does not impair vision (Table 77–2).

TABLE 77–1. SYSTEMIC MANIFESTATIONS OF WILSON DISEASE

LIVER DISEASE
- Jaundice, anorexia, hemolytic crisis, hepatitis, cirrhosis

NEUROLOGICAL DISEASE
- Extrapyramidal disorders or cerebellar dysfunction

PSYCHIATRIC DISORDERS
- Personality changes, clinical signs of schizophrenia, mania, depression, psychosis, neurosis, behavioral disturbance

BLOOD DISORDERS
- Hemolytic anemia, neutropenia, thrombocytopenia

KIDNEY DISORDERS
- Renal tubular acidosis, aminoaciduria, glycosuria, uricosuria, microhematuria, hypercalciuria, renal stones

JOINT DISTURBANCES/BONE DISEASE
- Arthritis, osteoarthritis, osteoporosis, pathologic fractures

TABLE 77–2. OCULAR MANIFESTATIONS OF WILSON DISEASE

- Kayser–Fleischer corneal pigment ring
- Sunflower cataract

DIAGNOSIS

■ Systemic

Wilson disease is an important diagnosis to make, although often difficult due to its rarity and varying clinical presentation. Signs and symptoms of neurologic, psychiatric, liver, blood, bone, and joint diseases may or may not be present. Diagnosis is conclusive when a similar syndrome is seen in a sibling or when the triad of liver disease, Kayser–Fleischer rings, and extrapyramidal motor disorder are found. However, manifestations of this disease may not always be this obvious and variants often confuse practitioners.

Wilson disease is responsible for approximately 20% of cirrhosis (chronic liver disease) between the ages of 4 and 16 years. Pediatricians, internists, and general practitioners should keep this diagnosis in mind when a younger patient is diagnosed with liver disease. Neurologists and psychiatrists must consider this disease in patients with extrapyramidal movement disorders, cerebellar symptoms, or both. Wilson disease should be considered in psychiatric patients with signs of liver or neurologic disease, and psychiatric patients who fail to respond to treatment or have a family history of the disease.

The standard laboratory tests are the measurement of serum copper and ceruloplasmin, and the 24-hour urinary excretion rate of copper. More than 150 µg/dL of serum copper, less than 20 mg/dL of ceruloplasmin, or more than 100 µg of urinary copper per 24 hours are considered diagnostic and will identify about 95% of adult cases. However, patients with Wilson disease may not have abnormal values for all of these tests. Laboratory results in children should be interpreted more carefully when the disease is suspected. High copper content in liver biopsy tissue early in the course of the illness is the most reliable diagnostic test. This has been recommended in every child with chronic liver disease and for those in whom Wilson disease is suspected but other tests are negative.

Detection of the disease in asymptomatic siblings is especially important. Appropriate tests include the 24-hour urinary copper level, serum ceruloplasmin assay, slit-lamp examination, and liver biopsy, if indicated. It can often be diagnosed and treatment instituted before illness occurs, thereby preventing the clinical manifestations.

■ Ocular

The Kayser–Fleischer ring is seldom noted in patients who are not symptomatic for neurologic disease. However, rarely a patient with an incorrect neurologic diagnosis may have the Kayser–Fleischer ring, thus leading to the correct diagnosis of Wilson disease.

TREATMENT AND MANAGEMENT

■ Systemic

Treatment of Wilson disease is aimed at the reduction of the body's copper balance by decreasing stored copper, and in most cases is lifelong (Table 77–3). D-Penicillamine, a copper-chelating (metal-binding) agent, is the most commonly used medication. Typical dosage is 250 mg four times per day on an empty stomach in adults. The patient is monitored daily for urinary copper excretion. One to three mg per day is the acceptable range. In most patients, neurologic signs improve with treatment; however, clinical improvement may not be seen for weeks to months in more severe cases, and in 25% of cases neurological symptoms actually worsen prior to improvement. Kayser–Fleischer rings will ultimately

TABLE 77–3. TREATMENT AND MANAGEMENT OF WILSON DISEASE

D-PENICILLAMINE
250 mg qid on empty stomach
- Indications: Initial treatment, maintenance treatment, presymptomatic patients, pregnancy
- Side effects
    Systemic: neurological worsening, toxicity, fever, rash, kidney dysfunction, decrease in blood platelets, zinc deficiency, taste and smell disorders, connective tissue disease, polyarthritis, lupus-like and myasthenia-like syndromes, aplastic anemia
    Ocular: optic neuritis, retinal hemorrhages, conjunctivitis, neuropathies

TRIENTINE
250 mg qid on empty stomach
- Indications: initial treatment, maintenance treatment, presymptomatic patients, pregnancy
- Side effects: lack of experience, not useful in patients failing to respond to penacillamine, lack of adequate research listing side effects, iron deficiency anemia, anorexia, abdominal pain, skin rash, rhabdomyolysis (disintegration of muscle)

ZINC ACETATE
50 mg tid on empty stomach
- Indications: maintenance treatment, presymptomatic patient, pregnancy
- Side effects: limited experience, dehydration, electrolyte imbalance, lethargy, dizziness, muscular incoordination, impairment of lymphocyte and neutrophil functions, increase in LDL cholesterol

DIETARY REDUCTION OF COPPER
- Indications: maintenance treatment in adjunct with medical treatment
- Side effects: limited experience, lack of clinical evidence supporting its use only at this time

disappear with treatment. Side effects from drug therapy include fever, rash, kidney dysfunction, and a decrease in blood platelets. Chronic D-penicillamine treatment may cause many other adverse systemic and ocular effects, including zinc deficiency, taste and smell disorders, connective tissue disease and polyarthritis, lupus-like and myasthenia-like syndromes, aplastic anemia, optic neuritis, retinal hemorrhages, conjunctivitis, and neuropathies. Prior to beginning D-penicillamine treatment, the following tests should be done: serum creatinine, creatinine clearance, blood urea nitrogen levels, urinalysis, complete blood count, and platelet count. During treatment, blood and renal status should continue to be monitored because of the toxic effects on bone marrow and the kidneys. It has also been recommended that a CT of the brain be obtained prior to initiation of treatment to provide baseline information about the extent of neurological damage. Other chelating agents (most commonly trientine hydrochloride) or prednisolone may be used to minimize side effects. It takes several weeks to months for D-pencillamine therapy to produce an effect on the neurological manifestations and liver disease. As a result, D-penicillamine therapy is less effective in patients with fulminant liver failure. Peritoneal dialysis and plasmaphoresis are the most effective treatments in cases of fulminant liver failure, but these are also often insufficient. Liver transplantation may ultimately be required for patients with irreversible liver insufficiency or fulminant hepatitis.

Changes in diet and eating habits also may be indicated. Dietary reduction of liver, mushrooms, cocoa, chocolate, nuts, and shellfish, as well as drinking and cooking with distilled water, are recommended.

Recently, oral zinc supplements (150 mg daily) have been used as an adjunct treatment in Wilson disease. Use of zinc for Wilson disease was initially considered when patients who were treated for sickle-cell anemia with zinc were found to be copper deficient. Zinc acts to block copper absorption in the intestinal cell mucosa. This in turn causes more copper to be excreted through the fecal route. Oral zinc therapy is not adequate alone because of its slow onset of action. When used with D-penicillamine, it helps reduce the body's copper more quickly (in the initial decoppering phase of treatment), and it decreases the amount of D-penicillamine needed for treatment, and possibly allows a more varied diet because it helps block the intestinal absorption of dietary copper. Zinc treatment is most promising in asymptomatic patients, and it has been suggested as the drug of choice in the treatment of pregnant patients. However, the use of zinc in the treatment of Wilson disease is still under research.

Genetic counseling is indicated in patients with Wilson disease and the siblings of these patients should be examined for liver or neurological disease, Kayser–Fleischer rings and copper levels in the body. Asymptomatic younger siblings should be carefully examined, because diagnosis can lead to appropriate treatment and a better prognosis.

■ Ocular

There is no ocular treatment for the Kayser–Fleischer ring or sunflower cataracts, as they pose no threat to visual function or the health of the eye.

CONCLUSION

Wilson disease is a rare disorder of copper metabolism and excretion, but it is fully treatable if recognized early. Its clinical manifestations are wide and variable, yet it is one of the few diseases in clinical medicine with a pathognomonic feature (the Kayser–Fleischer ring). Pediatricians, general practitioners, internists, neurologists, psychiatrists, and eyecare practitioners should be aware of this uncommon disease because most of its devastating effects can be avoided with early intervention.

REFERENCES

Affra RC. *Grayson's Diseases of the Cornea*, 3rd ed. St. Louis: Mosby Year Book; 1991.

Brewer GJ, Yuzbasiyan-Gurkan V, Lee DY. Use of zinc–copper metabolic interactions in the treatment of Wilson's disease. *J Am College Nutr.* 1990;9:487–491.

Cairns JE, Walshe JM. The Kayser–Fleischer ring. *Trans Ophthalmol Soc UK.* 1970;90:187–190.

Cartwright GE: Current concepts: Diagnosis of treatable Wilson's disease. *N Engl J Med.* 1983;298:1347–1350.

Crumley FE. Case study, pitfalls of diagnosis in the early stages of Wilson's disease. *J Am Acad Child Adolesc Psychiatr.* 1990;29:470–471.

Danks DM. Copper and liver disease. *Eur J Pediatr.* 1991;150:142–148.

Dobyns WM, Goldstein NP, Gordon H. Clinical spectrum of Wilson's disease (hepatolenticular degeneration). *Mayo Clin Proc.* 1979;54:35–42.

Emery AEH, Rimoin DL. *Principles and Practice of Medical Genetics.* New York: Churchill Livingstone; 1990;2.

Smithgal JM. The copper-controlled diet: Current aspects of dietary copper restriction in management of copper metabolism disorders. *J Am Diet Assoc.* 1985;85:609–611.

Starosta-Runinstein S, Young AB, Kluin K, et al. Clinical assessment of 31 patients with Wilson's disease. *Arch Neurol.* 1987;44:365–379.

Sternlieb I. Perspectives on Wilson's disease. *Hepatology.* 1990;12:1234–1239.

Tankanow RM. Pathophysiology and treatment of Wilson's disease. *Clin Pharm.* 1991;10:839–849.

Walshe JM. The physiology of copper in man and it's relation to Wilson's disease. *Brain.* 1967;90:149–176.

Wiebers DO, Hollenhorst RW, Goldstein NP. The ophthalmologic manifestations of Wilson's disease. *Mayo Clin Proc.* 1977;52:409–416.

Woods SE, Colón VF. Wilson's disease. *Am Fam Pract.* 1989;40:171–178.

78
Chapter

Gout

Esther S. Marks

Gout comprises a group of disorders generally characterized by hyperuricemia (elevated uric acid levels), leading to acute attacks of sodium urate crystal-induced inflammatory arthritis. This may be followed by the development of chronic aggregated deposits of these crystals (tophi) in and around the joints of the extremities, the skin, and in some cases the kidneys. Permanent joint and kidney damage may result.

Recognized for hundreds of years, gout was even referred to by the Greek physician Hippocrates in the fifth century BC. The name comes from the Latin word "gutta," meaning a drop. It was thought that drops of "humors" would flow into a joint, setting off an acute attack of inflammation (Jayson et al, 1974).

In the past, gout was associated with ocular inflammation termed gouty iritis. Under more recent scrutiny, this association has been seriously questioned. However, there clearly are ocular manifestations of gout, in particular bilaterally chronic red eyes.

EPIDEMIOLOGY

■ Systemic

In the United States the prevalence of gout varies with the source. Wyngaarden (1988) lists it as 130 to 370 per 100,000, with a positive family history in 6 to 18% of cases. It appears to be much more common in middle-aged men (95%) than in women (5%), who are almost always postmenopausal (Wyngaarden, 1988). However, some sources now list the frequency of gout in women to be as high as 15 to 30% of newly diagnosed cases. Women usually have a milder course of the disease (Macfarlane & Dieppe, 1985).

Gout represents 5% of all arthritis (Wyngaarden, 1988). It is associated with many other conditions such as obesity, diabetes mellitus, hyperlipidemia (especially hypertriglyceridema), hypertension, and atherosclerotic cardiovascular disease.

■ Ocular

Few epidemiological data are available in the literature on the prevalence or incidence of ocular manifestations of gout. The most commonly noted finding is chronic bilateral injection of the conjunctiva and episclera (Ferry et al, 1985).

NATURAL HISTORY

■ Systemic

In the human body, purine (a component of cell nuclei) metabolism results in uric acid as an end product. This is excreted almost exclusively by the kidneys. Hyperuricemia may be caused by either overproduction or underexcretion of uric acid. Overproduction may be due to a purine-rich diet, an inborn metabolic defect, or disorders characterized by increased cell turnover (eg, psoriasis, polycythemia vera, myeloid metaplasia, multiple myeloma, and acute leukemia (Boss & Seegmiller, 1979). Underexcretion of uric acid may be due to kidney abnormalities, drugs (thiazide diuretics, aspirin, ethambutol, alcohol, nicotinic acid), lead poisoning, and other conditions such as uncontrolled diabetes, starvation, exercise, hypothyroidism, and hyper- and hypoparathyroidism (Boss & Seegmiller, 1979). Other conditions, such as obesity, hyperlipidemia, atherosclerosis, and hypertension, have also been associated with gout (Kelley & Schumacher, 1993).

Patients may live with hyperuricemia for years without symptoms, until sodium urate crystals precipitate in and around a joint spontaneously, or triggered by dietary or alcoholic overindulgence, trauma, illness, or surgery. In an unsuccessful attempt to metabolize the indigestible crystals, engulfing leukocytes burst, releasing lysosomes and other enzymes into the joint and surrounding tissue. This results in a severe inflammatory reaction, acute gouty arthritis.

A single joint is affected in 75 to 90% of initial attacks, and more than 50% will involve the first metatarsophalangeal joint of the big toe—referred to as podagra (Wyngaarden, 1988). There are many theories as to why the big toe is so commonly affected. The most widely accepted theory is that crystal precipitation is favored in joints with lower temperatures and local degenerative changes. This is particularly true of the big toe, located distant from the heart and required to withstand strong forces (Jayson et al, 1974). The big toe is followed in frequency by the foot, ankle, knee, wrist, fingers, and elbow (Scott, 1980). Subsequent attacks may involve more than one joint and may affect even larger joints, such as the hip. As many as 60% of patients will have a second attack within the first year (Cardenosa & Deluca, 1990).

The acute attack often occurs at night, beginning with a feeling of discomfort in the joint, followed by significant swelling, redness, and tenderness. The patient may be awakened with pain so excruciating, that just the weight of a sheet on the joint is intolerable. Without treatment, the mild to moderate attack may last several hours to days, the severe attack sometimes weeks, but both fully resolve. The hyperuricemic patient then enters a symptom-free period of varying duration, referred to as intercritical gout. The self-limited nature of the acute attack of gout is somewhat of a mystery. One possible factor may be that the inflammation in the joint increases the local temperature, resulting in increased urate solubility (Kelley & Schumacher, 1993).

The patient may only experience one or two acute episodes, or develop multiple acute attacks of increasing duration and severity, until permanent joint damage occurs due to clumps of sodium urate crystals (tophi) forming within and around the joints and elsewhere (Figure 78–1). This is termed chronic tophaceous gouty arthritis (Table 78–1). About 20% of gout patients develop tophi, leading to a destructive arthritis (Scott, 1980). The skin over a

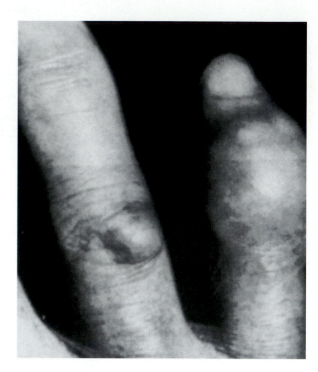

Figure 78–1. Tophus of fifth digit, with smaller tophus over fourth proximal interphalangeal joint. (*Reprinted with permission from Kelley WN, Schumacher HR. Gout. In: Kelley WN, Harris ED, Ruddy S, Sledge CB, eds.* Textbook of Rheumatology. *Philadelphia: Saunders; 1993:1295*).

TABLE 78–1. SYSTEMIC MANIFESTATIONS OF GOUT

ACUTE GOUTY ARTHRITIS
- Hyperuricemia
- Sodium urate crystal deposition in joint
- Most commonly affects big toe, foot, ankle, knee, wrist, fingers, elbow
- Significant swelling, tenderness, redness of joint
- Excruciating pain

INTERCRITICAL GOUT
- Hyperuricemia
- Asymptomatic

CHRONIC TOPHACEOUS GOUT
- Hyperuricemia
- Tophi deposition
    In and around joints leading to bony erosions, calcification, narrowing of joint space
    In skin of elbows, hands, cartilage of the ears— may ulcerate and discharge contents
    In kidney leading to urate nephropathy, acute uric acid nephropathy, nephrolithiasis, renal failure

tophaceous joint may become quite thinned to the point of ulceration, with discharge of the solid urates as a white chalky substance. Tophi may also occur in other tissues such as the skin of the elbows, hands, cartilage of the ears, and kidneys.

Kidney involvement is a common extra-articular manifestation of gout. It may take several forms. Gouty or urate nephropathy—the deposition of urate crystals in the interstitial tissue of the kidney—is not believed to contribute significantly to renal dysfunction in the majority of patients with gout. However, acute uric acid nephropathy—uric acid crystal obstruction of the collecting ducts and distal tubules—does lead to acute renal failure. This is especially common in patients with high cell turnover (eg, leukemias). Nephrolithiasis (uric acid kidney stones) occurs in about 1% of established gouty arthritis patients per year (Kelley & Schumacher, 1993). Renal damage from crystal or stone formation may lead to a failure to clear waste products, secondary hypertension, heart disease, or cerebrovascular accidents.

■ Ocular

Chronic bilateral conjunctival injection is the most commonly associated ocular manifestation of gout (Table 78–2). Described as "dusky red," the bulbar and palpebral injection has been reported to be aggravated by manipulation of the tissue during ocular examination. Unfortunately, it does not appear to be an indicator of blood urate levels, and interestingly does not necessarily subside when urate levels are lowered medically (Ferry et al, 1985). Episcleritis and scleritis have also been associated with gout.

Asteroid hyalosis (Figure 78–2) has recently been considered a possible ocular manifestation of gout. Safir and co-workers (1990), reported that 7 of 76 (9.2%) patients with asteroid hyalosis had gout, far exceeding the prevalence of gout in the general population (0.13 to 0.37%). Ferry and associates (1985) found that 3 out of 69 (4.3%) patients with gout had asteroid hyalosis. This also far exceeds the typically reported prevalence of asteroid hyalosis (0.042 to 0.50%) (Safir et al, 1990).

Uveitis was once believed to be strongly associated with gout. However, in a study of 69 patients with severe gout, Ferry and colleagues (1985) found no patients with uveitis.

TABLE 78–2. OCULAR MANIFESTATIONS OF GOUT

- Chronic bilateral conjunctival injection
- Episcleritis
- Scleritis
- Asteroid hyalosis
- Crystal deposition in cornea, sclera, lens, tarsal plates, extraocular muscles, tendons
- Elevated intraocular pressure (?)

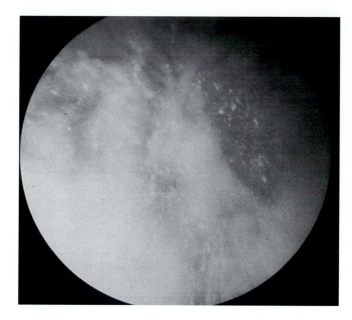

Figure 78–2. Asteroid hyalosis in a patient with gout.

Elevated intraocular pressure has also been reported although no studies have been able to substantiate this association.

Crystal and tophi deposition in ocular tissues, although rare, has been reported. It is theorized that this deposition occurs in poorly vascularized or avascular tissues such as the cornea, sclera, lens, tarsal plates, and extraocular muscle tendons (Bloch & Henkind, 1992). Corneal crystal deposition has been variably described in the epithelial and subepithelial layers.

DIAGNOSIS

■ Systemic

The diagnosis of gout includes a thorough history and physical examination in order to rule out other rheumatologic disorders such as pseudogout (a calcium crystal induced arthropathy), as well as to establish any associated conditions. The clinical presentation of hyperuricemia (serum urate concentration above 7 mg/100 mL) alone does not make the diagnosis. The presence of sodium urate crystals must be demonstrated from tophi or synovial fluid aspirated from affected joints. Analysis of renal function including a 24-hour urine collection for determining uric acid excretion is recommended.

Affected joints should be x-rayed to reveal the punched-out bony erosions characteristic of gout. Round or oval in shape, these erosions usually occur on the long axes of bones. There may also be an increase in density in the areas of soft tissue swelling due to repeated attacks, and eventual uniform narrowing of the joint space (Cardenosa & Deluca, 1990).

■ Ocular

There are no ocular manifestations pathognomonic for gout. However, gout should be considered in patients presenting with chronic bilateral conjunctival injection, recurrent episcleritis, or scleritis of unknown etiology. Asteroid hyalosis may also be a potential warning sign of gout.

TREATMENT AND MANAGEMENT

■ Systemic

The correct diagnosis of hyperuricemia and gout is critical, because the medications used to treat these disorders have potentially serious side effects. Some rheumatologists feel that gout is overdiagnosed or misdiagnosed by primary care physicians (Wolfe & Cathey, 1991). This may be partly due to equating hyperuricemia with gout and thus treating it as gout. Treatment is clearly warranted in symptomatic hyperuricemic patients with evidence of renal damage, frequent acute attacks, and chronic joint changes or tophi. However, treatment of the asymptomatic idiopathic hyperuricemic patient is questionable. Serum uric acid levels above 11 mg/100 mL warrant a 24-hour urine uric acid level test and close renal monitoring but do not require immediate treatment (Kelley, 1993).

The treatment of gout (Table 78–3) must address both the acute and chronic aspects of this disorder. An acute attack of gout requires rest and medication to reduce inflammation as quickly as possible. Colchicine is given until symptoms subside, usually within a few hours. If gastrointestinal toxicity occurs (nausea, diarrhea, vomiting),

indomethacin, phenylbutazone, or naproxen may be given instead. These medications do not prevent future attacks, alter the amount of uric acid in the body, or alter uric acid deposition. Therefore, once the acute attack is over, long-term or chronic treatment must be considered to prevent recurrent arthritis and tophaceous gout.

The medications for long-term treatment decrease serum uric acid either by increasing excretion from the kidney with uricosuric agents (eg, probenecid or sulphinpyrazone) or by decreasing the formation of uric acid with xanthine oxidase inhibitors (eg, allopurinol). Patients also should be instructed on proper diet. The strict exclusion of foods and alcohol is unnecessary and usually results in poor patient compliance; therefore, the key is moderation. Weight reduction is also recommended, as it may help lower plasma urate levels. If necessary, surgical removal of large tophi may be performed once serum uric acid levels are controlled. Patients on medications that alter uric acid metabolism may need to be closely monitored, or have their medications changed. For example, thiazide diuretics, which cause the undersecretion of uric acid, may need to be replaced with β-blockers or calcium channel blockers in patients with gout and hypertension.

■ Ocular

The available literature does not address treatment of the gout-related chronic bilateral conjunctival injection (see Table 78–3). Artificial tears may be used for symptomatic relief. Topical vasoconstrictors may be considered for cosmesis, but chronic use should be strongly discouraged to avoid rebound hyperemia. Episcleritis should be treated with standard modalities: warm/cold compresses, artificial

TABLE 78–3. TREATMENT AND MANAGEMENT OF GOUT

■ SYSTEMIC	■ OCULAR
ACUTE GOUTY ARTHRITIS	**CHRONIC BILATERAL CONJUNCTIVAL INJECTION**
• Rest *plus*	• Artificial tears prn *or*
• Colchicine 0.5 mg q1h, d/c after maximum 4–6mg *or*	• Topical vasoconstrictors—very limited use advised
• Indomethacin 25–100 mg po q4h until relieved then taper *or*	
• Phenylbutazone 150 mg qid × 24 hr then taper *or*	**EPISCLERITIS**
• Naproxen 1.5 g/d until symptoms subside	• Warm/cold compresses *plus*
	• Artificial tears qid *or*
CHRONIC TOPHACEOUS GOUT	• Mild topical steroids in moderate to severe cases (eg, prednisolone acetate 0.125% qid)
• Moderation of diet (eg, high-purine foods and alcohol) *plus*	
• Weight reduction *plus*	**SCLERITIS**
• Probenecid 250 mg bid increase to maximum 3 g/d *or*	• Topical steroids (prednisolone acetate 1% qid to q4h) *plus*
• Sulphinpyrazone 50 mg bid increase to 200–400 mg/d *or*	• NSAIDs (eg, indomethacin 75–100 mg po daily)
• Allopurinol 300 mg/d po increase to maximum 600 mg *plus*	• If severe *add* prednisone 60–80 mg daily, taper, and then discontinue after 2 weeks
• Surgical removal of large tophi if necessary	• If unresponsive, use immunosuppressives

tears, or if moderate to severe, topical steroids. Scleritis should also be treated with standard regimens: topical steroids combined with nonsteroidal antiinflammatory agents, oral steroids, and immunosuppressive agents if unresponsive to treatment.

Chronic bilateral conjunctival injection, recurrent episcleritis, or scleritis of unknown etiology may warrant a serum uric acid level test. The presence of asteroid hyalosis also may warrant evaluation for gout, especially in patients with other signs or symptoms of gout.

Treatment for gout appears to have little impact on the eyes. However, Liu and associates (1988) found that patients on long-term allopurinol therapy had anterior subcapsular lens changes including opacities and thinning of the anterior clear zone.

CONCLUSION

Historically, gout was considered almost exclusively a "disease of kings," caused purely by overindulgence in food and alcohol. Now recognized genetic and environmental factors, as well as changes in diet, have altered the face of gout worldwide. An eminently treatable disorder, gout should no longer be a cause of debilitating arthritis. Although relatively few ocular manifestations of gout exist, an alert eyecare provider may aid in the initial diagnosis.

REFERENCES

Becker MA. Rheumatology. *JAMA*. 1989;261:2287–2289.

Bloch RS, Henkind P. Ocular manifestations of endocrine and metabolic disease. In: Tasman W, Jaeger EA, eds. *Duane's Clinical Ophthalmology*. Hagerstown, MD: Harper & Row; 1992;5:20–21.

Boss GR, Seegmiller JE. Hyperuricemia and gout: Classification, complications and management. *N Engl J Med*. 1979;300: 1459–1468.

Cardenosa G, Deluca SA. Radiographic features of gout. *Am Fam Physician*. 1990;41:539–542.

Ferry AP, Safir A, Melikian HE. Ocular abnormalities in patients with gout. *Ann Ophthalmol*. 1985;17:632–635.

Fishman RS, Sunderman FW. Band keratopathy in gout. *Arch Ophthalmol*. 1966;75:367–369.

Jayson M, Dixon A. Gout and pseudogout. In: Jayson M, Dixon A, eds. *Understanding Arthritis and Rheumatism: A Complete Guide to the Problems and Treatment*. New York: Pantheon; 1974:105–117.

Kelley WN. Hyperuricemia. In: Kelley WN, Harris ED, Ruddy S, Sledge CB, eds. *Textbook of Rheumatology*. Philadelphia: Saunders; 1993;1:498–506.

Kelley WN, Schumacher HR. Gout. In: Kelley WN, Harris ED, Ruddy S, Sledge CB, et al, eds. *Textbook of Rheumatology*. Philadelphia: Saunders; 1993;2:1291–1336.

Liu CSC, Brown NAP, et al. The prevalence and morphology of cataracts in patients on allopurinol treatment. *Eye*. 1988; 2:600–606.

Macfarlane DG, Dieppe PA. Diuretic induced gout in elderly women. *Br J Rheum*. 1985;24:155–157.

Safir A, Dunn SN, Martin RG, et al. Is asteroid hyalosis ocular gout? *Ann Ophthalmol*. 1990;22:70–77.

Scott JT. Gout and other related forms of arthritis. In: Scott JT, ed. *Arthritis and Rheumatism*. Oxford: Oxford University Press; 1980:67–75.

Slansky HH, Kuwabara T. Intranuclear urate crystals in corneal epithelium. *Arch Ophthalmol*. 1968;80:338–344.

Wolfe F, Cathey MA. The misdiagnosis of gout and hyperuricemia. *J Rheum*. 1991;18:1232–1234.

Wyngaarden JB. Gout. In: Wyngaarden JB, Smith LH, eds. *Cecil Textbook of Medicine*. Philadelphia: Saunders; 1988:1161–1170.

Zell SC, Carmichael JM. Evaluation of allopurinol use in patients with gout. *Am J Hosp Pharm*. 1989;46:1813–1816.

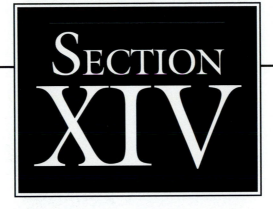

SECTION XIV

RENAL DISORDERS

79
Chapter

Wilms Tumor

Kelly H. Thomann

Wilms tumor (nephroblastoma) is a childhood malignancy of the kidney, almost always diagnosed prior to age 7 years. Once considered highly lethal, Wilms tumor is now one of the most responsive of all childhood cancers. The advancement of treatment modalities has led to a substantial improvement in survival rate, exceeding 90%. This increased survival rate has also been accomplished through the National Wilms Tumor Studies (NWTS 1,2, and 3), cooperative investigations that helped develop specific guidelines for the diagnosis and management of this tumor. NWTS-4 is currently ongoing, with one of its goals to determine the optimum radiation and chemotherapy treatment for specific stages of the disease.

Miller and associates (1964) noted the association of aniridia with Wilms tumor. Ocular manifestations other than aniridia are rarely encountered with Wilms tumor.

EPIDEMIOLOGY

■ Systemic

Wilms tumor is the most common malignant abdominal tumor in children, and accounts for 20% of all pediatric neoplasms. This tumor shows no racial, sexual, demographic or environmental predisposition. Wilms tumor occurs in 1 out of 100,000 children, with 500 cases per year diagnosed in the United States. It is almost always diagnosed in early childhood: 20% prior to age 2 years, 65% between 2 and 6 years, 14% between 6 and 10, and less than 1% after age 10. The median age at diagnosis is 39 months for unilateral tumors and 26 months for bilateral tumors. The left and right kidneys are affected equally, and about 5% of cases are bilateral.

■ Ocular

Aniridia is found in 1 out of 50,000 in the general population. Fraumeni and Glass (1968) reported the incidence of aniridia among children with Wilms tumor to be 6 in 440. It has also been reported that Wilms tumor occurs in 5 of 15 cases of sporadic aniridia and in 1 of 10 familial cases.

NATURAL HISTORY

■ Systemic

Genetic factors probably play a role in Wilms tumor. It is currently believed to occur in both hereditary and sporadic forms. The first NWTS established that the inherited form is actually much less common than previously believed, probably accounting for about one out of five cases. These patients more frequently have associated congenital anomalies.

The tumor originates in embryonal renal cells and grows from the kidney substance. It appears grossly as a large, white, soft mass arising from the kidney with an irregular surface and "pseudocapsule" surrounding it. It extends through the capsule of the kidney into the surrounding tissue, especially the perinephric fat. It may spread to the psoas muscle (located dorsally near the lumbar vertebral column, which helps to flex the trunk) as well as the pancreas, splenic hilum (a fissure on the spleen where nerves and vessels enter), and diaphragm. If the tumor is on the right side, it may extend to the liver and hepatic portal (the entrance of the portal vein and hepatic artery and exit of the hepatic duct). The tumor

589

varies in size, but is often very large when first diagnosed. It may grow rapidly or in spurts.

Congenital anomalies associated with Wilms tumor include genital abnormalities, hemihypertrophy, and central nervous system and musculoskeletal defects (Table 79–1). These are more commonly associated with bilateral tumors and the hereditary type. Wilms tumor will be diagnosed earlier in these patients because of the known association of this tumor and these anomalies.

Metastasis may occur via direct invasion to surrounding tissue or lymph nodes and hematogenously. The lung is the primary hematogenous site, probably because most metastases take a venous route. The liver may also be the site of hematogenous metastases, although less frequently. This tumor rarely metastasizes to the brain or bone, an important fact in the differential diagnosis from neuroblastoma (a malignant tumor of the nervous system, usually involving the spinal cord).

An unfavorable histologic pattern occurs in 12% of patients with Wilms tumor, and this is associated with a high relapse rate. Other factors associated with a poor prognosis include older age at diagnosis, bilaterality, and tumor size.

■ Ocular

Aniridia is generally attributed to an autosomal dominant gene with high penetrance. When Wilms tumor occurs in a patient with aniridia, it is called the aniridia–Wilms tumor syndrome and is due to a specific chromosomal deletion. These cases are sporadic rather than hereditary. The tumor component of aniridia–Wilms tumor syndrome is usually diagnosed at a younger age because of the known association with nephroblastoma. The syndrome shows no sex predilection and there is no difference in the pathological features or natural history of the tumor. Other ocular manifestations of the aniridia–Wilms tumor syndrome are consistent with those found in aniridia alone. These include cataracts, glaucoma, retinal atrophy, foveal hypoplasia, ptosis, dislocated lens, and micro-ophthalmia (Table 79–2).

Aniridia is a congenital hypoplasia of the iris. Although the name implies total absence of the iris, this rarely occurs, and the root is almost always present. Aniridia is often associated with corneal opacification, usually occurring after the age of 2 years. It begins as superficial vascularization of the cornea with opacification at the limbus, most often in the vertical meridian. The opacification progresses

TABLE 79–1. SYSTEMIC AND OCULAR CONGENITAL ANOMALIES ASSOCIATED WITH WILMS TUMOR

Aniridia–Wilms Tumor Syndrome

Systemic
Ear (pinna) and facial deformities
Mental retardation
Microencephaly
Ptosis
Blocked tear ducts

Ocular
Glaucoma
Cataracts
Circumferential corneal pannus
Nystagmus
Macular hypoplasia
Optic nerve hypoplasia
Anisocoria

Other Than Aniridia–Wilms Tumor Syndrome

Systemic
Musculoskeletal
  Hemihypertrophy
  Club foot
  Cleft lip–palate
  Retarded growth and development
  Skull or craniofacial anomaly
  Abnormalities of the pinna of the ear
Genitourinary
  Hypospadias (abnormality of male urethra)
  Cryptorchidism (failure of the testes to descend into the scrotum)
  Duplication of collecting system or ureter
  Kidney abnormalities
Central Nervous System
  Mental retardation
  Seizure disorder
  Microencephaly
  Hamartomas
Other
  Pigmented nevi/hemangiomas

Ocular
Esotropia
Congenital nystagmus
Eye muscle palsy

TABLE 79–2. MANIFESTATIONS OF ANIRIDIA

■ **SYSTEMIC**
- Pattern of inheritance autosomal dominant or sporadic
- Renal abnormality present in great majority of cases (polycystic kidney, nephroptosis, other)
- Wilms tumor (especially in sporadic cases)

■ **OCULAR**
- Corneal pannus
- Malformation of anterior chamber angle
- Partial dislocation of lens
- Lens coloboma
- Cataract
- Glaucoma
- White deposits in peripheral retina
- Macular aplasia
- Optic nerve hypoplasia
- Varying degrees of iris hypoplasia, from minimal hypoplasia to almost total lack

slowly and extends centrally, becoming a circumferential pannus. It may involve the visual axis and cause a decrease in vision.

Glaucoma develops in about one third of patients with aniridia, usually around adolescence. Most of these patients do not develop congenital glaucoma, evidenced by the lack of buphthalmos. This supports the belief that the anterior chamber angle undergoes changes in early life that subsequently lead to glaucoma.

Lamellar and diffuse cataracts are found in about one half of patients with aniridia. Nystagmus may also be associated with aniridia as well as macular hypoplasia and hypoplastic optic discs.

Visual acuity in patients with aniridia is usually about 20/200, although it may range from normal to total blindness.

Systemic congenital anomalies frequently occur in patients with the aniridia–Wilms tumor syndrome. Microencephaly, mental retardation, or delayed development occur in greater than one half of cases. Aniridia occurring without Wilms tumor does not show this frequency of other congenital anomalies.

Ocular abnormalities other than aniridia are rarely encountered in solitary Wilms tumor (see Table 79–1).

DIAGNOSIS

■ Systemic

The diagnosis of Wilms tumor is relatively straightforward. It is almost always diagnosed in infants and toddlers, and rarely in adults. Most children with Wilms tumor will present with a large asymptomatic mass in the abdomen or generalized enlargement of the abdominal area. The parent usually notices the mass when bathing or dressing the child, or it may be an incidental finding on a routine physical examination. Often no systemic symptoms will be present, and the child will play and act normal despite the large abdominal mass. This presentation is felt to be almost diagnostic for Wilms tumor.

Symptoms may be present at the time of tumor diagnosis. These include flank or abdominal pain in about 25% of patients; and fever, vomiting, or anorexia in about 10%. Clinical signs may include hematuria or elevated blood pressure secondary to increased renin, both of which occur in 25% of patients.

An examination of the abdomen will reveal a mass of renal origin in the flank that moves with breathing and is usually ballottable (feels as if it is floating when palpated). This is considered a good sign, because it supports a better prognosis for removal. Small, fixed tumors are often invasive and more difficult to remove. The abdominal examination should also look for distended abdominal vessels. These may indicate occlusion of the inferior vena cava by tumor thrombus. The physical examination and history

should attempt to detect any congenital anomalies associated with Wilms tumor (see Table 79–1).

Imaging studies are indicated to diagnose Wilms tumor as well as look for involvement of the opposite kidney. Computed tomography (CT) scan with contrast is currently the most precise method to assess the lesion, despite the contraindications associated with ionizing radiation and injection of contrast medium. Abdominal CT will show a renal mass, often distorting or deviating part of the kidney. Magnetic resonance imaging (MRI), which is noninvasive and does not use ionizing radiation, may replace CT in the future, but currently CT remains the primary study to be obtained. Intravenous urography (x-ray of the urinary tract after IV injection of an opaque medium that is rapidly excreted into the urine) is also useful in the diagnosis to assess kidney function.

Abdominal ultrasound may also be used to assess the mass, detect tumor thrombi in the renal veins, and delineate tumor extension into the inferior vena cava or right atrium. Four-view chest x-rays are used to detect metastasis into the lungs.

Laboratory testing should include complete blood count with differential and urinalysis to detect urine catacholamines. Hypokalemia, or elevated erythropoietin and plasma renin levels, may also be found. Other nonspecific biochemical abnormalities may include increased erythrocyte sedimentation rate, haptoglobin (a serum that binds free hemoglobin), abnormal serum proteins, and elevated fibrinogen levels.

The differential diagnosis of Wilms tumor includes hydronephrosis (distention of the pelvic and kidney area with urine secondary to ureter obstruction), neuroblastoma, and other tumors with abdominal enlargement or organomegaly such as leukemia, lymphoma, and hepatoma.

■ Ocular

Aniridia is evident on external inspection and obvious with biomicroscopy. Its presence should alert the practitioner to the possibility of Wilms tumor, especially if aniridia is not familial or if the patient displays other congenital anomalies. Diagnosis of ocular conditions associated with aniridia (cataracts, corneal opacification, glaucoma) will be evident on routine eye examination.

TREATMENT AND MANAGEMENT

■ Systemic

A child with Wilms tumor should be managed by a medical team with extensive experience in pediatric cancer, following NWTS protocol. The team should include a pediatric oncologist and radiation specialist, along with respiration, physical, and recreational therapists. Management of these children also includes supportive care through educational monitoring, psychological counseling, and psychosocial support for family, as well as the treatment of physical side effects.

Wilms tumor is now one of the most responsive of all childhood cancers, with a 5-year survival rate of about 90% when treated by standard NWTS protocol. The overall cure rate has increased through a combination of nephrectomy, chemotherapy, and irradiation, depending upon the tumor stage. Although other studies have shown that irradiation to the abdomen can cause future infertility in children, there have not been enough long-term data in Wilms tumor treatment to support this. Irradiation is only used when it will immediately benefit survival.

NWTS-1 clarified the grading of Wilms tumor and NWTS-2 further updated this classification (Table 79–3). Treatment and management is currently based upon this system, and will continue to be modified as new understanding is extrapolated from current Wilms tumor studies.

Surgery is the primary component in the management of these patients, with radiation and chemotherapy added if indicated according to the staging of the tumor (Table 79–4). The primary goal of surgery is to remove the entire tumor. About 5 to 15% of tumors are too large at diagnosis and can rupture during surgery. In these cases, preoperative chemotherapy is used to shrink the tumor.

Bilateral tumors do not always carry a poor prognosis; however, bilaterality should be detected before surgery to determine the best approach. Bilateral nephrectomy and renal transplant have not proven to be very successful.

During surgery, local structures are biopsied, and the opposite kidney is checked carefully along with the liver and the rest of the abdomen for metastases. The greatest risk during surgery is hemorrhage secondary to resection of the vena cava.

Radiation is used conservatively, to avoid growth retardation and secondary malignancies. The indications and type of radiation should follow the protocol put forth by the NWTS stage (see Table 79–3) and will be updated following NWTS-4.

■ Ocular

The management of patients with aniridia can be very difficult (Table 79–5). These patients are often visually

TABLE 79–3. STAGING SYSTEM FOR WILMS TUMOR

Stage I

Tumor limited to kidney and completely excised

Surface of renal capsule is intact

Tumor not ruptured before or during removal

No residual tumor apparent beyond the margins of resection

Stage II

Tumor extends beyond the kidney, but is completely removed

There is regional extension of the tumor (penetration through the outer surface of the renal capsule into the perirenal soft tissues)

Vessels outside the kidney substance are infiltrated or contain tumor thrombus

Tumor may have been biopsied, or there has been local spillage of tumor confined to the flank; no residual tumor apparent at or beyond the margins of excision

Stage III

Residual nonhematogenous tumor confined to the abdomen

    Lymph nodes on biopsy are found to be involved in hilus, periaortic chains, or beyond

    There has been diffuse peritoneal contamination by tumor, such as by spillage of tumor beyond flank before or during surgery, or by tumor growth that has penetrated through the peritoneal surface

    Implants are found on the peritoneal surface

    Tumor extends beyond the surgical margins either microscopically or grossly

    Tumor is not completely resectable because of local infiltration into vital structures

Stage IV

Hematogenous metastases

Deposits beyond stage III (eg, lung, liver, bone, brain)

Stage V

Bilateral renal involvement at diagnosis

An attempt should be made to stage each side according to the above criteria on the basis of the extent of disease before biopsy

TABLE 79–4. TREATMENT AND MANAGEMENT OF WILMS TUMOR[a]

1. Resection of lesion
   Prior chemotherapy when indicated (tumor too large for safe resection)
2. Chemotherapy/radiation at primary tumor site: depends upon staging at resection
   I.   Radiation not necessary because entire tumor resected; maintenance through actinomycin D and vincristine
   II. No gross residual remains but higher risk of microscopic residual; local irradiation is combined with actinomycin D and vincristine
   III. Gross postsurgical residual remains or tumor ruptured during surgery; when rupture minimal, actinomycin D and/or vincristine and tumor bed irradiation
   IV. Metastatic disease to lung—whole-lung irradiation and single 5-day course of actinomycin D, then maintenance with actinomycin D and vincristine
   V.   Postoperative radiation is considered and determined by histology and extent of residual lesion

[a] NWTS-3 protocol.

TABLE 79–5. MANAGEMENT OF ANIRIDIA AND ASSOCIATED OCULAR COMPLICATIONS

GENERAL
- Low-vision aids
- Sunglasses with ultraviolet protection
- Aperture contact lenses

CORNEAL OPACIFICATION
- Usually no treatment indicated
- Lamellar or penetrating keratoplasty

GLAUCOMA
- Standard medical treatment
- Goniotomy
- Trabeculotomy
- Trabeculectomy

CATARACTS
- Surgery, only if absolutely indicated

impaired initially and may progressively lose sight despite attempts to preserve vision.

Pupil-aperture contact lenses have not been successful because of the risk of decompensating an already abnormal cornea. Lamellar or penetrating keratoplasty may be done occasionally, although they are rarely successful. Cataract surgery is usually not indicated because the cataract is seldom the cause of significant visual acuity loss, and it is contraindicated because of the greater risks associated with the abnormal cornea.

The treatment of the glaucoma associated with aniridia is also problematic. Standard medical regimens are primarily used because surgery is difficult due to abnormal angle structures. If surgery is indicated, goniotomy is the initial procedure, because it may help prevent progressive peripheral iris adhesions that block the trabecular meshwork. Trabeculotomy, followed by trabeculectomy, are the next procedures performed, when indicated.

Standard low-vision aids including high-magnification and large-print materials are useful in these patients, as well as sunglasses with ultraviolet protection.

Conclusion

Improvements in technology have led to a broader understanding of Wilms tumor, and therefore, made it a more curable form of cancer. Although rare, eyecare practitioners should be aware of the positive correlation between aniridia and Wilms tumor.

References

Beckwith JB, Palmer NF. Histopathology and prognosis of Wilms' tumor. *Cancer*. 1988;41:1937–1948.

Breslow N, Beckwith J. Epidemiological features of Wilms' tumor: Results of the National Wilms' Tumor Study. *JNCI*. 1982;68:429–436.

Breslow N, Beckwith JB, Ciul M, Sharples K. Age Distribution of Wilms' tumor: Report from the National Wilms's Tumor Study. *Cancer Res*. 1988;48:1153–1157.

Breslow N, Sharples K, Beckwith JB, et al. Prognostic factors in non-metastatic, favorable histology Wilms' tumor. *Cancer*. 1991;68:2345–2353.

Duane TD, Jaeger EA, eds. *Duane's Clinical Ophthalmology*, vol 3. *The Developmental Glaucomas*. Philadelphia: Harper & Row; 1987.

Earley LE, Gottschalk CW. *Strauss and Welt's Diseases of the Kidney*. 3rd ed. Boston: Little, Brown; 2:1979.

Evans AE, Norkool P, Evans I, et al. Late effects of Treatment for Wilms' tumor. *Cancer*. 1991;67:331–336.

Exelby PR. Wilms' tumor 1991. Clinical evaluation and treatment. *Urol Clin North Am*. 1991;18:589–597.

Farewell VT, D'Angio GJ, Breslow N, Norkool P. Retrospective validation of a new staging system for Wilms' tumor. *Cancer Clin Trials*. 1981;4:167–171.

Fraumeni JF, Glass AF. Wilms' tumor and congenital aniridia. *JAMA*. 1968;206:825–828.

Grayson M. *Diseases of the Cornea*. 3rd ed. St. Louis: Mosby; 1991.

Green DM, Finkelstein JZ, Breslow NE, Beckwith JB. Remaining problems in the treatment of patients with Wilms' tumor. *Pediatr Clin North Am*. 1991;38:475–489.

Hammond GD, Bleyer A, Hartman JR, et al. The team approach to the management of pediatric cancer. *Cancer*. 1978;41:29–35.

Jakobiac FA. *Ocular Anatomy, Embryology and Teratology*. Philadelphia: Harper & Row; 1982.

Khan AB. Hypertension associated with increased renin concentrations in nephroblastoma. *Arch Dis Child*. 1991;66:525–526.

Miller RE, Fraumeni JF, Manning MD. Association of Wilms' tumor with aniridia, hemihypertrophy and other congenital malformations. *N Engl J Med*. 1964;270:922–927.

Pendergrass TW. Congenital anomalies in children with Wilms' tumor. *Cancer*. 1976;37:403–409.

Pizzo PA. *Cancer: Principles and Practice of Oncology*. 3rd ed. Philadelphia: Lippincott; 1989.

White KS, Kirks DR, Bool KE. Imaging of nephroblastomatosis: An overview. *Radiology*. 1992;182:1–5.

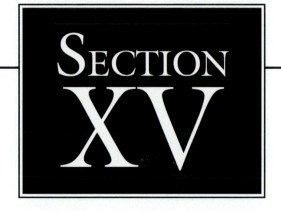

SECTION XV

NUTRITIONAL DEFICIENCIES

80
Chapter

Vitamin Deficiencies

Tanya L. Carter

Nutritional deficiencies can result in clinically evident ocular manifestations. They are more common in developing nations than in North America. Although the relationship between socioeconomic status and diet is the key factor in nutritional deprivation, other causes of deprivation must be considered, such as inadequate absorption, storage, and transport. Some nutritionists believe that the average American diet is deficient in many fundamental nutrients. Depleted soils, chemical fertilizers, pesticides, and processing and cooking styles are other factors that contribute to dietary nutritional deprivation. Additionally, food sensitivities, chemical imbalances, individual nutritional demands, and combining foods that are antagonistic may also cause deprivation. The recommended daily allowance (RDA) is the minimum amount below which nutritional problems may occur. Many nutritionists are now recommending a suggested optimal intake (SOI) that is usually well above the RDA. The therapeutic dose of a nutrient is usually 10 to 50 times the RDA. Therapeutic doses are gradually decreased upon resolution of signs and symptoms.

The six basic classes of substances that are considered essential nutrients are proteins, carbohydrates, fats, fiber, minerals, and vitamins. The next two chapters will focus on the more common vitamin and mineral deficiencies.

Vitamins are organic compounds that are necessary for normal growth, development, and life itself. They serve as components of enzymes that metabolize energy from food, as antioxidants, and as structural components of bones, teeth, and skin. They also play an important role in red blood cell formation, hormone function, the production of genetic material, and the proper function of the immune, gastrointestinal, respiratory, nervous, and muscular systems.

There are two categories of vitamins, fat-soluble (vitamins A, D, E, and K) and water-soluble (B-complex vitamins, vitamin C, and carotenes, folic acid, and bioflavonoids). Fat-soluble vitamins are stored in the body and therefore are more prone to reach toxic levels. The water-soluble vitamins are easily lost in cooking, and must be replenished daily because excesses are excreted in the urine. They are usually nontoxic except in extremely high quantities.

Free-radical pathology is an important concept in understanding the role of many vitamins and minerals in maintaining good health. A free radical is an atom or molecule that has an unpaired electron. Although essential for biological systems, they may be destructive. Free radicals are used to kill invading bacteria, release energy, and detoxify chemicals. Yet they can act to destroy cell membranes, genetic material, and enzymes, as well as to promote cross-linkage of collagen molecules. Vitamins A, C, and E and zinc serve as free-radical scavengers. Our bodies are burdened with an overabundance of free radicals due to pollution, radiation exposure, and unknowingly eating rancid foods. Thus it is possible that under conditions of stress, even a mild nutrient deficiency may affect the body's ability to perform.

■ VITAMIN A (RETINOL)

Vitamin A is a naturally occurring fat-soluble substance. It plays an important role in maintaining the integrity of epithelial membranes in many tissues, including the mucous membranes of the eyes, skin, and respiratory, gastrointestinal, reproductive, and genitourinary systems. Beta-carotene, the provitamin A, is an antioxidant. Retinol is necessary for normal cell growth, bone development, resistance to infection, and maintenance of ocular health.

EPIDEMIOLOGY

■ Systemic

The exact prevalence or incidence of vitamin A deficiency in developed countries is not known. In the United States, many nutritionists feel that the amount of vitamin A for optimal health is not obtained. Vitamin A deficiency is a common problem in underdeveloped countries like Asia, the Caribbean, India, Central and South America, and Africa. Children are more commonly affected and suffer from a high incidence of associated morbidity and mortality.

■ Ocular

Sommer (1982) reported vitamin A deficiency to be the leading cause of childhood blindness in many underdeveloped countries. It is estimated that 10 million children develop xerophthalmia yearly, of which a quarter million suffer from blindness. The mortality in untreated cases of xerophthalmia ranges between 50 and 90%. Even children with mild xerophthalmia are reported to die at a rate of three to nine times the norm.

According to Sommer (1989), there is evidence that a "subclinical" vitamin A deficiency involving conjunctival epithelium is more pervasive than clinical xerophthalmia.

NATURAL HISTORY

■ Systemic

The onset of vitamin A deficiency is insidious. As the disease becomes more advanced it will progress more rapidly, resulting in irreversible damage (Table 80–1). An early clinical sign of deficiency in children is the absence of the "spring growth spurt." Sommer (1989) proposed that vitamin A influences mortality, at least in part, by altering resistance to infections like measles, respiratory disease, and diarrhea. The mechanism for the altered resistance is possibly related to the disrupted epithelial linings of the respiratory, gastrointestinal, and genitourinary tracts that occur early in deficiency. Borderline deficiencies may manifest if compounded by illness, like measles or diarrhea, where the body's nutritional demand increases. Marked deficiency is more often seen in association with fad diets; diseases causing malabsorption (gastroenteritis, cystic fibrosis, celiac disease); problems with storage (liver disease); and deficiency in retinol-binding protein (RBP), which affects transport. Some diabetics may be at risk because they cannot convert carotene to vitamin A because of an increase in beta-lipoprotein, which is the major carrier of carotene. The conversion of carotene to vitamin A takes place in the liver and intestine. An increase in beta-lipoprotein leads to an increase in transport out of the intestine, which decreases its availablity for conversion. Other systemic manifestations include diseases producing hard, dry, flaky skin and hyperkeratosis (psoriasis, keratosis follicularis/Darier disease, ichthyosis) and problems with respiratory, gastrointestinal, and genitourinary function. The mucous membrane atrophy of these organs results in decreased resistance to infections. In particular, there may be an increased susceptibility to respiratory infections like pneumonia or tonsillitis. Severe chronic deficiency can result in death when cellular growth is inhibited, the lysosome membranes are disrupted, or there is an altered resistance to infection.

■ Ocular

Night blindness, a well-known consequence of vitamin A deficiency, is an early symptom experienced even in mild cases of deprivation (Table 80–2). Retinal, a form of vitamin A, is a component of the rod and cone visual pigment (rhodopsin and iodopsin, respectively). The onset of night blindness is insidious, with rod function affected earlier and to a greater extent than cone function. Initially, one may have trouble seeing in the dark or at dusk, which is a result of a lengthened dark adaptation time. In chronic cases the cones will be affected, leading to impairment of central acuity and defects in color vision. Also, bright lights in the dark may be momentarily blinding. Night blindness is usually reversible with oral supplements.

Hypovitaminosis A is a major cause of abnormal precorneal tear film. This results from a lack of vitamin A that subsequently affects the mucin-secreting goblet cells present in the conjunctival epithelium. Xerophthalmia is a term used to describe the spectrum of severe ocular manifestations that includes night blindness (nyctolopia), conjunctival and corneal xerosis, Bitot spot, and keratomalacia. Other associated findings include cataracts, glaucoma, and retinal pigment epitheliopathy. Early stages of vitamin A deficiency are often referred to as subclinical, because marked xerophthalmia is not present yet structural damage has occurred as evidenced by conjunctival cell cytology. As the disease progresses, severe ocular drying (xerosis) occurs.

TABLE 80–1. SYSTEMIC MANIFESTATIONS OF VITAMIN DEFICIENCIES

VITAMIN A
- Psoriasis
- Keratosis follicularis
- Ichthyosis
- Arrested growth
- Respiratory dysfunction
- Gastrointestinal dysfunction
- Genitourinary dysfunction
- Lowered resistance to infection

THIAMINE/B$_1$
- Beriberi
- Wernicke encephalopathy
- Korsakoff syndrome
- Learning disability
- Indigestion, anorexia, constipation
- Fatigue, weakness, neurosensory and motor deficits
- Cardiac dysfunction
- Depression
- Decreased mental alertness

RIBOFLAVIN/B$_2$
- Tissue hypoxia
- Glossitis
- Angular stomatitis
- Seborrheic dermatitis

NIACIN/B$_3$
- Glossitis
- Pellagra
- Diarrhea
- Dementia, memory loss, disorientation, psychosis, decreased mental alertness
- Chronic fatigue and weakness
- Headache
- Insomnia
- Anorexia

PYRIDOXINE/B$_6$
- Seborrheic dermatitis
- Glossitis

- Angular stomatitis
- Peripheral neuropathy
- Lymphocytopenia

VITAMIN B$_{12}$
- Macrocytic (dietary) anemia
- Pernicious (absorption defect) anemia
- Leukopenia
- Thrombocytopenia

VITAMIN C
- Tendency to bruise easily
- Petechial and broad-based hemorrhages into the skin
- Low resistance to infection
- Scurvy

VITAMIN D AND CALCIUM
- Muscular cramping and twitching
- Rickets
- Osteomalacia
- Hyperparathyroidism
- Inefficient blood coagulation
- Insomnia
- Sensitivity to pain
- Poor bone healing

VITAMIN E
- Skin wrinkling
- Poor wound healing
- Respiratory failure
- Myocardial infarction, stroke
- Neurological deficit
    Hyporeflexia
    Gait disturbance
    Ataxia
    Vertigo

At first a patient may present with typical dry eye symptoms along with conjunctival inflammation. As the disease becomes more severe and chronic, the classic signs of xerosis manifest as conjunctival looseness, folds, pigmentation, decreased luster, dry granular patches, and poor wetting (Figure 80–1). The loss of goblet cells leads to squamous cell metaplasia and epithelial keratinization. This forms a diffuse skin-like appearance that is not always reversible with therapy.

The Bitot spot is described as a sequela of conjunctival xerosis. It appears as an oval or triangular, shiny, gray spot and is usually found bilaterally near the temporal limbus. This overlies an area of conjunctival drying that contains desquamated keratin mixed with saprophytic gram positive bacilli. A foamy substance may be scraped from the surface, leaving a chalky conjunctival bed (Figure 80–2). The exact role that vitamin A plays in the development of the

TABLE 80–2. OCULAR MANIFESTATIONS OF VITAMIN DEFICIENCIES

VITAMIN A
- Dermatitis (eyelid)
- Dry eyes
- Xerophthalmia
- Night blindness
- Bitot spot
- Diffuse conjunctival infection
- Cataract
- Peripheral pigment epitheliopathy
- Macular degeneration
- Glaucoma[a]

VITAMIN B$_1$
- Restricted EOM motility, ophthalmoplegia
- Anterior or retrobulbar optic neuropathy
- Nystagmus

VITAMIN B$_2$
- Angular or seborrheic blepharoconjunctivitis
- Dermatitis (eyelid)
- Dry eyes
- Diffuse conjunctival injection
- Limbal injection
- Phlyctenular keratoconjunctivitis
- Corneal vascularization
- Keratitis/infiltrates
- Cataract
- Photophobia

VITAMIN B$_3$
- Dermatitis (eyelid)
- Hyperpigmentation, hyperkeratosis (eyelid)
- Madarosis
- Diffuse conjunctival injection
- Corneal epithelial erosions
- Photophobia

- Pigment maculopathy
- Optic neuropathy

VITAMIN B$_6$
- Blepharitis (angular or sebhorreic)
- Dermatitis (eyelid)
- Dry eyes

VITAMIN B$_{12}$
- Subconjunctival hemorrhages
- Retinal hemorrhages
- Cotton wool spots
- Retinal venous tortuosity
- Optic neuropathy

VITAMIN C
- Conjunctival petechial hemorrhages
- Recurrent subconjunctival hemorrhages
- Retinal hemorrhages
- Orbital hemorrhages
- Hyphema
- Glaumcoma[b]

VITAMIN D AND CALCIUM
- Band keratopathy
- Cataract
- EOM dysfunction

VITAMIN E
- Cataract
- Pigmentary retinopathy
- Macular degeneration
- EOM dysfunction
- Nystagmus
- Night blindness

[a] The exact role is still under investigation.
[b] Due to its role in maintaining or enhancing the use of vitamin A.

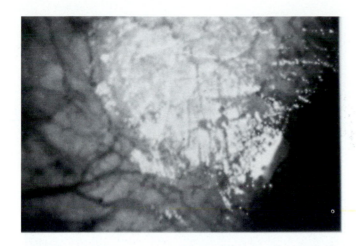

Figure 80–1. In vitamin A deficiency, a dry lusterless conjunctiva with a crocodile pattern and failure to wet the tears. *(Reprinted with permission from Fells P, Bors F, Ocular complications of self-induced vitamin A deficiency. Trans Ophthamol Soc UK. 1969;89:222.)*

Bitot spot is not entirely clear. Many have found Bitot spots in individuals who were not deficient in vitamin A. Also, in some there is no response to vitamin A therapy. However, some feel this may be due to chronic vitamin A deficiency resulting in irreversible squamous cell metaplasia.

Corneal xerosis may develop as the xerophthalmia progresses. A dry granular appearance with loss of luster and superficial punctate staining will occur early on. This is often described as "orange peel" or "pebble like" and can progress to marked keratinization. Scattered gray or yellow areas of opacification can form, which may coalesce, leading to "liquefactive" stromal necrosis and ulceration, termed keratomalacia. The changes that occur in keratomalacia are irreversible. Phthisis bulbi may be the final stage of this process.

The antioxidant property of beta-carotene is a factor in protecting the lens proteins from oxidation. It is well documented that nutritional factors play a role in the development of cataracts. Bhat (1983) found that the formation of insoluble lens proteins occurs earlier or faster in undernourished subjects.

Normally the RPE stores vitamin A for utilization by the photoreceptors. According to Fells and Bors (1969), retinal pigment epitheliopathy can occur in chronic vitamin A deficiency. The exact mechanism for the pigmentary disturbance is not well established. It appears as small, white intraretinal opacities and pigment mottling in the periphery (Figure 80–3).

Vitamin A may play a role in primary open-angle glaucoma. Krishna and Pramod (1982) found serum carotenoid levels significantly lower in patients with glaucoma compared with normals. It is speculated that lowered vitamin A levels increased the resistance to aqueous outflow due to decreased enzyme activity in the trabecular meshwork. Further research is needed to substantiate the role of vitamin A in glaucoma. People with a predisposition to glaucoma may need more vitamin A.

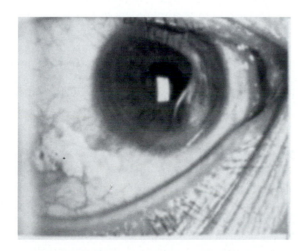

Figure 80–2. Nonresponsive Bitot spot in a 20-year-old man. The superior margin has a foamy appearance, the remainder has a cheesy appearance. *(Reprinted with permission from Sommer A, Emran N, Tjakrasudjatma S, Clinical characteristics of vitamin A responsive and nonresponsive Bitot's spots. Am J Ophthamol. 1980;90:163.)*

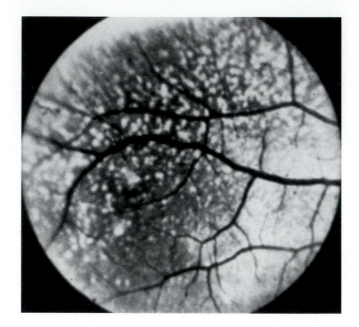

Figure 80–3. Photograph of superotemporal area of right fundus showing discrete white dots apparently deep to the vessels, secondary to vitamin A deficiency. *(Reprinted with permission from Fells P, Bors F, Ocular complications of self-induced vitamin A deficiency.* Trans Ophthamol Soc UK. *1969;89:225.)*

DIAGNOSIS

■ Systemic

The key to diagnosis is observation of the clinical signs and associated symptoms. These include dry, irritated skin, indigestion, problems with breathing, or frequent colds. The best diagnostic laboratory test is the serum vitamin A assay. Levels less than 20 μg/100 mL are considered deficient. Assessing the level of serum retinol-binding protein (RBP) is used to rule out transport of vitamin A as a source of deficiency.

■ Ocular

Symptoms of night blindness or difficulty driving during dusk can be supported by electroretinography (ERG) and dark adaptometry. The ERG response will show early loss of the a-wave followed by disappearance of the remaining waves. Genest (1967) reported that both a-waves and b-waves are equally affected by low serum vitamin A. ERG values return to normal if vitamin A therapy is implemented early on. Dark adaptation time is lengthened. Patients may also complain of being blinded after exposure to a bright light, such as the headlights of a car or a light turned on in a dark room. Dark-adaptometry can also be used to diagnose subclinical vitamin A deficiency.

The clinical signs of conjunctival xerosis, corneal xerosis, keratomalacia, Bitot spot, and retinal pigment epitheliopathy may be seen along with dry eye symp-

toms of burning, irritation, and lacrimation in vitamin A deficiency. An early dry eye condition can be diagnosed with the Schirmer test or staining using fluorescein and rose bengal. Impression cytology, an important tool in diagnosis, can determine if goblet cells are absent. Visual acuity and color vision deficits along with photophobia may also be evident.

TREATMENT AND MANAGEMENT

■ Systemic

The recommended mode of therapy for vitamin A deficiency is retinyl palmitate given orally (Table 80–3). If there is a problem with absorption, an intramuscular injection is suggested. Additionally, vitamin B-complex and systemic antibiotics are also recommended because of the role of vitamins B_2, B_3, and B_6 in maintaining mucous membranes and promoting tissue repair. Also, the disrupted epithelial linings of the respiratory, gastrointestinal, and genitourinary tracts can increase the incidence of infections.

■ Ocular

Retinal palmitate is given orally to reverse night blindness and conjunctival xerosis. The effective oral dose of vitamin A to treat corneal xerosis is that which causes a rapid increase in blood plasma levels (see Table 80–3). Conjunctival and corneal xerosis respond to systemic therapy in 1 to 4 days. The response to topical therapy occurs after weeks of

TABLE 80–3. TREATMENT AND MANAGEMENT OF VITAMIN DEFICIENCIES

VITAMIN A
- Oral: 200,000 IU retinyl palmitate × 2 days
- IM: 100,000 IU
- RDA: 1400–3300 IU: Infancy–10 years
  - 4000 IU: Female adult
  - 5000 IU: Male adult
  - 6000 IU: Pregnancy/lactation
- Vitamin A toxicity can occur with greater than 30,000 IU/d

BETA CAROTENE
- RDA: 2400 µg
- Night blindness
  - Oral: 30,000 IU/d × 2–3 weeks
- Conjunctival xerosis
  - Oral: 30,000 IU/day × 2–3 weeks
  - Topical: 0.01% retinoic ointment 1–3×/d
    - Vit-A-Drops 3–4×/d
- Bitot Spot
  - Oral: 200,000 IU
- Corneal xerosis
  - Oral: Dose that causes rapid increase in serum levels
  - Topical: See conjunctival xerosis
- Keratomalacia
  - See corneal xerosis

THIAMINE/B$_1$
- Oral: 500 mg/d
- RDA: 0.5 mg: Infants
  - 1.2 mg: Children
  - 1.5 mg: Adults
  - 1.6 mg: Pregnancy/lactation

RIBOFLAVIN/B$_2$
- Oral: 6 mg/d
- IM: 1 single 25-mg dose
- RDA: 0.6 mg: Infants
  - 1.2 mg: Children
  - 1.7 mg: Adults
  - 2.0 mg: Pregnancy
  - 2.2 mg: During lactation
- Cataract
  - 50–100 mg daily

NIACIN/B$_3$
- Oral: 50–250 µg nicotinamide/d
- RDA: 8 mg: Infants
  - 9 mg: Children
  - 20 mg: Adults

PYRIDOXINE/B$_6$
- Oral: 100–150 mg/d
- RDA: 1.2 mg: Children
  - 2.0 mg: Adults
  - 2.5 mg: Pregnancy/lactation

VITAMIN B$_{12}$
- RDA: 10 µg: Adolescents and adults
  - 15 µg: Pregnancy/lactation
- Not obtained from fruits or vegetables but mainly from meats and meat products
- Pernicious anemia
  - 1–30 µg parenteral injections/d followed by 100 µg IM monthly for life

VITAMIN C
- RDA: 35 mg: Infants
  - 40 mg: Children
  - 60 mg: Adults
- SOI: 150 mg/d
- During stress or sickness: 1000 mg/d
- Cataracts
  - 1000 mg/d in time release capsules
- Corneal ulcers
  - 1500 mg/d

VITAMIN D
- RDA: 400 IU
- Exposure to sunlight
- Ricketts
  - 2200 IU daily
- Osteomalacia
  - 1600 IU × 1 month

CALCIUM
- RDA: 400–600 mg: Infants
  - 800 mg: Children 1–10 years
  - 1300 mg: Adults and children 10–18 years
  - 1300 mg: Pregnancy/lactation
- The elderly may need higher amounts

VITAMIN E
- Oral: 400–1800 IU/d
- RDA: 5 IU: Infants
  - 10 IU: Children
  - 30 IU: Adults
- SOI: 30–400 IU/day

Reprinted with permission from Food and Nutrition Board Commission on Life Sciences National Research Council. Recommended Daily Allowances. Washington, DC: National Academy Press; 1989.

therapy. Sommer (1983) found that topical retinoic acid ointment in arachis oil speeds healing. However, due to the potential for scarring, this treatment is reserved for opacities that are on the visual axis. The effectiveness of Vit-A-Drops in vitamin A deficiency as well as other dry eye diseases is currently under investigation. Rengstorff and associates (1988) reported that Vit-A-Drops, which contain 5000 IU of retinol and polysorbate 80, are effective in the treatment of various dry eye disorders. Topical antibiotics may be indicated in cases of epithelial erosion. Keratomalacia is treated in the same manner as corneal xerosis; however, it may not necessarily respond to therapy. Bitot spot may be treated as well. Semba and colleagues (1990) reported cases of Bitot spots that showed a response in as soon as 2 weeks.

Beta-carotene can be obtained from fruits and vegetables, while good sources of vitamin A include animal liver, eggs, fish liver oils, and milk. Megadoses of vitamin A can be toxic because it is fat soluble. Up to approximately 30,000 IU daily is usually safe. The RDA as put forth by the Food and Nutrition Board is outlined in Table 80–3.

■ VITAMIN B$_1$

Vitamin B$_1$ (thiamine) is important to the normal functioning of the heart, muscles, digestive system, nervous system, and an individual's capacity to learn. It serves as a co-enzyme for converting carbohydrates into glucose and it is necessary for the synthesis of acetylcholine. The more common systemic manifestations of thiamine deficiency include beriberi, Wernicke encephalopathy, and Korsakoff syndrome. The ocular manifestations of deficiency include extraocular muscle palsies, optic neuropathy, and nystagmus.

EPIDEMIOLOGY

Thiamine deficiency is endemic in the Orient and Pacific Islands. It generally occurs in populations relying heavily on polished rice or unenriched white flour that has lost thiamine in the milling process. In North America, it is estimated that 5% of adults over 60 years of age are deficient because of poor dietary intake. The prevalence is even higher among the poor, the institutionalized, alcoholics, and patients with chronic GI syndromes. Fever, exercise, hyperthyroidism, pregnancy, and lactation increase thiamine requirement.

NATURAL HISTORY

■ Systemic
Thiamine deprivation may develop in a short period of time because depletion of body stores can occur in just 12 to 14 days. Signs of early deficiency may include impaired digestion of carbohydrates, anorexia, and constipation (see Table 80–1). Chronic deficiency can lead to beriberi syndrome, which is characterized by progressive peripheral neurosensory and motor deficits, cardiac decompensation, and personality changes. Cardiovascular and cerebral abnormalities

become evident in severe, chronic deficiency. Wernicke encephalopathy can result from severe, acute deficiency; however, it is more commonly found in association with chronic alcoholism or chronic malnutrition. This syndrome is characterized by dementia, somnolence, ataxia, ophthalmoplegia, and neurological dysfunction that may range from mild confusion to coma. Resolution of signs and symptoms may begin 24 hours after initiating therapy. Damage to the cerebral cortex can lead to Korsakoff psychosis and untreated cases can lead to death.

■ Ocular
Chronic thiamine deficiency can cause restricted extraocular muscle motility, anterior or retrobulbar optic neuropathy, and nystagmus (see Table 80–2). The optic neuropathy is due to an alteration in myelin sheath and ATP formation that results in axoplasmic flow stasis. There is a slow, progressive, bilateral, yet often asymmetric involvement of the optic nerves. Toxic optic neuropathy may arise as a result of increased vulnerability to toxicity from exogenous substances such as tobacco and alcohol. The administration of thiamine can improve the condition even if the alcohol and tobacco abuse continues. The ophthalmoplegia associated with Wernicke encephalopathy includes lateral rectus muscle weakness, impaired conjugate gaze, partial third-nerve palsies, ptosis, and nystagmus.

DIAGNOSIS

■ Systemic
Along with the signs already outlined, a patient with thiamine deficiency may complain of fatigue, weakness, muscle tenderness, paresthesia, loss of appetite, indigestion, palpitation, sleep disturbances, poor memory, irritability, and other personality changes. The best laboratory test for assessing thiamine status is the evaluation of the erythrocyte transketolase activity (a thiamine-dependent enzyme) after stimulation by thiamine pyrophosphate. A significant increase in enzyme activity reflects a thiamine deficiency. Direct serum thiamine assay is not a useful diagnostic tool because only small quantities of thiamine are found in the blood. Urinary microbial or chemical assays are not valuable for assessing thiamine status mainly because of problems obtaining a satisfactory sample size.

■ Ocular
Ocular diagnosis of thiamine deficiency is based on clinical observation of the signs and correlated symptoms. The most common complaint is a gradual decline in vision ("nutritional amblyopia"). The visual acuity loss is usually bilateral and rarely falls below 20/200. Pain behind the eye, diplopia, and

color vision defects also arise in deficiency states. Bilateral centrocecal scotomas are the classic visual field defects associated with nutritional optic neuropathy; however, central scotomas also have been reported. The scotomas may be more easily detected with colored targets, especially red.

TREATMENT AND MANAGEMENT

The recommended therapy for thiamine deficiency is oral daily dosing until resolution of signs and symptoms, followed by a daily maintenance dose that meets the RDA as outlined in Table 80–3. Good dietary sources include plant and animal tissue, whole-grain cereals, peas, beans, nuts, oranges, organ meats, legumes, and brewer's yeast.

■ VITAMIN B₂

Vitamin B₂ (riboflavin) is essential in the metabolism of carbohydrates, fatty acids, and amino acids. It is necessary for transporting hydrogen and assisting in the transfer of oxygen from plasma to the tissues. Riboflavin is important in tissue repair, formation of antibodies, maintaining mucous membranes, and enhancing the efficacy of vitamin D. It also plays a role in light adaptation and promoting ocular lens clarity. Deficiency can result in restricted cellular growth and tissue hypoxia resulting in dermatitis, glossitis, angular stomatitis, circumcorneal injection, superficial keratitis, corneal vascularization, and keratoconjunctivitis sicca.

EPIDEMIOLOGY

Riboflavin deficiency is more commonly found in underdeveloped countries. However, in the United States reports indicate that one third of women over age 65 and men over age 75 have diets deficient in vitamin B₂. As with thiamine deficiency, riboflavin deprivation is associated with low socioeconomic status, the elderly recluse, and chronic alcoholism because of inadequate dietary consumption. Other depleting factors include oral contraceptives, cooking styles, processed foods, exposure to UV light, and stress.

NATURAL HISTORY

■ Systemic
Signs of deficiency include a purplish-red, inflamed, or shiny tongue (glossitis), cracking in the corners of the lips (angular stomatitis), greasy skin, and seborrheic dermatitis

(see Table 80–1). Initially the corners of the mouth will be pale followed by hyperkeratosis, inflammation, and local ulceration, which progresses to cracks or fissures. The dermatitis commonly involves the nasolabial folds and forms a butterfly distribution involving the cheeks and skin around the ears. Sebrell and Butler (1950) have proposed the concept of a deficiency syndrome that is characterized by angular stomatitis, glossitis, seborrheic dermatitis, and corneal vascularization.

■ Ocular
One of the earliest signs of riboflavin deprivation is conjunctival injection, with subsequent proliferation and anastomosis of the limbal vessels followed by corneal vascularization (see Table 80–2). Prolonged deficiency can lead to keratitis sicca, interstitial infiltration, and even ulceration. The underlying causes for these ocular changes are tissue hypoxia and mucous membrane dysfunction. The corneal changes will respond to oral riboflavin therapy.

Phlyctenular keratoconjunctivitis, rosacea keratitis, and seborrheic and angular blepharoconjunctivitis also occur in association with riboflavin deficiency. Riboflavin and niacin are present with vitamin A in retinal tissue and are thought to work synergistically to produce efficient visual function. These B vitamins are implicated as necessary components for light adaptation; however, their exact role is not clear.

Biochemical evidence exists that supports the association between riboflavin deficiency and cataract formation in humans; however, its role is still controversial. Riboflavin serves as the coenzyme for glutathione reductase, which catalyses the reduction of oxidized glutathione in the lens. Researchers postulate that because oxidized glutathione is a free radical, its reduction may serve to protect the lens proteins against free radical damage. Additionally, studies have shown that glutathione reductase activity is decreased in cataractous lenses. Bhat (1987) supported this association with a study in which riboflavin deficiency was found in 81% of cataract patients and only 12.5% of control subjects.

DIAGNOSIS

■ Systemic
Diagnosis is based on the clinical signs and associated symptoms, which include dry irritated skin and sore tongue. The diagnostic laboratory tests are the serum erythrocyte fluorometric assay to measure the level of reduced glutathione, and the serum microbial assay utilizing an organism (*Tetrahymena thermophia*) that requires riboflavin for growth. Urine analysis will show deficiency if values fall below 27 μg/g creatinine for an adult. For

children between the ages of 1 and 15, values are considered deficient if they fall below 70 to 150 µg/g creatinine.

■ Ocular

Riboflavin deficiency should be considered when faced with the common ocular signs and corresponding symptoms. The patient will complain of irritation, lacrimation, and burning. Keratitis may lead to decreased visual acuity and photophobia. Corneal and conjunctival fluorescein and rose bengal staining may be present.

TREATMENT AND MANAGEMENT

The recommended therapeutic approach is a single intramuscular dose or daily oral doses until resolution of the signs and symptoms after which the RDA should be maintained as outlined in Table 80–3. To manage or prevent cataract formation some suggest much higher doses daily.

Good dietary sources of riboflavin include whole grains, brewer's yeast, nuts, organ meats, cheese, milk, and egg yolks.

■ VITAMIN B₃

Vitamin B₃ (niacin) is also known as nicotinic acid or nicotinamide. As a component of two important co-enzymes, it plays an essential role in electron transfer for cellular respiration. It also is necessary in the metabolism of carbohydrates, fats, proteins, and amino acids; proper functioning of the nervous system; and promoting healthy skin. To some extent, niacin may be synthesized by bacteria in the human intestine. Pellagra is a well-known consequence of niacin deficiency. It is characterized by cutaneous, gastrointestinal, mucosal, neurological, and mental disturbances. This classic deficiency syndrome is described as the three D's: dermatitis, diarrhea, and dementia. The associated dermatitis can involve the eyelids. Central nervous system involvement may manifest ocularly as external ophthalmoplegia and optic neuropathy.

EPIDEMIOLOGY

Niacin deficiency is still endemic in areas of the world that rely heavily on corn as their principal food source, because corn is deficient in nicotinic acid. In the United States, niacin deficiency is associated with the poor dietary intake of alcoholics, the elderly recluse, and the impoverished. Other sources of deficiency include malabsorption, as in gastrointestinal disease, stress, heavy coffee and refined sugar consumption, hyperthyroidism, infections, and medications, and the increased demands of pregnancy and lactation.

NATURAL HISTORY

■ Systemic

One of the earliest signs of niacin deficiency is glossitis (see Table 80–1). This begins as a burning sensation of the tongue followed by erythema and edema. As the disease progresses, the classic syndrome, pellagra, may develop, manifesting as dermatitis, diarrhea, and dementia. The skin will be erythematous followed by vesicle formation, crusting, scaling, and desquamation. The dermatitis tends to be most severe in sun-exposed areas. The diarrhea is caused by intestinal mucous membrane atrophy. Central nervous system involvement will manifest as neurasthenia, followed by dementia and psychosis, which are characterized by disorientation, memory loss, confusion, hallucinations, and distortions of perception. Later delirium may occur.

■ Ocular

Advanced stages of deficiency may result in eyelid dermatitis, hyperpigmentation, hyperkeratosis, inflammation, and madarosis (see Table 80–2). Additionally, conjunctival hyperemia, epithelial erosions, small lymphocytic and leukocytic infiltrates, optic neuropathy, and pigment maculopathy are signs associated with deficiency states. The optic neuropathy may be anterior or retrobulbar and typically is bilateral. Further neuronal involvement may manifest as external ophthalmoplegia.

DIAGNOSIS

■ Systemic

Diagnosis is based on the signs and their corresponding symptoms, which include chronic fatigue and weakness, hallucinations, and distortions of perception. The more common laboratory tests employed are the serum microbial assay that utilizes the *T. thermophilia* organism (which requires nicotinic acid for growth); and urine analysis that measures the level of N-methylnicotinamide (a metabolite of niacin). The normal daily excretion is at least 0.5 mg/g creatinine.

■ Ocular

Niacin deficiency should be suspected when classic dermatologic signs are found along with conjunctival, corneal, and retinal signs as previously outlined. Possible niacin deficiency should be considered in the presence of unexplained gradual loss of visual acuity ("nutritional amblyopia"). The acuity loss is usually bilateral and rarely progresses below 20/200. The patient may also complain of photophobia and aching behind the eyeball that worsens with strong light. Color vision testing may show dyschromatopsia, and visual field testing will show central or centrocecal scotomas.

TREATMENT AND MANAGEMENT

Niacin deficiency will respond to a daily oral therapeutic regimen of nicotinamide. Once resolution of signs and symptoms is achieved, at least the RDA, as outlined in Table 80–3, should be maintained. Parenteral therapy is necessary in the presence of malabsorption.

Good dietary sources of niacin include brewer's yeast, beef, kidney, liver, fish, poultry, soybeans, wheat germ, peanuts, and legumes.

■ VITAMIN B₆

Vitamin B_6 (pyridoxine) is a water-soluble co-enzyme that is primarily involved in the metabolism of nitrogen and tryptophan into nicotinic acid. It also is important in the metabolism of other amino acids. It is essential in maintaining the health of neuronal tissue, in antibody production, and possibly in bone development. Deficiency can cause problems similar to vitamins B_2 and B_3 deprivation. Low vitamin B_6 intake is implicated in the onset of cancer, coronary heart disease, eyelid dermatitis, and angular blepharoconjunctivitis.

EPIDEMIOLOGY

Exact incidence and prevalence of pyridoxine deficiency is not known; however, it is observed in association with chronic alcoholism, use of oral contraceptives, antihypertensive medications, postmenopausal estrogen, patients taking isonicotinic acid hydrazide (INH) to treat tuberculosis, and in those treated with L-dopa for Parkinson disease. Recent studies show a high prevalence of pyridoxine deficiency in the elderly.

NATURAL HISTORY

■ Systemic
Small amounts of vitamin B_6 are stored in the body and any excess is excreted in the urine; therefore adequate dietary intake is essential. Exposure to heat, sunlight or air causes rapid inactivation. Signs of pyridoxine deficiency include seborrhea-like lesions about the eyes, nasolabial folds, mouth, forehead, and behind the ears.

Glossitis, angular stomatitis, peripheral neuropathy, and lymphocytopenia may also be present (see Table 80–1).

■ Ocular
Eyelid dermatitis and angular blepharoconjunctivitis are reported in association with pyridoxine deficiency (see Table 80–2). The fissuring and cracking at the outer canthi are frequently associated with similar changes at the angles of the mouth. Periocular seborrheic dermatitis that does not respond to riboflavin or niacin therapy may respond to pyridoxine.

DIAGNOSIS

■ Systemic
Nausea, vomiting, weakness, insomnia, and irritability are signs and symptoms of vitamin B_6 deficiency. The most common diagnostic laboratory tests are the urine fluorometric assay of 4-pyridoxic acid (principal excreted metabolite of vitamin B_6), serum assay of alanine (SGPT) and aspartic (SGOT) transaminases, and the serum microbial assay utilizing *T. thermophilia*. Urine analysis is better at indicating short- versus long-term dietary intake, and reports indicate that it is not a reliable indicator of B_6 status. Vitamin B_6 deficiency causes decreased plasma SGPT and SGOT. The radioenzymatic serum assay will result in a mean B_6 level of 3.6 to 18.0 μg/L of whole blood.

■ Ocular
Ocular symptoms of vitamin B_6 deficiency include burning, irritation, and foreign body sensation.

TREATMENT AND MANAGEMENT

Vitamin B_6 deficiency is treated with an oral daily regimen until resolution of the signs and symptoms, followed by the RDA as outlined in Table 80–3. If angular blepharoconjunctivitis is present, differential diagnosis must also include the more common cause, *Staphylococcus aureus*.

Good dietary sources of vitamin B_6 include meats, brans, wheat germ, bananas, pears, cantaloupe, cabbage, peas, green leafy vegetables, brown rice, milk, and brewer's yeast.

■ VITAMIN B₁₂

Vitamin B_{12} (cobalamins) is essential for the production of normal red blood cells, white blood cells, platelets, detoxification of cyanide, and cellular replication. It is a co-enzyme in the initial stages of DNA synthesis and plays a major role in myelin sheath formation. The cobalamins are synthesized by microorganisms in water, soil, and the intestine of animals. They are not found in fruits and vegetables except in the legume nodules of root vegetables. Megaloblastic anemia is the major consequence of deficiency states, and pernicious anemia is the classic type of megaloblastic anemia. The most common ocular manifestation of vitamin B_{12} deficiency is optic neuropathy. Subconjunctival and retinal hemorrhages, cotton-wool spots, and congested vessels may be present in association with anemia.

EPIDEMIOLOGY

Vitamin B_{12} deficiency is predominately a disease of the elderly, strict vegetarians, and chronic alcoholism, because of poor dietary intake. Pernicious anemia more commonly occurs in 40- to 80-year-old northern Europeans of fair complexion because of an inherited disorder of absorption. It has also been reported in other races on rare occasions. Poor absorption may also arise due to stomach or intestinal disease, surgical resection of the small intestine, or competition for receptor sites from drugs like birth control pills and alcohol. Other depleting factors include inherited disorders of intracellular metabolism, as well as pregnancy and hyperthyroidism, which increase vitamin B_{12} requirements.

NATURAL HISTORY

■ Systemic

Vitamin B_{12} deficiency takes at least a few years to develop because the depletion of liver stores occurs gradually. Systemic manifestations of deficiency include anemia, leukopenia, and thrombocytopenia (see Table 80–1). In pernicious anemia, vitamin B_{12} is deficient because of an inherited absence of intestinal glycoprotein intrinsic factor necessary for absorption. Vitamin B_{12} anemias are characterized by large, irregular-shaped red blood cells that have a short lifespan. The characteristic symptoms of vitamin B_{12} deprivation include fatigue, weakness, dyspnea, sore tongue, paresthesia, vertigo, diarrhea, constipation, irritability, forgetfulness, impaired judgement, anorexia, syncope, headaches, fever, drowsiness, amenorrhea, tachycardia, palpitations, angina pectoris, and postural hypotension. Initially, this megaloblastic anemia may occur without any associated CNS involvement; however, later stages can manifest as a progressive peripheral neuropathy due to demyelination, muscle

weakness, and loss of tactile senses. Other signs include pallor of skin and fingernail beds, loss of hair or weight, depression, and if severe, cardiac failure. Death may occur if treatment is not initiated.

■ Ocular

Optic neuropathy may precede, coincide with, or follow the signs and symptoms of megaloblastic anemia (see Table 80–2). Optic neuropathy precedes anemia and neural involvement in one out of three cases. Early stages may manifest as bilateral retrobulbar neuropathy, which progresses to temporal pallor and eventually anterior optic atrophy. Damage to the myelin sheath is the primary mechanism for optic nerve involvement. Prognosis for recovery of visual loss and visual field defects is enhanced if therapy is initiated early in the course of optic nerve involvement; however, recovery is usually slow. Cases have been reported of recovery occurring after 10 months of therapy.

Vitamin B_{12} deficiency is commonly associated with "toxic optic neuropathy" due to tobacco abuse where the optic nerve becomes vulnerable to the toxicity from the cyanide. Alcohol abuse may also lead to vitamin B_{12} deficiency, because of associated malnutrition and interference by alcohol with B_{12} absorption. In this case the associated optic nerve involvement is known as nutritional optic neuropathy. See Chapter 82 for further discussion of this topic.

Retinal hemorrhages, cotton-wool spots, and congested/tortuous vessels may also appear in the presence of severe chronic anemia.

DIAGNOSIS

■ Systemic

Diagnosis of vitamin B_{12} deficiency is based on the clinical signs and symptoms, along with blood serum levels. If deficiency is suspected, one should obtain a serum microbial assay. The normal values range between 200 and 900 pg/mL. Serum levels may be normal due to the presence of a biologic inactive analog of vitamin B_{12} that will interfere with the assay. Urinary methylmalonic acid levels may also be used for diagnosis. Vitamin B_{12} anemia is diagnosed by obtaining a complete blood count (CBC). This will show reduced quantities of erythrocytes, white blood cells, and platelets. The hemoglobin and hematocrit levels will be decreased, while the mean corpuscular volume and mean corpuscular hemoglobin will be increased. A serum smear will reveal large oval RBCs and hypersegmented neutrophils. The Schilling test for gastrointestinal absorption should be obtained to specifically rule out pernicious anemia. In phase one of this test, vitamin B_{12} labeled with radioactive cobalt is given orally. Measurements are based on how much is recovered in the urine in 24 hours. Normal measurements usually range between 7 and 38%. In the second stage, intrinsic factor is added to the vitamin B$_{12}$ doses. A lower amount recovered in phase one versus phase two implies that the malabsorption is a result of a deficiency in the intrinsic factor. A bone marrow smear may show megaloblastic changes and erythroid hyperplasia secondary to an increase in the number of immature erythroid cells.

■ Ocular

Ocular diagnosis is based on direct observation of the retinal signs as previously outlined. The main complaint with optic nerve involvement will be a gradual decrease in visual acuity ("nutritional amblyopia"). Photophobia and pain behind the eyeball that is made worse by strong light has also been reported. This is believed to be caused by abnormal conduction within the nerve fibers due to myelin sheath dysfunction. The neural response becomes disseminated resulting in increased sensitivity. Color vision defects will occur, and perimetry or Amsler grid testing will show a central or central cecal scotoma. True "toxic amblyopia" from tobacco abuse may manifest with larger areas of the visual field affected.

The ocular manifestations of vitamin B$_{12}$ anemia include retinal hemorrhages, cotton-wool spots, venous dilation, and tortuosity. Peripheral capillary microaneurysms have also been reported.

TREATMENT AND MANAGEMENT

Dietary vitamin B$_{12}$ deficiency is treated by enhancing the diet with naturally occurring vitamin B$_{12}$ as well as with supplements (see Table 80–3). Vitamin B$_{12}$ is not found in plants except for in the roots of certain legumes that contain microorganisms that synthesize the B$_{12}$. It can be obtained from meats and meat products including red meat, fish, poultry, milk, and eggs. Only 10 to 20% of dietary vitamin B$_{12}$ is absorbed. The intake of iron and folic acid should be increased, because they too are involved in the production of red blood cells. Pernicious anemia is treated with parenteral injections of vitamin B$_{12}$. It is recommended that approximately 1–30 µg be given daily until levels increase followed by monthly injections for life. When managing nutritional optic neuropathy, the recommended therapy is to supplement the entire B complex rather than B$_{12}$ alone.

■ VITAMIN C

Vitamin C (ascorbic acid) is a water-soluble compound found in plasma, WBCs, and platelets. It is necessary in the formation of connective tissue and reducing capillary permeability. Along with the bioflavinoids, it also functions to strengthen capillaries, thereby minimizing the occurrence of hemorrhages. The presence of vitamin C enhances iron absorption and the ability to fight infection. It also promotes wound healing and healthy teeth, gums, and bones; converts food to energy; recycles vitamin E; and is one of the primary antioxidants. Scurvy, characterized by hemorrhages and abnormal formation of bones and teeth, is a well-documented consequence of vitamin C deprivation. In the eye, vitamin C deficiency has been associated with hemorrhages, cataracts, and possibly glaucoma.

EPIDEMIOLOGY

Although the classic vitamin C deficiency syndrome, scurvy, is rarely found today, various levels of deprivation often occur in the United States. Studies suggest that the prevalence of vitamin C deficiency is higher in the institutionalized elderly. This may be associated with food storage and cooking styles in institutions and a lack of interest in food.

NATURAL HISTORY

■ Systemic

Under normal circumstances, body stores can sustain periods of vitamin C deprivation for up to 3 to 4 months. During periods of increased stress, surgery, burns, smoking, and infection, the demand for vitamin C increases dramatically. Certain drugs like aspirin, antibiotics, cortisone, and oral contraceptives deplete body stores or increase the demand for this nutrient. The vitamin content of many foods is affected by cooking, processing, and storage. Vitamin C is particularly vulnerable, showing losses of up to 80%.

A subclinical vitamin C deficiency can exist prior to developing the classic signs and symptoms. This usually develops 2 to 3 months after the onset of dietary deficiency. The earliest clinical signs of vitamin C deficiency may include a tendency to bruise easily with petechial or ecchymotic hemorrhages into the skin, weakened hair or nails, and a low resistance to infection. In more advanced stages the classic deficiency syndrome known as scurvy may develop, resulting in arthritis; anorexia; nosebleeds; bleeding into the joints, muscles, and gums; impaired wound healing; ulcers; and impaired digestion. If untreated, death may occur. Prasad and Rama (1985) presented one of many reports suggesting that the antioxidant properties of vitamins A, C, and E and selenium may be necessary for preventing cancer because they reduce the formation and effectiveness of cancer-causing agents (see Table 80–1).

■ Ocular

There is an abundance of vitamin C in the eye. The normal aqueous humor level is 25 times that of plasma. The more common ocular manifestations of vitamin C deficiency are conjunctival petechial hemorrhages and recurrent subconjunctival hemorrhages (see Table 80–2). Prolonged deficiency may lead to retinal and orbital hemorrhages and hyphemas. Because vitamin C reduces capillary permeability and fragility, it is recommended in the management of diabetic retinopathy, macular degeneration, and central serous maculopathy. Some researchers have found that adequate levels seemed to decrease the risk of subcapsular cataracts via the role of vitamin C as an antioxidant. This association is supported by the fact that the normally high concentration of vitamin C in the lens decreases with cataract formation. The lack of vitamin C may slow healing of corneal ulcers and other wounds due to its role in collagen formation. Vimo and associates (1967) reported that megadoses of vitamin C (100 to 150 mg/kg 3 to 5 times daily) decreased intraocular pressure in patients with glaucoma. Lane (1980) observed that the average IOP was significantly lower in subjects with a mean daily intake of 1200 mg versus 75 mg. The significance of vitamin C as it relates to the onset or management of glaucoma is still under investigation. The most obvious problem is that megadoses often are not tolerated, and the duration and magnitude of the IOP decrease is limited.

DIAGNOSIS

■ Systemic

The symptoms of vitamin C deficiency may include weakness, headaches, shortness of breath, impaired digestion, and swollen or painful joints. Vitamin C status is directly assessed by measuring the serum and leukocyte ascorbic acid concentrations. Serum levels of less than 0.2 mg/dL are considered deficient. The urinary excretion test involves giving an oral dose of ascorbic acid and then measuring the amount released in the urine in 6 hours. Those with deficiency will excrete less of a given dose than those with adequate intake. Measuring urinary ascorbate levels is more effective to detect excesses of vitamin C than it is at detecting deficiencies.

■ Ocular

Observation of the clinical signs as previously outlined is the key to diagnosing ocular vitamin C deficiency. Retinal hemorrhages that involve the macula, hyphemas, or cataracts may lead to decreased vision.

TREATMENT AND MANAGEMENT

Some nutritionists suggest that the optimal intake should be greater than the RDA (see Table 80–3). This should be increased further when ill or during stress. Body stores are increased through ingestion of 500 mg daily. As a water-soluble nutrient, toxicity does not occur. However, by taking megadoses, the increased acidity can result in allergic reactions, diarrhea, or kidney stones. It is suggested that if supplements are taken, a buffered form should be used.

Todd (1987) reported successfully reversing cataracts with large daily doses in time-release capsules. Other studies report that megadoses will speed the healing of corneal ulcers.

Citrus fruits, papaya, cantaloupe, strawberries, green pepper, broccoli, spinach, tomatoes, sweet potatoes, and green leafy vegetables are good dietary sources of vitamin C.

VITAMIN D AND CALCIUM

Vitamin D is a fat-soluble micronutrient that is essential in the absorption and utilization of calcium and phosphorus. It primarily serves to elevate plasma levels of calcium and phosphorus by activating intestinal absorption, enhancing renal reabsorption, and mobilizing these minerals from the bone. In adults, the body's requirement is usually met by its own synthesis via exposure to ultraviolet radiation.

Calcium is a macromineral that constitutes about 85% of the mineral matter in bones as calcium phosphate. It is necessary for bone growth and metabolism, blood coagulation, healthy teeth, maintaining plasma pH balance, activating enzymes, controlling muscle contraction, neuromuscular excitability, and maintaining membrane permeability. It is a factor in efficient brain function, energy storage in muscles, and healthy digestive, circulatory, and immune systems. Vitamin D and the parathyroid hormones are the primary factors controlling calcium homeostasis.

Hypocalcemia and vitamin D deficiency are associated with rickets, osteomalacia, hyperparathyroidism, zonular cortical cataract, band keratopathy, conjunctival calcification, and impaired oculomotor function.

EPIDEMIOLOGY

The current practice of enriching food with vitamin D has made the incidence of deficiency very rare. However, vitamin D deficiency may still be found in countries where it is customary to be shielded from the sun (for example, due to certain clothing customs) or in breast-fed infants and those fed unfortified milk.

Up until the early 1900s, approximately 75% of children of working-class parents, in many industrialized countries, suffered from rickets. Today rickets will occasionally appear in children who are poverty stricken. Milder cases of calcium deficiency occur in association with hypoparathyroidism, nursing mothers, and poor dietary intake. Certain factors affect calcium absorption, such as the presence of phytic acid, commonly found in cereals, whole-meal breads, flour, and oatmeal. Calcium absorption is more efficient in males than in females, and the elderly may require a higher intake because inactivity, which often occurs with aging, causes skeletal demineralization.

NATURAL HISTORY

■ Systemic

A small drop in the concentration of serum calcium can lead to muscular cramping and uncontrolled muscle contractions known as tetany. Low serum calcium also leads to secondary hyperparathyroidism, because there is increased secretion of the parathyroid hormone, which in turn enhances mobilization of calcium from bone stores (see Table 80–1). Excessive parathyroid hormone causes phosphaturia, which interferes with bone calcification, resulting in rickets or osteomalacia. Rickets is a childhood disease caused by inadequate deposition of calcium lime salts in developing cartilage and newly formed bone. It is characterized by imperfect skeletal formation, enlarged odd-shaped head, thin skull, slight fever at night, free perspiration about head, pallor, slight diarrhea, enlargement of liver and spleen, and unhealthy teeth. Severe cases are marked by convulsions, hemorrhaging, and tetany. The prognosis is favorable, with deformity disappearing in 90% of treated cases. However, some bone deformities may require surgery. Osteomalacia is the adult form of rickets, which is metabolically identical to the form seen in children. However, because the longitudinal growth has stopped, only the shafts of the long and flat bones are affected. The bone mass is still of normal volume, but there is a loss of bone density. It is characterized by soft, pliable bones that become structurally deformed. Osteomalacia is most often related to diseases causing malabsorption like chronic pancreatitis, celiac disease, Crohn disease, gastric and small bowel resections, fistulas, chronic ulcerative colitis, and biliary obstruction. Other signs of vitamin D and calcium deficiency include insomnia, pale skin, sensitivity to pain, and poor healing of bone injuries.

■ Ocular

Zonular cortical cataracts may appear months or years after the onset of hypocalcemia (see Table 80–2). Typically they develop gradually, forming small, punc-

tate, discrete refractile opacities that are separated from the capsule by a clear zone. These are usually bilateral and seldom interfere with vision. Extraocular muscle deficits are also associated with later stages of deficiency.

Hyperparathyroidism is associated with band keratopathy and conjunctival calcification, because calcium is mobilized from the body reserve, resulting in calcium deposition into various body tissues.

DIAGNOSIS

Adults that are deficient in vitamin D or calcium will complain of rheumatic pains in the limbs, spine, thorax, and pelvis; progressive weakness; nervous system hyperirritability; depression; headaches; and insomnia. A child with rickets may exhibit restlessness, slight fever at night, free perspiration about the head, diffuse soreness and tenderness of the body, and headaches. Radiographs will show characteristic bony deformities or decrease in bone density. The status of vitamin D is indirectly measured by serum calcium, phosphorus, and alkaline phosphatase activity. Analysis will show normal or low plasma calcium (norms: 8.5 to 10.5 mg/dL), low phosphorus levels (below 2.5 mg/dL), and increased plasma alkaline phosphatase activity. A direct measure of the vitamin D status is now available which assesses the plasma level of the vitamin D metabolite, hydroxyvitamin D.

Normal serum calcium levels range from 8.9 to 10.1 mg/dL. Serum calcium is not a useful indicator of dietary calcium intake. Urinary calcium reflects intake to some extent, but further research is needed regarding the nature of this relationship. Hair analysis is a useful method for obtaining the average level of the body's mineral content over a several-month period. Trace elements are accumulated in hair at a rate 10 times higher than in blood serum or urine. The areas where it is most useful is in showing inefficient absorption and toxic levels of minerals such as calcium, magnesium, zinc, manganese, and chromium. This mode of diagnostic testing is often criticized because comparisons of data from different laboratories often show large variations. Also, hair and serum values do not always correlate well, because serum levels give an instantaneous picture of mineral status. Hair analysis indicates the average level over the last 2 to 3 months, yet it can be a useful addition to serum and urine analysis as a diagnostic tool.

TREATMENT AND MANAGEMENT

Exposure to sunlight along with oral vitamin D daily is the suggested therapy for rickets. Osteomalacia is treated with vitamin D for approximately one month followed by the normal daily requirement of vitamin D, calcium, and phosphorous, as outlined in Table 80–3.

Normally 800 to 1300 mg of calcium daily is sufficient to prevent deficiency. Only about 30 to 60% of the normal dietary calcium is absorbed. In cases of malabsorption, dietary fat should be restricted to 30 g daily.

Good dietary sources of vitamin D include beans, chard, cheese, egg yolk, milk, molasses, shellfish, tuna, salmon, cod liver oil, and watercress. Calcium can be obtained from rhubarb, nuts, beets, bran, green vegetables, cauliflower, carrots, dates, lemons, oranges, parsnips, pineapples, raspberries, rutabagas, milk, cheese, and yogurt.

■ VITAMIN E

There are seven naturally occurring forms of vitamin E. The most active form is tocopherol. Vitamin E is associated with the lipid fraction of cells and membranes. As an antioxidant it serves to protect vitamin A from oxidation and prevent lipid peroxidation of cell membranes. It also serves an important role in maintaining vascular health by protecting red blood cells from lysis, stabilizing blood vessel cell walls, reducing thrombin formation, and promoting healthy reproductive, neurological, and muscular systems. Sufficient quantities of vitamin E are necessary in people who exercise. This protects the fatty acids from oxidative destruction and provides the body with extra energy for muscle contractions.

The National Institutes of Health reported in 1983 that vitamin E was an essential nutrient in retinal function by preventing the oxidation of vitamin A and by preventing the peroxidation of photoreceptor lipoproteins. Its role in retinopathy of prematurity is well documented. Vitamin E deficiency is also implicated in cataract formation, eye movement abnormalities, pigmentary retinopathy, and central serous retinopathy.

EPIDEMIOLOGY

Clinical vitamin E deficiency has only been reported in premature infants and newborns, and in association with conditions causing malabsorption of lipids, cystic fibrosis, or biliary atresia (obstructive liver disease). Yet many more Americans may be deficient, because life styles that produce an abundance of free radicals will increase the need for vitamin E. The National Institutes of Health reported that the average American diet only contains approximately 10 IU daily. In addition, cooking over high heat and food processing leads to oxidation and loss of vitamin E. Also, vitamin E is lost in vegetable oils because it is taken out to be sold separately as a supplement.

NATURAL HISTORY

■ Systemic
Free-radical damage can affect many systems (see Table 80–1). In chronic deficiency there may be loss of the skin's elasticity. The vascular system may respond with strokes, hemorrhages, and poor wound healing, and there may be respiratory difficulties or an increased susceptibility to myocardial infarction. Rosenblum and associates (1981) reported the occurrence of a progressive neurological syndrome that is believed to occur if vitamin E is deficient during the development of the nervous system. This syndrome is characterized by hyporeflexia, gait disturbance, truncal ataxia, vertigo, transient loss of vision, decreased adduction, nystagmus on adduction, and limited superior gaze.

■ Ocular
Vitamin E deficiency can result in night blindness and visual dysfunction because one of its roles is to maintain the integrity of vitamin A (see Table 80–2). Because vitamin E is highly concentrated in the photoreceptor outer segments, it is thought to protect its photoreceptor membranes from oxidative damage. Therefore, when vitamin E is deficient, it may initiate the process of lipofuscin formation within the retinal pigment epithelial cell with subsequent damage to the RPE cell membrane. This may lead to inefficient metabolism of the rod and cone outer segments and cell death. The cell's contents are then deposited extracellularly in the form of drusen. Macular degeneration may develop if this process occurs in the macular region and other risk factors for macular degeneration are present (genetic traits, exposure to UV light, presence of cardiovascular disease, and cigarette smoking).

Berger and colleagues (1991) reported a generalized retinal pigment epithelium dropout and pigment clumping in chronic vitamin E deficiency in the presence of normal vitamin A levels (Figure 80–4). The mechanism for the occurrence of this pigmentary retinopathy is thought to be the same mechanism that causes macular degeneration.

In the presence of increased oxygen, vitamin E deficiency can enhance oxidative injury to retinal capillaries forming in the developing eye. This results in retinopathy of prematurity.

Jacques and co-workers (1988) and others have reported a statistically significant relationship between vitamin E deficiency and lens opacification. Because the oxidative process causes unfolding and cross-linkages with other proteins, they postulate that vitamin E serves to stabilize lens protein oxidation.

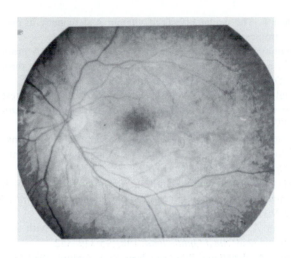

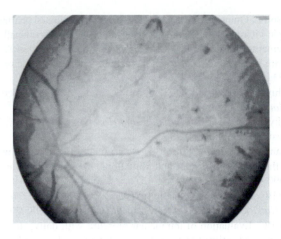

Figure 80–4. Widespread depigmentation, pigment clumping **A**, narrowing of retinal arterioles, and scalloped foci of pigment dropout within the vascular arcades, and loss of the foveal reflex **B**, secondary to vitamin E deficiency. *(Reprinted with permission from Berger AS, Tychsen E, Rosenblum JL, Retinopathy in human vitamin E deficiency.* Am J Ophthalmol. *1991;3:774.)*

The ocular manifestations of progressive neurologic dysfunction related to vitamin E deficiency include decreased adduction, nystagmus on adduction, and limited superior gaze.

DIAGNOSIS

■ Systemic
Systemic manifestations include hyperreflexia, gait disturbance, truncal ataxia, and vertigo. The available laboratory diagnostic tests are serum vitamin E levels and erythrocyte tocopherol levels.

■ Ocular
Ocular diagnosis of vitamin E deficiency is suspected when a patient complains of night vision problems, decreased visual acuity that is not correctable with a refractive prescription, transient loss of vision, and limited ability to adduct or elevate the eyes. Examination may reveal constricted and depressed visual fields, reduced color vision, increased dark adaptation threshold, or attenuated electroretinogram signals.

TREATMENT AND MANAGEMENT

Daily doses of vitamin E are recommended until resolution of the signs and symptoms, followed by RDA requirements (see Table 80–3), however, nutritionists rec-

ommend a larger suggested daily intake. Good dietary sources are green leafy vegetables, whole grains, vegetable and seed oils (safflower oil has the highest content), wheat germ, sweet potatoes, seeds, and peanuts.

REFERENCES

Berger AS, Tychsen E, Rosenblum JL. Retinopathy in human vitamin E deficiency. *Am J Ophthalmol.* 1991;3:774–775.

Day PL, Langston WC, O'Brien CS. Cataract and other ocular changes in vitamin G deficiency: An experimental study on albino rats. *Am J Ophthalmol.* 1931;14:1005–1009.

Fells P, Bors F. Ocular complications of self-induced vitamin A deficiency. *Trans Ophthalmol Soc UK.* 1969;89:221–228.

Frei B, England L, Ames BN. Ascorbate is an outstanding antioxidant in human blood plasma. *Proc Natl Acad Sci USA.* 1989;86:6377–6381.

Genest AA, Sarwono D, Gyorgy P. Vitamin A blood serum levels and electroretinogram in five to fourteen year old age groups in Indonesia and Thailand: A preliminary report. *Am J Clin Nutrition.* 1967;20:1275–1279.

Goodhart RS, Shils ME. *Modern Nutrition in Health and Disease.* 6th ed. Philadelphia: Lea & Febiger; 1980.

Hamilton HE, Ellis PP, Sheets RF. Visual impairment due to optic neuropathy in pernicious anemia: Report of a case and review of the literature. *Blood.* 1959;14:378–385.

Hittner HM, Rudolph AJ, Kretzer FL. Suppression of severe retinopathy of prematurity with vitamin E therapy: Ultrastructural mechanism of clinical efficacy. *Ophthalmology.* 1984;91:1512.

Jacques PF, Hartz SC, Chylack LT, et al. Nutritional status in persons with and without senile cataract: Blood vitamin and mineral levels. *Am J Clin Nutr.* 1988;48:152–158.

Johnson L, Quinn GE, Abbasi S, et al. Effect of sustained pharmacologic vitamin E levels on incidence and severity of retinopathy of prematurity: A controlled clinical trial. *J Pediatr.* 1989;114:827.

Ibrahim K, Kara RY, Zuberi SJ. Hypercarotenemia: A case report. *JPMA.* 1976;224–225.

Krishna SM, Pramod KS. Vitamin A and primary glaucoma. *Glaucoma.* 1982;4:226–227.

Kutsky R. *Handbook of Vitamins and Hormones.* New York: Van Nostrand Reinhold; 1973.

Lamand M, Favier A, Pineau A. Determination of trace elements in the hair: Significance and limitations. *Ann Biologie Clinique.* 1990;48:433–442.

Lane BC. Nutrition and vision. In: Bland J, ed. *1984–85 Yearbook of Nutritional Medicine.* New Canaan, CT: Keats; 1985:273.

Lane BC. Evaluation of intraocular pressure with daily, sustained closework stimulus to accommodation to lowered tissue chromium and dietary deficiency of ascorbic acid. PhD dissertation, 1980, New York University.

Lascari AD. Carotenemia. *Clin Pediatr.* 1981;20:25.

Maugh TH. Hair: A diagnostic tool to complement blood serum and urine. *Science.* 1978;202:1271.

Mueller JF, Vilter RW. Pyridoxine deficiency in human beings induced with desoxypyridoxine. *J Clin Invest.* 1950;29:193.

Murray MT. Iron: Deficiencies and supplements. *Health Counselor.* Nov/Dec 1991:31–33.

Paton D, Mclaren DS. Bitot spots. *Am J Ophthalmol.* 1960; 50:568.

Pihl RO, Parks M. Hair element content in learning-disabled children. *Science.* 1977;198:204–206.

Prasad K, Rama B. Nutrition and cancer. In: Bland J, ed. *1984–85 Yearbook of Nutritional Medicine.* New Canaan, CT: Keats; 1985.

Rapp J. Nutrition in the vision of children. *J Am Opt Assoc.* 1979;50:1107–1111.

Rengstorff RH, Krall CC, Westerhout DI. Topical anitioxidant treatment for dry-eye disorders and contact lens-related complications. *Afro-Asian J Ophthalmol.* 1988;7:81–83.

Rodger F. The ocular effects of vitamin A deficiency in man in the tropics. *Exp Eye Res.* 1964;3:367–372.

Rosenblum JD, Keating JP, Prensky AL, Nelson JS. A progressive neurologic syndrome in children with chronic liver disease. *N Engl J Med.* 1991;304:503.

Russel RM, Smith VC, Multack R, et al. Dark adaptation testing for diagnosis of subclinical vitamin A deficiency. *Lancet.* 1973;2:1161–1163.

Semba R, Sopandi W, Natadisastra M, Sommer A. Response of Bitot's Spot in Preschool Children to Vitamin A Treatment. *Am J Ophthalmol.* 1990;110:416–420.

Senile cataract and vitamin nutrition. *Nutr. Rev.* 1989;47:326–328.

Sommer A. New imperatives for an old vitamin (A). *J Nutrition.* 1989;119:96–100.

Sommer A. Treatment of corneal Xerophthalmia with topical retinoic acid. *Am J Ophthalmol.* 1983;95:349–352.

Sommer A. *Nutritional Blindness.* New York: Oxford; 1982:51–52.

Sommer A, Emran N, Tjakrasudjatma S. Clinical characteristics of vitamin A responsive and nonresponsive Bitot's spots. *Am J Ophthalmol.* 1980;90:160.

Sommer A, Quesada J, Doty M, Faich G. Xerophthalmia and anterior segment blindness among preschool children in El Salvador. *Am J Ophthalmol.* 1975;80:1066.

Sommer A, Sugana T, Djunaedi E, Green R. Vitamin A responsive panocular xerophthalmia in healthy adult. *Arch Ophthalmol.* 1978;96:1630–1634.

Sommer A, Tarwotjo I, Hussaini G, Susanto D. Increased mortality in mild vitamin A deficiency. *Lancet.* 1983;2:585–588.

Stern JJ. Nutrition in ophthalmology. In: Goodhart R, Shils M, eds. *Modern Nutrition in Health and Disease.* 5th ed. Philadelphia: Lea & Febiger; 1973:1009.

Todd GP. *Nutrition in Health and Disease.* Norfolk, VA: Donning; 1987.

Tomasi LG. Reversibility of human myopathy caused by vitamin E deficiency. *Neurology.* 1979;29:1182–1186.

Wohbach S, Howe P. Tissue changes following deprivation of fat soluble vitamin A. *J Exp Med.* 1925;42:753–777.

81
Chapter

Mineral Deficiencies

Tanya L. Carter

Minerals are important components of hormones and enzymes. They are vital for cellular function and also serve as building blocks for bones, teeth, muscles, plasma cells, and neuronal tissue. As electrolytes, they serve to control neuromuscular contractions and help maintain osmotic pressure as well as the acid–base balance of internal fluids. Minerals also play a role in the digestive and reproductive systems. Calcium (see Chapter 80), chloride, magnesium, potassium, phosphorus, sodium, and sulfur are classified as macrominerals; while copper, cobalt, chromium, fluorine, iodine, iron, manganese, selenium, and zinc are the trace minerals. The Senate Select Committee on Nutrition reported that 99% of the American population is deficient in at least one mineral.

■ IODINE

Iodine is important in the development and function of the thyroid gland and in manufacturing the hormone thyroxine, which controls the rate at which cells utilize energy from food. It also is essential in the proper functioning of the heart and immune systems as well as protein synthesis. Additionally, iodine deficiency is the most common cause of endemic goiter. Associated hypothyroidism may lead to photophobia, cataracts, eyelid edema, and optic neuropathy.

EPIDEMIOLOGY

Iodine deficiency is more prevalent in areas near freshwater lakes as opposed to those near the seacoast. In many highland areas of America, like states bordering Canada and areas between the Rocky and Appalachian Mountains, the soil is not rich in iodine and many people suffer from dietary deprivation. The process of putting iodine in salt has significantly decreased the incidence of deficiency. Yet it is estimated that approximately 200 million people throughout the world suffer from goiter caused by iodine deficiency.

NATURAL HISTORY

■ Systemic
Almost 80% of dietary iodine is absorbed by the thyroid gland and is bound with the amino acid tyrosine to form tri-iodothyronine (T3) and thyroxine (T4). The main function of these thyroid hormones is to control the basal metabolic rate. Iodine deficiency is one cause of goiter, characterized by thyroid enlargement and hypothyroidism (Table 81–1). Physical, sexual, and mental development may be inhibited, and there is lowered resistance to infection and lowered basal metabolism. Signs include obesity, dry skin, dry hair, poor complexion, unhealthy nails, low blood pressure, slow pulse, sluggishness of all functions, and nervous irritability.

■ Ocular
The ocular manifestations of hypothyroidism include photophobia, cataracts, periorbital or eyelid edema, and optic

TABLE 81–1. SYSTEMIC AND OCULAR MANIFESTATIONS OF IODINE DEFICIENCIES

- ■ **SYSTEMIC**
  GOITER/HYPOTHYROIDISM
  - Enlarged thyroid gland, obesity, dry skin and hair, poor complexion, unhealthy nails, sluggishness of all functions, nervous irritability, lowered resistance to infection, hypotension, slow pulse, inhibitions of physical, sexual, and mental development

- ■ **OCULAR**
  - Edema (periorbital or eyelid)
  - Photophobia
  - Cataract
  - Optic neuropathy

TABLE 81–2. TREATMENT AND MANAGEMENT OF IODINE DEFICIENCY

- • RDA: Infants: 40 µg
          Children: 50–120 µg
          Adults: 150 µg
          Pregnant: 200 µg

Reprinted with permission from Food and Nutrition Board Commission of Life Sciences National Research Council. Recommended Daily Allowances. Washington, DC: National Academy Press; 1989.

neuropathy (Table 81–1). See Chapter 18 for a more detailed discussion of this condition.

DIAGNOSIS

Iodine deficiency is diagnosed by assessing urinary iodine. Levels that are less than 25 µg/g creatine are considered deficient. In primary hypothyroidism, laboratory evaluation will show high levels of serum thyroid-stimulating hormone (TSH) and decreased levels of T3 and T4 hormones. It is important to remember that changes in the serum-binding protein levels will affect measured T3 and T4. T3 uptake reflects the level of unsaturated thyroid hormone binding sites. The ability of the thyroid gland to take up radioactive iodine is also used as a diagnostic tool.

TREATMENT AND MANAGEMENT

Table 81–2 describes the treatment and management of iodine deficiency. Good dietary sources of iodine include fresh seafish, seaweed, garlic, leafy greens, celery, tomatoes, radishes, carrots, onions, and iodized salt. If iodine deficiency is suspected, a referral to an endocrinologist or internist is recommended.

■ IRON

Iron is needed for the production of erythrocytes. It also binds oxygen to hemoglobin for transport to body tissues. The body has a high demand for iron, and this often is not satisfied by the average American diet. There are two different types of iron, nonheme (mainly from vegetables) and heme (from meat and fish), which is absorbed more efficiently. Microcytic anemia is produced in deficiency states. Iron deficiency is also associated with alterations in cellular function, growth, motor development, behavior, and cognitive function. The gastrointestinal and other organ systems are affected. Ocular manifestations may include subconjunctival or flame-shape retinal hemorrhages, retinal ischemia, and distended/tortuous veins.

EPIDEMIOLOGY

Iron deficiency is considered the most common chronic disease of humankind and the most common cause of anemia throughout the world. It is more prevalent in countries where there are meat shortages; however, it is estimated that at least 18 million people in the United States are iron deficient. The primary cause of iron deficiency is inadequate dietary intake, malabsorption, and chronic blood loss. In food, iron is bound to proteins and amino acids and must be reduced for absorption. Vitamin C and other gastric acids serve to reduce the complex, thereby enhancing absorption. Many components in foods, such as phytates (a carbohydrate in whole grains), fiber, egg yolks, and tea, may bind iron, thereby making it unavailable for absorption. This is true for many other minerals. Females are very susceptible to iron deficiency because of blood loss during menstruation and the high iron demand during pregnancy.

NATURAL HISTORY

■ Systemic

Early stages of iron deficiency result in malfunctioning of the iron-dependent enzymes involved in energy production and metabolism. Marginal deficiency can affect immune function, which can lead to an increased incidence and chronicity of infections such as candida albicans and colds. The long-term and final stage of iron deficiency is anemia (Table 81–3), which usually develops very gradually.

TABLE 81–3. SYSTEMIC AND OCULAR MANIFESTATIONS OF IRON DEFICIENCY

- **SYSTEMIC**
  - Microcytic anemia
    - Chronic fatigue
    - Dyspnea
    - Palpitations, tachycardia
    - Pale skin, opaque or brittle nails
    - Increased rate of infections
    - Lymphatic tissue shrinkage
  - Menorrhagia
  - Learning disabilities

- **OCULAR**
  - Subconjunctival hemorrhages
  - Retinal hemorrhages
  - Cotton wool spots
  - Retinal venous tortuosity
  - Retinal pallor

Chronic iron deficiency can also lead to menorrhagia (excessive menstrual flow). Signs of anemia include chronic fatigue, dyspnea, palpitation, tachycardia, pale skin, opaque or brittle nails, increased rate of infections, and lymphatic tissue shrinkage. Iron deficiency has also been implicated in learning disabilities because of the effect on brain function. It is associated with decreased attentiveness, narrower attention span, and decreased voluntary activity.

Ocular

Severe anemia can lead to subconjunctival and flame-shape retinal hemorrhages, cotton-wool spots, retinal pallor, and distended, tortuous veins (see Table 81–3).

DIAGNOSIS

Systemic

Iron deficiency is diagnosed through observation of the clinical signs and symptoms, which include chronic fatigue, shortness of breath, and headache. If deficiency is suspected, appropriate laboratory testing should be obtained. The more commonly used procedures include serum iron assay, serum ferritin assay, total iron-binding capacity (TIBC), percent serum transferrin saturation and complete blood count. The serum iron assay measures the amount of iron bound to transferrin (plasma iron-transport protein) The direct measurement of serum iron can be unreliable, because levels vary considerably over a short period of time. Serum ferritin is the chief iron-storage protein in the body and correlates with total body iron stores. Detecting low ferritin levels is specific for iron deficiency, because only two other conditions will cause a decrease in ferritin: hypothyroidism and ascorbate deficiency. Unfortunately, this test is not always available. The total iron binding capacity (TIBC) test is also used diagnostically. This is thought to be the most sensitive diagnostic test. The normal TIBC value ranges from 150 to 300 µg/dL. In deficiency states the TIBC value will increase from 350 to 500 µg/dL. TIBC is also used to determine the percentage of transferrin saturation (serum iron value divided by the TIBC). Normally, transferrin is about 30% saturated.

A complete blood count (CBC) includes an assessment of the number of red blood cells, hematocrit (Hct), and hemoglobin (Hgb), along with various morphologic indices that are used to differentiate the type of anemia. These indices include mean corpuscular volume (MCV), mean corpuscular hemoglobin (MCH), and mean corpuscular hemoglobin concentration (MCHC). A fall in the RBC count below 2.5 million/mm^3 is diagnostic for anemia. The MCV reflects the size of the red blood cells; those produced during iron deficiency are usually smaller (microcytic). An MCV of less than 80 µm^3 is diagnostic for microcytic cells. The Hct count is a measure of the number of cells in a given volume of blood. The Hct may drop by as much as 30% before signs or symptoms manifest. The Hgb status is reflected in the overall Hgb concentration and the MCH. MCH is a measure of the hemoglobin content of each RBC, which determines the color. The normal Hgb concentration is 12 to 16 g/dL of blood for females and 14 to 18 g/dL in males. MCH level below 26 pg is diagnostic and is termed hypochromic. MCHC is also a measure of chronicity. Normal MCHC levels range from 32 to 36%. The white blood cell count and function may also be altered in deficiency states.

Urinary iron tests are not useful because iron is not normally excreted in the urine. Hair analysis may be useful as a compliment to serum analysis; however, its validity is still questionable. Studies by Lamand and associates (1990) indicate that caution must be taken when using data from hair analysis because the environmental minerals will be absorbed by the hair and the different steps in the hair analysis process may modify the mineral composition.

TREATMENT AND MANAGEMENT

Most cases of iron deficiency are managed with oral ferrous sulfate or ferrous gluconate along with a balanced diet

TABLE 81–4. TREATMENT AND MANAGEMENT OF IRON DEFICIENCY

- RDA: Adult males: 10 µg
          Adult females: 18 µg
          Pregnant: 30–60 µg
- With malabsorption, the non-heme iron is more effective than ferrous sulfate salts.

Reprinted with permission from Food and Nutrition Board Commission of Life Sciences National Research Council. Recommended Daily Allowances. Washington, DC: National Academy Press; 1989.

(Table 81–4). In cases of poor absorption, nonheme iron is more effective than the ferrous sulfate salts. In severe deficiency, iron injections or transfusions may be necessary. Iron supplements are highly recommended and the demand usually is not met with the average diet, because only 10% of dietary iron is absorbed. In addition to initiating iron supplements, the exact cause of the iron deficiency should be determined to rule out a slow-bleeding cancer or ulcer. A referral to a hematologist or internist is recommended to best manage the anemia.

When treating iron deficiency, it is important to realize that after menopause, women build up their iron stores. Therefore, women who are taking supplements may develop an abundance of iron. Excess iron acts as a catalyst in certain reactions that produce free radicals, and it competes with chromium for blood protein-binding sites. A shortage of chromium may lead to various metabolic disorders such as an inability to maintain appropriate blood glucose levels.

Dietary sources of iron include egg yolks, leafy green vegetables, dried beans, peaches, apricots, dates, prunes, raisins, cherries, figs, and blackstrap molasses.

■ POTASSIUM

Potassium is an electrolyte that regulates osmotic pressure and helps maintain the alkaline pH of internal body fluids. The proper balance of potassium, calcium, and magnesium is necessary in the conduction of nerve impulses and for neuromuscular contractions. It is also necessary for the normal health of the adrenal glands and the generalized electrophysiology of cells. Low potassium intake has been associated with renal dysfunction, hypertension, possibly strokes, weakness of extraocular muscles, dry eyes, and deposits on contact lenses.

EPIDEMIOLOGY

There are no available data on the incidence and prevalence of potassium deprivation. However, adequate levels of

dietary potassium are most often easily maintained. Yet potassium deprivation does occur due to various disorders that produce excess urinary or gastrointestinal loss and dietary deficiency of meat and vegetables. The more common depleting factors include alcohol abuse, stress, laxatives, diarrhea, enemas, excess salt, diabetic acidosis, renal disease, and the widespread use of steroids and diuretics.

NATURAL HISTORY

■ Systemic

Potassium deficiency leads to functional and structural changes in the kidneys. Renal disease may develop after short periods of deprivation and severe, prolonged deficiency can lead to irreversible damage. Clinical signs include an inability to concentrate and acidify urine, nocturia, muscle weakness or paralysis, unhealthy-looking skin, slow-healing injuries, and edema (Table 81–5). These signs can occur rapidly and are easily reversible with oral potassium chloride. When the gastrointestinal system is the site for potassium loss, clinical signs and symptoms may not develop for many years. Current research shows that potassium has a role in preventing hypertension.

■ Ocular

Potassium deficiency is associated with fatigue and weakness of the extraocular muscles (see Table 81–5). Lane (1985) reported that potassium deficiency plays a role in contact lens coating, dry-eye syndrome, and oculomotor as well as accommodative dysfunction.

DIAGNOSIS

■ Systemic

Patients may complain of muscle weakness, irregular heartbeat, impaired neuromuscular function, poor reflexes, ner-

TABLE 81–5. SYSTEMIC AND OCULAR MANIFESTATIONS OF POTASSIUM DEFICIENCY

- **SYSTEMIC**
  - Renal disease
  - Hypertension
  - Possible strokes
  - Unhealthy skin
  - **Signs and Symptoms**
    Nocturia, muscle weakness, edema, slow-healing injuries, irregular heartbeat, poor reflexes, nervousness, lethargy, constipation, insomnia

- **OCULAR**
  - Dry eyes
  - Oculomotor and accomodative dysfunction

TABLE 81–6. TREATMENT AND MANAGEMENT OF POTASSIUM DEFICIENCY

- RDA: None
- SOI: 1.8–5.6 g/d

vousness, dizziness, lethargy, insomnia, and constipation. The more commonly utilized diagnostic laboratory tests are serum and urinary analysis. A basic blood chemistry analysis, which includes a fasting potassium assay, should be performed. Urinary analysis of electrolytes is usually of limited value because the wide range of water and electrolyte intake from the diet leads to a wide range of normal values. Hair analysis may be obtained as a complement to the serum and urinary analysis.

■ Ocular

The symptoms associated with potassium deficiency include burning, tearing, inability to successfully wear contact lenses, and diplopia.

TREATMENT AND MANAGEMENT

The Food and Nutrition Board does not report an RDA for potassium. Yet, some nutritionists suggest an optimal daily intake (Table 81–6). Good dietary sources include oranges, bananas, cantaloupes, avocados, dates, prunes, dried apricots, raisins, watermelon, whole grains, seeds, nuts, peas, beans, milk, fresh fish, beef, and poultry.

■ ZINC

Zinc is an important component of several enzyme systems that are involved in the metabolism of nucleic acids, proteins, carbohydrates, and alcohol. It is a co-enzyme that is required in DNA/RNA synthesis and vitamin A use. It serves as an antioxidant in protecting cell membranes against peroxidative damage. The ocular manifestations of zinc deficiency can include macular degeneration, optic neuropathy, low intraocular pressure, and possibly cataracts.

EPIDEMIOLOGY

Zinc deficiency in humans was first reported in 1961 in the Middle East in people whose diet was high in breads and low in animal protein. The Senate Select Committee on Nutrition reported that 85% of the population is deficient in zinc.

Factors that can lead to deficiency include poor dietary intake; stress; deficient soils used to grow food; excessive levels of copper and cadmium that compete with zinc for cellular sites; the use of EDTA in foods for chelation of certain metals; use of drugs and foods that contain phytic acid or fiber that will chelate zinc; excessive loss of body fluids as in perspiration and increased urination (often associated with alcohol abuse and diuretics); and diseases that affect zinc metabolism like alcoholic cirrhosis and acrodermatitis enteropathica (a disease of the skin of the extremities that is caused by a genetically determined malabsorption of zinc).

NATURAL HISTORY

■ Systemic
Zinc deficiency can manifest as atherosclerosis, failure to grow, anorexia, testicular atrophy, skin lesions, skin stretch marks, acne, psoriasis, opaque fingernails, brittle hair, and lowered levels of plasma vitamin A (Table 81–7). Zinc's role in protein synthesis has lead to the controversial association between zinc deficiency and learning disabilities. One theory of the effect of zinc on learning is that "active protein synthesis is required for new memory formation" (Yolton, 1981). Further research is required for this topic.

■ Ocular
The high concentration in ocular tissues has lead to much research regarding ocular findings (see Table 81–7). The literature varies on the importance of zinc in cataract formation. Animal studies found cataract development corre-

TABLE 81–7. SYSTEMIC AND OCULAR MANIFESTATIONS OF ZINC DEFICIENCY

- **SYSTEMIC**
  - Growth failure
  - Testicular atrophy
  - Skin disease: acne, psoriasis, opaque fingernails, brittle hair, skin stretch marks
  - Learning disability
  - Atherosclerosis
  - Lack of taste and smell

- **OCULAR**
  - Dry eyes
  - Cataracts
  - Macular degeneration
  - Optic neuropathy
  - Night blindness
  - Dyschromotopsia
  - Low IOP

lated with zinc-deficient diets. Todd (1987) found that 20 mg of zinc daily would reverse cataract in humans. Todd claimed a 67% success rate using zinc along with other vitamins. Other mineral deficiencies that have been associated with cataracts are calcium, chromium, magnesium, and selenium. These minerals are components of antioxidative enzymes and therefore have an antioxidative role.

Recent research suggest that macular degeneration may be associated with a lack of zinc-dependent enzyme. This enzyme is responsible for the metabolism of retinal byproducts by the RPE cells. Newsome and associates (1988) reported less visual loss in a group of patients with macular degeneration given 100 mg bid zinc sulfate supplements, and also noted that those who developed macular degeneration had a tendency toward zinc deficiency.

Because of the high concentration of zinc in the retina and optic nerve, there is speculation that zinc's role in axoplasmic transport may lead to optic neuropathy in deficiency states. Certain toxic optic neuropathies may be associated with zinc deficiency, because many of the associated drugs are zinc chelators. These toxic neuropathies begin with red/green dyschromatopsia and retrobulbar neuropathy in their early states.

Zinc's role in vitamin A metabolism may cause signs and symptoms that are common to vitamin A deficiency. Zinc helps maintain normal serum levels of vitamin A by mobilizing it from the liver. Zinc also plays a role in transforming retinol to retinaldehyde for utilization by the rods, thus playing a role in night blindness.

Low levels of zinc have been associated with low intraocular pressure. As a coenzyme of carbonic anhydrase, zinc is involved in aqueous production. Decreased zinc levels may lead to reduced carbonic anhydrase activity, thus lowering the IOP.

DIAGNOSIS

■ Systemic

Symptoms of zinc deficiency include lack of taste or smell, dry irritated skin, poor appetite, and fatigue. Normal serum zinc values range from 0.75 to 1.4 µg/mL. Dietary zinc deficiency may not result in lowered plasma levels because blood zinc is sensitive to a wide range of nondietary factors. The use of hair analysis as a diagnostic tool is becoming more widespread. Kobayashi and associates (1991) reported that marginal zinc deficiencies can be assessed through hair analysis.

■ Ocular

The corresponding symptoms associated with zinc deprivation are decreased visual acuity, dyschromatopsia, and night blindness.

TABLE 81–8. TREATMENT AND MANAGEMENT OF ZINC DEFICIENCY

- Oral:15–45 mg/d
- RDA: Infants 3 mg
  Children: 10 mg
  Adults: 20 mg
  Pregnant/lactation: 30 mg
- **Cataracts:** 20 mg/d
- **Macular degeneration:** 30 mg/d as preventative therapy
  100 mg/d therapeutic dose
- Must monitor closely because toxicity may occur with doses greater than 45 mg/d.
- Todd (1987) suggests 25,000 IU vitamin A, 400 IU vitamin E and vitamin C, 1000 µg Biotin, 50 mg L-glutathione, 1 tbsp lecithin granules, and reducing dietary fat.

TREATMENT AND MANAGEMENT

■ Systemic

Therapeutic daily doses of zinc are suggested in deficiency states (Table 81–8). This type of therapy should be closely monitored by a trained nutritionist, because zinc toxicity may occur with doses greater than 45 mg/d. Excessive zinc interferes with the metabolism of other minerals like iron and copper, and can distort the ratio of HDL/LDL cholesterol levels. Therefore it is recommended that iron and copper are given in conjunction with zinc therapy. Good dietary sources include milk, eggs, poultry, seafood, red meat, onions, peas, soybeans, mushrooms, whole grains, nuts, and seeds. Soils are often deficient in zinc, making supplements an important source.

■ Ocular

Specific treatment regimens relative to zinc have been outlined for the management of cataracts and macular degeneration (see Table 81–8). The recommended dosage of zinc for the treatment of macular degeneration varies among investigators. Todd (1987) suggests managing macular degeneration with a daily vitamin and mineral regimen (see Table 81–8), as well as reducing fat consumption as much as possible in order to reduce free-radical damage.

■ CONCLUSION

Good nutritional status is required for adequate biological function, and the ocular structures are no exception. Nutritional deficiencies are more common in the elderly, chronic illness, endocrine imbalances, inability to chew, physical handicaps, and fad diets, and in those impoverished and institutionalized. It is important to realize that it is prudent to maintain an overall good nutritional balance, because nutrients function interdependently and sometimes synergistically. Therefore, eyecare practitioners should be aware of the ocular manifestations of nutritional deficiency, and should consider obtaining a good nutritional history in addition to a medical history when indicated. If a deficiency is suspected, a referral for laboratory analysis and nutritional counseling should be considered. Before nutritional therapy is initiated, an evaluation from a family physician or internist should be obtained to rule out any contraindications or conflict with existing medical management.

REFERENCES

Bhat KS. Nutritional status of thiamine, riboflavin and pyridoxine in cataract patients. *Nutr Rep Int.* 1987;36:685–692.

Bhat KS. Distribution of HMW proteins and crystallins in cataractous lenses from undernourished and well-nourished subjects. *Exp Eye Res.* 1983;37:267–271.

Frei B, England L, Ames BN. Ascorbate is an outstanding antioxidant in human blood plasma. *Proc Natl Acad Sci USA.* 1989;86:6377–6381.

Goodhart RS, Shils ME. *Modern Nutrition in Health and Disease.* 6th ed. Philadelphia: Lea & Febiger; 1980.

Hamilton HE, Ellis PP, Sheets RF. Visual impairment due to optic neuropathy in pernicious anemia: Report of a case and review of the literature. *Blood.* 1959;14:378–385.

Ibrahim K, Kara RY, Zuberi SJ. Hypercarotenemia: A case report. *JPMA.* 1976;224–225.

Jacques PF, Hartz SC, Chylack LT, et al. Nutritional status in persons with and without senile cataract: Blood vitamin and mineral levels. *Am J Clin Nutr.* 1988;48:152–158.

Kobayashi S, et al. Determination of zinc in very small body hair samples by one-drop flame atomic absorption spectrophotometry. *Jpn J Hygiene.* 1991;46:762–768.

Kutsky R. *Handbook of Vitamins and Hormones.* New York: Van Nostrand Reinhold; 1973

Lamand M, Favier A, Pineau A. Determination of trace elements in the hair: Significance and limitations. *Ann Biologie Clinique.* 1990;48:433–442.

Lane BC. Nutrition and vision. In: Bland J, ed. 1984–85 *Yearbook of Nutritional Medicine.* New Canaan, CT: Keats; 1985:273.

Lane BC. Evaluation of intraocular pressure with daily, sustained closework stimulus to accommodation to lowered tissue chromium and dietary deficiency of ascorbic acid. PhD dissertation, 1980, New York University.

Lascari AD. Carotenemia. *Clin Pediatr.* 1981;20:25.

Leopold IH. Zinc deficiency and visual impairment. *Am J Ophthalmol.* 1978;85:871–874.

Maugh TH. Hair: A diagnostic tool to complement blood serum and urine. *Science.* 1978;202:1271.

Mueller JF, Vilter RW. Pyridoxin deficiency in human beings induced with desoxypyridoxine. *J Clin Invest.* 1950;29:193.

Murray MT. Iron: Deficiencies and supplements. *Health Counselor.* Nov/Dec 1991:31–33.

Newsome DA, Swartz M, Leone NC, et al. Oral zinc in macular degeneration. *Arch Ophthalmol.* 1988;106:192–198.

Paton D, Mclaren DS. Bitot spots. *Am J Ophthalmol.* 1960;50:568.

Pihl RO, Parks M. Hair element content in learning-disabled children. *Science.* 1977;198:204–206.

Prasad K, Rama B. Nutrition and cancer. In: Bland J, ed. *1984–85 Yearbook of Nutritional Medicine.* New Canaan, CT: Keats; 1985.

Rapp J. Nutrition in the vision of children. *J Am Opt Assoc.* 1979;50:1107–1111.

Rengstorff RH, Krall CC, Westerhout DI. Topical antioxidant treatment for dry-eye disorders and contact lens-related complications. *Afro-Asian J Ophthalmol.* 1988;7:81–83.

Rosenblum JD, Keating JP, Prensky AL, Nelson JS. A progressive neurologic syndrome in children with chronic liver disease. *N Engl J Med.* 1991;304:503.

Sommer A. Treatment of corneal xerophthalmia with topical retinoic acid. *Am J Ophthalmol.* 1983;95:349–352.

Sommer A. *Nutritional Blindness.* New York: Oxford; 1982: 51–52.

Sommer A, Quesada J, Doty M, Faich G. Xerophthalmia and anterior segment blindness among preschool children in El Salvador. *Am J Ophthalmol.* 1975;80:1066.

Stern JJ. Nutrition in ophthalmology. In: Goodhart R, Shils M, eds. *Modern Nutrition in Health and Disease.* 5th ed. Philadelphia: Lea & Febiger; 1973:1009.

Todd GP. *Nutrition in Health and Disease.* Norfolk, VA: Donning; 1987.

Yolton DP. Nutritional effects of zinc on ocular and systemic physiology. *J Am Optom Assoc.* 1981;52:409–414.

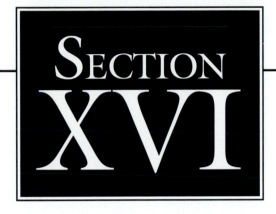

SECTION XVI

DRUG AND ALCOHOL ABUSE

82
Chapter

Drug and Alcohol Abuse

Tanya L. Carter

The manifestations of drug abuse are numerous and often resemble manifestations of other disease processes. Not only are illicit drugs abused, but licit drugs such as tobacco, alcohol, caffeine, and prescription medications when taken in excess can lead to adverse systemic and ocular affects. Factors that lead to adverse sequelae are direct toxicity from the drug itself, pharmacologic effects, associated nutritional deficiencies, and the mode of administration. The various substances used to dilute or "cut" the primary drug, such as talc, flour, cornstarch, and sugar, can lead to emboli. Additionally, ocular trauma may be self-inflicted due to adverse behaviors and altered states of consciousness while under the influence.

There are two patterns of drug abuse. One occurs from dependence after a course of extended medical therapy. The second results from experimentation, to obtain euphoria or other desired effects, which progresses to more intense involvement. Because there are numerous drugs that are abused, this chapter will be limited to some of the most commonly abused substances.

The epidemiology of drug abuse varies considerably over time. The particular substance that is being abused will go in and out of style. Cycles of popularity are a function of availability and cost. Additionally, the exact prevalence is often hard to ascertain, because most surveys rely on self-reporting and physicians do not routinely screen patients for substance abuse.

■ ALCOHOL

Ethanol or ethyl alcohol is an organic, volatile, flammable substance that is obtained, in its pure form, by fermentation and distillation of grain. It is present in fermented or distilled liquors and is used in preparing essences, tinctures, and extracts, as well as in manufacturing ether, ethylene, rubbing compounds, antiseptics, and other industrial products. It is also given intravenously to stop premature labor. Alcohol acts as a depressant to the central nervous system and causes potent psychoactive effects when taken in excessive amounts. Psychological and physiological dependence can occur. The physiological dependence, or physical dependence as it is often called, will result in withdrawal signs and symptoms.

Methanol is an organic, poisonous, volatile, and flammable liquid that is obtained from distillation of wood. It is also known as carbinol, methyl alcohol, or wood alcohol, and is more commonly found in bootleg whiskey. Unlike ethanol, it is not intended for human consumption. It is used as a solvent, as an additive for denaturing ethyl alcohol, as an antifreeze agent, in fuel, and in the preparation of formaldehyde.

EPIDEMIOLOGY

Alcohol holds the title of being the oldest and most frequently abused drug. According to the National Institute on

Drug Abuse (1990), approximately 102 million Americans over the age of 12 used alcohol. Use was defined as those who had a drink in the past month. This represented 51.2% of the household population. Ten million Americans were cited as heavy users, which is defined as having had 5 or more drinks per occasion on 5 or more days in the past 30 days. Heavy use most commonly occurrs between 18 and 25 years of age. An estimated 5 million Americans are alcoholics.

NATURAL HISTORY

■ Systemic

Alcoholism is a chronic, progressive, and potentially fatal disease. It is characterized by physiological dependence resulting in physical, emotional, and social changes that progressively worsen as the abuse continues. Tolerance is common, whereby higher and higher concentrations are needed for an effect. The exact mechanism for the onset of alcoholism is not fully understood. It is felt that psychological, physiological, sociological, and genetic factors play an important role. Much controversy surrounds exactly how genetics determines alcoholism. Recently, attention has been given to an association between a genetic mutation of the D2 dopamine receptor gene on chromosome 11 and alcoholism. However, many researchers, such as Comings (1991), Gelernter (1991), Parsian (1991), and their associates, feel that more than one loci is involved and the way in which alcoholism is expressed is influenced by environment and culture.

The main consequence of acute ethanol poisoning is irregularly descending CNS depression that causes peripheral vasodilation with flushing of the skin, rapid pulse, hypotension, tachycardia, hypothermia, polyneuritis, coma, and death from respiratory or circulatory failure (Table 82–1). The probable lethal dose for adults varies from one pint to more than one quart when ingested at one time. Acute intoxication also results in temporary mental disturbances, muscular incoordination (staggered gait, impaired reflex action), drowsiness, and stupor.

Chronic alcohol abuse affects many organs, particularly the liver, brain, peripheral nervous system, and gastrointestinal tract. Direct tissue toxicity causes cirrhosis of the liver, gastritis, pancreatitis, and neurological disorders such as tremulousness, hallucinosis, seizures, and delirium. Wernicke–Korsakoff syndrome occurs secondary to thiamine deficiency that is usually associated with chronic ethanol ingestion. This syndrome involves neurological and psychological dysfunction that is characterized by encephalopathy, loss of memory, disorientation, psychosis, polyneuritis, ataxia, delirium, insomnia, illusions, and hallucinations. Animal studies have shown changes in the

TABLE 82–1. SYSTEMIC MANIFESTATIONS OF ALCOHOL ABUSE

- Alcoholism
- Respiratory failure
- Circulatory failure
- Mental disturbances
- Liver cirrhosis
- Gastritis
- Pancreatitis
- Neurological disorders
- Wernicke–Korsakoff syndrome
- Skin flushing
- Tachycardia
- Muscular incoordination
- Drowsiness
- Stupor, delirium
- Tremulousness
- Seizures
- Hallucinations
- Emotional instability
- Slurred speech
- Poor comprehension
- Poor memory
- Irritability
- Bad judgement

optic nerve, lateral geniculate body, and dorsal nuclei in this syndrome. The associated nutritional deficiency is due to decreased food intake, poor choice of food, increased urination, and an increased nutrient requirement. Chronic alcoholism also interferes with absorption of certain nutrients. An example is the zinc chelator, tannin, that is often found in lower-quality red wines, which causes decreased zinc absorption and increased fecal elimination. The absorption of vitamin B_{12} is also altered, along with alcohol-destroying vitamin A. Absorption is also affected by associated gastrointestinal disease. Additionally, hepatitis and cirrhosis alter the nutritional storage capacity of the liver. Other consequences of nutritional deficiency are outlined in Chapters 80 and 81.

The manifestations of methanol abuse are more severe than those of ethanol abuse. The major consequence of methanol poisoning is a severe metabolic acidosis with progressive cerebral dysfunction, circulatory collapse, and respiratory failure. The signs and symptoms include exhilaration accompanied by headache, muscular weakness, weak and rapid pulse, rapid and shallow breathing, nausea, vomiting, and abdominal pain. Direct toxicity to the nervous system may lead to convulsions and coma. Respiratory failure can result in cyanosis (bluish, grayish, or dark purple discoloration to the skin) and death from a lack of oxygen and an excess of carbon dioxide in the blood. The probable lethal dose for adults is 500 to 5000 mg/kg body weight.

■ Ocular

Alcohol amblyopia is a well known consequence of chronic alcoholism (Table 82–2). It usually is associated with drinking excessively and steadily for many years. It is now known that the associated nutritional deficiency, primarily in the vitamin B complex—thiamine (B_1), niacin (B_3), B_{12} and folate—is the major underlying factor. Other nutrients that are involved are iodine, zinc, and vitamin A. Nutritional optic neuropathy may manifest initially as a bilateral, yet often asymmetric, retrobulbar neuropathy that progresses slowly to anterior optic atrophy. Visual acuity loss ranges from a mild decrease in acuity to amaurosis. The classic visual field defect is a centrocecal scotoma, yet central scotomas and occasional peripheral constrictions have also been reported. Prognosis for recovery of vision loss and visual field defects is a function of the severity of the loss and is enhanced if therapy is initiated early in the course of optic nerve involvement. Vitamin B complex therapy was found to improve the optic neuropathy in many instances despite continuation of the alcohol abuse. Nutritional deficiencies that are associated with alcohol abuse may also lead to cataracts, macular degeneration, and ophthalmoplegia. More details on the ocular manifestations of nutritional deficiencies can be found in Chapters 80 and 81.

True toxicity to the optic nerve also occurs in chronic alcohol abuse and is found mainly in association with methanol poisoning. Sharpe (1982) showed that the pathophysiology is related to myelin damage with axonal preservation in the retrolaminar portion of the optic nerve. The mechanism for this disturbance is thought to be due to anoxia. Toxic optic neuropathy will manifest in the same manner as nutritional optic neuropathy. Yet, methanol intoxication may present initially with disc edema, which can lead to optic atrophy. The initial amaurosis may occur suddenly and improve, and then increase again but with permanent vision loss. The central scotoma is large, dense, and irregular, and is not reversible. Methanol intoxication can also cause pupillary dilatation and sluggishness, optic nerve hyperemia, and retinal edema. These signs may manifest within 2 months of the visual acuity decline. Prognosis for visual recovery is poor when vision is severely affected. Temporary blindness attributed to ethanol is usually rare.

Acute ethanol intoxication can cause decreased speed of accommodation and disturbance of higher visual functions. Adams and Brown (1978) and others showed instances of decreased rate of recovery from bright light exposure (dazzling). Russell and associates (1980) reported transient changes in color vision with normal visual acuity. Howells (1956) reported the onset of nystagmus with a minimum of 50 mL of alcohol. Studies by Hogan and Linfield (1983) and others showed the possibility of induced esophoria, intermittent esotropia, and altered stereopsis with acute intoxication. Wilkinson and colleagues (1974) concluded that saccadic eye movements are slowed and pursuit movements become inefficient and jerky due to changes in cerebral function. Eye involvement has also been reported to be related to liver cirrhosis. Summerskill and Molnar (1962) reported a 12% incidence of lid retraction and lag in chronic alcoholics with cirrhosis versus 1% in noncirrhotic controls. Rapidis and colleagues (1975) reported chronic uveitis while Cavka (1963) reported yellowish sclera and telangiectasis with small arteriolar aneurysms and venular varices of the palpebral and bulbar conjunctiva.

DIAGNOSIS

■ Systemic

The diagnosis of alcohol as well as other drug abuse is often based on suspicion and guesswork. The abusers usually do not volunteer this information; however, a careful history is often revealing. Questioning patients about alcohol and other drug abuse should be approached gingerly. One technique put forth by Cohen and associates (1980) is to first ask about the use of coffee and cigarettes, and then about the use of any prescription drugs, alcohol, and finally illicit drugs. Suspicions should be raised in the presence of certain characteristic signs and symptoms such as changes in mood and emotional instability, impaired motor coordi-

TABLE 82–2. OCULAR MANIFESTATIONS OF ALCOHOL ABUSE

ETHANOL
- Nutritional optic neuropathy
    - Retrobulbar or anterior pallor
    - Centrocecal or central scotoma
    - Decreased vision
    - Color vision defects
- Nystagmus
- Esophoria
- Altered motilities
- Accommodative insufficiency
- Stereopsis deficit

METHANOL
- Toxic optic neuropathy
    - Anterior disc edema
    - Hyperemia
    - Optic atrophy
    - Centrocecal or central scotomas
- Decreased vision
- Retinal edema
- Mydriasis

nation, slurred speech, ataxia, sweating, nausea, vomiting, drowsiness, and stupor. Other diagnostic signs of alcohol abuse include a patient who has a history of difficulty maintaining employment or appears manipulative as well as evasive. Suspicions should be confirmed with urine and blood analysis. Urine testing will detect drug use within the preceding 7 days, while blood analysis can determine an approximate quantity of alcohol intake. Certain questionnaires such as the CAGE questionnaire or Brief Michigan Alcoholism Screening Test can be used as an indirect means of detecting alcohol use. The content of these questionnaires is outlined in Speicher (1989).

■ Ocular

In chronic alcoholism the patient may present with decreased acuity that ranges from mild blurring to total blindness. However, examination will usually reveal amblyopia rather than blindness. Occasionally, chronic alcoholics experience an acute amaurosis lasting 24 hours with no sound pathologic basis. Although methanol poisoning is associated more frequently with blindness, the patient usually does not survive to complain about it. Visual field changes that are due to direct toxicity may show larger areas of defects than nutritional optic neuropathy. Also, the visual field defect is smaller, more central, and steeper than in tobacco amblyopia. According to Harrington (1962), centrocecal defects will have the area of greatest density near fixation. Red-colored targets may more easily detect incipient scotomas. Other ocular symptoms include pain behind the eye, diplopia, red green dyschromatopsia, impaired depth perception, and near point blur. Knave and co-workers (1974) and others showed disturbances in the electroretinogram (ERG), while reduced dark adaptation in monkeys was reported by Van Norren and Padmos (1977). The diagnosis of alcohol-induced nutritional optic neuropathy should be one of exclusion. Orbital and cerebral CT scans or MRI are warranted to rule out compressive lesions, and laboratory tests should be done to rule out optic neuritis.

The presence of severe end-stage nystagmus, the onset of nystagmus prior to 45-degree lateral gaze, and jerky pursuits are signs used by the National Highway Traffic Safety Administration to help detect drivers who are intoxicated (Halperin & Yolton, 1986).

TREATMENT AND MANAGEMENT

Table 82–3 summarizes the treatment and management of alcohol abuse.

■ Systemic

In cases of acute intoxication, the stomach is immediately washed with a gastric lavage of tap water and 3% sodium

TABLE 82–3. TREATMENT AND MANAGEMENT OF ALCOHOL ABUSE

- ■ SYSTEMIC
  - ● **Acute**
    Gastric lavage
    Artificial respiration if necessary
    IV saline or lactate
    Hypertonic glucose
  - ● **Chronic**
    Rehabilitation programs
  - ● **Methanol**
    Oral ethanol combined with saline or bicarbonate

- ■ OCULAR
  - ● Discontinue alcohol
  - ● Vitamin A, B complex, zinc

bicarbonate. The airways are opened if necessary, with oxygen and artificial respiration. This should be followed by intravenous saline or lactate for circulatory collapse, dehydration, or acidosis. Aspiration of vomitus should be avoided. Hypertonic glucose or urea is given to relieve cerebral edema. Chronic alcoholism is primarily treated through rehabilitation programs, the most prominent organization being AA (Alcoholics Anonymous). Detoxification may require medical supervision due to the potentially severe withdrawal symptoms (delirium tremens).

A person suffering from methanol poisoning should immediately be given gastric lavage with 5% sodium bicarbonate. Acidosis is stabilized with 3% sodium bicarbonate intravenously at the rate of 1000 mL/h. Ten mL of oral ethanol is given to prevent the formation of toxic formic acid. Severe poisoning is treated with intravenous ethyl alcohol combined with bicarbonate or saline. The patient should also receive treatment for shock, mild external heat, and bed rest in a dimly lit room.

■ Ocular

The first step in reversing the ocular manifestations of alcohol abuse is to remove the alcohol. This should be followed by vitamin therapy including vitamin B complex, vitamin A, and zinc. It is recommended that a hematologist, internist, or nutritionist manage the nutritional deficiency.

■ TOBACCO

Tobacco is extracted from the nicotiana plant. The leaves are dried and used for smoking, chewing or snuff. Tobacco and tobacco smoke contain many substances such as nicotine, pyridine, picoline, cyanide, and carbon monoxide.

"Tar" is defined as total particulate matter collected by a filter after removing moisture and nicotine. The aromatic hydrocarbon in tar is the primary carcinogen. Nicotine is a highly toxic and addicting substance that causes transient stimulation and subsequent depression of the CNS, peripheral autonomic ganglia, and the skeletal muscle motor endplates. Smooth muscle cells are also excited. Nicotine is the most active constituent of tobacco and is responsible for the narcotic properties. Recently more emphasis has been placed on the health hazards associated with cigarette smoking such as lung disease, heart disease, and cancer.

Tobacco amblyopia is the main ocular manifestation of tobacco abuse. True "tobacco amblyopia" occurs on rare occasions and is most often associated with pipe and cigar smoking, followed by chewing tobacco or snuff, and lastly by cigarette smoking.

EPIDEMIOLOGY

■ Systemic
Even though the popularity of smoking cigarettes is subsiding, tobacco is still rated as the second most abused substance in the United States, with a high percentage of young smokers. The National Institute on Drug Abuse (1990) reported that approximately 53 million Americans were classified as current cigarette smokers, which represents 26.7% of the household population.

■ Ocular
Tobacco amblyopia usually occurs in men between the ages of 40 and 60. The prevalence of tobacco amblyopia is difficult to ascertain because much of the literature contain reports of "tobacco–alcohol" amblyopia without differentiating the two.

NATURAL HISTORY

■ Systemic
The systemic effects of chronic tobacco abuse are numerous (Table 82–4). They include bronchopulmonary disease (emphysema, lung cancer), cardiovascular disease, cancer (mouth, throat, lung), and allergies. Significant morbidity and mortality are classic end results. The reader is referred to the United States Department of Health, Education, and Welfare (1979) report for more complete details.

■ Ocular
Tobacco amblyopia is usually associated with prolonged use, yet most authors believe that the actual quantity does not

TABLE 82–4. SYSTEMIC MANIFESTATIONS OF TOBACCO ABUSE

- Cancer (mouth, throat, lung)
- Cardiovascular disease
- Bronchopulmonary disease (emphysema)
- Allergies
- Lack of appetite, digestive disturbance
- Insomnia
- Constipation
- Decreased sexual desire
- Fatigue
- Depression

influence the onset because reported tobacco use varies significantly (Table 82–5). There are various contradictions in the literature as to the histopathology of tobacco amblyopia. Yet, many authors conclude that the primary involvement is selective neuronal atrophy involving the macular and paramacular fibers in the optic nerve. The amblyopia is usually bilateral, yet often asymmetric, and develops gradually without progressing to a complete loss of vision. Reports of visual acuity loss have ranged between 20/30 and 5/200. The optic neuropathy is usually retrobulbar but may progress to temporal optic pallor. Few cases of pallor involving the entire papilla have been reported. Other signs may include pupillary constriction, centrocecal scotomas, and color vision defects. The visual field defects may be relative or absolute and are more easily detected with red targets. Harrington (1962) stated that the visual field defects in true tobacco amblyopia are characterized by bilaterality, are always centrocecal with sloping edges, are a similar shape in each eye, and have an area of increased density within the scotoma between fixation and the blindspot, which he believes to be unique to tobacco effects. A few cases of peripheral visual field constriction have been noted, although it is questionable whether these cases represent true tobacco amblyopia. Halperin and co-workers (1959) believed that the levels of carbon monoxide in cigarette smoke may impair night vision. Prognosis for visual recovery is favorable. Vision will usually improve with or without continued tobacco consumption; however, recovery is faster with discontinuation of smoking and/or improved

TABLE 82–5. OCULAR MANIFESTATIONS OF TOBACCO ABUSE

OCULAR MANIFESTATIONS
- Nutritional optic neuropathy
- Toxic optic neuropathy
- Miosis

nutritional intake. Recovery usually occurs in 2 to 10 months, although if smoking continues, recovery may take years. In some cases normal visual acuity and fields have occurred even in the presence of temporal optic nerve pallor.

There is general agreement among investigators that tobacco consumption alone does not explain the development of toxic amblyopia. The major concern is that amblyopia develops in a small percentage of smokers. Additionally, amblyopia is more frequently found in association with smokers who are heavy drinkers; hence the term "tobacco–alcohol amblyopia." Traquair (1931) and others believe that poor health, systemic disease, and malnutrition increases the retinal and optic nerve sensitivity to the toxic effects of tobacco. Foulds and associates (1969) also implicated a nutritional component in their belief that a causal relationship between vitamin B_{12} deficiency and tobacco amblyopia may be due to an inability to detoxify cyanide. Heaton and colleagues (1958) and others found depressed plasma B_{12} levels in various patients with optic neuropathy who showed ocular improvement with B_{12} therapy even if they continued smoking. Foulds and Pettigrew (1977) presented evidence that there is a defect in the metabolism of sulphur in patients with tobacco amblyopia. Sulphur is required to detoxify cyanide into thiocyanate (the nontoxic metabolite of cyanide). Those with tobacco amblyopia were found to have lower levels of thiocyanate than most tobacco smokers. Dietary supplements of sulphur-containing amino acids or parenteral inorganic sulfur resulted in increased levels of plasma and urinary thiocyanate and increased visual acuity despite continued smoking. Deficiencies in vitamin B_{12}, pyridoxine, and folic acid are also implicated due to their role in the metabolism of sulphur.

Most researchers agree that pipe and cigar smoking is associated with amblyopia more often than cigarettes. Leishman (1951) stated that this may be due to the possibility that in pipe smoking the tobacco is more likely to be swallowed causing an upset of gastric function resulting in metabolic disturbances, whereas cigarette smoking mainly involves inhalation into the lungs. A nutritional component may be correlated with the fact that pipes and cigars are smoked at an older age when nutritional status is also compromised. Also, pipe smoking has been found to impair B_{12} absorption.

DIAGNOSIS

■ Systemic

Diagnosing tobacco intoxication can be achieved by measuring urinary levels of thiocyanate, which are elevated in most smokers but will be deficient in those with tobacco amblyopia. Systemic symptoms may include a lack of appetite, digestive disturbance, insomnia, constipation, diminution of sexual desire, and a feeling of fatigue and depression.

TABLE 82–6. TREATMENT AND MANAGEMENT OF TOBACCO ABUSE

- ■ **SYSTEMIC**
  - Encourage elimination of tobacco use
  - **Nutritional therapy**
    Complete balanced diet with emphasis on vitamin B complex and folic acid
    300 mg thiamine/wk × 10 weeks
    1000 μg IV B_{12}/wk × 10 weeks

- ■ **OCULAR**
  - Same as systemic therapy

■ Ocular

Patients with tobacco amblyopia will usually complain of a gradual (weeks to months) decrease in acuity mainly for near-point tasks. They may also state that their vision is better in the dusk than in bright daylight and may experience color desaturation, especially to red targets. The key diagnostic factor is the characteristic visual field defect, which was outlined earlier in the Natural History section. If the typical defects are not evident, other disease processes must be ruled out. In this instance further testing with orbital and cerebral CT scans or MRI as well as blood analysis are recommended to rule out other sources of amblyopia. Support can be given by measuring plasma levels of sulfur-containing amino acids, red cell glutathione, vitamin B complex, and folic acid, along with assessing the overall nutritional state.

TREATMENT AND MANAGEMENT

Because there are various nutritional factors that are implicated in tobacco amblyopia, it is recommended that a complete balanced diet is achieved with special emphasis on supplemental vitamin B complex and folic acid. Suggested regimens are outlined in Table 82–6. Patients should be educated on abstinence from smoking tobacco.

■ DEPRESSANTS

Depressants represent a category of drugs that cause generalized CNS depression. Included in this class are the sedatives or hypnotics and antianxiety or tranquilizer agents. These drugs differ in their mode of action and in onset and duration of action. Depressants are commonly prescribed for medical use. Abuse most often occurs when one becomes habituated after chronic use; yet these drugs may purposely be sought after for their euphoric effects or to counteract the effect of various stimulant drugs.

BARBITURATES

Barbiturates are organic compounds that act by increasing the inhibitory activity of gamma-aminobutyric acid (GABA) in the central nervous system, thereby inhibiting the action of the sympathetic branch of the autonomic nervous system. This results in multiple organ system depression. Barbiturates are primarily used medically for their sedative and anticonvulsant capabilities as well as to treat certain types of epilepsy. The more commonly abused barbiturates include amobarbital (Amytal), pentobarbital (Nembutal), phenobarbital (Luminal), and secobarbital (Seconal). Because of the high potential for fatal overdose, safer sedative drugs (like benzodiazepines) are currently used instead of barbiturates. Although these drugs may cause fewer fatalities, there still is a high potential for abuse.

EPIDEMIOLOGY

Barbituric acid was first synthesized in 1863, but it was not until 1950 that abuse began. It is estimated that approximately 7 million Americans have used sedatives for nonmedical purposes at some point in their lifetime, which correlates to 3.7% of the U.S. population over the age of 12. Some 600,000 Americans were cited as current users by the National Institute on Drug Abuse (1990).

NATURAL HISTORY

■ Systemic
Small doses (30 to 50 mg) of the short- and intermediate-acting barbiturates will induce sedation while larger doses will induce sleep (Table 82–7). The side effects of moderate barbiturate poisoning are similar to alcohol intoxication. These include slurred speech, poor reflexes, poor comprehension, poor memory, stupor, irritability, and bad judgement. Severe poisoning causes depressed respiration, heart rate, blood pressure, and body temperature. Overdosing may also lead to confusion, ataxia, cyanosis, cardiovascular collapse, coma, and death secondary to respiratory arrest. The lethal dose is 50 to 500 mg/kg body weight when taken as a single dose. Psychological dependence develops with

therapeutic doses. This dependence leads to self-medication with larger doses, which causes physical dependence. The signs and symptoms of withdrawal secondary to the physical dependence include seizures, psychosis, restlessness, anxiety, tremors, and at times nausea and vomiting. Some may experience delirium during which exhaustion and cardiovascular collapse may occur.

■ Ocular
Barbiturate abuse mainly effects the oculomotor system (Table 82–8). Acute toxicity with high doses can cause subtle affects on pursuits in the form of cogwheel irregularities according to Holzman and associates (1975). Mild binocular instability or a more gross loss of oculomotor control during fixation and lateral gaze may also occur. This instability may progress to loss of the optokinetic response and elimination of the fast phase of induced vestibular nystagmus. There will be no response to caloric stimulation if coma ensues. Chronic abuse may lead to ptosis, blepharoclonus (fluttering of the eyelids after tapping between the eyebrows—called the glabellar tap test), and transient horizontal as well as vertical central positional nystagmus. Even moderate therapeutic doses can lead to weakening in convergence, sluggish pupillary responses, and variable pupil size. Poor perfusion from sympathetic inhibition is thought to lead to optic neuropathy.

DIAGNOSIS

■ Systemic
The state of euphoria will present as an elevated mood, decreased anxiety, and an increased feeling of energy and self-confidence. Some may also describe a floating feeling. Euphoria is followed by drowsiness, slurred speech, depressed mood, dizziness, vertigo, and headache. The appropriate laboratory tests to detect intoxication include analysis of blood and urine levels as well as obtaining an EEG, which may show nonspecific depression.

■ Ocular
In the early stages, the subtle oculomotor pursuit deficits may only be observable with electronystagmography. While tracking an OKN stimulus, the smooth pursuits will be replaced with jerky, saccadic movements. As blood levels increase, cogwheel-type movements may be more easily observed with the naked eye. The glabellar tap test can also be used in the diagnosis of barbiturate abuse. A normal response to tapping between the eyebrows will elicit only a few blinks, in contrast to a barbiturate user who will respond with fluttering of the eyelids. For those who

TABLE 82–7. SYSTEMIC MANIFESTATIONS OF THE ABUSE OF DEPRESSANTS

■ DEPRESSANT	■ MANIFESTATION
BARBITURATES Amobarbital (Amytal), pentobarbital (Nembutal), Phenobarbital (Luminal), Secobarbital	• CNS depression • Moderate to severe poisoning (similar to alcohol intoxication) • Euphoria • Overdose Confusion Ataxia Cyanosis Cardiovascular collapse Respiratory arrest
NON-BARBITURATES Chloral hydrate, methalqualone (Quaalude), paraldehyde (Paral), ethchlorvynol (Placidyl), glutehimide (Doriden)	• Sedation • Hypnosis • Weak pulse • Shortness of breath • Weakness • Nausea/vomiting • Euphoria shifting to anxiety, agitation, and hypochondriosis • Dizziness • Sleepiness
BENZODIAZEPINES Diazepam (Valium), chlorodiazepoxide (Librium), flurazepam (Dalmane), lorazepam (Ativan), oxazepam (Serax)	• Sedation • CNS depression • Similar to alcohol and barbiturate overdose • Muscle weakness

recover from coma, decreased visual acuity or bilateral blindness may be present (Roth, 1926). This visual disturbance will usually improve; however, permanent optic atrophy has been reported in some cases. Complaints of diplopia, dyschromatopsia, yellow or green tinge to vision, and visual hallucinations may occur. Dermatitis of the lids and conjunctivitis have been associated with barbiturate sensitization (Sattler, 1932).

TREATMENT AND MANAGEMENT

Acute barbiturate intoxication is initially managed by establishing open airway with artificial respiration, oxygen, and CO_2 inhalation (Table 82–9). The stomach should be washed via gastric lavage, with fluid as well as the electrolyte balance maintained. Once vital signs and kidney function are stabilized, urea is given to induce diuresis.

Current treatment modalities for chronic barbiturate abuse involve in- and outpatient programs for detoxification. Detoxification involves gradually decreasing the doses of the drug. Phenobarbital may be used for withdrawal because fatal doses of phenobarbital are much higher than toxic doses. This is followed by psychological and social rehabilitation. Close medical supervision is required because the withdrawal stages are severe and sometimes life threatening.

NON-BARBITURATE SEDATIVES AND HYPNOTICS

The non-barbiturate sedatives and hypnotics are a class of drugs that include chloral hydrate, ethchlorvynol (Placidyl), glutethimide (Doriden), methaqualone (Quaalude), and paraldehyde (Paral). These depressants inhibit the stimulation of the area of the cortex that is responsible for wakefulness and are commonly used to treat insomnia. Methaqualone (Quaalude) is no longer distributed for medical purposes in the United States because of the magnitude of its abuse. Paraldehyde (Paral) is a liquid polymer of acetaldehyde. It is useful in treating acute alcoholism and delirium tremens. Glutethimide (Doriden) and ethchlorvynol (Placidyl) are used more for their hypnotic ability. Additionally, ethchlorvynol is often used to dilute street drugs.

TABLE 82–8. OCULAR MANIFESTATIONS OF THE ABUSE OF DEPRESSANTS

■ **DEPRESSANT**

BARBITURATES
Amobarbital (Amytal), pentobarbital (Nembutal), phenobarbital (Luminal), secobarbital (Seconal)

NON-BARBITURATES
Choral hydrate, methalqualone (Quaalude), paraldehyde (Paral), ethchlorvynol (Placidyl), glutethimide (Doriden)

BENZODIAZEPINES
Diazepam (Valium), chlorodiazepoxide (Librium), flurazepam (Dalmane), lorazepam (Ativan), oxazepam (Serax)

■ **MANIFESTATION**
- Common
  - Oculomotor dysfunction
- Uncommon
  - Optic neuropathy
  - Lid dermatitis
  - Ptosis
  - Blepharoclonus
  - Nystagmus
  - Variable pupil size
  - Conjunctivitis

- See barbiturates, above
- No effect on accomodation

- Extraocular muscle dysfunction
- Allergic conjunctivitis

TABLE 82–9. TREATMENT AND MANAGEMENT OF THE ABUSE OF DEPRESSANTS

■ **SYSTEMIC**

BARBITURATES
- **Acute**
  - Artificial respiration
  - Gastric lavage
  - Induce diuresis
- **Chronic**
  - Detoxification/drug-free programs
  - Psychological and social rehabilitation programs

NON-BARBITURATES
- **Acute**
  - Artificial respiration
  - Gastric lavage
  - Give CNS stimulants (coffee, tea)
- **Chronic**
  - See barbiturates, above

BENZODIAZEPENES
- Like barbiturates, above; however, do not use phenobarbitals for the detoxification stage

■ **OCULAR**
- Discontinue drug abuse

EPIDEMIOLOGY

The prevalence of nonmedical use of sedatives is estimated at 7 million or 3.7% of Americans over the age of 12. Some 600,000 Americans were reported to be current users in 1990 by the National Institute on Drug Abuse.

Natural History

■ Systemic

Therapeutic doses of most of the drugs in this category induce sleep while allowing an almost normal sleep pattern in most patients (see Table 82–7). However, overdoses produce similar side effects to alcohol intoxication. Chloral hydrate depresses and eventually paralyzes the central nervous system. It is believed that the lethal dose in adults is 50 to 500 mg/kg body weight. Characteristic signs include weak pulse, shortness of breath, weakness, as well as nausea and vomiting due to gastric irritation. The signs of paraldehyde poisoning are similar to chloral hydrate except there may be odor on the breath. The effects of glutethimide (Doriden) and ethchlorvynol (Placidyl) overdoses are similar to chloral hydrate except Placidyl is especially dangerous since it is fat-soluble and resistant to excretion.

■ Ocular

Chronic chloral hydrate abuse causes nystagmus, blurred vision, cranial nerve palsies, decreased convergence, miosis, ptosis (which is also seen in therapeutic doses), and visual hallucination where objects appear smaller than their actual size (see Table 82–8). Ethchlorvynol (Placidyl) abuse causes visual and auditory hallucinations which may persist weeks after the drug is discontinued. Optic neuropathy, diplopia, transient vision blur, and nystagmus have also been reported. Vision loss that is due to optic neuropathy will recover upon discontinuing the drug. Glutethimide (Doriden) may cause diplopia, mydriasis, and nystagmus when excessive amounts are taken. Paraldehyde causes visual hallucinations especially upon withdrawal as well as pupillary miosis or mydriasis (associated with overdose). No documentation of the ocular side effects of methaqualone (Quaalude) can be found in the literature.

DIAGNOSIS

■ Systemic

The euphoric state from non-barbiturate sedative hypnotic drugs is similar to barbiturate intoxication except that mood may be unstable and manifest as rapid shifts from euphoria to sadness, irritability, anxiety, and agitation, along with hypochondriacal concerns. Patients may also report dizziness, generalized weakness, and sleepiness. Blood and urine samples will confirm the diagnosis and EEG may show a nonspecific depressant effect.

■ Ocular

Diagnosis is based on observation of the signs and symptoms as outlined in the natural history. Pertinent ocular history contributory to the diagnosis includes difficulty in sustaining near point tasks.

TREATMENT AND MANAGEMENT

Chronic abuse is managed in the same fashion as barbiturate therapy (see Table 82–9). Acute intoxication is treated with gastric lavage with coffee and tea except in paraldehyde poisoning. In this case, CNS stimulants are given by mouth, rectum, or by injection. Airway passages should be maintained with artificial respiration and oxygen.

BENZODIAZEPINES

Benzodiazepines are classified as minor tranquilizers that have a low incidence of effects outside of the CNS. They are the drugs of choice for relieving anxiety, tension, muscle spasms, and insomnia; inducing sedation; and preventing convulsions because they produce less physical and psychological dependence than barbiturates. Also they produce fewer adverse effects and deaths due to overdose. The more commonly used benzodiazepines include diazepam (Valium), chlordiazepoxide (Librium), flurazepam (Dalmane), lorazepam (Ativan), and oxazepam (Serax).

EPIDEMIOLOGY

According to The National Prescription Audit, the reduction of prescriptions written for all tranquilizers and sedatives, especially diazepam, has lead to a reduced potential for abuse. The estimated prevalence of nonmedical use of tranquilizers in 1990 was 9 million or 4.3% of the U.S. household population over the age of 12 (National Institute on Drug Abuse, 1990).

NATURAL HISTORY

■ Systemic

Prolonged therapeutic use of the benzodiazepines may lead to psychological and physical dependence. Side effects of therapeutic doses include drowsiness and respiratory depression that lasts 4 to 6 hours. Abuse produces effects that are similar to alcohol intoxication. Overdoses can lead to ataxia, slowed comprehension, orthostatic hypotension, irritability, delirium, coma, and death from respiratory arrest (see Table 82–7).

■ Ocular

The main ocular side effect is extraocular muscle involvement and allergic conjunctivitis (see Table 82–8). In general the benzodiazepines do not cause significant ocular autonomic effects (change in accommodation or pupil size). Chlordiazepoxide (Librium) may induce exophoria and decrease depth perception as well as saccadic velocity. Baird and associates (1968) reported elimination of the corneal blink reflex and slowed extraocular responses with diazepam doses of 7.2 mg/kg in adults and 4.0 mg/kg in children. Other possible manifestations include nystagmus and jerky pursuits.

DIAGNOSIS

■ Systemic

The symptoms of abuse are similar to alcohol and barbiturate intoxication. Blood and urine analysis are indicated to detect abuse. An EEG will show nonspecific depressant effects.

■ Ocular

Ocular diagnosis is assisted by complaints of difficulty with near-point tasks, diplopia, ocular irritation, itching, or tearing.

TREATMENT AND MANAGEMENT

The mode of therapy is similar to that for the barbiturates (see Table 82–9). Substitution with phenobarbital during the detoxification stage is not recommended because it has a similar duration of action and potential for dependency.

■ STIMULANTS

Stimulants are a category of drugs that augment the action of the neurotransmitter norepinephrine, thereby stimulating the sympathetic nervous system. They may also stimulate the release of dopamine in the brain. Stimulants are easily found in our society. Almost everyone has used stimulants in the form of caffeine present in coffee, tea, and cola beverages, or from nicotine in tobacco products. Stimulants are often used by athletes, students, and truck drivers because they increase short-term physical and mental performance. The more commonly abused stimulants include tobacco, amphetamines, metamphetamine, methylphenidate (Ritalin), phenmetrazine (Preludin), and cocaine. Because of the high potential for abuse, medical use of these drugs has declined considerably. However, newer drugs that are being used in place of amphetamines (especially appetite suppressants) have potential for abuse.

Amphetamines are synthetic stimulants used to elevate mood and to treat narcolepsy (inability to stay awake) as well as certain types of mental depression. They are sometimes used to treat obesity because they also act as an appetite suppressant. Amphetamines are also used to manage hyperkinesis "attention deficit disorder" in children, and athletes use them to enhance performance. Large doses are toxic, and chronic use has led to drug dependence. The more commonly used amphetamines include amphetamine sulfate (Benzedrine) and dextroamphetamine sulfate (Dexedrine). Amphetamine abuse usually begins after becoming habituated to a medical prescription, but it is often purposely sought after for its euphoric effect. Methamphetamines are a class of drugs that are chemically related to amphetamines. The more commonly used methamphetamine is methadrine, also known as "speed." Amphetamine and methamphetamines are usually taken orally or injected intravenously.

Methylphenidate (Ritalin) is a mild CNS stimulant. It is more often used, instead of amphetamines, to treat hyperkinesis in children because the adverse effects are milder. This drug is often abused by intravenous injection. Phenmetrazine (Preludin) is used to treat obesity. It is abused both orally and with intravenous injection. Like other injected drugs, there is a risk for emboli retinopathy and respiratory as well as cerebral complications.

Cocaine is derived from the leaves of the coca plant and is the most potent of the nonsynthetic stimulants. Cocaine was first used medically in the 1800s as a topical anesthetic. It blocks nerve conduction by inhibiting the reuptake of norepinephrine. Its use as an anesthetic has subsided because it is not metabolized as fast as other synthetic stimulants. Illicit cocaine is usually smoked or inhaled (snorted). On the street, cocaine is referred to as snow, coke, and crack. Crack is a "freebase" form of cocaine. It is prepared for smoking by heating with baking soda or ammonia, which serves to extract cocaine hydrochloride salt. This mixture is evaporated, leaving potent, pure crystals that are rolled into a cigarette form and smoked. Illicit cocaine is usually cut with other substances like sugars, talc, cornstarch, procaine, quinine, and amphetamines, which decreases its strength to about half the original potency.

EPIDEMIOLOGY

The estimated prevalence of stimulant use other than cocaine is approximately 13 million or 7% of Americans over the age of 12 (National Institute on Drug Abuse, 1990). Amphetamine abuse began around 1935, when amphetamines were readily found in nasal decongestants and other over-the-counter medications. Because of their limited therapeutic benefit, amphetamines are not used as often medically, thereby decreasing the potential for abuse. Amphetamines were more commonly abused in the 1960s but were replaced with cocaine in the 1970s. Illicit cocaine use was first reported in the mid-1700s. According to the National Institute on Drug Abuse (1990), approximately 6.2 million Americans used cocaine within the year preceding the survey, and 1.6 million were reported as current users. Many users are professionals. The emergence of "crack" has increased cocaine's street popularity mainly because for the first time it is relatively inexpensive ($5 to $10 per vial). The extent of crack use in the United States has been difficult to determine.

NATURAL HISTORY

■ Systemic

Stimulants affect the central nervous, peripheral nervous, and cardiovascular systems. All of the stimulants produce euphoria; increase energy, wakefulness, ability to concentrate, and feelings of sexuality; suppress appetite; and disrupt normal sleep patterns (see Table 82–10).

Specifically, amphetamine intoxication can cause excitement, talkativeness, hyperactive reflexes, vomiting, and severe anxiety that progresses to paranoia and toxic psychosis with increased dosages. These side effects usually last approximately 4 hours. As the dosage increases, the effects become altered. For example, the ability to concentrate turns into either a compulsion to repeat a task over and over or a total focusing of attention on the same object. Higher dosages may also lead to tachycardia, arrhythmias, delirium, convulsions, coma, cerebral hemorrhages, and death secondary to circulatory collapse. Psychological and physical dependence develop quickly. The lethal dose probably occurs with a dosage of 5 to 50 mg/kg body weight; however, it is known to vary. Full-blown amphetamine psychosis includes delusions of persecution and distortions of body images. Delusions may persist after the drug abuse has been discontinued. Withdrawal produces convulsions,

TABLE 82–10. SYSTEMIC MANIFESTATIONS OF THE ABUSE OF STIMULANTS

- Sympathomimetic
- Tachycardia
- Arrhythmias
- Hyperthermia
- Increased blood pressure
- Circulatory collapse
- CNS stimulant
- Nervous system effects
  - Euphoria
  - Increased energy
  - Excitement
  - Talkativeness
  - Hyperactive reflexes
  - Wakefulness
  - Headaches
  - Anxiety/paranoia
  - Confusion
  - Convulsions
  - Coma
  - Hallucinations
  - Needle tracks (pop scars)
  - Inflammation of the nasal mucosa

delirium, depressed mood, fatigue, hypotonia, and sleep disturbance. Methamphetamine has milder cardiac effects, while methylphenidate and phenmetrazine have lower levels of potency.

Cocaine's initial CNS stimulation results in euphoria, excitement, elevation of mood, feeling of power and intensity, increased concentration, increased physical and mental performance, excessive talking, and anxiety, which can progress to paranoia and toxic psychosis with long-term use. The initial CNS stimulation is followed by depression of higher nervous centers, resulting in depression, alterations in pulse, increased respiration, convulsions, collapse, and death from respiratory arrest. The lethal dose is thought to range between 30 mg and 1.2 g. Acute myocardial infarction and cardiac arrhythmias may also occur. Psychological dependence occurs faster with the crack version of cocaine, yet the cocaine abuser usually does not manifest physical dependence. Crack abuse also causes more frequent pulmonary and cerebrovascular complications. Stroke may occur secondary to acute elevation of blood pressure, cerebral vasospasm, rupture of an aneurysm or arteriovenous malformation, immuno-allergic vasculitis, and cardiogenic emboli, which are usually hemorrhagic rather than ischemic. Miller (1992) reported cases of perforated gastric ulcers in the crack abuser that were atypically located, and O'Donnel and associates (1991) reported a case of interstitial pneumonitis. Crack abuse may also lead to pneumomediastinum, pulmonary edema, and bronchiolitis. Normally the pulmonary involvement is relatively mild and reversible. The effects of inhaled, snorted, smoked, or swallowed cocaine usually last around 2 hours. Smoking cocaine has a higher incidence of toxicity than if inhaled or swallowed. Inhaled cocaine has effects similar to intravenous amphetamine. However, the more life-threatening side effects are not seen as often because cocaine is metabolized more rapidly.

■ Ocular

Stimulants have been found to cause lid retraction, mydriasis, decreased pupillary response to light, decreased accommodation, convergence insufficiency, color vision defects, posterior subcapsular cataracts, and visual hallucinations in the form of blue tinges to objects (Table 82–11.) Pupillary dilation may precipitate acute angle closure in the presence of narrow angles. Fraunfelder (1976) reported one case of blepharospasm and retinal venous thrombosis with ingestion of massive doses of amphetamines. Retinal vasoconstriction and microaneurysms have also been documented. Corneal erosions may be evident if cocaine is accidently rubbed on the cornea. This can occur when the powder is being prepared for smoking or during inhalation. Diaz-Calderon and associates (1991) reported a case of bilateral internuclear ophthalmople-

TABLE 82–11. OCULAR MANIFESTATIONS OF THE ABUSE OF STIMULANTS

Amphetamines, meta-amphetamine, methylphenidate (Ritalin), phenmetrazine (Preludin), cocaine

- **OCULAR MANIFESTATIONS**
  - Lid retraction
  - Mydriasis
  - Accommodative insufficiency
  - Convergence insufficiency
  - PSC
  - Retinal vasoconstriction and microaneurysms

TABLE 82–12. TREATMENT AND MANAGEMENT OF THE ABUSE OF STIMULANTS

- **SYSTEMIC**
  - **Acute**
    Clear airway passages
    Gastric lavage with tap water, activated charcoal, or induce vomiting if ingested orally
    Treat CNS symptoms with barbiturates
  - **Chronic**
    Detoxification and rehabilitation programs
- **OCULAR**
  - Discontinue drug abuse

gia secondary to ruptured arteriovenous malformation in the midbrain that was caused by smoking crack cocaine.

DIAGNOSIS

Systemic

Diagnosis is based on observation of patient signs and symptoms. A thorough case history may reveal a pattern of abuse. All stimulants can produce tremor of the hands and feet, restlessness, feeling of well being, alertness, power, and initially a feeling of increased mental capacity. Additionally, amphetamines and cocaine can cause dizziness, nausea, diarrhea, fever, palpitations, chest pains, headaches, confusion, hallucinations, dehydration, and dry mouth. The hallucinations involve the visual, auditory, and olfactory systems. Intake of stimulants can be assessed through blood and urine sampling. Needle tracks or "pop" scars in the skin may be evident with stimulants that are taken intravenously or subcutaneously. A pop scar is a depression in the skin that resembles a vaccination mark. Thrombophlebitis or toxic dermatitis may also be apparent at the injection site. Inflammation of the nasal mucosa may be diagnostic for abuse by inhalation. Withdrawal from amphetamines will manifest symptoms of prolonged sleep, lassitude, and depression.

Ocular

Ocular involvement is diagnosed by observation of the signs as outlined in the Natural History section, above. Specifically, the patient may report near-vision blur, near-point asthenopia, photophobia, perceptions of blue or yellow tinge to objects, and diplopia that is due to neuro-ophthalmoplegia.

TREATMENT AND MANAGEMENT

The initial step in treating severe overdose is to clear airway passages and stabilize the circulatory dysfunction (Table 82–12). Stimulants that are ingested orally are treated by gastric lavage with tap water and activated charcoal or vomiting is induced. CNS symptoms are treated with barbiturate therapy. Intravenous diazepam or barbiturates are administered for acute cocaine intoxication. Chronic abuse is managed with detoxification followed by inpatient or outpatient rehabilitation programs.

OPIATES

The opiates are classified as narcotic analgesics, which include any drug that is derived from or contains opium. Raw opium is a naturally occurring substance that is derived by air drying the juice from the poppy plant. There are twenty different alkaloids that contain up to 25% opium. The more commonly known alkaloids include morphine, codeine, heroin, and papaverine. Opiate receptors on cell surfaces interact with opiate drugs, resulting in sedation and anesthesia. The analgesic property of opiates is due to its action in the part of the brain that interprets the nerve message rather than by blocking transmission of the pain impulse. Thus, the subjective perception of pain is relieved, yet the ability to feel and have sensation is not altered. Opiates possess a significant potential for abuse because they also relieve anxiety and promote a feeling of well-being. Long-term use results in both a psychological and physiological dependence, thereby producing withdrawal signs and symptoms. Unfortunately, the physical dependence occurs with therapeutic dosages.

Morphine is a naturally occurring opiate that contains approximately 10% raw opium by weight, and is considered one of medicine's strongest analgesics. It is administered subcutaneously, intramuscularly, or intravenously. Morphine was used extensively in medicine until 1850, when its use declined due to the significant potential for opiate addiction and illicit use. Currently it is reserved for moderate to severe pain relief only when other non-narcotic analgesics are ineffective.

Codeine is a naturally occurring opiate that is less potent than morphine. It contains approximately 0.7 to 2.5% raw opium. It is commonly used in tablet or liquid form to relieve mild to moderate pain and as an antitussive (cough suppressant). Physical dependence usually does not result with typical therapeutic use.

Heroin is a semisynthetic derivative of morphine. It is produced by chemically mixing morphine with acetic acid. The name developed because it was thought to be the "heroic" cure for morphine addiction. However, heroin is three times as potent as morphine and the potential for addiction is greater than any other drug. Heroin can be administered orally, nasally ("snorting"), subcutaneously ("skin-popping"), or intravenously ("mainlining"), which is the preferred route. Most illicit heroin is cut with fillers.

There is a class of synthetic narcotic–analgesics known as opioids. This term signifies any drug whose pharmacologic actions resemble those of morphine. Opioids of common use include meperidine (Demerol), methadone (Dolophine), propoxyphene (Darvon), pentazocine (Talwin), fentanyl (Sublimaze), butophenol (Stadol), and nalbuphine (Nubain). These drugs are used medically as pain relievers and in relieving the symptoms of morphine and heroin withdrawal. Recently, some of these drugs have also become widely abused.

EPIDEMIOLOGY

The opium poppy plant is native to ancient civilizations in Asia. The East Indians typically confined its use to medical and ritual purposes, while the Chinese often smoked opium for social reasons. Abuse was first recorded in the 17th century, making it the second oldest abused drug after alcohol. Morphine was more commonly used in the West, because raw opium is not legally permitted in the United States. Morphine abuse was replaced by heroin in the 1960s. The National Institute on Drug Abuse reported an estimated 2 million users in 1990. This correlates to roughly 1% of the U.S. population over the age of 12. The use of heroin significantly decreased in the 1970s and was replaced by other analgesics like propoxyphene. However, heroin use is currently on the rise again because of a new form that is capable of being smoked, thereby creating a greater potential for abuse.

NATURAL HISTORY

■ Systemic

Opiate administration results in generalized CNS depression (Table 82–13). The effects and duration of action will depend on the mode of administration. The overall duration of action usually ranges from 3 to 6 hours. Acute intoxication produces an initial euphoria, heightened sense of well-being, loss of pain sensation, skin flushing, and itching. This is followed by drowsiness, inability to concentrate, lethargy, bradycardia, hypotension, a decrease in body temperature, constipation, and anxiety. Respiratory failure resulting in death can occur with 100 to 200 mg. This occurs because the CNS respiratory centers fail to respond effectively to varying levels of carbon dioxide, thereby decreasing the respiratory control mechanism. Opiates do not produce temporary psychosis. After injecting heroin, the initial response is a physical sensation that is described as a "rush," which is reported to be the most intense pleasure that can be experienced. Other side effects include depressed REM (rapid eye movement) sleep,

TABLE 82–13. SYSTEMIC MANIFESTATIONS OF OPIATE AND OPIOID ABUSE

- Opiates
  Raw opium, morphine, heroin, codeine, papverine

- Opioids
  Meperidine (Demerol), methadone (Dolophine), propoxyphene (Darvon), pentazocine (Talwin), fentanyl (Sublimaze), butophenol (Stadol), nalbuphine (Nubain)

- Euphoria
- Heightened sense of well-being
- Anxiety
- Apathy
- Hypochondriosis
- Floating feeling
- Loss of pain sensation
- Feeling of heaviness in extremities
- Skin flushing and itching
- Inability to concentrate
- Drowsiness
- Lethargy
- Bradycardia
- Hypotension
- Hypothermia
- Shallow breathing
- Constipation
- Respiratory failure
- Circulatory failure

TABLE 82–14. OCULAR MANIFESTATIONS OF OPIATE ABUSE

- Opiates include
    Raw opium
    Morphine
    Heroin
    Codeine
    Papaverine
- Pinpoint miosis
- Decreased IOP
- Nystagmus
- Accommodative excess
- Stevens–Johnson syndrome
- Excessive tearing

TABLE 82–15. TREATMENT AND MANAGEMENT OF OPIATE ABUSE

- ■ **SYSTEMIC**
    - **Acute**
        Clear airway passages
        Gastric lavage with potassium permanganate
        Keep patient awake
        Antagonist treatment (nalorphine)
    - **Chronic**
        Methadone detoxification for heroin addicts going through withdrawal
        Rehabilitation programs

- ■ **OCULAR**
    - Discontinue drug abuse

decreased libido, and altered menstrual cycle. Those abusing morphine and heroin may become hypochondriacal, apathetic, and easily bored with people. Severe withdrawal complications occur, such as hypertension, tachycardia, irritability, paresthesia, restlessness, depression, and sleep disturbance.

■ Ocular

The most prominent ocular manifestation of opiates is pupillary miosis, usually in the form of "pinpoint" pupils (Table 82–14). Other side effects include decreased intraocular pressure, nystagmus, blurred vision, increased accommodation, and Stevens–Johnson syndrome. Opiate withdrawal produces excessive tearing, irregularity in pupil size, paresis of accommodation, and occasional diplopia.

DIAGNOSIS

■ Systemic

Blood and urine toxicology screenings are used diagnostically. Over 90% of a dose is excreted in the urine within the first 24 hours, except for the long-acting drugs like methadone. Symptoms of opiate abuse are sometimes described as a floating feeling, and the extremities may feel heavy. Symptoms of withdrawal include abdominal cramps, muscle aches and spasms, chills, sweating, nausea, vomiting, and diarrhea. The presence of needle tracks in the skin or "pop" scars from subcutaneous injections will support the diagnosis. Other diagnostic signs are thrombophlebitis and toxic dermatitis over the injection site.

■ Ocular

The patient may report decreased vision secondary to pupillary miosis and alterations in accommodation. Extraocular muscle relaxation may result in diplopia.

TREATMENT AND MANAGEMENT

Acute overdose of orally ingested opiates is treated with gastric lavage utilizing potassium permanganate (Table 82–15). Artificial respiration and inhalation of oxygen with 5% carbon dioxide is necessary to maintain an open airway. The patient should be kept awake and the electrolyte balance maintained. Antagonists like nalorphine are used to block access to or displace opiates from the receptor sites. Methadone detoxification is commonly used to treat heroin addicts going through withdrawal. Low doses are thought to prevent the "drug hunger," while higher doses block the euphoric effects. Rehabilitation programs with psychotherapy are also recommended.

■ MARIJUANA

Marijuana and hashish are products of the cannabis (hemp) plant. Marijuana is prepared from the dried flowering tops, while hashish is prepared from the flowers, leaves, and stalks. Hashish is five to eight times more potent than marijuana. Delta-9-tetrahydrocannabinol (THC) is the main psychoactive component. THC alters the way in which sensory information gets into and is processed by the hippocampus. Although marijuana mainly affects the brain, resulting in psychological effects, other organs such as the respiratory, cardiovascular, and reproductive systems are also affected. Marijuana is not considered addictive, yet physical dependence has been reported with chronic, heavy use. The desired psychological effects of euphoria and detachment from reality are usually obtained by smoking a marijuana cigarette (commonly referred to as a "joint"). Cannabis is used as a herbal medication in several countries, but is not used medically in the United States, because of the inability to control the drug's potency and the variability of response. Current areas of medical research involving marijuana and other related compounds involve treating migraines, asthma, epilepsy, hypertension, and glaucoma.

EPIDEMIOLOGY

Marijuana is the third most commonly used recreational drug after alcohol and tobacco. Cannabis abuse began as early as the mid 1800s. According to the National Institute on Drug Abuse (1990), approximately 10 million Americans over the age of 12 used marijuana. This translates to roughly 5.1% of the population in this age category. This survey also reported that "since 1962 the percentage of Americans 18 to 25 years old who have used marijuana increased from 4% to 68%, while the percentage who have tried other drugs (cocaine, heroin, hallucinogens and inhalants) increased from 3% to 33%."

NATURAL HISTORY

■ Systemic
The systemic manifestations of marijuana use are dose dependent (Table 82–16). The effects occur rapidly and may peak within 10 to 30 minutes after inhalation. Acute intoxication causes an initial period of excitement, restlessness, talkativeness, and hyperactivity followed by calm and euphoria. Undesirable psychological effects in the form of altered perception and psychomotor coordination may impair machine-operating skills such as driving. Learning, memory, thinking, and comprehension may also be impaired, and there may be an altered sense of time. Mild changes in mood, or transient episodes of confusion, anxiety, and toxic delirium, may also occur. Eventually sleep is induced. Large doses may result in auditory or visual hallucinations within 20 to 30 minutes. Chronic, heavy use may cause behavioral disorders and CNS damage manifesting as epileptic seizures or dementia. There are no reported cases of death due to overdosing in the United States, probably because the content of THC in the marijuana that is produced in the United States is low (2.5 to 5.0 mg per cigarette).

TABLE 82–16. SYSTEMIC MANIFESTATIONS OF MARIJUANA ABUSE

- CNS damage (seizures, dementia)
- Psychological affects on the brain
- Hypotension or increased heart rate
- Respiratory disease
- Reproductive dysfunction (altered menstrual cycle and temporary infertility)
- **Initial**
  Excitement
  Restlessness
  Talkativeness
  Hyperactivity
- **Late**
  Calm, euphoria
  Detachment from reality
  Altered perception
  Psychomotor uncoordination
  Impaired learning, memory, thinking, and comprehension
  Changes in mood
  Anxiety
  Toxic delirium
  Auditory hallucinations
  Epileptic seizures
  Temporary infertility
  Heightened sexual arousal
  Enhanced sense of taste, touch, smell, hearing

The respiratory system is affected because marijuana smoke contains carcinogenic hydrocarbons. The cardiovascular system responds with hypotension, mild to moderate increase in heart rate, and sometimes tachycardia. Chronic use may alter the menstrual cycle and cause temporary infertility.

■ Ocular
The most prominent sign of marijuana use is conjunctival injection, which may be diffuse or ciliary (Table 82–17). The lids may also be congested. Some are of the opinion that mydriasis occurs in chronic use, while others report no pupillary involvement. An increase or decrease in tear production has also been reported. Acute intoxication may lead to nystagmus and blepharospasm. The cannabinol component in marijuana has a promising role in decreasing intraocular pressure. This association was first reported by Hepler and Frank (1971). They found a change in IOP varying from +4 to –45% in 13 volunteers in 1 hour after smoking 2 grams of marijuana. Others have confirmed the

TABLE 82–17. OCULAR MANIFESTATIONS OF MARIJUANA ABUSE

- Conjunctival hyperemia
- Lid congestion
- Mydriasis or miosis
- ↑ or ↓ in tear production
- Nystagmus
- Blepharospasms
- Decrease IOP
- Visual hallucinations

TABLE 82–18. TREATMENT AND MANAGEMENT OF MARIJUANA ABUSE

- **SYSTEMIC**
  - **Acute**
    Treat psychosis with supportive reassurance
  - **Chronic**
    Detoxification and rehabilitation programs

- **OCULAR**
  - Discontinue drug abuse

IOP-lowering effect. Flom and co-workers (1975) reported a 25% average decrease in intraocular pressure from baseline in non to moderate users, while heavy users demonstrated no drop in IOP after smoking the drug. The exact mechanism for the reduction in IOP is not fully understood. Experiments by Green and Pederson (1973) found a decrease in fluid secretion and increase in ultrafiltration. Purnell and Gregg (1975) felt that the IOP lowering was associated with the hypotonizing action of the drug, and therefore felt it to be mediated by the CNS. Unfortunately, the cannibinols were not found to be of clinical value in treating glaucoma in the United States, because of their psychoactive component and the inability to control the dosage. Also, Gaasterland (1980) pointed out that because the cannibinols lower blood pressure, any decrease in perfusion pressure to the optic nerve may create a situation whereby the IOP is lowered but vision loss is not prevented (because blood perfusion pressure to the eye as well as IOP are lowered). Nevertheless, a topical solution called Canasol, which contains cannabis sativa, is used in Jamaica as antiglaucoma therapy.

DIAGNOSIS

■ Systemic

Diagnosis of marijuana use may be obtained from a careful case history as outlined in the section on alcohol. Suspicion can be supported by blood toxicology screens; however, THC leaves the bloodstream rapidly. It is stored in body fats and has a half-life of 8 days. Besides euphoria, marijuana users may report feelings of relaxation, heightened sexual arousal, and a keen sense of hearing. The senses of taste, touch, and smell may appear to be enhanced. Some may also experience headaches.

■ Ocular

The visual hallucinations associated with marijuana use are described as brightly colored light flashes or amorphous forms that develop into shapes, faces, or scenes. Patients may also report symptoms of diplopia or photophobia with acute intoxication. CNS involvement can cause accommodative insufficiency leading to the complaint of near-vision blur. Dyschromatopsia, yellow vision, and heightened color perception is associated with chronic use.

TREATMENT AND MANAGEMENT

It is preferred that the systemic effects of intoxication are treated without any other medications (Table 82–18). Patients experiencing feelings of anxiety or paranoia are managed with supportive reassurance. Detoxification should be followed by drug rehabilitation programs.

■ HALLUCINOGENS

Hallucinogens are a class of drugs that distort one's perception of reality. True hallucinations (seeing things that are not there) usually do not occur; instead perceptions are altered. The three major classes of hallucinogens are the indolealkylamines (eg, LSD), phenethylamines (eg, mescaline), and phencyclidines (eg, PCP and angle dust). These substances are derived from a variety of sources such as the mushroom, cactus, and hemp plants. Hallucinogens act by stimulating the part of the sympathetic nervous system that affects the ascending reticular activating system. The exact basis for the hallucinatory effect has not been determined. Prolonged use leads to psychological dependence. Many hallucinogens are structurally similar to amphetamines.

Phencyclidines are sometimes categorized separately because they cause a wide variety of effects depending on dosage. They were originally used medically for their stimulant and anesthetic properties. Human medical use was discontinued because upon emerging from anesthesia, disorientation, agitation, delirium, and hallucinations can occur; phencyclidines are still used in veterinary medicine. Unfortunately, the illicit use of phencyclidines combined with other abused drugs frequently occurs.

Epidemiology

Hallucinogen abuse was first reported in the mid 1900s. There was widespread abuse in the 1960s, mainly of LSD. According to the National Institute on Drug Abuse (1990), 15 million or 7.6% of the population of the United States over the age of 12 was estimated to have used hallucinogens for nonmedical purposes over their lifetime, and 600,000 reported use in the last month. Phencyclidine (PCP or angle dust) was not well accepted on the street because of its unpredictable effects and high rate of undesirable effects. Studies show that phencyclidine use is more popular among young adolescents. The National Institute on Drug Abuse (1990) reported approximately 1 in 8 persons in the 18- to 25-year-old cohort and 1 in 20 in the 12- to 17-year-old cohort had used the drug at least once, and of those exposed to the drug, approximately 23% became chronic users.

Natural History

■ Systemic

Intoxication with hallucinogens mainly produces psychological effects such as altered perceptions (hallucinations), judgement, intellect, concentration, sense of time and space, and ultimately loss of contact with reality, severe anxiety, confusion, panic reactions, and paranoia (Table 82–19). Changes from one mental state to another may

TABLE 82–19. SYSTEMIC MANIFESTATIONS OF HALLUCINOGEN ABUSE

- Psychological effects on the brain
    Hallucinations
    Altered judgment, concentration, sense of time and
        space
    Confusion
    Anxiety, paranoia
    Aberrant behavior
    Delirium
- Toxic psychosis
- Sympathomimetic effects on the respiratory and
  cardiovascular systems
    Hypertension
    Tachycardia
    Circulatory collapse
    Hyperthermia
    ↑ respiratory rate
    Sweating
    Tremors
    Paresthesia
    Sleep disturbance
    Anorexia
    Slurred speech
    Irritability
    Floating feeling

occur quickly. Physiological effects include increased blood pressure, tachycardia, hyperthermia, increased respiratory rate, sweating, salivation, tremors, hyperactive reflexes, sleep disturbance, anorexia, slurred speech, nausea, and vomiting secondary to adrenomimetic action. Additionally, overdoses may produce irritability, delirium, convulsions, grand mal seizures, and circulatory collapse. The pharmacological effect has not been reported to cause fatalities and it is not clear whether there is a fatal dose. However, toxic psychosis may lead to aberrant behaviors resulting in self-inflicted injury. The onset of action can range from a few minutes to several hours after ingesting the drug, with an 8- to 10-hour duration of action.

Exposure to phencyclidine usually is in the powder form where 1 to 100 mg is sprinkled on marijuana or tobacco. Drug effects will usually last 4 to 6 hours with moderate doses. Low doses (2 to 5 mg) may cause mild depression, followed by stimulation. Approximately 10 mg will achieve the desired effect, which is described as a feeling of escape or detachment from the environment or dreamlike state of reality and illusion of invulnerability. Moderate doses may also cause elevated blood pressure, rapid pulse, anorexia, increased muscle rigidity, dulled sense of touch and pain, and occasional myoclonic jerks. Overdoses may additionally cause tachycardia, seizures, delirium, ataxia, respiratory depression, convulsions, coma, and death. The psychological side effects include bizarre sensations (eg, the feeling of walking on clouds), dramatic mood changes, slowed comprehension, poor memory, severe anxiety, combativeness, agitation, paranoid delusions, auditory and visual hallucinations (eg, body image changes), and acute episodes of schizophrenia. Users of phencyclidines may also exhibit facial grimacing or a blank stare and loss of sensitivity to pin pricking.

■ Ocular

Much emphasis is placed on the occurrence of spectacular hallucinations with the use of indolealkylamines like LSD. However, according to Krill and associates (1960) and Cohen and Ditman (1969), one will usually experience abnormal visual perceptions rather than true hallucinations (Table 82–20). The altered perceptions include changes in color vision; positive or negative afterimages; illusions of movement (objects may move in a wavelike fashion or melt); halos around objects; shimmering of images; micropsia or macropsia; metamorphopsia; teleopsia (perceptual disturbance involving an apparent increase in distances between objects); motion-perception defects like the "strobe light affect," where a moving object is seen in serial momentary stationary positions; and palinopsia (visual perseveration), whereby there is "streaking" of moving objects that is termed the trailing effect. One may also experience visual hallucinations in the form of intense colored geometric patterns that appear to move kaleidoscopically with an iridescent quality. The hallucination or altered visual perception episodes are not dose related, and flashbacks may

TABLE 82–20. OCULAR MANIFESTATIONS OF HALLUCINOGEN ABUSE

- Hallucinations (described as abnormal visual perceptions rather than true hallucinations)
  - Altered color perception
  - Positive or negative afterimages
  - Illusions of movement
  - Halos around objects
  - Shimmering images
  - Microposia
  - Macropsia
  - Metamorphopsia
  - Teleopsia
  - Palinopsia
  - Intense-colored geometric patterns
  - Words or images move around
- Solar retinopathy secondary to sun gazing
- Mydriasis
- **Phencyclidine**
  - Hallucinations in association with delirium
  - Ptosis
  - Decreased corneal reflexes
  - Irregular nystagmus in horizontal and vertical gaze
  - Papilledema and retinal hemorrhages in association with HTN encephalopathy

occur months to years after the drug is discontinued. Other ocular manifestations include pupillary dilation and lacrimation.

Phencyclidine abuse may result in visual hallucinations that are related to the delirium. Also, ptosis, paucity of spontaneous eye movement, and decreased corneal reflexes have been reported. Herskowitz and Oppenheimer (1977) reported a syndrome where primary gaze is normal but bursts of irregular nystagmus occur in the direction of vertical and horizontal gaze. Associated hypertensive encephalopathy may cause papilledema with retinal hemorrhages.

Solar retinopathy may occur in association with abuse of hallucinogens. It is typical for the drug user to stare at bright lights or the sun, which causes an exaggerated experience or "trip." It is felt that the mydriatic effect of the drug allows more light exposure, resulting in a thermal burn that occurs within 30 to 60 seconds. The maculopathy is described as a "honeycombed" or "hole-like" lesion.

DIAGNOSIS

■ Systemic

Blood and urine toxicology screenings are not widely available for the hallucinogens except for phencyclidines. Often a history of drug abuse must be coaxed from the patient. Therefore, the diagnosis often relies on observation of the

signs and symptoms. Patients may report a sense that time may seem to pass slowly, there is a feeling of oneness with the universe, a floating feeling, and a sense of unusual clarity of thoughts. Cerebellar involvement may cause symptoms of dizziness and poor coordination. Paresthesia, restlessness, and nausea may also be apparent, while overdoses will cause additional symptoms such as abdominal cramps, dry mouth, and vomiting.

■ Ocular

Some patients suffering from altered visual perceptions will present for an eye exam because of an interference with certain basic activities such as reading, driving, and watching television. They may complain that the words or images move around or merge together. Diagnosing these symptoms as secondary to drug abuse has to be one of exclusion; the symptoms are similar to those described in acquired nystagmus, intermittent strabismus, uncorrected hyperopia or presbyopia, and binocular instability. These symptoms can also occur with migraines, epilepsy, and intracranial lesions involving the temporal or parieto-occipital region (Hoffman, 1984; Klee & Willanger, 1966; Robinson & Watt, 1947; Swash, 1979). Thus, a complete history with neuroophthalmologic examination (perimetry, oculomotor function, CT scan or MRI, and EEG) is required. Blood and urine samples will be negative when flashbacks are occurring.

The diagnosis of solar maculopathy is based on observing the typical honeycombed or hole-like appearance. Fluorescein angiography may be normal early on with a late-stage choroidal fluorescence. Amsler grid testing and perimetry will show metamorphopsia and central scotomas. The patient will report blurred vision (usually around 20/40), which may improve after the initial presentation.

TREATMENT AND MANAGEMENT

Treatment is initiated by first stabilizing the vital signs (Table 82–21). The airway passages should be opened and

TABLE 82–21. TREATMENT AND MANAGEMENT OF HALLUCINOGEN ABUSE

- ■ **SYSTEMIC**
  - Stabilize vital signs
  - Open airway passages
  - Ice packs for hyperthermia
  - Reorient to reality with verbal cues and supportive reassurance in a quiet dim room
  - Antianxiety medications as needed

- ■ **OCULAR**
  - Discontinue drug abuse

ice packs administered to decrease hyperthermia. The psychosis is managed by reorienting the patient to reality with verbal cues and supportive reassurance. This should be carried out in a quiet, dimly lit room. The goal is to relieve the anxiety and not to contradict or direct the patient's illusions. Antipsychotic medications are not recommended because they can increase anticholinergic effects. However, antianxiety medications (diazepam, haloperidol, and so forth) are sometimes needed.

◼ INHALANTS

Inhalants refer to substances such as organic solvents, degreasers, and aerosol propellants that produce psychological and physiological effects when inhaled. These substances act as stimulants or depressants, and are easily obtained from common household products such as whipped cream aerosols, nail polish, glue, paint thinner, pan-coating sprays, transmission fluid, and room deodorizers. The desired chemicals within these substances include nitrous oxide, amyl nitrite, butyl nitrite, esters, acetone, aromatic hydrocarbons, alcohols, and many others. Nitrous oxide, which is commonly referred to as laughing gas, is a well-known inhalant. These substances are abused for their euphoric and excitatory effects. They are usually ingested by inhaling into a cloth that has been soaked or sprayed or by inhaling from a bag or balloon that has the chemical sprayed into it. A secondary danger from abusing inhalants is that they often contain compounds that are even more toxic than the chemical that produces the desired effect.

EPIDEMIOLOGY

Abuse of nitrous oxide as "laughing gas" was first reported as early as the 19th century. This was followed by sniffing gasoline in the 1950s and model airplane glue in the 1960s. In 1960, amyl nitrite abuse rose when it became available over the counter in ampules that were crushed and inhaled. Approximately 10 years later it was reclassified as prescription only, but was replaced with butyl nitrite. Butyl nitrite was packaged as a room odorizer or liquid incense and was easily available at drug paraphernalia stores. Around this time inhaling a variety of aerosol sprays containing alcohol also became popular. Currently inhalants are more commonly abused by adolescents and young adults (high school and college students in particular), probably because they are easier to obtain than alcohol for this age group. The National Institute on Drug Abuse (1990) reported approximately 10 million Americans who had used inhalants over their lifetime. This corresponds to 5% of the total U.S. population over the age of 12.

NATURAL HISTORY

◼ Systemic

The onset and duration of action is rapid because of the large surface area of the lungs. The chemicals are transported across the pulmonary capillary membrane. The systemic manifestations vary according to the chemical that is inhaled. The effects most often reported (Wilford, 1981) involve an initial cortical disinhibition followed by generalized CNS depression resulting in transient ataxia, slurred speech, vomiting, slow and shallow respiration, and local irritation to the mucous membranes that may present as watery discharge from the nose (Table 82–22). Mani-festations of acute intoxication with low doses may also include laryngospasm or airway freezing due to rapid vaporization as well as obstruction of the passage of oxygen across the capillary membrane. Unpleasant breath odor may also be apparent. Inhaling certain substances like hydrocarbons or fluoroalkene gases may cause respiratory depression, arrhythmias, loss of consciousness, and sudden death. Other physiological changes that occur from certain substances involve myocardial, hepatic or renal toxicity, bone marrow suppression, and encephalopathy. The psychological effects may resemble the early stages of alcohol intoxication or they may take on the characteristics of anesthesia. There may be signs of impulsiveness, excitement, hyperactivity, and exhilaration or feelings of numbness or weightlessness. Cerebral involvement can progress to mental confusion, clumsiness, cognitive and perceptual impairments, delirium, and sometimes irreversible brain damage. Altered behavior may result in recklessness that causes self-inflicted injury or danger. Death may also occur from asphyxiation due to an intense inhalation from a bag or ingestion of other toxic ingredients.

TABLE 82–22. SYSTEMIC MANIFESTATIONS OF INHALANT ABUSE

- Generalized CNS depression
- Laryngospasms
- Airway freezing
- Respiratory depression
- Arrhythmias
- Euphoria; drunkeness (transient ataxia, slurred speech, clumsiness); vomiting
- Watery discharge from the nose; breath odor
- Loss of consciousness; excitement; impulsiveness, hyperactivity; mental confusion; cognitive and perceptual impairments
- Insomnia; delirium; hallucinations

TABLE 82–23. OCULAR MANIFESTATIONS OF INHALANT ABUSE

- Conjunctival hyperemia and irritation
- Corneal epithelial erosion due to direct contact
- Visual hallucinations
- Blurry vision
- Diplopia
- Lacrimation

TABLE 82–24. TREATMENT AND MANAGEMENT OF INHALANT ABUSE

- ■ **SYSTEMIC**
  - Stabilize vital signs
  - Treat psychosis with supportive reassurance (ie, talk patient down) in a quiet, safe environment
- ■ **OCULAR**
  - Discontinue drug abuse

■ Ocular

Inhalants are irritating to the conjunctiva and cornea resulting in conjunctival hyperemia and lacrimation (Table 82–23). Direct contact can lead to corneal epithelial erosion and edema. The effects are of short duration and are reversible.

DIAGNOSIS

■ Systemic

Diagnosis is based on the signs and symptoms. A user may experience symptoms of drunkenness with inability to concentrate, unsteady gait, sleepiness, confusion, and impaired judgements. Other consequences include headaches, dizziness, insomnia, delusions of unusual strength and ability to fly, auditory hallucinations, and feelings of giddiness. Chemicals that are typically found in inhalants may be evident in the urine or with a breathalizer test.

■ Ocular

Symptoms of ocular involvement include blurry vision, diplopia, lacrimation, and visual hallucinations and distortions of visual perceptions.

TREATMENT AND MANAGEMENT

The only method of treating an acute state of intoxication is to first control the vital signs, followed by supportive assurance (eg "talking" the patient down). It may be necessary to provide an environment that is calming and will protect the patient from self-inflicted injury (Table 82–24).

■ CONSEQUENCES OF INTRAVENOUS DRUG ABUSE

There are a variety of systemic and ocular manifestations of intravenous drug abuse (Tables 82–25 and 82–26). The problems are not only related to the drug itself, but to the foreign

particulate material that is used to "cut" the drug. These may overwhelm the immune system, resulting in inability to effectively respond to infection. Also the particles themselves can cause vascular occlusions. Additionally, infections may arise secondary to aseptic techniques, drug contamination, and sharing injection needles. Table 82–27 summarizes treatment and management of intravenous drug abuse.

ACQUIRED IMMUNE DEFICIENCY SYNDROME

By far, AIDS is the most serious consequence of intravenous drug abuse. Needle sharing is common with IV drug

TABLE 82–25. SYSTEMIC MANIFESTATIONS OF INTRAVENOUS DRUG ABUSE

SYSTEMIC MANIFESTATIONS
- Pulmonary emboli
- Cerebrovascular emboli
- **Fungal Infection**
  Disseminated
  Endocarditis
  Circulating immune complexes resulting in arthritis, mucocutaneous vasculitis, glomerulonephritis
- **Bacterial Infection**
  Disseminated
  Endocarditis
  Circulating immune complexes

SIGNS AND SYMPTOMS
- **Of Pulmonary Emboli**
  Dyspnea, chest pain
- **Of Cerebrovascular Emboli**
  Transient ischemia attacks, hemiplegia, other neurologic sequelae
- **Of Fungal Infection**
  Fever, malaise, joint pain
- **Of Bacterial Infection**
  See fungal infection, above
  Petechia on skin, palms, soles of feet; nodules on fingers and toes; clubbing of fingers; needle tracks; thrombophlebitis; dermatitis overlying site of injection

TABLE 82–26. OCULAR MANIFESTATIONS OF INTRAVENOUS DRUG ABUSE

AIDS
- CMV retinitis and other ocular manifestations of AIDS

TALC EMBOLI
- Talc retinopathy
  - Tiny cluster of yellow-white glistening crystals
  - Microaneurysms
  - Hemorrhages
  - Venous tortuosity
  - Retinal ischemia
  - No effect on vision unless macular ischemia is present

FUNGAL INFECTION
- **Fungal endopthalmitis**
  - Focal chorioretinitis
    - Retinal white cotton-like exudates
    - Decreased acuity
    - Photophobia
    - Ocular pain
  - Uveitis
  - Papillitis
  - Vitritis

BACTERIAL INFECTION
- **Bacterial endophthalmitis**
  - Retinitis
    - Retinal white cotton-like infiltrates with fluffy borders extending into the vitreous
    - Roth spots
    - Candle-wax drippings
    - Blurry vision
    - Photophobia
    - Ocular pain
  - Vasculitis
  - Lid swelling
  - Conjunctival edema, injection, or petechiae
  - Corneal edema
  - Uveitis
  - Papillitis
  - Vitritis

users and is a risk factor for transmitting the human immunodeficiency virus (HIV). The numerous systemic and ocular manifestations of AIDS are described in Chapter 58.

TALC RETINOPATHY

Talc retinopathy occurs as a result of embolization of talc, cornstarch, or other particles to the retina after intravenous injection of drugs that contain these substances as fillers and binders. Often tablets that are normally used for oral consumption are crushed, dissolved in boiling water, and administered intravenously. Unfortunately some of the substances are insoluble and remain in suspension. Most of the talc and cornstarch particles are larger than 5.0 μm. This is a sufficient size for occlusion, because capillary diameter is typically 3.5 to 5.0 μm. The pulmonary and cerebral vasculature also traps the larger particles.

EPIDEMIOLOGY

Data outlining the prevalence or incidence of talc retinopathy was not found in the literature.

NATURAL HISTORY

■ Systemic
Pulmonary vascular embolization causes direct occlusion to the small pulmonary vessels or induces endothelial proliferation and granulomas with secondary occlusion of the capillaries, arterioles, and arteries. Initially there is obstruction of blood flow to the distal lung, with subsequent constriction of the air spaces and airways. Later, there can be loss of the alveolar surfactant (a lipoprotein that maintains alveolar stability), and pulmonary hypertension. Complete pulmonary infarction rarely occurs, because the lung has multiple pathways for obtaining oxygen. Occlusions of the cerebral vasculature may lead to transient ischemic attacks, strokes, and cerebral hemorrhages with the resultant neurological sequelae.

■ Ocular
Prolonged use of intravenous drugs that are filled with talc can result in choroidal and/or retinal intracapillary emboli. They appear as multiple, tiny clusters of yellow or white glistening crystals that are usually situated in the perifoveal arcade (Figure 82–1). Microaneurysms, hemorrhages, and venous tortuosity may also form. Retinal ischemia may develop, leading to neovascularization, vitreal hemorrhages, and subsequent nonrhegmatogenous retinal detachment. Peripheral talc retinopathy, although less common, can result in neovascularization at the border between perfused and nonperfused retina that resembles sickle-cell retinopathy. The classic sequelae will follow in the form of fibrotic scarring and subsequent retinal detachment.

DIAGNOSIS

■ Systemic
Pulmonary complications may present with sudden dyspnea (difficulty breathing). Chest pain is not evident unless

TABLE 82–27. TREATMENT AND MANAGEMENT OF INTRAVENOUS DRUG ABUSE

■ **SYSTEMIC**
AIDS
- See text

TALC EMBOLI
- Discontinue intake of particles
- Refer to internist or pulmonary specialist to manage complications of pulmonary involvement
- Refer to internist or neurologist to manage cerebral complications

FUNGAL INFECTION
- **Disseminated**
  Oral ketoconazole, flucytosine, or IV miconazole or amphotericin B
- **Endocarditis**
  Bed rest
  Antifungal agents
  Prophylactic antibiotics

BACTERIAL INFECTIONS
- **Disseminated**
  High-dose, oral, broad-spectrum antibiotics
  Begin treatment prior to culture results and modify as needed
- **Endocarditis**
  High-dose, oral, broad-spectrum antibiotics
  Begin treatment prior to culture results and modify as needed

■ **OCULAR**
TALC EMBOLI
- Discontinue intake of particles
- Refer to internist or pulmonary specialist to manage complications of pulmonary involvement
- Refer to internist or neurologist to manage cerebral complications

FUNGAL INFECTION
- **Endophthalmitis**
  Commence treatment before diagnosis is confirmed
  Intravitreal injection of amphotericin B or miconazole
  Pars plana vitrectomy with or without intraocular or systemic antifungals
  Corticosteroid treatment is controversial

BACTERIAL INFECTION
- **Endophthalmitis**
  100 µg gentamicin and 2.25 mg cefazolin in 0.1 mL solution
  or
  Daily subconjunctival injection of 40 mg gentamicin and 1.25 mg cefazolin
  or
  1 mg/kg intravenous or intramuscular gentamicin

  The above, every 8 hours for 10–14 days
  and
  Fortified topical eyedrops with gentamicin (9.1 mg/mL) and 50 mg/mL cefazolin every 1 hour
  Topical cycloplegics
  After 24 hours of antibiotic therapy, topical, subconjunctival and systemic steroids initiated: 40–80 mg oral prednisolone daily, tapered quickly in 7–14 days
  Vitrectomy recommended in advanced cases or if response is not noted within 36–48 hours of administering above regimen

infarction has occurred. Diagnosis is confirmed with a chest x-ray (that may show a parenchymal infiltrate), pulmonary angiography, and pulmonary function tests. However, retinal signs may sometime precede positive laboratory findings. Cerebral involvement is diagnosed by observing the typical signs and symptoms. Cerebral angiography will show scattered areas of nonperfusion as well as narrowing and fragmentation of arterioles and capillaries.

■ Ocular

Usually early manifestations of talc retinopathy will not pose any problems for the patient. However, if macular ischemia occurs, it may result in decreased visual acuity. Fluorescein angiography will show precapillary arteriolar occlusions, capillary nonperfusion, and vascular leakage. Perimetry or Amsler grid testing may show central scotomas. Fundus photography

utilizing a green filter may highlight the emboli. Focal electroretinography (ERG) will show a reduced amplitude of the foveal signal. Color vision testing as well as dark adaptometry will be normal. Talc retinopathy can be distinguished from drusen and fundus albipunctatus with fluorescein angiography. The perifoveal microvascular occlusions will be absent in these instances. Hematologic testing and the presence of glistening particles will distinguish emboli induced peripheral changes from those seen in sickle-cell retinopathy.

TREATMENT AND MANAGEMENT

Management of talc complications mainly involves discontinuation of the particle intake. Referral should be made to

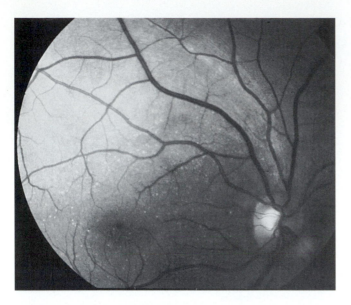

Figure 82–1. Talc retinopathy. *(Courtesy of the Optometry Service, FDR VA Hospital, Montrose, NY.)*

an internist to detect and manage complications of pulmonary involvement, and to a neurologist, if indicated, to rule out and manage cerebral complications.

FUNGAL INFECTION

Fungal infections occur more often when sharing dirty, unsterilized needles and when the proper aseptic precaution of cleaning the skin prior to intravenous injection is not followed. *Candida* is the most common fungal organism that is responsible for both systemic and ocular involvement. Because *Candida* is ubiquitous in the general environment and frequently cultured from the mouth, gastrointestinal tract, and genitourinary tract, other risk factors (like immunodeficiency) may lead to opportunistic infections. *Aspergillus* is the second most common fungal infection found in intravenous drug users; however, only a few cases have been reported. It too is ubiquitous in the environment and is commonly cultured from dust, air, and the respiratory tract. Endocarditis is a frequent complication of parenteral drug addiction, with the endocardium of the aortic and mitral valves most often affected. Disseminated fungal infection may also occur on rare occasions. Endophthalmitis associated with intravenous drug abuse develops as a result of invasion of the organism into the eye from the bloodstream, metastasis from other tissues, or septic emboli from infected heart valves that lodge intraocularly. Usually, however, no associated systemic disease is found.

EPIDEMIOLOGY

Approximately 10 to 15% of the cases of endocarditis associated with intravenous drug abuse are due to *Candida*. Yet, infection with multiple organisms is common.

NATURAL HISTORY

■ Systemic

Infectious endocarditis associated with IV drug abuse develops acutely. This disease is characterized by vegetations growing on valves or other parts of the endocardium. Often the organism is localized on sterile vegetations of platelets and fibrin that are already present. These vegetations may occlude the valve orifices or stimulate an immune reaction, with subsequent scar formation resulting in conduction abnormalities. Pieces of the vegetation may break off, forming emboli to the brain, kidney, spleen, liver, extremities, and lung with subsequent infarction. Myocarditis may develop from coronary artery emboli, extension of the infection to the myocardium with abscess formation, or immune complex vasculitis. Circulating immune complexes may also result in glomerulonephritis, arthritis, and mucocutaneous vasculitis. There is a high rate of mortality associated with endocarditis if left untreated. However, fewer cases of mortality are reported with intravenous drug abuse than with cases associated with immunodeficiency.

■ Ocular

Ocular manifestations may occur weeks after the use of intravenous drugs. Ocular involvement may range from a localized lesion (abcess of suppurative and granulomatous inflammatory material) to full-blown endophthalmitis. Both *Candida* and *Aspergillus* will give similar signs that are characterized by a choroidal or chorioretinal white cotton-like circumscribed exudate (Figure 82–2). An overlying vitreal haze is usually present when the predisposing factor is IV drug abuse. The lesion typically originates in the choroid. It can progress to the RPE and eventually extend into the overlying retina. Lesions are approximately 1 mm in diameter and are most often found in the posterior pole. Uveitis, papillitis, vitritis, and Roth spots (white-centered hemorrhages) may also develop. Visual prognosis is improved if treatment is initiated early on, but poor once the vitreous is involved. Phthisis bulbi may result in intractable cases.

Fungal endophthalmitis occurs and progresses at a much slower rate than bacterial endophthalmitis. Embolization from the heart valves in infectious endocarditis may result in retinal and conjunctival hemorrhages and central or branch retinal artery occlusion.

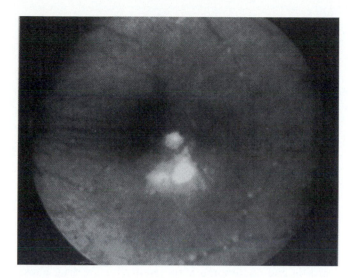

Figure 82–2. Candida retinitis. *(Courtesy of Dr. Scott Richter.)*

DIAGNOSIS

■ Systemic

Endocarditis and endophthalmitis in an otherwise healthy person should raise the suspicion of possible drug abuse. Blood and urine toxicology testing should be obtained to detect the presence of abused substances, antibody titers, circulating immune complexes, and fungal organisms. Blood cultures for fungal organisms may be negative because multiple samples are often needed to enhance fungal growth. Rheumatoid factor will be positive in approximately 50% of cases after 6 weeks. An echocardiogram is needed to visualize the internal cardiac structures. The presence of needle tracks and thrombophlebitis as well as dermatitis overlying the injection site are supportive signs. Diagnostic symptoms of endocarditis will generally start 2 weeks after the acute infection and include fever, malaise, and on occasion joint pain. Unlike other causes of endocarditis, heart murmurs are usually absent in cases associated with IV drug abuse.

■ Ocular

One should suspect fungal endophthalmitis based on the presence of characteristic signs and symptoms and a history of intravenous drug abuse. The patient may complain of blurry vision, photophobia, and generalized ocular pain. A systemic workup may be negative, because disseminated fungal infection may not show up concurrently with endophthalmitis. Vitreous or anterior chamber cultures are considered mandatory when fungal endophthalmitis is suspected. It is believed that vitreous culture is better than anterior chamber paracentesis.

TREATMENT AND MANAGEMENT

■ Systemic

The therapy of choice to treat disseminated systemic infections is to administer oral ketoconazole. Other agents that are used are oral flucytosine and intravenous miconazole or amphotericin B. Acute endocarditis is managed with bed rest, antifungal agents, and prophylactic antibiotics.

■ Ocular

There are many variations as to how to manage fungal endophthalmitis. However, it is generally agreed that treatment should commence even before the diagnosis is confirmed. For those who do treat with antifungal agents, intravitreal injection is required, because systemic administration does not result in sufficient penetration into the vitreous. Amphotericin B or miconazole are usually the agents of choice. Pars plana vitrectomy may also be performed with or without intraocular or systemic antifungal agents. The safety and efficacy of this regimen is still questionable. The use of topical or systemic corticosteroids is controversial.

BACTERIAL INFECTIONS

Bacterial infections associated with IV drug abuse usually arise from microorganisms on the skin. Disseminated infection and endocarditis are life-threatening consequences. As in fungal endocarditis, infection produces vegetations on the endocardium with the heart valve being the major site of infection. Endophthalmitis associated with IV drug abuse develops due to spread from an endogenous site of infection.

EPIDEMIOLOGY

Fifty percent of endocarditis cases associated with IV drug abuse are caused by *Staphylococcus*, while *Streptococcus* makes up about 15% of the cases. However, infection with multiple organisms is common. Ocular manifestations of bacterial infection are less common than fungal infections in IV drug users.

NATURAL HISTORY

■ Systemic

Staphylococcus aureus usually causes acute endocarditis. This characteristically develops on a normal heart valve, is rapidly destructive, produces metastatic foci, and can cause fatality in 6 weeks if left untreated. *Streptococci* is more commonly associated with subacute endocarditis. It characteristically occurs on a damaged heart valve, does not produce metastases, and there is a longer onset of fatality if left untreated (sometimes up to a year). The clinical features are similar to fungal endocarditis in that vegetations can lead to occlusion of valve orifices, development of immune reactions, scar formation with valvular stenosis, and myocardial involvement from coronary artery emboli, myocardial abscesses, or immune complex vasculitis. Emboli to the pulmonary, cerebral, renal, liver, and peripheral vasculature may occur with resultant infarction. Other manifestations include glomerulonephritis, arthritis, mucocutaneous vasculitis, skin petechiae, nodules on the finger or toes, small hemorrhages on the palms and soles of the feet, and clubbing of the fingers in chronic cases. Prognosis for recovery is good in treated cases; however, fatality may occur from heart failure, rupture of mycotic aneurysm, or renal failure. See Chapter 4 for a more detailed discussion.

■ Ocular

Endophthalmitis may present acutely with rapid progression. Signs are usually evident in the first 24 to 48 hours. The posterior chamber is the site most involved, with retinitis the most common ocular manifestation. The retinal lesions may be found centrally or peripherally and are characterized by a white cotton-like infiltrate with fluffy borders extending into the vitreous. Roth spots may occur in 5% of cases. A "candle-wax" vasculitis similar to that found in sarcoidosis may also be evident. Advanced cases will manifest with lid swelling, conjunctival edema, injection, petechiae, corneal edema, uveitis (often with hypopyon), papillitis, and vitritis. Banks and co-workers (1973) reported 3 cases of unilateral, purulent panophthalmitis in 28 heroin addicts. Prognosis is enhanced if treatment occurs early and prior to vitreal involvement.

Embolization from the heart valves in endocarditis can result in retinal and conjunctival hemorrhages, and central or branch retinal artery occlusion, resulting in retinal edema and ischemia.

DIAGNOSIS

■ Systemic

The diagnosis of bacterial infection is based on blood assays of antibody titers to the organism, serum titers to teichoic acid (a cell-wall antigen in *S. aureus*), circulating immune complexes, and the presence of microorganisms. Bacteremia (widespread dissemination by way of the bloodstream) may be evident. Rheumatoid factor is positive in approximately 50% of cases in 6 weeks after onset. An echocardiogram

may not always detect the vegetations. Diagnostic symptoms include fever, malaise, and possibly joint pain.

■ Ocular

Retinitis will mainly cause decreased acuity. Severe endophthalmitis involving the uvea will cause blurry vision, photophobia, and pain. A vitrectomy with culture should be performed for confirmation, because many of the therapeutic medications are toxic.

TREATMENT AND MANAGEMENT

■ Systemic

High concentrations of broad-spectrum antibiotics, especially directed at *S. aureus*, are used to treat bacterial endocarditis and bacteremia associated with IV drug abuse. Therapy is initiated prior to knowing the results of culture and altered as needed once results are available. Good results are seen with parenteral penicillin, gentamicin, cephalosporin, and vancomycin given for long durations.

■ Ocular

The management of bacterial endophthalmitis, although controversial, usually involves administering intravitreal, subconjunctival, topical, and systemic broad-spectrum antibiotics simultaneously (see Table 82–27).

■ QUININE

Quinine is an alkaloid that is derived from cinchona bark. Oral quinine sulphate or bisulfate is mainly used to treat nocturnal muscle cramps and malaria. It also has mild analgesic and antipyretic properties but it is not used for this purpose. Hemorrhoids and varicose veins are sometimes treated with a mixture of quinine and urea hydrochloride. It is described in this chapter on drug abuse because it is commonly used to cut heroin. Although the side effects of quinine abuse on vision and hearing usually occur with large doses, effects from smaller amounts have been reported that are thought to be due to hypersensitivity reactions.

NATURAL HISTORY

■ Systemic

Effects of long-term therapeutic doses are characterized by mild allergic, CNS, gastrointestinal, cardiovascular, and auditory failure (Table 82–28). The typical signs and symptoms include tinnitus, nausea, vomiting, headache, abdominal pain, diarrhea, vertigo, fever, pruritus, skin rashes, and ventricular fibrillations on occasion. Smaller doses may result in similar signs and symptoms in people who are hypersensitive. Additionally, angio-edema, asthma, thrombocytopenia, hypoprothrombinemia, hemolytic anemia, and

TABLE 82–28. SYSTEMIC MANIFESTATIONS OF QUININE ABUSE

- CNS depression
  Lethargy, irritability, drowsiness, confusion
- Gastrointestinal, cardiovascular, respiratory, and auditory failure
  - Tinnitus, partial deafness
  - Nausea, vomiting
  - Headache
  - Abdominal pain
  - Diarrhea
  - Vertigo
  - Fever
  - Ventricular fibrillations
  - Asthma
- Allergy
  Pruritis, skin rashes, angioedema
- Anemia
- Muscle twitching

circulatory failure may manifest. Overdoses may cause severe effects in the form of partial deafness, cardiac depression, circulatory collapse, respiratory arrest, syncope, coma, and death. Eight grams is the average lethal dose.

■ Ocular

The most prominent feature of quinine poisoning is an acute loss in vision (moderate blur to complete blindness) that spontaneously begins to recover gradually with residual visual acuity deprivation. Typically the patient will wake up with an acute, significant loss of vision 1 day after drug use (Table 82–29). Usually there is partial recovery of central vision, sometimes within a few days, with residual peripheral visual field constriction. As little as 0.8 g of quinine was reported by Lincoff (1975) to cause this response. The

TABLE 82–29. OCULAR MANIFESTATIONS OF QUININE ABUSE

- Presumed retinal ganglion cell toxicity and secondary neuropathy
  Acute moderate to severe loss in vision with partial recovery
  Cherry red spot
  Arterial narrowing
  Dilated pupils that are not reactive to light or accommodation
  Photophobia
  Diplopia
  Color vision defects
  Night blindness
  Residual peripheral visual field constriction
- Iris edema and ischemia

exact mechanism for the visual involvement is controversial because the fundus may appear normal during the initial stage of acute blindness, and there is a progressive onset of subsequent retinal changes even when vision has started to improve. Additionally, angiography, ERG, VER, and EOG findings are not consistent. Nevertheless, quinine is believed to cause direct toxicity to the retinal ganglion cells and secondary atrophy of the rods and cones. There is preservation of the macular fibers, which allows for recovery of visual function. The retinal signs usually develop after the initial acute loss of vision and are characterized by edema, arterial attenuation, and at times, a macular cherry red spot indicating generalized retinal infarction with preservation of the macular fibers. Also, optic atrophy develops gradually. The pupils are dilated and nonreactive to light or accommodation. The pupil involvement is thought to be correlated with the optic neuropathy as well as the occurrence of iris edema and ischemia. The pupillary response usually recovers gradually but will remain sluggish.

DIAGNOSIS

■ Systemic

Observation of the characteristic signs and symptoms as outlined in the natural history should raise the suspicion of possible quinine toxicity. In addition the patient may report dizziness, lethargy, irritability, drowsiness, confusion, and muscle twitching. Diagnosis is confirmed with laboratory assessment of plasma quinine levels. Toxic levels are considered to be 10 mg/L or more. Evidence of intravenous drug abuse should enhance the suspicion.

■ Ocular

In addition to the typical pattern of vision loss, the patient may report residual photophobia, diplopia, defects in color vision, and night blindness. ERG will usually become progressively abnormal, which may persist after intervention. The VEP will show abnormal latency and waveform and EOG amplitudes have also been reduced in some cases. Visual fields are helpful to differentiate other types of toxic optic neuropathy because there will usually be recovery of the central visual field defect with residual peripheral constriction.

TREATMENT AND MANAGEMENT

■ Systemic

Acute poisoning is treated with gastrointestinal aspiration and lavage. The vital signs and symptoms should be managed closely until the drug is eliminated, which usually occurs in a few hours. Unfortunately, there is no antidote known to counter the side effects (Table 82–30).

TABLE 82–30. TREATMENT AND MANAGEMENT OF QUININE ABUSE

- ■ **SYSTEMIC**
  - Gastric aspiration lavage
  - Stabilize vital signs
  - No antidote to counter side effects

- ■ **OCULAR**
  - Oral vasodilators
  - Intravenous, retrobulbar, or subconjunctival adrenocorticotropic hormone
  - CO_2 inhalation and globe massage have been used to prevent vasoconstriction; however, this treatment is controversial

■ Ocular

Therapy to prevent vision loss is attempted with oral vasodilators (to inhibit vasoconstriction); intravenous, retrobulbar, or subconjunctival adrenocorticotropic hormone; carbon dioxide inhalation; and globe massage. However, it is not clear whether these therapeutic measures are beneficial, because recovery usually occurs spontaneously and the onset of retinal vascular attenuation is not believed to be contributory.

CONCLUSION

Drug and alcohol abuse is a serious social problem in the United States. The widespread use of illicit drugs, and misuse of prescription drugs, makes it increasingly likely that primary eyecare practitioners will encounter a variety of drug-related problems among their patients. Because many of the signs and symptoms are similar to other disease processes and often drug abusers do not volunteer this information, it is important to include drug abuse in the differential diagnosis.

REFERENCES

Adams AJ, Brown B. Marijuana, alcohol, and combined drug effects on the time course of glare recovery. *Psychopharmacology.* 1978;56:81–86.

Apter JT, Pfeiffer CC. Effect of hallucinogenic drugs on the ERG. *Am J Ophthalmol.* 1956;42:206–210.

Baird HW, Bileggi AJ. Diminished corneal reflexes after diazepam. *Lancet.* 1968;2:106.

Banks T, Flectcher R, Ali N. Infective endocarditis in heroin addicts. *Am J Med.* 1973;55:444–451.

Bard LA, Gills JP. Quinine amblyopia. *Arch Ophthalmol.* 1964;72:328–331.

Brown GC, Brown RH, Brown MM. Peripheral proliferative retinopathies. *Int Ophthalmol.* 1987;11:41–50.

Carroll FD. Toxicology of the optic nerve. In: Srinivasan BD, ed. *Ocular Therapeutics.* Kinderhook, NY: Masson; 1980:139–143.

Cavka V. New Ophthalmological symptoms in cirrhosis of the liver. *Jugoslav Oftal Arh.* 1963;1:5–44.

Cohen S, Ditman KS. Prolonged adverse reactions to lysergic acid diethylamide. *Arch Gen Psychiatr.* 1963;8:475–480.

Colasanti BK. Contemporary drug abuse. In: Graig CR, Stitzel RE, eds. *Modern Pharmacology.* 2nd ed. Boston: Little, Brown; 1986:610–630.

Comings DE, Comings BG, Muhleman D, et al. The dopamine D2 receptor locus as a modifying gene in neuropsychiatric disorders. *JAMA.* 1991;266:1793–1800.

Diaz-Calderon E, Del Brutto OH, Aquirre R, Alarcon TA. Bilateral internuclear ophthalmoplegia after smoking "crack" cocaine. *J Clin Neuro-ophthalmol.* 1991;11:297–299.

Fisher JH. The influence of nicotin on ganglion cells: Its bearing on the pathology of tobacco amblyopia. *Ophthalmol Rev.* 1901;20:151–159.

Flom Mc, Adams AJ, Jones RT. Marijuana smoking and reduced pressure in human eyes: Drug action or epiphenomenon? *Invest Ophthalmol Vis Sci.* 1975;14:52–55.

Ford Foundation. *Dealing with Drug Abuse: A Report to the Ford Foundation. The Drug Abuse Survey Project.* New York: Praeger; 1973.

Foulds WS, Chisholm IA, Stewart JB, Wilson TM. The optic neuropathy of pernicious anemia. *Arch Ophthalmol.* 1969;82:427–432.

Foulds WS, Pettigrew AR. The biochemical basis of the toxic amblyopias. In: Perkins ED, Hill DW, eds. *Scientific Foundations of Ophthalmology.* London: Heinemann; 1977:50–54.

Fraunfelder FT. *Drug-induced Ocular Side Effects and Drug Interactions.* Philadelphia: Lea & Febiger; 1976.

Friberg TR, Gragoudas ES, Regan CDJ. Talc emboli and macular ischemia in intravenous drug abuse. *Arch Ophthalmol.* 1979;97:1089–1091.

Gaasterland DE. Efficacy in glaucoma treatment: The potential of marijuana. *Ann Ophthalmol.* 1980;12:448–450. Editorial.

Gelernter J, O'Malley S, Risch N, et al. No association between an allele at the D2 dopamine receptor gene (DRD2) and alcoholism. *JAMA.* 1991;266:1801–1807.

Glaser JS. Topical diagnosis: Prechiasmal visual pathways. In: Tasman W, Jaeger EA, eds. *Duane's Clinical Ophthalmology.* Philadelphia: Lippincott; 1991;2:69–74.

Grant WM. *Toxicology of the Eye.* 3rd ed. Springfield, IL: Thomas; 1986.

Green K, Pederson JE. Effect of delta-tetrahydrocannabinol on aqueous dynamics and ciliary body permeability in the rabbit. *Exp Eye Res.* 1973;15:499.

Gunn M. Toxic amblyopia. *Tr Ophthalmol Soc UK.* 1887;7:67–71.

Halperin E, Yolton RL. Is the driver drunk? Oculomotor sobriety testing. *J Am Optometric Assoc.* 1986;57:654–657.

Halperin MH, McFarland RA, Niven JI, Roughton FJ. The time course of the effects of carbon monoxide on visual thresholds. *J Physiol.* 1959;146:583–593.

Harrington DO. Amblyopia due to tobacco, alcohol and nutritional deficiency. Differential diagnosis with special reference to the character of the visual field defect. *Am J Ophthalmol.* 1962,53:967–972.

Heaton JM, McCormic AJA, Freeman AG. Tobacco amblyopia; A clinical manifestation of vitamin B_{12} deficiency. *Lancet.* 1958;2:286–290.

Hepler RS, Frank IR. Marihuana smoking and intraocular pressure. *JAMA.* 1971;217:1392.

Herskowitz J, Oppenheimer EY. More about poisoning by phencyclidine (PCP, angel dust). *N Engl J Med.* 1977;297:1405.

Hoffman JA. LSD flashbacks. *Arch Gen Psychiatr.* 1984;41:631–632.

Hogan RE, Linfield PB. The effects of moderate doses of ethanol on heterophoria and other aspect of binocular vision. *Ophthalmic Physiol Opt.* 1983;3:21–31.

Holzman PS, Levy DL, Uhlenhuth EH, et al. Smooth pursuit eye movements, and diazepam, CPZ, and secobarbital. *Psychopharmacologia.* 1975;44:111–115.

Howells DE. Nystagmus as a physical sign in alcoholic intoxication. *Br Med J.* 1956;1:1405–1406.

Hutchinson J. Statistical details of four year experience in respect to the form of amaurosis supposed to be due to tobacco. *Ophthalmol Hosp Res.* 1873;7:169–185.

Kaye D. Infective Endocarditis. In: Wilson JD, Braunwald E, Isselbacher KJ, et al, eds. *Harrison's Principles of Internal Medicine.* 12th ed. New York: McGraw-Hill; 1991:508–512.

Klee A, Willanger R. Disturbances of visual perception in migraine. *Acta Neurol Scand.* 1966;42:400–414.

Knave B, Persson HE, Nilsson SE. A comparative study on the effects of barbiturates and ethyl alcohol on retinal functions. *Acta Ophthalmol.* 1974;52:254–259.

Krill AE, Wieland AM, Ostfeld AM. The effect of two hallucinogenic agents on human retinal function. *Arch Ophthalmol.* 1960;64:724–733.

Leishman R. Gastric function in tobacco amblyopia. *Tr Ophthalmol Soc UK.* 1951;71:319–327.

Levi L, Miller NR. Visual illusions associated with previous drug abuse. *J Clin Neuro-ophthalmol.* 1990;10:103–110.

Limaye SR, Goldberg MH. Septic submacular choroidal embolus associated with intravenous drug abuse. *Ann Ophthalmol.* 1982;14:518–522.

Lyncoff MH. Quinine amblyopia. *Arch Ophthalmol.* 1955;53:382–384.

Mclane NJ, Carroll DM. Ocular manifestations of drug abuse. *Surv Ophthalmol.* 1986;30:298–313.

McLaren D. *Nutritional Ophthalmology: Malnutrition & the Eye.* New York: Academic Press; 1980.

Menezo JL, Martinez-Costa R, Marin F, Cortes-Vizcaino V. Tuberculous panophthalmitis associated with drug abuse. *Int Ophthalmol.* 1987;10:235–240.

Michelson JB, Freedman SD, Boyden DG. *Aspergillus* endophthalmitis in a drug abuser. *Ann Ophthalmol.* 1982;14:1051–1054.

Michelson JB, Friedlaender MH. Endophthalmitis of drug abuse. *Int Ophthalmol Clin.* 1987;27:120–126.

Michelson JB, Robin HS, Nozik RA. Nonocular manifestations of parenteral drug abuse. *Surv Ophthalmol.* 1986; 30:314–320.

Miller TA. Crack and gastroduodenal perforation. *Gastroenterology.* 1992;102:1431–1432.

Moser KM. Pulmonary thromboembolism. In: Wilson JD, Braunwald E, Isselbacher KJ, et al, eds. *Harrison's Principles of Internal Medicine.* 12th ed. New York: McGraw-Hill; 1991:1090–1096.

National Institute on Drug Abuse. *National Survey on Drug Abuse.* Rockville, MD: U.S. Department of Health and Human Services; 1990.

National Institute on Drug Abuse. *Marihuana and Health. Sixth Annual Report to the U.S. Congress.* Rockville, MD: U.S. Department of Health, Education and Welfare; 1976.

National Institute on Drug Abuse. *White Paper on Drug Abuse. A Report to the President from the Domestic Council Drug Abuse Task Force.* Rockville, MD: U.S. Department of Health, Education, and Welfare; 1975.

Nicotine. In: Gosselin RE, Smith RP, Hodge HC, eds. *Clinical Toxicology of Commercial Products.* 5th ed. Baltimore: Williams & Wilkins; 1984:311–313.

O'Donnell AE, Mappin FG, Sebo TJ, Tazelaar H. Interstitial pneumonitis associated with "crack" cocaine abuse. *Chest.* 1991;100:1155–1157.

Parsian A, Todd RD, Devor EJ, et al. Alcoholism and alleles of the human D2 dopamine receptor locus: Studies of association and linkage. *Arch Gen Psychiatr.* 1991;48:655–663.

Parsons JH. Action of nicotin upon nerve cells. *J Physiol London.* 1901;26:38–39.

Pettigrew AR, Fell GS. The simplified colorimetric determination of thiocyanate in biological fluids, and its application to investigation of the toxic amblyopias. *Clin Chem.* 1972;18:996–998.

Purnell WD, Gregg JM. Delta-9-tetrahydrocannabinol, euphoria and intraocular pressure in man. *Ann Ophthalmol.* 1975;7:921–923.

Quinine. In: Gosselin RE, Smith RP, Hodge HC, eds. *Clinical Toxicology of Commercial Products.* 5th ed. Baltimore: Williams & Wilkins; 1984:355–361.

Rapidis P, Andreanos D, Krystallis A. Uveal manifestations of chronic alcoholism. *Arch Soc Ophthalmol Grece Nord.* 1975;22:398–406.

Reynolds JE. *Martindale The Extra Pharmacopoeia.* 29th ed. London: Pharmaceutical Press; 1989:518–520.

Robinson PK, Watt AC. Hallucinations as remembered scenes as an epileptic aura. *Brain.* 1947;70:440–448.

Roth JH. Luminal poisoning with conjunctival residue. *Am J Ophthalmol.* 1926;9:533–534.

Russell RM, Carney EA, Feiock K, et al. Acute ethanol administration causes transient impairment of blue-yellow color vision. *Alcohol Clin Exp Res.* 1980;4:396–399.

Sharpe JA. Methanol optic neuropathy: A histopathological study. *Neurology.* 1982;32:1093–1100.

Silvette H, Haag HB, Larson PS. Tobacco amblyopia: The evolution and natural history of a "tobaccogenic" disease. *Am J Ophthalmol.* 1960;50:71–100.

Speicher CE. *The Right Test: A Physician's Guide to Laboratory Medicine.* John Dyson, ed. Philadelphia: Saunders; 1989:29–37.

Srinivasan BD. Bacterial endophthalmitis. In: Srinivasan BD, ed. *Ocular Therapeutics.* Kinderhook, NY: Masson; 1980:59–63.

Summerskill WHJ, Molnar GD. Eye signs in hepatic cirrhosis. *N Engl J Med.* 1962;226:1244–1248.

Swash M. Visual perseveration in temporal lobe epilepsy. *J Neurol Neurosurg Psychiatr.* 1979;42:569–571.

Thomas CL, ed. *Taber's Cyclopedic Medical Dictionary.* Philadelphia: Davis; 1993:2398–2417.

Traquair HM. Toxic amblyopia. *Trans Ophthmol Soc UK.* 1931;50:372–385.

Traquair HM. Tobacco amblyopia. *Lancet.* 1928;2:1173–1177.

Urey JC. Some ocular manifestations of systemic drug abuse. *J Am Opt Assoc.* 1991;62:832–841.

U.S. Department of Health, Education, and Welfare. Public Health Services. *Smoking and Health. A Report of the Surgeon General.* Washington, DC: HEW; 1979.

Van Norren D, Padmos P. Influence of anesthetics, ethyl alcohol, and freon on dark adaptation of monkey cone ERG. *Invest Ophthalmol Vis Sci.* 1977;16:80–83.

Walsh FB. *Clinical Neuro-ophthalmology.* 2nd ed. Baltimore: Williams & Wilkins; 1957:1180–1230.

Wilford BB: *Drug Abuse, A Guide for the Primary Physician.* Chicago: American Medical Association; 1981.

Wilkinson IMS, Kime R, Purnell M. Alcohol and human eye movement. *Brain.* 1974;97:785–792.

Witherspoon CD, Feist FW, Morris RE, Feist RM. Ocular self-mutilation. *Ann Ophthalmol.* 1989;21:255–259.

I
Appendix

Ocular Manifestations of Systemic Disease

	Lids, Lashes, Adnexa	Conjunctiva, Sclera	Cornea	Iris, Uvea, Ciliary Body, Anterior Chamber	Lens	Vitreous
Acquired immuno-deficiency syndrome	Molluscum contagiosum, herpes zoster ophthalmicus, Kaposi sarcoma	Nonspecific conjunctivitis, Kaposi sarcoma, microvasculo-pathy	Ocular surface disease; HSV, HZV, and microsporidial keratitis, fungal and bacterial ulcers	Primary HIV uveitis		
Addison disease, *see* Adrenal dysfunction						
Adrenal gland dysfunction	Pigmentation (Addison disease)	Pigment of conjunctiva (Addison disease)		Increased IOP (Cushing syndrome)		
Albinism	White lashes, poliosis			Light blue to brown irides, iris transillumination		
Alzheimer disease						
Anemia		Conjunctival pallor/hemor-rhage, subcon-junctival hemorrhage		Hyphema (aplastic)		Blood in vitreous from retinal internal limiting membrane breaks
Ankylosing spondylitis				Iridocyclitis		
Aplastic anemia, *see* Anemia						
Arnold Chiari malformations, *see* Chiari malformations						
Arteriosclerosis						

Optic Nerve	Macula	Retina, Choroid	Extraocular Muscles, Eye Movements	Higher Cortical Function	Other
Neuritis, neuropathy, papilledema		Noninfectious retinopathy, CMV retinitis, syphilitic retinitis	3,4,6 CN palsy, abnormal saccades, abnormal pursuits, and eye movements	Visual field defects	Pupil abnormalities, lymphoma
Chiasmal compression (Cushing syndrome, adrenal insufficiency), papilledema (neuroblastoma)		Hypertensive retinopathy (Cushing syndrome, primary aldosteronism, pheochromocy-toma)			Exophthalmos (Cushing syndrome), Horner syndrome (neuroblastoma), proptosis with ecchymosis (neuroblastoma)
	Hypoplasia	Small capillary free zone in posterior pole, prominent choroidal vessels	Nystagmus	Bihemispheric VEP asymmetries	Reduced VA
Degeneration			Impaired ocular motility	Visuospatial disorientation, agnosia, apraxia, hallucinations, optic ataxia	Dyschromatopsia, decreased contrast sensitivity
Pallor (aplastic, pernicious), swelling (aplastic), neuropathy (pernicious)		Dilated/tortuous veins, hemorrhages (retinal/preretinal), exudates, cotton-wool spots, pallor of fundus, retinal edema, CRVO	CN palsies (iron deficient)		
		Hyalinization of arterioles, broadening of arterial light reflex, copper to silver wire appearance, CRVO/BRVO, hypoperfusion retinopathy			

	Lids, Lashes, Adnexa	Conjunctiva, Sclera	Cornea	Iris, Uvea, Ciliary Body, Anterior Chamber	Lens	Vitreous
Atopic dermatitis	Prominent lower eyelid fold, pruritis, foreign-body sensation, blepharitis, thickened lid margins	Keratoconjunctivitis, symblepharon	Superficial punctate keratitis, increased susceptibility to herpes simplex, keratoconus	Uveitis, ocular hypertension	Cataracts	
Behçet syndrome	Ulcerative eyelid lesions	Conjunctivitis, episcleritis, scleritis	Keratitis	Bilateral granulomatous anterior uveitis, hypopyon, iris neovascular-ization, posterior synechiae, secondary glaucoma	Cataracts	Cells, hemorrhage
Cancer, *see* specific type						
Cardiac disorders, *see* specific valvular disease						
Cerebrovascular disease				Anterior segment ischemia (carotid disease)		
Chiari malformations			Exposure keratitis			
Chlamydia	Edematous lids, lid deformities (late complication), pseudoptosis	Follicular/papillary conjunctivitis, dry eye	Ulceration and scarring secondary to trichiasis (trachoma), superior keratitis, vascularization, limbal swelling, micropannus (inclusion conjunctivitis)	Mild anterior uveitis		
Chronic progressive ophthalmoplegia	Ptosis					
Cicatricial pemphigoid	Severe dry eye, entropion, trichiasis	Chronic conjunctivitis, symblepharon, ankyloblepharon, shrinkage	Vascularization			
Crohn disease, *see* Inflammatory bowel disease						

Optic Nerve	Macula	Retina, Choroid	Extraocular Muscles, Eye Movements	Higher Cortical Function	Other
		BRVO, RD, central serous choroidopathy			
Papillitis, papilledema, atrophy	Edema, hemorrhage	Focal retinal lesions, RD, RPE hypertrophy, retinal atrophy, CRVO/BRVO, peripheral vasculitis, choroidal vasculitis, sheathing	CN 3,4,6 palsies		
		Plaques, emboli, cotton-wool spots, asymmetric retinopathy, hypoperfusion retinopathy (carotid disease)	Motility abnormalities (vertebrobasilar disease)	Bilateral hemianopsia (vertebrobasilar disease), transient visual obscuration (carotid disease)	Horner syndrome (vertebrobasilar disease)
Papilledema			CN 6 palsy, INO, nystagmus		
		Pigmentary retinopathy	Ophthalmoplegia		Orbicularis oculi weakness, reduced saccadic velocity

	Lids, Lashes, Adnexa	Conjunctiva, Sclera	Cornea	Iris, Uvea, Ciliary Body, Anterior Chamber	Lens	Vitreous
Cushing syndrome, *see* Adrenal dysfunction						
Diabetes	Decreased tear production, periorbital edema		Decreased sensitivity, abrasions, erosions, slow and defective re-epithelialization	Rubeosis iridis, ectropion uveae, neovascular glaucoma, increased incidence of COAG	Premature or diabetic cataract	
Diffuse large-cell Lymphoma			Keratic precipitates	Posterior or anterior uveitis, hypopyon, neovascular glaucoma		Vitritis
Drug and alcohol abuse, *see* Tables 82–2, 82–5, 82–8, 82–11, 82–14, 82–17, 82–20, 82–23, 82–26, and 82–29						
Dysproteinemias, *see* Waldenstroms macroglobuline-mia, multiple myeloma						
Ehlers–Danlos syndrome	Prominent epicanthal folds	Blue sclera	Microcornea, keratoconus or globus, haze at Bowman membrane, rupture with minimal trauma		Ectopia lentis	
Erythema multiforme	Lid edema, focal ulcerations, dry eye	Conjunctival pseudo or true membranes, scarring		Iritis, iridocyclitis		
Erythema nodosum				Uveitis (if associated with systemic inflammatory disease)		
Fabry disease, *see* Sphingolipidoses						
Gaucher disease, *see* Sphingolipidoses						
Giant-cell arteritis				Rubeosis irides with secondary glaucoma		
Gout	Crystal deposition in tarsal plates	Chronic bilateral conjunctival injection, episcle-ritis, scleritis, crystal deposition in sclera	Crystal deposition		Crystal deposition	Increased incidence of asteroid hyalosis

Optic Nerve	Macula	Retina, Choroid	Extraocular Muscles, Eye Movements	Higher Cortical Function	Other
	Edema	Diabetic retinopathy (nonproliferative/ proliferative)	3,4,6 CN palsy		Decreased accommodation, fluctuating vision or refraction, tritan color defect
Optic nerve sheathing		Exudative RD, subretinal infiltrates	CN palsies (with CNS involvement)		Blurred vision
		RD, angioid streaks, vitreoretinal degeneration	Strabismus		Myopia
AION		CRAO	CN 3,6 palsy	Cortical blindness (occipital infarction)	Ocular pain
			Crystal deposition in EOM tendons		

	Lids, Lashes, Adnexa	Conjunctiva, Sclera	Cornea	Iris, Uvea, Ciliary Body, Anterior Chamber	Lens	Vitreous
Guillain–Barré syndrome	Ectropion, ptosis, lagophthalmos		Keratoconjunctivitis sicca, exposure keratitis, neurotrophic ulceration			
Hansen disease	Brow/lash loss, thickened lids, ptosis, ectropion, lagophthalmos, dacryoadenitis, dacryocystitis	Palpebral and limbal lepromas, episcleritis, scleritis, staphyloma or scleromalacia	Hypesthesia, beaded and thickened corneal nerves, neurotrophic keratitis, secondary infection, pannus or avascular interstitial keratitis	Iris pearls, iris atrophy with miotic pupil, acute or chronic anterior uveitis, secondary glaucoma	Secondary cataract	
Herpes simplex	Blepharitis	Conjunctivitis	Epithelial or stromal keratitis, trophic ulcer	Uveitis, secondary glaucoma		
Herpes zoster	Skin lesions, ptosis, secondary *Staphylococcus aureus* infection, complications secondary to scarring, dacryoadenitis, canaliculitis	Conjunctivitis, mucous membrane lesions, conjunctival vesicles, petechial hemorrhages, episcleritis, scleritis	Punctate epithelial keratitis, pseudodendrite, anterior stromal infiltrates, mucous adherent plaques, keratouveitis, disciform keratitis, neurotrophic keratitis, exposure keratitis, scarring	Iritis, pupil distortion, iris atrophy, cyst formation, hypopyon, heterochromia irides, anterior chamber hemorrhage, hypotony, acute or chronic glaucoma	Cataract	
Histoplasmosis						
HIV, *see* AIDS						
Homocystinuria				Blue irides, iridodonesis, secondary glaucoma	Ectopia lentis, phakodonesis, congenital cataracts	
Hyperlipidemia	Xanthelasma		Arcus			
Hypertension						
Hyperthyroidism, *see* Thyroid dysfunction						

Optic Nerve	Macula	Retina, Choroid	Extraocular Muscles, Eye Movements	Higher Cortical Function	Other
Papilledema			External ophthalmoplegia		
			Retinitis		
			CN 3,4,6 palsy		Ophthalmic division of CN 5 involved: frontal, lacrimal, nasociliary; Horner syndrome; light-near dissociation; proptosis
	Exudative maculopathy	Circumpapillary choroiditis, peripheral atrophic choroidal scars, linear streak lesions			
Atrophy, staphyloma		CRAO, RD, peripheral retinal degeneration	Strabismus		Progressive myopia
		Lipemia retinalis			
Bilateral disc edema		Retina: vasoconstriction, sclerosis, exudation; choroid: Elschnig spots, Siegrist spots, BRVO/CRVO, BRAO/CRAO, macroaneurysm			

	Lids, Lashes, Adnexa	Conjunctiva, Sclera	Cornea	Iris, Uvea, Ciliary Body, Anterior Chamber	Lens	Vitreous
Hypothyroidism, *see* Thyroid dysfunction						
Inflammatory bowel disease		Episcleritis (Crohn disease), scleritis		Uveitis (Crohn disease)		
Intracranial tumors						
Iron deficient anemia, *see* Anemia						
Juvenile rheumatoid arthritis			Band keratopathy	Uveitis, secondary glaucoma	Cataract	
Kawasaki disease		Bilateral conjunctival hyperemia, subconjunctival hemorrhage	Superficial punctate keratitis	Bilateral iridocyclitis		Opacities
Kearns–Sayre syndrome	Ptosis		Clouding of endothelium			
Leprosy, *see* Hansen disease						
Leukemia	Lacrimal gland infiltration, dacryocystitis, infiltration of lid, exophthalmos	Infiltrates, swelling, subconjunctival hemorrhage, necrosis secondary to ischemia, episcleritis	Sterile peripheral corneal ulcers	Infiltration, iris color change, pseudo hypopyon		Infiltrates
Lyme disease	Periorbital edema	Conjunctivitis, episcleritis	Keratitis	Granulomatous iritis		Vitritis
Marfan syndrome	Down-slanting palpebral fissures	Blue sclera		Iridodonesis, Reiger anomaly, deep anterior chamber angle, heterochromic irides, hypoplastic iris dilator, transillumination defects, secondary glaucoma	Ectopia lentis	

Optic Nerve	Macula	Retina, Choroid	Extraocular Muscles, Eye Movements	Higher Cortical Function	Other
Papilledema			CN 3,4,6, palsy	Visual field defects	Pupil abnormality, color vision defect
Bilateral disc edema		Chorioretinal inflammation			
		Salt-and-pepper retinopathy, peripapillary changes, visible choroid vessels	Progressive ophthalmoplegia with ptosis		
Infiltrates, papilledema		Infiltrates, serous sensory RD, RPE changes, cystoid retinal edema, drusen, dilated tortuous veins, yellowing of the vascular reflex, hemorrhages, cotton-wool spots, microan-eurysm, periph-eral retinal neo-vascularization	Extraocular muscle infiltrates		
Optic neuropathy, optic neuritis, bilateral disc edema, pseudotumor cerebri		Retinitis	CN 3,4,6 palsies		Photophobia, facial nerve palsy
		RD, peripheral retinal degenerations	Strabismus		Amblyopia, anisometropia, enophthalmos, colobomas

	Lids, Lashes, Adnexa	Conjunctiva, Sclera	Cornea	Iris, Uvea, Ciliary Body, Anterior Chamber	Lens	Vitreous
Metastases of systemic malignancies	Ptosis	Conjunctival erythema				Floaters
Multiple myeloma	Orbital bone involvement	Sludging of blood, iridescent crystalline deposits	Iridescent crystalline deposits	Ciliary body cysts		
Multiple sclerosis				Granulomatous uveitis		
Myasthenia gravis	Ptosis, lid twitch, incomplete lid closure		Decreased corneal sensitivity			
Myopathies, *see* Oculopharyngeal muscular dystrophy, Kearns–Sayre syndrome, Chronic progressive ophthalmoplegia						
Myotonic dystrophy	Ptosis				Opacity	
Neuroblastoma, *see* Adrenal dysfunction						
Neurofibromatosis	Neurofibromas of lids, café au lait spots on lids	Neurofibromas, schwannomas	Neurofibromas, schwannomas, corneal nerve thickening, decreased sensitivity, exposure keratitis	Iris: Lisch nodules, hamartoma of anterior chamber, congenital glaucoma, neovascular glaucoma	Cataracts	
Niemann–Pick disease, *see* Sphingolipidoses						
Nutritional deficiency, *see* Tables 80–2 and 81–2						

10

Optic Nerve	Macula	Retina, Choroid	Extraocular Muscles, Eye Movements	Higher Cortical Function	Other
			Diplopia	Visual field defects	Decreased vision, headaches / head pain, proptosis
Compression		Retinopathy		CN 3,4,6 palsy secondary to compression	
Optic neuritis			INO/BINO, impaired smooth pursuits or saccades, nystagmus		Uhtoff sign
			Ophthalmoplegia, diplopia		Blurred vision, orbicularis weakness, decreased accommodation
			Nystagmus, pseudo internuclear ophthalmoplegia, convergence difficulties, saccadic quiver		
	Pigment changes	Peripheral pigment changes, epiretinal membrane	Motility disturbances, exotropia / exophoria, convergence insufficiency		Hypotony, orbicularis oculi weakness, poor Bell phenomenon
Nerve or chiasmal gliomas					Orbital meningiomas, neurofibromas, schwannomas, CN 5,7 palsy

	Lids, Lashes, Adnexa	Conjunctiva, Sclera	Cornea	Iris, Uvea, Ciliary Body, Anterior Chamber	Lens	Vitreous
Oculopharyngeal muscular dystrophy	Ptosis					
Osteogenesis imperfecta		Blue sclera	Corneal collagen irregularities	Congenital glaucoma	Dislocation, zonular cataract	Subhyaloid hemorrhage
Paget disease	Epiphora secondary to lacrimal duct obstruction			Glaucoma		
Parathyroid disease (Pth dx)		Conjunctival calcification (hyper Pth dx)	Band keratopathy (hyper Pth dx), pannus (hyper Pth dx), keratocon-junctivitis (hypo Pth dx)		Polychromatic cataract (hypo Pth dx)	
Parkinson disease	Blepharospasm, blepharoplegia, Myerson sign, Wilson sign					
Pernicious anemia, see Anemia						
Pheochromocytoma, see Adrenal dysfunction						
Pituitary dysfunction						
Polyarteritis nodosa		Conjunctival hyperemia, inflammation, scleritis		Iridocyclitis		
Polycythemia		Dilated/tortuous conjunctival vessels				
Polymyalgia rheumatica						
Pseudotumor cerebri						

Optic Nerve	Macula	Retina, Choroid	Extraocular Muscles, Eye Movements	Higher Cortical Function	Other
			Ophthalmoplegia		
Compression		Choroidal sclerosis			Partial color blindness
Neuropathy		Angioid streaks	EOM palsy		Exophthalmos
Papilledema (hypo Pth dx)					
			Abnormal saccades and/or pursuits, convergence insufficiency		Decreased contrast sensitivity, abnormal VEP
Compression of optic nerve, chiasm, or tract, optic atrophy			Compression of CN 3,4,6		Compression of first or second division of trigeminal nerve
Bilateral disc edema, ischemic optic neuropathy		Ischemic retinopathy, choroidal vasculitis	EOM palsy		Photophobia, intraocular pain, decreased visual acuity, exophthalmos
Florid color, edema		Deep purple hue of fundus, small, scattered superficial and deep hemorrhages; retinal edema; darkened, dilated, tortuous veins; bilateral CRVO		Cerebrovascular insufficiency with secondary amaurosis fugax, visual field loss	
AION (when associated with giant-cell arteritis)					Diplopia and / or transient visual obscuration (when associated with giant-cell arteritis)
Papilledema			CN 6 palsy		

	Lids, Lashes, Adnexa	Conjunctiva, Sclera	Cornea	Iris, Uvea, Ciliary Body, Anterior Chamber	Lens	Vitreous
Pseudoxanthoma elasticum			Nonspecific opacities, keratoconus, wrinkles in Descemet membrane		Subluxation, cataract	
Psoriatic arthritis		Mucopurulent conjunctivitis, episcleritis		Anterior uveitis		
Reiter syndrome		Conjunctivitis		Uveitis, secondary glaucoma	Cataract secondary to chronic uveitis	Vitritis secondary to chronic uveitis
Rheumatoid arthritis		Episcleritis, scleritis (non or necrotizing)	Keratitis sicca, filamentary keratitis, secondary bacterial keratitis, furrowing of peripheral cornea			
Rosacea	Blepharitis, meibomianitis, disrupted tear film, hordeola, chalazia	Conjunctival hyperemia	Punctate keratitis, epithelial erosions, vascularization, thinning, ulceration, perforation	Anterior uveitis		
Rubella (congenital)			Clouding, microcornea	Miotic / irregular pupil, iridocyclitis, transillumination defects, glaucoma	Cataract	
Sarcoidosis	Granulomatous lid lesions, lacrimal gland enlargement	Conjunctival granulomas	Keratoconjunctivitis sicca	Anterior uveitis, secondary glaucoma	Secondary cataract	Vitreal opacities
Scleroderma	Lagophthalmos, tightening of lids, ptosis, decreased tear production	Conjunctival microvascular abnormalities	Keratoconjunctivitis sicca	Anterior uveitis	Early cataracts	
Sickle hemoglobinopathies		Conjunctival sickling		Focal iris atrophy, microhyphema, rubeosis irides		Hemorrhage
Sjögren syndrome			Keratitis sicca, filamentary sicca, bacterial keratitis			

Optic Nerve	Macula	Retina, Choroid	Extraocular Muscles, Eye Movements	Higher Cortical Function	Other
Drusen, optic atrophy secondary to optic nerve drusen		Angioid streaks, drusen, peripheral punched-out lesions	EOM paralysis		Exophthalmos
	Edema secondary to chronic uveitis				
Pallor		Retinal pigment changes and folds, subretinal neovascularization	Nystagmus		Microophthalmia
Neovascularization of disc, direct optic nerve infiltration, papilledema secondary to intracranial lesions, optic atrophy		Periphlebitis or posterior uveitis with perivenous sheathing and exudates, retinal vein occlusion (rare), neovascularization of retina, choroidal granulomas	CN palsy		
Bilateral disc edema, neuropathy		Hypertensive retinopathy, choroidopathy			
Optic disc sign		Retinopathy (nonproliferative to proliferative), choroidal vascular occlusion, retinal arteriolar occlusion, arteriolo-venous anastomoses, retinal detachment			

	Lids, Lashes, Adnexa	Conjunctiva, Sclera	Cornea	Iris, Uvea, Ciliary Body, Anterior Chamber	Lens	Vitreous
Spasmus nutans						
Sphingolipidoses		Conjunctival angiokeratoma (Fabry disease), pigmented pingueculae (Gaucher disease)	Verticellata (Fabry disease), corneal opacification (Niemann–Pick disease)		Posterior cataracts (Fabry disease), lenticular opacities (Niemann–Pick disease)	
Sturge–Weber syndrome	Nevus flammeus of eyelid	Anomalous vessels of episclera and conjunctiva	Buphthalmos (with glaucoma at less than 3 years of age)	Iris heterochromia, glaucoma		
Syphilis	Gumma of lids and orbit, blepharoptosis	Conjunctivitis, episcleritis, scleritis, gumma of conjunctiva and sclera	Interstitial keratitis, gumma of cornea	Iris capillary abnormalities, anterior uveitis, gumma of iris and ciliary body, secondary glaucoma	Cataracts, dislocation	Vitritis
Systemic lupus erythematosus		Nonspecific conjunctivitis, scleritis	Keratoconjunctivitis sicca, stromal / marginal infiltrates, ulceration, vascularization, superficial punctate keratitis, pannus	Nongranulomatous uveitis		Hemorrhage
Tay–Sach disease, *see* sphingolipidoses						

Optic Nerve	Macula	Retina, Choroid	Extraocular Muscles, Eye Movements	Higher Cortical Function	Other
			Strabismus, pendular nystagmus		Amblyopia
	Cherry red spot (Tay–Sachs disease, Niemann–Pick type A & B)	Retinal angiokeratoma (Fabry disease), retinal white spots (Gaucher disease)	Ocular motor apraxia (Gaucher disease), eye movement paralysis (Gaucher disease), supranuclear gaze paresis (Niemann–Pick disease)		
Papilledema secondary to intracranial malformation		Choroidal hemangioma, serous / exudative retinal detachment, retinal pigmentary atrophy / retinitis pigmentosa, choroidal coloboma, atrophic chorioretinitis, retinoblastoma		Homonymous hemianopsia secondary to intracranial malformation	
Neuritis, papillitis, perineuritis, neuroretinitis, optic atrophy, papilledema	Edema, stellate maculopathy, disciform detachment	Retinitis, chorioretinis, retinal pigment epithelitis, vasculitis, choroiditis, serous/exudative RD, subretinal neovascularization, retinal necrosis, CRAO, CRVO	CN 3,4,6 palsy	Arteritis with stroke-like effects to any part of the visual pathways	Pupil abnormalities: Argyll–Robertson, tonic pupil
Neuritis, neuropathy, atrophy		Vasculitis, arterial occlusions, neovascularization, RD	EOM palsies, INO nystagmus	Visual field loss, cortical blindness	Pupil abnormality

	Lids, Lashes, Adnexa	Conjunctiva, Sclera	Cornea	Iris, Uvea, Ciliary Body, Anterior Chamber	Lens	Vitreous
Thyroid dysfunction	Lid retraction, lid lag, lagophthalmos, proptosis, wide-eye stare (hyperfunction); madarosis, periorbital myxedema (hypofunction)	Edema (hyperfunction)	Exposure, photophobia (hyperfunction)	Increased IOP (hyperfunction)		
Toxocariasis						Vitritis, white mass/granuloma, vitreous bands
Toxoplasmosis	Ptosis (congenital)			Anterior uveitis		Vitritis
Tuberculosis	Granulomas of lid	Granulomas of conjunctiva and sclera, conjunctivitis, scleritis	Granulomas of cornea, phlyctenular keratoconjunctivitis, interstitial keratitis	Granulomas of uvea, uveitis with or without retinal vasculitis		
Tuberous sclerosis	Adenoma sebaceum of eyelids, poliosis			Iris hypopigmentation		
Ulcerative colitis, *see* Inflammatory bowel disease						
Valvular heart disease		Conjunctival petechiae (bacterial endocarditis)				
Varicella	Eyelid vesicular lesions	Conjunctivitis, limbal/conjunctival vesicles	Superficial punctate keratopathy, stromal disciform keratitis			
Vogt–Koyanagi–Harada disease	Poliosis, lacrimation	Perilimbal vitiligo	Keratic precipitates	Bilateral uveitis, posterior synechiae, iris nodules, iris neovascularization, secondary glaucoma	PSC cataracts	Cells

Optic Nerve	Macula	Retina, Choroid	Extraocular Muscles, Eye Movements	Higher Cortical Function	Other
Blurred margins (hyperfunction)			Restriction, diplopia (hyperfunction)		
Distorted optic nerve	Hypertrophic macula, macular granuloma	Retinitis, choroiditis, retinal traction, retinal folds, tortuous / dilated vessels			Endophthalmitis
Neuritis / papillitis		Retinochoroiditis, retinal tears, retinal detachment, chorioretinal scars	Nystagmus, strabismus (congenital)		Microophthalmia, enophthalmos
Granuloma, optic neuropathy					Granulomas of orbit
Astrocytic hamartoma, papilledema		Astrocytic hamartoma, pigment epithelial defects			Atypical coloboma
Neuritis (bacterial endocarditis)		Embolic CRAO, BRAO, Roth spots (bacterial endocarditis)	CN 3,4,6 palsy (bacterial endocarditis)		
Papilledema	Edema, scarring	Vessel sheathing, bilateral serous non-rhegam-atogenous retinal detachment, chorioretinal scarring, diffuse RPE depigmenta-tion, subretinal neovasculariza-tion			Blurred vision, photophobia, ocular pain

	Lids, Lashes, Adnexa	Conjunctiva, Sclera	Cornea	Iris, Uvea, Ciliary Body, Anterior Chamber	Lens	Vitreous
Von Hippel–Lindau disease						
Waldenström macroglobulinemia		Sludging of blood				
Wegener granulomatosis	Dacryocystitis or adenitis, nasolacrimal duct obstruction, eyelid erythema and edema	Episcleritis, scleritis	Subepithelial infiltrates, marginal infiltrates, circumlimbal ulceration / furrowing, exposure keratitis	Uveitis		
Wilm tumor			Pannus	Aniridia	Cataracts	
Wilson disease			Kayser–Fleischer pigment ring		Sunflower cataract	
Wyburn–Mason syndrome	Ptosis	Dilated conjunctival vessels secondary to orbital AVM				Hemorrhage secondary to retinal AVM

Optic Nerve	Macula	Retina, Choroid	Extraocular Muscles, Eye Movements	Higher Cortical Function	Other
Optic nerve or peripapillary angioma, papilledema secondary to CNS angioma		Angiomatosis retinae	CN palsy or nystagmus secondary to CNS angioma		
Compression		CRVO		EOM palsy secondary to compression of nerve	
Compression		Diffuse vasculitis, venous congestion, disseminated ischemic retinitis, retinal and choroidal detachments	Eye movement restrictions		Proptosis, orbital granulomatosis and vasculitis
Glaucoma, Hypoplasia	Hypoplasia		Nystagmus, EM palsy, esotropia		Anisocoria
Arteriovenous malformation, papilledema secondary to CNS AVM	Hemorrhage secondary to retinal AVM	Retinal arteriovenous malformation, BRVO / CRVO secondary to retinal AVM, ischemia secondary to retinal AVM	CN palsies secondary to orbital AVM		Proptosis secondary to orbital AVM

II
Appendix

Selected Laboratory Diagnostic Tests

Test Name	Reference Range[a]	Units
Hematologic Tests		
Complete blood count with differential (CBC w/diff)		
White blood cell count (WBC)	$4.0\text{--}11.0 \times 10^3$	Cells/mm^3
Red blood cell count (RBC)	$3.8\text{--}5.4 \times 10^6$	Cells/mm^3
Hemoglobin (Hgb or HG)	11.5–16.0	g/dL
Hematocrit (HCT)	35.0–48.0	%
Mean corpuscular volume (MCV)	75–100	μm^3
Mean corpuscular hemoglobin (MCH)	27–35	pg
MCH concentration (MCHC)	31–37	%
WBC differential		
Neutrophils	47–75	%
Lymphocytes	18–46	%
Monocytes	0–12	%
Eosinophils	0–6	%
Basophils	0–2	%
Platelet count	$140\text{--}450 \times 10^3$	Cells/mm^3
Clotting indices		
Prothrombin time (PT)	10.3–13.3	Sec
Partial thromboplastin time (PTT)	22.9–34.9	Sec
Erythrocyte sedimentation rate (ESR)		
Laboratory (Westegren)	0–15 (males)	mm/hr
	0–20 (females)	mm/hr
Clinical rule of thumb	≤ age/2 (males)	mm/hr
	≤[age + 10]/2 (females)	mm/hr
Lymphocyte evaluation		
% T cells, CD$_2$	74–92	%
% T-helper, CD$_4$	33–62	%
% T-suppressor, CD$_8$	12–38	%
CD$_4$ / CD$_8$	0.9–3.0	
CD$_2$ abs count	700–2700	Cells/μL
CD$_4$ abs count	410–1572	Cells/μL
CD$_8$ abs count	116–961	Cells/μL
Sickle preparation	Neg	
Hemoglobin electrophoresis		
Hgb A$_1$	96–98	%
Hgb A$_2$	0–4	%
Hgb F	0–2	%
Hgb S	0	%
Hgb C	0	%
Serum/Blood Chemistries		
Glucose	65–115	mg/dL
Blood urea nitrogen (BUN)	7–25	mg/dL
Creatinine	0.6–1.5	mg/dL
Sodium	135–145	mEq/L
Potassium	3.5–5.3	mEq/L
Chloride	96–109	mEq/L
Ferritin	10–350	mg/mL
Total iron-binding capacity (TIBC)	250–450	mg/dL
Iron	42–135	mg/dL
Calcium	8.5–10.8	mg/dL
Phosphorus	2.5–4.5	mg/dL
Albumin	3.5–5.0	g/dL
Total protein	6.0–8.5	g/dL
Uric acid	3.0–8.0	mg/dL
Alkaline phosphatase	38–126	IU/L
CO$_2$	22–31	mmol/L

Test Name	Reference Range[a]	Units
Total bilirubin	0–1.2	mg/dL
SGOT (AST)	5–40	IU/L
SGPT (ALT)	7–56	IU/L
LDH	0–240	IU/L
Cholesterol	133–199	mg/dL
Triglycerides	35–150	mg/dL
HDL cholesterol	30–90	mg/dL
LDL cholesterol	0–130	mg/dL
VLDL cholesterol	5–40	mg/dL
Glucose tests		
Fasting blood sugar (FBS)	65–115	mg/dL
Glycosylated hemoglobin (HgbA$_{1c}$)	3.9–6.7	%
2-hour postprandial glucose	<120	mg/dL
Oral glucose tolerance test (OGTT)		
1/2 hr	<200	mg/dL
1 hr	95–177	mg/dL
2 hr	80–160	mg/dL
3 hr	65–135	mg/dL
Angiotensin-converting enzyme (ACE)	10–50	Units/L
Serum lysozyme	2.8–15.8	µg/mL

Endocrine Function Tests

Thyroid profile		
Free thyroxine index (FTI)	4–13.2	
T$_3$ radioimmunoassay (T$_3$RIA)	80–200	mg/dL
T$_4$	4.5–11.5	µg/mL
T$_3$ resin uptake (T$_3$RU)	25–35	% Uptake
Thyroid-stimulating hormone (TSH)	0.6–4.6	µU/mL
Prolactin	1.0–19.2	mEq/L
Parathyroid hormone	20–70	mIEq/L

Serological Tests

Antinuclear antibodies (ANA)	Neg (<1:20)	
Lupus erythematosus preparation	No cells seen	
Rheumatoid factor	Neg (<1:20)	
Serum acetylcholine receptor antibody	Neg (≤0.03)	nmol/L
Anti-scleroderma antibody	Neg	
Sjögren antibody	Neg	
Immunoglobulins (Ig)		
IgG	800–1700	mg/dL
IgA	100–490	mg/dL
IgM	50–320	mg/dL
Human leukocyte antigen (HLA) disease associations		
Ankylosing spondilitis	B27	
Reiter syndrome	B27	
Graves disease	B27	
Multiple sclerosis	B27 + Dw2 + A3 + B18	
Myasthenia gravis	B8	
Psoriasis	A13 + B17	
Toxocariasis titer		
Enzyme-linked immunosorbent assay (ELISA)	<1:8	
Cytomegalovirus (CMV) index		
ELISA IgG	0.0–0.79	

Test Name	Reference Range[a]	Units
Toxoplasmosis titer or index		
ELISA IgG	0.0–0.79 *or*	
	<1:16 neg	
	>1:256 recent infection	
	>1:1024 active infection	
	Note: For ocular infection, simply looking for any strength titer (positive result), therefore even 1:1 is considered positive	
Human immunodeficiency virus (HIV)		
ELISA	Neg	
Western blot	Neg	
Lyme index		
ELISA IgG and IgM	<0.80 neg	
	0.80–0.99 borderline	
	≥1.00 positive	
Syphilis		
Rapid plasma reagin (RPR)	NR	
Venereal disease research laboratory (VDRL)	NR	
Fluorescent treponemal antibody absorption (FTA-Abs)	NR	
Purified protein derivative (PPD)	Skin induration ≥ 10 mm positive	
	5–9 mm equivocal	
	<5 mm neg	
Cerebrospinal Fluid Tests		
Glucose	40–75	mg/dL
Protein	10–40	mg/dL
Cells	0–5 lymphocytes	cells/mm³
Opening pressure	70–180	mmH₂O
IgG	2–4	mg/dL
IgA	0.15–0.6	mg/dL
IgM	<0.10	mg/dL
Urinalysis		
Specific gravity	1.003–1.030	
Appearance	Clear	
Color	Yellow	
pH	4.5–8.0	
Protein/albumin	Neg	
Ketone/acetone	Neg	
Glucose	Neg	
Blood	Neg	
Leukocyte esterase	Neg	
Nitrite	Neg	
Bilirubin	Neg	
Urobilinogen	Neg (or trace)	

[a] Values vary with age, sex, medications, disease, and laboratory. Abs count, absolute count; Neg, negative; NR, nonreactive.

III
Appendix

Selected Medical Abbreviations

AAO	Awake, alert, and oriented		HCTZ	Hydrochlorthiazide
AD	Alzheimer disease		HCVD	Hypertensive cardiovascular disease
AIDS	Acquired immunodeficiency syndrome		HIV	Human immunodeficiency virus
AION	Anterior ischemic optic neuropathy		H/O	History of
ALL	Acute lymphocytic (lymphoid) leukemia		HPI	History of present illness
ALT	Argon laser trabeculoplasty		HSV	Herpes simplex virus
AMA	Against medical advice		HTN	Hypertension
AMD (ARMD)	Age-related macular degeneration		HX	History
AML	Acute myelogenous (myeloid, myelocytic) leukemia		HZO	Herpes zoster ophthalmicus
			HZV	Herpes zoster virus
ARC	AIDS-related complex		IBD	Inflammatory bowel disease
ASA	Aspirin		ICA	Internal carotid artery
ASHD	Arteriosclerotic heart disease		ICCE	Intracapsular cataract extraction
AVM	Arteriovenous malformation		ICP	Intracranial pressure
AZT	Zidovudine		IDDM	Insulin-dependent diabetes mellitus
BM	Bone marrow or bowel movement		IDU	Idoxuridine
BP	Blood pressure		INH	Isoniazid
BPH	Benign prostatic hypertrophy		INO	Internuclear ophthalmoplegia
CA	Carcinoma		KS	Kaposi sarcoma
CABG	Coronary artery bypass graft		LBP	Lower back pain
CAD	Coronary artery disease		LOC	Loss of consciousness
CC	Chief complaint		LP	Lumbar puncture or light perception
CHF	Congestive heart failure		MAI	*Mycobacterium avium-intracellulare*
CLL	Chronic lymphocytic (lymphoid) leukemia		MD	Myotonic dystrophy
			MG	Myasthenia gravis
CML	Chronic myelogenous (myeloid, myelogenous) leukemia		MI	Myocardial infarction
			MID	Multi-infarct dementia
CMV	Cytomegalovirus		MRI	Magnetic resonance imaging
C/O	Complain of		MS	Multiple sclerosis
COPD	Chronic obstructive pulmonary disease		MVA	Motor vehicle accident
CT	Connective tissue or computer tomography		MVP	Mitral valve prolapse
			NIDDM	Non-insulin-dependent diabetes mellitus
CVA	Cerebrovascular accident		NKA	No known allergies
DJD	Degenerative joint disease		NKAM	No known allergies to medications
DM	Diabetes mellitus		NPH	Neutral protamine hagedorn (insulin)
DTR	Deep-tendon reflexes		NSAID	Nonsteroidal antiinflammatory drug
ECCE	Extracapsular cataract extraction		NTG	Nitroglycerin
ECG/EKG	Electrocardiogram		OA	Osteoarthritis
EEG	Electroencephalogram		OBS	Organic brain syndrome
EKC	Epidemic keratoconjunctivitis		ODM	Ophthalmodynamometry
EMB	Ethambutol		OPG	Ocular plethysmography
EMG	Electromyogram		OPPG	Ocular pneumoplethysmography
EOG	Electro-oculogram		OX3	Oriented times three
ERG	Electroretinogram		PAT	Paroxysmal atrial tachycardia or preadmission testing
ETOH	Alcohol			
FMH	Family medical history		PCN	Penicillin
FU	Follow up		PCP	*Pneumocystis carinii* pneumonia
FX	Fracture		PE	Physical examination
GCA	Giant-cell arteritis		PFT	Pulmonary function test
GDM	Gestational diabetes mellitus		PMD	Private medical doctor
HA	Headache		PMI	Past medical illness
HASHD	Hypertensive arteriosclerotic heart disease		POD	Postoperative day
			PRN	As often as necessary
HCT	Hematocrit		PTSD	Post-traumatic stress disorder

PUD	Peptic ulcer disease
PVD	Peripheral vascular disease
RA	Rheumatoid arthritis
RAPD	Relative afferent pupillary defect
RIND	Reversible ischemic neurologic deficit
ROS	Review of systems
RTC	Return to clinic
SLE	Systemic lupus erythematosus
SOAP	Subjective, objective, assessment, plan
SOB	Shortness of breath
S/P	Status post
STD	Sexually transmitted disease

SX	Symptoms
TB	Tuberculosis
TIA	Transient ischemic attack
TURP	Transurethral resection of prostate
URI	Upper respiratory infection
US	Ultrasonography
UTI	Urinary tract infection
VEP	Visually evoked potential
VER	Visually evoked response
WU	Workup
XR	X-ray

Prescription Abbreviations

sig	Let it be marked
disp	Dispense
sol	Solution
ung	Ointment
susp	Suspension
gtt	Drop
tab	Tablet
cap	Capsule
i	1
ii	2
iii	3
iv	4
po	By mouth
npo	Nothing by mouth

iv	Intravenous
im	Intramuscular
q	Every
qhs	Every evening
qod	Every other day
qd	Once per day
bid	Twice per day
tid	Three times per day
qid	Four times per day
q2h	Every 2 hours
prn	As needed
otc	Over the counter
stat	Immediately
ac	Before meals
pc	After meals

Index